Rheumatology and Immunology

Volume 4 of
THE SCIENCE AND PRACTICE OF CLINICAL MEDICINE

John M. Dietschy, M.D.
Editor-in-Chief

Professor of Internal Medicine
University of Texas
Southwestern Medical School
Attending Staff
Parkland Memorial Hospital
Dallas, Texas

Rheumatology and Immunology

Edited by
Alan S. Cohen, M.D.

Conrad Wesselhoeft Professor of Medicine
Boston University School of Medicine
Director, Division of Medicine and Thorndike Memorial Laboratory
Boston City Hospital

Director, Arthritis Center of Boston University
Head, Arthritis and Connective Tissue Disease Section
Boston University Medical Center
Boston, Massachusetts

GRUNE & STRATTON, INC.

A Subsidiary of Harcourt Brace Jovanovich, Publishers
New York   San Francisco   London

Grune & Stratton, Inc.
111 Fifth Avenue
New York, New York 10003

Distributed in the United Kingdom by
Academic Press, Inc. (London) Ltd.
24/48 Oval Road, London NW 1

Library of Congress Catalog Number 79-52766
International Standard Book Number 0-8089-1118-X

Printed in the United States of America

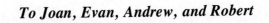

To Joan, Evan, Andrew, and Robert

Contents

Contents

DIFFERENTIAL APPROACH TO MAJOR IMMUNOLOGIC SYNDROMES

SPECIFIC IMMUNOLOGIC DISEASES

Acknowledgments

I would like to thank Lorraine Nangle for her invaluable assistance in organizing this complex and multiple-authored text. I would also like to thank Joan Cohen for her patience and understanding during the process of editing this volume.

Preface

Rheumatology is a young medical subspecialty that has grown to maturity only in the past 20 years. The disorders that afflict the musculoskeletal system are multiple, varied, and often serious, and the number of persons with such disorders is enormous, now estimated at over 31 million. Several studies have shown that musculoskeletal disorders are often *the* most common cause of symptoms that lead patients to physicians' offices. Several years ago the fiscal impact of arthritis was estimated to be over 13 billion dollars due to loss of wages, loss of productivity, and various social factors, as well as the obvious direct medical costs. In addition to their prevalence and the cost of treating them, these disorders have a great impact on the quality of life because of the loss of mobility, pain, and general disability that may result. Finally, due to the ubiquitous presence of the target organ, i.e., connective tissue (blood vessels, joints, muscle and bone), the rheumatic diseases can present not only to the internist but to the ophthalmologist, urologist, orthopedist, and virtually every medical and surgical subspecialist as well.

For these reasons it behooves students, residents in training, primary care physicians (be they internists, family practitioners, or pediatricians), and indeed medical subspecialists to have a basic knowledge of the clinical and scientific aspects of rheumatology. *The Science and Practice of Clinical Medicine* has attempted to stress straightforward pathophysiology plus the clinical aspects of medicine throughout the series. This approach lends itself especially well to a volume on rheumatology and immunology, since these multiple disciplines interact. Because of the obvious strong impact the latter discipline has had on rheumatology and vice versa, the text has been divided into a major section on rheumatology, plus a smaller section on immunology.

The rheumatology section is devoted to a discussion of the basic principles, including a regional approach to common musculoskeletal disorders. Following this is a succinct analysis of the basic aspects of connective tissue biochemistry, basic epidemiology, and so forth. Diagnostic procedures in these disorders overlap considerably (i.e., synovial fluid analysis and tests for rheumatoid factors and the antinuclear antibodies); therefore the next major subdivision is devoted to this area. The section on diagnostic procedures is followed by an approach to the differential diagnosis of the rheumatic diseases. The specific articular and connective tissue diseases are then discussed in classical fashion. Each author is an expert in the field on which he or she is writing, and the format utilizes a small number of general references rather than exhaustive documentation.

A similar format is followed in the section on immunology; that is, basic immunologic concepts, differential diagnosis, and specific diseases. Many of the so-called autoimmune diseases are included in the rheumatology text and are not repeated in the latter section. Allergy, as it overlaps the rheumatic disease area, is also included, but diseases such as asthma are to be found in Volume 2 on pulmonary diseases.

Due to the nature of rheumatology, with its overlapping disease syndromes, and because the etiology of a number of these diseases is unknown, as well as for didactic reasons, there are sections of the book that deal with similar disorders through different approaches (i.e., vasculitis and immune complex disease) in the belief that where etiology and pathogenesis are not known with certainty, several conceptual approaches are reasonable.

Rheumatology has many frontiers that are actively being pushed back, many diseases that have been defined only in recent years. It is our hope that this text will, in a modest fashion, enable interested medical persons to approach these diseases with a better understanding of their scope and pathogenesis and of the science and practice of the rheumatic disorders.

Alan S. Cohen, M.D.

Contributors

William P. Arend, M.D.
Associate Professor of Medicine
University of Washington
School of Medicine
Chief, Arthritis Section
Veterans Administration Hospital
Seattle, Washington

Peter Barland, M.D.
Professor of Medicine
Albert Einstein College of Medicine
Attending Physician
Montefiore Hospital and Medical Center
Bronx, New York

John Baum, M.D.
Professor of Medicine, Pediatrics, and Preventive
    Medicine and Community Health
University of Rochester
School of Medicine and Dentistry
Physician and Pediatrician
Strong Memorial Hospital
Rochester, New York

William P. Beetham, Jr., M.D.
Assistant Professor of Medicine
Harvard Medical School
Department of Medicine
Lahey Clinic Foundation
Chief of Rheumatology
New England Deaconess Hospital
Boston, Massachusetts

J. Claude Bennett, M.D.
Professor of Medicine
Professor and Chairman, Department of Microbiology
Director, Division of Clinical Immunology and
    Rheumatology
University of Alabama
Medical School
Birmingham, Alabama

Rodney Bluestone, M.B., M.R.C.P.
Professor of Medicine
University of California at Los Angeles
School of Medicine
Chief, Rheumatology Section
Wadsworth Veterans Administration Hospital
Los Angeles, California

Alfred Jay Bollet, M.D.
Professor and Chairman, Department of Medicine
State University of New York
Downstate Medical Center
Physician-in-Chief
State University Hospital
Brooklyn, New York

Peter H. Byers, M.D.
Acting Assistant Professor of Pathology and Medicine
University of Washington
School of Medicine
Seattle, Washington

John J. Calabro, M.D.
Professor of Medicine and Pediatrics
University of Massachusetts
Medical School
Director of Rheumatology
Worcester City Hospital
Worcester, Massachusetts

Juan J. Canoso, M.D.
Associate Professor of Medicine
Boston University
School of Medicine
Chief, Rheumatology Section
Boston Veterans Administration Hospital
Boston, Massachusetts

Beverly A. Carpenter, M.D.
Assistant Professor of Medicine
University of Cincinnati
Medical Center
Assistant Director of Internal Medicine
Jewish Hospital
Cincinnati, Ohio

Edgar S. Cathcart, M.B., D.Sc.
Professor of Medicine
Boston University
School of Medicine
Chief, Arthritis Section
University Hospital
Boston, Massachusetts

Leonard Chess, M.D.
Associate Professor of Medicine
Director, Division of Rheumatology
Columbia University
College of Physicians and Surgeons
New York, New York

Charles L. Christian, M.D.
Professor of Medicine
Cornell Medical School
Acting Chairman, Department of Medicine
New York Hospital-Cornell Medical Center
New York, New York

Joseph J. Combs, Jr., M.D.
Assistant Professor of Medicine
Mayo Medical School
Mayo Clinic
Rochester, Minnesota

Eugene A. Davidson, Ph.D.
Professor and Chairman, Department of Biological
   Chemistry
Pennsylvania State University
Milton S. Hershey Medical Center
Hershey, Pennsylvania

John S. Davis IV, M.D.
Professor of Medicine
University of Virginia
School of Medicine
Charlottesville, Virginia

John L. Decker, M.D.
Chief, Arthritis and Rheumatism Branch
National Institute of Arthritis, Metabolism, and
   Digestive Diseases
National Institutes of Health
Bethesda, Maryland

Edward K. Dunham, M.D.
Assistant Clinical Professor of Medicine
Harvard Medical School
Director, Allergy Clinic
Beth Israel Hospital
Boston, Massachusetts

George E. Ehrlich, M.D.
Professor of Medicine
Temple University
School of Medicine
Chief of Rheumatology
Albert Einstein Medical Center and
Moss Rehabilitation Hospital
Philadelphia, Pennsylvania

Gary R. Epler, M.D.
Assistant Professor of Medicine
Boston University
School of Medicine
Division of Pulmonary Medicine and Thoracic Services
University Hospital
Boston, Massachusetts

Wallace V. Epstein, M.D.
Professor of Medicine
University of California at San Francisco
School of Medicine
San Francisco, California

Baher S. Foad, M.D., F.A.C.P.
Assistant Clinical Professor of Medicine
University of Cincinnati
Medical School
University of Cincinnati Medical Center
Cincinnati, Ohio

Michael M. Frank, M.D.
Clinical Director, National Institute of Allergy and
   Infectious Diseases
Chief, Laboratory of Clinical Investigation
National Institutes of Health
Bethesda, Maryland

Edward C. Franklin, M.D.
Professor of Medicine
Chairman, Rheumatic Diseases Study Group
New York University
School of Medicine
Director, Irvington House Institute
New York University Medical Center
New York, New York

Don L. Goldenberg, M.D.
Associate Professor of Medicine
Boston University
School of Medicine
Associate Director of Medicine
Boston City Hospital
Boston, Massachusetts

Duncan A. Gordon, M.D., F.R.C.P.(C.)
Professor of Medicine
University of Toronto
School of Medicine
Director, Rheumatic Disease Unit
Toronto Western Hospital
Toronto, Ontario
Canada

Edward D. Harris, Jr., M.D.
Professor of Medicine
Dartmouth Medical School
Director, Arthritis Center
Dartmouth-Hitchcock Medical Center
Hanover, New Hampshire

Evelyn V. Hess, M.D., F.A.C.P.
McDonald Professor of Medicine
University of Cincinnati
Medical School
Director, Division of Immunology
University of Cincinnati Medical Center
Cincinnati, Ohio

Gary S. Hoffman, M.D.
Assistant Professor of Clinical Medicine
Columbia University
College of Physicians and Surgeons
New York, New York
Attending Physician
Mary Imogene Bassett Hospital
Cooperstown, New York

Karen A. Holbrook, Ph.D.
Assistant Professor
Department of Biological Structure
University of Washington
School of Medicine
Seattle, Washington

Stephen W. Hosea, M.D.
Senior Investigator
Laboratory of Clinical Investigation
National Institute of Allergy and Infectious Diseases
National Institutes of Health
Bethesda, Maryland

Gene G. Hunder, M.D.
Associate Professor of Medicine
Mayo Medical School
Mayo Clinic
Rochester, Minnesota

Joseph H. Korn, M.D.
Assistant Professor of Medicine
University of Connecticut
School of Medicine
University of Connecticut Health Center
Farmington, Connecticut

E. Carwile LeRoy, M.D.
Professor of Medicine
University of South Carolina
School of Medicine
Director, Division of Rheumatology and Immunology
Medical University of South Carolina
Charleston, South Carolina

Robert A. Lewis, M.D.
Instructor in Medicine
Harvard Medical School
Assistant Physician
Robert B. Brigham Hospital
Boston, Massachusetts

Mart Mannik, M.D.
Professor of Medicine
Head, Division of Rheumatology
University of Washington
School of Medicine
Seattle, Washington

Alfonse T. Masi, M.D., Dr.P.H.
Professor and Head, Department of Medicine
Peoria School of Medicine
University of Illinois
College of Medicine
Methodist Medical Center of Illinois
Peoria, Illinois

Daniel J. McCarty, M.D.
Professor and Chairman, Department of Medicine
Medical College of Wisconsin
Milwaukee, Wisconsin

James L. McGuire, M.D.
Instructor in Medicine
Southwestern Medical School

Junior Attending Staff in Internal Medicine
Parkland Memorial Hospital
Dallas, Texas

Thomas A. Medsger, Jr., M.D.
Associate Professor of Medicine
University of Pittsburgh
School of Medicine
Active Staff
Presbyterian–University Hospital
Pittsburgh, Pennsylvania

Robert F. Meenan, M.D.
Assistant Professor of Medicine
Boston University
School of Medicine
Associate Director, Multipurpose Arthritis Center
Boston City Hospital
Boston, Massachusetts

John A. Mills, M.D.
Associate Professor of Medicine
Harvard Medical School
Physician
Massachusetts General Hospital
Boston, Massachusetts

Gregory R. Mundy, M.D.
Associate Professor of Medicine
University of Connecticut
School of Medicine
Division of Endocrinology and Metabolism
University of Connecticut Health Center
Farmington, Connecticut

J. D. O'Duffy, M.D.
Associate Professor of Medicine
Mayo Medical School
Division of Rheumatology
Mayo Clinic
Rochester, Minnesota

Raymond E. H. Partridge, M.D.
Associate Professor of Medicine
Tufts University
School of Medicine
Physician
Tufts-New England Medical Center
Boston, Massachusetts

Carl M. Pearson, M.D.
Professor of Medicine
University of California at Los Angeles
School of Medicine
Director, Division of Rheumatology
University of California at Los Angeles Medical Center
Los Angeles, California

Mark B. Pepys, M.B., Ph.D., M.R.C.P.
Senior Lecturer in Medicine
Departments of Medicine and Immunology
Royal Postgraduate Medical School
Consultant Physician
Hammersmith Hospital
London, England

Robert H. Persellin, M.D.
Professor of Medicine
University of Texas
Head, Division of Rheumatology
University of Texas Health Science Center
San Antonio, Texas

Sheldon R. Pinnell, M.D.
Professor of Medicine (Dermatology)
Duke University Medical Center
Durham, North Carolina

Richard M. Pope, M.D.
Assistant Professor of Medicine
University of Texas
Division of Rheumatology
University of Texas Health Science Center
San Antonio, Texas

Donald Resnick, M.D.
Associate Professor of Radiology
University of California at San Diego
School of Medicine
Chief, Department of Radiology
Veterans Administration Hospital
San Diego, California

Michael J. Reza, M.D.
Assistant Clinical Professor of Medicine
University of California at Los Angeles
School of Medicine
Associate Director, Clinic for Neuromuscular Disorders
University of California at Los Angeles Medical Center
Los Angeles, California

Dwight Robinson, M.D.
Associate Professor of Medicine
Harvard Medical School
Associate Physician
Massachusetts General Hospital
Boston, Massachusetts

Ross E. Rocklin, M.D.
Professor of Medicine
Tufts University
School of Medicine
Chief, Allergy Division
New England Medical Center Hospital
Boston, Massachusetts

Gerald P. Rodnan, M.D.
Professor of Medicine
University of Pittsburgh
School of Medicine
Active Staff
Presbyterian–University Hospital
Pittsburgh, Pennsylvania

Alan Rubinow, M.D.
Assistant Professor of Medicine
Boston University
School of Medicine
Physician-in-Charge, Allergy Clinic
Boston City Hospital
Boston, Massachusetts

C. O. Samuelson, M.D.
Associate Professor of Medicine
University of Utah
College of Medicine
University of Utah Medical Center
Salt Lake City, Utah

Frank R. Schmid, M.D.
Professor of Medicine
Chief, Section of Arthritis–Connective Tissue Diseases
Northwestern University
Medical School
Chicago, Illinois

H. Ralph Schumacher, M.D.
Associate Professor of Medicine
University of Pennsylvania
School of Medicine
Director, Rheumatology–Immunology Center
Veterans Administration Hospital
Philadelphia, Pennsylvania

Robert S. Schwartz, M.D.
Professor of Medicine
Tufts University
School of Medicine
Tufts-New England Medical Center
Boston, Massachusetts

Gordon C. Sharp, M.D.
Professor of Medicine
Director, Division of Immunology and Rheumatology
University of Missouri
Medical School
Columbia, Missouri

John T. Sharp, M.D.
Professor of Clinical Science (Medicine)
University of Illinois
School of Clinical Science at Urbana-Champaign
Chief, Medical Service
Danville Veterans Administration Hospital
Danville, Illinois

Albert L. Scheffer, M.D.
Associate Clinical Professor of Medicine
Harvard Medical School
Director, Allergy Clinic
Peter Bent Brigham Hospital
Boston, Massachusetts

Lawrence E. Shulman, M.D., Ph.D.
Associate Professor of Medicine
Johns Hopkins University
School of Medicine
Baltimore, Maryland
Associate Director, Arthritis, Bone, and Skin Diseases
   Branch
National Institute of Arthritis, Metabolism, and
   Digestive Diseases
National Institutes of Health
Bethesda, Maryland

Martha Skinner, M.D.
Associate Professor of Medicine
Boston University
School of Medicine
Assistant Visiting Physician
Boston City Hospital
Boston, Massachusetts

J. Donald Smiley, M.D.
Professor of Internal Medicine
Southwestern Medical School
University of Texas Health Science Center
Director, Section of Rheumatology and Clinical
    Immunology
Presbyterian Hospital of Dallas
Dallas, Texas

Mary Betty Stevens, M.D.
Associate Professor of Medicine
Johns Hopkins University
School of Medicine
Director, Rheumatology Division
Good Samaritan Hospital
Baltimore, Maryland

John D. Stobo, M.D.
Associate Professor of Medicine
University of California at San Francisco
School of Medicine
Head, Section of Rheumatology/Immunology
Moffitt Hospital
San Francisco, California

Norman Talal, M.D.
Professor of Medicine
University of California at San Francisco
School of Medicine
Chief, Immunology and Arthritis Section and Clinical
    Immunology Laboratory
Veterans Administration Hospital
San Francisco, California

Eng M. Tan, M.D.
Professor of Medicine
University of Colorado
School of Medicine
Head, Division of Rheumatic Diseases
University of Colorado Medical Center
Denver, Colorado

Charles D. Tourtellotte, M.D.
Professor of Medicine
Temple University
School of Medicine
Chairman, Section of Rheumatology
Temple University Hospital
Philadelphia, Pennsylvania

Frank J. Twarog, M.D., Ph.D.
Assistant Clinical Professor of Pediatrics
Harvard Medical School
Associate in Allergy
Children's Hospital Medical Center
Boston, Massachusetts

Heinz W. Wahner, M.D.
Professor of Laboratory Medicine
Mayo Medical School
Section of Diagnostic Nuclear Medicine
Mayo Clinic
Rochester, Minnesota

Thomas A. Waldmann, M.D.
Chief, Metabolism Branch
National Cancer Institute
National Institutes of Health
Bethesda, Maryland

Stanley L. Wallace, M.D.
Professor of Medicine
State University of New York
Downstate Medical Center
Associate Director of Medicine
Chief of Rheumatology
Jewish Hospital and Medical Center of Brooklyn
Brooklyn, New York

John R. Ward, M.D.
Professor of Medicine
University of Utah
College of Medicine
Chief, Arthritis Division
University of Utah Medical Center
Salt Lake City, Utah

Peter A. Ward, M.D.
Professor and Chairman
Department of Pathology
University of Connecticut
Health Center
Farmington, Connecticut

Stephen I. Wasserman, M.D.
Associate Professor of Medicine
University of California at San Diego
Medical School
San Diego, California

Robert B. Zurier, M.D.
Associate Professor of Medicine
University of Connecticut
School of Medicine
Division of Rheumatic Diseases
University of Connecticut Health Center
Farmington, Connecticut

Rheumatology and Immunology

REGIONAL STRUCTURE AND FUNCTION: BASIC PRINCIPLES IN RHEUMATOLOGY

Articular Structures

HANDS, WRISTS, AND ELBOWS

Juan J. Canoso

I. Hands and Wrists
   A. Anatomy
      1. Bones and Joints
         a. Wrist
         b. Fingers
      2. Muscles and Innervation
      3. Anatomic Landmarks
   B. Physical Examination
   C. Abnormal Findings
      1. Deformities
         a. Ulnar Drift
         b. Boutonniere Deformity
         c. Swan-Neck Deformity
         d. Thumb Deformities
      2. Tenosynovitis
         a. Flexor Tenosynovitis
         b. Dorsal Tenosynovitis
         c. DeQuervain's Tenosynovitis
      3. Dupuytren's Contracture
      4. Nerve Compression Syndromes
         a. Carpal Tunnel Syndrome
         b. Ulnar Tunnel Syndrome at the Wrist (Guyon's Canal)
         c. Ulnar Nerve Compression Distal in the Palmar Space
II. Elbows
   A. Anatomy
      1. Bones and Joints
      2. Muscles and Innervation
      3. Anatomic Landmarks
   B. Physical Examination
   C. Abnormal Findings
      1. Epicondylitis
         a. Lateral Epicondylitis (Tennis Elbow)
         b. Medial Epicondylitis (Golfer's Elbow)
      2. Subcutaneous Olecranon Bursitis
      3. Nerve Compression Syndromes
         a. Cubital Tunnel Syndrome
         b. Posterior Interosseous Nerve Syndrome

HANDS AND WRISTS

The structural and functional complexity of the hand is reflected in a range of pathology that cannot be comprehensively discussed within the limits of this chapter. Only certain aspects of the normal and abnormal hand with particular relevance to the rheumatic diseases will be considered.

Anatomy

Bones and joints. *Wrist.* At the distal end of the ulna there is a tough fibrocartilaginous plate, known as the triangular articular disc, which covers the ulnar head. This disc plate and the distal end of the radius articulate with the proximal row of carpal bones at the radiocarpal or wrist joint. This, like the midcarpal, is an ellipsoid joint in which all motions except rotation are possible. In contrast, little motion occurs at the carpometacarpal (CMC) joint, in which the articular surfaces are relatively flat. An exception is the CMC joint of the thumb, in which a saddle configuration of the trapezium corresponds to a saddle configuration of the metacarpal base, thus allowing motion in two planes that are oriented at 45° to the planes of motion of the fingers. The functional value of the thumb, which has been estimated as at least one-half the value of the entire hand, is dependent upon the motion and stability of the CMC joint.

Arthrography shows infrequent (10–20 percent) communication between the distal radioulnar joint and the radiocarpal joint, and between the radiocarpal joint and the midcarpal joint. In contrast, communication between the midcarpal joint and the CMC is frequent, with the exception of the CMC of the thumb, which remains separate by being enclosed in a tough capsule even when destructive processes of the carpus, such as rheumatoid arthritis, have produced confluence of all other wrist joints.

Fingers. The metacarpophalangeal (MCP) joints are ball and socket structures. Their capsule is reinforced anteriorly by a fibrocartilaginous plate which is firmly attached to the proximal phalanx but loosely connected to the metacarpal. The transverse metacarpal ligament unites the fibrocartilaginous plates of the medial four MCP joints. Laterally, the capsule is reinforced by eccentrically placed collateral ligaments which become taut

1

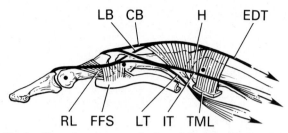

Fig. 1. Normal extensor mechanism of the digits: EDT, extensor digitorum tendon; H, extensor hood; LB, lateral band; CB, central band; TML, transverse metacarpal ligament; IT, interosseous tendon; LT, lumbrical tendon; FFS, fibrous flexor sheath; RL, retinacular ligament. (Modified by permission of author and publisher from Tubiana R: Lésions traumatiques de l'appareil extenseur au niveau des doigts, in Verdan C (ed): Chirurgie des Tendons de la Main. Paris, Expansion Scientifique, 1976.)

in flexion and lax in extension, an arrangement that in normal individuals prevents lateral movement of the finger when the MCP joint is flexed at 90°. Finally, the interphalangeal (IP) joints of the fingers are hinges which only allow flexion and extension.

Muscles and innervation. Wrist motion is mainly exerted by ulnar and radial flexors and extensors of the

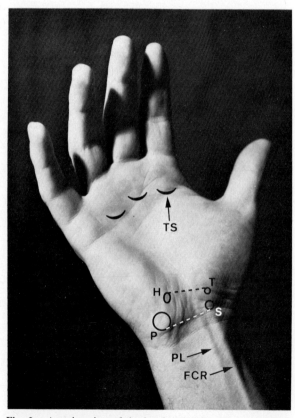

Fig. 2. Anterior view of the hand and wrist: TS, entrance of flexor tendon into flexor synovial sheath; dotted lines outline the distal and proximal edges of the flexor retinaculum; H, hook of hamate; T, crest of trapezium; P, Pisiform; S, tubercle of scaphoid; PL, tendon of palmaris longus—the median nerve runs deep to PL; FCR, tendon of flexor carpi radialis.

carpus, whereas motion of the digits involves the coordinated action of long flexors, extensors, and small muscles of the hand (the thenar, hypothenar, interossei, and lumbrical muscles). Flexion of the digits results from simple pull of the flexor muscles, particularly the profundus, supplemented by the superficialis when greater strength is needed. Extension is a much more complex function that requires coordinated action of long extensors, intrinsic muscles, and the retinacular ligament, a structure that links the anterior aspect of the proximal phalanx to the dorsal aspect of the distal phalanx and couples the passive motion of proximal and distal IP joints.

A consideration of the structure and function of the extensor hood is central to the understanding of the extensor mechanism in general and the action of the intrinsic muscles in particular. This roughly triangular membranous structure covers and reinforces the MCP joint dorsally, and near the proximal interphalangeal (PIP) joint it splits into three bands. The central band inserts at the base of the middle phalanx; the lateral bands, after merging at the dorsum of the middle phalanx, insert at the base of the distal phalanx. Tendinous contributions to the extensor hood include the tendon of the extensor digitorum, of which the hood itself is an expansion, and the tendons of the intrinsic muscles (interossei and lumbricals). As can be seen in Figure 1, the pull of the intrinsic muscles passes anteriorly to the MCP joints and posterior to the PIP and distal interphalangeal (DIP) joints. Therefore, their contraction will bring the MCP joints into flexion and the PIP and DIP joints into extension. In addition, the dorsal interossei are so inserted that their contraction spreads the digits away from the third digit, while the palmar interossei bring the digits together. In the thumb an expansion of the tendon of the extensor pollicis longus, joined laterally by the tendon of the abductor pollicis brevis and medially by the adductor pollicis, forms a triangular arrangement that resembles the extensor hood of the fingers.

All of the small muscles of the hand are supplied by the nerve root T_1, whose fibers are carried by the ulnar and median nerves. The ulnar innervates the hypothenar muscles, interossei, lumbricals 3 and 4, adductor pollicis, and sometimes part of the flexor pollicis brevis. The abductor pollicis brevis, opponens pollicis, and all or part of the flexor pollicis brevis are innervated by the median. Thus ulnar nerve injury produces paralysis and atrophy of most of the intrinsic muscles of the hand. Due to loss of action of the intrinsic muscles, which, as explained above, flex the MCP joints and extend the PIP and DIP joints, ulnar palsy results in extension of the MCP joints and flexion of the PIP and DIP joints from unbalanced action of long flexors and extensors.

Anatomic landmarks. Anteriorly, the flexor retinaculum, which bridges the concavity of the carpus and limits the carpal tunnel anteriorly, extends from the pisiform and hook of hamate medially to the tubercle of scaphoid and crest of trapezium laterally (Fig. 2). The proximal edge of the flexor retinaculum corresponds to

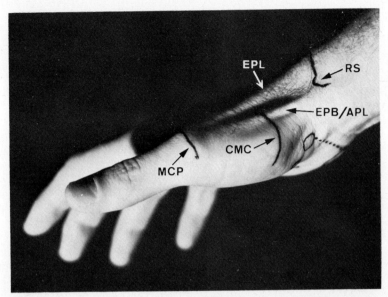

Fig. 3. Radial aspect of the wrist. The "anatomic snuffbox" is limited anteriorly by the extensor pollicis brevis (EPB) and abductor pollicis longus (APL) tendons in a common tendon sheath. The critical relation of the radial styloid (RS) to this sheath is shown. The extensor pollicis longus (EPL) tendon bounds the snuffbox posteriorly. CMC is the first carpometacarpal joint, and MCP is the first metacarpophalangeal joint.

the distal crease of the wrist. In the distal forearm and perpendicular to the crease, two tendons can be readily identified—the lateral corresponding to the flexor carpis radialis and the medial to the palmaris longus (absent in 10 percent). These two tendons allow the mapping of the median nerve, which as it enters the carpal tunnel runs medial to the flexor carpi radialis and deep to the palmaris longus tendons. Further down the palm, the proximal palmar crease corresponds to the entrance of the flexor tendon of the index finger into its synovial sheath, while the distal crease keeps a similar relation with the tendon sheaths of digits 3 and 4.

In the radial side the "anatomic snuffbox" is outlined anteriorly by the tendons of the extensor pollicis brevis and abductor pollicis longus, which run, enclosed in a common tendon sheath, above the radial styloid (Fig. 3). Posteriorly, it is outlined by the tendon of the extensor pollicis longus. Ulnar deviation of the wrist allows palpation of the scaphoid. The trapeziometacarpal joint (CMC joint of the thumb) is identified immediately distal to the scaphoid.

Posteriorly, the head of the ulna and its styloid process and the dorsal tubercle of the radius (Lister's tubercle) can be readily identified (Fig. 4). The latter is the point at which the tendon of the extensor pollicis longus turns laterally. Gentle flexion of the wrist facilitates the palpation of the radiocarpal and midcarpal joints.

Physical Examination

In the history, a brief review of activities of daily living concerning the hand, such as the ability to turn door knobs, hold a cup, button and unbutton clothes, and handle a fork and knife is of utmost importance. Ques-

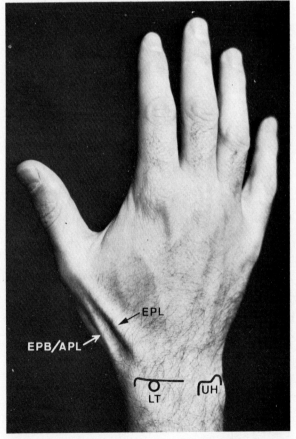

Fig. 4. Posterior aspect of hand and wrist: EPB, extensor pollicis brevis; APL, abductor pollicis longus; EPL, extensor pollicis longus; LT, Lister's tubercle; straight line, the radiocarpal joint; UH, distal ulnar head. Radially, the tendinous boundaries of the "anatomic snuffbox" are shown.

Table 1
Range of Motion of Wrist, Thumb, and Fingers

Joint		Maneuver	Degrees
Wrist		Flexion	75
		Extension	70
		Abduction (radial deviation)	20
		Adduction (ulnar deviation)	35
Thumb			
	CMC	Flexion	15
		Extension (radial abduction)	20
		Abduction (palmar abduction)	60
		Adduction	0
	MCP	Flexion	55
		Extension	10
	IP	Flexion	80
		Extension	15
Fingers			
	MCP	Flexion	90
		Extension	45
		Abduction/adduction*	
	PIP	Flexion	100
		Extension	0
	DIP	Flexion	80
		Extension	0

*Variable, 0 at 90° flexion.

tions are asked regarding the presence of pain, weakness, stiffness, paresthesiae, and color changes, as well as their exact location and circumstances.

A careful inspection is made of the following: nails; skin; alignment of forearm, wrist, and fingers; normal contours; and muscle bulk in interosseous spaces and thenar and hypothenar eminences. Pitting or detachment (onycholysis) of the nails, ulcerations, scars, rashes, swelling, atrophies, and deformities are recorded.

A functional assessment of thumb and fingers is more important than detailed goniometric measurements. Precise goniometry is important in the wrist and, under certain circumstances, in the thumb and fingers (Table 1). In general, motion of the fingers and thumb is normal when all can reach the palm in flexion and can be returned to their extended position, and when the tip of the thumb can reach the tip of all other digits (opposition). This is also an excellent estimation of the precision motion of the hand. Abduction and adduction are measured in centimeters as the maximal span from the tip of the thumb to the tip of the little finger. Impaired thumb function is expressed as the distance in centimeters from its tip to the MCP joint of the little finger.

Flexion and extension of fingers occur in the sagittal plane, but similar motions of the thumb are recorded in the frontal plane (despite the fact that anatomically the axis of flexion at the thumb CMC joint is not at 90° with the axis of flexion of the MCP joints of digits 2–5, but at 45°). Thus, in extension, the thumb is maximally deviated toward the radial side in the plane of the hand, and flexion brings its tip close to MCP 5. In abduction, the thumb moves anteriorly and becomes almost vertical to the

plane of the hand, while adduction returns it to the radial side of the index finger.

Flexor lags are recorded in centimeters from the tip of the digit to the palm, and extensor lags in centimeters from the tip of the digit to the plane of the dorsum of the hand. It is important to remember that lags due to tendon rupture, loss of gliding within sheaths, or peripheral neuropathy lead to a disproportionate loss of active motion while passive motion can be normal. In contrast, loss of motion due to articular disease leads to equal loss of active and passive motion.

The integrity of long flexors is tested by attempting flexion of the digit while the middle phalanx (the proximal phalanx in the thumb) is held in extension. Ruptures of extensor tendons produce a variable degree of extension lag which relates to the number of tendons ruptured. If rupture of only one tendon has occurred (usually in the dorsum of the wrist in rheumatoid and other synovitis), distal intertendinous connections tend to mask the loss by transferring pulling forces from neighboring tendons. Rupture of two or more tendons negates this phenomenon and obvious deformity results.

Extensor lags can occur in the absence of ruptured extensor tendons in three situations. The first results from MCP synovitis leading to volar subluxation and contracture of the intrinsic muscles. The second is also due to MCP synovitis, but here the extensor tendons slip into the ulnar valleys, on occasion deeply enough to become weak flexors. Finally, posterior interosseous nerve palsy (discussed below) can be confused with extensor tendon rupture.

Abnormal intrinsic muscle tension is tested by holding the proximal phalanx in extension (thereby stretching the intrinsic muscles further) while the middle phalanx (distal in the thumb) is passively brought into flexion. Tight intrinsic muscles make the flexion difficult or impossible.

Finally, the integrity of the collateral ligaments of the MCP joints is tested by attempting to abduct and adduct the digit while the proximal phalanx is kept at 90° flexion. Only tears of one or both ligaments will allow such motion to occur.

Synovitis is identified by pain on motion (particularly at the extremes of motion), weakness, swelling, increased warmth, local tenderness, and decreased range of motion. In IP joints the sole evidence of synovitis may be pain on lateral compression of the joint. In IP and MCP joints, small effusions are best appreciated by four-finger palpation—two at the sides, one dorsal, and one palmar to the joint. Swelling is unusual at the wrist and the only finding may be a weak grip and deep tenderness at the radiocarpal joint.

Pain resulting from eroded joint surfaces occurs throughout the range of motion of the joint, is generally associated with bony crepitation, and is aggravated by longitudinal compression of the joint.

The power grip can be assessed with a dynamometer or tested with an ordinary sphygmomanometer, in which the rubber part of the calf is folded twice and the cotton flap rolled around it. The apparatus is calibrated at 20 mm Hg and the patient is asked to squeeze the cuff maximally three times. The results are averaged and noted as grip strength.

Abnormal Findings

Deformities. Ulnar drift. In this deformity, usually bilateral, the digits have undergone an ulnar angulation at the MCP joint. A common association is volar (anterior) subluxation of the base of the proximal phalanx. Its pathogenesis is a subject of controversy. Some important factors include (1) weakening of the capsule and ligaments secondary to chronic MCP synovitis, (2) normally greater ulnar and volar strain exerted by the flexor tendons, and (3) flexion of ring and little finger CMC and MCP joints upon completion of tightening of power grip, resulting in an ulnar pull along the line of the transverse metacarpal ligament (which, as mentioned before, relates to the base of the proximal phalanges 2–5 through its volar plate attachment).

Rheumatoid arthritis is the most common cause of ulnar drift, but it has also been observed in systemic lupus erythematosus, rheumatic fever, Parkinson's disease, congenital deformities, and as a result of certain occupations such as carpentry.

Boutonniere deformity. This deformity is characterized by flexion at the PIP joint and hyperextension at the DIP joint (Figure 5). It is due to chronic synovitis of the PIP joint, which causes weakening of the central slip of the extensor tendon and palmar dislocation of the lateral bands. When this occurs, the lateral bands act as flexors rather than extensors of the PIP joint. Boutonniere deformity is seen in 15–30 percent of patients with rheumatoid arthritis, in other chronic synovitis such as psoriatic arthropathy, and as a result of trauma or burns.

Swan-neck deformity. This deformity consists of hyperextension of the PIP joint, and flexion of the DIP joint (Figure 6). Unlike ulnar drift and boutonniere deformity, which result from disease in one joint, swan-neck deformity can occur due to disease at the DIP, PIP, MCP, or extensor and flexor tendon, muscle imbalance as seen in certain neurologic disorders, and heritable disorders of the connective tissue, particularly the Ehlers-Danlos syndrome.

Rupture or stretching of the extensor tendon as it inserts in the distal phalanx leads to DIP flexor deformity (mallet finger), which may lead to compensatory hyperextension of the PIP joint. Chronic synovitis may stretch the volar capsule at the PIP joint and rupture of the superficial flexor tendon may lead to hyperextension of the PIP joint with secondary flexor deformity at the DIP joint. The most complex mechanism, often found in rheumatoid arthritis, is MCP synovitis leading to volar subluxation and flexor deformity and tightening of the intrinsic muscles. The latter produces hyperextension of the PIP joint; the flexor deformity of the DIP joint then develops as a secondary or compensatory mechanism. Maneuvers to detect intrinsic muscle tightening have been described

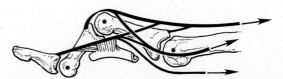

Fig. 5. Boutonniere deformity. (Modified by permission of author and publisher from Tubiana R: Lésions traumatiques de l'appareil extenseur au niveau des doigts, in Verdan C (ed): Chirurgie des Tendons de la Main. Paris, Expansion Scientifique, 1976.)

above. Loss of hand function in swan-neck deformity is directly related to loss of PIP joint flexibility, which in turn may be functional or due to structural damage.

Thumb deformities. These may include flexor deformity of the MCP joint with hyperextension of the IP joint, or hyperextension of the MCP joint (usually associated with lateral instability) with flexor deformity of the IP joint. If the MCP and IP joints of the thumb are considered equivalent to the PIP and DIP joints of other digits, deformities of the thumb with flexion of the MCP joint are equivalents of the boutonniere deformity, and those with hyperextension of the MCP joints are equivalents of the swan-neck deformity (Lister). Nalebuff has classified the thumb deformities in types I–IV according to the pattern of deformity and the joint primarily responsible for the deformity. Type I is the common boutonniere deformity due to MCP synovitis, while in the rare type II the primary damage is at the CMC joint. The swan-neck deformity of type III is due to synovitis of the CMC joint, whereas in type IV the same final deformity is due to synovitis at the MCP joint.

Another important thumb deformity is the "square hand," due to degenerative joint disease of the trapeziometacarpal joint. Here, evidence of synovitis affecting other joints is lacking and associated Heberden's nodes can be prominent. Pain and weak grip result from this process, which may be difficult to distinguish from early de Quervain's tenosynovitis. Maneuvers to differentiate the two are discussed below.

Tenosynovitis. Flexor tenosynovitis. Inflammatory and/or hyperplastic changes in flexor tendon sheaths may occur as a result of repetitive trauma, chronic synovitis, acute or chronic infection, or for no obvious reason. In addition to the features suggestive of tendon sheath dis-

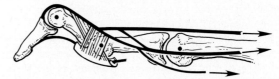

Fig. 6. Swan-neck deformity. (Modified by permission of author and publisher from Tubiana R: Lésions traumatiques de l'appareil extenseur au niveau des doigts, in Verdan C (ed): Chirurgie des Tendons de la Main. Paris, Expansion Scientifique, 1976.)

ease described above, tenderness along the tendon sheath, various degrees of swelling, and locking of the finger in flexion (trigger finger) often occur.

In digits 2, 3, and 4 the flexor tendon sheaths extend from the distal phalanx to approximately the flexor creases of the palm, but the sheath of the flexor pollicis longus extends to the carpal tunnel, and in 70 percent of people the sheath of the flexor tendon of the fifth digit merges into the tendon sheaths of the carpal tunnel. Thus at the carpal tunnel two distinct tendon sheaths can be identified: one corresponds to the flexor pollicis longus and the other is a folded structure common to the flexor digitorum tendons and the median nerve. Due to the toughness of the flexor retinaculum, wrist flexor tenosynovitis is associated with little if any swelling. The most important findings are a weak grip and evidence of median nerve dysfunction (carpal tunnel syndrome as described below).

Flexor tenosynovitis is common in rheumatoid arthritis. Several digits are often involved and there is a high correlation between digital flexor tenosynovitis, wrist flexor tenosynovitis expressed as the carpal tunnel syndrome, and dorsal tenosynovitis. In the idiopathic form, digital flexor tenosynovitis usually involves only one digit, the trigger phenomenon is common, and again, there is high association with fibrotic proliferation at other sites such as carpal tunnel syndrome, de Quervain's tenosynovitis, and Dupuytren's contracture.

Dorsal tenosynovitis. This is a common finding in rheumatoid arthritis but it can also occur in other chronic synovitides, such as psoriatic arthrophathy. Clinically, it is characterized by a painless, boggy swelling in the dorsum of the wrist. Deep tenderness or pain on motion of the wrist is an indication of concomitant wrist synovitis. The danger of dorsal tenosynovitis lies in possible rupture of the extensor tendons of the digits, usually the fifth and the fourth. Although it is not possible to predict which patients with dorsal tenosynovitis will have this complication, rupture of one tendon usually presages rupture of another. Two other processes can lead to extensor tendon rupture in patients with rheumatoid arthritis: rupture of the extensor pollicies longus at Lister's tubercle (usually in association with tenosynovitis), and attrition of the fifth, fourth, and sometimes the third extensor tendons against a dorsally subluxed, roughened ulnar head.

DeQuervain's tenosynovitis. This syndrome encompasses the clinical findings resulting from nonspecific inflammatory and proliferative changes in the common tendon sheath of the extensor pollicis brevis and abductor pollicis longus. Occupational trauma is important; it often occurs in electricians, typists, and other individuals whose activities require repetitive flexion of the thumb and abduction of the wrist. The patient presents with pain in the radial aspect of the wrist that is exacerbated upon any movement of the thumb. The pain often radiates to the thumb and the distal forearm. There is exquisite

tenderness at the radial styloid, and ulnar deviation of the wrist while the flexed thumb is tucked inside the remaining four fingers elicites excruciating pain (Finkelstein's sign). The tendon sheath itself may be thickened, and the crepitus may be felt on motion of the thumb.

Several conditions should be carefully considered in the differential diagnosis, and the possibility of a fortuitously or causally related association should be kept in mind. Wrist synovitis is excluded by free wrist motion and absence of deep tenderness at the articular line. Degenerative disease of the CMC joint of the thumb is excluded by the absence of pain and crepitation upon gentle passive torque motion of the joint. A negative Tinel's sign (see below) mitigates against the presence of carpal tunnel syndrome.

DeQuervain's tenosynovitis responds well to a local corticosteroid injection (this should distend the sheath) and a thumb splint. Recurrences are quite unusual and can be treated by tenosynovectomy. Distension of this tendon sheath, sometimes causing an hourglass appearance due to the impression of the extensor retinaculum, and a granular content should raise the suspicion of tuberculosis. Acute tenosynovitis with redness and heath is often an accompaniment of disseminated gonococcal or meningoccal infection.

Dupuytren's contracture. The thick palmar fascia is continuous with the tendon of the palmaris longus and the distal edge of the flexor retinaculum proximally, and it splits distally into four slips which merge with the fibrous digital sheaths of the flexor tendons. Its surface is firmly bound to the skin by anteroposterior fibers intermingled with fat and areolar tissue, which act as a cushion and allow a firmer grip. Dupuytren's contracture develops as fibrous hyperplasia sets in the palmar fascia and the fibrofatty tissue anterior to it, resulting in a fibrotic retraction of the palmar skin often associated with flexor deformity of the ring and sometimes the little finger. Nodules may form in the palmar skin and may be the sole manifestation of the disease. In some cases Dupuytren's contracture is associated with one or more of the following: fibrotic knuckle pads, nodular thickening of the plantar fascia, and fascial thickening in the penis (Peyronie's disease).

The etiology of Dupuytren's contracture is unknown. It is seen predominantly in males. A high prevalence of the condition has been found in older individuals, alcoholics, epileptics, and patients with pulmonary tuberculosis. It has occurred in the wake of a bout of shoulder–hand syndrome, and some cases of shoulder–hand syndrome have followed fasciectomy for Dupuytren's disease.

Fortunately, most cases do not require treatment. Local corticosteroid infiltrations are usually of no avail. If severe deformity develops or if there is functional loss of the hand, surgical intervention may be indicated.

Nerve compression syndromes. Carpal tunnel syndrome. This common syndrome results from compression of the median nerve within the tight confines of the carpal tunnel. As mentioned above, the contents of the tunnel include the median nerve, the flexor tendons of the thumb and digits, and their synovial sheaths. Any one of these, in addition to the osteoligamentous boundaries of the tunnel, can develop volumetric changes that may cause compression and dysfunction of the median nerve.

Thus, carpal tunnel syndrome may result from synovitis (rheumatoid arthritis, systemic lupus erythematosus, or rubella arthritis), instertitial swelling (pregnancy, oral contraceptives, hypothyroidism, or acromegaly), proteinaceous deposits (amyloidosis), hypertrophic neuropathy (leprosy or idiopathic), or anomalous muscle bellies (lumbricals, flexor digitorum superficials, or palmaris profundus), as well as ganglia, osteophytes, fracture (common), tophi, and osteoid osteoma of carpal bones.

Classically, nocturnal paresthesia with or without pain occurs in the sensory distribution of the median nerve (radial side of the palm, palmar surface of the thumb, and index and middle fingers), progressing to continuous symptoms, decreased grip and dexterity, and atrophy of the superficial muscles of the thenar eminence. In some patients, however, pain and paresthesias are perceived in the arm or the shoulder. Tapping over the median nerve (Fig. 2) will reproduce the symptoms (Tinel's sign), or holding the wrist in flexion (Phalen's maneuver) will reproduce the symptoms, usually within 1 minute.

The final documentation of carpal tunnel syndrome requires nerve conduction studies (particularly the sensory conduction which is affected earlier by pressure on the nerve) and an electromyogram. While these tests are definitive, they may not be needed in clear-cut cases treated conservatively. When surgery is contemplated, however, they are mandatory to rule out definitively peripheral neuropathy or radiculopathy as the cause of symptoms.

Conservative treatment of carpal tunnel syndrome includes a resting splint, systemic measures directed to the cause of the compression (diuretics if edema, antiinflammatory agents if synovitis), and local injection of corticosteroids. Upon failure of these procedures, surgery may be needed to avoid permanent nerve damage. If surgery is performed, it is of utmost importance not just to decompress, but also to obtain a tissue sample which in obscure cases can afford a final diagnosis.

Ulnar tunnel syndrome at the wrist (Guyon's canal). This syndrome is infrequently encountered except as a result of trauma or pressure from a ganglion or an anomalous muscle. Weakness and atrophy of the ulnar-innervated muscles ensues, which is particularly noticeable at the interossei. Numbness in the small and ring fingers is unusual.

Ulnar nerve compression distal in the palmar space. Rarely, a deep-seated ganglion may produce this syndrome characterized by selective atrophy of the first interosseal space.

ELBOWS
Anatomy
Bones and joints. At the elbow the distal end of the humerus meets the proximal end of the radius and ulna. Whereas the radius has a concave facet which corresponds to the convexity of the capitulum the trochlear notch of the ulna articulates with the trochlea of the humerus in a typical hinge arrangement. In addition, the head of the radius, held in place by an annular ligament, articulates with a notch in the lateral aspect of the coronoid process of the proximal end of the ulna at the proximal radioulnar joint, which widely communicates with the elbow joint. The articular capsule of the elbow is reinforced by strong medial and lateral collateral ligaments.

Muscles and innervation. The most important flexors of the elbow are the brachialis and biceps brachii (innervated by the musculocutaneous, roots $C_{5,6}$) and the brachioradialis (radial, $C_{5,6}$). Extension is predominantly exerted by the triceps brachii (radial, $C_{6,7,8}$). The main supinators are the supinator (radial, $C_{5,6}$) and biceps brachii, while the strongest pronator is the pronator quadratus (anterior interosseous, C_8, T_1).

Anatomic landmarks. Important landmarks in the lateral aspect of the elbow held at 90° flexion (Fig. 7) include the olecranon process at its tip, and proximal and lateral to it the prominence of the lateral epicondyle in which the wrist extensors insert. Anterior to the lateral epicondyle the radial head can be readily palpated, especially during pronation/supination. Medially, the olecranon process is again identified at the tip, and proximal and medial to it is the medial epicondyle, which is the main insertion of the wrist flexors. The ulnar nerve can be rolled under the fingers in the cleft between the olecranon process and the medial epicondyle; it is contained in the cubital tunnel, the floor of which is the medial ligament of the elbow, and the roof of which is a ligament that extends from the medial epicondyle to the medial aspect of the olecranon process. When the elbow is fully extended the pit lateral to the olecranon process corresponds to the radiocapitular joint.

Physical Examination
The elbow is a hinge that can only be flexed and extended. Pronation and supination occur as the head of the radius pivots on the capitulum, while its distal end crosses the ulnar head anteriorly, medially in pronation and laterally in supination. When the elbow is extended a lateral angulation (valgus) of the axis of the forearm in relation to the axis of the humerus develops, the "carrying angle." Upon progressive flexion, however, this angle changes into a varus angulation. The range of motion of the elbow and the radioulnar joints is shown in Table 2.

Abnormal Findings
Loss of active and passive extension and loss of flexion are common findings in rheumatoid arthritis, other synovitides, and articular disorders such as chondrocalcinosis. In mild or early forms of rheumatoid arthri-

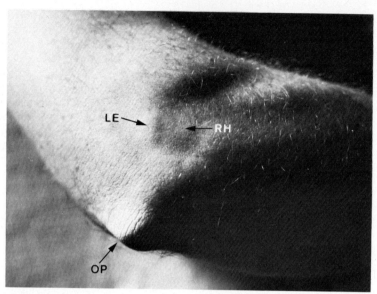

Fig. 7. Lateral view of the elbow. At its tip, the olecranon process (OP) is seen. Above and lateral to it, the lateral epicondyle (LE) is seen and is readily palpable. The proximal radial head (RH) can be palpated just distal to LE.

tis painful loss of the last degrees of extension, perhaps in association with minimal loss of motion and tenderness of the wrist joint, may be the only physical indication of the disease. Synovial effusions are often first noted laterally in the space between the olecranon process and the lateral epicondyle. While loss of extension results in minor functional loss, marked loss of flexion can interfere with essential activities such as feeding.

Elbow instability, subluxation of the proximal radioulnar joint, and posterior subluxation of the ulna are unfortunate complications of persisting rheumatoid synovitis.

Epicondylitis. *Lateral epicondylitis (tennis elbow).* This common condition (by no means confined to tennis players) is characterized by pain in the lateral aspect of the elbow which often radiates to the lateral aspect of the forearm and sometimes to the upper arm. The diagnosis is established by finding an area of exquisite tenderness at or just distal to the lateral epicondyle. The pain is reproduced by extension of the wrist against resistance.

Several mechanisms have been considered as re-

sponsible for this condition, including increased pain perception in an area normally tender, muscle attachment strain, minute tendinous tears, and calcific deposits and cartilage fibrillation at the head of the radius. However, none has explained all cases and it is possible that the pathogenesis and lesion may vary with the individual and the stage of the disease.

Fortunately, most cases of lateral epicondylitis respond to restriction of the offending activity and its course is one of slow, spontaneous resolution after weeks to months (and occasionally longer). Rest, isometric arm exercises, and local corticosteroid infiltration relieve the majority of patients. Tennis players may benefit from a larger grip on the racket, rackets that absorb more stress, warming up before playing, and stopping before becoming overtired. Surgical treatment is usually successful but is reserved for cases resistant to conservative therapy in which severe pain persists.

Medial epicondylitis (golfer's elbow). This is a mirror image of the tennis elbow, in that pain is present at the medial epicondyle and is increased by flexion of the wrist against resistance. Therapy is similar to that for tennis elbow.

Subcutaneous olecranon bursitis. The subcutaneous olecranon bursa (not to be confused with a bursa deep to the triceps tendon insertion in the olecranon process) is a disclike, flattened synovial sac with a minute amount of fluid, superficially located at the tip of the elbow. Its floor corresponds to the posterior aspect of the olecranon process, and the overlying skin is lax and virtually painless upon prick or puncture. Subcutaneous olecranon bursitis presents in pathognomonic fashion as a cystic swelling at the tip of the elbow. As a synovial

Table 2
Range of Motion of Elbow and Radioulnar Joints

Joint	Maneuver	Degrees
Elbow*	Flexion	145
	Extension	0
Radioulnar	Pronation	70
	Supination	85

*Carrying angle (radial deviation of forearm in full extension) 10°.

structure, the olecranon bursa is subject to most conditions that may affect diarthrodial joints, but with some peculiarities.

Acute cases may exhibit redness, warmth, tenderness, and pitting edema along the subcutaneous border of the ulna; subacute and chronic cases are usually painless. When inflammation is severe full flexion of the elbow may be prevented by mounting pain as the skin is increasingly taut in the final arc of flexion. Extension, however, is not impaired—an important clue to exclude concurrent elbow synovitis.

Cases of acute olecranon bursitis are usually due to sepsis or gout or are idiopathic (probably traumatic). Since clinical differentiation between these common etiologies is not possible, bursal aspiration is indicated. Bursal fluid analysis should be performed with the same attention to detail as synovial fluid analysis, including careful search for crystals and organisms (gram stain and appropriate cultures).

Septic subcutaneous olecranon bursitis usually follows trauma with a break of the skin; gram-positive cocci are often demonstrated in the fluid and cultures usually yield staphylococci and, less often, streptococci. In the absence of fever and clinical indications of bacteremia, those cases are treated with sling or needle or surgical drainage, depending upon the presence of inspissated fluid or evidence of loculation, and systemic antibiotics are administered orally for 10 days to 2 weeks.

Acute gouty bursitis is discussed elsewhere. Interestingly, the bursal fluid cell count in acute bursal gout is often low (below 5000 cells/mm³). A detailed search for crystals should be undertaken in sediment of spun specimens, lest crystals be missed.

In acute idiopathic olecranon bursitis crystals are not found on compensated polarized microscopy and cultures are negative. Despite the severe inflammation present, the cell count is low (below 5000/mm³), in association with a poor mucin clot.

Upon subsidence of acute idiopathic bursitis, and after aspiration in chronic cases, the bottom of the bursa is usually granular and often nodular, with nodules of up to 7 mm in diameter. Rheumatoid nodules and tophi, however, often occur at the roof of the bursa and can be displaced in all directions.

Subacute and chronic effusions associated with rheumatoid arthritis and other connective tissue disorders should be treated systemically, with local protection against pressure. They often persist, however. If not painful or unsightly, these chronic effusions, similar to idiopathic chronic effusions, are best left alone. Local steroid injection is successful in most cases but carries a slight risk of secondary infection. Bursectomy is curative.

Nerve compression syndromes. *Cubital tunnel syndrome.* Paresthesias, hypoesthesia, and sometimes weakness and atrophy of the intrinsic muscles of the hand may result from compression of the ulnar nerve at the cubital tunnel. This compression can be physiologic (as seen in some individuals after sleeping with the elbow in flexion, narrowing the cubital tunnel) or pathologic, either due to extrinsic pressure or to the presence of a space-occupying lesion within the canal. Extrinsic compression has often followed a faulty posture in the operating room, when the ulnar nerve was damaged by pressure on an armboard. Space-occupying lesions include rheumatoid synovitis, ostophytes, ganglia, aberrant muscles, and hypertrophic neuropathy as in leprosy.

Most patients with cubital tunnel syndrome experience pain and paresthesias in the ulnar distribution when the nerve is tapped and also upon forceful flexion of the elbow. Nerve conduction studies are helpful in accurately localizing the level of the lesion and radiopaque compressive lesions can be demonstrated by x-ray studies of the cubital canal. Treatment includes avoidance of external pressure and, if progressive deficit is noted, surgical decompression.

Posterior interosseous nerve syndrome. This deep branch of the radial nerve can be compressed by elbow joint synovitis. As a result of the compression, weakness of the long extensors ensues leading to paralytic flexion of the third, fourth, and fifth digits at the metacarpophalongeal joint. This can simulate extensor tendon rupture. However, passive flexion of the wrist will extend the MCP ruling out tendon rupture (tenodesis effect). Since the extensor carpi radialis receives its innervation above the site of compression, attempted dorsiflexion of the wrist will bring the wrist into radial deviation in the neutral position, which is diagnostic. An additional clue to this diagnosis is the presence of severe synovitis at the elbow, whereas extensor tendon rupture is usually associated with dorsal tenosynovitis or dorsal subluxation of the ulnar head at the wrist.

REFERENCES

Canoso JJ: Idiopathic or traumatic olecranon bursitis. Clinical features and bursal fluid analysis. Arthritis Rheum 20:1213, 1977

Dorwart BB, Schumacher HR: Hand deformities resembling rheumatoid arthritis. Semin Arthritis Rheum 4:53, 1974

Flatt AE: The Care of the Rheumatoid Hand (ed 2). St. Louis, Mosby, 1974

Gray RG, Gottlieb NL: Hand flexor tenosynovitis in rheumatoid arthritis. Arthritis Rheum 20:1003, 1977

Hueston JT, Tubiana R (eds): Dupuytren's Disease. New York, Grune & Stratton, 1974

Kuczynski K: Upper limb, in Passmore R, Robson JS (eds): A Companion to Medical Studies, vol 1 (ed 2). Oxford, Blackwell, 1976, pp 231–2345

Lapidus PW, Guidotti FP: Stenosing tenovaginitis of the wrist and fingers. Clin Orthop 83:87, 1972

Lister G: The Hand: Diagnosis and Indications. Edinburgh, Churchill Livingstone, 1977

Millender LH, Sledge CB (eds): Symposium on Rheumatoid Arthritis. Orthop Clin North Am 6:601, 1975

Murley AHG: The painful elbow. Practitioner 215:36, 1975

Phalen GS: The carpal-tunnel syndrome. Clinical evaluation of 598 hands. Clin Orthop 83:29, 1972

Priest JD, Jones HH, Nagel DA: Elbow injuries in highly skilled tennis players. J Sports Med 2:137, 1974

Stein H, Dickson RA, Bentley G: Rheumatoid arthritis of the elbow. Ann Rheum Dis 34:403, 1975

Tubiana R: Lésions traumatiques de l'appareil extenseur au niveau des doigts, in Verdan C (ed): Chirurgie des Tendons de la Main. Paris, Expansion Scientifique, 1976

Wadsworth TG: The external compression syndrome of the ulnar nerve at the cubital tunnel. Clin Orthop 124:189, 1977

SHOULDERS AND NECK

William P. Beetham, Jr.

Pain involving the neck often extends into the shoulder and upper extremity. Symptoms in these areas are common and may arise from cervical lesions, musculoskeletal disorders of the shoulder, or compression syndromes of the thoracic outlet, or they may be referred from more distant sites. A knowledge of the function and anatomy of the neck and shoulders is essential to the clinician who must evaluate pain and disability involving these areas. It is the purpose of this chapter to review the anatomy and function of the neck and shoulders and to describe a systematic clinical approach to symptoms in this area with special emphasis on a thorough physical examination. Throughout the chapter joint anatomy will be correlated with the techniques of physical examination used to detect and to localize disease within or outside the joint.

ANATOMY
Cervical Spine

The unique structure of the cervical spine provides support for the head by means of the coordinated action of muscle, ligaments, and bones and also allows extensive mobility. The neck has the greatest range of motion of the entire spine.

Atlas and axis. The cervical spine contains seven vertebrae. The upper two cervical vertebrae have a special structure. The *atlas,* or first cervical vertebra, consists of an anterior and posterior arch with enlarged lateral masses. The ring of bone formed by these arches encloses the odontoid process of the axis anteriorly and the spinal canal posteriorly. Transverse ligaments attach the odontoid process to the atlas. The atlas articulates with the skull by means of two atlantooccipital joints, which are specialized for flexion and extension. The *axis,* or second cervical vertebra, has a bony projection known as the dens or odontoid process, which extends from the upper portion of its vertebral body. The atlas articulates with the axis through a midline joint formed between the odontoid process and the anterior arch of the atlas and also through a pair of lateral joints. These atlantoaxial joints allow rotation of the skull and atlas on the odontoid process.

Vertebrae. The remaining cervical vertebrae consist of an anterior portion, which is the vertebral body, lateral masses containing the pedicles and facets, and the laminae and posterior spines (Fig. 1). The vertebral body and adjacent intervertebral discs comprise the weight-bearing area. The pedicle and lamina on each side fuse together posteriorly, forming a bony arch which encloses the spinal cord. A bony spinous process projects posteriorly from the laminae in the midline. The seventh cervical and first thoracic vertebrae have spinous processes that are especially prominent at the base of the back of the neck. A lateral process, known as the transverse process, arises from the lamina on each side. These bony projections are the sites of muscle attachments and supporting ligaments.

Apophyseal joints. Each vertebra has four articular processes which arise from the lateral masses. One process projects downward and outward on each side of the vertebra and one process projects upward and inward from each side of the vertebra to form a pair of true or diarthrodial joints between adjacent vertebrae (Fig. 1). These articulations are the apophyseal joints and are also known as the posterior articular facets. They contain articular cartilages and synovial membranes. The opposing articular surfaces formed between the inferior process of one vertebra and the superior process of the next lower vertebra help to stabilize the vertebrae and prevent forward displacement of the upper vertebra on the lower one.

Uncovertebral joints (joints of von Luschka). The lower five cervical vertebrae contain bony projections that arise along the posterolateral aspect of the vertebral bodies. An articulation occurs between the upward bony ridge on the superior surface of the vertebral body and the beveled inferior surface of the adjacent vertebral body (Fig. 1). These articulations are not present in the remainder of the vertebral column. They have been given various names, including uncovertebral joints, lateral interbody joints, and joints of von Luschka. The anatomy and function of these articulations are controversial. Most anatomists believe these articulations do not contain articular cartilages, synovial membranes, or joint capsules and therefore do not function as true joints. They are actually pseudoarthroses. The bony ridges formed by these articulations protect the intervertebral discs along the posterolateral aspect of the vertebral body. Osteophyte formation at the uncovertebral joints may encroach on the intervertebral foramen and nerve root.

Intervertebral discs. The vertebral bodies of C_2 through C_7 are separated by a fibrocartilagenous intervertebral disc and thin cartilagenous plates. The cartilagenous plates are located between the vertebral body and the disc. The outer layers of the disc are composed of tough, concentrically arranged fibers (annulus fibrosus) that enclose the soft, gelatinous center (nucleus pulposus). The vertical height of the cervical disc is two times greater anteriorly than posteriorly. The wedge shape of these discs helps form the normal lordotic curve of the cervical spine. The elasticity of the disc allows both lateral and vertical compression. This helps to absorb shock on the spinal column and distributes the weight of the body more evenly.

Spinal nerves. There are eight pairs of spinal nerves in the cervical region of the spine. The first leaves the spinal canal between the occipital bone and the atlas, and the eighth leaves between the seventh cervical and first thoracic vertebrae. Each nerve is connected to the spinal cord by a ventral and dorsal root. The dorsal root is the sensory branch, and the ventral root is the motor branch. Both of these roots merge into a mixed spinal nerve before passing obliquely through the intervertebral foramen (Fig. 1). The foramen is bounded above and below by the pedicles of adjacent vertebrae. The inner aspect of the foramen is formed by the uncovertebral and lateral aspect of the vertebral body. The outer wall of the fora-

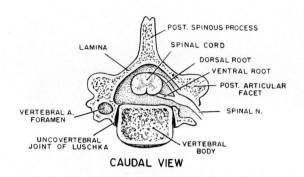

CAUDAL VIEW

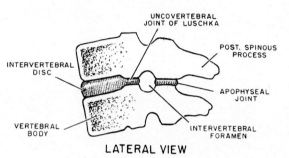

LATERAL VIEW

Fig. 1. Typical cervical vertebra (C_{3-7}).

men is formed by the apophyseal joint. The motor portion of the nerve lies close to the uncovertebral joint and the sensory portion is located near the posterior articulation, making them susceptible to injury from derangement in either area.

Vertebral artery. The vertebral artery is the first branch of the subclavian artery. It passes through the foramina in the transverse processes of the sixth through the second cervical vertebrae and supplies blood to the brain (Fig. 1). Degenerative change in the vertebrae may cause compression of the artery.

Shoulder Joint and Pelvic Girdle

Glenohumeral joint and pelvic girdle. The glenohumeral or shoulder joint is a ball and socket joint capable of great mobility. It is formed by the articulation of the humeral head with the glenoid cavity of the scapula (Fig. 2). The scapula is a large, flat, triangular bone that forms part of the shoulder girdle. It is attached posteriorly to the chest wall by muscles. The scapula is divided posteriorly by a spine into the supraspinatus and infraspinatus fossae. The spine extends laterally to form the acromion, which projects anterolaterally over the glenoid cavity. The acromion also forms the summit of the shoulder and articulates with the distal end of the clavicle. The clavicle constitutes the anterior portion of the shoulder girdle and assists in holding the arm away from the body. The coracoid process arises from the neck of the scapula near the glenoid cavity and projects anteriorly. The scapular borders, acromion, clavicle, and coracoid process are all clinically palpable.

Articular capsule and synovial membrane. The articular capsule of the shoulder encloses the glenohumeral joint and is very loose and lax, allowing marked mobility

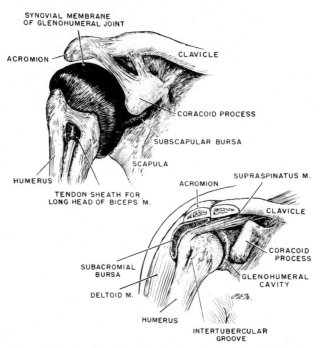

Fig. 2. Anterior views of the shoulder joint showing the relationship of the subacromial bursa and synovial membrane of the glenohumeral joint to adjacent bony structures.

of the joint. The synovial membrane lines the inner surface of the capsule and has two outpouchings: one functions as a bursa for the subscapularis muscle and the other extends along the bicipital groove of the humerus forming a sheath for the tendon of the long head of the biceps muscle (Fig. 2).

Muscles and rotator cuff. The shoulder joint is enclosed by a group of powerful muscles and tendons that strengthen the joint and adjacent capsule. The tendons of the supraspinatus, infraspinatus, and teres minor muscles insert into the greater tuberosity of the humerus, and the tendon of the subscapularis muscle inserts into the lesser tuberosity. Together these four muscles and tendons are known as the rotator cuff of the shoulder and help prevent displacement of the humerus from the glenoid cavity, stabilizing the joint. Each of the four tendons is incorporated into the fibrous articular capsule that encloses the shoulder joint before their insertions. The capsule is reinforced anteriorly by the subscapularis tendon, superiorly by the supraspinatous tendon, and posteriorly by the teres minor and infraspinatus tendons.

Bursae. The subacromial bursa is a large structure that lies below the acromion and superficial to the rotator cuff and articular capsule (Fig. 2). The subdeltoid bursa is a lateral extension of the subacromial bursa. It lies beneath the deltoid muscle. When the arm is elevated, the bursa and underlying supraspinatous tendon become compressed by the acromion. A tear of the rotator cuff is likely to produce a communication between the bursa and glenohumeral cavity. A communication between the bursa and joint cavity exists in about 25 percent of older adults. The subcoracoid bursa separates the coracoid

process from the capsule of the shoulder. Several other bursae are located in the region of the shoulder but are not significant clinically.

Acromioclavicular and sternoclavicular joints. The acromioclavicular and sternoclavicular joints are both true diarthrodial joints containing articular cartilage and synovial membranes. The sternoclavicular joint is separated into two distinct cavities by a fibrocartilaginous disc. Any movement of the shoulder girdle involves these joints and is associated with scapular motion. When these articulations are abnormal, palpation over the joints may reveal swelling or tenderness. Pain involving these joints can often be aggravated by motion of the shoulder girdle.

PHYSICAL EXAMINATION
Neck

Inspection and palpation. Inspection may reveal important clues. An abnormally low hairline, webbing of the lateral tissues, and a midline pore or tuft of hair may be signs of associated spine anomalies or malformations. The contours of the neck and shoulder are inspected from both front and back. The hostile, anxious individual often tightens the neck muscles. Poor posture associated with slumping or rounding of the shoulders and forward protrusion of the head causes muscular strain. Muscle spasm in the neck is associated with stiffness and straightening of the cervical spine, which loses its normal lordotic curvature. In torticollis, the head is laterally flexed or rotated by contraction of muscles including the sternocleidomastoid, which may become hypertrophic on the involved side. The neck should also be palpated for areas of tenderness or masses, such as tumors, cysts, thyroid enlargement, lymph nodes, and abscesses. Inspection and palpation supplement each other and often can be performed together. They should be followed by an evaluation of joint motion.

Cervical motion. The neck is capable of a wide range of motion. The head can be bent forward for flexion and backward for extension. It can be rotated to each side as if looking over the shoulder. Lateral movement is evaluated by tipping the patient's head sideways, bringing the ear close to the shoulder. The patient with a painful neck may elevate the shoulder girdle instead of bending the neck in an effort to avoid painful neck motion by substituting scapular swing. This may create a false impression of good motion.

The range of motion in the neck is dependent on the composite movement between all vertebrae. Normal motion is determined by the compressibility of the intervertebral discs, shape and angulation of articular surfaces, and laxity of ligamentous structures. Flexion and extension occur primarily between the atlas and skull. Most of the rotation in the neck takes place in the atlantoaxial joints. The other cervical joints allow flexion, extension, lateral bending, and rotation. Lateral motion of the neck, however, occurs primarily in the lower portion of the cervical spine.

Normally the cervical spine permits about 45° of flexion, 55° of extension, 40° of lateral bending, and 70° of rotation. Any acute disorder which produces muscle spasm may restrict motion of the cervical spine temporarily. Chronic inflammatory or degenerative disease of the spine, such as ankylosing spondylitis, causes permanent loss of motion. Rigidity of the neck may represent meningeal irritation due to meningitis or subarachnoid hemorrhage, increased muscle tone as in Parkinsonism, or loss of bony mobility as in ankylosing spondylitis.

Shoulder

Patterns of pain (palpation). A thorough physical examination can often help establish the cause of pain and limitation of motion in the shoulder. There are three basic patterns of pain in the shoulder: referred pain; disease within the shoulder joint; and involvement of muscles, tendons, and bursae which lie outside the shoulder joint. Careful localization of pain and tenderness by palpation is an essential part of the shoulder examination.

Referred pain. Referred pain is caused by disease that lies outside the shoulder joint in a region that has innervation in common with the shoulder. For example, angina or disease under the diaphragm may be referred to the shoulder. Pain due to degenerative joint or disc disease in the cervical spine is commonly referred to the region of the shoulder. Radicular pain resulting from nerve root impingement may extend down the arm into specific fingers and cause decreased stretch reflexes, muscular weakness, and numbness or tingling in the fingers. Cervical syndromes are usually associated with pain and stiffness in the neck muscles. When shoulder pain is referred from other areas, motion of the shoulder is usually normal unless there is secondary adhesive capsulitis.

Disease within the shoulder joint. Pain in the shoulder due to disease within the shoulder joint itself is relatively uncommon but may occur in rheumatoid arthritis and less frequently in degenerative joint disease, especially when there has been previous injury. This type of pain is usually diffuse and difficult to localize. The pain is often aggravated by motion of the arm and is associated with limitation of motion in the shoulder.

Involvement of muscles, tendons, bursae. The third and by far the commonest cause of pain near the shoulder is involvement of structures that lie outside the joint itself, such as muscles, tendons, and bursae. The subacromial bursa, which lies below the acromion and underneath the deltoid muscle, is commonly involved along with the underlying supraspinatus tendon (Fig. 2). Inflammation of this bursa or underlying tendon causes pain and tenderness in the region of the shoulder. The pain extends into the upper arm but usually not the lower arm. The patient with acute bursitis or tendinitis of the shoulder tends to hold the arm at the side because abduction of the arm is very painful. When the arm is raised over the head, the subacromial bursa and supraspinatus tendon are squeezed between the humerus and acromion causing pain. Before the shoulder is examined by palpation, the patient should be asked to point to the area of greatest pain or tenderness with the hand of the uninvolved extremity. This is often very helpful since the patient's description of the pain may be misleading. Often an exquisitely tender area can be consistently localized by palpation in the region of the deltoid muscle over the anterior and anterolateral aspect of the shoulder joint. If the inflammatory reaction is mild or chronic, the pain is likely to be diffuse or vague and cannot be accurately localized by palpation.

Bicipital tenosynovitis. Bicipital tenosynovitis may cause pain in the shoulder. It is characterized by inflammation of the tendon and tendon sheath of the long head of the biceps muscle. Rolling of the bicipital tendon under the examiner's fingertips is extremely painful when this condition is present. The tendon is located in the groove near the anterior aspect of the humeral head (Fig. 2). Accentuation of pain when the patient's forearm is supinated against resistance with the elbow flexed at 90° is known as Yergason's sign and is helpful in confirming the diagnosis.

Inspection. Both shoulders should be inspected for evidence of swelling, muscle atrophy, asymmetry, and fasciculations. Visible distention of the articular capsule resulting from synovitis or fluid in the shoulder joint is relatively uncommon and when present produces soft tissue swelling over the anterior aspect of the joint. Swelling of the subacromial bursa may cause localized fullness in the region of the deltoid muscle, which may be distended further by partial elevation of the arm. When the shoulder is dislocated anteriorly, the lateral aspect of the shoulder appears flat, losing its rounded appearance. Dislocation of the shoulder posteriorly produces flatness of the anterior aspect of the shoulder. Bilateral periarticular swelling

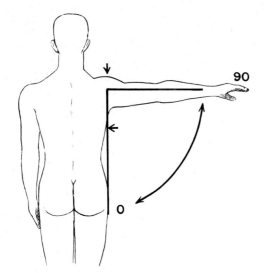

Fig. 3. Range of abduction for normal shoulder joint with scapula fixed by applying pressure in areas marked by arrows.

may occur in the region of the shoulder as a conspicuous feature of amyloid disease and is known as the shoulder pad sign.

Shoulder motion. The next method of evaluating the shoulder consists of measuring the range of motion in the shoulder. The shoulder is the most movable joint in the body. Motion of the shoulder is complicated because it not only occurs in the glenohumeral joint but also involves a combination of synchronous movements at the acromioclavicular, sternoclavicular, and scapulothoracic articulations. The glenohumeral joint permits flexion (forward movement of the arm), extension (backward move-

ment of the arm), abduction (elevation of the arm from the side), adduction (lowering the arm to the side), external rotation (turning the arm outward), internal rotation (turning the arm inward), and circumduction (a combination of all these motions). In addition, the other shoulder girdle joints allow elevation or shrugging of the shoulder girdle above the resting position, depression or lowering the shoulder girdle below the resting position, forward protrusion of the shoulder girdle, and backward retraction of the shoulder girdle.

Active motion. Most of the motion in raising the arm to 90° is done in the shoulder joint (glenohumeral joint), but above 90° most of the motion is performed by swinging the scapula. Scapula swing is associated with elevation or a shrugging motion of the shoulder. In order to evaluate abduction of the shoulder joint it is necessary to prevent scapula swing by stabilizing the scapula. This can be done by fixing the scapula posteriorly with one hand or by pressing down on the shoulder to prevent any shrugging or shoulder elevation. Normally the shoulder is capable of 90° of abduction with the scapula stabilized (Fig. 3).

A simple method of evaluating shoulder motion is to have the patient raise both arms above the head with the elbows extended and touch the palms of the hands together (Fig. 4). This will demonstrate pain, weakness, and limitation of motion. This maneuver also evaluates abductors and rotators and is an excellent general screening test for involvement of the shoulders. Do not let the patient bend the elbows or bring the arms forward in flexion because this can create a false appearance of good shoulder motion. This is an active form of shoulder motion because the patient is using his own muscles. Active

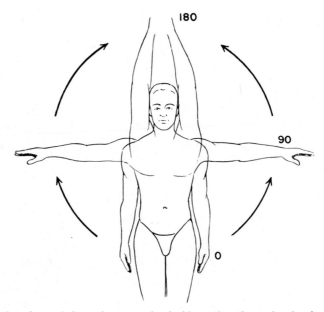

Fig. 4. Abduction of extended arms in arc over head with rotation of scapulae showing range of motion for normal shoulder joints.

range of motion in the shoulder can be tested further by asking the patient to place one hand behind the back for internal rotation and to place one hand behind the head for external rotation.

Active elevation of the arm over the head is painful when tendinitis, bursitis, or a partial tear of the rotator cuff is present. The pain is most severe in the arc from 60° to 120° because the inflamed tendon is compressed between the humerus and acromion arch at this level.

Passive motion. If the patient is unable to raise his arms over his head sideways, the shoulders should be examined further by evaluating the range of passive motion in the shoulder. Passive movement of the shoulder should be tested by having the patient rest his arm on the examiner's arm with muscles completely relaxed. Movement should be evaluated slowly with good support of the arm to prevent decreased motion from painful muscle spasm. Evaluation of internal and external rotation of the shoulder is performed with the examiner at the side of the patient. The patient may be sitting or standing. The scapula normally participates in rotation of the shoulder and does not need to be stabilized when testing rotation. With the forearm held horizontally and the elbow bent at a right angle, the forearm is moved upward for external rotation and downward for internal rotation (Fig. 5). The horizontal position of the forearm is a neutral or 0° position. The normal shoulder is capable of 90° of external rotation and 90° of internal rotation. Evaluation of passive motion in the shoulder should routinely include abduction with the scapula stabilized and internal and external rotation without stabilization of the scapula. If the patient cannot raise his arm actively over his head but the examiner can move the patient's arm normally passively, it suggests the involvement lies outside the shoulder joint in a painful muscle, tendon, or bursa.

Adhesive capsulitis (frozen shoulder). If the joint is limited in passive motion as well as active motion, either disease in the shoulder joint itself or more commonly adhesive capsulitis is present. The end result of chronic pain in the shoulder, regardless of cause, is often adhesive capsulitis or a frozen shoulder. Adhesive capsulitis is due to tightening of the joint capsule and adjacent ligaments resulting in decreased motion of the shoulder. A patient with extensive adhesive capsulitis can appear to move the shoulder joint but actually is only capable of scapular swing and elevation or depression of the shoulder girdle. Normal passive range of motion should eliminate a diagnosis of adhesive capsulitis.

Rupture of rotator cuff. Rupture of the rotator cuff may cause pain and limitation of motion in the shoulder. This is often associated with trauma or strain of the arm and shoulder and is likely to occur suddenly. If the tear is complete, there is inability to abduct the arm from the side, and the head of the humerus tends to become subluxed; however, the arm can be held in abduction when elevated to 90° by the action of the deltoid muscle. Incomplete rotator cuff tears are more difficult to diag-

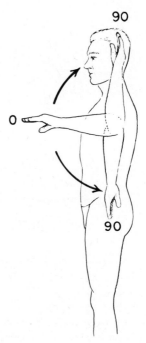

Fig. 5. Range of internal and external rotation for normal shoulder joint.

nose and commonly cause tenderness over the deltoid muscle resembling tendinitis or bursitis of the shoulder.

Shoulder–hand syndrome. The shoulder–hand syndrome is a form of reflex neurovascular dystrophy associated with pain and limitation of motion in the shoulder and involvement of the hand. In the early stages the hand becomes swollen and edematous. In later stages, there is often muscle atrophy and flexion contractures of the fingers.

NEUROVASCULAR COMPRESSION SYNDROMES OF THE SHOULDER GIRDLE AND THORACIC OUTLET
Definition and Anatomy

The subclavian artery, subclavian vein, and brachial plexus are subject to pressure at several potential sites of compression as these structures leave the neck and pass into the region of the shoulder. Compression of this neurovascular bundle may cause pain, paresthesias, or vasomotor disturbances affecting the upper extremity. Various compression syndromes have been described at specific sites but usually produce similar symptoms in the involved extremity. Since the tests used to evaluate the various thoracic outlet syndromes are not completely specific and may also occur in asymptomatic individuals, an exact anatomic diagnosis is not always possible. Excessive use of the arm in an unusual position may predispose to these syndromes as does hyperabduction of the arm during sleep.

The subclavian artery and brachial plexus may be compressed by a hypertrophied scalenus anticus muscle, a cervical rib, or an anomalous first thoracic rib (Fig. 6).

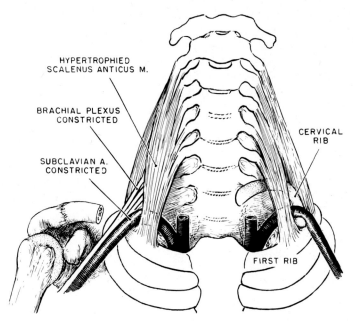

HYPERTROPHIED
SCALENUS ANTICUS M.

BRACHIAL PLEXUS
CONSTRICTED

CERVICAL
RIB

SUBCLAVIAN A.
CONSTRICTED

FIRST RIB

Fig. 6. Anterior view of thoracic outlet showing relationship of emerging nerves and blood vessels to the scalenus anticus muscle and cervical rib. The bony structures of the shoulder girdle are also included to show that depression of the shoulder or elevation of the arm can also compress the neurovascular bundle.

The costoclavicular syndrome is characterized by compression of the subclavian artery and brachial plexus in the space between the first thoracic rib and the clavicle. Hyperabduction of the arm may compress the neurovascular bundle in the angle formed by the insertion of the pectoralis minor muscle and the coracoid process.

Maneuvers for Recognition

The Adson maneuver is performed with the patient sitting. The patient's arms should be by the sides. The radial pulse is felt while the patient takes a deep breath, extends the neck, and turns the head toward the arm being examined. Diminution or obliteration of the radial pulse during this procedure indicates a positive result. Sometimes a systolic bruit may be heard just above or below the medial portion of the clavicle while the radial pulse is decreased. The test may be positive in either the cervical rib or scalenus anticus syndromes. It may also occur in asymptomatic patients.

The costoclavicular maneuver is performed in the sitting position with the patient's arms resting on the legs. The radial pulse is felt while the patient's shoulders are thrust backward and downward as in an exaggerated military posture. The test is positive when the radial pulse is decreased or obliterated. This test is often positive in asymptomatic individuals. A systolic bruit may be heard over the subclavian artery when the radial pulse is decreased but disappears when the pulse is obliterated. The costoclavicular syndrome is probably the commonest form of the thoracic outlet syndrome.

Hyperabduction of the arm may cause the radial pulse to be diminished or obliterated. If the pulse is decreased but not obliterated, a systolic bruit may be heard above or below the clavicle. If these maneuvers are positive in an asymptomatic individual they are not clinically significant.

NEUROLOGIC EVALUATION OF THE SHOULDERS, NECK, AND UPPER EXTREMITIES

Cervical nerve root compression often causes pain in the region of the scapula, shoulder, and arm that must be differentiated from lesions in the shoulder. Therefore, a neurologic evaluation of the upper extremity is essential in all patients with symptoms in the shoulder and arm.

Radicular pain of the lower cervical nerve roots may be intensified by extension of the head, especially when the head is turned toward the side opposite the involved extremity. This is particularly true of intervertebral disc rupture at C_{5-6} and C_{6-7}, but the pain of disc rupture at C_7-T_1, is usually not exacerbated by neck movement. In contrast, pain arising from shoulder involvement is aggravated by shoulder motion rather than neck motion. Pain from C_5 to C_8 nerve roots characteristically involves the arm and frequently involves the shoulder blade. The pain tends to radiate from the upper medial portion of the scapula, passing across the shoulder to the outer aspect of the arm. The location of the arm pain depends on the level of the nerve root involved, and sometimes the pain radiates into the pectoral region.

Since cervical disc disease and bony spur formation affect C_6 and C_7 nerve roots (C_{5-6} and C_{6-7} interspaces) most frequently, compression of these nerve roots will be described in more detail. Involvement of the C_6 root causes pain and subjective sensory symptoms over the radial aspects of the forearm, thumb, and index finger. Patients with C_7 radiculopathy often have pain and subjective sensory symptoms over the dorsum of the wrist and the index, middle, and ring fingers. Although patients with nerve root compression frequently complain of subjective numbness and paresthesias, objective sensory loss rarely occurs. The upper extremity should also be examined for motor weakness and reflex changes. Radiculopathy of the C_6 root is usually associated with weakness and sometimes atrophy of the biceps muscle and diminution of the biceps reflex, whereas radiculopathy of the C_7 root is associated with weakness and sometimes atrophy of the triceps muscle and diminution of the triceps reflex. A midline cervical disc protrusion or severe spondylosis may cause myelopathy with long tract signs.

Marked weakness of neck and shoulder girdle muscles is characteristic of polymyositis. Painful muscle spasm can create a false impression of weakness if the patient gives way during testing because of pain rather than decreased muscular strength.

CLINICAL MANIFESTATIONS OF RHEUMATIC DISEASE

Although pain may be localized to the cervical spine or shoulder joint, often symptoms in these locations are more diffuse and include both areas. Some disorders may be primarily confined to the neck, such as uncomplicated cervical spondylosis, whereas other disorders may primarily affect the shoulder area, as in a tear of the rotator cuff. Systemic diseases, such as rheumatoid arthritis and ankylosing spondylitis, may affect both the neck and shoulder. Pain in the neck and shoulder may also be referred from more distant sites due to intrathoracic disease, angina pectoris, or disease under the diaphragm. Pain arising from cervical spine involvement is usually aggravated by neck motion whereas pain arising from the shoulder is exacerbated by shoulder motion. The differential diagnosis is discussed in more detail in the section on Shoulder and Neck Pain in the fascicle on Differential Approach to Major Rheumatic Syndromes.

REFERENCES

Beetham WP Jr, Polley HF, Slocumb CH, et al: Physical Examination of the Joints. Philadelphia, Saunders, 1965

Cailliet R: Neck and Arm Pain. Philadelphia, Davis, 1964

Cailliet R: Shoulder Pain. Philadelphia, Davis, 1966

Fager CA: Diagnosis of cervical nerve root compression. Med Clin North Am 47:463, 1963

Jackson R: The Cervical Syndrome. Springfield, Ill, Thomas, 1971

Katz WA: The shoulders and neck in the diagnosis of rheumatic diseases, in Katz WA (ed): Rheumatic Diseases: Diagnosis and Management. Philadelphia, Lippincott, 1977, pp 90–113

Steinbrocker O: The painful shoulder, in Hollander JL, McCarty DJ Jr (eds): Arthritis and Allied Conditions (ed 8). Philadelphia, Saunders, 1972, pp 1461–1502

LOWER BACK, HIP JOINT, AND PELVIC GIRDLE

Raymond E. H. Partridge

I. Lower Back
    A. Anatomy
       1. Lumbar Spine
       2. Apophyseal Joints
       3. Intervertebral Discs
       4. Ligaments
       5. Sacrum and Coccyx
       6. Spinal Cord and Spinal Nerves
       7. Spinal Muscles
    B. Physical Examination
       1. Normal Function
       2. Normal Motion
    C. Abnormal Findings
       1. Deformities
          a. Scoliosis
          b. Kyphosis and Lordosis
          c. Spondylolisthesis
       2. Lumbar disc herniation
       3. Lumbosacral strain

II. Hip Joint and Pelvic Girdle
    A. Anatomy
       1. Pelvis
       2. Sacroiliac Joint
       3. Hip Joint
       4. Muscles
       5. Blood Vessels
       6. Nerves
    B. Physical Examination
       1. Gait
       2. Inspection
       3. Normal Examination
       4. Motion
       5. Muscle Power
    C. Abnormal Findings
       1. Bursitis
          a. Trochanteric Bursitis
          b. Iliopectineal Bursitis
          c. Ischiogluteal Bursitis
       2. Femoral Head Abnormalities
          a. Slipped Femoral Capital Epiphysis
          b. Ischemic Necrosis
          c. Transient Osteoporosis
       3. Toxic Synovitis

LOWER BACK

Back pain constitutes one of the commonest problems seen by the practicing physician, particularly among the working population. A basic understanding of the anatomy and function of the lumbar spine, pelvis, and hips is essential for accuracy of diagnosis and planning of treatment. The vertebral column serves as the axis of the body and, together with the muscles, ligaments, and joints, is structured to support weight bearing, posture, and locomotion. The intimate relationship between the spinal column and the spinal cord and nerve roots means that both nervous and musculoskeletal systems have to be considered when analyzing pain and deformity of the back and lower limbs. Symptoms may also be referred from adjacent anatomic sites and a thorough assessment of the back and hips includes careful general symptomatic enquiry of all organ systems and examination of breasts, abdomen, peripheral blood vessels, rectum, and genitourinary organs.

Anatomy

Lumbar spine. In the fetus the vertebral column has the shape of a C with lumbar kyphosis, but at the time of birth the lumbar spine is nearly straight (Fig. 1). The anterior convexity, or lordosis, of the lumbar region develops on weight bearing, allowing balance of the body on the sacrum. The curves of the spine are maintained on weight bearing by muscular contraction and by the shape of the vertebral bodies and intervertebral discs.

In the elderly, the lumbar spine may lose its lordosis as a result of anterior compression of vertebral bodies from osteoporosis and of dessication of the intervertebral discs. The structure and size of the vertebrae are in keeping with their role in weight bearing, so that the vertebrae become heavier and more massive from the cervical spine downwards—they are largest in the lumbar region. Each of the five lumbar vertebrae consists of a kidney-shaped body of cancellous, spongy bone covered by compact bone, and a vertebral arch enclosing the spinal canal. The vertebral arch consists of two pedicles projecting posteriorly from the upper half of the vertebral body with two laminae that are directed posteromedially to form the roof of the canal. A large thick spinous process projects dorsally from the midline of the roof. Projecting laterally from the junction of pedicles and laminae are the flat, winglike transverse processes, which slant laterally and upward. The pedicles have notches on the upper and lower borders that form part of the boundary of the intervertebral foramina, through which the spinal nerves leave the spinal canal. The foramina are triangular in shape with progressive narrowing of the lateral angle in the fourth and fifth vertebrae. The fifth lumbar and first sacral nerve roots lying in the narrow lateral recess are more susceptible to pressure from protrusion of intervertebral discs than are the higher lumbar roots.

Apophyseal joints. The four articular facets of each vertebra arise from the junction of pedicle and lamina. The concave, superior facets are directed dorsomedially and the convex inferior facets dorsolaterally; the superior facets of each vertebra articulate with the inferior facets of the vertebra above to form the apophyseal joints. These are true diarthroidal joints that have hyaline cartilage and synovial membrane and are surrounded by rather lax articular capsules. The upper lumbar facets lie in a sagittal plane, permitting flexion and extension, but little rotation. The lumbosacral articulation is more coronal in position, but rotation is limited by the iliolumbar

ligaments. The pars interarticularis lies between the superior articular process and the lamina. A bony defect in the pars (spondylolysis) may lead to forward displacement of the superior vertebrae (spondylolisthesis) if present bilaterally.

Intervertebral discs. The intervals between the vertebrae are amphiarthrodial joints of fibrocartilage, the intervertebral discs. The lumbar discs account for about one-third of the height of the lumbar spine. The discs are thicker anteriorly than posteriorly and contribute to the lumbar lordosis and lumbosacral angle. A thin layer of compact cortical bone on the vertebral body is covered by a thin layer of hyaline cartilage that fills the central concavity. The cartilage plate extends to the raised compact epiphyseal ring of bone anteriorly and laterally, and to the vertebral margin posteriorly. The annulus fibrosus is a concentric series of fibrocartilagenous lamellae with consecutive layers of oblique fibers crossing in different directions at angles of between 30° and 60° alternately. The peripheral fibers extend over the edge of the cartilage to insert into the vertebral body (Sharpey's fibers). The deepest fibers blend with the cartilage at the edge of the discs.

The annulus encloses the nucleus palposus, which is closer to the posterior margin of the disc. Annulus and nucleus blend together without a definite structural interface. The nucleus consists of a network of collagen fibers in a polysaccharide gel with a very high water content; a number of cells resembling histiocytes and chondrocytes are interspersed in the matrix. Vascular and neural elements are absent. The nucleus exhibits properties of a viscid fluid under pressure, but there is considerable elastic recoil. The intervertebral discs absorb vertical pressure and distribute it evenly over the annulus, which may deform and permit motion between the vertebrae. The nucleus may bulge in either direction but usually does so posteriorly due to its position and the weakness of the posterior annulus. After the third or fourth decade the disc gradually loses fluid, and by the sixth or seventh decade the nucleus may become fibrocartilage.

Ligaments. The discs and vertebral bodies are covered anteriorly and posteriorly by two ligaments. The anterior longitudinal ligament is a broad, strong band of fibers extending from the body of the atlas to the sacrum. In the lumbar area the ligament covers the anterior part of the vertebral body and is attached firmly at the epiphyseal ring. The posterior longitudinal ligament lying between the posterior aspect of the vertebrae and the dura is of variable width, being narrower over the vertebral bodies and wider over the discs. The lateral extensions over the discs are thinner than the central band, creating weak areas that may be the site of dorsolateral protrusion of the nucleus palposus. Other ligaments are present that contribute greatly to the strength and stability of the vertebral column. The vertebral laminae are joined by the tough ligamentum flavum, which extends laterally as far as the articular capsule. The supraspinous ligament is a strong fibrous cord extending along the tips of the spinous

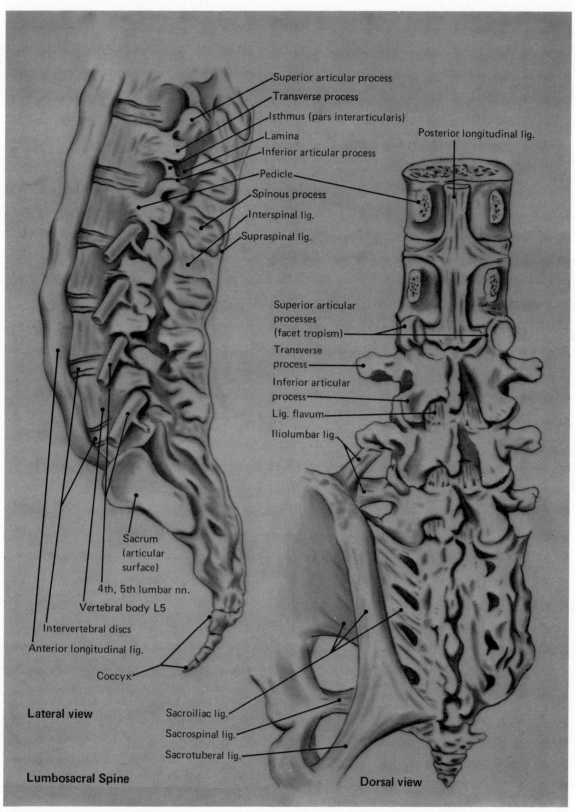

Superior articular process

Transverse process

Isthmus (pars interarticularis)

Lamina

Inferior articular process

Pedicle

Spinous process

Interspinal lig.

Supraspinal lig.

Posterior longitudinal lig.

Superior articular processes (facet tropism)

Transverse process

Inferior articular process

Lig. flavum

Iliolumbar lig.

Sacrum (articular surface)

4th, 5th lumbar nn.

Vertebral body L5

Intervertebral discs

Anterior longitudinal lig.

Coccyx

Lateral view

Sacroiliac lig.

Sacrospinal lig.

Sacrotuberal lig.

Lumbosacral Spine

Dorsal view

Fig. 1. Lumbosacral spine. (Adapted from an original painting by Frank H. Netter, M. D., from *Clinical Symposia,* copyright 1973 by CIBA Pharmaceutical Company, Division of CIBA-GEIGY Corporation.)

processes from C_7 to the medial sacral crest. The interspinous ligaments that decussate as they pass from the root of one spinous process to the tip of the next are strong in the lumbar region.

Sacrum and coccyx. The sacrum consists of five fused vertebrae in the shape of a triangle with the base upward. It is broadened by large transverse processes into a lateral fused mass of bone on each side. It is concave and smooth on the pelvic surface, where there are transverse ridges representing lines of fusion of the vertebral bodies. Laterally anterior sacral foramina are present for the ventral rami of the sacral nerves. Dorsally the spinal processes fuse to form the sacral crest over the sacral canal. The caudal portion of the sacral canal terminates in an inverted U-shaped opening, the sacral hiatus, from a failure of fusion of the last sacral laminae. Anatomic anomalies of this area are common. The coccyx consists of four fused vertebral bodies articulating with the apex of the sacrum.

Spinal cord and spinal nerves. In the spinal canal the spinal cord ends at the first or second lumbar vertebra (conus medullaris) and the tapered fibrous end of the cord (filum terminale) is attached to the periosteum of the coccyx. The conus migrates to this level because skeletal growth is greater than neural growth. The spinal nerves therefore slope inferiorly from their origin to the foramina, forming a parallel group of nerve roots, the cauda equina. The outer layer of the three coverings of the spinal cord, the dura mater, is separated from the vertebral bodies by a layer of epidural fat in which there is a rich venous plexus. The arachnoid membrane is loosely attached to the dura, and between the arachnoid and the pia mater enveloping the cord the subarachnoid space contains the cauda equina.

Each spinal nerve is formed by a dorsal (sensory) and ventral (motor) root uniting as they exit through the intervertebral foramen just beyond the dorsal root ganglion. The dural arachnoid sheath and subarachnoid space extend out beyond the ganglion, forming the "nerve root sleeve" which anchors the dura by attachment to the foramen. Each nerve passes through the upper part of the intervertebral foramen and is numbered for the body of the vertebra above (i.e., the first lumbar root exits below the first lumbar vertebra). This is above the level of the disc, so disc protrusion is more likely to compress the root of the next lowest nerve (i.e., protrusion of the fifth lumbar disc will compress the first sacral root more commonly than the fifth lumbar root).

The structure of a nerve root differs from that of a peripheral nerve. In a peripheral nerve a connective tissue sheath, the epineurium, offers protection from mechanical pressure, and the perineurium around small nerve fascicles forms a diffusion barrier to irritants and resists tensile forces. Groups of fibers cross from one fasciculus to another, giving a longitudinal plexus formation to the nerve. The fibers in the nerve root, in contrast, run in nonplexiform parallel strands, perineurium is absent, and the epineurium is poorly developed, thus the root is more susceptible to mechanical pressure.

After emerging from the intervertebral foramen each spinal nerve divides into a posterior and anterior primary ramus. The posterior primary rami remain separate and innervate the back muscles and a portion of the overlying skin. The anterior primary rami of the lumbar and sacral nerves enter into plexus formation, the lumbosacral plexus, from which the nerves of the lower limb are derived. The lumbar plexus is formed from union of the first four lumbar nerves and divides into the obturator nerve, supplying the adductor muscles of the thigh and the femoral nerve innervating the iliacus and quadriceps muscles. The sacral part of the plexus is formed from the fifth lumbar and first three sacral nerves, with branches from the fourth lumbar and fourth sacral, and lies on the anterior part of the sacrum. The greater part of the plexus forms the sciatic nerve, which leaves that plexus through the greater sciatic notch to pass into the posterior midline aspect of the thigh.

Spinal muscles. The musculature of the spine must be considered with regard to its function of providing spinal stability and spinal motion. The sacrospinalis or erector spinae group are extensors, lateral flexors, and stabilizers of the vertebral column. They originate from the sacrum and adjacent portion of the iliac crest and continue cranially, dividing in the upper lumbar region into a complex series of longitudinal subgroups anatomically divided on the basis of origin, insertion, length, and direction. The multifidus muscles are well developed in the lumbar region, originating from the dorsal margin of the articular processes to insert into the spinous process two to four vertebrae above. Other small muscles present are the interspinales, intertransversarii, and rotators.

Physical Examination

Physical examination of the lumbar spine cannot be considered in isolation. In addition to posture, gait, and spinal motion a careful evaluation of the lower limbs and a full neurologic examination must be performed, together with rectal, pelvic, abdominal, and breast examinations.

Symptomatic inquiry regarding pain, deformity, and function is an essential preliminary to examination (discussed more fully in the chapter on Low Back and Hip Pain in the fascicle on Differential Approach to Major Rheumatic Syndromes), and observation should be made of abnormalities in gait and posture as the patient enters the examining room. The subject must be adequately undressed for examination to visualize the spine, buttocks, and legs. The patient should be examined initially in the standing position both from the side and the back to observe posture. The bony landmarks are helpful in identifying structures in clinical examination. An imaginary line between the iliac crests transects L_4. The vertebrae may be counted from the prominence of C_7 spine downward and the coccyx is palpable in the gluteal crease near the anal orifice. The sacroiliac joints are located beneath overlying dimples in the skin at the level of the posterior superior iliac spine. The skin should be inspected for cafe au lait spots (which might indicate neurofibromatosis), ecchymoses, psoriatic patches (particularly between the buttocks), a midline hairy patch over L_5 suggestive of spina bifida, and scars.

In the normal posture, the spine is straight on inspection from the back, the pelvis and shoulders even, and the head centrally placed. A plumb line dropped from the C_7 spine to the floor should fall along the cleft between the buttocks. There is a natural thoracic kyphosis and lumbar lordosis that can be assessed visually for increase or decrease. Some increase in lumbar lordosis may be seen in normal women. Placing of the fingers on the iliac crests, which should be level, will allow assessment of pelvic tilt. This may be due to scoliosis, leg length discrepancy, or flexion–adduction deformity of one hip with prominence of the buttock. Muscle wasting of the buttock, hamstrings, and gastrocnemius is assessed best in the standing position.

Motion of the lumbar spine takes place at the apophyseal joints and to a limited extent at the discs; the range between individual vertebrae is small. Spinal motion is measured in forward flexion, lateral flexion to each side, extension, and rotation. Forward flexion is tested by asking the patient to bend forward and touch the toes; however, much of this movement takes place at the hips, allowing some patients with a rigid lumbar spine to perform this action, while others with normal spinal motion cannot because of tight hamstrings. True spinal movement is assessed by measuring the distance between C_7 and S_1 in erect and flexed positions (Schober test, Fig. 2). The increase in length in a normal adult is about 10 cm. The test can also be used to measure segmental motion in the lumbar spine utilizing the distance between T_{12} and S_1. Gross reduction in the Schober test is characteristic of ankylosing spondylitis. The spine normally extends 25°–30°, with most of the motion occurring in the lumbar region. Lateral flexion is symmetric, normally 30°–35° on each side. Unilateral limitation by pain with radiation into the buttock or leg may indicate lumbar disc disease, and marked limitation bilaterally is characteristic of ankylosing spondylitis. Rotation of the spine is almost entirely thoracic, the lumbar spine contributing less than 5°.

Palpation with the finger tips should be done to identify pain sites over the spinous processes, interspinous ligaments, renal angle, sciatic notch, and sacroiliac joints. Light percussion with the fist or reflex hammer over the spine from C_7 downward produces severe pain over a vertebra in cases of tumor, infection, or neural impingement. Chest expansion is measured at the nipple line on maximum inspiration and expiration; normal adult expansion is 5–6 cm. Limited chest excursion with back pain is common in young patients with ankylosing spondylitis.

The rest of the examination can be performed with the patient lying on a couch. Gaenslen's test is helpful in

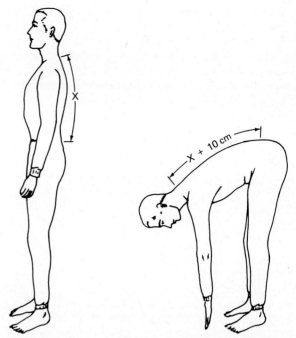

Fig. 2. Schober test. Measure the distance (x) between T_1 and S_1 with spine erect and fully flexed. The normal increase in an adult is 10 cm.

differentiating between sacroiliac and lumbosacral lesions. While one hip and knee are acutely flexed, the other hip is forcibly extended as the limb hangs over the side of the couch; there is pain on that side if the sacroiliac joint is involved. For the "pump handle" test the hip and knee are flexed and the thigh and pelvis are pushed toward the opposite shoulder. Pain in the sacroiliac joint is a positive sign. Both of these tests require a normal hip joint for their interpretation.

From a supine position the straight leg can usually be elevated to about 90°, although tight hamstrings may cause discomfort. Pain produced in the back or leg with limited straight leg raising suggests nerve root irritation on that side; the pain is enhanced by dorsiflexion of the foot (Lasègue's sign). Leg raising on the unaffected side may cause referred pain on the involved side by tugging the compromised root against a protruding disc. Limitation of straight leg raising can be voluntary. If there is doubt about the genuineness of the sign, ask the patient to sit up and forward. If he is able to do so without flexing the knees the possibility of malingering or functional overlay must be considered. The femoral stretch test for high lumbar root lesions is performed with the patient in the prone position. Each knee is flexed in turn to stretch femoral nerve roots, causing pain in patients with high lumbar disc lesions.

A full neurologic examination of the lower limbs must be done if a nerve root lesion is suspected. Muscle power is tested by asking the patient to contract maximally each muscle group against resistance. Knee extension (L_{3-4}), foot dorsiflexion (L_{4-5}), plantar flexion (S_{1-2}), and eversion (L_5, S_1) are tested with the patient in a supine position. With the patient prone the power of hip extension (gluteus maximus, L_5, S_{1-2}) can be checked.

The dermatomes of the lower limb are mapped and the reflexes tested. Diminution of sensation at the side of the foot (S_1) and a reduced or absent knee jerk (L_{3-4}) or ankle jerk (S_{1-2}) are indicative of root lesions.

Abnormal Findings

Deformities. Scoliosis.   Scoliosis is an abnormal deviation of the spine laterally, described according to the direction of the convexity. Compensatory curves are usually present. A postural scoliosis with pelvic tilt occurs as a result of leg length discrepancy or unilateral hip deformity and will correct on forward flexion of the spine either in a sitting or standing position.

A structural scoliosis cannot be actively or passively straightened and the curve will accentuate on forward flexion with rib prominence on one side (producing a unilateral rib "hump") from vertebral rotation. Spasm of the erector spinae muscles unilaterally after back trauma will produce lumbar scoliosis. The extent of vertebral rotation and the degrees of curvature are measured radiologically.

By far the commonest type of scoliosis is the adolescent idiopathic variety occurring during the period of rapid growth from the age of 10 onward. It is eight times more common in girls than boys and a family history is often obtainable. A right thoracic curve occurs in 90 percent of these children. Untreated, the scoliosis may gradually worsen, but it usually stops progressing when growth ceases, although curves of over 60° may continue to increase. The scoliosis is painless during adolescence but degenerative changes developing in the spine later in life are a common cause of back pain. Total lung capacity and vital capacity become reduced and correlate with the severity of the curvature. Arterial hypoxemia is noted with curvatures over 65°; respiratory infections and cor pulmonale may increase mortality.

A structural scoliosis also develops after poliomyelitis and during Marfan's syndrome, Ehlers-Danlos syndrome, and a variety of neuromuscular disorders. Congenital scoliosis resulting from a hemivertebra or a failure of vertebral separation is severe.

Kyphosis and lordosis.   Flattening of the lumbar lordosis is seen in osteoarthritis and lumbar disc disease and is characteristic of ankylosing spondylitis. An increase of lumbar lordosis is seen secondary to fixed flexion deformity of the hips, which must be screened for motion. Lumbar lordosis with a hollow at the base of the spine and prominence of the sacrum may indicate spondylolisthesis. A regular fixed thoracic kyphosis is seen in senile osteoporosis from anterior vertebral wedging, and an angulated gibbus of the spine is usually a result of fracture, old pyogenic infection, or tuberculosis.

A rigid thoracic kyphosis and exaggerated lumbar lordosis (Scheuermann's juvenile kyphosis) is seen equally in male and female adolescents as a cause of progressive spinal deformity and pain. An associated scoliosis is present in 30–40 percent of cases. Roentgenograms may show vertebral wedging, Schmorl's nodes (protrusion of nucleus palposus into the vertebral body), and vertebral end-plate irregularity. A flexible postural kyphosis must be distinguished from this condition.

Spondylolisthesis.   A bilateral defect of uncertain origin in the pars interarticularis (spondylolysis) will allow a forward slip of one vertebra on another (usually the fifth lumbar on the first sacral). Malformed laminae are common and spina bifida is 13 times more frequent than expected. Forward slipping starts at the age of 5 or 6 and is most rapid during adolescence, but it is usually asymptomatic at this age, although strenuous activity may initiate pain. Hamstring spasm causes impairment of straight leg raising and a waddling gait may be seen. Lumbar lordosis increases and a depression can be palpated in the lumbar region. Progressive slipping in adults causes chronic lumbar pain with radicular radiation, hamstring spasm, and neurologic deficits. Spondylolisthesis is seen in lateral roentgenograms, but the effect in the pars is best appreciated in the oblique view.

Pseudospondylolisthesis is a stable forward slip of a vertebra from a number of causes, including osteoarthritis of the apophyseal joints and a congenital elongation of the isthmus between the laminae and superior articulations.

Lumbar disc herniation.   Most herniations of the nucleus palposus occur posterolaterally since the annulus is weakest in this position. There is usually associated trauma, although this may be minor. The L_{4-5} and L_5–S_1 discs are involved most frequently, followed by L_{3-4}. Low back pain is the earliest symptom, resulting from ligament and periosteal stretching, and is followed by radiation of the pain along a dermatome, caused by compression of a nerve root. Coughing or sneezing (Valsalva) aggravates the pain. Spasm of the paraspinous muscles will cause limited motion and lumbar scoliosis toward the side of the sciatica (medial compression of the root) or away from the sciatica (lateral compression of the root). The sciatic or femoral stretch test is positive. Root compression is manifested by sensory change along a dermatome, motor weakness of the muscles innervated by the nerve root, and tendon reflex inhibition. By following the procedures for physical examination previously described the involved root or roots can be determined. Leg pain may be the only symptom, or may become the predominant symptom if the nucleus becomes completely extruded (relieving pressure on the annulus).

A midline disc protrusion causes compression of the cauda equina, with low back and perineal pain, bladder dysfunction, and widespread bilateral sensory and motor loss in the extremities.

The discs become dehydrated and narrower with aging, causing degenerative changes. Osteophytes and articular facets encroach upon the intervertebral foramina, causing nerve root impingement.

Lumbosacral strain. Acute lumbosacral strain following unusually heavy lifting or acute spinal torsion is commonest in 25–50-year-old men. Pain is usually centered over L_{4-5} and S_1 and radiates to either side of the spine. Spasm of the paraspinous muscles is present, causing limitation of lumbar motion. Abnormal neurologic signs are absent and the sciatic stretch test is negative. The structures involved are difficult to determine and may involve paraspinous muscles, ligaments, or annulus without significant nuclear protrusion.

Chronic or recurrent lumbar pain is seen most commonly in women. Poor posture, increased lumbar lordosis, obesity, ligamentous relaxation after pregnancy, and minor leg length discrepancy may be predisposing factors. Other symptoms of chronic ill health and fatigue may be present. The symptoms are aggravated by prolonged standing at working surfaces ill adjusted for height. A full examination, including a rectal and pelvic exam is necessary to exclude underlying disease. Gynecologic problems are only occasionally the cause of this type of backache.

HIP JOINT AND PELVIC GIRDLE
Anatomy

Pelvis. The hemipelvis consists of three bones—the ilium, ischium, and pubis—which fuse at maturity. The ilium forms the superior, wide portion of the pelvis and the upper free edge (iliac crest) gives attachment to the abdominal muscles and sacrospinalis. The crest curves anteriorly to end in a prominence easily palpable beneath the skin, the anterior superior iliac spine. The inferior portion of the ischium is capped by a large bony prominence, the ischial tuberosity, that is palpable in the buttock if the hips are flexed. Between the medial aspect of the tuberosity and gluteus maximus muscle is the ischial bursa. The pubic bones are joined anteriorly at the pubic symphysis, which consists of an interpubic disc of fibrocartilage reinforced by strong ligaments. All three bones are involved in the formation of the acetabulum, which is directed laterally, downward, and forward.

Sacroiliac joint. The sacroiliac articulation is a synovial joint between the surfaces of the sacrum and ilium connected by powerful ligaments. The articular surfaces are irregular and lock together to provide stability for transmission of weight bearing from the vertebral column to the pelvic girdle and lower limb. Movement at the sacroiliac joint is minimal, although it increases during pregnancy as a result of ligamentous laxity.

Hip joint. The hip joint is a ball-and-socket joint between the head of the femur and the acetabulum (Fig. 3). There is an excellent range of motion in all directions with great stability provided by the depth of the acetabulum and the strength of the capsule and associated ligaments; dislocation occurs only with great force. The acetabulum is deepened by a fibrocartilaginous rim attached to its edge, the labrum. The acetabular cartilage forms an incomplete ring, with the thickest cartilage located superiorly for weight bearing. The deep fossa of the acetabulum is deficient in cartilage and is occupied by fat covered with synovial membrane. The femoral head is completely covered with cartilage (thickest superiorly and thinnest at the periphery), except over a pit (visible radiologically) for the ligament of the head. The fibers of the capsule with heavy ligamentous reinforcements anteriorly and posteriorly tend to tighten when the hip is extended, thus helping to maintain posture with little muscular effort.

The head of the femur is joined to the main shaft by the femoral neck, which does not lie parallel to the frontal plane but projects obliquely anteriorly to it at an angle of 5°–15°. If the angle of anteversion is increased beyond 15° a "toe-in" gait may be seen in children with increased internal rotation. In the frontal plane the femoral neck makes an angle of 120°–135° with the shaft of the femur. When the angle decreases below 120° the condition of coxa vara, which may be congenital or secondary to an underlying growth disorder, results in a gait abnormality.

Where the femoral neck joins the body of the femur a lateral protruberance, the greater trochanter, projects upward and is separated by the multilocular trochanteric bursa from the gluteus maximus and iliotibial band. Between the anterior superior iliac spine and the pubic tubercle the inguinal ligament forms the base of the femoral triangle, which is bounded medially by the adductor longus and laterally by the sartorius. From its lateral border medially the triangle contains the femoral nerve, femoral artery, femoral vein, and a lymph node. The hip joint can be aspirated by locating the femoral artery 1 inch below the inguinal ligament and inserting a needle 1 inch lateral to this point.

Muscles. The hip flexors, psoas major and iliacus, are innervated by the second, third, and fourth lumbar roots and insert into the lesser trochanter. Gluteus maximus, the principal hip extensor, arises from the ilium and sacrum to form the rounded contour of the buttock and inserts into the linea aspera of the femur and the iliotibial band. The powerful adductor muscles on the inner side of the thigh, adductors longus, brevis, and magnus, and the gracilis muscle arise from the inferior pubic ramus and insert into the medial side of the femur. They are innervated by the obturator nerve (L_{2-3-4}). Abduction is effected by the gluteus medius and minimus, which arise from the wing of the ilium to insert into the greater trochanter. The glutei also stabilize the pelvis when the foot of the opposite side is raised from the ground. The anterior fibers and the tensor fascia lata are internal rotators of the hip joint. External rotation is performed by the gluteus maximus, sartorius, and a number of small muscles inserted into the greater trochanter, the internal and external obturators, pyriformis, gemelli, and quadratus femoris.

Blood vessels. The arterial supply of the lower limb comes from the external iliac artery, which crosses into the thigh as the femoral artery and then divides into superficial and deep branches. The deep femoral artery is the main source of blood to the thigh and hip. The medial and lateral retinacular vessels along the femoral neck supply the femoral head. Interruption of these vessels by

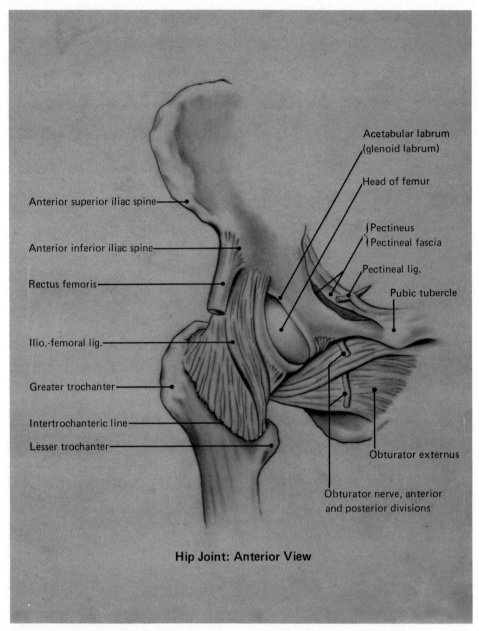

Fig. 3. Anterior view of hip joint. (Redrawn by permission from Grant: An Atlas of Anatomy, 1962. Courtesy of Williams & Wilkins, 1962.)

injury or inflammation may cause aseptic necrosis of the femoral head.

Nerves.   The hip joint is supplied by branches from sciatic, obturator, and femoral nerves. Pain may be felt posteriorly, anteriorly in the groin, or along the anterior thigh. Because there is a common innervation with the knee joint, disease of the hip may present initially as knee pain.

Physical Examination

Gait.   Evaluation of the gait is an important part of hip examination although a gait abnormality is not necessarily pathognomonic for any specific neuromuscular dis-

order. Examination should be carried out with the subject undressed and include observation from behind, from the front, and from each side. Normal gait should have rhythm and symmetry. The gait cycle has two phases: a weight-bearing or stance phase occupying 70 percent of the cycle, and a swing phase of 30 percent. The stance phase begins when the forward heel strikes the ground, continues as the body rolls forward onto the ball of the foot, and ends with toe push-off. The weight-bearing hip is on 25° of flexion at the beginning of the stance phase and hyperextends 20° at toe push-off. The pelvis rotates slightly by gluteus medius action to bring the center of gravity over the weight-bearing hip and to allow the free leg to swing through.

During normal gait there is a period of double support when the two extremities are in contact with the ground simultaneously. The external moment of force acting on the hip joint increases from midstance to toe push-off (hip extension) until the body weight is shifted at time of double support, when the force drops to zero. Vertical and lateral motion of the pelvis during a gait cycle results in center of gravity displacement by about 2 inches. The width of a normal walking base is 2–4 inches.

There are many causes of an abnormal gait, including pain, weakness, deformity, spasticity, ataxia, and hysterical conversion reactions. Several different types of gait may be observed that are characteristic of disease of the hip and of the associated muscles. Hip pain will produce a slow antalgic gait with incomplete loading of the painful hip and a shortened stance phase. With a stiff or ankylosed hip the leg will swing through by rotation of the entire pelvis on the opposite hip. A Trendelenburg gait results from weakness of the gluteus medius, which may be due to deformity of the upper end of the femur (coxa vara) or neuromuscular disease. The hip on the side of the swinging through leg will not rise and the trunk leans markedly to the side of the weight-bearing limb.

The gluteus maximus shortens at the time of heel strike to slow the forward momentum of the trunk and to arrest hip flexion. If the muscle is weak the patient compensates by checking his stride by lurching backward. This produces the gluteus maximus lurch or extensor-thrust gait. A short-leg gait, which may result either from true leg shortening or apparent shortening because of pelvic tilt, will produce a tip-toe gait on the affected side with a flexed knee on the unaffected side. Analysis of gait is often difficult as a patient with a flexed painful hip with limited motion and muscle wasting may show a composite gait with several features, but assessment should be made of the character and duration of the swing and stance phases on each side.

The problems of femoral anteversion may be assessed best by examination of gait. Increased anteversion will cause a toe-in gait in order to cover the femoral head completely during weight bearing; femoral retroversion will give a toe-out gait with the patellae pointing laterally.

Inspection. The standing patient should be inspected for the presence of any fixed deformity of the hip, asymmetry, muscle wasting, swelling, or pelvic tilt. Note also any abnormal rotation of the leg, the position of the patella, and whether the feet are flat on the floor. Pelvic tilt may be due to an adduction contracture of the hip; in order to uncross the legs, the pelvis on the affected side is raised, causing apparent limb shortening. An abduction contracture of the hip will cause apparent limb lengthening, with a compensatory pelvic raise on the opposite side. A full examination of the spine must be done as previously described to assess the contribution of spinal deformity, particularly scoliosis, to pelvic tilt.

Swelling of the hip joint is usually masked by the thickness of the soft tissues, but swelling in the femoral triangle may be due to a psoas abscess with hip flexion from psoas muscle spasm; swelling over the sacroiliac joint may be seen with tuberculous abscess. Prominence of the greater trochanter is usually a result of pelvic tilt, but may be described by the patient as a swelling. The presence of buttock, quadriceps, and hamstring wasting should be noted. Postural stability is examined in the standing position. Normally, when a person is standing on one leg the pelvis on the opposite side is tilted upward by action of the gluteus medius and minimus (Trendelenburg test). The test is positive if the hip on the non-weight-bearing side fails to rise as a result of gluteus muscle weakness, gluteal inefficiency (coxa vara), or gluteal inhibition from hip pain.

Further physical examination is performed with the patient recumbent. The presence of fixed deformities should be observed; the common fixed hip deformity is flexion/external rotation. The patient may compensate for a fixed flexion deformity by pelvic rotation and increased lumbar lordosis. Determination of leg length and the distinction between true shortening of the affected limb and apparent shortening from fixed hip deformity with pelvic tilt is important. If there is a fixed adduction or abduction contracture of the hip the good leg must be adducted or abducted by the same amount before measurement is made. True leg length is measured from the anterior superior iliac spine to the tip of the medial malleolus.

Apparent leg length is measured from the xiphisternum to the medial malleolus. In apparent shortening the limb is not altered in length but appears short as a result of adduction contracture of the hip. If true shortening is present it must be determined if the shortening is above or below the greater trochanter. A simple test to determine whether the deformity is above the greater trochanter is to draw an imaginary line between the anterior superior iliac spine and the ischial tuberosity. Normally the greater trochanter can be palpated below that line (Nelaton's line). If the trochanter is above the line an abnormality of the femoral neck or hip joint can be suspected. Occasionally apparent shortening may be due to an increase in the length of the opposite limb. This effect may be seen in conditions resulting in hypervascularity of the limb, such as neurofibromatosis or arteriovenous malformations, or as a result of overgrowth from monarticular juvenile rheumatoid arthritis.

Motion of the hip joint should be accurately measured. The examiners hand rests on the anterior superior iliac spine during the examination to check that motion is not being performed at the pelvis, giving a false impression of hip motion. The patient lies supine and holds the opposite hip in full flexion to flatten lumbar lordosis. If a fixed flexion deformity of the hip is present the limb rises from the table and the angle of fixed flexion deformity is recorded. The hip is then flexed, with the examiner using a hand to check that no pelvic movement occurs. The normal range of flexion is 110°–120°. Abduction is measured in extension and flexion. The normal range of abduction in extension is 40° and in flexion 75° (it is greater in children). The leg is crossed to the opposite side to measure adduction (normally 30°). Normal legs cross about midthigh. Internal and external rotation in extension and 90° of flexion are usually similar—about 45°. Patrick's test can be performed with the knee and hip flexed and externally rotated with the foot resting on the opposite knee. Hip pain caused by a sharp depression of the knee in this position is indicative of hip synovitis. Extension is measured with the patient in a prone position; each leg is lifted and the range is compared (normal range 20°–30°). Loss of full extension is a very early sign of hip synovitis.

Muscle power of hip flexors, extensors, abductors, and adductors is tested by asking the patient to perform the respective movements against resistance and feeling the tone in the contracting muscle. Apparent loss of power may be due to pain on active joint motion, but with weakness due to pain the initial strength of contraction is good with a sudden "break" in the contraction due to pain.

The hips cannot be examined in isolation. Full examination of the spine and lower limbs is essential and a rectal and pelvic examination should be performed.

Abnormal Findings

Bursitis. A number of bursae have been identified in relation to the hip joint. Three of these are clinically important: the trochanteric, iliopectineal, and ischiogluteal bursae. The bursae around the hip may be subject to acute or chronic inflammation; it is often idiopathic or a result of mild trauma, but it may occur during the course of inflammatory joint disease. Sepsis is rare in this group. The symptoms of bursitis may be confused clinically with arthritis of the hip.

Trochanteric bursitis. The trochanteric bursa lies between the gluteus maximus tendon and the lateral surface of the greater trochanter. The bursa may be involved during the course of rheumatoid arthritis but the inflammation is usually nonspecific. Calcification within the bursa may sometimes be seen radiologically. Pain is present over the posterolateral aspect of the trochanter and may radiate down the lateral side of the thigh to the knee on walking. The patient is frequently awakened at night by pain caused by lying on the affected side. There is tenderness by direct palpation over the trochanter but swelling is rare. Hip movements are usually normal, but there may be pain and guarding on flexion and internal rotation of the hip. If inflammation is severe the leg is held in external rotation to reduce gluteus maximus tension.

Iliopectineal bursitis. The iliopectineal bursa overlies the iliopubic junction and the hip joint. Anteriorly the bursa is covered by the iliopsoas muscle. It communicates with the hip joint in 15 percent of normal people. The femoral nerve is nearby and may be irritated by bursitis. Pain is present over the lateral border of the femoral (Scarpa's) triangle and is elicited by forced flexion or extension of the hip, both of which stretch the

iliopsoas, with pain referred to the anterior thigh and the knee. Adduction of the hips in flexion usually causes acute pain by squeezing the bursa. A swelling may be present in the triangle, which must be differentiated from a femoral hernia and a psoas abscess, and aspiration of bursal fluid for analysis and culture is essential for management. Sepsis, tuberculosis, and acute hemorrhage from trauma can affect the bursa and there may be extension of synovitis from the hip joint in rheumatoid arthritis and pigmented villonodular synovitis.

Ischiogluteal bursitis. The ischiogluteal bursa lies between the tuberosity of the ischium and the gluteus maximus. Bursitis is usually traumatic, produced by prolonged sitting on hard surfaces. The pain is worse on sitting and may radiate into the back of the thigh, mimicking sciatica. Acute and severe bursitis can occur, causing constant pain at night. Swelling may be present on inspection and the bursa is tender to palpation over the ischium when the hip is flexed.

Nonspecific bursitis around the hip is usually responsive to the intrabursal injection of steroid.

Femoral head abnormalities. *Slipped femoral capital epiphysis.* Epiphysiolysis with separation of the epiphysis from the metaphysis at the epiphyseal plate is most common in the femur. It is a condition of adolescence before epiphyseal closure, occurring predominantly in males (60–80 percent) between the ages of 10 and 18 and a year or two earlier in females. Affected adolescents tend to be tall and thin or obese with a Frohlich-type habitus and genital underdevelopment. Fifteen percent of cases are bilateral but synchronous onset in both hips is rare. The periosteal–perichondral covering tears, allowing the femoral head to slide backward and downward with some rotation of the head, resulting in a coxa vara deformity. The cause is uncertain; there is usually no history of trauma and histology only shows disruption of the epiphyseal plate. Possible etiologic factors include a change in the position of the epiphyseal line from horizontal to oblique during adolescence and a thinning of the periosteum that occurs naturally in the years prior to epiphyseal closure, making the epiphysis more susceptible to shearing stress. An excess of growth hormone and decreased sex hormone have been shown to decrease the resistance of the epiphysis to shearing stress.

Pain in the hip and knee and a limp are the presenting symptoms. An external rotation deformity of the hip occurs on walking, with slight flexion deformity and limitation of external rotation and abduction. There is usually a little shortening with prominence of the greater trochanter. If the slip is severe a Trendelenburg gait may develop. In 2–3 years the slip will become stable with femoral neck remodeling and union of the epiphysis to the femoral neck in the new position. Late in the disease cartilage necrosis may occur but ischemic necrosis is unusual. The alteration of weight-bearing surfaces predisposes the patient to osteoarthritis of the hip in later life.

Ischemic necrosis. A mechanical interruption of the blood supply to the femoral head causes a bone infarct or avascular necrosis. Subchondral fractures occur early with subsequent collapse, sclerosis, and flattening of the femoral head. After the necrotic phase, revascularization occurs with resorption of dead tissue, pseudocyst formation, and repair. The surface cartilage initially remains intact with a depression where the head joins the neck resulting from pressure by the outer rim of the acetabulum, but later cartilage degeneration and osteoarthritis develop.

There are many causes, including femoral neck fracture, caisson disease, sickle cell disease and other hemoglobinopathies, and Gaucher's disease. The occurrence of avascular necrosis during corticosteroid administration and in chronic alcoholics is believed to be from fat emboli. A variety of avascular necrosis of the ossification center of the femoral head occurs in children between the ages of 2 and 11 (Legg-Perthes disease). Boys are affected more often than girls in a ratio of 4:1 and 90 percent of cases are unilateral. Capsular thickening with compression of the retinacular vessels or increased pressure from synovial effusion have been suggested as etiologic factors. At this age there is little anastomosis between the metaphyseal and epiphyseal arteries. Remodeling results in widening of the femoral neck and enlargement of the femoral head (coxa magna), which may remain flattened.

Transient osteoporosis. Episodes of spontaneous pain on weight bearing associated with radiologically apparent rarefaction of the femoral head after 4–6 weeks and spontaneous resolution after 6–18 months are the characteristics of transient osteoporosis. The episodes may be isolated, but further attacks involving the knee, ankle, and foot may occur with local heat and swelling. A bone scan shows increased uptake of the affected area of bone, indicating osteoblastic activity. The cause is unknown, but unusual muscular exertion has been recorded in some patients immediately prior to onset.

Toxic synovitis. This is a benign self-limiting synovitis occurring between the ages of 3 and 20 years. Eighty percent of cases are boys who present with fever of up to 101°F (occasionally higher), hip pain, flexion and external rotation contracture, and limp. Radiographs show widening of the medial joint space and distension of the capsular shadows. The etiology is unknown but may be traumatic or viral. Symptoms last 7–21 days with complete resolution. Laboratory studies are usually not helpful, although a mild leukocytosis may be present and aspiration of the joint may be necessary to exclude infection. Follow-up radiographs must be taken to rule out Legg-Perthes disease.

REFERENCES

Adams JA: Transient synovitis of the hip in children. J Bone Joint Surg 45B:471 1963

Cozen L: Trochanteric bursitis. Am J Orthop 7:70, 1965

Hutcheson BC, Freeman CE: Iliopectineal bursitis. A cause of hip pain frequently unrecognized. Am J Orthop 4:220, 1962

James JIP: Idiopathic scoliosis. Clin Orthop 77:57, 1971

Morris JM: Biomechanics of the spine. Arch Surg 107:418, 1973

Rothman RH, Simeone FA: The Spine. Philadelphia, Saunders, 1975

Swartout R, Compere EL: Ischiogluteal bursitis. The pain in the arse. JAMA 227:551, 1974

Swezey RL: Transient osteoporosis of the hip. Arthritis Rheum 13:858, 1970

Turner RH, Bianco AJ: Spondylolysis and spondylolisthesis in children and teenagers. J Bone Joint Surg 53A:1298, 1971

KNEES, ANKLES, AND FEET

John J. Calabro

I. Knees
   A. Anatomy
     1. Bones and Joints
     2. Muscles and Ligaments
     3. Bursae
     4. Blood and Nerve Supply
   B. Physical Examination
     1. Normal Function
     2. Pain
     3. Inspection
     4. Palpation
     5. Range of Motion
   C. Knee Disorders
     1. Internal Derangements
     2. Osteochondritis Dissecans
     3. Popliteal (Baker's) Cysts
     4. Prepatellar and Anserine Bursitis
     5. Caisson Disease

II. Ankles and Feet
   A. Anatomy
     1. Bones and Joints
     2. Muscles and Ligaments
     3. Bursae
     4. Blood and Nerve Supply
   B. Physical Examination
     1. Normal Function
     2. Inspection
     3. Palpation
     4. Range of Motion
   C. Ankle and Foot Disorders
     1. Static Disabilities of the Feet
     2. Sympathetic Reflex Dystrophy
     3. Tarsal Tunnel Syndrome
     4. Foot Bursitis, Tendinitis, and Fasciitis
     5. Morton's Neuroma
     6. March (Stress) Fracture

The knees, ankles, and feet are fundamentally weight-bearing structures. As instruments of support and locomotion, they excel among those of all other animal species. Consequently, derangements of these structures seriously compromise the life style of humans so afflicted. This chapter describes the anatomy and function of these structures in relation to clinical problems that may be encountered.

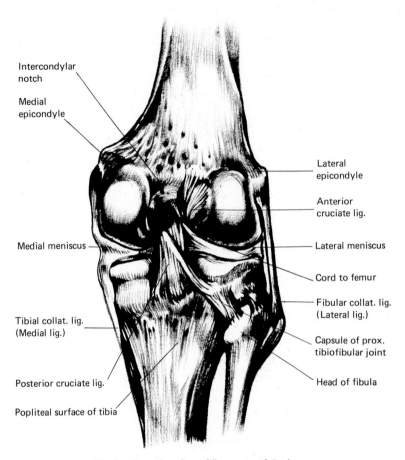

Intercondylar notch

Medial epicondyle

Lateral epicondyle

Anterior cruciate lig.

Medial meniscus

Lateral meniscus

Cord to femur

Fibular collat. lig. (Lateral lig.)

Tibial collat. lig. (Medial lig.)

Capsule of prox. tibiofibular joint

Posterior cruciate lig.

Head of fibula

Popliteal surface of tibia

Fig. 1.   Posterior view of ligaments of the knee.

KNEES

The knee, the largest joint of the body, is used to carry and propel the body. It is a common site of injury, especially in athletes, and of chronic rheumatic disorders, such as rheumatoid and osteoarthritis. Most disorders of the knee can be diagnosed by a thorough history and physical examination, aided by additional diagnostic procedures such as synovial fluid analysis, x-rays, arthrography, and arthroscopy. Occasionally surgical exploration and biopsy may be needed. A knowledge of the basic anatomy and function of this complex articular structure is essential to an understanding of knee problems.

Anatomy

Bones and joints.   The knee consists of the articulating surfaces of the femur and tibia, the proximal end of the fibula, and the patella, a sesamoid bone within the quadriceps tendon. It is a compound condylar joint composed of three distinct articulations: the medial femorotibial, the lateral femorotibial, and the patellofemoral. Anatomically, it contains articulating hyaline cartilages that cover the femoral and tibial condyles, wedge-shaped fibrocartilaginous menisci that act as cushions or shock absorbers, a thin layer of synovium that lines the capsule, and the joint capsule. The capsule attaches to the epiphyses of the femur and tibia and has the capacity to distend in response to increases in its contents. The large supra-

patellar pouch tends to accumulate excess fluid, and joint effusions are best detected as lateral bulges in this area.

Muscles and ligaments.   Knee motion and stability are controlled by several major muscles and ligaments. The quadriceps muscles, of which the medial vastus is the most prominent, extend the knee, while the hamstrings flex the knee. The sartorius and gracilis muscles, both originating from the pelvis, also contribute to extension of the knee. External rotation of the tibia and fibula on the femoral condyles is accomplished by the biceps femoris, while internal rotation is achieved primarily by the popliteus and semitendinosus muscles. The gastrocnemius muscle, which originates proximal to the femoral condyles and inserts distally at the Achilles tendon, not only limits hyperextension of the knee but also promotes plantar flexion of the foot. During weight bearing and motion, the knee is stabilized by a number of muscles, including the popliteus, biceps, tensor fascia femoris, and the iliotibial band.

Knee ligaments of major importance are the articular capsule, the ligamentum patellae, the medial and lateral collateral ligaments, and the anterior and posterior cruciate ligaments (Fig. 1). The articular capsule is a thin, fibrous membrane that is strengthened by the fascia lata, tendons, and ligaments supporting the joint. The ligamentum patellae is the extension of the common tendon of the quadriceps which attaches from the patella to the tibial tuberosity. The infrapatellar fat pad lies below the patella between the ligamentum patellae and the synovial membrane. The collateral ligaments provide lateral and medial support to the knee while the two cruciate ligaments render anteroposterior support.

Bursae. Of the many bursae in the knee, the largest is the semimembranous bursa, located in the medial popliteal space. It is superficial in position, and deeper to it is the medial gastrocnemius bursa. A lateral gastrocnemius bursa communicates with the joint space. Bursae surrounding the gastrocnemius head may fuse to form a composite bursa which when distended is referred to as a popliteal cyst or Baker's cyst. Additional superficial bursae include a large prepatellar bursa between the skin and patella which has no communication with the joint space, a small superficial infrapatellar bursa between the skin and patellar ligament, a deep infrapatellar bursa beneath the patellar ligament, and the anserine bursa on the medial aspect of the knee between the tibial collateral ligament and tendons of the sartorius, gracilis, and semitendinosus muscles.

Blood and nerve supply. The knee receives its blood supply from the popliteal artery, the descending branch of the lateral femoral circumflex artery, and the recurrent branch of the anterior tibial artery. The nerve supply of the knee is derived from the femoral nerve, the saphenous nerve, the obturator nerve, and the tibial and common peroneal branches of the sciatic nerve through genicular branches that accompany corresponding arteries.

Physical Examination

As with all joints, the examination of the knee involves a routine that includes inspection, palpation, and assessment of range of motion. It is critically important to examine both knees, even when the patient complains of problems in only one. In the normal knee, the anatomic configuration and landmarks are maintained and the range of motion is normal.

Normal function. The key to an understanding of normal function is the realization that the knee is not a simple-hinge joint and that its movement is helicoid or spiral in character.

The chief movements of the knee are flexion and extension. Some rotation occurs with flexion, and a slight degree of medial rotation of the femur is needed for extension. As the knee joint passes from full flexion to full extension, the medial condyle of the femur can roll farther than the lateral condyle. During extension, the two femoral condyles revolve on the tibia and its menisci. The posterior cruciate ligament greatly restricts the forward roll of the condyles and causes them to spin. In effect, the movement is of the hinge type with the addition of some forward roll. During extension, turning of the lateral femoral condyle is arrested by the lateral meniscus and anterior cruciate ligament. Extension continues while the medial femoral condyle is completing its final spin and roll, but the femur must rotate medially on its long axis to permit this. The pivot around which it rotates is the anterior cruciate ligament. At the same

time, the lateral femoral condyle, which is no longer rolling, and the lateral meniscus, whose sharp anterior margin is locked to it by its groove, slide forward together on the tibia, moving as one structure. The medial femoral condyle then completes the process of extension at the same time as the entire femur undergoes rotation. When these movements are achieved, the anterior border of the medial meniscus then fits into the curved groove on the femoral condyle.

The muscles and ligaments of the knee have three primary functions. The first is to maintain posture by stabilizing the leg when standing. The second is kinetic, to move the joint to the limits allowed by its configuration. The third is propulsive, to move the leg on the thigh against resistance.

Normally, the knee extends to a straight line of 0° and can hyperextend up to 15°. The knee can be flexed passively by the examiner or actively by the subject to 135°–150°.

Pain. A careful history of the character of pain and of associated symptoms often provides important diagnostic clues to the major causes of knee pain (Table 1). Diffuse pain, for example, occurs from capsular distention, while localized pain results from tendinitis, bursitis, or meniscus tear. Knee pain radiating to the calf is often due to popliteal distension. Intense pain after climbing is a feature of chondromalacia patellae, while intermittent pain with locking may be due to a loose body within the joint. Pain is usually absent in a neuropathic (Charcot's) joint. Early morning stiffness of one or more hours duration is characteristic of rheumatoid arthritis, while gelling, or stiffness after prolonged inactivity, is common in osteoarthritis.

Inspection. The knees should be inspected for evidence of abnormalities or instability with and without weight bearing. On weight bearing the knees may be angulated. Lateral angulation is genu varum or bowlegs, while medial angulation is genu valgum or knock knees. Anterior angulation of the knee is a flexion contracture or limitation of extension, while backward bowing from hyperextension is genu recurvatum. Walking may reveal a limp, locking, buckling, or a contracture.

The knees are also inspected with the patient first supine and then prone. Normal landmarks and depressions are lost to bulges from synovial thickening or effusion or from bony spurs. There may be swelling of the suprapatellar and infrapatellar areas, as well as the popliteal fossa behind the knee. Massive distention may produce a popliteal or Baker's cyst, which is usually more prominent when the knee is extended. A popliteal cyst may dissect downward into the posterior leg muscles resulting in swelling of the calf. The anterior aspect of both thighs should be inspected for evidence of atrophy of the quadriceps femoris muscle. Atrophy of the quadriceps and other muscle groups is common with prolonged disuse of the knee.

Palpation. The soft tissues are palpated with the finger tips for their consistency, thickness, warmth, tenderness, and swelling. Swelling from synovitis is fluc-

Table 1
Major Causes of Knee Pain

Rheumatic disorders	Metabolic disorders
Acute arthritis	Hyper-, hypothyroidism
Chronic arthritis	Hyperparathyroidism
Connective tissue disorders	Acromegaly
Bursitis, tendinitis, tenosynovitis	Ochronosis
Popliteal (Baker's) cyst	Hemachromatosis
Structural disorders	Neoplastic and related disorders
Traumatic	Pigmented villonodular synovitis
Postural	Primary and secondary tumor
Developmental	Secondary hypertrophic osteoarthropathy
Ankle and foot deformities	Lymphoma, leukemia
	Multicentric reticulohistiocytosis
Vascular diseases	
Thrombophlebitis	Neurologic disorders
Vascular insufficiency	Peripheral neuritis, sciatica
Intermittent claudication	Multiple sclerosis
Peripheral edema	Tabes dorsalis
Anterior tibial syndrome	
	Miscellaneous
Hematologic disorders	Osteomyelitis
Hemophilia	Osteonecrosis
Hemoglobinopathies	Osteochondritis dissecans
	Chondromalacia patellae
	Osgood-Schlatter's disease
	Hemangioma
	Caisson disease

tuant or boggy in contrast to the firmness of adjacent soft tissues. The synovial membrane may be fluctuant and distended if excessive synovial fluid is present. Abnormalities of the synovial membrane are usually felt more easily over the medial than over the lateral aspect of the knee. Ballottement of the patella is possible when large joint effusions are present. This is performed by compression of the suprapatellar pouch with the left hand while rocking the patella against the femur anteroposteriorly with the forefinger of the right hand. Another test, useful for detection of even minimal effusion, is the bulge sign. The medial aspect of the knee is stroked and pressure is applied cephalad with one hand to express the synovial fluid from the area. The examiner then taps the lateral aspect of the knee with the other hand. If synovial fluid is present, a distinct fluid wave or bulge will appear on the medial aspect of the knee. The posterior aspect of the knee is also palpated for evidence of abnormalities, including fluctuant synovial swelling or a popliteal cyst.

The prepatellar bursa is easily palpable when distended. On the other hand, it may be difficult to palpate small bursae, such as the anserine, even when enlarged. Localization of palpable swelling and tenderness to the region of the bursa helps to differentiate bursal from synovial involvement. When both occur simultaneously, careful palpation may help to distinguish one from the other.

The articular margins and bones of the knee should be palpated for abnormalities and tenderness, such as exostoses due to osteoarthritis. Palpation of the patella

may disclose abnormalities such as chondromalacia. If pushing the patella against the femur elicits tenderness or a grating sensation, there may be derangement of the patellofemoral surface. While patellofemoral grating or crepitus may be a sign of osteoarthritis or chondromalacia patellae, it is also noted in healthy subjects.

Range of motion. Flexion contractures or limitation of extension may result from chronic afflictions of the knee such as rheumatoid arthritis. A catch or jerky motion on passive flexion and extension suggests loose bodies in the joint space. Increased mobility found on adducting and abducting the leg on the femur in a rocking fashion suggests a tear of the medial or lateral collateral ligament. Abnormally increased forward excursion of the tibia on the femur indicates instability of the anterior cruciate ligament, whereas increased posterior mobility and excursion signify instability of the posterior cruciate ligament.

Knee Disorders

The causes of knee pain are multiple and diverse (Table 1). Consequently, the knee may be the major site of involvement in a variety of conditions, including the connective tissue diseases, endocrine and metabolic disorders, hematologic and neoplastic diseases, and structural and vascular disorders.

While symmetric swelling of knees is typical of rheumatoid arthritis, it may occur in a host of other inflammatory and noninflammatory disorders. Synovial fluid analysis aids in distinguishing inflammatory from noninflammatory disorders but is even more critical with swelling of a single knee, primarily to rule out infectious arthritis. Knee swelling may be the initial manifestation of ankylosing spondylitis that may precede by years the development of back complaints and other features of spondylitis. Similarly, recurrent knee synovitis may be the sole expression of enteropathic or psoriatic arthritis years before typical gastrointestinal or cutaneous manifestations, respectively, disclose the true nature of the underlying arthritis.

Internal derangements. Most injuries of the knee are caused by disruption of the rotator mechanism. When bearing weight, the tibia rotates laterally as the knee extends and rotates medially when the knee flexes. If this synchrony is prevented forcibly, as by the weight of the falling body, the rotator mechanism of the knee may be deranged.

Local tenderness of the medial or lateral aspect of the joint space between the tibia and the femur and below the femoral condyles suggests a tear or some other disorder of the meniscus. On the other hand, tenderness along the ligamentous attachments over the medial or lateral femoral condyles extending above the region of the joint space suggests a disorder of the collateral ligaments. Lesions of the collateral ligaments may be differentiated from those of the menisci by eliciting pain on abduction and adduction of the tibia with the femur stabilized. Evidence of a tear in the posterior portion of either meniscus can be gleaned by the presence of McMurray's sign. When the knee is moved from full flexion to extension, a palpable and sometimes audible snapping occurs when the torn meniscus moves in and out of place.

Instability of the knee involves the collateral ligaments more frequently than the cruciate ligaments. Stability of the collateral ligaments may be tested with the knee in full extension. The examiner fixes the femur with the left hand while grasping the ankle with the right hand and then attempts to adduct and abduct the leg on the femur in a rocking fashion. Normally, there is no appreciable motion. Increased mobility indicates relaxation or tear of the medial or lateral collateral ligament. To check for instability of the cruciate ligaments, the patient is examined in a sitting position with the knee flexed to 90°. The femur is held fixed while the examiner attempts alternately to pull and push the tibia forward and backward. Normally, there is little or no excursion of the leg on the femur. Increased forward excursion of the tibia signifies instability of the anterior cruciate ligament, while increased posterior excursion signals instability of the posterior cruciate ligament.

Osteochondritis dissecans. This is a local disorder of subchondral bone most commonly found in the knees of adolescents and young adults. A devitalized fragment of bone and its articular cartilage demarcates from its original site, usually on the lateral position of the medial femoral condyle. There is mild discomfort, aggravated by exercise, and with separation of the fragment instability of the knee occurs. By forcing the tibia into internal rotation while extending the knee from 90° of flexion, at about 30° the patient complains of pain which is promptly relieved by external rotation of the tibia.

Popliteal (Baker's) cysts. These cysts may originate from accumulations of fluid in a noncommunicating bursa, from distention of a bursa by fluid from a disorder of the knee, and from posterior herniation of the joint capsule in response to increased intraarticular pressure. A popliteal cyst must be differentiated from a normal fat pad, aneurysm, tumor, infection, and varicosities. If a popliteal cyst dissects into the posterior aspect of the leg, the calf reveals a fluctuant fullness or firm induration. If dissection of a popliteal cyst is acute, it may mimic phlebitis with localized heat, redness, and a positive Homan's sign. Diagnosis may be confirmed by arthrography or aspiration of synovial fluid from the indurated calf area.

Prepatellar and anserine bursitis. Prepatellar bursitis (housemaid's knee) is manifest as tender swelling between the skin and lower patella or patellar tendon resulting from prolonged kneeling. Pain is usually minimal without direct pressure to the swollen area. Anserine bursitis is characterized by tenderness and swelling localized to the medial aspect of the knee between the medial collateral ligament and the tendons of the sartorius, gracilis, and semitendinous muscles. Patients often complain of pain when climbing stairs.

Caisson disease. Workers subjected to sudden decompression from pressurized chambers, such as the caissons used in tunnel construction, may experience acute throbbing pain in the extremities, commonly known as "the bends." Because nitrogen is highly soluble in lipid, the fatty marrow of long bones is especially susceptible to injury. Nitrogen bubbles obstructing terminal arteries may cause avascular necrosis, particularly of the proximal tibia and femoral epiphyses. There is minimal or no knee pain until collapse of necrotic bony trabeculae occurs. On x-ray examination, caisson disease resembles avascular necrosis and bone infarction due to other causes, such as sickle cell disease and other hemoglobinopathies.

ANKLES AND FEET
Anatomy

Bones and joints. The ankle (supratalar or talocrural) is a hinge joint for flexion and extension formed by the talus (astragalus) and distal tibia. The distal tibiofibular joint is composed of the convex fibular surface and the concave tibial surface without an intervening articular cartilage. The superior (trochlear) surface of the talus articulates with the tibia and is anchored on each side by the malleoli to render stability to the ankle. Beneath the talus lies the subtalar (talocalcaneal) joint and anteriorly are the talonavicular and calcaneocuboid joints. These promote supination and pronation of the foot. The capsular ligament is a weak structure, especially anteriorly and posteriorly, that is stabilized by strong ligamentous attachments. Synovium lines the capsule and is most extensive anteriorly.

The bones of the foot form two longitudinal groups,

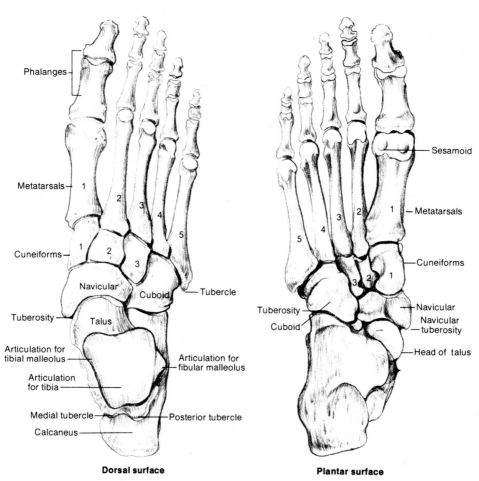

Fig. 2. Bones of the feet.

a medial and a lateral (Fig. 2). The medial group, which receives most of the body's thrust through the tibia, comprises the talus, navicular, three cuneiforms, three medial metatarsal bones, and the medial phalanges. The lateral group consists of the calcaneus, cuboid, and two lateral metatarsal bones and their phalanges.

The talocalcaneal and talonavicular joints are the only joints of the foot in which considerable movement takes place. The subtalar (talocalcaneonavicular) joint is a large articulation between the talus above and the calcaneus and navicular below and in front. The talonavicular segment of this joint is of the ball and socket type. The lower part of the head of the talus articulates with the spring (plantar calcaneonavicular) ligament, which is of importance in maintaining the longitudinal arch. The midtarsal joint is supported by the long and short plantar ligaments that separate the posterior and anterior parts of the foot. The tarsal tunnel lies between the medial malleolus and the calcaneus, roofed by the flexor retinaculum. Several tendons and the posterior tibial nerve pass through the tunnel. Nerve entrapment from tenosynovitis (tarsal tunnel syndrome) can produce symptoms comparable to those of the carpal tunnel syndrome that occurs at the wrist.

The joints distal to the midtarsal joint include the

intertarsal, tarsometatarsal, intermetatarsal, metatarsophalangeal (MTP), and the interphalangeal joints. These joints form the arches of the foot. They have tight capsules and little motion, unlike the corresponding joints of the hand. The MTP and interphalangeal joints are fashioned and supplied with ligaments like the corresponding joints of the hand. The deep transverse metatarsal ligaments (ligaments of the metatarsal heads) extend to the hallux, unlike the corresponding ligaments of the hand which leave the pollex free. The small intertarsal joints (between cuboid, navicular, and cuneiforms), the tarsometatarsal joints, and the joints between the bases of the metatarsals may be considered together as side-to-side and end-to-end joints. The side-to-side joints have strong plantar ligaments that act as transverse ties. The end-to-end joints have strong plantar ligaments, weak dorsal ligaments, and in some instances, collateral ligaments.

Muscles and ligaments. The ankle joint receives strong support posteriorly from the flexor hallucis longus tendon. The medial and lateral sides of the ankle joint are strongly reinforced by the deltoid ligament medially and the lateral ligament. The deltoid (internal lateral) ligament is a fan-shaped band originating on the medial malleolus and attaching to the navicular, talus, sustentaculum tali, and calcaneonavicular ligament. The tendons of the tibialis posterior and flexor digitorum muscles reinforce it. The lateral ligament has three main bands. The anterior band stretches from the lateral malleolus to the lateral surface of the neck of the talus. The medial band (calcaneofibular ligament) extends from the malleolus to the lateral surface of the calcaneus. The posterior band (talofibular ligament) tightly binds the fibula and talus.

The foot has three arches which are joined in the shape of a cone, the base of which is formed by the metatarsals. The medial longitudinal arch includes the calcaneus, the talus, the navicular, the three cuneiforms, and the three medial metatarsals. The lateral longitudinal arch comprises the calcaneus, the cuboid, and the two outer metatarsals. The transverse arch is wedge shaped because of the contour of the bones, which include the middle and lateral cuneiforms and the second, third, and fourth metatarsals. When the arch gives way, the metatarsal heads are lowered, promoting the formation of painful calluses.

The tendon of the tibialis anterior muscle inserts into the first cuneiform and the base of the first metatarsal. The extensor hallucis longus tendon lies in front of the ankle and passes forward, inserting on the dorsal aspect of the big toe. The tendons of the extensor digitorum longus muscle are directed to the four outer toes. The extensor digitorum brevis tendon can be felt on the posterolateral aspect of the dorsum of the foot. The peroneus brevis tendon passes forward under the lateral malleolus to insert into the tuberosity of the fifth metatarsal.

The soleus muscle, originating from the proximal tibia and fibula, joins the tendon of gastrocnemius to reach the back of the calcaneus as the Achilles tendon. Extending forward from the calcaneus and sending supporting slips to each of the digits is the plantar aponeurosis, a strong fibrous band that provides major support to the longitudinal arch.

Bursae. No bursae communicate with the ankle joint. Numerous bursae occur about the feet and ankles, notably at pressure points, such as the first and fifth MTP joints. There are several bursae in the heel, one between the skin and Achilles tendon (Achilles tendon bursa), one between the Achilles tendon and the calcaneus (retrocalcaneal bursa), and one between the skin of the sole and the caudal portion of the calcaneus (subcalcaneal bursa). These are frequently involved in rheumatoid and other forms of inflammatory joint disease.

Blood and nerve supply. The ankle and foot receive their blood supply primarily from branches of the anterior and posterior tibial arteries. The veins of the dorsum of the foot are arranged in the shape of a fan and are usually visible. The saphenous veins arise from the marginal veins of this group. Branches of the anterior and posterior tibial nerves provide the nerve supply of the ankle and foot.

Physical Examination

Normal Function. The ankle and foot have the dual roles of supporting and propelling the body. A normal foot maintains integrity through muscular equilibrium. The foot performs the will of the muscles, which in turn perform the will of the individual either to stand erect or to perform some phase of locomotion. In walking, the triceps surae (two heads of the gastrocnemius and the soleus) raise the heel from the ground and cause plantar flexion of the ankle at the end of the stance phase. In advancing the leg or swing phase, the four anterior crural muscles enable the foot to clear the ground by causing dorsiflexion. In the act of locomotion, the weight of the body is transmitted to the talus through the tibia, while leverage from metatarsals raises and lowers the weight load. Toes, designed to dig in, assist in propelling the body forward. During walking, the heel absorbs shock which is then transmitted smoothly throughout the foot. In running, the forefoot absorbs shock and then transmits it posteriorly.

Movement of the ankle (talocrural) joint is confined primarily to plantar flexion and dorsiflexion, which are normally about 45° and 20°, respectively. Inversion and eversion of the foot occur primarily at the subtalar joint. Supination or inversion of the foot occurs when the sole of the foot is turned inward. Pronation or eversion of the foot occurs when the sole of the foot is turned outward. Normally, inversion is about 30° and eversion about 20°.

The first MTP joint of the great toe flexes about 35° and extends 70°, while the second to fifth MTP joints flex and extend about 40°. The proximal interphalangeal joints normally do not extend beyond the neutral position indicated by 0° but can flex to about 50°. Movement of the distal interphalangeal joints varies but extension is roughly 20°–30° and flexion is 40°–50°.

From the description above, it is clear that the foot and ankle act as a delicately balanced propulsive unit that can produce major alterations in gait when affected by disease or other alterations. Consequently, examination of the ankle and foot requires a methodical approach so as not to omit important details. For completion, inspection of shoes for points of wear should also be included.

Inspection. The ankle and foot should be inspected not only in a non-weight-bearing position but also with the patient standing and walking. Both ankles and feet are compared from the front, back, and sides for evidence of swelling, atrophy, deformities, skin and nail changes, edema, nodules, or other abnormalities. Abnormal positions of the foot, such as pes planus (flat feet), should be noted. Detection of corns, calluses, and bunions provides important clues to other deformities.

The foot and ankle are inspected for the presence of either local or diffuse swelling. Diffuse swelling may signal pitting edema from congestive heart failure, Sudeck's atrophy (see Ankle and Foot Disorders), or scleroderma. Edema fluid elicits pitting on direct pressure while swelling from synovitis does not, unless the two coexist. Effusion or synovial swelling involving the ankle (talocrural) joint produces swelling or fullness over the anterior aspect of the joint. Swelling behind the malleoli is often a clue to heel involvement. Inflammation of forefoot supporting ligaments results in their stretching, producing metatarsal spread (spreadfoot), which is a common feature of the rheumatoid foot.

The gait is usually affected by afflictions or deformities of the ankle and foot. Outward displacement of the forefoot, as seen in rheumatoid arthritis, produces a toe-out gait. The patient avoids painful ankle and foot motion by rolling the foot from the lateral to the medial side, thereby replacing the normal heel-to-toe gait. The toe-in (pigeon-toed) gait results from inward displacement of the forefoot. It may be congenital but may also be secondary to ankle and foot deformities.

Inspection of the skin and nail often provides important diagnostic clues. Erythematous papules and pustular lesions of the sole may signify Reiter's syndrome or psoriasis. Onycholysis of toenails also occurs in both Reiter's syndrome and psoriatic arthritis. Pitting of the toenails, however, is a feature of psoriatic arthritis and not of Reiter's syndrome. The peripheral circulation may be impaired in many of the rheumatic and connective tissue disorders. In polyarteritis and scleroderma, for example, ischemic ulcerations of the digits are not unusual. Raynaud's phenomenon may affect the feet as well as the hands, as does induration of the skin (sclerodactyly) from scleroderma.

Inspection of shoes for points of wear (pressure points) may reveal foot deformities. For example, excessive wearing of the innersole is indicative of a pes planus deformity.

Palpation.   The ankle and foot joints may be palpated with the patient seated, then lying supine as well as prone. If ankle swelling or effusion is present, it usually occurs anteriorly because the synovial membrane is most extensive here. Warmth and tenderness from synovitis may also be present. Swelling or tenderness behind the malleoli usually reflects heel involvement. Causes include osseus spurs, tendinitis, bursitis, fasciitis, periostitis, tumors, or strains from trauma of ligaments and other soft tissues. Achillotendinitis and/or bursitis produce local tenderness and induration in back of the heel. Rheumatoid nodules may also occur at this site, as may calluses, tophi, and fibrous nodules. Heel pain may also be due to bony spurs or periostitis behind or on the under surface of the calcaneus. These occur in response to soft tissue inflammation, such as plantar fasciitis, and are particularly notable in Reiter's syndrome and rheumatoid arthritis. Asymptomatic calcaneal spurs disclosed on x-ray are not uncommon, however, particularly in the elderly.

The intertarsal and then the MTP joints are palpated between the examiner's thumb on the dorsum of the foot and his fingers on the plantar surface. Swelling, tenderness, and warmth may be detected in the presence of synovitis. Tenosynovitis appears as a superficial linear swelling unlike the more diffuse swelling of synovitis. MTP joint tenderness can be elicited by squeezing the metatarsal heads together between the thumb on one side of the foot and the fingers on the other side. In turn, tenderness of each MTP joint can be evaluated by firm palpation of each joint between the thumb and forefinger. The proximal and distal interphalangeal joints of the toes are palpated for swelling, tenderness, and warmth.

Combined inspection and palpation may disclose changes in skin color, texture, and temperature, as well as hair loss, nail changes, and edema. The dorsalis pedis and posterior tibial pulses are easily palpable, except that the latter are normally absent in 10 percent of people. Diminished or absent pulses and trophic changes of the skin or nail occur with peripheral vascular diseases, but also with hepatic, renal, metabolic, neurologic, or other disorders.

Range of motion.   Limitation of ankle and foot motion may result from chronic disorders of the foot. When pronounced, associated deformities and abnormalities of gait soon follow. It is important to clarify, however, whether abnormalities of gait are due to local deformities or to lesions of peripheral nerves or the central nervous system.

Ankle and Foot Disorders

There are a host of disorders that can affect the ankle and foot (Table 2). Clearly, the most common are static disabilities resulting from undue stress, obesity, faulty shoes, or as secondary effects of derangements of the hip, knee, or spine. Most forms of chronic arthritis and connective tissue disorders may also involve the ankle and foot. Most initial attacks of acute primary gout occur in the first MTP joint, instep, or heel area. Moreover, the most common site for tophaceous deposits of sodium urate are in the capsule and bones of the first MTP joint. Osteoarthritis of the ankle or foot is usually secondary to previous injury, congenital deformity, underlying chronic arthritis, or foot disabilities. Osteochondritis or avascular necrosis of any of the metatarsal heads may occur during periods of active growth.

Static disabilities of the feet.   Foot strain from excessive body weight and/or occupational stress constitutes one of the most common causes of painful feet and leg cramps. Pronation of the longitudinal and transverse arches results, along with depression of the talar head and valgus deformity of the heel. These abnormalities may be noted only with weight bearing.

Flattening of the longitudinal arch results in flat feet (pes planus), which may be congenital or acquired, causing pain, fatigue, and a limp. Pes cavus is an abnormal elevation of the longitudinal arch, also congenital or acquired. In talipes equinus the foot is held in plantar flexion. It often results from contracture of the Achilles tendon and is common in bedridden patients. Inward or outward deviation of the heel denotes talipes varus or talipes valgus, respectively. Inversion (supination) of the foot results when the sole is turned inward, while eversion (pronation) occurs when the sole is turned outward. Adduction of the foot is inward displacement of the forefoot, abduction is outward displacement of the forefoot. Deformities of adduction and inversion (varus) or abduction and eversion (valgus) are often combined (talipes equinovarus) and may also be associated with knee abnormalities such as genu varum.

The most common deformity of the great toe is hallux valgus. Lateral deviation of the great toe results in abnormal rotation and prominence of the first MTP joint and overlapping or underlying of the second toe. Hallux

Table 2
Major Causes of Ankle and Foot Pain

Rheumatic disorders	Vascular disorders
Acute arthritis	Raynaud's disease
Chronic arthritis	Arteriosclerosis
Connective tissue disorders	Buerger's disease
Bursitis, tendinitis, tenosynovitis	Dependent edema
Tarsal tunnel syndrome	
	Neurologic disorders
Static disabilities	Peripheral neuritis
Foot strain	Central nervous system
Flat feet (pes planus)	disease
Pes cavus	Tabes dorsalis
Talipes equinus, varus, valgus	
Hallux valgus, ridigis	Miscellaneous
Hammer toe, cockup toe	Osteomyelitis
Calcaneal spurs	Osteochondritis
March fracture	Sudeck's atrophy
Corn, bunion, callus	Morton's neuroma
	Paget's disease
	Primary and secondary
	tumor

rigidis is complete fixation of the first MTP joint. A hammer-toe deformity includes hyperextension of the MTP joint and plantar flexion of the proximal interphalangeal joint. A cockup deformity of the toe is dorsal displacement of the proximal phalanx on the metatarsal head, resulting in metatarsal head depression toward the sole and subluxation of the MTP joint.

The above deformities may be due to a variety of causes, including rheumatoid and other forms of chronic arthritis. Common pathomechanical factors include occupational stress, obesity, and poorly fitting shoes. Foot deformities result in undue pressure (microtrauma) from shoes and thus enhance the development of superimposed painful corns, bunions, and calluses.

Sympathetic reflex dystrophy. This disorder, also known as Sudeck's atrophy, is due to an imbalance of the autonomic outflow to the extremity. It is manifest by exquisite pain, stiffness, hyperemia, and marked swelling of the entire foot so that patients cannot bear weight. Diffuse and mottled demineralization (osteoporosis) is disclosed on x-ray of the involved foot.

Tarsal tunnel syndrome. This condition, resulting from compression of the posterior tibial nerve, is not recognized as often as its counterpart (carpal tunnel syndrome) in the wrist. Symptoms include burning pain and paresthesias of the toes and sole which are usually worse at night. Palpation of the medial side of the ankle may reveal tenderness or fusiform swelling over the posterior tibial nerve. Tapping the nerve may reproduce symptoms, as may sustained finger pressure. The diagnosis can be confirmed by nerve conduction studies.

Foot bursitis, tendinitis, and fasciitis. Inflammation of a bursa or tendon occurs frequently at the heel, bunion (first MTP), and bunionette (fifth MTP) areas. Achillotendinitis or achillobursitis produces pain in back of the heel, while plantar fasciitis produces pain on the under surface of the heel. These often result from excessive foot abuse

or stress but are frequent manifestations of acute or chronic inflammatory disorders of the foot.

Morton's neuroma. A fibrous neuroma may form at the junction of the medial and lateral plantar nerves. Firm palpation may disclose tenderness or a palpable tumor between the third and fourth metatarsal heads. It is usually unilateral and more frequent in women. Clinically, the disorder is characterized by severe burning pain of the anterior portion of the foot, usually between the third and fourth digits, that occurs with walking while wearing shoes. Pain is relieved by rest and removing the shoe.

March (stress) fracture. A transverse fracture of the metatarsal bone, most frequently the second or third, may result from excessive walking (marching) or prolonged abuse of the feet. Local forefoot pain and swelling are the major complaints. Examination discloses local swelling and tenderness at the site of the fracture. Diagnosis is confirmed by x-ray, which may be normal initially until callus forms several weeks later.

REFERENCES

Basmajian JV: Joints of lower limb, in Grant's Method of Anatomy. Baltimore, Williams & Wilkins, 1975, pp 364–387

Beetham WP, Polley HF, Slocumb CH, Weaver WF: Physical Examination of the Joints. Philadelphia, Saunders, 1965, pp 143–192

Calabro JJ: A critical evaluation of the diagnostic features of the feet in rheumatoid arthritis. Arthritis Rheum 5:19, 1962

Goodgold J, Kopell HP, Spielholz NI: The tarsal-tunnel syndrome: Objective diagnostic criteria. N Engl J Med 273:742, 1965

Heffet AJ: Anatomy and mechanics of movement of the knee joint, in AJ Heffet (ed): Disorders of the Knee. Philadelphia, Lippincott, 1974, pp 1–17

Moll JMH, Wright V: Measurement of joint motion. Clin Rheum Dis 2:3, 1976

Wilson JN: A diagnostic sign in osteochondritis dissecans of the knee. J Bone Joint Surg 49-A:477, 1967

Pain

Stanley L. Wallace

Pain is almost universally present in the rheumatic diseases. Joint pain is the most common presenting complaint when the patient with arthritis comes to the physician. Joint pain also contributes strongly to patient disability; it is a major factor in depression among patients with rheumatic diseases. An adequate understanding of rheumatic pain can contribute to diagnosis and to optimal treatment.

One of the problems in the study of pain in the joints is that patients are impoverished in the language they can use to describe their suffering. This makes it difficult for the physician to distinguish one variety of pain from another. In general, pain has five characteristics; intensity, duration, and the quality of the pain are the most important to diagnosis. The significance of the pain to the patient and the psychic response to the painful stimulus, the other characteristics, are useful factors in evaluating any patient's joint pain. Articular pain, like visceral pain, is recognized by the patient as being "deep," i.e., beneath the skin. The pain is generally not well localized within the specific joint, and its borders are poorly delineated. Further compounding this problem is the fact that adjacent structures (bursae, muscles, etc.) are frequently also involved with inflammation in many of the rheumatic disorders, and pain may arise from these structures as well.

Intensity of pain correlates roughly with the degree of painful stimulus; in inflammatory disease it is approximately proportional to the severity of inflammation. Even here, however, where a linear relationship between inflammation and pain might be expected, there are exceptions. The pain of acute gout (see below), for example, is generally more severe than in other disorders with equivalent gross manifestations of inflammation (i.e., similar joint fluid white blood cell counts or equal degrees of synovial fluid hyaluronate depolymerization).

The duration of pain—the episodicity or persistence of the entire inflammatory process in the joint—is an important factor to consider in differential diagnosis. The quality of articular pain is generally thought to be similar to that of most visceral pain—dull and aching. This is not completely true; there are clear differences in the quality of pain among various joint diseases (see below), the mechanisms of which are not completely understood. Ultimately, all joint pain, no matter what the origin or character, is mediated through the articular nervous system.

INNERVATION OF THE JOINT

Macro- and microdissection studies in experimental animals show that the joint is supplied by two groups of articular nerves, but there is significant variability from species to species, from individual to individual, and from joint to joint. In general, the primary articular nerves serve the joints directly, while the accessory articular nerves arise from the nerve supply of adjacent muscles and are more variable in number and distribution.

The nerve supply of the cat knee can be used as the archetype for the understanding of joint innervation. There are three primary articular nerves in the cat knee: the posterior, lateral, and medial. The posterior, which is the largest, arises from the posterior tibial nerve and is distributed mainly to the posterior capsule of the knee joint, the posterior fat pads, the oblique and cruciate ligaments, and the annular ligaments surrounding the menisci.

The medial articular nerve in the cat knee is a branch of the saphenous nerve. It supplies the medial surface of the articular capsule, the medial collateral ligament, the medial part of the annular ligament attached to the medial meniscus, the patellar ligament, the patellar periosteum, and the infrapatellar fat pad. The lateral articular nerve is less constant and usually is a branch of the lateral popliteal nerve. It innervates the joint capsule and the lateral collateral ligament.

Accessory articular nerves arising from nerves in muscle are extremely variable in the cat. In general, these nerves arise more often from muscles above the knee joint than below it and are present in extensor muscles of the joint rather than flexor. They help innervate the joint capsule, the various ligaments, the fat pads, and the patellar periosteum.

The nerve endings present in the tissues of the cat's knee joint (innervated by the articular nerves just described) are classifiable morphologically into four types. The first three are mechanoreceptors; the type IV endings include some that serve as pain receptors and others have vasomotor functions. Some observers feel that the mechanoreceptor endings may also serve a nociceptive function.

The type IV endings are often found in networks, or sometimes as free nerve terminals, throughout the fibrous capsule, the adjacent periostea of the tibia, fibula, and patella, the ligaments and tendons of the joint, the articular fat pads, and the adventitial sheaths of all the small arteries and arterioles. It must be emphasized that these nerve endings are *absent* from synovia and menisci, except in the walls of the small vessels serving these tissues.

The sensory impulses from joints are transmitted along the primary sensory neurones, through the posterior roots, and into the posterior horn of the spinal cord. The secondary sensory neurones cross to the opposite side of the spinal cord within one or two segments and combine to form the lateral spinothalamic tract, which terminates in the posterolateral nucleus of the thalamus. The third sensory neurone carries the impulse from the thalamus to the cortex of the postcentral convolution, but the significance of the cortical connection is not clear. Electric stimulation of this locus in the cortex does not produce pain.

JOINT PAIN IN DISEASE

The precise and immediate mechanisms of joint pain in the various articular diseases are not as yet known. Among the participants in the inflammatory process that may ultimately play some role in the induction of pain are the following: various immunologic reactions; granulocytes and their lysosomal and phagosomal enzymes; other tissue proteinases; monocytes and macrophages and their products; platelets; the kinin system; complement and its fractions; the components of the alternate pathway; and prostaglandins, histamine, serotonin, and other low molecular weight mediators of inflammation. Presumably, the locus at which any or all of these substances or cells may work to induce pain is the perivascular network of nerve endings in subsynovial tissue and in the joint capsule.

Two articular diseases will exemplify the problems in moving from these hypothetical mechanisms to actual pain in the clinical situation. The pain of acute gout differs from the pain of other arthritides in intensity, quality, and emotional environment associated with the attack. A sense of profound or intolerable heat is often felt and of crushing or oppressive weight of the affected joint. Irritability of temper is proverbial in the gouty patient during an attack; he or she is likely to be irascible, choleric, cantankerous, morose, and querulous. Finally, the pain is disproportionate to the degree of inflammation seen in the joint, as noted above. Perhaps lysosomal membrane disruption by the urate crystal, with consequent cell death and release of both lysosomal and cytoplasmic enzymes into the synovial fluid, leads to a higher concentration or a different pattern of such enzymes than in other diseases. Joint fluid kinin levels are also highest

in gout and may contribute to the characteristic pain. One proposal has suggested that Hageman factor, kallikrein, kinins, complement, lysosomal hydrolases, and histamine could interact or jointly contribute to aspects of acute gouty inflammation, including perhaps the intensity and quality of the pain.

Pain in rheumatoid arthritis is less intense, more aching, more persistent, and more frequently associated with depression. Its major characteristic, however, is its almost invariable association with stiffness. The location of morning stiffness as arising in the joint rather than in adjacent tissues is not universally accepted. Nevertheless, rheumatoid joint pain and stiffness generally wax and wane together; local intraarticular therapy that relieves joint inflammation relieves both pain and stiffness, at least in that joint.

The initiation of tissue injury in the synovium in rheumatoid arthritis starts with the immune complex and the activation of complement. Biologically active complement components are present in rheumatoid synovial fluid. The immune complexes provoke further tissue injury by reacting with polymorphonuclear leukocytes and synovial wandering cells. Polymorphonuclear leukocyte lysosomal enzymes contribute to inflammation. Some parts of these and other inflammatory pathways in rheumatoid arthritis ultimately must lead to the characteristic pain and stiffness.

REFERENCES

Freeman MAR, Wyke B: The innervation of the knee joint. An anatomical and histological study in the cat. J Anat 101:505, 1967

Kellermeyer RW, Naff GB: Chemical mediators of inflammation in acute gouty arthritis. Arthritis Rheum 18:765, 1975

Kellgren JH: Pain, in Copeman WSC (ed): Textbook of the Rheumatic Diseases, 4th ed. Edinburgh, Livingstone, 1969, p 19

Connective Tissue

SYNOVIAL MEMBRANE

Peter Barland

The anatomic structures located between apposing bones that allow for movement and growth are referred to as joints. Three types of joints are generally recognized: fibrous, cartilaginous, and diarthrodial. In fibrous joints the bones are united by collagenous ligaments and little if any motion is possible. Fibrous joints usually ossify after the growth and development of the skeleton are completed. In cartilaginous joints the bones are separated by either hyaline cartilage or fibrocartilage. In the adult cartilaginous joints occur principally in the axial skeleton and, while allowing for only small amounts of motion,

they are capable of absorbing a large amount of pressure. Neither fibrous nor cartilaginous joints are invested with a synovial membrane. In diarthrodial joints the ends of the apposing bones are covered by hyaline articular cartilage and are separated by a fluid-filled synovial space that is encapsulated by the synovial membrane (Fig. 1). The term *synovial* was used by Paracelsus to describe the egg-white, gelatinous quality of the fluid found in the diarthrodial joint.

ANATOMY

The synovial membrane is the vascular connective tissue that encloses the synovial cavity. It lines all the intraarticular surfaces except those composed of hyaline cartilage, either in the form of articular cartilage or intraarticular discs or menisci. Intraarticular ligaments such

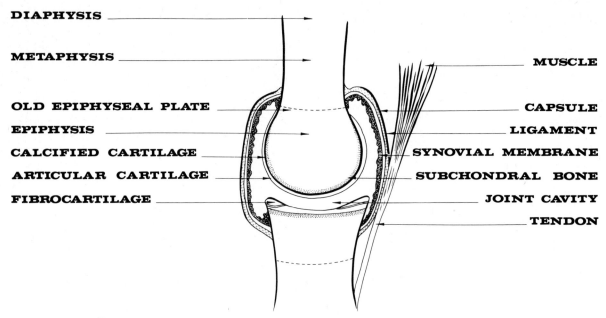

DIAPHYSIS

METAPHYSIS

OLD EPIPHYSEAL PLATE

EPIPHYSIS

CALCIFIED CARTILAGE

ARTICULAR CARTILAGE

FIBROCARTILAGE

MUSCLE

CAPSULE

LIGAMENT

SYNOVIAL MEMBRANE

SUBCHONDRAL BONE

JOINT CAVITY

TENDON

Fig. 1. Normal diarthrodial joint showing the relationship between the synovial membrane and the other principal anatomic components. (Reprinted by permission of authors and publisher from Hamerman and Schubert: The diarthrodial joint, an essay. Am J Med 33:558, 1962.)

as the cruciate ligaments of the knee are also covered by synovial tissue. Tissue similar to the synovial membrane also lines bursae and tendon sheaths in which viscous fluid similar to synovial fluid is found. The synovial membrane joins with the apposing bones at the junction of the articular cartilage and the periosteum. At this point the synovium is also in continuity with the marrow space of the subchondral bone. There is a gradual transition between the synovial membrane and the fibrous outer capsule of the joint, which forms a tough but flexible connection between the articulating bones. The capsule may be thickened in some areas to form ligaments which provide additional strength against mechanical stress. The collagenous fibers of the capsule merge with the metaphysial periosteum of the articulating bones and also penetrate into the cortical bone (Sharpey's fibers), thereby further strengthening the union between the articulating bones.

The blood vessels that supply the joint also supply the subchondral bone. Usually several arteries enter the joint where the synovial membrane and capsule join the periosteum and form an anastomosing circumferential arterial network. The multiple interconnecting sources of arterial blood supply assure the synovial membrane of adequate blood flow regardless of the position of the joint with accompanying compression and stricture of blood vessels. There is also an extensive lymphatic system draining the synovial membrane.

Most of the innervation of the joint consists of pain and proprioceptive fibers that terminate in the joint capsule. The proprioceptive fibers are important in musculoskeletal kinesthetics. The pain fibers are stimulated by stretching of the capsule and lead to reflex contraction of the muscles that flex or adduct the distended joint while

also mediating reflex relaxation of the reciprocal extensor muscles. These reflex mechanisms may be responsible for the flexion contractures and extensor muscle atrophy that rapidly develop around chronically distended joints. Very few nerves actually enter the synovial membrane. While some of these appear to be pain fibers, most of the intrasynovial nerves are part of the autonomic nervous system and function in regulating vascular resistance and blood flow within the synovium.

Recent observations indicate an important role for prostaglandins and cyclic nucleotides in the metabolic activity of synovial tissue. Since these inter- and intracellular mediators are affected by autonomic neurotransmitters, the nervous supply of the synovium may also contribute to the regulation of several cellular functions in the synovium in addition to vasoconstriction and vasodilatation.

Embryology and Development

The structures of the diarthrodial joint are formed between the fourth and sixth weeks of embryonic development. The synovial membrane evolves as a condensation of primitive mesenchymal cells which are situated between the chondrogenic zones that develop into the articular cartilages. While movement of the primordial limb appears to be required for normal joint development the inducers responsible for differentiation of these structures are not known. In the differentiation of the skeletal system the final structure of the various tissues is largely determined by the nature of the extracellular matrix synthesized by the resident mesenchymal cells. The extracellular matrix of hyaline cartilage is characterized by collagen fibers with a single type of polypeptide subunit embedded in macromolecular complexes composed of sulfated and nonsulfated proteoglycans. The synovial fluid can be considered to be the specific extracellular matrix produced by the superficial cells of the synovial membrane. The principal characteristic of synovial fluid is its high concentration of a nonbranching high molecular weight anionic polysaccharide, hyaluronate, which is probably linked covalently to a small protein component. The synovial fluid is noticeably devoid of fibrillar components. Before we can examine how the composition of synovial fluid is regulated we must first describe the histologic and cytologic features of the cells of the synovial membrane.

Histology.   The synovial membrane is a pink glistening tissue lining the joint space. Under the microscope one sees a superficial cellular layer, one to three cells in depth, resting on a vascular network (Fig. 2). The deeper portions of the synovial membrane vary from areolar to adipose tissue depending on the particular synovial region selected for study. With aging, there is an increasing amount of fibrous tissue in the deeper synovium and some atrophy of the superficial cellular layer. The nuclei of the superficial cells are located at one pole of the cell and their cytoplasm is extended into long arborizing processes which intertwine to form a network facing the synovial fluid. These superficial cells are referred to as the synovial lining cells. They do not form a true histologic membrane since they are not separated from the underlying connective tissue by a continuous basement membrane and there are no recognizable cellular connections or junctions.

Scanning electron microscopy has shown large gaps between the lining cells exposing portions of the deeper synovial tissue. These observations clearly dispel the idea that these cells with their intercellular matrix form a continuous barrier against diffusion of material into or out of the synovial fluid. The scanning electron microscope also reveals that the synovial membrane consists of a series of parallel folds which probably represent an adaptation of this structure to the considerable expansion and contraction involved in joint motion. The spaces between the synovial lining cells contain an amorphous material, which stains faintly and inconsistently with metachromatic dyes, and fine fibrils that usually run parallel to the cell processes. Typical collagen fibers are notably absent from the intercellular matrix of the lining cells.

ULTRASTRUCTURE

Ultrastructurally, the synovial lining cells can be differentiated into two types, frequently referred to as A and B. Approximately two-thirds of the cells in the normal human synovium are of the B type and are characterized by a highly developed rough endoplasmic reticulum, the intracisternal spaces of which are frequently dilated. There is, in addition, an extensive Golgi apparatus as well as small dense secretory granules, numerous pinocytotic vesicles, and numerous cytoplasmic filaments along the inner aspect of the plasma membrane (Fig. 3). Ultrastructurally, these cells closely resemble active fibroblasts and functionally are the major source of the extracellular synovial matrix analogous to the chondroblasts, fibroblasts, and osteoblasts found in other forms of connective

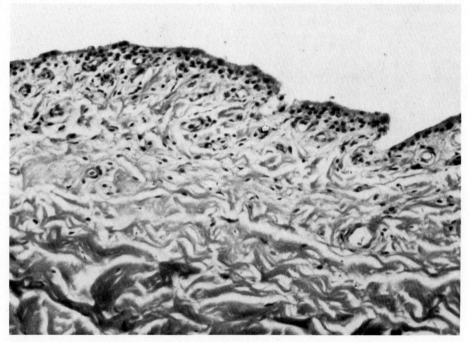

Fig. 2.   Photomicrograph of normal human synovial membrane. The lining cells form a cellular layer 0–3 cells deep with their cytoplasmic processes most superficial. No basement membrane separates the lining cells from the underlying areolar connective tissue containing collagen fibers, small blood vessels, and perivascular histiocytes. A dense collagenous tissue is seen in the deepest portion of the synovial membrane; this layer merges with the capsule of the joint.

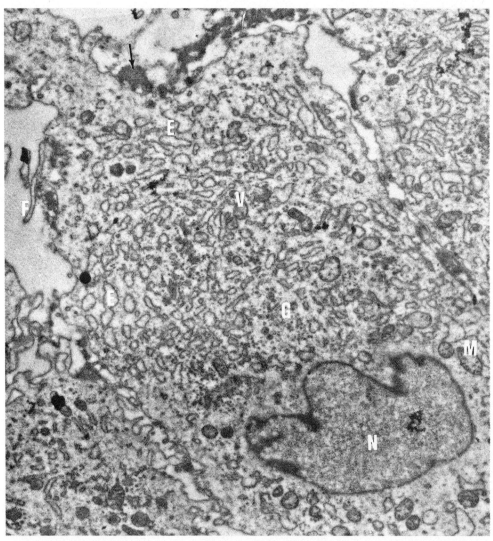

Fig. 3. Electron micrograph of type B lining cell from normal human synovial membrane. The nucleus (N) is eccentric and irregular in outline. There is abundant rough endoplasmic reticulum (E), the cisternae of which are often dilated by a material of low electron opacity. There is a well-developed Golgi apparatus (G), several cytoplasmic mitochondria (M), and small vacuoles (V). Much dense amorphous material is present in the extracellular matrix in close proximity to the cell membrane (arrow). Numerous pinocytotic vesicles are seen adjacent to the cell membrane. A filopodium (F), probably arising from a type A lining cell, is seen in close proximity to the surface of the B cell (× 15,000). (Reproduced by permission of the authors and publisher from Barland P, Novikoff AB, Hamerman D: Electron microscopy of the human synovial membrane. J Cell Biol 14:207, 1962.)

tissue. The type B cells are seen to predominate in the early embryo before the vascularization of the synovial membrane. After chemical synovectomy the B cells regenerate from proliferating undifferentiated cells of the subchondral bone marrow, whereas A cells are seen only after revascularization of the synovium. In the normal synovium mitotic activity is rarely seen in the B cells, suggesting that these cells are long lived and have a highly differentiated function. Further evidence of a high metabolic state in the B cells is their intense staining for several enzymatic activities, including succinic dehydrogenase, lactic dehydrogenase, and NADH and NADPH dehydrogenase. When synovial explants are placed in tissue culture the B cells undergo rapid mitosis and mi-

grate out from the explants to form monolayers which continue to synthesize hyaluronate in large amounts while maintaining much of their oxidative enzyme activity. In addition to hyaluronate the synovial monolayer cultures synthesize a substance immunologically related to cartilage protein polysaccharides. The biochemical nature and in vivo function of this material has not been defined.

The type A synovial lining cells account for approximately one-third of the cells present in the intimal layer of the normal synovium. These cells are characterized by the presence of numerous large cytoplasmic vacuoles frequently containing electron-dense and membranous structures and a well-developed, often multicentric Golgi

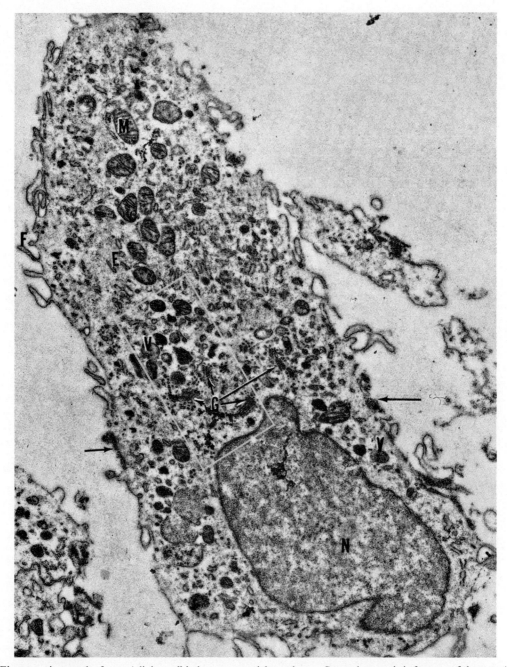

Fig. 4. Electron micrograph of type A lining cell in human synovial membrane. Some characteristic features of the type A cell can be observed. A prominent Golgi apparatus (G) is situated near the basally located nucleus (N). The cell membrane is extended into numerous fingerlike filopodia (F). The cytoplasm contains numerous mitochondria (M) and many membrane-bound vacuoles of differing size, the contents of which vary in density and fine structure (arrows) ($\times$ 13,500). (Reproduced by permission of the authors and publisher from Barland P, Novikoff AB, Hamerman D: Electron microscopy of the human synovial membrane. J Cell Biol 14:207, 1962.)

apparatus. The cell membrane of the A cells is extended into numerous fingerlike structures that have been named *filopodia* (Fig. 4). In addition, coated vesicles and thickened depressions of the plasma membrane with radiate striations into the subjacent cytoplasm are present in the A cells. These cells have the ultrastructural features of macrophages in active interchange with the extracellular material. The demonstration of acid phosphatase activity in the vacuoles of these cells as well as the uptake of thorotrast and ferritin by the A cells after intraarticular injection documents their phagocytic activity.

The A cells probably arise from monocytic cells in the circulation since they are not seen in the embryo or the regenerating synovial membrane until after the synovium has become vascularized. It is likely that these cells can migrate into the deeper synovium, where they may remain for long periods of time. Indeed, one of the most remarkable properties of these A cells is their ability to retain phagocytized and adsorbed materials. Elemental gold has been identified in the lysosomal granules of these synovial macrophages for as long as 23 years after a course of chrysotherapy. The synovial macrophages have also been found to retain antigenically active egg albumin on their surface membranes for at least 1 month after intraarticular injection. This capacity for antigens to persist on the surface of the synovial macrophages in an immunogenic form has provided the basis for the production of an experimental immune arthritis in rabbits and may offer an explanation as to why the human synovium is the site of so many chronic immunoinflammatory conditions. Studies using synovial organ cultures indicate that the A cells have surface receptors for the Fc chains of immunoglobulins and for complement components—properties similar to those found in circulating monocytes. These A cells do not appear to divide in routine explant cultures of the synovial membrane and probably correspond to some of the glass-adherent cells obtained after proteolytic treatment of the synovial membrane.

Cells with ultrastructural features of both A and B synovial lining cells have been described by several observers. However, these cells usually account for only a small number of the lining cells and no distinct function has been ascribed to these cells. It seems doubtful that these cells are precursors of the type A and B lining cells since they are not seen more frequently in embryonic or regenerating synovium. It is also unlikely that these intermediate cells represent transitional forms between the other two types of lining cells because phagocytized material such as elemental gold remains localized within the A cells over prolonged periods of time and is not found at all in the B lining cells. More likely, these intermediate cells represent morphologic expressions of different functional states of either the A or B cells or both. In the author's opinion the A and B synovial lining cells are developmentally, functionally, and morphologically distinct.

BLOOD SUPPLY AND VASCULAR PERMEABILITY

Immediately beneath the synovial lining cells is an extensive network of capillaries and venules. The ultrastructural relationships between the lining cells, the joint space, and the underlying connective tissue is shown in Fig. 5. The rate of blood flow through this synovial plexus can be measured by the rate of disappearance of Xenon −133 from the synovial fluid. Several mechanisms or factors appear to be capable of modulating this blood flow under experimental conditions. These factors include autonomic nerve stimulation, histamine, prostaglandins E_1 and E_2, and intraarticular pressure. Investigation as to which of these factors is operative in vivo is an important area for future study. In the human synovium the cytoplasm of the endothelial cells lining these capillaries is quite attenuated, but "fenestrae" (holes in the cytoplasm covered only by a single membrane or diaphragm) are not present as they are in the rabbit synovium. These endothelial cells and their surrounding basement membrane and perivascular histiocytes represent the principal barrier for the diffusion of plasma proteins and particulate materials into the synovial fluid. Those proteins which exit from the intravascular compartment do so through gaps between the endothelial cells. Some of these proteins are recaptured via pinocytosis by the endothelial cells or are trapped in the perivascular histiocytes. Once past these barriers the proteins rapidly enter the synovial space.

The rate at which an individual plasma protein enters the synovial space is largely dependent upon the "Stokes radius" of the protein molecule (a measure dependent on the size and shape of a molecule in physiologic solutions). High molecular weight molecules, such as IgM and α_2 macroglobulin, and highly asymmetric molecules, such as fibrinogen, are present in very low concentrations in normal synovial fluid, whereas albumin is present in concentrations approaching that of plasma. Although the large domain of solute occupied by the hyaluronate molecules in synovial fluid also limits the concentrations of proteins in synovial fluid, this factor appears to play a secondary role in determining the concentrations of plasma proteins present in the joint space. The synovial capillaries are also particularly permeable to inert particles such as 300-Å colloidal carbon, which, when injected intravenously, can be found in the synovial space and in the type A lining cells within 30 minutes—well before they are found in most other extravascular compartments. This ready permeability may contribute to the predilection of the synovium and joint space as a site for the localization of systemic infections as well as circulating immune complexes.

Proteins and other macromolecules leave the synovial space predominantly by way of the lymphatic system, whereas particulate material is removed by phagocytosis by the type A lining cells or is retained in collagenous areas of the joint for prolonged periods of time. Oxygen and nutrients such as electrolytes, amino acids, sugars, and fatty acids required for the survival of the articular cartilage, as well as the waste products of chondrocyte metabolism, pass into and out of the synovial cavity from the intravascular space by a process of diffusion. There is no evidence of an energy-requiring active transport system such as exists in membranes where the cells are connected by tight junctions. With aging there is increasing fibrosis and decreased blood flow to the synovium. These changes may impair the passage of nutrients to the chondrocytes of the articular cartilage thereby contributing to the degenerative changes seen in this tissue with aging. Similarly, the increased intraarticular pressure accompanying joint effusion causes a rapid fall in the partial pressure of oxygen and a fall in the pH of synovial fluid which may be detrimental to the articular cartilage.

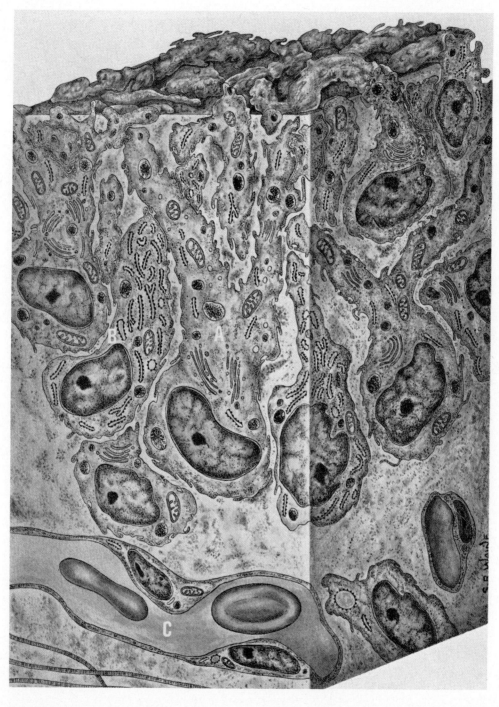

Fig. 5. Surface of the normal human synovial membrane showing the relationship of the lining cells to the joint space (top) and the underlying capillaries, perivascular cells, and connective tissue. The cytoplasmic processes branch and overlap as they approach the synovial cavity, but they do not form a continuous layer so that large gaps exist between the processes, providing direct access between the joint space and the sublining cell extracellular matrix. (Reproduced by permission of the authors and publisher from Barland P, Novikoff AB, Hamerman D: Electron microscropy of the human synovial membrane. J Cell Biol 14:207, 1962.)

Relatively undifferentiated histiocytic cells are present surrounding the larger capillaries and venules. Although these cells have received little attention there is recent evidence suggesting that these perivascular cells synthesize and secrete prostaglandins and a plasminogen activator that may play important roles in normal joint function. An occasional mast cell and fibroblast are also present in the subintimal synovial tissue and numerous

Table 1
Biochemical Products of the Normal Human Synovial Membrane

Product or Activity	Synovial Cell of Origin				
	B Lining Cell	A Lining Cell	Endothelial and Perivascular Cells	Mast Cell	Subsynovial Fibroblast
Hyaluronate	+				
Substance immunologically related to cartilage protein–polysaccharide	+				
Plasminogen activator		?+	?+		
Fibrinogenolysin		+			
Procollagenase		+			
Proteoglycan protease		?+			
Prostaglandin E$_2$			+		
Collagen					+
Elastin					+
Histamine				+	

collagen and elastic fibers are found in the extracellular matrix. Some of the products synthesized by the normal synovium either in vivo or in vitro and the cells that are probably responsible for their production are listed in Table 1.

BIOCHEMICAL PRODUCTS OF SYNOVIAL MEMBRANE

Hyaluronate

The high viscosity of synovial fluid essential to its lubricant properties is almost entirely dependent upon its content of hyaluronate, which is synthesized in all likelihood by the type B synovial lining cells. Immunofluorescent studies of normal synovial membrane utilizing antisera to hyaluronate–protein complexes show intense straining of the lining cell layer. Monolayer cell cultures derived from the B cells continue to synthesize large amounts of hyaluronate. The hyaluronate appears to be assembled from uridine diphosphate sugars in the Golgi apparatus of these monolayer cultures and is later localized in vacuoles which transport the protein–polysaccharide to the plasma membrane. Although the mechanisms that control the rate of hyaluronate production in vivo are not yet well understood, there is some evidence in vitro that mediators such as bradykinin, connective tissue–activating peptides, and prostaglandin E$_1$ act through cell membrane cyclic nucleotides to stimulate synovial fibroblast cultures to synthesize hyaluronate. However, the relationship between prostaglandin stimulation and hyaluronate production is not a simple one. In the presence of continued high levels of prostaglandin E, as may be encountered in some inflammatory synovial fluids, the synovial fibroblasts become refractory to stimulation by these mediators, leading to a reduction in cyclic AMP levels and a fall in hyaluronate synthetic rates.

Plasminogen Activator

In addition to hyaluronate, the normal synovial membrane secretes a plasminogen activator into the synovial fluid. This protease may prevent fibrin formation in the synovial space, which might otherwise both impair joint function and provoke an inflammatory reaction. There is some histochemical evidence to suggest that the endothelial cells and the perivascular histiocytes are the cells responsible for the production of plasminogen activator. In the rheumatoid synovial membrane, plasminogen activator activity is significantly reduced due in part to the presence of enzyme inhibitors in the rheumatoid membrane. This reduction in plasminogen activator activity may contribute to the prominent fibrin deposits seen in rheumatoid synovitis. Besides plasminogen activator acting on serum plasminogen to form plasmin, the normal synovial membrane appears to produce a protease capable of directly degrading fibrinogen without the formation of fibrin degradation products. The latter protease activity is inhibitable by heparin.

Collagenase

Another important product of the synovial membrane is collagenase. While this enzyme activity is measured at greatly enhanced levels in synovial explants from rheumatoid and other inflammatory forms of synovitis, low levels of activity have also been detected in normal appearing human synovium and in normal rabbit synovium. The synovial cells responsible for the synthesis and secretion of collagenase in vivo are not known. In vitro, however, collagenase is secreted by large stellate cells that can be isolated from synovial membranes by proteolytic digestion. The collagenase-synthesizing cells are glass adherent and long lived and possess phagocytic activity, which suggests that they are derived from the type A lining cells. Monolayer cultures that grow out from synovial explants, probably from proliferating B cells, do not secrete detectable amounts of collagenase.

The collagenase produced by the synovial cells is released in the form of a zymogen or proenzyme that is not readily bound to serum protease inhibitors but does bind to collagen fibers. The latent collagenase must be activated by a second protease in order to express its collagenolytic activity. Plasminogen activator, another product of the synovial membrane, appears to be particularly effective in converting procollagenase to its active form in the presence of normal serum. It has not been established whether the collagenase system has a physiologic role in the normal synovial membrane. Possibly it prevents collagen from accumulating in the synovial fluid and the extracellular matrix of the synovial lining cells, or it may act in concert with other degradative enzymes in controlling the turnover of normal articular cartilage.

Proteoglycan Protease

It seems very likely that the synovial membrane also secretes enzymes or proenzymes capable of digesting the core protein present in the proteoglycans of articular cartilage. The enzymes appear to be active at neutral pH. Thus, explants of normal human synovial tissue incubated in vitro with slices of articular cartilage cause the leaching of proteoglycan subunits from the cartilage. This reaction does not require direct physical contact between the synovium and the cartilage. The enhanced activity of these proteoglycan-degrading enzymes as well as the enhanced collagenolytic activities seen in rheumatoid synovia may be important factors in the dissolution of articular cartilage that frequently accompanies rheumatoid arthritis.

Prostaglandins

Many of the activities of the synovial membrane, including blood flow, vascular permeability, and hyaluronate production can be modulated by the short-lived extremely potent fatty acid hormones known as the prostaglandins. It is therefore not surprising to learn that the synovial membrane and synovial cells in culture are a rich source of prostaglandin synthetase and prostaglandin production. Immunofluorescent studies of normal human synovium using antisera to prostaglandin E demonstrate the major site of fluorescent staining to be the endothelial and perivascular cells. Since protaglandins have a very short intracellular storage phase these immunofluorescent studies may be depicting the hormones attached to receptor sites rather than the cells that produce the hormones. Progress in this area of synovial membrane biochemistry seems certain to lead to a clearer understanding of how synovial membrane function is regulated in normal and pathologic conditions.

Proteolytic Enzymes

In addition to the synthesis of hyaluronate, which appears to be required for joint lubrication, the normal synovial membrane produces numerous proteolytic enzymes that have the potential for irreversibly degrading the articular cartilage. This capacity for self-destruction may reflect the need for the joint space to dissolve rapidly or remove any clot or cartilage fragments which may form inside the joint as a result of the frequent trauma inherent in joint motion. The presence of such foreign bodies in the synovial fluid would seriously impair joint function. The proteolytic activity of the synovial membrane is found in its large number of macrophages, derived in all likelihood from the pool of circulating monocytes. These cells carry the potential for several immunoinflammatory reactions, such as virus attachment, antigen processing, complement component production, cell-mediated immune responses, and immune complex absorption and phagocytosis. All of these activities have been demonstrated in the inflamed synovium. These properties may contribute to the large number of immunologic and inflammatory conditions that can localize in the human diarthrodial joint.

REFERENCES

Anderson H: Development, morphology and histochemistry of the early synovial tissue in human foetuses. Acta Anat 58:90, 1964

Barland P, Novikoff AB, Hamerman D: Electron microscopy of the human synovial membrane. J Cell Biol 14:207, 1962

Castor CW, Lewis RB: Connective tissue activaton, X. Current studies of the process and its mediators. Scand J Rheumatol [Suppl] 12:41–54, 1975

Gardner DL: Pathology of the Connective Tissue Diseases. Baltimore, Williams & Wilkins, 1965

Hamerman D, Barland P, Janis R: The structure and chemistry of the synovial membrane in health and disease, in Bittar EE, Bittar N (eds): The Biological Basis of Medicine, vol 3. New York, Academic Press, 1969, pp 269–309

Hamerman D, Schubert M: Diarthrodial joints, an essay. Am J Med 33:555, 1962

Harris ED Jr, Cohen GL, Krane SM: Synovial collagenase: Its presence in culture from joint disease of diverse etiology. Arthritis Rheum 12:92, 1969

Henrickson RC, Cohen AS: Light and electron microscopic observations of the developing check interphalangeal joint. J Ultrastruct Res 13:129, 1965

Krey PR, Cohen AS: Fine structure analysis of rabbit synovial cells I. Normal synovium and changes in organ culture. Arthritis Rheum 16:324, 1973

Krey PR, Scheinberg MD, Cohen AS: Fine structure analysis of rabbit synovial cells II. Fine structure and rosette-forming cells of explant and monolayer cultures. Arthritis Rheum 19:581, 1976

Kushner I, Somerville JA: Permeability of human synovial membrane to plasma proteins: Relationship of molecular size and inflammation. Arthritis Rheum 14:560, 1971

Newcombe DS, Ishikawa Y: The effect of anti-inflammatory agents on human synovial fibroblast prostaglandin synthetase. Prostaglandins 12:849, 1976

Webb FW, Ford PM, Glynn LE: Persistence of antigen in rabbit synovial membrane. Br J Exp Pathol 52:31, 1971

Werb Z, Mainardi CL, Vater CA, Harris ED Jr: Endogenous activation of latent collagenase by rheumatiod synovial cells. N Engl J Med 266:1017, 1977

COLLAGEN CHEMISTRY

Sheldon R. Pinnell

Collagen is the major structural macromolecule and accounts for 30–40 percent of the total protein found in the human body. Collagen's role in weight-bearing tissues such as bone and cartilage relies on its remarkable tensile strength; a fiber 1 mm in diameter is capable of supporting 20–30 kg. Collagen provides a framework for cells, functions in the compartmentalization of tissues, and serves as the major structural component of the various conduits of the body (e.g., blood vessels, gastrointestinal tract). It is active in embryonic induction, differentiation of tissues, and epithelial–mesenchymal interactions. In addition, collagen is essential in the repair of tissue injury and it is important in some very specialized functions of the body, including light transmission (cornea and lens capsule), fluid exchange (pulmonary alveolus and renal glomerulus), and platelet aggregation. Recently, studies have shown that collagen is synthesized not only by mesenchymal cells, but also by epithelial cells. During synthesis, collagen undergoes an unusual number of intra- and extracellular enzymatic modifications. A precise orchestration of these multiple modifications is necessary for the resultant functional protein; disorder in any of these steps may result in disease. This chapter will include a discussion of each of these modifications which can then be used as a framework for the consideration of diseases in subsequent chapters.

COLLAGEN STRUCTURE
Collagen Molecule

The shape of the collagen molecule is quite unusual when compared to other proteins (Fig. 1); it exists as an extremely long, thin rod (3000 Å by 15 Å). Each molecule is made up of three individual polypeptide chains (α chains), each of which contains approximately 1000 amino acids and extends the entire length of the molecule. The amino acid sequence of the collagen α chain is unique in that each third amino acid is glycine; the polypeptide chain can be represented as (Gly–X–Y) repeating subunits. Proline is frequently found in position X and 4-hydroxyproline in position Y. The presence of these pyrrolidine residues causes each α chain to adopt a special type of helical structure (polyproline II) which is different from the more common α helix of globular and other fibrous proteins. The three helical α chains are wrapped around each other in a ropelike manner to form a triple-stranded super helix. The presence of glycine in each third position is essential for this helical structure. Glycine has no side chains and is positioned on the inside of the three-stranded molecule; it holds the chains together by hydrogen bonding to peptide bonds on adjacent chains (NH···O=C).

Microfibril and Fibril

The next order of structure is the microfibril. Individual molecules are precisely oriented one to another in

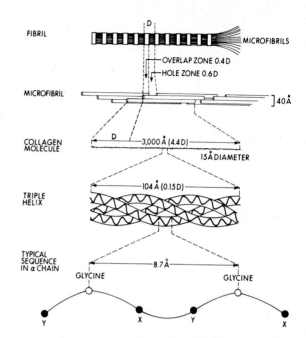

Fig. 1. Collagen structure. The collagen fibril is an aggregation of many microfibrils. One model for the microfibril has individual molecules arranged as a pentafibril; the molecules are quarter-staggered one to another. The collagen molecule is composed of three individual polypeptide chains (α chains) that wrap around each other in a triple helix. The helix is made possible because each third amino acid in the polypeptide chain is glycine. (Modified by permission of the authors and publisher from Prockop, Guzman: Hosp Practice 12:62, 1977.)

the same direction staggered at a distance (D) of 680 Å. The molecule is 4.4 D long with a space or hole region of 0.6 D before the start of the next molecule. Regular spacing of overlap zones and hole regions results in the banding patterns seen by electron microscopy. A model has been proposed of the microfibril in which five molecules, quarter-staggered one to another, are positioned as the strands of a spiraling five-stranded rope. In cross section the diameter of the microfibril is approximately 40 Å. At subsequent levels of structure, microfibrils are wrapped around each other to produce fibrils and fibrils coil around one another to produce ever-enlarging fibers (to more than 3000 Å diameter). At a higher level of organization, fibers can be parallel (tendon), orthogonal (cornea), tubular (around blood vessels), or random bundles (bone and skin).

MOLECULAR HETEROGENEITY

Detailed structural studies have revealed the presence of several different collagen α chains that have their own primary structure and are the products of separate genes (Table 1). Each molecular species maintains the basic three-chain collagen structure, which is further modified to serve its own unique function in tissue. A few tissues consist predominantly of a single type of collagen (type I in bone and tendon; type II in cartilage). Most tissues, however, contain a mixture of type I and type III

Table 1
Genetically Distinct Human Collagens

Type	Molecular Composition	Tissue Distribution	Characteristic Features
I	$[\alpha_1(I)]_2\alpha_2$	Bone, tendon, dermis, ligament, lung, heart valve, fascia, uterus, scar, cornea, liver, dentin	Most prevalent form of collagen in the body; hybrid molecule containing two chain types
II	$[\alpha_1(II)]_3$	Cartilage, nucleus pulposus, notochord	Relatively high content of hydroxylysine and glycosylated hydroxylysine
III	$[\alpha_1(III)]_3$	Cardiovascular tissue, dermis, lung, liver, intestine, uterus, leiomyoma	Contains interchain disulfide linkages
IV	$[\alpha_1(IV)]_3$	Basement membranes	Probably heterogeneous; contains high content of hydroxylysine and glycosylated hydroxylysine; probably contains globular regions; contains interchain disulfide linkages
AB	Unknown	Fetal membranes, muscle	Hybrid molecule containing two chain types; relatively rich in hydroxylysine; may be basement membrane

collagens. Basement membrane collagen has not been entirely characterized and it is likely to be heterogeneous.

COLLAGEN BIOSYNTHESIS

Collagen is synthesized in precursor form, designated *procollagen,* with peptide extensions on the amino- and carboxy-terminal ends of the collagen molecule (Fig. 2). These extensions increase the size of each α chain by about 50 percent and are thought to (1) provide increased solubility in order to facilitate transcellular and transmembrane movement of the protein, (2) prevent intracellular fibrillogenesis, and (3) provide proper registration and alignment of the three procollagen chains in the molecule and facilitate rapid formation of the triple helix. Each species of procollagen chain is synthesized from its own messenger RNA.

Procollagen Structure

Our structural understanding of the pro-α_1 (I) collagen chain is more complete than that of other procollagen chains (Fig. 2). The collagen domain (collagen molecule) consists of a helical region consisting of 1011 residues $[(Gly-X-Y)_{337}]$ and short nonhelical extensions at the aminoterminal (16 residues) and carboxy-terminal (25 residues) ends through which collagen cross-linking takes place. An amino-terminal domain consists of a globular region of approximately 100 residues containing intrachain, but not interchain disulfide linkages. This globular subunit is followed by a short helical region of repeating Gly-X-Y subunits (about 50 residues), followed by a short, nonhelical segment of 8 residues which links to the collagen domain. The carboxy-terminal domain consists

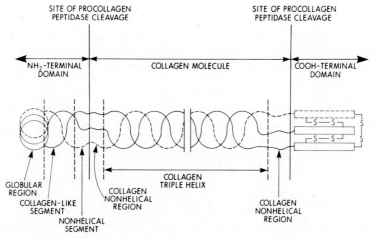

Fig. 2. Type I procollagen molecule is composed of two pro-α_1 (I) chains (solid lines) and one pro-α_2 chain (broken lines). Structural details of the pro-α_1 (I) chain are provided in the text. Procollagen is converted to collagen in the extracellular space following cleavage of amino- and carboxy-terminal extension peptides by specific procollagen peptidases. (Modified by permission of the authors and publisher from Prockop, Guzman: Hosp Practice 12:65, 1977.)

of a globular subunit (about 330 residues) containing interchain and probably intrachain disulfide linkages. The helical region of the amino-terminal domain contains small amounts of hydroxyproline. Compounds that are characteristic for the carboxy-terminal domain include tryptophan, mannose, and N-acetylglucosamine.

Hydroxyproline, Hydroxylysine, and Hydroxylysine Glycoside Biosynthesis

4-Hydroxyproline and hydroxylysine are unusual amino acids that are unique to collagen and collagenlike proteins. Each is formed as a result of posttranslational enzymatic hydroxylation of certain prolyl and lysyl residues already incorporated into the collagen polypeptide chain. Each hydroxylating enzyme is membrane bound and hydroxylates suitable prolyl and lysyl residues as the enlarging polypeptide chain enters the cisternae of the rough endoplasmic reticulum. Both prolyl and lysyl hydroxylases require as cofactors and cosubstrates molecular oxygen, ferrous ion, α-ketoglutarate, and ascorbic acid. Although the precise role of each of these substances is unknown, oxygen appears to be incorporated into the hydroxyl group of hydroxyproline and hydroxylysine; during the reaction α-ketoglutarate is stoichiometrically converted to succinate. Ascorbic acid serves as a reducing agent for the reaction and may be important in the activation of inactive precursors of the enzyme(s). Prolyl and lysyl hydroxylases are capable of modifying prolyl and lysyl residues only when these occur in the Y position of the repeating Gly–X–Y triplet. An exception to this general rule occurs in the nonhelical extension peptides of the collagen molecule, where hydroxylysine residues are formed that are essential in cross-linking of collagen.

Hydroxyproline comprises about 10 percent of the amino acid composition of the collagen molecule and is known to be essential for stabilization of the triple-helical structure necessary for the molecule to function as a rigid rod. Hydroxylysine is essential for collagen cross-linking. Galactose is added through o-glycosidic linkage to the hydroxyl group of certain hydroxylysyl residues by a specific collagen galactosyl transferase. In turn, glucose is added to certain of these galactosyl hydroxylysyl residues by a specific collagen glucosyltransferase. These glycosyltransferases require Mn^{2+}, are membrane bound, and act on the collagen polypeptide chain before the helix is formed. Although the precise function of glycosylated hydroxylysyl residues is unknown, they are thought to be important in regulation of fibril formation and collagen cross-linking.

Molecular Assembly and Secretion

Following the completion of pro-α chain synthesis, three completed chains are assembled into a molecule, interchain disulfide linkages form in the carboxy-terminal domain, and the triple-helix assembles. The completed procollagen molecule passes into Golgi vacuoles for secretion out of the cell. Microtubules are probably involved in this process since colchicine and vinblastine are capable of interfering with procollagen secretion.

Procollagen Processing and Fibril Formation

Following secretion from the cell and extracellular transport to its connective tissue site, procollagen is processed by stepwise removal of the amino-terminal and carboxy-terminal extension peptides by specific endopeptidases that have been designated *procollagen peptidase(s)*. Although the ultimate fate of the collagen extension peptides is unknown, a role in feedback inhibition of collagen biosynthesis has been proposed. Procollagen to collagen conversion may also be coupled to fibril formation.

Cross-Linking

Collagen strength ultimately depends on cross-linking of collagen molecules one to another. Collagen cross-linking occurs as a series of covalent reactions between lysyl- and hydroxylysyl-derived side chains (Fig. 3). Lysyl or hydroxylysyl side chains in the short, nonhelical amino- or carboxy-terminal extension peptides of the collagen molecule are oxidized and deaminated to aldehydes (allysine or hydroxyallysine, respectively) by lysyl oxidase, a copper-dependent enzyme. The resulting aldehydes are capable of reacting with helical hydroxylysyl and occasionally lysyl side chains to produce aldimine linkages. If the cross-link has been derived from hydroxyallysine and hydroxylysine, Amadori rearrangement can take place to a more stable ketoamine. Cross-links derived from glycosylated hydroxylysyl residues have been demonstrated, but a precise understanding of the effect of glycosylation on cross-link stability is not yet known.

Collagen solubility is reduced by intermolecular cross-linking. With aging, collagen solubility and aldimine cross-links diminish. Although aldimine cross-links have been presumed to be further modified in cross-link biosynthesis, an additional form has never been identified. Recently, it has been suggested that the aldimine linkage is stabilized by oxidation to a peptide linkage. Although histidine-containing intermolecular cross-links have been proposed, their identification may result as an artifact of borohydride reduction which is used to stabilize cross-links for identification.

An additional type of collagen cross-link is known to link two of the three α chains within the type I collagen molecule to form β chains. Two allysine residues occurring in amino-terminal, nonhelical peptides join to form an aldol condensation product. Since these cross-links do not link molecules, their precise effect on stability is not known.

COLLAGEN TURNOVER

Collagen-containing connective tissues are constantly being remodeled. In some cases turnover may be rapid, such as in wound healing and the postpartum resorption of the uterus. In general, the triple helix of the collagen molecule is quite impervious to proteolytic attack. Specific collagenases, however, are capable of cleaving the collagen molecule into two pieces, an amino-terminal 75 percent fragment and a carboxy-terminal 25 percent fragment. At physiologic temperatures, the triple

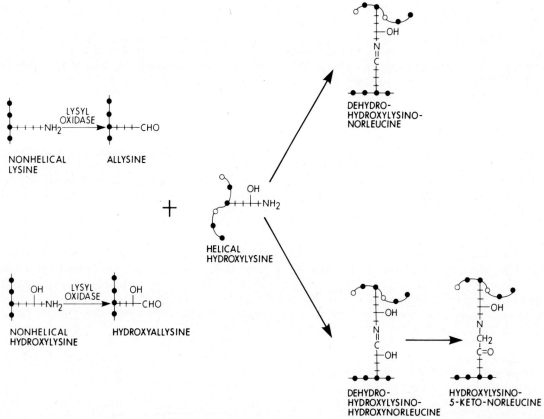

Fig. 3. Intermolecular collagen cross-linking. Lysyl and hydroxylysyl residues in short, nonhelical amino- and carboxy-terminal ends of the collagen molecule are converted to aldehydes (allysine and hydroxyallysine) by lysyl oxidase. This conversion probably occurs following formation of the microfibril. Aldimine linkages spontaneously form between these nonhelical aldehydes and helical hydroxylysyl residues. The aldimine cross-link derived from hydroxyallysine and hydroxylysine can rearrange to form a more stable ketoamine.

helical structure of the fragments is no longer stable and following denaturation the chains can be further degraded by tissue proteinases. The nature of the collagen substrate that is degraded is important (e.g., granulocyte collagenase attacks type I collagen preferentially (15:1) in comparison to type III collagen). Cross-linking appears to stabilize collagen against degradation by collagenase. Mammalian collagenases are synthesized as zymogens and are inhibited by such serum proteins as α_2 macroglobulin and α_1 antitrypsin.

Collagen turnover has traditionally been measured by determining hydroxyproline excretion in urine. Collagen contains large amounts of this unique amino acid, which is easily measured colorimetrically. Since hydroxyproline is not reutilized in collagen biosynthesis, its presence in urine has been interpreted as resulting from collagen breakdown. Unfortunately, such studies are imprecise and insensitive measures of collagen metabolism. As collagen chains are degraded and hydroxyproline is released, it is rapidly metabolized by hydroxyproline oxidase. Hydroxyproline that is excreted into the urine is predominantly peptide bound (about 95 percent). In addition, the Cl_q component of complement contains

appreciable amounts of hydroxyproline. Its turnover (4.5 mg/kg/day) must also be taken into consideration in any calculations relying on urinary hydroxyproline excretion.

REFERENCES

Bornstein P, Traub W: The chemistry and biology of collagen, in Neurath H, Hill RL (eds): The Proteins, 3rd ed. (in press)
Pinnell SR: Disorders of collagen, in Stanbury JB, Wyngaarden JB, Fredrickson DS (eds): The Metabolic Basis of Inherited Disease, 4th ed. New York, McGraw-Hill, 1978, pp 1366–1394
Ramachandran GN Reddi AH: Biochemistry of Collagen. New York, Plenum Press, 1976

COLLAGENASES

Edward Day Harris, Jr.

Collagen is the most abundant protein in the body and the principal structural component of bone, cartilage, tendons, and ligaments. As described in the preceding chapter, collagen molecules have an intrinsic stability conferred by the tight packing of amino acid residues in helical configuration of single α polypeptide chains (molecular weight ~95,000 daltons). These α chains form a triple-helical complex with two other α chains. In vivo, each of these completed molecules (molecular weight ~290,000 daltons) aggregates with many others to form fibrils. Most studies suggest that fibrils are composed of microfibrils of five collagen molecules arranged in a quarter-staggered overlap to one another, and that these microfibrils in turn aggregate longitudinally and laterally with others to form fibrils. The insoluble, fibrillar arrangement of collagen confers stability upon individual molecules; in solution, for example, the single collagen molecules denature to gelatin at temperatures greater than 37°C, whereas in the insoluble fibrillar state the denaturation temperature is significantly higher (>50°C).

Additional stability for collagen fibrils is provided by posttranslational insertion of covalent cross-links among molecules. Although the chemistry of these cross-links has been worked out in detail, their physiologic role is less well understood. It is likely, however, that a major function of cross-links is modulation of susceptibility to enzymatic degradation. Recently formed, immature fibrils are more susceptible to collagenolysis than are mature collagen bundles.

In normal processes of connective tissue metabolism, a baseline level of collagen formation and resorption takes place at all times. During phases of growth and tissue repair (healing of wounds and bone fractures, postpartum resorption of uterus) this is accentuated. In chronic proliferative and inflammatory diseases of joints, resorption of normal connective tissue is excessive, and collagen breakdown is a major component of this excess. Study of collagenases, their mode of action, and factors regulating synthesis, release, activation, and activity give insight into pathogenesis of these lesions, and perhaps will offer new concepts of therapy for these diseases.

Collagenase is an enzymatic activity that catalyzes degradation of native collagen in fibril form under physiologic conditions. This definition may include proteinases that cleave cross-links between collagen fibrils extracellularly and enzymes (cathepsins) that degrade fragments of collagen fibrils intracellularly within phagolysosomes at acidic pH, as well as enzymes that cleave the helical collagen molecule in the neutral pH range found in extracellular tissue spaces.

MECHANISMS OF COLLAGENOLYSIS

The sequence of collagen breakdown from the initial attack on fibrillar substrate to the last degradation of peptide fragments from denatured α chains undoubtedly involves many enzyme systems. There are two that are rate limiting: one is the first step of depolymerization of insoluble aggregates; the other is the cleavage of the triple helix of single molecules at the characteristic site three-quarters from the amino-terminus. After hydrolysis between residues 772 and 773 of the helical portion, the two reaction products quickly denature at physiologic pH and temperature and are degraded by many proteinases both within cells and in extracellular tissues (Table 1).

Starkey and Barrett have demonstrated that leukocyte elastase, a serine proteinase present in large quantities in azurophilic granules of these cells, has specificity to cleave the nonhelical cross-linked region of collagen molecules. This produces monomeric collagen, which could be more susceptible to specific collagenases that attack the helical region as well as being prone to solubilization and subsequent denaturation without specific cleavage. The melting temperature (the collagen–gelatin transition temperature) of collagen in solution is approximately 37°C. Therefore, any molecule solubilized from fibril form, even though intact, begins irreversible denaturation. As few as 0.1 cross-links/mole of collagen induces resistance to collagenase within collagen fibrils.

Table 1
Sequential Degradation of Collagen

Step	Substrate	Enzyme	Mechanism
I	Cross-linked fibril	Elastase or other enzymes	Cleavage of cross-link regions (the nonhelical termini of collagen) to produce collagen monomers
	Monomeric collagen (aggregated in fibril form)	Tissue or PMN leukocyte collagenase	Cleavage of peptide bond of 3 helical chains (between residues 772 and 773: Gly–Ileu or Gly–Leu)
	Monomeric collagen (solubilized from fibril or cleaved into 2 fragments by collagenase)	Elastase, plasmin, gelatinases (extracellular)	Hydrolysis of multiple peptide bonds of gelatin formed as soluble monomers or fragments undergo thermal denaturation at physiologic temperatures
		Cathepsin B, collagenolytic cathepsin (intracellular)	Hydrolysis of multiple peptide bonds of gelatin pinocytosed by phagocytic cells
	Gelatin fragments	PZ-peptidases (di- and tri-peptidases)	Cleavage of low molecular weight fragments of gelatin to peptides which are excreted in urine or completely metabolized
II	Cross-linked fibrils	Collagenase and/or elastase	Formation of collagen fibril fragments that can be phagocytosed and degraded within phagolysosomes by cathepsin B and collagenolytic cathepsin

CELLULAR FUNCTION AND
COLLAGENOLYSIS IN ARTHRITIS

Two factors increase potential for excessive collagenolysis within chronically inflamed joints: an increase in the total number of cells producing collagenase and an increased production of enzyme by each cell (Table 2). Cells responsible for production of enzyme can be classified as those in either the inflammatory phase or the proliferative phase of these diseases.

Polymorphonuclear Leukocytes

Polymorphonuclear leukocytes (PMN) are trapped within joint spaces after being drawn there by multiple chemotactic factors. A precursor form of collagenase is released from specific granules of PMN. It is activated by many diverse proteinases, including a proteinase described in synovial fluid from rheumatoid patients. The PMN collagenase is probably less well inhibited by α_2 macroglobulin than are macrophage and fibroblast enzymes, and for unknown reasons it is incapable of effective cleavage of type III collagen. Exposure of PMN to opsonized antigen–antibody complexes or tissue debris for phagocytosis induces latent collagenase release.

Table 2
Factors Affecting Rate of Collagenolysis within Joints

I. Cause increased rates of collagenolysis
   A. Increased temperature: change from 33° to 36°C augments the rate of collagenolysis fourfold
   B. Saturation of plasma/synovial fluid inhibitors of collagenase (α_2 macroglobulin, β_1 anticollagenase) by excess of proteinases
   C. Depletion of tissue inhibitors of collagense (from cartilage, tendons)
   D. Increase in general proteinase activity: plasmin activates latent collagenase
   E. Presence of factors stimulating collagenase synthesis
      1. Proteinases: low concentration
      2. Products of activated lymphocytes (lymphokines)
      3. Phagocytosis by cells of poorly digestible material (e.g., iron granules, membrane components)
      4. Low molecular weight mediators?? (e.g., prostaglandins)
      5. Membrane-active agents capable of producing multinucleate giant cells (e.g., lysolecithin); giant cells are associated with increased collagenase production

II. Cause decreased rates of collagenolysis
   A. Lower intraarticular temperatures
   B. Mineralized connective tissue
   C. Intermolecular cross-links
   D. Increased tissue levels of collagenase inhibitors (e.g., endogenous tissue inhibitors, circulating α_2 macroglobulin, β_1 anticollagenase)
   E. Type II collagen: in articular cartilage resists degradation by collagenases from multiple mammalian sources
   F. Type III collagen: resists degradation by PMN leukocyte collagenases
   G. Non-collagen matrix proteins (e.g., fibronectin)

Synovial Cells

Synovial cells, particularly in rheumatoid disease, are heterogeneous. Along with lymphocytes and plasma cells, there are bone marrow-derived macrophages, mesenchymal cells (e.g., synovial cells), and endothelial cells. Macrophages and synovial cells grown as separate lines of cells from numerous experimental animals each produce collagenase, neutral proteinase, elastase, and plasminogen activator. The collagenase is in latent form and can be activated by numerous proteinases as well as by nonenzymatic means. In rheumatoid joints a leading candidate for the proteinase that activates latent synovial collagenase is plasmin. This serine proteinase is activated readily by plasminogen activator from plasminogen which is abundant in inflammatory exudates. Isolated rheumatoid synovial cells produce enormous quantities of collagenase. Synthesis has been localized primarily to "dendritic" or "stellate" cells found in cultures of cells adherent to culture dishes. These may be macrophages or mesenchymal cells altered by the chronic inflammatory process. Factors responsible for the induction of enzyme by rheumatoid cells may include exposure to poorly digestible debris (including red cells and fibrin), soluble products of activated monocytes, and low concentrations of proteinases.

INHIBITORS OF COLLAGENASE

Chelating agents (e.g., EDTA, 1,10-phenanthroline) and compounds with active sulfhydryl groups inhibit the activity of collagenase. Calcium ions are a requisite for the stability of the collagenase as a catalyst. Reversible inhibition of collagenase activity is caused in vivo by tissue inhibitors (<40,000 daltons) that are similar to an inhibitor released by collagenase-producing cells. The principal irreversible inhibitor of collagenase in vivo is probably α_2 macroglobulin. Once the enzyme has been bound by α_2 macroglobulin it is inactive against high molecular weight substrates (e.g., collagen) until the α_2 macroglobulin itself is destroyed or denatured by thermal or acid treatment, neither of which is likely to occur in vivo. Another serum protein, β_1-anticollagenase, accounts for a small amount of inhibitory activity in vivo. Of the drugs tested in cell systems to date, only corticosteroids have been effective in inhibiting the synthesis and release of collagenase from cells. It has been shown that 1×10^8 M dexamethasone is sufficient to inhibit collagenase production and release from macrophages; this is in the range of concentration needed to saturate steroid receptors on macrophage cell membranes and can be achieved by pharmacologic levels in vivo. Corticosteroids also inhibit prostaglandin and plasminogen activator release by these cells.

In rheumatoid arthritis the hypertrophied synovial membrane may recruit periosteal and perichondral cells and begin to invade cartilage from the periphery at the cartilage–bone junction. A new interface, the pannus–cartilage junction, is created. Latent collagenase is released from cells. The availability of just a small amount of proteinase is needed to activate the extracellular, latent collagenases released by cells and adherent to collagen substrates. Occasionally, in very aggressive disease, there is evidence that insoluble fragments of fibrils are broken free from insoluble aggregates and are phagocytosed and degraded intracellularly. Most degradation of collagen probably occurs extracellularly, however, and this is related to intimate contact between cells and substrate.

REFERENCES

Gross J: Aspects of the animal collagenases, in Ramachandran GN, Reddi AH (eds): Biochemistry of Collagen. New York, Plenum, 1976, pp 275–312

Harris ED Jr: Mammalian collagenases, in Barrett AJ (ed): Proteinases in Mammalian Cells and Tissues. New York, Elsevier/North Holland, 1977, pp 249–284

Harris ED Jr, Krane SM: Collagenases. N Engl J Med 291:557, 1974

Harris ED Jr: Role of collagenases in joint destruction, in Sokoloff L (ed): The Joints and Synovial Fluid. New York, Academic Press, 1978, pp 243–266

PROTEOGLYCANS

Eugene A. Davidson

It is generally considered that the connective tissues of the body contain cellular and fibrous elements embedded or resident in an amorphous matrix commonly referred to as *ground substance*. The major components of this supporting environment are complex macromolecules containing a number of polysaccharide chains covalently attached to a polypeptide backbone. These entities are termed *proteoglycans*, in part to call attention to their unusual structure and to distinguish them from the large number of glycoproteins normally found in the circulation. Salient differences are summarized in Table 1. The proteoglycans may be further organized into aggregate elements with physical properties unique to the complex and more than the sum of the component parts. Some of the activities ascribed to proteoglycans include maintenance of hydration level, ion binding, collagen fiber orga-

nization, control of calcification, and diffusion barrier. The proteoglycan molecules have presented a number of challenging structural and organizational problems, few of which have been solved to a satisfactory level of detail. The ensuing discussion is based largely on work carried out with cartilage. Extrapolation to other tissues is tenuous but may still provide the best guide for understanding the role of these substances.

SACCHARIDE COMPONENTS

The carbohydrate side chains of the proteoglycans of connective tissues, termed *glycosaminoglycans*, have several features in common: the presence of a hexosamine (either glucosamine or galactosamine), a repeating disaccharide unit, and ester sulfate. The latter group is usually, although not exclusively, present on the amino sugar and is largely responsible for the ion-binding properties and extended domain of the macrostructure. Although considerable similarities exist in the saccharide structures, tissue distributions clearly indicate that they have differing functions, although specific biologic roles have generally not been established. Structural data are summarized in Table 2 and tissue locales in Table 3.

There are two glycosaminoglycans absent from the tabular list. These are hyaluronic acid and heparin. The former, a nonsulfated high molecular weight (10^5–10^6 or greater) repeating polymer of D-glucuronic acid and N-acetyl-D-glucosamine is present in most connective tissues. It appears to function as a lubricant and shock absorber in joints and as an organizing element in cartilage. The properties of high hydration capacity and extended domain may be responsible for both of these effects. However, hyaluronic acid does not appear to be present in covalent association with protein and the details of its biosynthesis are still obscure in that membranous systems and lipid-bound intermediates may be involved. In contrast, heparin has a highly sulfated structure similar to that of heparan sulfate, has physiologic functions rather than structural ones (anticoagulant, lipase activator), and is covalently associated with protein. It is primarily a cellular or circulatory component found in high concentrations in mast cells, liver capsule, and hog gastric mucosa.

Table 1
Differences between Proteoglycans and Glycoproteins

Feature	Glycoprotein	Proteoglycan
Percent by weight (carbohydrate)	2–15	60–90
Size of saccharide chains (monosaccharide units)	Branched, 2–5 different sugars, 2–12 monosaccharides	Linear, repeating disaccharide, 20–120 monosaccharides
Charge density	Zero to 2 per chain	1–2 per monosaccharide unit
Linkage to protein	Mainly N-glycosidic to amide nitrogen of asparagine	0-Glycosidic, primarily to serine hydroxyl
Linkage sugar	N-Acetylglucosamine	Xylose
Molecular weights	15,000–250,000	10^5–10^6 or higher
Aggregation/organization tendency	None	Marked

Table 2
Structure of Glycosaminoglycans

Saccharide	Amino Sugar	Alternating Monosaccharide	Linkage Regions Sugars
Chondroitin 4-sulfate (C4S)	N-Acetylgalactosamine 4-0-sulfate β 1→4	D-Glucuronic acid	Xylose, galactose
Chondroitin 6-sulfate (C6S)	N-Acetylgalactosamine 6-0-sulfate β 1→4	D-Glucuronic acid	Xylose, galactose
Dermatan sulfate* (DS)	N-Acetylgalactosamine 4-0-sulfate β 1→4	L-Iduronic acid and/or D-glucuronic acid	Xylose, galactose
Heparan sulfate† (HepS)	Glucosamine (N-acetyl, 6-0-sulfate and N-sulfo) α 1→4	L-Iduronic acid and/or D-glucuronic acid	Xylose, galactose
Keratan sulfate I‡ (KSI)	N-Acetylglucosamine 6-0-sulfate β 1→4	D-Galactose (6-0-sulfate)	
Keratan sulfate II§ (KSII)	N-Acetylglucosamine 6-0-sulfate β 1→4	D-Galactose (6-0-sulfate)	Mannose, N-acetylgalactosamine

*The uronic acid in dermatan sulfate is primarily L-iduronic acid with about 10–20 percent D-glucuronic present. The latter tends to be located near the protein backbone.

†A highly complex and variable structure. The proportion of N-acetyl to N-sulfate varies, as does the ratio of the two uronic acids. Occasional sulfated iduronic residues are also present, as are disulfated and nonsulfated amino sugars. There appears to be a near continuum of structural features ranging from low N-sulfate to molecules where this feature predominates and the final architecture is similar to that of heparin.

‡A low level of sulfated galactose residues are present.

§Reports of the presence of fucose and N-acetylneuraminic acid suggest that this molecule is a hybrid glycoprotein.

LINKAGE REGION

The covalent attachment site of the glycosaminoglycans is usually the hydroxyl group of specific serine residues in the polypeptide chain. A linkage trisaccharide, galactosyl–galactosyl-xylose is generally present with a uronosyl residue initiating the repeating saccharide chain at the terminal galactose site. As long as the serine residues have neither a free amino nor a free carboxyl group, the entire saccharide chain may be cleaved by treatment under alkaline conditions. Removal of the α hydrogen leads to a β elimination, converting the serine residue to dehydroalanine. In the presence of sodium borohydride, the eliminated chain is stabilized by reduction of the terminal xylose to xylitol and the generated dehydroalanine loci are concurrently reduced to alanines. This reaction permits a quantitative assessment of the number of saccharide chains present in a proteoglycan and provides a handle for measurement of the number average molecular weights of the eliminated chains (amino sugar to xylitol ratio). There is some evidence that

Table 3
Glycosaminoglycans in Tissue

Glycosamino-glycan*	Tissue	Molecular Weights† of Polysaccharide Chain
C4S	All cartilage, skin, bone	14,000–30,000
C6S	Cartilage, skin, aorta, nucleus pulposus, umbilical cord	10,000–30,000
DS	Skin, tendon, ligaments, heart valves, blood vessel walls	25,000–40,000
HepS	All connective tissues, cell membranes	6,000–?‡
KSI	Cornea	10,000
KSII	Skeletal tissues	<10,000

*See Table 2 for definitions of abbreviations.

†The chain molecular weights depend on the tissue of origin and exhibit polydispersity of varying degree within the same proteoglycan molecule. The C4S of costal cartilage and DS of skin have been studied in greatest detail. A higher molecular weight C4S (80,000–100,000) has been isolated from tumor cells.

‡Recent reports have suggested that a very high molecular weight HepS is present in several cell types and may be associated with the plasma membrane.

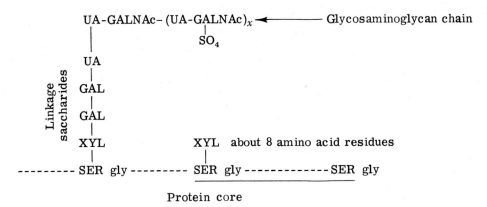

Fig. 1. Cartilage proteoglycan structure showing the linkage region saccharides and approximate spacing of attachment sites.

the attachment of the initial uronosyl residue is catalyzed by a different enzyme than that involved in the synthesis of the main segment of the saccharide chain. Most biosynthetic information is derived from studies with cartilage (C4S and C6S). Data on dermatan sulfate, heparin sulfate, and the keratan sulfates are fragmentary and incomplete.

PROTEOGLYCAN STRUCTURE

In view of the fact that these macromolecules are difficult to obtain in undergraded form, they have marked aggregation behavior, and they may exhibit both internal and population heterogeneity, detailed structures cannot be written. A number of models have been proposed and common features are summarized in Figures 1 and 2. Several points deserve comment.

1. More than one type of glycosaminoglycan chain *may* be attached to a single polypeptide backbone. In such cases, the differing chain types are not randomly distributed but rather appear to be present in clusters.

2. The glycosaminoglycan chains may differ in mo-

lecular weight, thus providing internal polydispersity within a single molecule.

3. In a given tissue, the C4S proteoglycan, for example, need not exhibit uniformity in terms of serine loci substituted. Thus the number of glycosaminoglycan chains per polypeptide may vary, thereby imposing a molecular heterogeneity. In any case, all serines are never substituted.

4. Although Figure 2 suggests equal distribution of the saccharide chains along the polypeptide core, this is only established for one region of one cartilage proteoglycan and may not be uniform. Electron microscopic studies of proteoglycan aggregates are suggestive of a uniformly high density of glycosaminoglycan chains but fine structure detail is simply not seen at the level of resolution available.

5. The aggregate structures generally assumed to be present in connective tissue are subject to modification by cathepsin action or other enzymatic attack. The resulting products neet not degrade completely, thus allowing for the continued presence of a variety of processed proteoglycans. It is not known whether such postsynthetic modification is part of a normal biologic sequence prior or subsequent to secretion from cells.

6. Superimposed on the above is the ability of cartilage proteoglycans to interact noncovalently with an organizing element such as hyaluronic acid. Such interaction leads to the formation of aggregates of enormous nominal molecular size. This complicates problems such as extraction, assessment of homogeneity, and understanding the nature of proteoglycan interaction with formed tissue elements.

DISTRIBUTION IN TISSUES

Highly structured regions such as cartilage may contain more than one-third of their dry weight as proteoglycan. The complex collagen fiber array present prevents ready extraction of the proteoglycan unless conditions are employed that denature or otherwise disrupt the collagen structure. Extractants currently employed include 3 *M* magnesium chloride and 4 *M* guanidinium chloride,

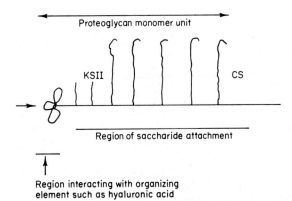

Fig. 2. Structure of a proteoglycan monomer unit. The number and type of the polysaccharide chains varies, as does their molecular weight. The molecular weight of the monomer ranges from 10^5 to 10^6. Disulfide bridges may stabilize the conformation of the region responsible for interactions with hyaluronate.

both of which solubilize about three-quarters of the proteoglycan present in bovine nasal septum cartilage. The
residual collagen network appears denatured (electron
microscopic observation) and the remaining proteoglycan
cannot be brought into solution without collagenase treatment. It must be realized that material extracted with
high concentrations of guanidinium salts or with metal
chlorides in 6 M urea may represent a denatured species.

There has been continual speculation about a possible covalent association between proteoglycan and collagen, especially with increasing age of a tissue. The known
cross-linking reactions of collagen do not exclude this
possibility, but definitive isolation of a linked structure or
fragment thereof has not been accomplished.

The increasingly refractory behavior of cartilage proteoglycan with advancing age involves more than just
stiffening of the fibrous matrix. There are distinct age-
related changes in the proteoglycan composition of most
connective tissues. Thus, in human costal cartilage the
ratio of C6S to C4S rises from 1 at birth to about 10 in the
sixth decade. During the same period the KSII content
increases from zero to about 60 percent of the total
saccharide fraction. Documented aging changes of comparable magnitude also occur in nucleus pulposus. These
time-dependent changes suggest that some continuous
remodeling of the matrix occurs. This, of necessity, involves degradation and removal of some components and
biosynthesis and secretion of new ones. The possibility
exists that preformed proteoglycans of one type (C4S, for
example) may serve as a template for the addition of C6S
or KSII chains, but such conversions have not been
demonstrated.

Purification of solubilized proteoglycan generally
takes advantage of the high buoyant density of the saccharide portion as compared to the protein. Thus, equilibrium density gradient centrifugation in cesium chloride
followed by a second gradient in the presence of a dissociating agent such as guanidinium chloride separates proteoglycan from noncovalently associated material such as
hyaluronic acid and one or more glycoproteins that may
play some functional role in aggregate assembly. The
proteoglycan isolated in such a fashion exhibits little
tendency to self-associate but maintains its ability to be
organized by hyaluronic acid. Since the molecular weight
of hyaluronate may be quite large (10^5 and greater) and
effective interaction between hyaluronate and proteoglycan requires a decasaccharide segment, a single molecule
of the former may assemble 50 or more proteoglycan
"monomers" to produce macroassemblies of enormous
molecular weight and domain. (*Domain* refers to the
excluded volume or space occupied, clearly a function of
conformation.) The highly charged nature of the proteoglycan aggregate leads to an extended conformation,
which can be visualized by electron microscopy. While
an overview of aggregate properties may be readily attained from such morphologic studies, this remains restricted to cartilage since even gross structural features

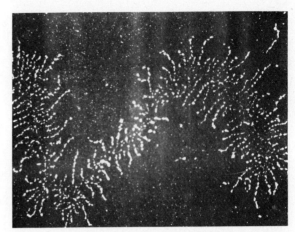

Fig. 3. Electron micrograph of cartilage proteoglycan aggregate. (From Rosenberg et al: J Biol Chem 248:3681, 1973.)

are unclear for proteoglycans present in most, if not all,
other tissues (Fig. 3).

FORMED ELEMENTS AND CALCIFICATION

Morphologic, structural, and functional observations
clearly show a specific interaction between proteoglycans
and collagen. There appear to both conformational and
charge effects. Dermatan sulfate and heparan sulfate
have the greatest effects on collagen fiber formation; the
former is generally associated with larger fibers. The
proteoglycans have been suggested to function in some
organizing capacity and the formation of collagen fibrils is
clearly accelerated in the presence of glycosaminoglycans. The saccharide chains, when examined by x-ray
diffraction of thin films, exhibit largely helical structure.
Thus, the charged groups have a distinct periodicity and
the potential to order selected regions of a polypeptide in
a regular manner. The recognition that several types of
collagen are present in different tissues combined with
the diverse nature of the proteoglycans allows for loose
or ordered fiber assays. Further study is needed to define
these interactions.

It has been known for some time that the matrix
component of calcifying tissue is largely removed when
mineralization occurs. The deposition of the hydroxyapatite crystals may require prior localized sequestration of
calcium ions, pH alteration, and liberation of phosphate
from selected substrates. The high charge density and
documentable calcium affinity of cartilage proteoglycan
suggest that this component is responsible for cation
acquisition and that disaggregation of the macrostructure
by cathepsin-catalyzed proteolysis may serve to release
calcium in locally high concentrations. The polysaccharide chains, freed of their restricting protein, may diffuse
from the tissue as bone deposition takes place. It has
been proposed that cathepsin D is the protease responsible for routine catabolism of proteoglycans in cartilage
but its involvement in calcification has not been
documented.

NONCARTILAGINOUS TISSUES

As indicated, proteoglycans from loci other than cartilage have been little studied. A few reports on DS proteoglycans suggest that they are of lower molecular weight than those from cartilage, contain proportionately more protein, and are more difficult to extract. In tissues where three of four different glycosaminoglycans have been identified, the types of proteoglycan present are generally not known. The multiple possibilities for hybrid structures offer little prospect that defined components will be isolated and characterized in detail.

DEGRADATION AND END-PRODUCT CATABOLISM

The major pathway for proteoglycan breakdown clearly involves proteolysis of the protein core as the initial step. The products thus produced (e.g., by cathepsin D action) are peptide fragments containing several as yet undegraded saccharide chains. These appear to diffuse out of the tissue, to enter the circulation, and to be cleared by the liver and spleen. Further breakdown takes place within lysosomes and requires a series of glycosidases and sulfatases, one for each of the structural types involved. In general, saccharide chains are degraded from the nonreducing end with sulfate cleavage a prerequisite to glycosidase action. The variety of mucopolysaccharidoses that have been described (Hurler's, Hunter's, etc.) involve defects in one or another of these enzymes.

REFERENCES

Balazs EA (ed): Chemistry and Molecular Biology of the Intercellular Matrix, vols 1–3. New York, Academic Press, 1970
Vogel HS (ed): Connective Tissue and Aging, vol 1. Amsterdam, Excerpta Medica, 1973
Whelan WJ (ed): Biochemistry, series 1, vol 5: Biochemistry of Carbohydrates. London, Butterworths, 1975

PROSTAGLANDINS

Dwight Robinson

The prostaglandins and thromboxanes are a group of unsaturated fatty acid derivatives with potent physiologic effects in every organ system. Certain prostaglandins are known to promote or modify inflammatory reactions, and it has been proposed that they may play a role in the pathogenesis of inflammatory rheumatic diseases. Furthermore, the inhibition of prostaglandin synthesis by antiinflammatory drugs appears to account for many of the pharmacologic effects of these agents.

The structures and biosynthesis of the most important prostaglandins are outlined in Figure 1. The fatty acid precursor of these prostaglandins, arachidonic acid, is stored in membranes in cells primarily as phospholipids. Various stimuli, such as tissue injury, lead to the

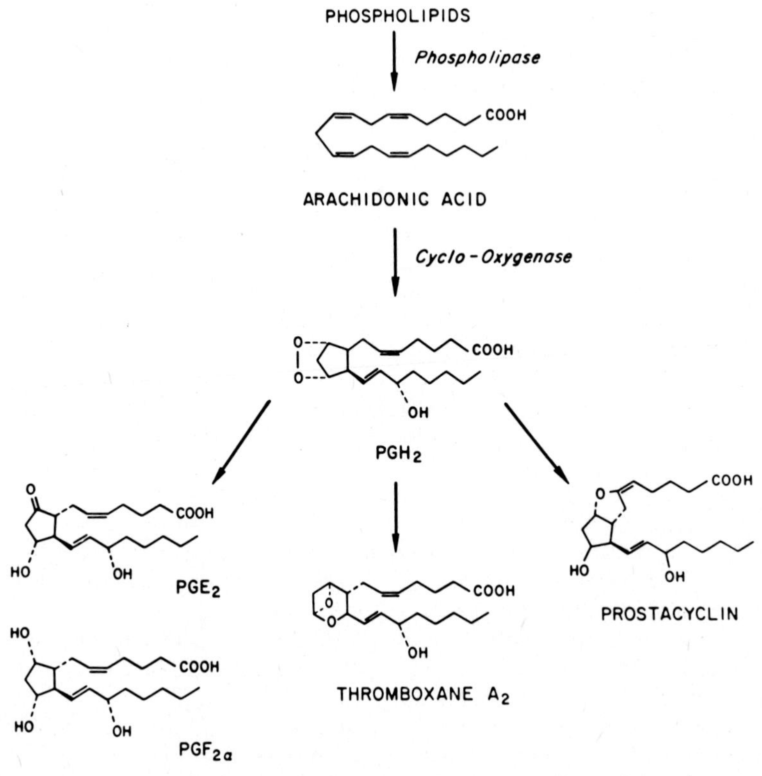

Fig. 1.   Pathway of biosynthesis of some important prostaglandins and thromboxane A_2.

release of free arachidonic acid by the enzyme phospholipase. Arachidonic acid is a substrate for the enzyme cyclooxygenase, which forms the endoperoxide intermediate PGH_2. This compound has physiologic activity itself, but, more important, it is acted upon by several isomerases to form either the classic prostaglandins PGE_2, and $PGF_2\alpha$, thromboxane A_2, or prostacyclin. All the prostaglandins are unstable in tissues or in the circulation and are rapidly converted to inactive metabolites.

FUNCTIONS

The physiologic effects of prostaglandins are numerous and vary with the specific prostaglandin and with different tissues. Many effects are related to the activity of these compounds in either contracting or relaxing smooth muscle in several tissues, including blood vessels, bronchi, and gastrointestinal and uterine muscles. The prostaglandins are also active in stimulating cyclic nucleotide synthesis. Prostaglandin functions are thus so varied that it is difficult to generalize, but a few functions that seem relevant to inflammation are summarized in Table 1. Some prostaglandins appear to be antagonistic to each other. An example occurs in platelet function, where thromboxane A_2, produced by stimulated platelets, promotes platelet agglutination, while prostacyclin, synthesized by blood vessel endothelium, inhibits platelet agglutination. In general, the type of prostaglandins synthesized by any given tissue is related to the specific isomerases present (Fig. 1), and this in turn will determine the specific responses of that tissue to a burst of prostaglandin synthesis.

INFLAMMATION

There is a substantial body of evidence supporting the concept that prostaglandins of the E type, e.g., PGE_2, are mediators of inflammation. The F prostaglandins appear to have little importance but recently prostacyclin has been found to have inflammatory effects. The evidence that the E prostaglandins act as mediators of inflammation includes the following findings: (1) the E prostaglandins cause inflammation when injected; (2) they act synergistically with other mediators to produce manifestations of inflammation; (3) they have been found in elevated concentrations in inflammatory exudates; and (4) the biosynthesis of prostaglandins is strongly inhibited by antiinflammatory drugs.

In spite of this evidence that the PGE_1 and PGE_2 are inflammatory mediators, there is also evidence that under some circumstances they may *inhibit* inflammation. Much of the latter evidence centers around the interactions of PGE with cyclic nucleotides. It is well established that many factors that lead to elevation of AMP levels in tissues are associated with inhibition primarily of several immune-mediated reactions, such as histamine release in immediate hypersensitivity reactions. Elevated AMP levels have also been associated with the inhibition of lymphokine release and other aspects of cellular immunity.

Recent work with experimental models has indicated that suppression of cellular immunity by PGE_1 and PGE_2

Table 1
Prostaglandin Functions Related to Inflammation

Prostaglandin	Function
PGE_2	Vasodilator
	Increases cAMP
	Stimulates bone resorption
$PGF_2\alpha$	Vasoconstrictor
	Increases cGMP
Thromboxane A_2	Vasoconstrictor
	Stimulates platelet agglutination
	Decreases cAMP
Prostacyclin (PGI_2)	Vasodilator
	Inhibits platelet agglutination
	Increases cAMP

may be significant in disease states. It has been demonstrated that the glomerulonephritis of NZB/NZW hybrid mice, an experimental model for human systemic lupus erythematosus, may be alleviated by administration of PGE_1. Daily subcutaneous injections of PGE_1 into NZB/NZW mice over a period ranging from 6 to 52 weeks of age resulted in a dramatic reduction in mortality due to prevention of the progression of immune complex–mediated glomerulonephritis in these animals. It was proposed that PGE_1 alleviated a deficiency in T lymphocyte suppressor function, but there is no direct evidence to support this mechanism. Regardless of the mechanisms involved, PGE_1 *suppressed* the progressive inflammatory glomerulonephritis which leads to death in untreated animals.

A convincing demonstration that PGE_2 may suppress certain aspects of cellular immunity has been provided by in vitro experiments. Human peripheral blood mononuclear cells (lymphocytes and monocytes) were shown to include a suppressor cell fraction which suppressed lectin-induced mitogenesis in vitro. The suppression of lymphocyte transformation was accounted for by PGE_2 secretion by a fraction of the mononuclear cell population. These experiments suggest that reactions of cellular immunity may be inhibited in man by exposure to PGE_2, but the role of this regulatory mechanism in rheumatic diseases remains to be established.

ANTIINFLAMMATORY DRUGS

Most nonsteroidal antiinflammatory drugs, including aspirin, indomethacin, phenylbutazone, phenylalkanoic acids, and others, are potent inhibitors of prostaglandin synthesis. It is also well established that there is a good correlation between the potency of antiinflammatory effects of these drugs and their potency in inhibiting prostaglandin synthesis. This has led to the hypothesis that all of the important pharmacologic effects of these drugs can be accounted for by their inhibition of prostaglandin synthesis. More recently, it has also been established that corticosteroids are potent inhibitors of prostaglandin synthesis by several types of cells and tissues. It seems likely that at least some of the antiinflammatory effects of corticosteroids are related to prostaglandin synthesis inhibition.

The mechanism of inhibition of prostaglandin synthesis by the nonsteroidal drugs is direct inhibition of the microsomal enzyme, cyclooxygenase (Fig. 1). Corticosteroids do not inhibit cyclooxygenase directly, but evidence has been presented suggesting that corticosteroids may inhibit the phospholipase step. However, the mechanism has not been established.

BONE RESORPTION

PGE_1 and PGE_2 stimulate osteoclastic bone resorption in vitro, and there is evidence that PGE_2 may act as a mediator of bone resorption in both neoplastic and rheumatoid disease in humans. It has been shown that two transplantable tumors in experimental animals cause hypercalcemia on a humoral basis by secretion of large quantities of PGE_2. It has also been shown that hypercalcemia associated with human neoplasms may be accompanied by evidence of increased PGE_2 secretion. Hypercalcemia in several of these patients returned to or toward normal levels with the administration of prostaglandin synthesis inhibitors (indomethacin or aspirin), suggesting that the hypercalcemia was related to excessive osteoclastic bone resorption mediated by PGE_2.

In rheumatoid arthritis there is frequently erosion of juxtaarticular bone adjacent to the rheumatoid synovial pannus, suggesting that the inflammatory pannus is elaborating a factor that promotes excessive local bone resorption. Utilizing an in vitro model we have shown that rheumatoid synovial tissue explants maintained in tissue culture release large amounts of a bone resorption–stimulating activity into the culture media. The bone resorption–stimulating activity was all accounted for by PGE_2 secreted by rheumatoid synovia. On the basis of this model system it was postulated that secretion of PGE_2 by rheumatoid synovial pannus stimulates excessive osteoclastic bone resorption in adjacent juxtaarticular bone. This may account for the familiar juxtaarticular bone erosions in rheumatoid arthritis. It follows that adequate suppression of prostaglandin synthesis by antiinflammatory drugs may reduce or prevent bone destruction in rheumatoid arthritis.

REFERENCES

Ferreira SH, Vane JR: New aspects of the mode of action of nonsteroidal anti-inflammatory drugs. Ann Rev Pharmacol 14:57, 1974

Goodwin JS, Messner RP, Bankhurst AD, et al: Prostaglandin producing suppressor cells in Hodgkin's disease. N Engl J Med 297:963, 1977

Kantrowitz F, Robinson DR, McGuire MB, Levine L: Corticosteroids inhibit prostaglandin production by rheumatoid synovia. Nature 258:737, 1975

Ramwell PW (ed): The Prostaglandins, vols 1–3, New York, Raven Press, 1973–1977

Robinson DR, Tashjian AH Jr, Levine L: Prostaglandin stimulated bone resorption by rheumatoid synovia. A possible mechanism for bone destruction in rheumatoid arthritis. J Clin Invest 56:1181, 1975

Samuelsson B, Paoletti R (eds): Advances in Prostaglandin and Thrombaxine Research, vols 1, 2. New York, Raven Press, 1976

Zurier RB, Sayadoff DM, Torrey SB, Rothfield NF: Prostaglandin E_1 treatment of NZB/NZW mice. I. Prolonged survival of female mice. Arthritis Rheum 20:723, 1977

Epidemiology

Alfonse T. Masi and Thomas A. Medsger, Jr.

BASIC EPIDEMIOLOGIC CONCEPTS

Epidemiology (*epi,* upon; *demos,* people; *logy,* science) is the science that deals with the distribution and control of disease in a population and with those factors determining or associated with the presence or absence of the disease. Although applied mainly to epidemic and contagious diseases in the past, this approach is being used increasingly for the study of many chronic endemic disorders. Among the rheumatic diseases, epidemiology has made major contributions to improved understanding and control of acute rheumatic fever. This discipline encompasses a broad range of studies, e.g., those of descriptive frequency, hypothesis-testing, and experimental trials, all conducted in populations, and its methodology interfaces with many fields, e.g., clinical, laboratory, and public health. Active interchange among epidemiologists, clinicians, and laboratory workers is essential for the best understanding of complex relationships revealed in such population studies.

INCIDENCE AND PREVALENCE

Incidence is the *rate* of occurrence of *new* cases of disease in a defined risk population during a given period of observation. Its determination requires longitudinal or sequential observation of a population over at least two points in time. *Prevalence* is the *ratio* (percent or proportion) of cases existing in a population at risk at a given point in time, e.g., point prevalence, or occurring during a specified interval of time, e.g., period prevalence. Point prevalence can be determined in a single survey by examination or interview and period prevalence by retrospective or longitudinal methods in one or more surveys.

Incidence rate multiplied by the average duration of disease equals prevalence. Thus, prevalence reflects both the risk of acquiring a disease and the influence of factors (e.g., sex, race, and socioeconomic status) that may affect its average duration. Incidence rates are more sensitive and specific indicators of the risk of acquiring disease than are prevalence frequencies; they are superior for inferring mechanisms of etiology or host predisposition.

SENSITIVITY AND SPECIFICITY RELATIONSHIPS

Sensitivity is defined as the proportionate frequency of diagnosis (or test positivity) among persons who truly have the attribute. *Specificity* is the proportionate frequency of *not* having the diagnosis (or test negativity) among persons who truly do *not* have the attribute (Table 1). A sensitive test will have a low proportion of false-negatives and a specific test will have a low proportion of false-positives. If a disease or attribute is uncommon, e.g., systemic lupus erythematosus or a positive LE cell test, the number of persons with false-positive criteria or tests may exceed true positives by severalfold, even with tests of high sensitivity and specificity.

MULTIFACTORIAL CONTRIBUTIONS TO ETIOLOGY

Most chronic acquired diseases are now believed to result from the interaction of multiple factors related to the host, the environment, and, at times, infecting agents (Fig. 1). Multifactorial mechanisms of disease often obscure recognition of the primary determining factor(s) by virtue of complex interactions and sequences of events. Epidemiology contributes to a broad perspective of disease and to synthetic concepts that can help rationalize theories of etiology and pathogenesis.

GLOBAL PERSPECTIVES OF ARTHRITIS PREVALENCE

The prevalence of musculoskeletal disorders in the United States was last assessed in the 1976 National Health Interview Survey of over 40,000 households among the civilian noninstitutionalized population (Table 2). Such statistics are based upon conditions reported in health interviews and may differ from those determined from examination surveys or medical records. Underre-

Table 1
Sensitivity and Specificity Measures

Test or Criteria	True or Standard Classification		Total
	Yes	No	
Positive	a	b	a + b
Negative	c	d	c + d
Total	a + c	b + d	a + b + c + d

Sensitivity equals a/a + c; specificity equals d/b + d.

porting of conditions tends to be found during health interviews, but self-diagnosis or misdiagnosis also occurs, with a usual net effect of lower than actual frequencies. The statistics also apply to conditions persisting for at least 3 months. The total reported prevalence of arthritis and rheumatic diseases among noninstitutionalized persons was 31.4 million (15.0 percent). The prevalence of arthritis or rheumatism among the institutionalized population is significantly higher and has been estimated to be 33.2 percent. The high prevalence in the institutionalized population is not surprising in view of the striking positive relationship of arthritis with increasing age.

Sex Distribution

Over all ages, arthritis prevalence (excluding gout) was reported almost twice as frequently by females as males, with the female preponderance greater in the youngest than in the oldest adult groups. No consistent or impressive sex difference was reported for nonarticular rheumatism, bursitis, or tenosynovitis. Males outnumbered females in displacement of intervertebral disc (1.3:1) and more so for gout (2.0:1). The latter sex ratio is

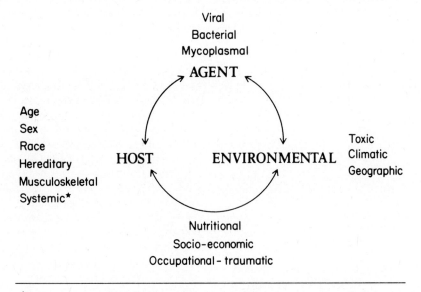

*e.g., circulatory, endocrinologic, immunologic, metabolic, neurologic, psychologic

Fig. 1. Factors contributing to arthritis: holistic model of disease. (Modified by permission of the authors and publisher from Hollander and McCarty (eds): Arthritis and Allied Conditions. Philadelphia, Lea & Febiger, 1979.)

Table 2
Preliminary Prevalence Data for Arthritis from 1976 Public Health Service Household Interview Survey

Arthritis Conditions (ICDA Codes)*	Millions	Percent of Population	Percent of Population by Age		
			Under 45	45–65	65+
Arthritis, not elsewhere classified (710–715)	24.6	11.7	2.7	25.6	43.7
Gout (274)	1.6	0.8	0.2	1.8	2.4
Rheumatism, nonarticular and unspecified (716, 717.0, 717.1, 717.9, 718)	0.8	0.4	0.1	0.7	1.6
Synovitis, bursitis, and tenosynovitis (731)	4.0	1.9	1.0	4.4	3.0
Other diseases of musculoskeletal system, not elsewhere classified†	0.4	0.2	0.1	0.3	0.3
Totals	31.4	15.0	4.1	32.8	51.0

*ICDA is International Classification of Diseases Adapted, 8th revision.
†728, 729, 732, 733.0, 733.2, 733.3, 733.6, 733.9, 734.

surprising in view of clinical series of gout indicating a greater male ratio of approximately 7:1.

Residence and Socioethnic Distributions

Arthritis prevalence does not differ impressively in major U.S. geographic regions. Rural versus urban residence and age seem to explain the slight regional differences, with higher reporting by persons living outside standard metropolitan areas. Arthritis prevalence increased, however, with decreasing family income and education of the head of family after adjustment was made for age. A similar relationship was found for nonarticular rheumatism, but not for displaced intervertebral disc, bursitis, or tenosynovitis. For gout, its prevalence correlated positively with income. Arthritis reporting was similar among whites and all other races combined.

Global population frequencies of arthritis contribute relatively little to determining disease mechanisms. They illustrate the scope of the problem, however, and emphasize certain clinically recognized relationships between age and sex and the frequency of various types of rheumatic disorders.

REFERENCES

Cobb S: The Frequency of the Rheumatic Diseases. American Public Health Association Monograph. Cambridge, Harvard University Press, 1971

Lawrence JS: Rheumatism in Populations. London, Heinemann, 1977

Masi AT, Medsger TA: Epidemiology of the rheumatic diseases, in Hollander JL, McCarty DJ (eds): Arthritis and Allied Conditions (ed 9). Philadelphia, Lea & Febiger (in press)

National Center for Health Statistics: USPHS Publ No 92, Series 10, DHEW Publ No 92, DHEW Publ No (HRA) 75-1519, 1974

Reynolds MD: Prevalence of rheumatic diseases as causes of disability and complaints by ambulatory patients. Arthritis Rheum 21:377, 1978

EPIDEMIOLOGY OF RHEUMATOID ARTHRITIS AND JUVENILE RHEUMATOID ARTHRITIS

The lack of known etiology and absence of specific disease definition presents a thorny dilemma to investigators seeking to measure the population frequency or natural course of rheumatoid arthritis. The disease may follow a variable, nonspecific pattern for months or years before becoming "typical." Although advanced stages of disease are more reliably diagnosed, they represent a minority and biased segment of the total spectrum. In an attempt to establish standardization, criteria have been developed for rheumatoid arthritis and other rheumatic diseases.

RHEUMATOID ARTHRITIS
Diagnostic Criteria

Two sets of widely utilized criteria for adult rheumatoid arthritis (RA) are currently available for clinical or population studies. A committee of the American Rheumatism Association (ARA) has proposed a set of 11 symptoms, signs, and laboratory examination criteria for RA, as well as specific exclusions that increase the diagnostic specificity. Categories of possible, probable, definite, and classic RA were defined, with increasing degrees of certainty of diagnosis, respectively. A minimum duration of clinical manifestations of 6 weeks is required for the definite and classic categories, and 4 weeks for the probable. The criteria were designed for reporting purposes and not as an aid to physicians in making a diagnosis in an individual patient. Criteria for definite RA yielded a sensitivity of 0.70 and a specificity of 0.91 compared with clinical judgement. A revision of these criteria (Rome, 1961) made them more suitable for definition of active RA and more easily applicable in epidemiologic surveys. The second set of criteria proposed for population studies (New York, 1966) emphasized the pattern of affected joints, demanding involvement of a distal extremity joint (hand, wrist or foot) and symmetry of a joint pair. The New York criteria listed no exclusions or restrictions on duration of joint manifestations.

Both the ARA (or Rome) and New York criteria have been compared in the same population or clinical study groups. In Sudbury, Mass., 118 of 4552 adults examined (2.6 percent) met ARA criteria for probable or definite classification versus only 17 (0.4 percent) who satisfied the stricter physical examination requirement of the New York criteria. On reexamination after 3–5 years, rather low proportions of the original ARA probable and definite groups (15 and 53 percent, respectively) retained an ARA classification of at least probable disease. Eleven (65 percent) of the original New York criteria positive patients continued to satisfy these criteria, all but one of whom also met ARA criteria.

One must recognize the limitations of syndromic criteria, yet strive to achieve a high degree of classification accuracy until the complete disease spectrum and its etiology can be defined.

Age and Sex Distribution

Population surveys concur in the generally increasing prevalence of RA with age, especially in women, reaching a peak in the oldest age groups. Although the overall sex ratio is almost three females to one male, this significant female preponderance results mainly during the childbearing ages, with a sex ratio of incidence of about 5:1. The sex ratios for onset in childhood and among the elderly are approximately 1:1. These results suggest a role of sex-hormone factors in the onset or course of RA.

Ethnic and Geographic Distribution

All races may develop RA. Despite current limitations in methodology and language translation difficulties, most studies indicate a prevalence of definite disease (by ARA criteria) of 0.3–1.0 percent in adults, with extremes ranging from 0.1 percent in a native Bantu tribe to 3.0 percent in a survey in Heinola, Finland. Neither climate nor geography seem to be the determining factor.

Personal–Social and Psychologic Factors

Studies of marital partners and viral serologic data do not indicate infectious agent associations in RA. In American men, a distinct trend was found toward increasing prevalence of RA with decreasing levels of education and lower levels of family income. Whether or not socioeconomic factors influence the risk of RA and related conditions, no question exists that these diseases impose a heavy economic and personal burden. The role of personality factors is controversial since it has not yet been possible to determine whether the observed patterns result from the disease or predispose to its onset.

Familial Occurrence

Population surveys have not generally revealed strong evidence of familial aggregation or concentration of RA. Family studies of probands with seropositive erosive arthritis, however, reveal a sixfold increased prevalence of this type of disease among siblings or dizygotic twins versus controls. In monozygotic twins,

the concordance is over 30 times the expected frequency and the data are consistent with a polygenic pattern of inheritance. Such results suggest host predisposition to more progressive RA and are supported by recent reports of a lymphocyte-defined surface antigen marker (Dw4) found in increased frequency among adult, white, seropositive, erosive RA patients versus controls (i.e., 60 versus 20 percent, respectively).

Course of Disease

Although the course of RA remains largely unpredictable, all studies concur on the poorer prognosis of patients with serum rheumatoid factor and bone erosions. Females tend to have more chronic and progressive disease than males. The course of disease tends to correlate with the number of joints involved by pain/tenderness or swelling during the early months, particularly the upper extremity joints. Since RA is a systemic disease, it is not surprising that mortality should be greater than expected in the general population. Increased mortality seems to occur in persons of all ages, especially those with younger onset. A relatively high frequency of death due to respiratory infection has been noted.

JUVENILE RHEUMATOID ARTHRITIS
Diagnostic Criteria

Chronic forms of idiopathic juvenile-onset arthritis represent a challenging area of classification, including juvenile rheumatoid arthritis (JRA), juvenile forms of ankylosing spondylitis (and related HLA-B27 associated disorders), and a number of other conditions in which arthritis may be a manifestation. Methodologic problems prevail similar to those described above for adult RA; the definition of disease influences the epidemiologic characteristics observed.

The current proposed revision of JRA criteria (1977) requires persistent arthritis of one or more joints for more than 6 weeks if excluding diagnoses have been eliminated. Within this framework, patients may be further classified according to manifestations found during the first 6 months after onset, i.e., systemic, pauciarticular, or polyarticular JRA. As yet, no specific population survey criteria for chronic juvenile-onset arthritis have been proposed.

Population Frequency

The National Health Interview Survey in 1969 indicated a prevalence of chronic arthritis in children of 0.8 per 1000, which is similar to an estimate of 0.6 per 1000 derived from a survey of school children in Taplow, England. No population estimates of the incidence of JRA are available except for those derived from hospitals or specialty clinics, which suggest 10 new cases per 100,000 juveniles annually; they may be suspected of being underestimates.

Age and Sex Distribution

Overall, the female to male ratio reported in JRA is about 1.5:1 and is significantly less than that of RA in young and middle-aged adults, but varies with the onset pattern. The sex ratio in systemic onset (Still's type) JRA is approximately equal, with the great majority having onset before 10 years of age. Pauciarticular-onset JRA seems to include at least two subgroups, those with and those without chronic, often asymptomatic, iridocyclitis. In patients with iridocyclitis, the average onset age is under 3 years, with girls predominating over boys in a ratio of about 3:1. In the pauciarticular group without iridocyclitis, the sex ratio is equal but consists of two heterogeneous subgroups. In one, girls predominate with an average onset age of 5 years. In the other, boys predominate with an average onset age of 10 years and a high proportion of HLA-B27 positivity or radiographic evidence of sacroiliitis. The latter group is presumably not JRA but rather juvenile onset spondyloarthropathy. Polyarticular-onset JRA usually begins after age 10, and females predominate in a ratio of about 5:1, as in young-adult onset RA.

Racial and Ethnic Distribution

Few data are available on the relative racial or ethnic distribution of JRA, but several studies hint at its rarity among orientals. An increased frequency has been reported in some North American Indian tribes, but they have been found to have a high frequency of HLA-B27; the question exists as to whether such children have JRA or juvenile spondyloarthropathy.

Course of Disease

Although the prognosis in JRA is better than in adult RA, functional capacity tends to decrease on the average with increasing length of follow-up. Long-term mortality ranges from about 1 to 3 percent in U.S. series to 5 percent in England and Europe. In Europe, renal insufficiency, essentially always secondary to amyloidosis, accounts for approximately one-half the deaths as opposed to only 13 percent in the United States. Interestingly, the sex ratio of fatal JRA cases is equal.

In earlier family studies of juvenile arthritis patients, a higher than expected frequency of sacroiliitis and ankylosing spondylitis was found among relatives, especially males. In light of recent B27 discoveries, it may now be assumed that such associations involve primarily spondyloarthritis syndromes rather than JRA per se.

JRA AND ADULT RA: CONTINUUM OR SEPARATE DISEASES?

It is now realized that the labels *JRA* or *JCP* (i.e., *juvenile chronic polyarthritis,* a term which is more popular in England), have been applied in the past to more than one disease process. After more careful disease classification, the concept is developing that various clinical syndromes affecting both children and adults, such as seropositive RA and ankylosing spondylitis, constitute a biologic spectrum regardless of onset age. Studies comparing early patterns of seropositive and seronegative RA in juveniles and young adults tend to support a unified concept of disease across all ages. Questions remain as to why particular clinical patterns, e.g., systemic onset (Still's type) disease, occur most frequently, although not exclusively, in the youngest ages and why the frequency of rheumatoid factor increases with age, both in juveniles and adults. These phenomena seem to represent age-related responses to the same disease rather than separate diseases manifesting in different age groups.

REFERENCES

Bennett PH, Burch TA: New York symposium on population studies in the rheumatic diseases: New diagnostic criteria. Bull Rheum Dis 17:453, 1967

JRA Criteria Subcommittee of the Diagnostic and Therapeutic Criteria Committee of the American Rheumatism Association Section of The Arthritis Foundation: Current proposed revision of JRA criteria. Arthritis Rheum 20 [Suppl]:195, 1977

Lawrence JS: Heberden Oration, 1969. Rheumatoid arthritis— Nature or nurture? Ann Rheum Dis 29:357, 1970

Lawrence JS: Rheumatism in Populations. London, Heinemann, 1977

Masi AT, Medsger TA: Epidemiology of the rheumatic diseases, in Hollander JL, McCarty DJ (eds.): Arthritis and Allied Conditions (ed 9). Philadelphia, Lea & Febiger, (in press)

Ropes MW, Bennett FA, Cobb S: 1958 revision of diagnostic criteria for rheumatoid arthritis. Arthritis Rheum 2:16, 1959

Schaller JG, Hanson V: Proceedings of the First ARA Conference on the Rheumatic Diseases of Childhood. Arthritis Rheum 20 [Suppl 2]:145–636, 1977

EPIDEMIOLOGY OF SPECIFIC TYPES OF ARTHRITIS

The epidemiology of the remaining rheumatic diseases can not be fully reviewed in this chapter. We have focused attention upon those major syndromes and classic studies that illustrate a variety of epidemiologic methods and concepts. Certain other important disorders such as rheumatic fever and infectious agent arthritis are covered elsewhere and are excluded from this discussion.

HLA-B27 ASSOCIATED ARTHRITIS SYNDROMES

Even prior to the landmark HLA-B27 discoveries, a spectrum of clinically related, overlapping spinal and peripheral arthritis syndromes was suspected of having genetic predisposition. It is now quite evident that the frequency of HLA-B27 differs in various racial groups and that the prevalence of ankylosing spondylitis and related spondyloarthritis syndromes parallel such frequencies, although these disorders can occur in the absence of this particular cell surface antigen. Interestingly, over 90 percent of whites with ankylosing spondylitis have B27, whereas only about half of nonrelated black cases are positive.

Ankylosing Spondylitis

The frequency of ankylosing spondylitis varies greatly in different populations, ranging from a virtual absence in Australian aboriginals or black Africans to a 4.2 percent prevalence in adult male Haida Indians. The absolute frequency also depends upon the disease definition, i.e., whether one is referring to the obvious classic, progressive, deforming disease or a more ill-defined spectrum of patients with radiologic sacroiliitis, with or without spinal or peripheral joint mainifestations. Earlier population studies of whites using clinical and radiographic criteria indicate a prevalence of ankylosing spondylitis of about 1 per 1000 adults with a male preponderance of at least 3:1. Since the discovery of HLA-B27, however, several clinical surveys of volunteer populations have revealed a higher frequency of "definite" and "possible" ankylosing spondylitis, ranging in B27 positive individuals from about 20 percent in one U.S. study of males and females to about 2 percent in a Hungarian study (3.0 percent in males and 0.6 percent in females). Approximately 8 percent of whites are HLA-B27 positive.

A semantic question is whether or not roentgenographic sacroiliitis and mild clinical involvement of the back should be classified as ankylosing spondylitis. Although two sets of criteria for population studies of ankylosing spondylitis have been proposed, considerable variability has been found in the determination and interpretation of symptoms of pain and stiffness in the dorsolumbar spine.

Ankylosing spondylitis is typically diagnosed in young adult males; the average age of onset is about 25 years. The ratio of males to females usually ranges from 3:1 to 9:1 in different studies. Onset may occur in juveniles, and peripheral arthritis is the initial symptom in about one-half. Such patients may be considered initially to have pauciarticular JRA and represent approximately 10 percent of children seen for chronic arthritis.

Reiter's Syndrome

Although once considered to be relatively rare, Reiter's syndrome, defined as the triad of arthritis, urethritis, and conjunctivitis, is now considered a common cause of arthritis in young adult males and perhaps the leading cause of noninfectious arthritis admissions to military hospitals. It has been reported both in epidemics, following bacillary dysentery, and as endemic or sporadic events following nongonococcal venereally acquired urethritis.

In Finland, during World War II, 0.2 percent of those affected in a shigella dysentery epidemic in the summer of 1944 were found to have Reiter's syndrome. Although it is rare in women, they seemed to be relatively more frequently affected in postdysenteric disease (10 percent in Finland) than in postvenereal diseases according to a survey of sporadic Reiter's cases (1 percent). A more recent epidemic occurred aboard an American naval vessel in June 1962; 10 sailors developed Reiter's syndrome among 602 cases of shigella dysentery (1.5 percent). Five of the Reiter's cases were located after 10 years and HLA typed; the four with chronic active arthritis had B27 and the fifth with mild remittent arthritis had a cross-reacting antigen, HLA-B7. With at least 4 of the 10 cases having this HLA type, an attack rate of Reiter's syndrome among shigella-infected B27 young adult males was estimated at about 20 percent.

Familial predisposition to Reiter's disease has been suggested by reports of several pairs of brothers with this condition and additional familial occurrences in the Reiter's patients following the Finnish epidemic. Family studies of sporadic Reiter's syndrome probands showed that rheumatoid arthritis and polyarthritis occurred in relatives and spouses in an expected frequency. Clinical spondylitis and radiologic changes of sacroiliitis, as defined by Rome criteria, however, were two to eight times as frequent among relatives as in a population control sample. None of the spouses showed any evidence of spondylitis.

Other HLA-B27 Associated Arthritis Conditions

Ulcerative colitis and granulomatous enteritis patients develop clinical spondylitis at a risk estimated to be 30-fold greater than in the general population, and approximately 60 percent of such spondylitis patients are HLA-B27 positive. However, neither asymptomatic roentgenographic sacroiliitis nor peripheral arthritis alone, occurring during the course of chronic inflammatory bowel disease, is associated with B27.

Spondylitis is also a well-recognized complication of approximately 2 percent of the psoriatic population, with 60–70 percent of such persons having B27. Controlled family studies of Reiter's syndrome and psoriatic arthritis indicate genetic relationships between these disorders. Thirteen percent of male relatives of Reiter's syndrome probands had psoriasis, as did 12 percent of the male relatives of the psoriasis probands, compared to only 1 percent of the population controls. Although radiographic evidence of sacroiliitis was not excessive in the psoriasis families, unlike that found in Reiter's relatives, the psoriasis relatives had more peripheral polyarthritis than the controls. Studies indicated that persons developing psoriatic arthritis have both psoriatic and arthritic familial predispositions, whereas persons with psoriasis alone do not show familial aggregation of arthritis. Such findings may now be better interpreted in the light of HLA typing results; psoriatic peripheral arthritis correlates with Bw38 and Bw17, sacroiliitis with B27, and psoriasis alone with A13.

SYSTEMIC LUPUS ERYTHEMATOSUS

The full spectrum of systemic lupus erythematosus (SLE) and its frequency in the population have been difficult to determine because of its remarkable variability in presentation and evolution. A subcommittee of the Diagnostic and Therapeutic Criteria Committee of the ARA proposed preliminary criteria for the classification of SLE in 1971 consisting of 14 types of manifestations. Any 4 or more of the manifestations found to be present, serially or simultaneously, would be sufficient for purposes of classifying patients as having SLE in clinical trials, population surveys, and other such studies. The preliminary criteria yielded 90 percent sensitivity in patients with clinically unequivocal SLE, 99 percent specificity against rheumatoid arthritis, and 98 percent specificity against other diseases. Evaluation of the sensitivity of the criteria was encouraging in several additional series, but it remains to be demonstrated whether these criteria will discriminate equally well against other connective tissue diseases.

Population studies became feasible after the discovery of the LE cell phenomenon and other distinguishing serologic methods. It is difficult to know if the increasing prevalence reported with time reflects mainly greater awareness, improved survival, or true increase in occurrence. In the long-term studies of the epidemiology of SLE in New York City, the first estimates of incidence in the early 1950s were about 0.4 per 100,000 population, which increased to 1.0 by the mid-1950s, and subsequently to over 3.0 by 1965 when last estimated in this population. Recently a study of health plan subscribers among residents of San Francisco City and County revealed an annual incidence of 7.4 cases per 100,000 population. The surprising statistic from this study was an overall prevalence of one SLE case per 1969 persons. In women 15–64 years of age, the prevalence was 1 case per 700, and in black women of this age, 1 per 245! The peculiarly increased predisposition of black women of childbearing age has been confirmed in mortality analyses as well. Several American Indian tribes had an annual incidence of SLE in excess of 10 per 100,000 population, with an estimated incidence of 31.3 for the full-blooded Sioux, but the populations upon which these data are based are relatively small.

Both clinical and epidemiologic studies have shown females to be more susceptible to SLE, particularly during the younger adult ages. The overall female to male ratio (5:1) varies with age, being greatest (8:1) during the childbearing years and considerably less (2:1) under age 10 and over age 60. No impressive change is seen with age in the low occurrence of SLE in males. Sex hormone factors are thus suggested as contributing to the onset or pathogenesis of SLE, which is supported by reports of SLE associated with Klinefelter's syndrome (karyotype XXY).

A further preponderance of black versus white females of about 3:1 has been noted in several populations. Insufficient data have been gathered to indicate important frequency correlations with latitude or geography, and no socioeconomic factors have been implicated.

Reports of familial occurrence of SLE have become impressive in number, suggesting familial aggregation. If real, it appears to operate at a generally low level, whether environmental, genetic, or infectious agent factors might be contributing.

Survival rates from the time of first SLE diagnosis have improved over the years—from the earlier hospital-based studies indicating a 4-year 50 percent survival to more recent clinic-based reports suggesting a 10-year 90 percent survival. Interpretations of such marked differences are complex and unresolved at present. Age, race, and sex factors do not appear to alter survival significantly, but involvement of the kidneys and central nervous system are generally considered poor prognostic features.

SYSTEMIC SCLEROSIS
(SCLERODERMA)

The term *scleroderma* encompasses a heterogeneous group of localized and systemic processes causing hardening of the skin, whereas *systemic sclerosis* implies a generalized disorder of connective tissues affecting both skin and internal organs.

A subcommittee of the Diagnostic and Therapeutic Criteria Committee of the ARA recently reported preliminary clinical findings from a multicenter prospective study of scleroderma criteria. Proximal scleroderma, that is, typical cutaneous involvement proximal to the digits, was considered a major criterion. It was found in 91 percent of systemic sclerosis patients and less than 1 percent of comparison patients (SLE, polydermatomyositis, and primary Raynaud's phenomenon). Localized scleroderma patients were excluded from analysis as were those with certain systemic rheumatic conditions frequently causing skin induration, such as "overlap" syndrome and eosinophilic fasciitis. Minor criteria were also identified, i.e., sclerodactyly (hardening of digits), digital pitting scars, basilar pulmonary fibrosis, and colonic sacculations found on barium enema. Either one major or two or more minor criteria were found in 97 percent of patients with definite systemic sclerosis but in only 3 percent of the comparison patients. Further evaluation of these preliminary clinical criteria is needed to assess their general applicability.

Because of its rarity, hospital and death certificate ascertainment have provided essentially all of the available frequency data as opposed to population surveys. Systemic sclerosis is unusual in childhood and in males before age 35. Incidence and mortality rise steadily with age. Females predominate over males in an overall ratio of about 3:1, and, as in SLE, the female to male ratio is considerably higher from age 15 to 44 compared with older age groups. Among women, blacks have a significantly greater incidence and mortality than whites.

In one national study of U.S. male veterans, incidence and mortality did not differ importantly by major geographic regions, after adjusting for hospital utilization factors, and no difference was found in regard to urban or rural residence location. Scleroderma patients were more likely to be employed as laborers or in other less skilled occupations, as well as to consume large amounts of alcohol. Suggestions have been made that scleroderma may be more common among miners or others chronically exposed to silica dust, and a sclerodermalike occupational acroosteolysis has been described in workers exposed to unfinished plastics (polyvinyl chloride). The importance of these relationships to the pathogenesis of systemic sclerosis is obscure.

Reports of the familial occurrence of systemic sclerosis remain limited, and HLA studies have been inconclusive.

Life-table analysis has revealed a median survival of almost 7 years from first hospital diagnosis in two series of patients (Fig. 1). Prognosis was significantly worse in males, older patients, and those with kidney, heart, or lung involvement at first evaluation. Heavy use of alcohol or cigarettes adversely affected survival in individuals without initial circulatory organ involvement.

POLYMYOSITIS
(DERMATOMYOSITIS)

These members of the connective tissue disease family are characterized by chronic, idiopathic, degenerative and inflammatory alterations of striated muscle, skin, and various internal organs.

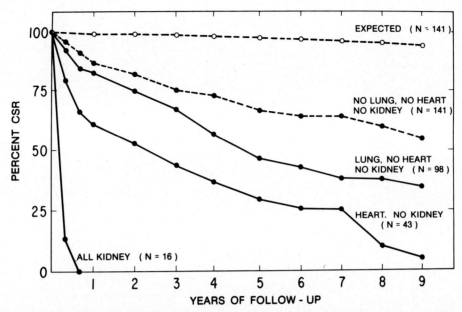

Fig. 1. Observed cumulative survival rates (CSR) for scleroderma patients with lung, heart, or kidney involvement and observed and expected SCR for scleroderma patients with none of these involvements at first hospital diagnosis (Memphis, Tenn., and Pittsburgh, Pa., patients). (Adapted by permission of author and publisher from Mesdger TA, Masi AT, Rodnan GP, et al: Survival with systemic sclerosis. Ann Intern Med 75:373, 1971.)

No official criteria have as yet been proposed for the classification of polymyositis, but combinations of clinical and laboratory features have been suggested for purposes of epidemiologic classification of cases, with appropriate exclusions of other forms of myopathy. Proposals for subclassification of polymyositis have been made over the years, for reasons of additional specificity, but lumping has been preferred by other authors. The more commonly used groupings include childhood dermatopolymyositis, adult dermatomyositis, adult polymyositis, and dermatopolymyositis associated with either malignancy or other connective tissue disease.

A bimodal age distribution is apparent, both in clinical series and incidence as well as in mortality studies. Childhood (ages 10–14) and adult (ages 45–64) peaks occur, with a paucity of patients diagnosed during young adulthood. This pattern contrasts with that of SLE in females, where the peak incidence occurs in the 15–44-year-old age group. Interestingly, in polymyositis, a significant female excess was noted from ages 10 to 19, again suggesting a sex hormone contribution to onset during adolescence. As in SLE, the total incidence was four times greater in black than in white females. The overall female to male sex ratio is 2:1 and tends to be greater in polymyositis patients with clinical features overlapping with other connective tissue diseases.

Polymyositis is reported in all climates and among a wide variety of races. No impressive frequency difference has been found by socioeconomic factors nor has evidence been provided for temporal–spatial clustering of cases. Among juvenile cases, however, a disproportion-

ate number had onset in the months of February, March, or April, suggesting a nonspecific precipitating factor during the colder months.

An overall 47 percent mortality at 7 years after initial diagnosis was found for polymyositis, as for scleroderma, but there was a relatively more rapid early death rate of 28 percent at the end of 2 years (Fig. 2). Poorer prognosis was associated with coexisting malignancy, older onset age, maleness, the presence of marked muscle weakenss, dysphagia, and aspiration pneumonia at first evaluation. Several recent reports suggest an excellent outlook in childhood-onset disease. In one study, blacks had a poorer survivorship than whites, which was attributed to greater dysphagia and muscle weakness on admission.

Various malignancies have been reported to occur in adults, chiefly with dermatomyositis, suggesting a greater than chance association; the relative frequency of this complication in polydermatomyositis is approximately 10 percent or less, but increases with age, especially in males.

Table 1 is a summary of the essential epidemiologic features of the connective tissue diseases and tends to emphasize the female preponderance over males, especially in the childbearing ages, and the particular susceptibility of black females.

HYPERURICEMIA AND PRIMARY GOUT

In contrast to rheumatoid arthritis, SLE, and most other connective tissue diseases, gout mainly affects adult males. The risk of developing hyperuricemia, which, in turn, predisposes to gout, depends on a com-

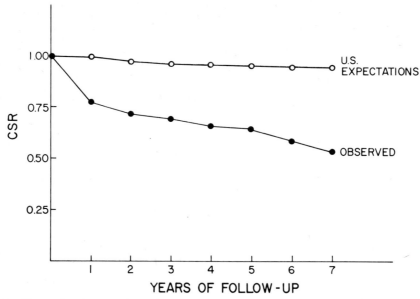

Fig. 2. Observed and expected cumulative survival rates (SCR) from first hospital diagnosis in 124 polymyositis patients (Memphis and Shelby County, Tenn., hospitals, 1947–1968). (Reproduced by permission of author and publisher from Medsger TA, Robinson H, Masi AT: Factors affecting survivorship in polymyositis. A life-table study of 124 patients. Arthritis Rheum 14:251, 1971.)

plex interaction of multiple factors, e.g., diet, environment, age, sex, and heredity. Primary gout was originally believed to be rare among native races living in their original habitat. At present, however, with changing life styles gout is frequently seen in orientals, Filipinos, Polynesians, and U.S. blacks.

In U.S. and most European populations, the normal mean serum uric acid (SUA) for males is about 5 mg/dl by non-autoAnalyzer methods, but higher mean levels have been found in South Pacific populations prone to gout. Mean SUA levels rise during childhood, with similar values in boys and girls. Starting at ages 15–19 years, the average male values exceed those of females, with the maximum difference of almost 1.5 mg/dl achieved in the 20–24-year-old age group. The mean female values further increase after age 40, reaching within about 0.5 mg/dl of the male values after the menopause. Such age and sex relationships suggest hormonal influences, but the mechanisms of such factors have not been demonstrated. Recently, a number of inborn errors of uric acid metabolism have been described, some of which are associated with hyperuricemia and clinical gout. Partial enzyme-defi-

Table 1
Epidemiologic Characteristics of Connective Tissue Diseases

	Rheumatoid Arthritis	Systemic Lupus Erythematosus	Systemic Sclerosis	Polymyositis/ Dermatomyositis
Annual Incidence (per million)	1000	75	10	10
Sex ratio, all ages (female:male)	2.5:1	5:1	2.5:1	2:1
Race ratio, both sexes (black:white)	1:1	4:1	2:1	3:1
Childhood diagnosis (%)	5–10	10	1	20
Incidence pattern	Increases with age, especially in females; F:M sex ratio of 6:1 in sero-positives of 15–45 years, and 1:1 in first and oldest decades.	Highest in females of 20–40 years; F:M sex ratio of 8:1 at 20–40 years and 2:1 in first and oldest decades.	Increases with age, especially in females; rare in children and males under age 35	Childhood and adult peaks seen
Five-year survival (%)	95+	90+	60	60

ciency states had been predicted to account for some considerable portion of the hyperuricemic population, but this does not appear to be the case.

Recent proposed preliminary criteria for the classification of the acute arthritis of primary gout include: (1) the presence of characteristic urate crystals in the joint fluid, and/or (2) a tophus proven to contain urate crystals, and/or (3) the presence of 6 of 12 other clinical, laboratory, and radiographic findings. The combination of criteria was highly sensitive and specific. Slight modifications were made for epidemiologic survey purposes.

The prevalence and incidence of gout correlate closely with the levels of SUA in the population but also seem to be increased in relatives of gouty patients whether such individuals were initially determined to be hyper- or normouricemic. Family history of gouty arthritis is especially correlated with onset of gout in premenopausal women; in one study, over one-half provided such a history. Women seem to be relatively protected from gout by virtue of their lower mean SUA levels over a longer life period than males, rather than some other innate factor, although data on this point are relatively limited.

DEGENERATIVE JOINT DISEASE

Osteoarthritis is considered the commonest joint disease among white populations, based on the presence of symptomatic and nonsymptomatic roentgenographic degenerative changes (i.e., osteoarthrosis). Approximately 30 percent of persons with radiographic evidence of degenerative joint changes complain of pain at such sites and would thus be considered to have osteoarthritis.

All degrees of radiographic evidence of osteoarthrosis of the extremities increase steadily with age to over 80 percent among elderly persons, as determined in the 1960–1962 National Health Examination Survey. Moderate or severe involvement is almost twice as prevalent in females. In surveys, differences between populations are apparent in overall frequency of osteoarthrosis and occasionally in the particular joints affected. In general, epidemiologic surveys have tended to confirm the association of osteoarthrosis with mechanical factors such as "wear and tear" and a number of body measurements.

Studies of the prevalence of radiographic evidence of osteoarthrosis in families and twins of index cases indicate that it is also influenced by genetic factors. The increased frequencies do not fit simple mendelian inheritance patterns and may be determined by multiple genes.

REFERENCES

Acheson RM, Collart AB: New Haven survey of joint diseases. XVII. Relationships between some systemic characteristics and osteoarthrosis in a general population. Ann Rheum Dis 34:379, 1975

Bennett PH, Burch TA: New York symposium on population studies in the rheumatic diseases: New diagnostic criteria. Bull Rheum Dis 17:453, 1967

Brewerton DA: Joseph J. Bunim Memorial Lecture. HLA-B27 and the inheritance of susceptibility to rheumatic diseases. Arthritis Rheum 19:656, 1976

Cohen, AS, Reynolds WE, Franklin EC, Kirka JP, Ropes M, Shulman L, Wallace SL: Preliminary criteria for the classification of systemic lupus erythematosus. Bull Rheum Dis 21:643, 1971

Fessel WJ: Systemic lupus erythematosus in the community. Incidence, prevalence, outcome, and first symptoms; The high prevalence in black women. Arch Intern Med 134:1027, 1974

Lawrence JS: Rheumatism in Populations. London, Heinemann, 1977

Masi AT, Medsger TA: Epidemiology of the rheumatic diseases, in Hollander JL, McCarty DJ, (ed.): Arthritis and Allied Conditions (ed 9). Philadelphia, Lea & Febiger (in press)

Masi AT, Rodnan GP, Medsger TA, et al: Clinical criteria for early-diagnosed systemic (SS): Preliminary results of the ARA multicenter cooperative study (abstract). Arthritis Rheum 21:576, 1978

Medsger TA, Dawson WN Jr, Masi AT: The epidemiology of polymyositis. Am J Med 48:715, 1970

Medsger TA, Masi AT: Epidemiology of systemic sclerosis (scleroderma). Ann Intern Med 74:714, 1971

Medsger TA, Masi AT, Rodnan GP, et al: Survival with systemic sclerosis (scleroderma). Ann Intern Med 75:369, 1971

Medsger TA, Robinson H, Masi AT: Factors affecting survivorship in polymyositis. A life-table study of 124 patients. Arthritis Rheum 14:249, 1971

National Center for Health Statistics: USPHS Publ No 1000, Series 11, No. 15. Washington, DC, US Government Print Office, 1966

National Center for Health Statistics: USPHS Publ No 1000, Series 11, No 17. Washington, DC, US Government Printing Office, 1966

Siegel M, Lee SL: The epidemiology of systemic lupus erythematosus. Semin Arthritis Rheum 3:1, 1973

Wallace SL, Robinson H, Masi AT, Decker JL, McCarty DJ, Yu T: Preliminary criteria for the classification of the acute arthritis of primary gout. Arthritis Rheum 20:895, 1977

Wright V, Moll JMH: Seronegative Polyarthritis. New York, Elsevier/North-Holland, 1976

Wyngaarden JB, Kelley WN: Gout and Hyperuricemia. New York, Grune & Stratton, 1976

Functional Assessment and Disability

George E. Ehrlich and Robert F. Meenan

The maintenance of functional capacity is a major aim of rheumatology practice. Drug therapy, by controlling pain and inflammation, certainly plays a significant role in reducing functional losses. Many patients with arthritis, however, will develop important limitations despite appropriate drug therapy. Thus assessment of function is an important area of exploration for the physician who treats such patients. A frank inquiry into what the patient can do, what the patient cannot do but wants to do, what the patient aims for, and even what the patient will settle for often provides a template for therapeutic approaches.

SCALES

Functional assessment is a complex task, and a variety of scales have been developed to facilitate the process. However, none is totally satisfactory for use with most of the patients with articular disease who are seen in ambulatory practice. One group of scales, for example, is designed to assess the seriously disabled person. One of these, the Barthel index, is used in rehabilitation programs to test the ability to feed one's self, to move from wheelchair to bed and return, to attend to personal hygiene, to get on and off the toilet, to bathe, to walk on a level surface, to ascend and descend stairs, to dress and undress, and to control bowel and bladder. The Katz Activities of Daily Living scale, another widely used measure of function, assesses similar activities. These scales are useful for evaluating rehabilitation programs, especially for inpatients, but not for noting minor limitations that may seriously compromise function.

Many articular disorders actually produce only minor differences from a person's premorbid capabilities; they may represent a summation of multiple but mild deficits, or a major deficit at only a single joint. In either case, these differences may seriously compromise function without limiting the basic daily activities measured by the Barthel and Katz scales, for although these scales are quite detailed, they focus on one extreme of the disability spectrum.

Another group of scales is designed to cover the broad range of disability found in arthritis patients. The best known of this group is the American Rheumatism Association (ARA) Functional Classification developed by Steinbrocker and co-workers in 1949. This scale contains four functional classes:

Class I: Complete, able to carry on all usual duties without handicaps.

Class II: Adequate, carries out normal activities despite discomfort or limited motion in one or more joints.

Class III: Limited, able to perform only some of the activities of usual occupation or self-care.

Class IV: Incapacitated, largely confined to bed and chair.

A similar five-point scale has been developed in Great Britain by the Medical Research Council.

CONSIDERATIONS IN EVALUATION

These broad disability scales have proven especially useful in epidemiologic surveys, where large numbers must be categorized. They are not very helpful in clinical practice, however, where a detailed functional assessment of the individual patient is required. The categories are so broad and so dependent on the notion of usual occupation that they group patients with a wide range of disability who may need very different therapeutic approaches.

As an example, minor functional deficits in the hands may leave a truck driver fully able to perform his duties while disabling a jeweler who requires fine movements of the fingers. A painful hip or knee with limited motion may make a stevedore unemployable but permit full employment for the desk-bound executive. The trucker and the executive would be included in ARA class II; the jeweler and the stevedore in class III; however, each has a different set of functional problems which needs to be assessed and acted upon.

Functional evaluation of the patient with arthritis should also explore performance in areas other than self-care and occupation. Mobility, hobbies, and sexuality, for example, are areas of great concern for many patients. Driving, sitting in a back seat, or using public transit may be difficult for many patients and may severely limit the range of their activities. Hobbies are frequently an important part of a full life, and disabilities in this area, especially with physical hobbies, may appear early in the disease course. Limitations of sexual function may be particularly troublesome for patients of all ages, even though they are rarely discussed. These problems may be due to pain, limited motion, or psychologic barriers.

No special skills or measurement techniques are required to perform therapeutically relevant functional assessments in arthritis. All the physician needs is an interest in the total patient and the willingness to invest some time in exploring certain key areas of everyday living. Once the functional needs of the patient have been identified, a wide variety of resources are available to assist the patient and the physican in dealing with those needs. Local chapters of the Arthritis Foundation and its central office in Atlanta provide information and access to support groups. Occupational therapists can suggest an array of ingenious self-help devices. Physical and rehabilitation therapists offer the possibility of intensive, goal-directed therapy programs. Services for the home-bound are available through the Visiting Nurse Association and other community agencies.

In summary, functional assessments are a vital component of clinical practice in rheumatology. When dealing with patients who have arthritis, it is just as important to identify and alleviate functional problems as it is to select the appropriate drug. The wise physician combines the two approaches in his efforts to enhance the quality of life for his patients with arthritis.

REFERENCES

Convery FR, Minteer, MA, Amiel D, Connett KL: Polyarticular disability: A functional assessment. Arch Phys Med Rehabil 58:494, 1977

Ehrlich GE: Total Management of the Arthritic Patient. Philadelphia, Lippincott, 1973

Katz S, Ford AB, Moskowitz RW, Jackson BA, Jaffe MW: Illness in the aged: The Index of ADL. JAMA 185:914, 1963

Mahoney FI, Barthel DW: Functional evaluation: The Barthel Index. Md State Med J 14:61, 1965

Steinbrocker O, Traeger CH, Batterman RC: Therapeutic criteria in rheumatoid arthritis. JAMA 140:659, 1949

DIAGNOSTIC PROCEDURES

Synovial Fluid

Alan S. Cohen and Martha Skinner

NORMAL SYNOVIAL FLUID

Paracelsus applied the name *synovial* to this fluid because of its viscosity and apparent resemblance to egg white. It is a clear pale yellow or straw-colored viscous liquid that in the normal state does not clot. Synovial fluid differs from serous cavity fluids, which are plasma ultrafiltrates, and cerebrospinal fluid, which is mostly a secretory product of the choroid plexuses. Although the distribution of electrolytes and most nonelectrolytes between plasma and joint fluid is in equilibrium and indicates that joint fluid is to a large degree a dialysate of plasma, there is little question that hyaluronic acid at least is uniquely produced by the synovial membrane and added to the joint fluid (see chapter on Synovial Membrane and chapter on Proteoglycans in fascicle on Regional Structure and Function). A generally acceptable figure for the level of hyaluronate in normal synovial fluid is 0.3 g/dl.

The presence of this large asymmetric hyaluronic acid molecule in the synovial fluid itself influences the further composition of the fluid. Hyaluronic acid may significantly affect the partition of diffusible solutes between solutions that contain it and buffer solutions; that is, the steric structure of the hyaluronate may obstruct some solute passage through the water surrounding the molecules. In this concept of excluded volume, the size and shape of the molecule play an important role. For example, one would expect small molecules not to be excluded and large ones, such as fibrinogen and macroglobulins, to be excluded. The quantity and physical state of hyaluronate produced under pathologic conditions may well be primary determinants of the nature of the remainder of the contents of the synovial fluid.

The amount of synovial fluid in a joint averages 1.1 ml (range 0.13–3.5 ml). Normal synovial fluid is relatively acellular with a mean total white cell count of 63/mm³ (range 13–180) even in the face of marked peripheral blood leukocytosis. Red blood cells generally are absent unless introduced in the process of arthrocentesis. Mononuclear cells (monocytes, lymphocytes, and phagocytes) predominate, with a mean polymorphonuclear leukocyte count of 6.5/mm³. The total protein of normal synovial fluid is considerably less than that of serum and amounts to about 1.8 g/dl.

Although it has long been assumed that the absence of clotting in normal synovial fluid was due to the lack of fibrinogen, studies on normal bovine synovial fluid have indicated that prothrombin, factor V, factor VII, tissue thromboplastin, and antithrombin are also lacking. It has been shown that the Hageman factor and plasma thromboplastin antecedent (factor XI), primarily in inactive form, are present in normal synovial fluid in concentrations comparable to those found in plasma. It is also significant that human synovial tissue and fibrous capsular tissue have been shown to contain only traces of or no tissue thromboplastin, and an activator of plasminogen of the tissue type is present in variable and low concentrations in these tissues. These findings, together with the evidence for fibrinogenolysis, would explain why blood that is shed into the synovial space fails to clot.

SYNOVIAL FLUID ANALYSIS

In the past few years, there has been a growing appreciation of the fact that synovial fluid analysis may provide far more than nonspecific data indicating inflammation or its absence. For example, it has become clear that the appearance of certain crystals in the fluid may be pathognomonic of one disease state or another, and obviously the presence of bacteria indicates infection. There has been an increasing awareness that the synovial compartment may in itself hold some of the clues to the pathogenesis and perpetuation of chronic joint disease if not to its specific etiology. Thus arthrocentesis and meticulous synovial fluid analysis, supplemented occasionally by biopsy of the synovial membrane, are undoubtedly an integral part of the diagnostic and therapeutic evaluation of any rheumatic complaint with an associated effusion. Pathologic synovial fluid will be described and the various diagnostic procedures that may be carried out will be assessed in the following paragraphs.

ARTHROCENTESIS

There are no absolute contraindications to synovial fluid aspiration, and its examination in a patient with a disorder associated with a joint effusion should be regarded as a mandatory part of the routine laboratory workup. The only significant complication of joint aspiration is infection, which with careful aseptic techniques is exceedingly rare. The diagnostic and, by implication, prognostic value of joint aspiration is the chief reason for the procedure. Aspiration may also have substantial therapeutic effect, however, as in massive effusions of any type, suppurative effusions, hemophilic effusions, and others. In some cases arthrocentesis is carried out and followed by instillation of medication or by a biopsy procedure depending upon specific indications. The usual approach to the joint space is from the extensor surface, where major blood vessels and nerves are sparse and the synovial pouch is most superficial.

To obtain equilibrium of glucose and possibly other substances (lipids) between the plasma and synovial fluid, the patient should be fasting for at least 6 hours and preferably longer. If the patient is not fasting, the sugar determinations are of little value, unless unequivocally low. The area to be aspirated is carefully washed several times with soap and water and then swabbed with iodine; this is followed by several alcohol washes. The alcohol is allowed to air dry. After the area has been draped with sterile towels, a small amount of Xylocaine is injected intracutaneously and subcutaneously.

The joint most commonly aspirated is the knee. This may be approached either 1–2 cm laterally or medially and 1–2 cm above the patella with the knee in a position of extension. From this location one may enter the suprapatellar quadriceps pouch with ease or the joint space under the patella as indicated by the size of the effusion. Some physicians prefer to approach the space through the patellar ligament with the knee held in a position of 90° flexion.

The aspiration needle is inserted through skin and subcutaneous tissue. It then usually meets a small amount of resistance when the capsule is penetrated; this occasionally produces a twinge of pain. Finally, it passes easily through the synovial membrane into the joint cavity. If the fluid is not readily obtained, the needle may be moved slightly or rotated gently, for sometimes it becomes plugged by a fold of synovial membrane or debris in the space.

As much fluid as is possible is obtained from the joint and allocated in the appropriate test tubes as soon as it is withdrawn. A portion (0.5 ml) is placed in a sterile tube containing heparin for culture both aerobically and anaerobically. If gonococcal arthritis is suspected, chocolate agar or Thayer-Martin media should be inoculated. If tuberculosis is suspected, several additional milliliters of synovial fluid should be placed in this tube for guinea pig inoculation.

All essential studies can be performed on a small quantity of fluid (1 ml) placed in a nonsterile tube with anticoagulant (heparin). This fluid is used for cytology, white cell count and differential, and gram stain. When enough fluid is available, a quantity is placed in a nonsterile tube with no anticoagulant for mucin determination and examination for crystals and inclusions. If necessary, these tests can be performed on the heparinized fluid

sample. A portion of synovial fluid (2 ml) is also placed in a nonsterile tube with potassium oxalate for sugar analysis. A simultaneous blood sugar should be obtained for comparison.

Cultures should be obtained on all synovial fluids even when a patient with a known articular disease is having an arthrocentesis for reasons other than diagnosis. Thus indolent infections, such as tuberculosis, will not be missed, for it is known that the occasional case of septic arthritis will not have red, hot, and inflamed joints, which make the clinical diagnosis highly suspect. In addition, in the rare case of iatrogenic infection due to the procedure, it is vital to know that infection was not previously present. Finally, there is much evidence that patients with preexisting articular disease (especially rheumatoid arthritis) are prone to develop superimposed infectious arthritis.

EXAMINATION OF SYNOVIAL FLUID
Gross Appearance

The procedure of synovial fluid analysis (Table 1) begins literally the moment the specimen appears in the syringe at the time of aspiration. It is important to note the color of the fluid, particularly whether the fluid is initially bloody and whether it becomes so during the procedure due to trauma. In the traumatic tap the blood may clot or be unevenly distributed through the tube; however, the amount of blood usually decreases as the procedure continues, or in rare instances, when the tissues are traumatized late in the tap, blood suddenly appears or increases. In the bloody atraumatic tap, the synovial fluid usually is frankly bloody, does not change in appearance throughout the procedure, usually does not clot, and upon centrifugation may leave a xanthochromic supernatant. However, the latter is difficult to interpret because of the yellow appearance of normal synovial fluid.

Table 1
Collection and Analysis of Synovial Fluid

Sterile tube containing heparin
   Culture aerobically and anerobically
   Inoculate chocolate agar if gonococcus suspected
   Guinea pig inoculation if tuberculosis suspected
   Cultures for fungi if indicated
   Gram stain

Nonsterile tube containing heparin
   Color, viscosity, turbidity
   Cytology, white blood cell count and differential
   May be used for mucin test and crystal examination

Nonsterile tube with no anticoagulant
   Color, clot, viscosity, turbidity, supernatant
   Mucin determination
   Examination for crystals and inclusions
   Special studies: rheumatoid factor, complement, antinuclear
      antibody, protein, quantitative hyaluronic acid, quantitative
      lipid studies, HBsAg

Nonsterile tube with potassium oxalate
   Sugar analysis

In addition to the color of the fluid, note should be made as to whether it is clear, turbid, or grossly purulent. When the fluid pours easily and forms drops from the syringe with the ease of water, the viscosity is low. When it forms a tenacious string several inches in length before breaking, the viscosity is high. Normal synovial fluid has a high viscosity. The presence or absence of a clot should be observed as well as the viscosity.

Bacteriology

Appropriate cultures are carried out using fluid in the sterile tube containing heparin, and organisms may be concentrated in a sediment by spinning at 2000–5000 rpm in a clinical centrifuge for 15–30 minutes. This sediment also should be used for gram stain or Ziehl-Neelsen staining procedures in the direct examination for bacteria. Such smears are occasionally difficult to interpret because of precipitated hyaluronic acid. The immediate observations of pathogens, however, may save 24 hours in the treatment of pyogenic arthritis (a disease in which prognosis is directly related to speed of diagnosis and treatment) and therefore is a desirable procedure.

Routine Cytology

The synovial fluid that has been collected in anticoagulant is shaken for at least 4 minutes for thorough mixing, then is drawn up to the 0.5 mark in the white cell pipette. This is diluted to the 1.1 mark with the normal saline solution containing a small amount of methylene blue (to aid in differentiation of cell types) and shaken. It is essential to use the saline diluent and not the usual white cell diluent containing acetic acid, for the latter precipitates the hyaluronic acid–protein complex. If large numbers of erythrocytes are present in the fluid, affecting the accuracy of the white cell count, these may be lysed by the use of hypotonic (0.3 N) rather than normal saline. Red blood cells and white blood cells are counted in the hemocytometer chamber in the standard fashion (count cells in the four corner squares and multiply by 50), but the high-power ($\times 40$) objective should be used.

The preparation of the smears on coverslips is performed in the standard way for peripheral blood with minor modifications. If the nucleated count (white cell count) is over 5000/mm^3, a coverslip smear may be made directly from the anticoagulated synovial fluid. When the nucleated cell count is lower, the synovial fluid should be spun in a clinical centrifuge for 10 minutes at 2000–3000 rpm, the supernatant removed, and the sediment resuspended in a small quantity (10 drops or 0.5 ml) of the anticoagulated fluid or supernatant. A drop is then placed on a coverglass, and the preparation is pulled. The smear should be thin because in thick preparations the hyaluronic acid tends to blur the cell types in drying. The smear is air dried and stained with Wright's stain. Usually polymorphonuclear leukocytes, small lymphocytes, and large monuclear cells are recognizable, although occasionally vacuolization occurs in the preparation and possibly in vivo. At times lupus erythematosus (LE) cells may be detected on direct examination of synovial fluid smears even when LE preparations made from peripheral blood are negative. Unidentified cells should be described and so classified, and it should be remembered that in a rare case malignant cells may be found.

Although the white cell count and differential are not specific diagnostic parameters, they are among the most important laboratory aids in distinguishing different types of synovial fluids, at least within certain broad groupings. The major pitfall to be avoided in this simple procedure is the use of an acid diluent before the cell count. When this occurs and a precipitate from the hyaluronate forms, it traps white cells and the count is markedly reduced, often by as much as 50 percent.

The normal synovial fluid is remarkably acellular, containing under 200 white blood cells/mm^3 and no red cells. The percent of polymorphonuclear cells is also quite low, almost invariably under 25 percent of the total. Quantitative and qualitative changes in the leukocytes present in the fluid provide an indication of the magnitude of the inflammation in the surrounding synovial fluid. It is useful to classify all fluids as inflammatory or noninflammatory, a classification generally determined by the total white cell count and percent of polymorphonuclear cells (Table 2).

Noninflammatory effusions. These synovial fluids usually have average total white cell counts of about 1000/mm^3 occasionally as high as 2000/mm^3, and almost never exceeding 5000/mm^3. Polymorphonuclear leukocytes usually average under 30 percent. The synovial membrane in these conditions shows little if any evidence of inflammation; hence their categorization as noninflammatory. The disorders in this category include degenerative joint disease and traumatic arthritis.

Noninfectious mild inflammatory effusions. This particular group of disorders shows only minimal synovial membrane inflammation, and the joint fluids likewise often appear to be benign. The mean total white count is about 3000/mm^3 or less, and rarely is it higher than 5000/mm^3. The percent of polymorphonuclear cells usually averages under 30 percent. The disorders in this category often include systemic lupus erythematosus, scleroderma, and others.

Noninfectious severe inflammatory effusions. In these diseases the degree of synovial reaction varies from moderate to severe, and the total white count averages 14,000–21,000/mm^3. Although the total count rarely exceeds 50,000, in an occasional case of rheumatoid arthritis or gout it may do so, and indeed counts of over 100,000/mm^3 have been recorded in both disorders. Polymorphonuclear cells usually constitute over 50 percent of the white cells and not infrequently rise to 90 percent of the total white cell population. There is a rough correlation of apparent severity of the clinical symptoms and overt inflammatory process to the amount of the white cell count; i.e., severe acute disease is often associated with high counts, but there are exceptions to this generalization. The disorders in this category usually include rheumatoid arthritis, gout, pseudogout, rheumatic fever, and others.

Table 2
Classification of Major Diagnostic Categories of Articular Disease According to Their Average Synovial Fluid Findings

Diagnosis	Appearance	Total WBC/mm^3 Average (Range)	Polymorphonuclear Leukocytes (%)	Mucin Test	Crystals	Synovial Fluid–Blood Glucose Differential (mg/100 ml)
Normal	Clear yellow	200 (0–200)	7	Good	—	0
Group I: noninflammatory effusions						
Traumatic arthritis	Clear or bloody	1,500 (50–6,500)	20	Good	—	5
Degenerative joint disease	Clear or turbid	600 (50–3,750)	13	Good	—	5
Group II: noninfectious mild inflammatory effusions						
Systemic lupus erythematosus	Clear or slightly turbid	2,860 (0–8,600)	13	Good	—	5
Group III: Noninfectious severe inflammatory effusions						
Gout	Turbid	21,500 (100–160,000)	70	Poor	Monosodium urate	11
Pseudogout	Slightly turbid	14,200 (50–75,000)	68	Fair	Ca pyrophosphate dihydrate	
Rheumatic fever	Slightly turbid	17,800 (0–60,000)	50	Good–Fair	—	6
Rheumatoid arthritis	Turbid	19,000 (250–80,000)	66	Fair–Poor	—	30
Group IV: Infectious inflammatory effusions						
Reiter's (presumed infectious)	Turbid	18,500 (100–43,000)	60	Poor	—	16
Acute bacterial	Very turbid	80,000 (150–250,000)	90	Poor	—	91
Tuberculous	Turbid	20,000 (2,500–100,000)	60	Poor	—	70

The values in this table represent mean values from our laboratory and in selected instances from the appropriate literature.

Infectious effusions. The highest synovial fluid white counts occur in fluids infected with bacteria. Counts of over 100,000/mm^3 are almost invariably associated with acute infection. On the other hand, counts of under 50,000 may be found in infectious arthritis, and one must always be alert to this possibility. The counts in tuberculosis effusions are, on the whole, lower than in other specific joint infections. In Reiter's syndrome with associated effusions the count is variable, although it is usually elevated. In fluids infected with bacteria the percentage of polymorphonuclear leukocytes is quite high and usually constitutes over 90 percent of the white cells.

Although many of the common viral diseases are associated with frank arthritis and joint effusions, rela-

tively few synovial fluid analyses have been reported. The cases reported have been in patients with rubella arthritis, chicken pox associated arthritis, and hepatitis Bs antigen (Hbs-Ag) associated arthritis (see section on Infectious Arthritis in fascicle on Specific Articular and Connective Tissue Diseases). The white counts have varied widely; some have shown counts of under 5000 cells and many mononuclear cells, whereas some have shown counts of 10,000–40,000 cells with many polymorphonuclear cells.

Viscosity

The viscosity is determined primarily by the amount and the degree of polymerization of the hyaluronic acid of the synovial fluid. When drops of synovial fluid form long

(2 inches or more) tenacious strings on falling from a syringe or pipette, viscosity is usually normal. When the fluid forms drops like water, viscosity is very low.

Clot Formation

Normal synovial fluid does not clot due to the absence of fibrinogen and a variety of other clotting factors. Clots do occur, however, in pathologic fluids, and their size is roughly proportional to the severity of the inflammation. They have been graded in size as small (1+), moderate (2+), and large (3+) by estimating the clot size in relation to the volume of synovial fluid in the test tube. When the clot occupies one-fourth of the fluid volume, for example, it is graded as 1+; one-half of the volume, 2+; and so forth. The 3+ clots usually form soon after withdrawal of the synovial fluid, while the 1+ clots may not form for many hours.

Hyaluronic Acid

Synovial fluid hyaluronic acid can be measured by a variety of techniques, including a turbidimetric method, digestion and analysis for hexosamine, digestion and analysis for uronic acid, and analysis by a qualitative "mucin" test. The qualitative mucin test is simple to perform and reasonably reproducible, needs no special apparatus, and generally suffices as an estimate of the degree of polymerization of synovial fluid hyaluronate. The method below is suggested as part of the routine synovial fluid examination.

One ml of the joint fluid being tested is added to 4 ml of 2 percent acetic acid, mixed rapidly with a glass rod, and read promptly. When the mucin (hyaluronic acid–protein complex) is normal, a tight ropy mass forms in a clear solution. This is qualitatively called a "good" mucin. A softer mass with some shreds in solution constitutes a "fair" mucin, whereas a "poor" result shows shreds and small soft masses in a turbid solution. Finally, some fluids may result in only a few clumped flecks of mucin suspended in a cloudy solution—i.e., a "very poor" mucin test. In general, the more inflamed the joint, the worse the mucin test; fluids from rheumatoid joints often have "fair" mucin tests, infected joints have "poor" tests, while noninflammatory effusions demonstrate "good" mucin tests. For routine interpretation a written description of the results of the mucin test should always accompany the final grading.

It is occasionally important to determine after aspiration whether or not synovial fluid has indeed been obtained. For example, after aspirations of tendon sheaths or Baker's cysts, in which the cyst contents may be very inspissated, or after aspirations of swelling in which it is not clear whether the abnormality is articular or periarticular, the results may suggest a "dry tap." In such cases, or when there is a question of whether the syringe contains only tissue fluid or local anesthetic, it is helpful to know whether the synovial space has or has not been entered. The presence of hyaluronic acid and the sensitivity of qualitative methods of its analysis make it possible to detect synovial fluid in extremely small amounts. As little as 3 μg of hyaluronic acid (contained in only 0.5 μl

of synovial fluid) may be readily identified either by precipitation with diluted acetic acid or by staining with metachromatic dye.

In the former method, the material coating the barrel of the syringe, or only the aspirating needle, may be expelled directly into a test tube or the dried contents flushed into the tube with a small amount of saline or water. Two percent acetic acid (0.25 ml) is added, and the solution is mixed gently by flicking the tube with the finger. It is then examined alongside a control tube for the presence of turbidity or a mucin clot. Sensitivity is enhanced by the addition of two drops of 1 percent albumin solution. No interference arises from contamination with blood or local anesthetics, such as Xylocaine.

A similar quantity of synovial fluid, confined by evaporation with a hair dryer to a spot 0.5 cm in diameter on Whatman's filter paper (No. 44), will show distinct metachromasia in comparison with a control spot of normal saline after staining for 2 minutes with 0.25 percent aqueous toluidine blue. Metachromasia will be optimal after air drying for 5–10 minutes.

Glucose

Parallel samples for serum glucose should always be obtained. Under normal fasting conditions the level of glucose in synovial fluid parallels that in the serum. Unless the patient is fasting, the synovial fluid sugar determination is of little value unless markedly low (less than 40 mg/dl) since the entrance and exit of glucose from the joint space is apparently not a simple matter of diffusion alone. For example, 2–3 hours after eating the synovial fluid sugar may be higher than that of the serum.

With increasing inflammation, the fasting synovial fluid glucose falls significantly below the serum level; therefore, when severe inflammation of an infectious origin is suspected, a marked serum–synovial fluid difference may be of greater diagnostic assistance. Noninflammatory effusions, on the other hand, show no differences between serum and synoval fluid effusions. In mild inflammation, differences of up to 10 mg/dl of glucose may occur. In more severe noninfectious inflammation (e.g., rheumatoid arthritis), however, the difference may be no greater than 20–30 mg/dl, even when the synovial fluid leukocyte count exceeds 50,000/mm^3. In acute infections a synovial fluid serum glucose difference of over 50 mg/dl is not uncommon, and in some instances the amount of glucose in the joint fluid is so low that it cannot be measured.

Synovial Fluid Proteins

Techniques of analysis for synovial fluid proteins are numerous and almost identical with standard methods for demonstration of serum proteins. The major precaution that should be taken to ensure good separation of the various protein fractions is pretreatment with hyaluronidase to eliminate the hyaluronic acid present.

Rheumatoid factors may be found in synovial fluid in titers comparable to or slightly lower than those present in the sera of patients with rheumatoid arthritis. In fact, in some instances patients with negative serology have been observed to have rheumatoid factor in their synovial fluid, thus suggesting its local manufacture. On the other hand, some patients with the factors in their serum do not demonstrate them in their synovial fluid.

Antinuclear antibodies have been demonstrated in a variety of synovial fluids and studies have shown that the nuclear antigen or DNA content of synovial fluids is elevated regardless of the diagnosis. DNA particles have also been demonstrated histochemically in synovial fluid. Further studies, however, indicated that DNA, chiefly in the native form, can be demonstrated by immunodiffusion against specific antisera in synovial fluids from patients with a variety of diseases. Thus, the presence of DNA in synovial fluid may represent a nonspecific sequel to cell breakdown.

Concentrations of complement components in the joint space are the result of flow rates into and out of the space as well as any synthesis or catabolism that may occur locally. In the case of rheumatoid arthritis serum complement levels are usually normal or elevated. Synovial fluid levels, however, are often profoundly depressed, particularly in patients with positive tests for rheumatoid factor. The intraarticular depletion of whole complement activity has been found to be proportional to the titer of rheumatoid factor in the serum or synovial fluid. Studies have demonstrated depressions of C1 in some patients and marked reductions of C4 and C2 in most patients with seropositive disease. In synovial fluids of seronegative patients only C4 was depleted significantly. Low levels of synovial fluid complement have also been observed occasionally in bacterial arthritis, gout, and pseudogout. In addition, elevated synovial fluid levels of complement have been found in gout and pseudogout, in ankylosing spondylitis, and especially in Reiter's syndrome, in which they appear to be directly related to the severity and the duration of inflammation.

Cryoproteins have been found in rheumatoid and nonrheumatoid synovial fluids. The latter have generally been devoid of complement and consisted predominantly of fibrinogen, with DNA and IgG present but less frequently. It should be emphasized that rheumatoid synovial fluids contain a complex mixture of cryoprotins consisting of mixed immunoglobulins, bound complement components, DNA, and rheumatoid factors.

C-reactive protein (CRP) has been demonstrated experimentally in synovial fluid when inflammation was induced. Another observation is the presence of an iron-binding protein, lactoferrin, in synovial fluid. Its presence is associated with inflammation, and the level seems to correlate with the degree of leukocytosis.

Large amounts of fibrin are occasionally found in synovial fluids of patients with rheumatoid arthritis although the reason is not clear. Fibrinogen is found in inflammatory but not in normal fluids. Plasminogen and the plasminogen proactivator, however, are found in both normal and diseased fluids.

The vasoactive peptides, kinins, have also been implicated in synovial inflammation. Articular cartilage, cartilage extracts, and chondroitin sulfate have been shown to generate kininlike activity in plasma, presumably by activation of Hageman factor, and kinins have been demonstrated in synovial fluids from acutely inflamed joints.

Prostaglandin B, which arises from prostaglandins E and A, has been found to be elevated in synovial fluids of patients with inflammatory synovitis when compared to the levels in synovial fluids of patients with degenerative joint disease.

Crystals

One of the most significant and useful observations in recent years is that crystals of various types can be found free and in the cells of synovial fluid. By direct and especially by polarizing microscopy these crystals can be specifically identified and their appearance has been related to the inflammatory process.

Crystals that can cause inflammation (i.e., monosodium urate, calcium pyrophosphate dihydrate, and possibly calcium hydroxyapatite) are 0.5 to 20.0 μm in length, minimally soluble in water, and capable of being phagocytized by mononuclear and polymorphonuclear cells during the inflammatory response. At the height of the response, the majority of the crystals are intracellular, though the extracellular proportion increases as inflammation subsides. Other crystals, such as those of cholesterol, which are not so clearly related to inflammation, have also been observed in synovial fluid, and it is to be expected that more will be described in future studies.

To demonstrate crystals, a drop of synovial fluid (not collected in oxalate, since oxalate itself is birefringent), preferably from a fluid that has not clotted, is placed on a glass slide, covered with a thin glass coverslip, and examined with the polarizing microscope. The preparation should be scanned under low and then high power for extracellular and intracellular birefringent crystals. Birefringent or anisotropic materials are those that exhibit two refractive indices when plane-polarized light passes through them (Fig. 1). When the refractive index for light vibrating parallel to a given axis is greater than the index for light perpendicular to it, the birefringence is termed *positive* with respect to the axis and vice versa. Such systems are common in biologic materials; hence the usefulness of this procedure. When crystals are observed, the retardation plate (first-order red plate compensator) is inserted in the polarizing microscope between the crossed Nicol prisms (analyzer and polarizer). If, when the crystals are at right angles to the plane of slow vibration of light throughout the plate, they appear blue while those parallel are yellow, the phenomenon is termed *negative* birefringence. On the axis of the polarizer or analyzer the crystals are extinguished (their color blends in with that of the background).

Monosodium urate cyrstals demonstrate strong negative birefringence, are long (average 8–10 μm), and have a needlelike appearance (Fig. 2). They may be seen extracellularly or within polymorphonuclear or mononuclear cells. They are seen almost invariably in effusions associ-

USE OF FIRST-ORDER RED COMPENSATOR
(RETARDATION PLATE)

Long axis of monosodium urate crystals aligned parallel to direction of slow ray of compensator

Long axis of calcium pyrophosphate crystals aligned parallel to direction of slow ray of compensator

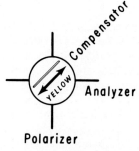

Color: yellow (negative birefringence)

Color: blue (positive birefringence)

Fig. 1. Polarization miscroscopy in synovial fluid analysis.

ated with acute gout and are virtually of pathognomonic significance (see section on Crystal-induced Arthritis: Gout in fascicle on Specific Articular and Connective Tissue Diseases). The fact that they may be observed in gouty joint fluids between attacks suggests that multiple factors contribute to the acute attack. The intracellular proportion of crystals is highest during the acute attack.

A second type of crystal, found both intracellularly and extracellularly, has been identified as calcium pyrophosphate dihydrate (CPPD) and is clearly associated with articular chondrocalcinosis and the acute arthritis called "pseudogout" (see chapter on Pseudogout in fascicle on Specific Articular and Connective Tissue Diseases). Crystals of this kind are elongated (often parallelopiped), are broader than urate crystals, may show an

apparent "line" running through them, and average 8–10 μ in length (Fig. 3). In the polarizing microscope they exhibit a weak positive birefringence. They have a high association with acute attacks of arthritis in patients having x-ray evidence of articular cartilage calcification (chondrocalcinosis). The crystals may be extracellular or within mononuclear or polymorphonuclear leukocytes.

A third type of crystal, identified as calcium hydroxyapatite, has been found in synovial fluid as well as in bursal and peritendinous exudates in calcific tendinitis. The crystalline material gives a chalky appearance to the synovial fluid and by light microscopy is extracellular, amorphorus, and often in clumps. These crystals are very difficult to see on standard light microscopy due to their small size.

Cholesterol crystals have also been observed in joint fluids. They are birefringent and have a rhombic structure with punched-out corners. These crystals are much larger than monosodium urate and CPPD crystals; they are not phagocytized by neutrophils and are usually seen in effusions of long duration. They do not appear to be related to an acute inflammatory reaction. On occasion, patients with crystal-induced synovitis have been found to have monosodium urate crystals as well as CPPD crystals.

Iatrogenic crystal-induced inflammation can occur following the injection of corticosteroid esters such as hydrocortisone acetate, prednisolone tertiary butyl acetate, etc. These synthetic esters are sparingly soluble microcrystals that initiate a mild to severe inflammatory reaction known as the "postinjection flare."

Cellular Inclusions

It is known that the synovial space contains considerable debris even when inflammation is minimal, and

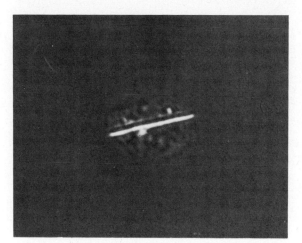

Fig. 2. Intracellular monosodium urate crystal.

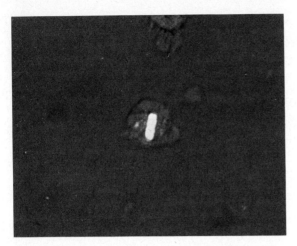

Fig. 3. Intracellular calcium pyrophosphate dihydrate crystal (CPPD).

that a large proportion of the cells in the synovial fluid have phagocytic potential. The inclusions that may be observed in most synovial fluid cells are assumed to represent phagocytized debris of diverse origins. Early observations of inclusion-bearing cells or ragocytes in synovial fluid indicated that these cells were present in large numbers in rheumatoid synovial fluids. They clearly are nonspecific, however, and occur in other inflammatory diseases such as rheumatic fever, Reiter's syndrome, septic arthritis, and scleroderma, whereas noninflammatory fluids obtained from patients with degenerative joint disease and traumatic arthritis rarely show inclusion cells. In rheumatoid arthritis as well as in other inflammatory diseases, cytoplasmic inclusions of synovial leukocytes stain positively with fluorescein-labeled antisera to IgG, IgM, IgA, components of the complement system, and nucleoprotein.

Although cells in the synovial lining may produce rheumatoid factor, only a very rare patient has a rheumatoid factor–positive synovial fluid in the presence of negative serology. In fact, synovial fluid may be negative in the face of high serum titers for rheumatoid factor. Thus, the number of inclusions cells in the synovial fluid is not specific for any disease, nor does the demonstration of rheumatoid factor in inclusions prove to be of practical diagnostic value in the great majority of patients. Inclusion cells can be estimated in a wet preparation of synovial fluid and recorded as another parameter of inflammation.

A variety of enzymes have been demonstrated in synovial fluid (see chapter on Synovial membrane in fascicle on Regional Structure and Function). Normal synovial membrane secretes a plasminogen activator that may prevent fibrin formation in the synovial space. This enzyme is significantly reduced in rheumatoid synovial fluid. The enzyme collagenase is found in normal synovial fluid but is at elevated levels in rheumatoid arthritis. In addition, enzymes that digest the protein core of pro-

teoglycans are believed to exist. The general increases in these synovial fluid enzymes in inflammatory types of arthritis are probably significant factors in the damage which occurs to articular cartilage.

Lipids

Lipid analysis is not a routine part of the joint fluid examination; however, analyses for cholesterol, phospholipids, neutral fats, and triglycerides on fasting fluids can be carried out in a clinical chemistry laboratory as they are on serum specimens. It appears that synovial fluid contains little lipid under normal circumstances but when it is associated with inflammatory (particularly rheumatoid) effusions the content rises markedly. The cholesterol content may be exceedingly high, and cholesterol crystals are not infrequently present.

Miscellaneous

Gross blood (not that from a traumatic arthrocentesis) is occasionally found in synovial fluid. A red cell count may be carried out as it is on whole blood. Bloody effusions are associated with hemophilia, pigmented villonodular synovitis, tumors of joints, some traumatic and neuropathic arthritides, and fractures adjacent to joints. Recurrent hemarthroses (and metal particles) have also been reported after prosthetic knee arthroplasty.

Fibrils may be noted in synovial fluids by light microscopy and may be drived from a variety of sources. Collagen is present, as has been shown by both electron microscopy and hydroxyproline analysis, although collagen fibers cannot be easily distinguished from fibrin in synovial fluid by either phase or polarization microscopy.

Many other measurements of substances in joint fluid have been carried out, but few are part of the routine joint fluid analysis. Studies of the penetration of various drugs into this space are of particular interest. Analyses of salicylates, adrenal corticosteroids, and antimicrobial agents are all of interest in particular disease states and undoubtedly will be important as synovial fluid takes its rightful place as one of the more useful and readily accessible body fluids for clinical, chemical, and research studies.

REFERENCES

Cohen AS, Brandt KD, Krey PR: Synovial fluid, in Cohen AS (ed): Laboratory Diagnostic Procedures in the Rheumatic Diseases, 2nd ed. Boston, Little, Brown, 1973, pp 1–62

Goldenberg DL, Cohen AS: Arthritis as a medical emergency, in Cohen AS, Freidin RB, Samuels MA (eds): Medical Emergencies: Diagnostic and Medical Procedures from Boston City Hospital. Boston, Little, Brown, 1977, pp 245–254

Oster G: Birefringence and dichroism, in Oster G, Pollister AW (eds): Physical Techniques in Biologic Research, vol 1. New York, Academic Press, 1955

Ropes MW, Bauer W: Synovial Fluid Changes in Joint Disease. Cambridge, Harvard University Press, 1953

Ruddy S, Austen KF: Complement and its components, in Cohen AS (ed): Laboratory Diagnostic Procedures in the Rheumatic Diseases, 2nd ed. Boston, Little, Brown, 1973, pp 131–157

Rheumatoid Factors

John S. Davis IV

Circulating proteins that react with antigenic sites on immunoglobulin G (IgG) molecules are characteristically found in patients with rheumatoid arthritis. These "antiantibodies" or "antiimmunoglobulins" have been named *rheumatoid factors* (RF) simply because of their association with rheumatoid arthritis. They have also been found with varying frequency in patients with most of the connective tissue diseases, many chronic and subacute infections, and a variety of miscellaneous disorders, and in many apparently healthy persons, particularly the elderly. Though initially RF were thought to reside exclusively in the IgM fraction, subsequent studies have shown that they exist in all major immunoglobulin classes.

HISTORY

Antibodies reacting with an individual's own immunoglobulins were first detected by Cecil, Nichols, and Stainsby in 1931; they found high titers of "streptococcal agglutinators" while using sera from certain patients with rheumatoid arthritis. In actuality, the streptococci were coated with IgG antistreptococcal antibody, and the RF were reacting with the IgG coat, thereby agglutinating the bacteria. Such an agglutination reaction is the principle for most of the subsequently devised tests.

Waaler and Rose later showed that sheep red blood cells "sensitized" with rabbit antibody to those cells could be agglutinated by a substance frequently found in the serum of patients with rheumatoid arthritis. In 1956, Singer and Plotz described a more practical assay using latex particles coated with human IgG. Subsequent studies showed that RF could agglutinate a variety of particles (e.g., bentonite and tanned red blood cells) coated with IgG obtained from numerous sources. Though a number of additional tests have been introduced, the latex fixation test still remains the most useful screening procedure.

CHARACTERISTICS

RF will react with the Fc portion of IgG molecules from a multitude of animal species; they react best with human or rabbit IgG. Serum RF have a rather weak avidity for native or undenatured IgG, and though they combine with the Fc portion of both native and aggregated IgG, they are best detected (for physicochemical reasons) by IgG that has undergone some conformational change.

RF usually exist in serum in a fraction detected on ultracentrifugation as a 22 S peak. These 22 S peaks will dissociate into 7 S and 19 S components when the sera are exposed to substances that can interfere with the interaction of antigens and antibodies. All of the agglutinating activity resides in the 19 S component, since RF will combine with 7 S IgG material from normal as well as diseased individuals (and IgG from other species).

It is not clear why the interaction of RF with IgG is so weak. The binding strength (avidity) is consistent with that seen in a variety of cross-reacting systems; it would also be consistent with the concept that more avid RF are already bound in vivo to insoluble or fixed IgG, possibly to IgG antibody that has already reacted with its own antigen. Thus the "free" RF found in serum and synovial fluid may simply be residual material.

IgG RF have also been extensively described and studied. Complexes have been found that are intermediate between 7 S and 19 S; when dissociated and reduced to their 7 S components many of them have RF activity. These 7 S RF are much more difficult to study than 19 S molecules because they are not good agglutinators and because they have the property of reacting with "self;" they may have important biologic functions.

IgA RF were first described in 1964. With the more recent observation that RF also exist in the IgD class, it becomes even more evident that RF are a broad group of antibodies with a wide range of specificities for IgG. It would appear that the vast majority of RF show primary reactivity for areas of the IgG molecule near or related to antigenic determinants on the Fc fragment of human or animal IgG. Other antiimmunoglobulins have specificities for sites on light chains as well as areas on heavy chains that have been revealed by proteolytic digestion.

RF react best with human IgG subclasses 1, 2, and 4 and very poorly with subclass 3. The shared antigen in those three subclasses is called *Ga autoantigenic determinant* and may have peculiar significance in the induction of RF in human disease. IgM RF can fix complement.

Monoclonal RF have also been described; some of these factors have been found in patients with Waldenstrom's macroglobulinemia. Some monoclonal RF have been associated with serum precipitins forming at low temperatures; these appear to be complexes of IgG and RF. The binding specificities of these monoclonal proteins seem to be somewhat different than those of the polyclonal factors seen in most disease states; these antiimmunoglobulins have been particularly useful as detectors of circulating immune complexes in a variety of systems.

METHODS OF MEASUREMENT

A variety of methods have been developed for measuring RF. The most commonly used test today is the latex slide agglutination test, in which latex particles coated with aggregated human 7 S IgG are agglutinated on a slide, usually at a 1:20 dilution of human serum (Fig. 1). A gross estimate of titer can be achieved by further serial dilutions of the serum. This test is a modification of the original latex tube test, in which the latex particle is agglutinated in solution, centrifuged, and the pattern in-

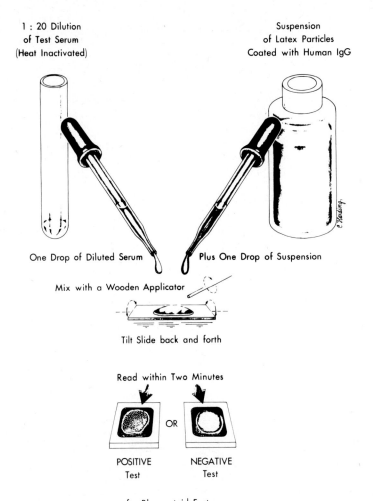

1 : 20 Dilution
of Test Serum
(Heat Inactivated)

Suspension
of Latex Particles
Coated with Human IgG

One Drop of Diluted Serum   Plus One Drop of Suspension

Mix with a Wooden Applicator

Tilt Slide back and forth

Read within Two Minutes

POSITIVE   NEGATIVE
Test   Test

for Rheumatoid Factors

Fig. 1.   Steps in the measurement of rheumatoid factor by the latex slide agglutination test.

terpreted according to various standards and controls. The tube dilution test has the advantage of being considerably more sensitive than the slide test, but it is more cumbersome to perform.

The sensitized sheep cell agglutination test (Waaler-Rose test) is still employed in many laboratories. Sheep cells coated with rabbit 7 S antibody to these erythrocytes are agglutinated by certain RF. It is important first to remove any anti-sheep cell antibodies from sera by suitable absorption so as not to produce false-positive test reactions. One must use fresh sheep cells that are standardized each day before use. This necessity for fresh cells makes the test somewhat awkward to perform on a routine basis, but the assay may have more specificity for the RF of rheumatoid arthritis.

A flocculation test using bentonite particles (instead of latex) coated with aggregated human IgG is still used in certain centers. However, there is no good evidence that the bentonite test has any advantage over the latex test.

A variety of other tests are also available in some laboratories. Formalinized and "tanned" sheep cells can be coated with aggregated human IgG; these cells are then agglutinated by RF. This test is very sentitive, but the assay is somewhat more difficult to perform than the latex tests and may not lead to any practical advantage in routine studies.

Another procedure that has enjoyed some vogue in recent years is the sensitized human cell agglutination test. Rh-positive, human red cells are coated with specific IgG (Ripley) antibody to the Rh antigen. According to some workers this test (like the Waaler-Rose) has increased specificity for patients with rheumatoid arthritis, but, unfortunately, Ripley serum is no longer available.

A radioimmunoassay for IgM RF has been developed. Torrigiani has advocated a method using insolubilized IgG as an immunoabsorbent from which RF can be eluted and characterized. Immunodiffusion tests have also been developed, employing both double (Ouchterlony) and single (Mancini) diffusion methodologies.

Serum to be tested for RF is best heated at 56°C before assay, since at least one labile complement component (Clq) can also agglutinate particles coated with

IgG, thus resulting in false-positive reactions; prozone phenomena are also seen.

BIOLOGIC FUNCTIONS

Controversy enshrouds possible roles of RF in rheumatoid arthritis and other disease states. Since so many elderly people produce RF, it is possible that it is a normal supplementary response mechanism to prolonged or repeated antigenic exposure. This would be consistent with the finding of RF in large numbers of Africans exposed to chronic parasite infestation. Thus RF may appear in patients with rheumatoid arthritis as a consequence of chronic inflammation or chronic infection; it might simply be an epiphenomenon.

About 70 percent of patients with rheumatoid arthritis have detectable RF. Patients without RF ("seronegative") appear to have a somewhat more benign disease. Systemic complications tend to occur more frequently in patients with RF, particularly those with very high titers; this observation suggests a pathogenetic role.

Since RF react with autologous IgG, RF could modify many of the functions of this immunoglobulin. As noted above, RF itself can fix complement, but under certain circumstances RF can block complement fixation by its IgG substrate. This balance between inhibition and augmentation of complement binding might have critical consequences in vivo.

RF can precipitate many soluble immune complexes such as DNA/(human)anti-DNA. Thus, RF might perform a critical function by making soluble complexes insoluble, thereby leading to problems or benefits for the individual, depending on the localization and subsequent metabolism of the complex. For instance, in the joint space RF might play a detrimental role by localizing soluble immune complexes which are then phagocytosed with the resultant release of lysosomal enzymes and tissue destruction. Contrariwise, the net effect of such localization might be to keep the soluble complexes from gaining entry to the circulation, where they might become damaging to such target organs as the kidney and lung.

Soluble complexes already in the circulation might react with RF and become insoluble; the result could be more effective clearance by the reticuloendothelial system. Tissue-fixed RF might even adsorb circulating immune complexes, leading to local problems (e.g., vasculitis) but less target organ disease (e.g., nephritis).

At the present time, there is increasing interest in the role of RF in lymphocyte modulation. Since some lymphocytes are coated with IgG, RF might react directly with this surface globulin; RF might even act as cell surface receptors.

With recent evidence that suppressor T cells are triggered by IgG-containing complexes (whereas helper T cells are activated by IgM-containing complexes), one could envision an extremely important modulating role for RF. If IgG complexes function in the feedback system by turning off further antibody production, RF (by coating these complexes with IgM) might instead promote activation of the antibody response. This hypothetical role, of course, would not hold for IgG and IgA RF, which might function quite differently.

It seems likely that RF play an important function in immune regulation. Peripherally they could greatly increase the thrust and potency of an antibody effect, especially in regard to clearance of antigen. Centrally, as a feedback modulator, they might also help maintain antibody production, particularly where there are less than optimal numbers of antibody-producing cells. By responding to the continual "pressure" of antigens with RF (as well as with specific antibody), the host would be maintaining the production of specific IgG antibody by inhibiting the suppression that would otherwise normally occur.

CLINICAL OBSERVATIONS

RF are clearly not specific for any disease entity; there is a correlation with age. Furthermore, not only is there documentation that approximately 5 percent of healthy subjects have RF, but some "normal persons" have very large amounts of these factors. RF are rarely demonstrable in children, even those with long-standing juvenile rheumatoid arthritis. There is some increased association of RF with urban (versus rural) residence, but not with any race or either sex.

RF may herald the appearance of rheumatoid arthritis or may appear late in the disease course. As mentioned previously, strongly positive tests for RF tend to correlate with the presence of nodules and a more relentless progressive course. Some patients with very large amounts of RF have developed hyperviscosity syndromes (with severe central nervous system problems); other patients may develop severe peripheral neuropathy, gangrenous ulcerations, and generally malignant disease. Some studies have shown that RF can be found at the site of severe vascular lesions in patients with rheumatoid arthritis. Production of RF occurs in plasma cells in and around affected joints, and high titers may be found in synovial fluid. Immunofluorescent studies of rheumatoid synovia have demonstrated deposits of IgG and IgM. Some of this material probably represents IgG/IgG RF or IgG/IgM RF which has been phagocytosed or become bound to local tissue. Many rheumatoid synovial cells will bind fluorescein-conjugated aggregated human IgG demonstrating the presence of RF on their surface.

A study in a rheumatic disease hospital in Finland did not reveal more serum RF in hospital employees than in a control group. In a number of identical twins of which only one has had rheumatoid arthritis, only the arthritic individual has been "seropositive."

About 10 percent of patients with juvenile rheumatoid arthritis have easily demonstrable RF. In careful studies looking for IgG RF, however, a much higher percentage of positives may be found. RF are found in about 30 percent of lupus erythmatosus patients and a small percentage of patients with polyarteritis nodosum and scleroderma. In Sjögren's syndrome and Felty's syndrome close to 100 percent of patients may have RF.

When tests for RF are positive early in patients with

rheumatoid arthritis they usually remain so indefinitely. Titers do not tend to fluctuate with disease activity, though the titer may fall with sustained remission. (Recent studies suggest that titers of RF may fall after treatment with penicillamine, gold, and various immunosuppressive drugs.)

The finding of RF in infectious diseases such as subacute bacterial endocarditis is of considerable interest. One study suggests that RF may be found in as many as 50 percent of such patients. These RF rarely react with rabbit antibody in the Waaler-Rose test. They tend to disappear completely after successful treatment of the infection. The transient appearance of RF after especially heavy prophylactic vaccination in army recruits has been noted.

An enigma is the remarkable association of rheumatoid arthritis (usually mild) and agammaglobulinemia. By definition, these patients should not have RF, but subcutaneous nodules have been described! Relatives of patients with acquired agammaglobulinemia may have an increased incidence of RF.

REFERENCES

Joshn PM, Faulk WP: Rheumatoid factor: Its nature, specificity, and production in rheumatoid arthritis. Clin Immunol Immunopathol 6:414, 1976
Williams RC: Rheumatoid factors and other serum components associated with rheumatoid arthritis, in: Rheumatoid Arthritis as a Systemic Disease. Philadelphia, Saunders, 1974, pp 154–176

Antinuclear Antibodies and the LE Cell Phenomenon

Eng M. Tan

NATURE OF ANTINUCLEAR ANTIBODIES AND THE LE CELL PHENOMENON

The initial discovery that opened the field of antinuclear antibodies was the report by Hargraves and associates of the lupus erythematosus (LE) cell phenomenon. Following this initial discovery, two important observations stimulated further work in this area. The first was the report by Haserick that the serum factor causing the LE cell phenomenon was present in the gamma globulin fraction of serum and was presumably an antibody. The other observation was made simultaneously in several laboratories, including those of Kunkel, Ceppellini, and Friou, that the LE cell factor was an antibody reactive with deoxyribonucleoprotein material. Subsequent studies have shown that the LE cell factor is only one of many serum autoantibodies that react with nuclear, cytoplasmic, and cell membrane antigens.

PATTERNS OF NUCLEAR STAINING

The term *antinuclear antibodies* (ANA) has become universally accepted because of common usage by many investigators, although the more correct terminology would be *autoantibodies* or *antibodies to nuclear antigens*. Traditionally, ANA is used in the literature to signify antibodies to nuclear antigens detected by the immunofluorescent technique. Organ sections have been used as substrates for detection of ANAs by this technique and different patterns of nuclear staining can be produced by the sera of patients with systemic lupus erythematosus (SLE). The four major patterns of nuclear staining (Fig. 1) include nuclear rim or peripheral staining, speckled nuclear staining, homogeneous nuclear staining, and nucleolar staining. Although these patterns of nuclear staining appear to be easily differentiated from each other, a number of features concerning the patterns of nuclear staining will be described. First, sera from patients with SLE often contain multiple antibodies which react with different nuclear antigens. Thus, patterns of nuclear staining may often be mixed patterns rather than distinctly of one type or another. Second, these different antibodies may be present in different concentrations in serum and on serial dilution different patterns of nuclear staining may be observed. Third, the patterns of nuclear staining illustrated in Figure 1 are patterns observed when using organ sections as substrate. Many commercial enterprises are now marketing ANA kits that use tissue culture cells as substrate. The patterns of nuclear staining on such cells may be different from those observed on organ sections, because tissue culture cells frequently contain concentrations of antigens different from those in cells of organs.

NATURE OF VARIOUS ANTIBODIES

With the combined use of several immunologic techniques, including immunofluorescence, complement fixation, immunodiffusion, and hemagglutination, the immunologic specificities of different ANA have been identified. They can be divided into those antibodies that are reactive with DNA, deoxyribonucleoprotein, histones, and nonhistone (acidic) nuclear proteins (Table 1).

Antibodies to DNA can be further subdivided into three main classes of antibody specificities. Antibodies that are reactive only with double-stranded DNA and not with single-stranded DNA have been reported but appear to be extremely rare and their clinical relevance is unknown. The second major group of antibodies to DNA are those that react in immunologic identity between double- and single-stranded DNA. By immunodiffusion tests, these antibodies appear to be reacting with antigenic determinants present in common on double- and single-stranded DNA. This type of antibody usually demonstrates a nuclear rim pattern of staining by immunofluorescence. High titers of this type of antibody are present in patients with SLE and this feature is often associated with nephritis. Antibodies to single-stranded DNA are

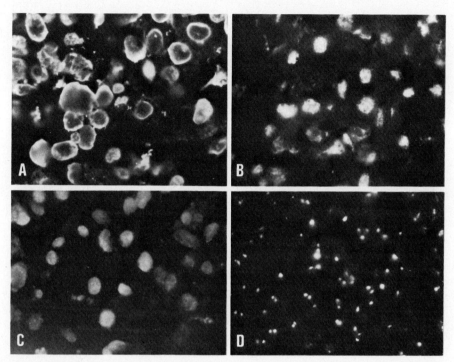

Fig. 1. Indirect immunofluorescent technique used to demonstrate antibodies to nuclear antigens; substrate was tissue section of mouse kidney. **A.** Nuclear rim pattern produced by antibodies to native DNA and nucleohistones. **B.** Speckled pattern produced by antibodies to nonhistone proteins. **C.** Homogeneous pattern produced by antibodies to histones. **D.** Antibodies in SLE sera producing nucleolar staining have not been analyzed.

Table 1
Autoantibodies to Nuclear Antigens

Antigenic Specificity	Characteristics of Antigenic Determinants	Immunofluorescent Pattern	Clinical Features
DNA			
Double-stranded DNA	Double-stranded helix essential	Not known	Very few reported; clinical significance unknown
Double- and single-stranded DNA	Common antigenic determinant on DS- and SS-DNA	Nuclear rim staining	High titers in SLE; often associated with nephritis
Single-stranded DNA	Purines and pyrimidines on DNA and RNA	No staining of nuclei in organ sections	Present in rheumatic and nonrheumatic (infectious) diseases
Deoxyribonucleoprotein	DNA–histone complex	Rim or homogeneous nuclear staining	"LE cell factor"
Histones	H1, H2A, H2B, H3, and H4	Rim or homogeneous nuclear staining	"LE cell factor;" high prevalence in drug-induced LE
Nonhistone (acidic) nuclear proteins			
Sm antigen	DNA-binding protein	Speckled nuclear staining	Highly specific for SLE
Nuclear RNP	RNA–protein complex	Speckled nuclear staining	Present in SLE, mixed connective tissue disease, and other rheumatic diseases
SS-B antigen	Nonhistone protein	Speckled nuclear staining	Present in SLE and Sjögren's syndrome
Blastoid cell nuclear antigen	Nonhistone protein of "activated" cells	Speckled nuclear staining	Present in few patients with SLE

those that are reactive with purines and pyrimidines on nucleic acids and are therefore often cross-reactive antibodies between single-stranded DNA and single-stranded RNA. Because purines and pyrimidines are not "exposed" and available for reactivity on double-stranded DNA, this type of DNA antibody is not reactive with the latter. By immunofluorescence no staining of nuclei is obtained on organ sections, but in tissue culture cells staining of dividing chromosomes is seen in cells undergoing mitotic division. This type of antibody is present in both rheumatic and nonrheumatic diseases, particularly in those nonrheumatic diseases characterized by chronic infectious processes.

Antibodies to deoxyribonucleoprotein have been studied extensively and have been shown to be the LE serum factor. The presence of antibody to deoxyribonucleoprotein is almost always detectable in those patients who have positive LE cells. The antibody has been shown to be reactive with DNA–histone complex, and by immunofluorescent staining a rim or homogeneous pattern of nuclear staining is observed.

Antibodies to histones are also present in the sera of approximately 35 percent of patients with SLE. However, antibodies to histones are present in almost all (96 percent) patients with LE-like disease induced by the ingestion of drugs such as procainamide and hydralazine. Antibodies to histones almost always demonstrate rim or homogeneous patterns of nuclear staining. The ability to recognize antibodies to histones has, in practice, been extremely useful in differentiating between patients with drug-induced LE and patients who spontaneously develop SLE.

Antibodies to the nonhistone (acidic) nuclear proteins have received intensive interest in recent years because it has been demonstrated that some of these antibodies may be used for diagnostic purposes to differentiate between rheumatic diseases. For example, anti-body to Sm antigen, which has been shown to be a DNA-binding protein and gives a speckled nuclear staining pattern, is highly specific for SLE. It has been suggested that this is a "marker" antibody for SLE. Antibody to another nonhistone nuclear protein is antibody to a nuclear RNA–protein complex. This antibody is also present in patients with SLE, but a characteristic of this antibody is its high association with mixed connective tissue disease. This antibody also gives a speckled pattern of nuclear staining. Indeed, all antibodies to the nonhistone or acidic nuclear proteins give speckled patterns of nuclear staining. Antibodies to two other nonhistone nuclear protein antigens are also seen in the sera of patients with SLE. They are antibody to the SS-B antigen and antibody to a blastoid cell nuclear antigen. Antibody to SS-B antigen is present in SLE but has a higher association with Sjögren's syndrome.

It is clear to a student of this disease that SLE is characterized by a multitude of antibodies to nuclear antigens. However, autoantibodies to other intracellular antigens have also been reported (Table 2). These include antibodies to nucleolar antigens that can be detected by immunofluorescence in a low percentage of patients with SLE. At the present time nothing is known about the clinical significance of antinucleolar antibodies in SLE.

Antibodies to ribosomal ribonucleoprotein have been reported to be present in a high incidence in SLE patients with renal disease. This antibody gives cytoplasmic and nucleolar staining. The antigen is present in the ribosomal fraction of cytoplasm. In addition, antibodies to the Ro and La antigens have been reported. Some sera containing antibodies to Ro and La antigens appear not to have ANA and therefore no nuclear staining is observed. These patients have been reported to have clinical features of SLE, and it has been suggested that they might be patients with SLE who are negative for ANA. Antibodies to single- and double-stranded RNA

Table 2
Autoantibodies to Other Intracellular Antigens

Antigenic Specificity	Characteristics of Antigenic Determinants	Immunofluorescent Pattern	Clinical Features
Nucleolar antigens	Several antigens present but none characterized	Nucleolar staining	Not known in SLE; also present in Raynaud's disease and scleroderma
Cytoplasmic antigens			
Ribosomal RNP	RNA–protein complex of ribosomes	Cytoplasmic and nucleolar staining	? High incidence of renal disease
Ro antigen	Cytoplasmic protein devoid of RNA	Not known	Not known
La antigen	Cytoplasmic RNA–protein not present in ribosomes	Not known	Not known
Other antigens			
Single-stranded RNA	Poly A, poly U, and other polynucleotides	Not known	Not known
Double-stranded RNA	Poly A–poly U, poly I–poly C	Not known	Not known

have been reported in the sera of patients with SLE. No specific patterns of immunofluorescent staining have been correlated with these antibodies, and, generally, the clinical significance of these antibodies is not known.

REFERENCES

Hargraves MM, Richmond H, Morton R: Presentation of two bone marrow elements: The "tart" cells and the "LE" cell. Mayo Clin Proc 23:25, 1948

Haserick JR, Lewis LA, Bortz DW: Blood factor in acute disseminated lupus erythematosus. I. Determination of gammaglobulin as specific plasma fraction. Am J Med Sci 219:660, 1950

Mattioli M, Reichlin M: Heterogeneity of RNA protein antigens reactive with sera of patients with systemic lupus erythematosus. Arthritis Rheum 17:421, 1974

Robbins WE, Holman HR, Deicher H, Kunkel HG: Complement fixation with cell nuclei and DNA in lupus erythematosus. Proc Soc Exp Biol Med 96:575, 1957

Sharp GC, Irwin WS, May CM, Holman HR, McDuffie FC, Hess EV, Schmid FR: Association of antibodies to ribonucleoprotein and Sm antigens with mixed connective tissue disease, systemic lupus erythematosus and other rheumatic diseases. N Engl J Med 295:1149, 1976

Tan EM, Kunkel HG: Characteristics of a soluble nuclear antigen precipitating with sera of patients with systemic lupus erythematosus. J Immunol 96:464, 1966

Tan EM, Schur P, Carr RI, Kunkel HG: Deoxyribonucleic acid (DNA) and antibodies to DNA in the serum of patients with systemic lupus erythematosus. J Clin Invest 45:1732, 1966

CLINICAL SIGNIFICANCE AND METHODS OF DETECTION OF ANTINUCLEAR ANTIBODIES AND THE LE CELL PHENOMENON

Since antinuclear antibodies (ANA) are present in many systemic rheumatic diseases, the single observation that a serum is positive for ANA will not contribute much information helpful in the diagnosis or in following response to treatment. Current techniques of detection and the clinical significance of their findings are discussed in this chapter.

CLINICAL SIGNIFICANCE

With the techniques available at present, further information concerning specificities of ANA should be obtained. As a first step, the laboratory reporting a positive ANA should also state the titer of ANA and the pattern of nuclear staining, including changes of pattern, if observed. This is particularly important in the context of the clinical information that is available to the attending physician. A low titer of ANA may not be clinically relevant in an elderly person who has arthritis as a minor complaint but may be extremely relevant in a young female patient with obscure musculoskeletal symptoms. There is no simple answer to the question, "At what titer could an ANA be considered significant?" It should be realized that there probably is no such entity as a false-positive ANA but that a low-titered ANA may not always be clinically pertinent to the patient's problem at that time.

Table 1
Prevalence of Certain Antinuclear Antibodies in Rheumatic Diseases

Disease	Antibodies to		
	Native DNA	Sm antigen	Nuclear RNP
Systemic lupus erythematosus	35/50 (70)*†	14/50 (28)	13/50 (26)
Rheumatoid arthritis	12/30 (40)	0/30 (0)	3/30 (10)
Sjögren's syndrome	8/28 (29)	0/28 (0)	1/28 (3)
Scleroderma	15/27 (55)	0/27 (0)	6/27 (22)
Dermatomyositis	5/20 (25)	0/20 (0)	0/20 (0)
Discoid lupus	8/16 (50)	0/16 (0)	4/16 (25)
Mixed connective tissue disease	6/12 (50)	1/12 (8)	12/12 (100)
Control	4/96 (4)	0/25 (0)	0/25 (0)

*Numbers in parentheses are percentages.

†Mean titer of native DNA antibody in SLE is significantly higher ($p < 0.01$) than mean titer in all other rheumatic diseases.

It has become quite clear that ANA of certain specificities appear to be segregated in some rheumatic diseases. For example, antibody to the Sm antigen has been detected in 28 percent of patients with SLE (Table 1), while in more than 200 other patients with different rheumatic diseases, only one patient (with the mixed connective tissue disease) had antibody to Sm antigen. As mentioned previously, antibody to this antigen may represent a "marker" antibody for SLE and may be extremely helpful for diagnostic purposes. In addition, SLE patients with anti-Sm antibody have been reported to constitute a subset of SLE cases characterized by chronic hypocomplementemia, skin lesions, and mild renal disease. Antibody to nuclear RNP is present in many rheumatic diseases, including SLE, discoid lupus, and scleroderma, and in a lower percentage in other diseases such as rheumatoid arthritis and Sjögren's syndrome. In the mixed connective tissue disease, however, antibody to nuclear RNP is present in all patients. In several reported studies, patients with the mixed connective tissue disease have had extremely high titers of antibodies to nuclear RNP and an absence of antibodies to other nuclear antigens.

Seventy percent of patients with SLE were found to have antibodies to native DNA (Table 1). However, patients with other rheumatic diseases were also found to have antibodies to native DNA. It is important to point out that in rheumatic diseases other than SLE, antibodies to native DNA may be present in low titers in contrast to the higher titers present in patients with SLE.

Studies by several laboratories have shown that ANA present in the blood have the capacity to bind with antigens in the circulation. This results in the formation of soluble antigen–antibody complexes that start a chain of inflammatory events, one of which is the binding of complement to the complex and the release of inflammatory

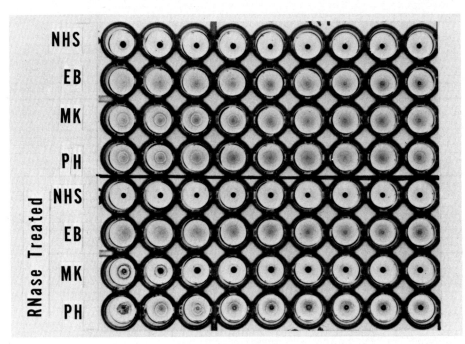

Fig. 1. Hemagglutination technique used to detect antibodies to Sm antigen and nuclear RNP (sometimes called ENAs). The upper set of wells shows reactions observed using red cells coated with both Sm and nuclear-RNP antigens; the lower set of wells, with red cells coated only with Sm antigen (after ribonuclease treatment of coated red cells). NHS, normal human serum, showing no reaction with either type of red cell; EB, serum containing antibody to Sm; MK, serum containing antibody to nuclear-RNP; PH, serum containing antibodies to both antigens with antibody to nuclear RNP present in higher concentration than antibody to Sm.

peptides from complement breakdown products. The final result of this inflammatory mechanism is the production of immune complex–mediated vasculitis. One of the organs most commonly affected is the kidney, where the clinical picture of glomerulonephritis evolves. The immune complex system that is of most clinical significance comprises DNA and antibody to DNA. Other antigen–antibody complexes, particularly those involving the nonhistone nuclear protein antigens, are also known to be involved but may be of less importance. Two of the important aims of therapy in SLE are the suppression of the level of circulating antibody to native DNA and the suppression of circulating immune complexes.

METHODS

The use of the indirect immunofluorescent technique for the detection of antibodies to nuclear antigens has already been described. Some of the other important new developments in this area have been the following. Radioimmunoassay methods have been developed for the detection of antibodies to DNA. Two methods are in general use by several laboratories and both employ radio-labeled DNA from mammalian, bacterial, or viral origins. Either the Farr (ammonium sulfate precipitation) technique or a membrane filter technique is used to detect antibodies binding to labeled DNA. One of the variabilities with this technique is the use of different sources of labeled DNA by different laboratories with the result that levels of binding to DNA considered significant vary from one laboratory to another. A standardized labeled DNA preparation is not yet available. An immunofluorescent method for the detection of antibodies to native DNA has been recently introduced with the use of an organism, *Crithidia luciliae*. This organism has a kinetoplast that contains native DNA reported to be free of histones and nonhistone proteins. The use of *C. luciliae* for the detection of antibodies to native DNA is becoming more widespread. A minor limitation is the fact that the technique is less sensitive than radioimmunoassay.

The hemagglutination technique has been used for detection of antibodies to certain nonhistone nuclear antigens. One assay for which this is used has been called antibody to extractable nuclear antigen(s) (ENA). Although there was initial confusion concerning the content of ENA, it is now clear that this material contains several nonhistone nuclear antigens, including Sm antigen and nuclear RNP. In the hemagglutination method, sheep red cells are coated with both Sm and nuclear RNP antigens in one assay and, simultaneously, another assay is done with red cells coated only with Sm antigen (Fig. 1). The ribonuclease-treated red cells that are coated only with Sm antigen are shown in the lower portion of this figure. Serum EB reacts to the same titer with Sm-RNP-coated red cells and with Sm-coated red cells. However, serum MK reacts with Sm-RNP-coated red cells but is negative with Sm-coated red cells. The interpretation here is that EB serum contains antibody to Sm antigen, whereas MK serum contains antibody to nuclear RNP antigen, which is the antigen that is sensitive to ribonuclease. Some sera, like PH, contain both antibodies and are reactive at higher titer with RNP and at lower titer with Sm antigen.

REFERENCES

Aarden LA, De Groot ER, Feltkamp TE: Immunology of DNA. III. Crithidia luciliae, a simple substrate for the determination of anti-dsDNA with the immunofluorescence technique. Ann NY Acad Sci 254:505, 1975

Notman DD, Kurata N, Tan EM: Profiles of antinuclear antibodies in systemic rheumatic diseases. Ann Intern Med 83:464, 1975

Acute Phase Phenomena

Mark B. Pepys

ACUTE PHASE PROTEINS AND ERYTHROCYTE SEDIMENTATION

The *acute phase response* or *reaction* is the name given to a characteristic increase in the concentration of some plasma proteins that occurs within hours to days of most forms of acute tissue damage, including physical or chemical trauma, infection, infarction, intoxication, immunologic injury, pregnancy, and the puerperium. Similar changes, the magnitude of which often parallels disease activity, persist during chronic inflammation, such as that associated with chronic infection, collagen disease and other nontransmissible inflammatory conditions, and malignant neoplasia. The functions of many of the acute phase reactants are not known, nor are the mechanisms by which the reaction is mediated, though in some cases elevated plasma levels are known to reflect increased synthesis.

ACUTE PHASE PROTEINS

The plasma proteins that increase in concentration in an acute phase response are known as *acute phase reactants*. They include C-reactive protein (CRP), fibrinogen, some protease inhibitors, some transport proteins, most complement components, and various other proteins of unknown function (Table 1). At the same time as the acute phase protein concentrations rise the levels of certain other plasma proteins may fall, particularly albumin, transferrin, α and β lipoproteins, inter-α-trypsin inhibitor, and properdin (Table 1); the concentration of α_2 macroglobulin tends to remain constant. There may be a transient initial fall after an acute episode before the levels of most acute phase proteins rise over the first day or so to attain maximal concentrations that are usually between 150 and 500 percent of normal. The rate of change and peak concentration differ significantly and independently between different acute phase proteins, in different acute clinical situations, and in different individuals after the same episode. There may also be different patterns of elevation of various proteins in different chronic diseases.

In infections and in conditions with abnormal immunologic function a distortion of the normal plasma protein pattern additional to and distinct from the acute phase reaction may be produced by elevated concentrations of

Table 1
Plasma Protein Profile in the Acute Phase Reaction

Proteins	Increased	Decreased
Coagulation proteins	Fibrinogen Prothrombin Factor VIII Plasminogen	
Protease inhibitors	α_1 Antitrypsin α_1 Antichymotrypsin	Inter-α-antitrypsin
Transport proteins	Haptoglobin Hemopexin Ceruloplasmin	Transferrin
Complement proteins	C1s, C1INH C2, factor B C3, C4, C5 C$\overline{56}$	Properdin
Miscellaneous	C-reactive protein (CRP) α_1-acid glycoprotein Gc globulin Cold-insoluble globulin Serum amyloid A-related protein (SAA)	Albumin Prealbumin α_1 Lipoprotein β Lipoprotein

immunoglobulins. These may contribute largely to the indirect assays of plasma protein profile, such as erythrocyte sedimentation rate (ESR) and plasma viscosity.

Elevation of CRP is the most constant and dramatic feature of the acute phase reaction both to different stimuli and in different individuals. CRP is exceptional among the acute phase proteins in several respects. Its concentration is low in normal healthy individuals (median in adults, 580 ng/ml, interquartile range 68 ng to 2.0 μg/ml), but rises rapidly within hours of an acute insult and may exceed 500 μg/ml in very active acute or chronic inflammation. With recovery it falls toward normal more rapidly than the other acute phase proteins. These properties, and the fact that the degree of elevation is much greater in some diseases than in others, make CRP the most useful single acute phase protein to measure in clinical conditions.

The serum amyloid A–related protein (SAA), which is thought to be the precursor of the major fibril protein AA of secondary amyloid, has recently been described as an acute phase reactant (see the section on Amyloidosis in the fascicle on Specific Articular and Connective Tissue Diseases). The normal plasma concentration is about 10 ng/ml and it may rise to over 2.5 μg/ml, starting within hours of onset of an acute episode. It is also elevated in apparently healthy old age as well as in pregnancy, chronic infections, chronic inflammatory diseases, and malignancy. Its significance in clinical management remains to be established.

The mechanisms by which diverse events can stimulate acute phase responses are not known. Postoperatively the time course of the acute phase reaction follows that of negative nitrogen balance, but manipulation of nitrogen balance does not affect it. The processes by which many of the acute phase proteins increase in concentration are also not known, though in the case of CRP, fibrinogen, haptoglobin, and ceruloplasmin increased hepatic synthesis is responsible.

Even where activities such as protease inhibition, transport, or coagulation are recognized, the precise in vivo role of the acute phase reaction is poorly understood. CRP binds in vivo to phospholipids that are ubiquitous in cell membranes and it interacts with the complement system, lymphocytes, phagocytic cells, and platelets. It may therefore participate in inflammatory or repair reactions, or both. The existence, in other species as phylogenetically distant as the teleosts, of proteins structurally homologous with CRP, and with the same binding specificity for choline phosphatides, supports the idea that CRP has an important function.

ERYTHROCYTE SEDIMENTATION

Sedimentation of erythrocytes proceeds very slowly in blood from healthy individuals because the negative zeta potential of erythrocytes prevents their aggregation. Increased concentrations of plasma proteins attenuate the zeta potential so that rouleaux formation occurs and these aggregates sediment more rapidly. Asymmetric macromolecules, such as fibrinogen and immunoglobu-

lins, exert a disproportionately large effect on the dielectric coefficient of plasma and hence on ESR. The same protein changes increase plasma viscosity, but the enhancement of sedimentation rate by erythrocyte aggregation greatly exceeds the retarding effect exerted by increased plasma viscosity per se. This is also true when transfused macromolecules that agglutinate red cells, such as dextrans and polyvinylpyrrolidone, are responsible rather than plasma proteins. However, extreme hyperviscosity of plasma in some cases of dysproteinemia, such as myeloma, can rarely prevent erythrocyte sedimentation.

At constant red cell concentration the relative contributions of the plasma proteins to the ESR are fibrinogen 10, α_2 globulins 5, γ globulins 2, and albumin 1. CRP concentration within the range observed in vivo has no effect on ESR. Under conditions in which IgG levels are not appreciably raised, ESR correlates best with the concentrations of fibrinogen, α_1-acid glycoprotein, α_2 macroglobulin, and α_1 antitrypsin, caeruloplasmin, and IgM. In dysproteinemic syndromes, such as myeloma, macroglobulinemia, cryoglobulinemia, cold agglutinin disease, and others, elevation of the ESR may result from the high concentration of the abnormal protein even when the levels of acute phase reactants are normal.

Reduction of the hematocrit increases ESR, probably by accelerating aggregation and reducing frictional forces between the sedimenting aggregates. Elevation of the hematocrit may cause abnormally low or retarded erythrocyte sedimentation, although in polycythemia vera this can occur even with a normal hemoglobin concentration. The shape, size, and hemoglobin content of the erythrocytes can all alter the ESR; for example, in sickle cell disease the ESR is reduced and cannot be used as an index of intercurrent illness.

MEASUREMENT OF ESR

The measurement of ESR is probably the test most widely used in screening for organic disease and in monitoring progress of inflammatory disease. A number of methods are available but the International Committee for Standardization in Hematology has proposed a standard procedure based on the Westergren method. Anticoagulated blood is diluted with one-quarter of its volume of sodium citrate and permitted to sediment in a 300-mm glass tube held vertically. The distance from the surface meniscus to the tip of the sedimenting column of red cells after 1 hour is recorded as the ESR. A large number of technical variables must be controlled to provide reproducible and valid results, but the procedure is nonetheless relatively simple.

In the alternative Wintrobe method undiluted blood sediments in a 100-mm tube. This method is more sensitive than the Westergren method to minimal elevations of asymmetric macromolecules in the plasma. On the other hand, when the Westergren ESR exceeds 50 mm/hr the Wintrobe ESR is anomalously low in up to 25 percent of cases. For mild elevations of ESR the Wintrobe method may be adequate, particularly as it can be corrected for the effect of hematocrit by the Hynes-Whitby curves. For moderately and grossly elevated ESR and for monitoring activity in chronic disease the Westergren procedure is preferable, even though there is no adequate method of correcting for anemia. The ESR can be measured in neonates using capillary blood and miniaturized techniques that correlate well with the standard Wintrobe method.

An alternative to the ESR is the recently described zeta sedimentation ratio (ZSR), which is a measure of the closeness with which red cells in whole blood will approach each other under a standardized stress. Anticoagulated blood in a vertical capillary tube is centrifuged in a special apparatus which subjects the erythrocytes to four cycles of alternate compaction and dispersion. The hematocrit of the blood in the portion of the tube containing red cells at the end of this procedure is called ZSR. Its value is affected, as is ESR, by sickle cells or marked poikilocytosis but it is independent of anemia and increases linearly with increasing plasma concentrations of fibrinogen and/or gamma globulin over the clinical range. There are also technical advantages over ESR measurement, and although extensive clinical experience is not yet available, the ZSR has been found to be useful in management of rheumatic disease.

Measurement of plasma viscosity has not been widely adopted for routine clinical purposes. It is not technically difficult and correlates better than does the ESR with concentrations of fibrinogen and alpha and gamma globulins. It also has the advantage over ESR and ZSR of not being affected by numbers or morphology of red cells.

REFERENCES

Aronsen KF, Ekelund G, Kindmark CO, Laurell CB: Sequential changes of plasma proteins after surgical trauma. Scand J Clin Lab Invest 29 [Suppl 124]:127, 1972

Bull BS, Brailsford JD: The zeta sedimentation ratio. Blood 40:550, 1972

Bull BS, Brecher G: An evaluation of the relative merits of the Wintrobe and Westergren sedimentation methods, including hematocrit correction. Am J Clin Pathol 62:502, 1974

Hutchinson RM, Eastham RD: A comparison of the erythrocyte sedimentation rate and plasma viscosity in detecting changes in plasma proteins. J Clin Pathol 30:345, 1977

International Committee for Standardization in Hematology: Reference method for the erythrocyte sedimentation rate (ESR) test on human blood. Br J Haematol 24:671, 1973

Johansson BG, Kindmark CO, Trell EY, Wollheim FA: Sequential changes of plasma proteins after myocardial infarction. Scand J Clin Lab Invest 29 [Suppl 124]:117, 1972

Pepys MB, Dash AC, Fletcher TC, Richardson N, Munn EA, Feinstein A: Analogues in other mammals and in fish of human plasma proteins, C-reactive protein and amyloid P-component. Nature 273:168, 1978

Rosenthal CJ, Franklin EC: Variation with age and disease of an amyloid A protein–related serum component. J Clin Invest 55:746, 1975

CLINICAL SIGNIFICANCE OF ACUTE PHASE PHENOMENA

The pathophysiologic significance of the acute phase response is not clear, nevertheless it has considerable clinical importance. The nonspecificity of the reaction makes its measurement a useful screening test for physical disease while the correlation with disease activity provides a monitor of progress and therapy. Quantitation of acute phase changes in the plasma is simple and can be made either indirectly by their effect on erythrocyte sedimentation or on plasma viscosity, or directly by estimating the concentration of individual proteins.

SIGNIFICANCE OF ABNORMAL ESR

The normal values used by Westergren were 1–3 mm/hr for men and 4–7 mm/hr for women. These have been broadened to 0–10 mm/hr for men and 0–15 mm/hr for women, and indeed certain studies suggest that the upper limit of normal increases with age. While the aforementioned levels are commonly used, several analyses of large numbers of sera suggest a normal of up to 15 for men or 25 for women up to age 50; and normals of up to 20 for men and up to 30 for women over age 50. Healthy women taking oral contraceptives frequently have ESR levels above normal.

Apart from technical errors, an abnormally low ESR (0–1 mm/hr) has characteristically been associated with a number of different conditions (Table 1), but in 95 percent of cases none of these are present: 40 percent of individuals in a hospital practice with low ESR have no detectable organic disease; in 15 percent slight elevation of hemoglobin may be responsible; and the remainder have a variety of unrelated disorders.

Elevation of ESR above normal is to be expected whenever there is an acute phase reaction or an elevation of plasma immunoglobulin or both, thus covering a very broad spectrum of disease. However, a raised ESR is not invariable in organic disease; in some cases it may not rise because sedimentation is impaired in association with

Table 1
Conditions Associated with Low ESR

Red cell abnormality
  Polycythemia
  Hemoglobinopathy
  Hereditary spherocytosis
  Pyruvate kinase deficiency

Plasma protein abnormality
  Hypofibrinogenemia
  Hyperproteinemia with hyperviscosity (myeloma, etc.)

Cardiac insufficiency
  Congestive cardiac failure
  Cyanotic congenital heart disease

Miscellaneous
  Severe cachexia
  Increased serum bile salt concentration
  Antiinflammatory drug therapy

Table 2
Conditions Associated with High ESR (≥100 mm/1 hr)

Disorder	Incidence in Different Series* (%)		
	A	B	C
Infection	53	44	
Connective tissue disease	33	24	25
Neoplasia	14	12	58
Renal disease		6	8
Miscellaneous		14	
Undetermined			6

*A, Payne, 1968; B, Cheah and Ransome, 1971; C, Zacharski and Kyle, 1967.

an intercurrent condition (Table 1), or because the usual alteration of plasma proteins concomitant with inflammation and tissue damage does not take place. A contrasting clinical situation is the presence of a raised ESR in the absence of any obvious cause. If the level is modest up to one-third of cases return to normal within 4–6 weeks, and further investigation or the emergence of symptoms with passage of time reveals a cause in most of the remainder. The frequency of different diagnoses established in such patients obviously varies with the nature of the clinical practice.

Among patients in general hospital practice who have gross elevation of ESR of 100 mm/hr or more (Table 2) about one-half have infections, usually of the respiratory or urinary tracts. Up to one-third have some form of connective tissue disease (most commonly rheumatoid arthritis), about 15 percent have neoplasms (usually metastatic malignancy, and including myeloma and other dysproteinemias), and up to 10 percent have some form of renal disease. About 5 percent have miscellaneous other conditions, leaving a final 5 percent in whom a diagnosis is not rapidly established by investigation or in whom it is apparently unrelated to the degree of ESR elevation.

In a referral center the pattern of diagnostic categories may tend to vary. In one series, for example (Table 2), over one-half the patients with ESR greater than 100 mm/hr suffered from malignancy (the commonest forms being lymphoma, large bowel carcinoma, breast carcinoma, and myeloma); proportionately less had banal bacterial infections. Among the few patients in whom a diagnosis is not rapidly established a cause emerges in the majority, but in most reported series there remain very occasional individuals in whom serious illness fails to develop despite ESR elevation persisting for as long as 10 years.

CLINICAL APPLICATIONS OF ESR AND CRP MEASUREMENT

Measurement of ESR is valuable in screening for organic disease and in monitoring progress and activity in chronic conditions. However, in addition to the variables that can affect or distort the result, which have been discussed here, there are many technical factors that can

prejudice its validity and reliability. It is noteworthy that most of them are eliminated by the use of either ZSR or plasma viscosity to monitor alterations in the plasma protein profile. Although not unduly complex, neither method has yet achieved widespread application.

The ESR and alternative procedures that also depend on the combined effect of all the plasma proteins suffer the disadvantages from a clinical viewpoint of responding relatively slowly to pathologic change or amelioration and of correlating rather crudely with activity of disease. Quantitation of CRP, the prototype acute phase reactant, is probably superior in these respects in many diseases. It also has the advantage as a screening test that any elevation into the range detectable by simple immunochemical assay (> 1 μg/ml) is abnormal. Elevation due to a trivial cause soon resolves owing to the rapid rates of rise and fall of plasma CRP in relation to disease activity.

For diagnostic and monitoring purposes precise immunochemical assay (Laurell or Mancini methods), rather than the older, less sensitive semiquantitative techniques, seems to be valuable in several clinical situations (Table 3); it may be extended by the recent resurgence of interest in CRP. CRP levels correlate better with disease activity in rheumatic fever, rheumatoid arthritis, and Crohn's disease than ESR or any other single indicator. CRP concentrations are also significantly greater for comparable degrees of disease activity in Crohn's disease than in ulcerative colitis. In SLE, CRP rises only slightly beyond the normal range even in severe active and progressive disease; but if there is an intercurrent infection the CRP responds promptly, and this may be valuable for differential diagnosis and therapy. Infections in general, particularly but not exclusively bacterial, cause profound elevations of CRP. In neonates, a raised CRP level is useful in confirming bacterial meningitis and/or septicemia and in detecting persistence or recurrence after therapy. In children, CRP is higher in pyelonephritis than in cystitis and differentiates the two better than other available tests. Following the CRP is probably the most sensitive means of detecting and monitoring postoperative complications involving inflammation, such as infection or thromboembolism. Finally, there is some evidence that when CRP returns to normal after treatment of some forms of malignant disease, its subsequent elevation may precede clinical and other signs of recurrence.

Table 3
Clinical Applications of C-Reactive Protein Measurement

Assessment of disease activity in rheumatic fever, rheumatoid arthritis, and Crohn's disease

Detection and monitoring of postoperative inflammatory complications

Detection of infection in systemic lupus erythematosus

Detection and monitoring of neonatal septicemia and/or meningitis

Level diagnosis in symptomatic bacterial urinary tract infection in childhood

Amos RS, Constable TJ, Crockson RA, Crockson AP, Mc-Conkey B: Rheumatoid arthritis: Relation of serum C-reactive protein and erythrocyte sedimentation rates to radiographic changes, Br Med J 1:195, 1977

Cheah JS, Ransome GA: Significance of very high erythrocyte sedimentation rates (100 mm or above in one hour) in 360 cases in Singapore. J Trop Med Hyg 74:28, 1971

Fischer GL, Gill C, Forrester MG, Nakamura R: Quantitation of "acute-phase proteins" postoperatively. Value in detection and monitoring of complications. Am J Clin Pathol 66:840, 1976

Honig S, Gorevic P, Weissmann G: C-reactive protein in systemic lupus erythematosus. Arthritis Rheum 20:1065, 1977

Payne RW: Causes of grossly elevated erythrocyte sedimentation rate. Practitioner 200:415, 1968

Pepys MB, Druguet M, Klass HJ, Dash AC, Mirjah DD, Petrie A: Immunological studies in inflammatory bowel disease, in Knight J (ed): Immunology of the Gut, Ciba Foundation Symposium 46. Amsterdam, Elsevier/Excerpta Medica/North-Holland, 1977, p 283

Sabel KG, Hanson LA: The clinical usefulness of C-reactive protein (CRP) determinations in bacterial meningitis and septicemia in infancy. Acta Paediatr Scand 6:381, 1974

Zacharski LR, Kyle RA: Low erythrocyte sedimentation rate: Clinical significance in 358 cases. Am J Med Sci 250:280, 1965

Zacharski LR, Kyle RA: Significance of extreme elevation of erythrocyte sedimentation rate. JAMA 202:264, 1967

Synovial Membrane Biopsy

Don L. Goldenberg

TECHNIQUES OF SYNOVIAL MEMBRANE BIOPSY

The synovial membrane is a highly vascular connective tissue that lines the inner surface of joint capsules, yet does not cover the articular cartilage (see the chapter on Synovial Membrane in the fascicle on Basic Structure and Function). Normally, the membrane consists of one to three surface layers of cells that resemble fibroblasts and are oriented radially from the joint space. There is a dense capillary network just below these cells. The tissue subjacent to this surface varies greatly in thickness. It usually is loose areolar fatty connective tissue but may be sclerotic and fibrous. There is evidence that aging affects the structure of a normal synovial membrane and dense fibrous subsynovial structure is more typical in the membranes of older patients. The normal synovial membrane contains few, if any, polymorphonuclear or mononuclear leukocytes except those that occasionally surround blood vessels.

Although it has long been appreciated that the histopathologic examination of synovial tissue can be diagnostically important, surprisingly few investigators have routinely examined a portion of the synovium in biopsy or autopsy studies. Until rather recently, open surgical biopsies were necessary to evaluate the synovial membrane. With the availability of closed synovial biopsy techniques, more has been learned about the synovial membrane and the value of its examination in the diagnosis of the rheumatic diseases.

OPEN BIOPSY

Synovial membrane biopsy may be performed by a closed or open surgical technique. The open surgical biopsy is carried out under local anesthesia and should be utilized in the evaluation of arthritis of the hip, sacroiliac joint, shoulder, or small joints of the hands or feet that are difficult to biopsy by the closed technique. This surgical technique also has the advantage of providing larger samples and allowing the surgeon to identify selected areas for biopsy that appear grossly abnormal.

CLOSED BIOPSY

Closed synovial membrane biopsy was described initially in 1932 but became a more realistic tool in 1963 with the introduction of a small-caliber biopsy needle (Parker-Pearson). This needle is now routinely used for closed synovial membrane biopsies of the knee. Such a biopsy can be performed by one person. Strict asepsis should be maintained, however, and therefore an assistant is usually necessary. The most commonly biopsied joint is the knee. After skin cleaning, a local anesthetic agent is injected 1 cm lateral and 1 cm superior to the outer lateral edge of the patella. The biopsy needle is passed into the joint and attached to a syringe. Any synovial fluid obtained is removed and sent for the appropriate microbiologic, cytologic, and chemical studies (see the chapter on Synovial Fluid Analysis in the fascicle on Diagnostic Procedures). At this point, some authors suggest distending the joint capsule with the injection of saline, although we have generally not found this necessary. The Parker-Pearson needle is then directed into the retropatellar space with the knee extended. The trochar is removed and the biopsy needle is inserted through the center of the 14-gauge needle. The needle at first is pointed superiorly and then is redirected in various positions. Tissue is drawn into the hooked portion of the needle by suction or by pressing the assistant's gloved hand over the needle hook, pushing the tissue into the cutting edge. Generally, three to four small biopsies are obtained from various sites.

Biopsy specimens should be fixed in formalin. If gout or pseudogout is suspected, a portion of the specimen should also be fixed in absolute alcohol to preserve any crystals. If joint infection is suspected, a portion of the membrane should be cultured. Some laboratories also obtain tissue for electron microscopy.

Closed synovial membrane biopsies of the ankle,

wrist, and elbows are also easy to perform and the procedure can be integrated with routine arthrocentesis. Generally, there is minimal morbidity, except for slight local pain and tenderness at the biopsy site. Rarely, a hemarthrosis may complicate the procedure. Patients are advised to rest the joint for 24 hours following the biopsy. The procedure can be done in an ambulatory or hospital setting.

Recently, synovial membrane biopsy through the arthroscope has been reported to be a valuable procedure. This may eventually be an acceptable alternative to open biopsies since it allows the operator to visualize directly the area of biopsy, yet does not require an open surgical procedure.

REFERENCES

Labowitz R, Schumacher HR: Articular manifestations of SLE. Ann Intern Med 74:911, 1971
Polley HF, Bickel WW: Punch biopsy of synovial membrane. Ann Rheum Dis 10:277, 1951
Schumacher HR, Kulka JP: Needle biopsy of the synovial membrane—Experience with the Parker-Pearson technique. N Engl J Med 8:416, 1972

APPLICATIONS OF SYNOVIAL MEMBRANE BIOPSY

There are usually no specific synovial membrane findings in the common rheumatic diseases. Occasionally, however, a synovial membrane biopsy and histopathologic evaluation will be the most definitive means of establishing a diagnosis (Table 1). Applications of synovial membrane biopsy in the diagnosis and evaluation of rheumatic diseases will be discussed in this chapter.

DIAGNOSTIC APPLICATIONS

Although it is generally not necessary to culture the synovial membrane in bacterial arthritis, tuberculous and fungal arthritis are often diagnosed only with synovial

Table 1
Specific Histopathologic Characteristics Demonstrated in Certain Rheumatic Diseases

Rheumatic Disease	Characteristic
Bacterial and fungal arthritis	Demonstrate organism in sections or with culture
Tuberculosis	Demonstrate organism in section or culture; caseating granuloma with giant cells
Hemochromatosis	Iron in synovial lining cell
Ochronosis	Fragments of pigmented cartilage
Pigmented villonodular synovitis	Villous hypertrophy, hemosiderin deposits with numerous giant cells
Primary and metastatic cancer	Malignant cells in the synovium
Gout	Monosodium urate crystals
Pseudogout	Calcium pyrophosphate dihydrate crystals

membrane culture and histologic examination (see the section on Infectious Arthritis in the fascicle on Specific Diseases). The synovial membrane culture is positive in greater than 90 percent of cases of tuberculous arthritis. Similarly, typical histologic findings of caseation, granulomas, and giant cells are demonstrated in over 90 percent of such cases. Atypical mycobacteria and fungal microorganisms are also recovered from cultures or seen on sections of synovial membrane more often than they are recovered from the examination of the synovial fluid.

Noncaseating granuloma may be demonstrated in the synovial membrane from patients with sarcoidosis and may help to confirm the clinical diagnosis. Rarely, sarcoidosis presents with arthritis without pulmonary or other extraarticular symptoms. The synovial biopsy then will yield the most useful diagnostic information.

Amyloid arthritis, though rare, may resemble rheumatoid arthritis. If there is any suspicion of amyloid joint disease, the synovial membrane should be biopsied and the pathologist alerted to the possibility so that Congo red stain, electron microscopy, and other appropriate studies will be completed. Most amyloid synovial membranes have revealed little inflammatory cell infiltrate or lining cell proliferation. Amyloid has been demonstrated as a superficial deposit overlying the synovial lining cells, scattered within the deeper tissue, and surrounding blood vessels. Most reports are of amyloidosis complicating multiple myeloma, although we have seen small deposits of amyloid surrounding blood vessels in rheumatoid synovial membranes.

Hemochromatosis and ochronosis are both complicated by arthritis, including calcium pyrophosphate dihydrate crystal deposition disease. The synovial membrane histopathology is of diagnostic value in both of these instances. The most helpful synovial membrane abnormality in hemochromatosis is the demonstration of iron in the synovial lining cells on Prussian blue stain. Iron may also be deposited in the deeper synovium in rheumatoid arthritis and other chronic inflammatory conditions, but the predominance of iron in the superficial lining cells is more characteristic of hemochromatosis and hemophilia. In rheumatoid arthritis, hemarthrosis and pigmented villonodular synovitis iron deposits occur predominantly in macrophages in tissue deep to the surface. Ochronosis may be diagnosed on gross inspection of involved joints by the blackish discoloration of the synovium and cartilage. Fragments of pigmented cartilage called "chards" can be demonstrated in light microscopic sections. Unusual, foamy appearing giant cells have been demonstrated in the joint in disorders of lipid metabolism as well as in the unusual disorder, multicentric reticulohistocytosis.

Benign and malignant tumors involving the synovium often reveal characteristic histopathologic changes. Synovial chondromatosis can be diagnosed by the presence of islands of metaplastic cartilage scattered throughout the subsynovial connective tissue. Pigmented villonodular synovitis reveals characteristic villous hypertrophy, heavily laden with hemosiderin and giant cells. Lymphoproliferative disorders as well as metastatic cancer to the synovium may initially be diagnosed with synovial membrane biopsy. Leukemic infiltration of the synovium accounts for the synovitis associated with leukemia, which may resemble juvenile rheumatoid arthritis. Similarly, metastatic invasion of the synovium may be difficult to distinguish from inflammatory synovitis unless a synovial biopsy is performed and the malignant cells are demonstrated in the synovium (Fig. 1).

EVALUATION OF COMMON
RHEUMATIC DISEASES

The role of synovial membrane biopsy in the evaluation of most common rheumatic diseases is less appreciated. The only example of specific synovial membrane characteristics in the common rheumatic diseases is the demonstration of monosodium urate crystals in gout and calcium pyrophosphate dihydrate crystals in pseudogout, and possibly the lymph follicle seen in rheumatoid arthritis. Crystals, however, are generally demonstrated in the synovial fluid so that synovial membrane examination is not usually necessary. There are a few reports of the demonstration of monosodium urate crystals in the synovial membrane when the crystals were not identified in the synovial fluid.

There are no pathognomonic synovial membrane findings in rheumatoid arthritis or the seronegative spondyloarthritides. The typical features of the rheumatoid synovium include vascular congestion and edema, mononuclear cell infiltration, and synovial lining cell proliferation. Giant cells and granuloma are occasionally present. These features, however, are also found in a variety of inflammatory disorders, especially Reiter's disease, psoriatic arthritis, and juvenile rheumatoid arthritis. Although lymphoid follicles may rarely be demonstrated in the synovium of these rheumatoid variants, the demonstration of lymphoid follicles in the synovial membrane is characteristic of rheumatoid arthritis (Fig. 2).

The synovial membrane characteristics of systemic lupus erythematosus (SLE), scleroderma, and degenerative joint disease, while not specific, can be diagnostically helpful. The synovial membrane in SLE generally reveals only minimal synovial lining cell hyperplasia and scattered mononuclear cell infiltration, but shows dense surface fibrin deposits and perivascular mononuclear cell infiltrates. On exceedingly rare occasions a pathognomonic hematoxylin body may be seen. The characteristic synovial membrane findings in scleroderma reveal marked superficial fibrin deposits but very little proliferation of lining cells or blood vessels. The synovial membrane in degenerative joint disease generally is normal in appearance although occasionally vascular congestion or fibrous atrophy are present.

Various authors have debated the utility of synovial membrane biopsies as a helpful diagnostic procedure due to the lack of specificity noted above. Satisfactory specimens are obtained from closed biopsy in over 90 percent of cases. A specific diagnosis following closed synovial

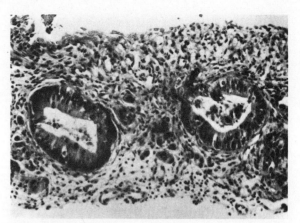

Fig. 1. Synovial membrane demonstrating malignant adenocarcinoma, metastatic to the synovium from the colon. H & E. × 150.

membrane biopsy has been obtained in as few as 30 percent of cases in one series to as many as 65 percent cases in another.

In a recent review of the synovial membrane biopsies of 29 patients with rheumatoid arthritis, 17 with degenerative joint disease, 13 with pseudogout, 13 with SLE, 10 with acute bacterial arthritis, and 8 with gout, the procedure was felt to be quite helpful. Specific diagnostic information included the findings of crystals in the synovia of gout and pseudogout (Fig. 3) and bacteria in infected membranes (Fig. 4). Lymphoid follicles were found only in rheumatoid synovial membranes. Most other light microscopic characteristics such as the amount of surface fibrin deposits, vascular edema, blood vessel proliferation, and modest synovial lining cell proliferation and leukocyte infiltration were typical of all of the synovial membranes. When features were systematically evaluated and graded for extent or severity of change, however, even more significant diagnostic information could be gained from the biopsies.

Although surface fibrin deposits were seen in mem-

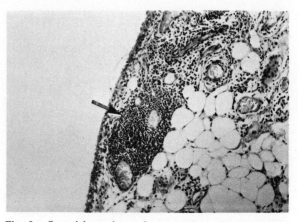

Fig. 2. Synovial membrane from a patient with rheumatoid arthritis demonstrating a lymphoid follicle (arrow). H & E. × 76.

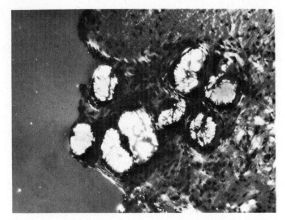

Fig. 3. Synovial membrane from a patient with pseudogout demonstrating birefringent crystalline deposits viewed under polarized microscopy. H & E. × 130.

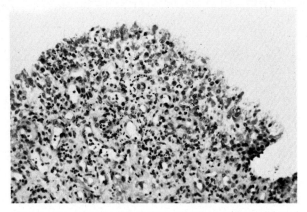

Fig. 4. Synovial membrane from a patient with gonococcal arthritis demonstrating synovial lining cell disorganization (arrow) and diffuse infiltration of polymorphonuclear leukocytes. H & E. × 125.

branes from each of the six rheumatic diseases, the fibrin deposits were more often present and more extensive in SLE than in the other diseases. Intense synovial lining cell proliferation (Fig. 1) was most common in rheumatoid arthritis. Modest, scattered mononuclear leukocytes were seen in membranes from each of the six categories, but extensive infiltrates were again more often seen in the rheumatoid membranes. Marked polymorphonuclear leukocyte infiltrates were present only in the membranes from patients with bacterial arthritis. Therefore, although definitive findings are not generally present, synovial biopsy can yield important diagnostic information provided careful histopathologic evaluation is performed.

Many laboratories are now more often incorporating synovial membrane histopathology into a variety of investigative activities. Histochemical stains, immunologic techniques, electron microscopic analysis, and enhanced microbiologic tools have expanded the role of synovial membrane examination such that the biopsy has become an important procedure in the study of rheumatic diseases.

REFERENCES

Gardner DL: The Pathology of Rheumatoid Arthritis. Baltimore, Williams & Wilkins Company, 1972

Goldenberg DL, Cohen AS: Synovial membrane histopathology in the differential diagnosis of rheumatoid arthritis, gout, pseudogout, systemic lupus erythematosus, infectious arthritis and degenerative joint disease. Medicine (Baltimore) 57:239, 1978

Radiology of Joints

Donald Resnick

The correct interpretation of skeletal radiographs in patients with articular disorders depends upon knowledge in two fundamental areas: (1) basic roentgenographic alterations that are characteristic of specific articular diseases; and (2) typical locations or "target sites" at which these alterations are apparent.

BASIC ROENTGENOGRAPHIC ALTERATIONS

Knowledge in this area requires an understanding of the pathogenesis and pathology of articular disorders. Recognizing, for example, that rheumatoid arthritis is initially associated with synovial inflammation, the physician can predict early roentgenologic signs in this disease such as soft tissue swelling (reflecting synovial fluid production, capsular distention, and soft tissue edema) and periarticular osteoporosis (reflecting regional hyperemia). Subsequently, synovial inflammatory tissue or "pannus" attacking cartilage and subchondral bone accounts for radiographically detectable symmetric joint space loss and marginal and central osseous erosions.

Similar pathologic aberrations in rheumatoid "variant" disorders, such as psoriasis, Reiter's syndrome, and ankylosing spondylitis, account for radiographic changes that simulate those of rheumatoid arthritis, although in "variant" disease, the absence of osteoporosis and the presence of bony proliferation and intraarticular bony ankylosis may aid in specific roentgenologic diagnosis. In osteoarthritis, altered stress in localized areas of the joint produces predictable pathologic abnormalities in cartilage and subchondral bone which are associated with radiographic findings such as asymmetric joint space loss, subchondral cysts and sclerosis, and osseous excrescences or osteophytes. In gout, monosodium urate deposits appear in synovium, cartilage, bone, and soft tissue. The resulting roentgenographic findings are asymmetric soft tissue masses, eccentric osseous erosion with adjacent bony proliferation, preservation of articular space, and lack of osteoporosis. In osteonecrosis, interruption of blood supply to subchondral bone results in its deterioration and necrosis, whereas overlying cartilage, obtaining most of its nutrition from adjacent synovial fluid, maintains its integrity. On the roentgenogram, bony cysts, collapse, fragmentation, and sclerosis appear in association with a relatively normal articular space.

TARGET SITES

For unexplained reasons, certain articular disorders affect certain articulations and spare others. Knowledge of characteristic "target sites" in each articular disease provides invaluable aid in interpretating joint radiographs. Typical distributions include symmetric alterations of the hands, wrists, feet, and knees in rheumatoid arthritis, asymmetric changes in the feet, hands, wrists and elbows in gout, and interphalangeal and weight-bearing joint predilection in osteoarthritis.

Knowledge in both of these areas alerts the radiologist as to what to look for and where to look for it. It places him in a unique position to aid the clinician in evaluating his patient with arthritis and, in many instances, to offer a single specific and correct diagnosis.

RHEUMATOID ARTHRITIS

Initial roentgenographic changes in rheumatoid arthritis frequently appear in the hand, wrist, and foot. The articulations of the hand most characteristically involved are the proximal interphalangeal joints, particularly the third, and the metacarpophalangeal joints, particularly the second and third. Distal interphalangeal joint alterations are an uncommon and minor feature of this disease. At the proximal interphalangeal and metacarpophalangeal articulations, symmetric soft tissue swelling, periarticular osteoporosis, diffuse loss of joint space, and "marginal" erosions are apparent (Fig. 1A). The latter appear as scalloped or pocketed osseous defects at the joint margins. Their distribution reflects the location of vulnerable areas of the joint where bone is not covered by protective cartilage. This allows abnormal synovium quick access to underlying bone. In the wrist, typical sites of early osseous erosions are the ulnar styloid, apposing portions of the distal radius and ulna, the midbody of the scaphoid, and the radial styloid, triquetrum, and pisiform. Soft tissue swelling along the outer aspect of the distal ulna relates to tendonitis and tenosynovitis, particularly in the extensor carpi ulnaris tendon and sheath. The changes of rheumatoid arthritis are soon apparent in all of the compartments or areas of the wrist joint, including the radiocarpal, inferior radioulnar, midcarpal, pisiform–triquetral, common carpometacarpal, and first carpometacarpal articulations.

In the foot, changes predominate at the metatarsophalangeal joints. Early erosions are apparent as radiolucencies that predilect the medial aspect of the metatarsal heads, although soft tissue swelling and osseous erosion on the lateral aspect of the fifth metatarsal head may be

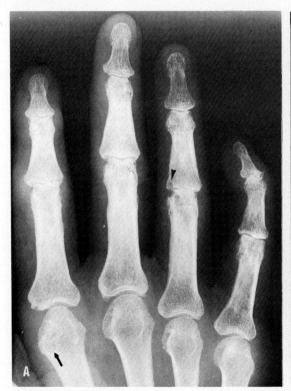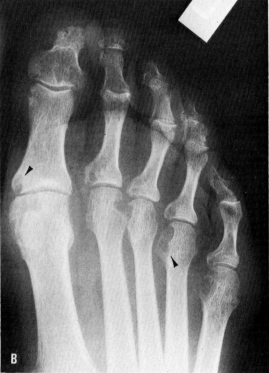

Fig. 1. Adult-onset rheumatoid arthritis. **A.** Typical findings in the hand are involvement of the metacarpophalangeal and proximal interphalangeal articulations, osteoporosis, erosions, and uniform loss of joint space. Note the marginal location of the erosive changes (arrowhead) and the predilection for involvement of the radial aspect of the metacarpal heads (arrow). **B.** In the foot, erosions predominate at the metatarsophalangeal joints (arrowheads). The interphalangeal joint of the great toe is also abnormal.

an initial manifestation of the disease (Fig. 1B). Additional sites of abnormality in the foot are the interphalangeal joint of the great toe, the articulations of the midfoot, and the calcaneus. An erosion on the posterosuperior aspect of the calcaneus is particularly characteristic, related to retrocalcaneal bursitis. Superficial plantar calcaneal erosions and well-defined plantar calcaneal spurs may also be observed.

Late changes in the hands, wrists, and feet reflect continued bone and cartilage destruction and tendon and ligament disease. Inflammatory changes in periarticular tissues such as tendons and ligaments result in joint laxity, altered muscle action and typical subluxations and deformities. Roentgen findings include ulnar deviation and volar subluxation of the phalanges at the metacarpophalangeal joints, radial deviation at the radiocarpal compartment of the wrist, carpal malalignment, and fibular deviation and plantar subluxation of the phalanges at the metatarsophalangeal joints. In general, rheumatoid arthritis produces fibrous ankylosis, rather than bony ankylosis, of the joint, although carpal and tarsal bony masses are not infrequent.

Knee involvement in rheumatoid arthritis is characterized by symmetric loss of joint space in the medial and lateral femorotibial compartments. Additional findings in the patellofemoral compartment indicate tricompartmental alteration in the rheumatoid knee. Marginal erosions appear on the femur and tibia and large joint effusions may be seen. The latter can result in synovial herniations or cysts, particularly in the popliteal region. These synovial cysts may cause soft tissue swelling on the posterior aspect of the knee. They are well demonstrated during knee arthrography as radiodense contrast material passes from the knee joint into the cyst itself.

The hip is not a common site of radiographic abnormality in rheumatoid arthritis, but when it is involved typical roentgenographic changes are observed. Uniform loss of articular space produces migration of the femoral head with respect to the adjacent acetabulum. This migration occurs along the axis of the femoral neck. Acetabular protrusion may allow the femoral head to protrude into the pelvis. Marginal and central erosions occur, particularly in the femoral head, and the resulting radiolucencies within bone may not appear to communicate with the articular space. These sharply marginated "pseudocysts" are more frequent in large joints such as the elbow, hip, and knee than in small joints of the hands and feet. Continued erosion of the femoral head may produce a peculiar blunted end to the proximal femur which is diminished in size and no longer appears to fit into the protruded acetabulum.

Although rheumatoid arthritis commonly results in abnormality in many articulations of the appendicular skeleton, the axial skeleton may also be altered, particularly the articulations of the cervical spine. In this location, changes occur in the apophyseal, atlantoaxial, and discovertebral joints as well as in adjacent structures such as the spinous processes of the vertebrae. Bony erosions predominate about apophyseal joints, anterior and posterior aspects of the odontoid process, and vertebral body end-plate regions. In the latter location, irregular vertebral body outlines are associated with loss of disc space. The presence of both disc space loss and vertebral body erosions and the absence of osteophytosis suggest the diagnosis of rheumatoid arthritis in the cervical spine. Forward subluxation of the atlas with respect to the axis is common and is exaggerated on lateral radiographs of the cervical spine obtained during neck flexion. Subaxial subluxations are also characteristic and the resulting radiographic picture of the cervical spine is termed the "step-ladder" appearance.

Elsewhere in the axial skeleton, superficial erosions and bony sclerosis may be seen at the sacroiliac joints. These changes are infrequent and mild and may be asymmetric or unilateral in distribution as compared to the more frequent, extensive, and symmetric sacroiliac joint alterations in ankylosing spondylitis. Abnormalities in the thoracolumbar spine are unusual.

In summary, the characteristic radiographic abnormalities in rheumatoid arthritis are symmetry of joint involvement, fusiform soft tissue swelling, periarticular osteoporosis, uniform loss of joint space, marginal erosions, "pseudocystic" lesions, and deformities. Extensive bone proliferation in the form of sclerosis, osteophytes, and periostitis is uncommon in rheumatoid arthritis, being more typical of other disorders such as osteoarthritis and rheumatoid "variant" diseases.

RHEUMATOID ARTHRITIS: JUVENILE-ONSET

Recently it has become apparent that many children previously diagnosed as having juvenile rheumatoid arthritis actually suffer from other conditions. The term *juvenile chronic polyarthritis* has been introduced as a general term to include a variety of disorders in children such as juvenile-onset rheumatoid arthritis, juvenile-onset ankylosing spondylitis, intestinal arthropathies, and other diseases. The present discussion focuses on children who appear to have juvenile-onset rheumatoid arthritis.

Juvenile-onset rheumatoid arthritis presents in a variety of ways; in some patients it produces changes simulating those of adult-onset disease, whereas in others abnormalities are readily differentiated from those occurring in adults. Unlike adult-onset rheumatoid arthritis, juvenile-onset disease may be associated with linear subperiosteal bone apposition, particularly in the phalanges, metacarpals, and metatarsals, reflecting the ease with which the less adherent periosteal membrane of the child is lifted from the parent bone and stimulated to produce new bone. Furthermore, preservation of joint space, intraarticular bony ankylosis, and disturbances of bone maturation and growth are features more typical of juvenile-onset rheumatoid arthritis.

Monoarticular disease, frequently of the knee, or polyarticular disease may be apparent. Wrists, knees, ankles, and cervical spine are commonly involved. In the

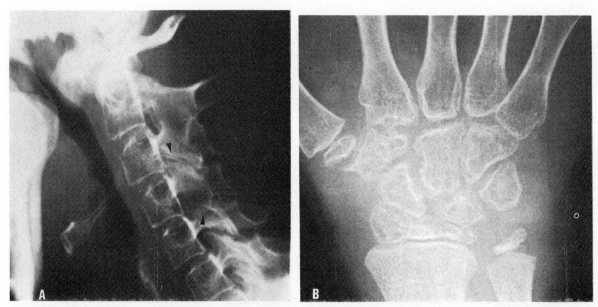

Fig. 2. Juvenile-onset rheumatoid arthritis. **A.** Cervical spine alterations are narrowing and osseous fusion of apophyseal joints (arrowheads), hypoplasia of vertebral bodies and intervertebral disc spaces, and atlantoaxial subluxation. Note also the undergrowth of the mandible. **B.** Osteoporosis, joint space narrowing, and irregular carpal ossification centers are apparent.

latter area, bony ankylosis of multiple apophyseal joints, and hypoplastic vertebral bodies and intervertebral discs are recognizable radiographic changes (Fig. 2A). Subluxation in the cervical spine simulates that occurring in adult-onset disease. Subluxation in children may also be seen in small joints of the hands and feet and in large joints such as the hip.

Typical growth disturbances in juvenile-onset rheumatoid arthritis include enlargement and irregularity of ossification centers such as the distal femur, carpal, and tarsal bones, and undergrowth of the mandible (Fig. 2B).

ANKYLOSING SPONDYLITIS

This disease affects both synovial and cartilaginous joints as well as tendon and ligament attachments to bone; it also predilects the axial skeleton. Particularly characteristic is involvement of the sacroiliac, apophyseal, and costovertebral synovial articulations and fibrocartilaginous joints such as the symphysis pubis, discovertebral junction, and sternomanubrial articulation. Extraaxial joint abnormality is not infrequent, particularly in the "root" joints such as the hip and shoulder.

The sacroiliac joint is frequently the earliest site of abnormality (Fig. 3A). Bilateral and symmetric sacroiliac joint alterations are most characteristic, although initially unilateral or asymmetric changes may be apparent. Changes predominate on the ilial aspect of the articulation. Blurring and indistinctness of subchondral bone, adjacent reactive bone sclerosis, and superficial osseous irregularity are seen. The joint space may at first appear widened, although joint space narrowing is common. Partial or complete intraarticular bony ankylosis of the sacroiliac joint may eventually result with disappearance of bone eburnation. The ligamentous portion of the sacro-

iliac space above the true sacroiliac joint is frequently blurred in appearance and may ossify. Additional pelvic alterations are irregularity and sclerosis of the symphysis pubis and "fraying" related to superficial erosions and proliferation of the iliac crests, ischial tuberosities, and trochanters.

In the spine, changes are initially seen at the thoracolumbar and lumbosacral junctions. Anterosuperior and anteroinferior corner erosions of the vertebral bodies are associated with reactive sclerosis of adjacent bone. Resultant loss of bone at the anterior vertebral margins produces a "squared-off" appearance, most apparent in the lumbar region, and adjacent bone eburnation results in the "shiny corner" configuration. Thin vertical bridges of bone, termed *syndesmophytes*, extend from one vertebral body to the next, representing ossification within the peripheral fibers of the annulus fibrosus of the intervertebral disc (Fig. 3B). These bony excrescences may become thicker and more widespread, leading to the appearance of the "bamboo" spine. Concomitantly, changes about the apophyseal joints include joint space narrowing, sclerosis, and bony ankylosis. Additional alterations in the posterior elements of the thoracolumbar spine are ossification of the inter- and supraspinous ligaments. The combination of ankylosis about multiple apophyseal joints on either side and ossification within these posterocentral ligaments may lead to the detection of three vertical radiodense lines on frontal radiographs of the spine, the "trolley-track" sign. Osteoporosis, disc space narrowing, discal calcification, and progressive kyphosis are seen at late stages of the disease. Trauma may lead to fractures through the ankylosed vertebral column. These fractures, which extend through the anterior and

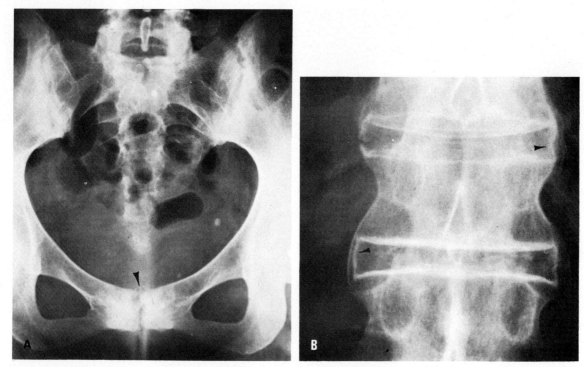

Fig. 3. Ankylosing spondylitis. **A.** Bilateral symmetric sacroiliac joint changes include bone sclerosis, mainly of the ilium, and joint space narrowing. Osteitis pubis (arrowhead) is also seen. **B.** Syndesmophytes appear as thin slender vertical osseous bridges extending between vertebral bodies (arrowheads).

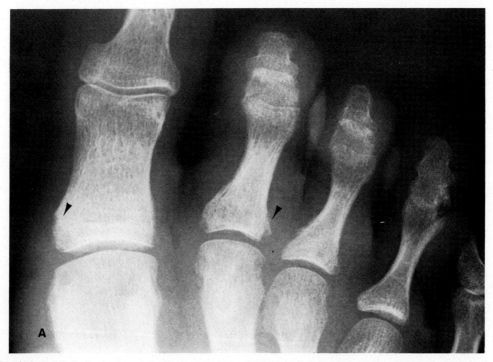

Fig. 4. Psoriasis and Reiter's syndrome. **A.** Bony proliferation is characteristic in both of these disorders. Observe irregular bony excrescences about involved metatarsophalangeal and interphalangeal joints (arrowheads). **B.** In psoriasis (facing page), large broad asymmetric outgrowths of the spine are characteristic (arrowhead).

posterior aspects of the vertebrae and/or disc, frequently do not heal well, creating a pseudarthrosis.

In the cervical spine, diagnostic alterations are joint space narrowing, sclerosis, and bony ankylosis of multiple apophyseal joints. These changes, which resemble the changes of juvenile-onset rheumatoid arthritis, are associated with typical findings of the anterior portion of the vertebral column, including syndesmophyte formation. Atlantoaxial subluxation, spinous process erosions, and resorption of the anterior aspect of the lower cervical vertebrae are additional findings.

Although the preceding discussion might indicate that the course of axial involvement in ankylosing spondylitis is constant and relentless, this is not the case. Occasional patients with ankylosing spondylitis develop sacroiliac changes without spinal involvement; the converse, spinal changes without sacroiliac abnormality, is distinctly unusual. Women with ankylosing spondylitis may demonstrate extensive sacroiliac joint and cervical spine changes without significant thoracolumbar disease.

The extraaxial articulations may be affected in ankylosing spondylitis, particularly the hip and shoulder, although additional joints may also be involved. Findings superficially resemble those of rheumatoid arthritis, although symmetry, osteoporosis, extensive erosions, and deformities are less frequent in ankylosing spondylitis than in rheumatoid arthritis. Hip involvement in ankylosing spondylitis may lead to a characteristic roentgenographic picture with symmetric loss of joint space and osteophytosis. Osteophytes first develop at the superolateral aspect of the femoral head and progress in the form of a collar of new bone which extends across the femoral head–femoral neck junction.

"Reankylosis" related to excessive heterotopic ossi-

fication has been reported following total hip arthroplasties in patients with ankylosing spondylitis.

It should be noted that a similar radiographic picture of sacroiliitis and spondylitis accompanies certain bowel disorders such as ulcerative colitis, regional enteritis, and Whipple's disease.

PSORIATIC ARTHRITIS AND
REITER'S SYNDROME

Roentgenologic manifestations are fundamentally similar in these two rheumatoid "variant" disorders. General radiographic features include the absence of osteoporosis and the presence of exuberant subchondral and subperiosteal new bone formation. The latter feature, which is also apparent with peripheral joint involvement in ankylosing spondylitis, is characterized by irregular bony excrescences at the margins of joint and linear or fluffy periosteal bone proliferation (Fig. 4A). This bone proliferation is unusual in rheumatoid arthritis and, when present, suggests the diagnosis of a rheumatoid variant condition.

The pattern of joint involvement in psoriasis is variable; some patients reveal polyarticular disease simulating the distribution of rheumatoid arthritis, whereas others demonstrate predilection for the distal interphalangeal joints of the fingers. Mono- or pauciarticular disease and arthritis mutilans are additional patterns of disease in psoriasis. Asymmetric disease is common. Terminal interphalangeal joint changes of the hands in psoriasis result in erosions with resorption of considerable portions of adjacent bone, widening of the articular space, "cup and saucer" appearance, intraarticular bony ankylosis, and resorption of terminal tufts. The degree of osseous resorption is greater than in rheumatoid arthritis and involves the shafts as well as the ends of the bones. In the

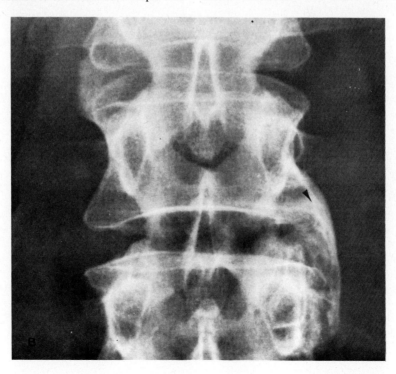

foot, selective involvement of the interphalangeal joint of the great toe may be seen, and posterior and plantar calcaneal erosions are associated with considerable new bone formation.

In Reiter's syndrome, an asymmetric lower extremity distribution is most common. Upper extremity changes are mild; it is rare to observe widespread destruction of multiple articulations in the hand and wrist. As in psoriasis, selective involvement of the interphalangeal joint of the great toe and calcaneus may be observed.

In both psoriatic arthritis and Reiter's syndrome, sacroiliac joint and spine changes may be apparent, although widespread involvement of the spine is more frequent in psoriasis. In both disorders, the most common pattern of sacroiliac joint abnormality is bilateral symmetric disease, simulating the findings of ankylosing spondylitis. However, both diseases may be associated with unilateral or asymmetric sacroiliac joint abnormalities in some patients, findings which are unusual in ankylosing spondylitis. These sacroiliac articular abnormalities include erosions and sclerosis. Bony ankylosis of the sacroiliac joint is less common in these disorders than in ankylosing spondylitis. In the spine, particularly in psoriatic arthritis, large asymmetric osteophytes are seen which differ considerably from the syndesmophytes of ankylosing spondylitis (Fig. 4B). These bony outgrowths are bulky in appearance and are most common in the lower thoracic and upper lumbar areas. Additionally, paravertebral ossification in some·patients occurs at a considerable distance from the vertebral column, producing a distinctive radiographic picture. Vertebral body erosions, sclerosis, and "squaring," and apophyseal joint ankylosis are not so common in these rheumatoid variant diseases as they are in ankylosing spondylitis. Cervical spine changes in psoriasis include paravertebral ossifications and osteophytes, and atlantoaxial joint subluxation.

DEGENERATIVE JOINT DISEASE (OSTEOARTHRITIS)
Appendicular Disease

Degenerative joint changes are particularly frequent in the interphalangeal joints of the hand, the first metatarsophalangeal joint, and the large weight-bearing articulations of the lower extremity, the knee, and the hip. In the hand, abnormalities are most common in the distal interphalangeal joints but also occur in the proximal interphalangeal and metacarpophalangeal articulations. Changes may be isolated in the distal or proximal interphalangeal joints but are rarely isolated in the metacarpophalangeal joints. Articular space narrowing is associated with subchondral sclerosis and osteophytosis. Osteophytes are frequently best observed on oblique and lateral radiographs as dorsal bony excrescences. The resulting expanded bone surfaces are closely apposed. At the metacarpophalangeal joints, uniform joint space narrowing and beaklike osteophytes are seen; erosions are not a feature of osteoarthritis of the metacarpophalangeal joints, as opposed to their common occurrence in rheumatoid arthritis. In the wrist, degenerative joint disease

occurs on the radial aspect at the first carpometacarpal and trapezioscaphoid areas (Fig. 5A). Degenerative changes elsewhere in the wrist, in the absence of accidental or occupational trauma, are unusual and should suggest other diagnoses.

In the foot, degenerative joint changes predominate at the first metatarsophalangeal (frequently in association with hallux valgus deformity) and the first tarsometatarsal joints, although isolated changes elsewhere in the midfoot are occasionally observed.

Osteoarthritis of the hip is associated with nonuniform loss of articular space. In most patients, this joint space loss is maximun on the weight-bearing superior surface of the articulation (Fig. 5B). Sclerosis and cyst formation occur on apposing portions of acetabulum and femur. These cysts are pyriform in shape with a thin rim of sclerosis. Osteophytes develop at both the lateral and medial areas of the joint but are most prominent on the medial portion of the femoral head. Rarely, patients with osteoarthritis of the hip develop significant loss of medial articular space with relative sparing of the superior aspect of the articulation. In both patterns of osteoarthritis, "buttressing" or new bone formation is prominent along the medial aspect of the femoral neck.

In the knee, osteoarthritis is characterized by an asymmetric loss of joint space. More commonly, medial femorotibial space loss predominates with relative sparing of the lateral femorotibial space (Fig. 5C). This may be associated with genu varum. In addition, patellofemoral space narrowing, evident on lateral radiographs is usually combined with loss of articular space in medial or lateral femorotibial spaces.

Although the joints of the appendicular skeleton listed above—interphalangeal, first carpometacarpal, trapezioscaphoid, first metatarsophalangeal, hip, and knee—are those most characteristically altered in osteoarthritis, it should be remembered that degenerative changes may be noted in any joint that has been previously altered by developmental or acquired abnormality. This variety of degenerative joint disease, secondary osteoarthritis, may complicate epiphyseal dysplasias, inflammatory arthritis such as rheumatoid arthritis, gout, hemophilia, trauma, or postsurgical change. Furthermore, patients with ochronosis and acromegaly develop cartilage abnormalities that predispose to secondary osteoarthritis.

Erosive osteoarthritis is a term applied to a variety of degenerative joint diseases associated with considerable inflammation and extensive subchondral destruction of bone. Erosions may predominate in the central portion of the joint rather than in the marginal areas, which are characteristic sites of erosion in rheumatoid arthritis and related disorders. Osteophytes are also apparent. Common sites of involvement in erosive osteoarthritis are the same as those involved in typical osteoarthritis and include the distal and proximal interphalangeal joints of the fingers and the first carpometacarpal and trapezioscaphoid areas.

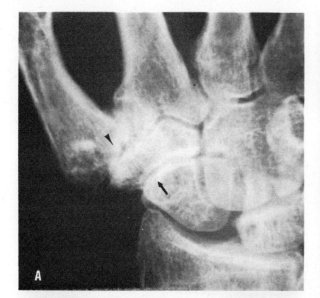

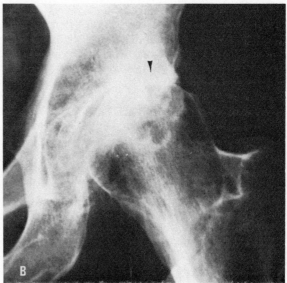

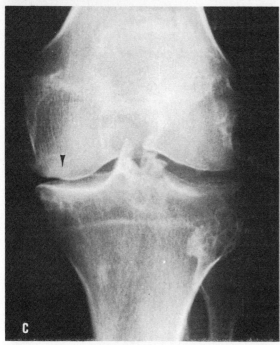

Fig. 5. Degenerative joint disease: appendicular skeleton. **A.** Degenerative disease of the wrist produces joint space narrowing, sclerosis, and osteophytes at the first carpometacarpal (arrowhead) and trapezioscaphoid (arrow) areas. **B.** In the hip, joint space narrowing is usually asymmetric in distribution and predominates on the superior aspect of the articulation (arrowhead). Note bony sclerosis, cysts, osteophytes, and "buttressing" or thickening along the medial aspect of the femoral neck. **C.** Observe asymmetric joint space narrowing with predilection for the medial femorotibial space (arrowhead). Findings include sclerosis, osteophytosis, and "sharpening" of the tibial spines.

narrowing, sclerosis, and occasional bony ankylosis are most frequent in the cervical spine, although they are also apparent in the thoracic and lumbar segments.

Two basic types of degenerative processes involve the discovertebral articulations. Intervertebral osteochondrosis relates to abnormalities of the central portion of the intervertebral disc, the nucleus pulposus, characterized by desiccation and dehydration of this structure. This disorder, which is extremely common, produces roentgenologic signs that include "vacuum" phenomena (radiolucent collections of gas overlying the intervertebral disc), disc space loss, and vertebral body marginal sclerosis. Spondylosis deformans probably results from degenerative changes in the outer portion of the disc, the anulus fibrosus. Breakdown in normal connections between the anulus and vertebral body allows anterolateral disc herniation, elevation of the anterior longitudinal ligament, and spinal osteophytes. These osteophytes, which may reach considerable size, occur a few millimeters from the superior and inferior edges of the vertebrae at the site of attachment of the anterior longitudinal ligament to the anterolateral surface of the vertebral body. They are associated with relative preservation of disc height. In the thoracic region, they predominate on the right side. It is suggested that the pulsatile aorta inhibits their formation on the left side.

Another condition associated with exuberant spinal

Axial Skeleton

Osteoarthritis may develop in synovial joints of the axial skeleton such as the sacroiliac and apophyseal joints. In the former location, unilateral or bilateral abnormalities occur, and ilial alterations predominate. Joint space loss is associated with a well-defined subchondral bone margin, as opposed to the frayed irregular appearance characteristic of ankylosing spondylitis. Condensation of subchondral bone produces a thin well-defined line of sclerosis, usually in the ilium. Osteophytes are most common at the superior and inferior limits of the articulation, creating radiodense shadows that may simulate sclerotic metastatic foci. In the apophyseal joints, osteophytes has been described under a variety of names including (senile) ankylosing hyperostosis of the spine, and Forestier's disease. Recent documentation of considerable extraspinal manifestations suggests that diffuse idiopathic skeletal hyperostosis (DISH) may be a more appropriate name for this disorder. The etiology of this condition remains unknown. It may be closely aligned to spondylosis deformans, although osteophytes are larger in size and greater in number and there appear to be ligamentous changes as well. The roentgenographic appearance in cases with extensive ossification is diagnostic: linear flowing ossification along the anterolateral aspect of the spine, particularly in the lower thoracic region; bumpy spinal contour; radiolucencies between the deposited bone and subjacent vertebrae; and radiolucent disc extensions (Fig. 6). The degree of ossification is greater than that observed in ankylosing spondylitis; furthermore, apophyseal and sacroiliac joint erosion and bony ankylosis do not occur in DISH. Preservation of intervertebral disc height is also characteristic, differing from the disc space loss typical in intervertebral osteochondrosis. Extraspinal manifestations of DISH include osseous excrescences at sites of tendon and ligament attachment to bone (iliac crest, ischial tuborosity, trochanters, calcaneus, patella, and ulnar olecranon), para-

articular osteophytes (sacroiliac and hip joints) and ligamentous ossification (iliolumbar and sacrotuberous ligaments).

GOUT

General radiographic features of gouty arthritis differ from those of rheumatoid arthritis; in gout, one notes the absence of both osteoporosis and symmetric joint involvement and the presence of asymmetric soft tissue masses with or without calcifications adjacent to or at a distance from joints, intra- and extra-articular erosions, and proliferative changes. Soft tissue masses or tophi may occur anywhere but are most common in the foot and ankle, the extensor surface of the forearm, and about the olecranon and infrapatella bursae. Particularly characteristic is the appearance of thin spicules of bone extending around soft tissue masses, termed the "overhanging edge" sign. These spicules represent elevated and displaced segments of cortical bone. Also characteristic is the presence of a relatively normal articular space despite osseous erosion, although in the late stages of the disease joint space narrowing is common. Bony ankylosis is occasionally observed in long-standing disease.

Gout produces changes that predilect the articulations of appendicular skeleton. In the foot, involvement of the first metatarsophalangeal joint is most typical, although any articulation may be altered, including the proximal and distal interphalangeal joints. Similarly, in

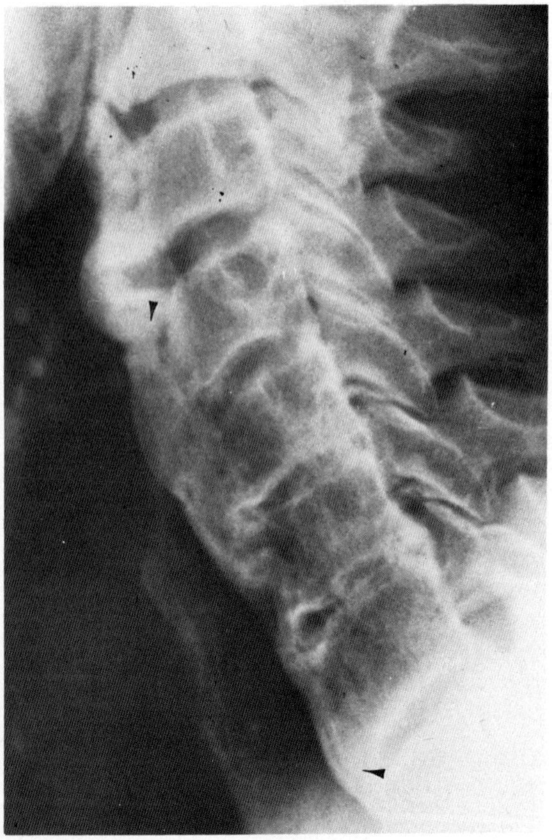

Fig. 6. Diffuse idiopathic skeletal hyperostosis. In the cervical spine extensive "flowing" ossification along the anterior aspect of the vertebral column is observed (arrowheads).

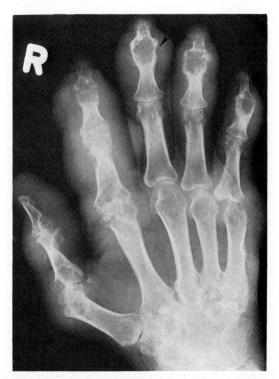

Fig. 7. Gout. Abnormalities include the absence of osteoporosis and the presence of asymmetric soft tissue masses, eccentric and central intra- and extraarticular osseous erosions, and joint space narrowing. Note significant involvement of the distal interphalangeal joints (arrowhead).

the hand and wrist, changes may be noted in any articulation, including the distal interphalangeal joints (Fig. 7). Pancompartmental involvement of the wrist in gout may simulate changes of rheumatoid arthritis, although in the former disease, the absence of typical marginal erosions and the presence of bony proliferation allow accurate diagnosis. Elbow abnormalities are also frequent in gout, whereas axial skeletal changes are unusual. Occasional patients with long-standing gouty arthritis develop large erosions about sacroiliac joints which may be unilateral or bilateral in distribution. Involvement of the spine or hip is rare in gout, although some reports suggest a relationship between gouty arthritis and osteonecrosis of the femoral head.

CALCIUM PYROPHOSPHATE DEPOSITION DISEASE

Calcium pyrophosphate deposition disease is a common disorder related to the presence of calcium pyrophosphate dihydrate crystals in and around joints. It is associated with two characteristic radiographic signs: (1) intra- and periarticular calcifications; and (2) structural joint changes, simulating osteoarthritis, termed *pyrophosphate arthropathy*.

The most common form of calcification is fibro or hyaline cartilage calcification, termed *chondrocalcinosis*. It should be emphasized that chondrocalcinosis limited to one joint may not indicate deposition of pyrophosphate crystals, but rather the accumulation of other crystalline deposits. Chondrocalcinosis of two or more articular sites usually indicates calcium pyrophosphate dihydrate crystal deposition. The latter deposits are most frequently observed in the fibrocartilage of the knee, wrist, and symphysis pubis. Fibrocartilage calcification appears as thick shaggy central articular radiodensities; hyaline cartilage calcification produces thin linear radiodensities that parallel the osseous surface (Fig. 8).

Articular calcification is also noted in synovial and capsular tissue. Capsular calcification produces curvilinear radiodensities that span the articulation, particularly in the elbow and metatarsophalangeal joints. Tendon and

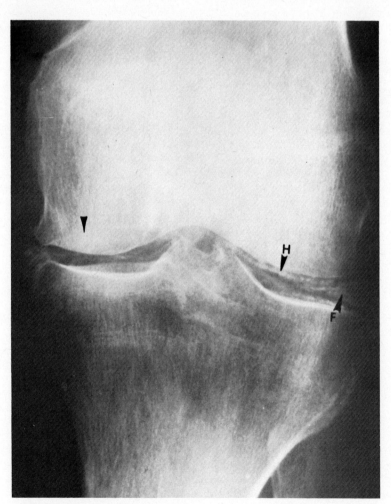

Fig. 8. Calcium pyrophosphate deposition disease. In the knee observe fibro (F) and hyaline (H) cartilage calcification (chondrocalcinosis). Mild medial femorotibial joint space narrowing is seen (arrowhead).

ligament calcification is also observed, especially in the rotator cuff and Achilles and quadriceps tendons. These deposits produce single or multiple linear densities that may attach to or be separated from the underlying bone. Soft tissue calcification is also occasionally noted.

Pyrophosphate arthropathy is most frequent in the knees, wrists, and metacarpophalangeal joints and is associated with joint space narrowing and bone eburnation which is identical to changes of osteoarthritis. Specific characteristics of pyrophosphate arthropathy that differ from those of degenerative joint disease are a predilection for joints rarely involved in osteoarthritis (elbow, shoulder, and wrist), extensive subchondral cyst formation, collapse and fragmentation of subchondral bone, and variable osteophyte formation. The peculiar distribution of pyrophosphate arthropathy should be stressed. Involvement of the radiocarpal compartment of the wrist is rarely observed in osteoarthritis; "degenerative" changes in this location suggest the diagnosis of pyrophosphate arthropathy whether or not adjacent calcification can be detected. Furthermore, isolated involvement of the patellofemoral compartment of the knee and talonavicular area of the midfoot are helpful in diagnosing pyrophosphate arthropathy.

Collapse and fragmentation of bone in calcium pyrophosphate deposition disease may be so rapid and extensive as to suggest the diagnosis of neuroarthropathy, although neurologic deficits may not be apparent in these individuals. Intraarticular osseous bodies are common in calcium pyrophosphate deposition disease and may be so numerous as to suggest the diagnosis of idiopathic synovial osteochondromatosis (see below).

Patients with primary hyperparathyroidism and hemochromatosis may demonstrate roentgenologic findings identical to those of idiopathic calcium pyrophosphate deposition disease. In hyperparathyroidism, subperiosteal (phalanges, lamina dura of teeth, tibia) and subchondral resorption (sacroiliac and acromioclavicular joints, symphysis pubis) allow accurate diagnosis.

NEUROARTHROPATHY

Neuroarthropathy resembles osteoarthritis with a vengeance. It is associated with disorders that interfere with normal pain and proprioceptive sensation about joints. These articulations lose their built-in protective mechanisms so that recurrent trauma leads to bone fragmentation, sclerosis, subluxation, and malposition. In most instances, neuroarthropathy is monoarticular in distribution. Changes may appear relatively acute and relentlessly progress. The most common diseases leading to neuroarthropathy are tabes dorsalis, diabetes mellitus, and syringomyelia.

The distribution and, to a lesser extent, the appearance of articular abnormality in neuroarthropathy depend upon the specific underlying disorder. Tabes dorsalis produces changes that predilect the large joints of the lower extremity such as the hip and knee. Diabetes mellitus produces alterations of the intertarsal, tarsometatarsal, and metatarsophalangeal joints. Syringomyelia characteristically involves the joints of the upper extremity.

All these disorders may be associated with changes in the vertebral column.

Soft tissue swelling in neuroarthropathy may be extensive, related to persistent or recurrent effusions. Osteoporosis is not apparent and, in fact, extensive osteosclerosis is frequently observed (Fig. 9). Intraarticular fractures lead to multiple intraarticular osseous fragments. Hypertrophic changes include bizarre osteophyte formation. Subluxation may be noted, whereas bony ankylosis is rare. In the spine, fragmentation and sclerosis of vertebral bodies, disc space loss, and huge hypertrophic spurs are seen. In some patients, particularly those with diabetes mellitus, resorption rather than hypertrophy of bone is seen. Tapering of bone ends or "penciling" is noted in these individuals and coexisting infection is very common.

INFECTION

Articular abnormalities may complicate infections caused by pyogenic, tuberculous, and fungal organisms and the pattern of roentgenographic alteration is somewhat dependent upon the offending organism. Juxtaarticular osteoporosis is characteristic of tuberculous and fungal infection, whereas it is unusual in pyogenic disease. Furthermore, the joint space may be maintained until late in the course of articular infection caused by tuberculosis and fungal organisms, whereas early joint space narrowing is typical of pyogenic arthritis.

Initial abnormalities in pyogenic infection include soft tissue swelling, rapid destruction of cartilage and bone, and reactive new bone formation. These osseous and cartilaginous changes become evident on the radiograph within 7–10 days of the onset of symptoms. The eventual radiographic picture in pyogenic arthritis will depend upon the specific organism and the effectiveness of antibiotic therapy.

Tuberculosis may affect any joint, particularly the knee and hip, as well as the vertebral column. Soft tissue swelling, regional osteoporosis, marginal osseous erosions, and eventual joint space loss are apparent. Reactive bone formation may be minimal. These radiographic changes are similar to those accompanying fungal disorders.

OSTEONECROSIS

An interruption of blood supply to subchondral bone producing osteonecrosis may be seen in a variety of conditions; it may be noted following trauma or irradiation, or in association with hemoglobinopathies, exogenous or endogenous steroid overload, diseases such as systemic lupus erythematosus, Caisson's disease, pancreatitis, and alcoholism. Findings are most commonly observed in the femoral head, proximal humerus, and distal femur. Cartilage is maintained, as it derives its nutrition from synovial fluid. Radiographic findings include maintenance of joint space, subchondral linear radiolucencies and cystic lesions, and bone eburnation, collapse, and fragmentation (Fig. 10). With extensive collapse of bone, incongruity of apposing osseous surfaces leads to secondary degenerative arthritis with narrowing of articular space.

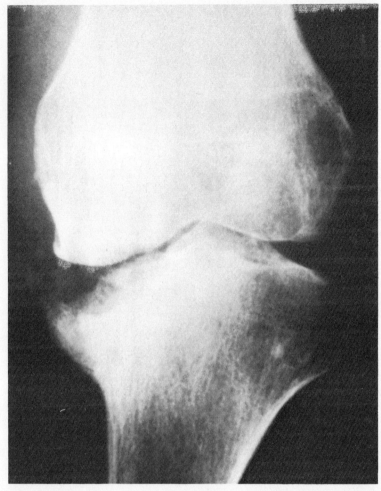

Fig. 9. Neuroarthropathy. Note collapse and fragmentation of the tibial plateaus and extensive bone sclerosis.

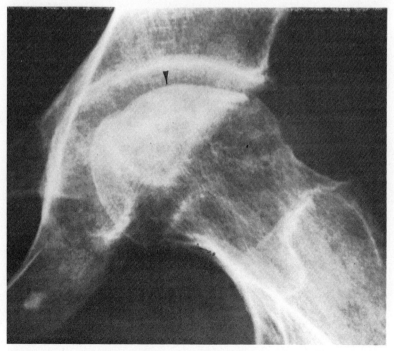

Fig. 10. Osteonecrosis. Significant collapse of the femoral head is observed (arrowhead). The joint space is maintained.

103

PRIMARY NEOPLASMS

Primary neoplasms of joints are rare. Two conditions are worthy of note; whether or not either represents a true neoplasm is a matter of debate.

Pigmented villonodular synovitis is a condition associated with monoarticular villonodular proliferation of synovial tissue, most frequently apparent in the knee, hip, and elbow. Radiographic changes are soft tissue swelling, which may be nodular in outline, and osseous erosion, particularly in "tight" articulations such as the hip (Fig. 11). Osteoporosis and joint space narrowing may be absent.

Idiopathic synovial osteochondromatosis is characterized by cartilaginous metaplasia of synovial tissue in a single joint such as the knee, elbow, or hip. Roentgenologic findings are soft tissue swelling and multiple intraarticular radiodensities of variable size representing calcification and ossification of synovial tissue (Fig. 12). Osteoporosis, joint space narrowing and osseous erosion may be late findings.

MISCELLANEOUS DISORDERS
Hemophilia

This disease is associated with recurrent hemarthrosis. The most commonly involved joints are the knees, ankles, and elbows. Acutely, joint effusion produces a relatively radiodense shadow about the articulation. Repeated hemorrhage leads to osteoporosis, degeneration of articular cartilage, subchondral cystic lesions, bony hypertrophy, and deformities (Fig. 13). The combination of osteoporosis, joint space narrowing, and bony hypertrophy in hemophilia simulates the findings of juvenile-onset rheumatoid arthritis, and differentiation of roentgenographic changes in the two conditions may be

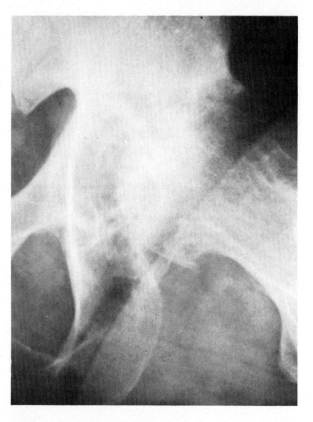

Fig. 11. Pigmented villonodular synovitis. Findings are joint space narrowing and multiple cystic lesions of acetabulum and femoral head.

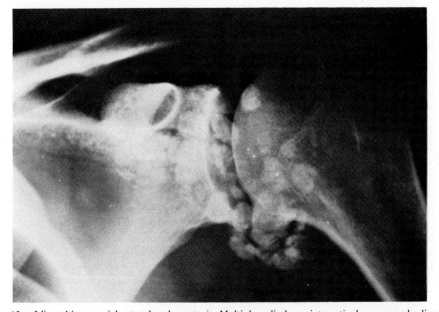

Fig. 12. Idiopathic synovial osteochondromatosis. Multiple radiodense intraarticular osseous bodies are seen. A large osteophyte is apparent on the medial aspect of the humeral head.

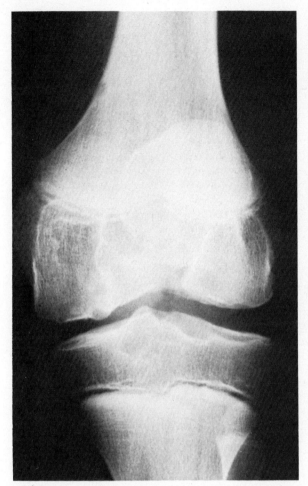

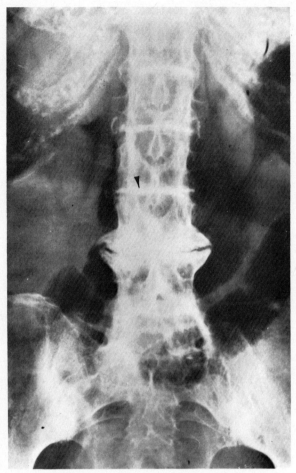

Fig. 13. Hemophilia. There is bony overgrowth of the epiphyses of the distal femur and proximal tibia. Cystic lesions are also seen. Note osseous irregularity of subchondral bone.

Fig. 14. Ochronosis. Widespread discal calcification is seen (arrowhead). Also observe spinal osteophytes and sacroiliac joint narrowing and sclerosis.

difficult. Subchondral cysts in hemophilia may be numerous and large, and massive intraosseous defects or pseudotumors may be seen. Bony enlargement, as in juvenile-onset rheumatoid arthritis, is most common about the knee. As much of the pathologic and radiographic picture of hemophilia relates to repetitive intraarticular bleeding, similar alterations may be seen in other conditions associated with such hemorrhage, including other bleeding diatheses and even synovial hemangiomas.

Ochronosis

Ochronosis results in an accumulation of homogentistic acid and its polymer in various tissues of the body, including cartilage, synovium, and bone. The abnormally pigmented cartilage is subject to deterioration, with resulting denudation of cartilaginous tissue. A degenerativelike arthropathy may appear. Radiographic findings in ochronosis are widespread discal calcification, loss of intervertebral disc height, and osteoporosis of vertebral bodies (Fig. 14). Degenerative joint disease with articular space narrowing, reactive bone formation, and osteophytosis may be noted in the hips, shoulders, and knees. Intraarticular osseous bodies are frequently apparent.

SUMMARY

Limitation of space has allowed a discussion of the radiographic features of only the more important articular disorders. It is apparent that proper interpretation of these features requires an understanding of the pathogenesis and pathology of the disease and a knowledge of the specific sites or "target areas" that are most frequently affected in each disease. This understanding and knowledge allow accurate diagnosis in many patients with arthritis and lead to earlier and more appropriate therapy.

REFERENCES

Ahlback S: Osteoarthrosis of the knee. A radiographic investigation. Acta Radiol [Suppl] (Stockh) 277:7, 1968

Ansell BM, Kent PA: Radiological changes in juvenile chronic polyarthritis. Skeletal Radiol 1:129, 1977

Dwosh IL, Resnick D, Becker MA: Hip involvement in ankylosing spondylitis. Arthritis Rheum 19:683, 1976

Feldman F, Johnson AM, Walter JF: Acute axial neuroarthropathy. Radiology 111:1, 1974

Forestier J, Rotes Querol J: Senile ankylosing hyperostosis of the spine. Ann Rheum Dis 9:321, 1950

Milgram JW: Synovial osteochondromatosis. A histopathological study of thirty cases. J Bone Joint Surg 59A:792, 1977

Resnick D: Patterns of migration of the femoral head in osteoarthritis of the hip. Am J Roentgenol 124:62, 1975

Resnick D: Rheumatoid arthritis of the wrist. The compartmental approach. Med Radiogr Photogr 52:50, 1976

Resnick D: The radiographic manifestations of gouty arthritis CRC Crit Rev Diagn Imaging 9:265, 1977

Resnick D, Feingold ML, Curd J, Niwayama G, Goergen TG: Calcaneal abnormalities in articular disorders. Radiology 125:355, 1977

Resnick D, Niwayama G: On the nature and significance of bony proliferation in "rheumatoid variant" disorders. Am J Roentgenol 129:275, 1977

Resnick D, Niwayama G, Coutts RD: Subchondral cysts (geodes) in arthritic disorders: Pathologic and radiographic appearance of the hip joint. Am J Roentgenol 128:799, 1977

Resnick D, Niwayama G, Goergen TG: Degenerative disease of the sacro-iliac joint. Invest Radiol 10:608, 1975

Resnick D, Niwayama G, Goergen TG, Utsinger PD, Shapiro RF, Haselwood DH, Wiesner KB: Clinical, radiographic and pathologic abnormalities in calcium pyrophosphate dihydrate deposition disease (CPPD): Pseudogout. Radiology 122:1, 1977

Resnick D, Shaul SR, Robins JM: Diffuse idiopathic skeletal hyperostosis (DISH): Forestier's disease with extraspinal manifestations. Radiology 115:513, 1975

Schmorl G, Junghanns H, in: Besemann EF (ed): The Human Spine in Health and Disease (ed 2). New York, Grune & Stratton, 1971, pp 141, 186, 354

Scott PM: Bone lesions in pigmented villonodular synovitis. J Bone Joint Surg 50B:306, 1968

Radioisotopic Assessment of Articular Structures

J. Desmond O'Duffy and Heinz W. Wahner

Joint scintigraphy was introduced in the 1960s by Weiss and Alarcón-Segovia, who showed that uptake of radioiodinated albumin and technetium-99 m (^{99m}Tc) pertechnetate was increased in inflamed joints as compared to normal ones. The localization of these isotopes in inflamed joints results from increased synovial vascularity associated with synovitis. The two isotopes currently used most often for joint scintigraphy are ^{99m}Tc-pertechnetate and ^{99m}Tc-diphosphonate. Whereas ^{99m}Tc-pertechnetate is 90 percent bound to serum protein, ^{99m}Tc-diphosphonate is a bone-seeking nuclide.

The essential features of the two types of radiopharmaceuticals are shown in Table 1. Although acceptable levels of total body radiation dosage are used, joint scans should probably be avoided in children and pregnant women.

^{99m}Tc-PERTECHNETATE IMAGING

To block uptake of the isotope by the thyroid gland, patients are premedicated with 250 mg of oral sodium perchlorate. ^{99m}Tc-Pertechnetate is not suited to scanning of joints of the axial skeleton. The hip joints cannot readily be imaged by ^{99m}Tc-pertechnetate because of interference from adjacent soft tissues and from activity in the bladder. Examples of normal and abnormal joint images are illustrated in Figure 1.

In the normal joint, uptake is not detected in amounts exceeding background radiation of adjacent tissues. In synovitis two phases of increased activity are recognized: an early "vascular" phase within minutes, and a delayed phase at 1–2 hours, which is thought to represent binding of nuclide to protein in the inflammatory exudate. Although the former mechanism predominates, the distinction is not important because uptake remains abnormal in inflamed joints for hours.

Abnormal scintigrams with ^{99m}Tc-pertechnetate correlate well with clinically apparent synovitis and may even exceed the accuracy of the physician in designating palpable synovitis. At times, abnormal joint scans predict sites where clinically apparent synovitis later develops. Any inflamed joint may produce a positive scintiscan. Studies of rheumatoid arthritis, gout, septic arthritis, and numerous other inflammatory arthropathies have been carried out. Abnormal uptake is lessened or normalized by effective treatment and scans have been useful for following the effects of treatment in rheumatoid arthritis.

Despite methodologic advances, joint scanning by ^{99m}Tc-pertechnetate has not yet found a prominent place in the practice of rheumatology. The chief reasons for this appear to be as follows: (1) The abnormal uptake is nonspecific. Abnormal scans are found in such nonarticu-

Table 1
Features of Technetium Radiopharmaceuticals

Isotope	Scan Begins	Isotope Half-Life (hr)	Usual i.v. Dose (mCi)	Total-Body Irradiation Dose (mrad/mCi)
^{99m}Tc-Pertechnetate	10 min	6	1–10	12
^{99m}Tc-Diphosphonate	2–4 hr	6	15	10

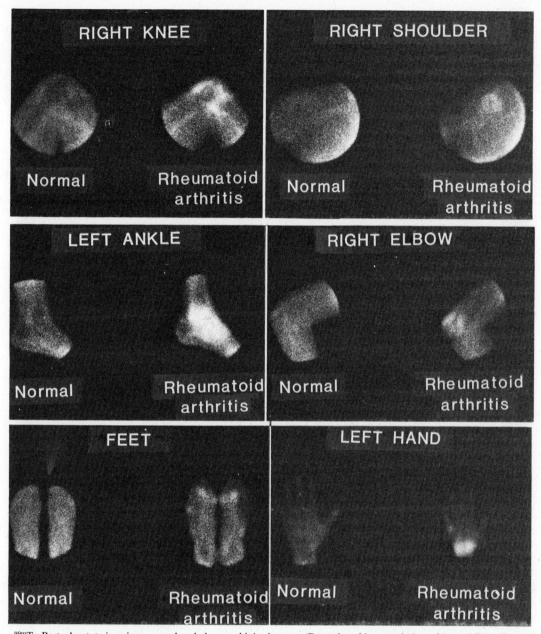

Fig. 1. ^{99m}Tc-Pertechnetate imaging: normal and abnormal joint images. (Reproduced by permission of the publisher from Wahner and O'Duffy: Mayo Clin Proc 51:525, 1976.)

lar states as Sudek's atrophy, shoulder–hand syndrome, and other conditions with increased vascularity. Positive scans are frequent over joints with mild osteoarthritis, thus interfering with the evaluation of other forms of synovitis. (2) The diagnosis of most rheumatic diseases by conventional clinical and radiologic methods is not difficult. (3) These scans involve an associated total-body irradiation burden.

Nevertheless, there are certain instances in which ^{99m}Tc-pertechnetate joint scanning is useful. In early rheumatoid arthritis, scans may show abnormal uptake where clinical findings are absent or doubtful. In polymyalgia rheumatica, clinical examination of joints is often

unrewarding, but abnormal scintigrams of shoulder joints are common. In psychogenic rheumatism, a normal scintigram reassures both patient and physician.

^{99m}Tc-DIPHOSPHONATE SCINTIGRAPHY

This is performed 2–4 hours after injection of 15 mCi of ^{99m}Tc-labeled diphosphonate. Diphosphonate is commercially available and is labeled just before use. Thyroid blockage is unnecessary. Because of the better target to background ratio, deeply located joints such as hips and spine can be evaluated.

The increased uptake of ^{99m}Tc-phosphate compounds by inflamed joints is thought to result from their chemadsorption onto hydroxyapatite crystals at juxtaarticular cancellous bone, which in most joint diseases becomes abnormally vascular. However, synovial vascularity is also likely to contribute to abnormal uptake. A drawback to joint scanning with radioactive phosphates is that normal joints show increased uptake as compared to background. Furthermore, positive images are obtained in degenerative joint disease when synovitis is not apparent. Therefore, the sensitivity of ^{99m}Tc-phosphate radiopharmaceuticals appears too great for practical application in the diagnosis of synovitis of peripheral joints.

Nevertheless, there are at least two conditions affecting the axial skeleton in which ^{99m}Tc-labeled phosphates have proven useful. In early ankylosing spondylitis, sacroiliac joint scans with ^{99m}Tc-phosphates may show abnormal uptake before clinical or roentgenologic abnormalties are apparent. Osteonecrosis of the femoral head either in children or adults may also be detected by ^{99m}Tc-labeled phosphates. In osteonecrosis, the decreased uptake over the area of dead bone contrasts with normal or increased uptake of the surrounding bone. Other possible indications are in patients with suspected loosening or infection of a joint arthroplasty, and in the preoperative evaluation of arthroplasty of the osteoarthritic knee. In the latter instance, the pattern of increased uptake of the diphosphonate may guide the surgeon as to the choice of operation, that is, arthroplasty versus osteotomy.

REFERENCES

Hoffer PB, Genant HK: Radionuclide joint imaging. Semin Nucl Med 6:121, 1976

Lentte BC, Russell AS, Percy JS, Jackson FI: The scintigraphic investigation of sacroiliac disease. J Nucl Med 18:529, 1977

McCarty DJ, Polcyn RE, Collins PA, Gottschalk A: ^{99m}Technetium scintiphotography in arthritis: I Technique and interpretation. Arthritis Rheum 13:11, 1970

Wahner HW, O'Duffy JD: Peripheral joint scanning with technetium pertechnetate, application in clinical practice. Mayo Clin Proc 51:525, 1976

Arthrography (Synoviography)

Gene G. Hunder and Joseph J. Combs, Jr.

Arthrography, namely, roentgenography of a joint after injection of a contrast material, is a widely used procedure. It is most commonly performed to visualize radiolucent intraarticular and periarticular structures. In some instances, the injection of air or carbon dioxide in addition to contrast medium produces better outlines (double-contrast technique). Tomography has been combined with arthrography to focus on a particular region of a joint.

Arthrography is relatively easy to perform and standard radiology equipment can be used. The examination may be repeated if follow-up is necessary. There are few complications except for mild discomfort during the procedure or for a short time afterward, and occasional transient eosinophilic synovitis. Contraindications include allergy to iodine, a hemorrhagic diathesis, and infection.

PROCEDURE

Before injecting the contrast material, the overlying skin is cleansed as for any arthrocentesis. For most joints the needle should be introduced under fluoroscopic guidance. If the needle is in the joint, the contrast medium will be seen to run into the cavity away from the tip of the needle. Visualization is improved by aspirating excessive joint fluid before the contrast material is injected. Currently employed contrast agents are commercial preparations used for excretory urography such as meglumine diatrizoate. Enough contrast medium is injected to distend the joint slightly. In a double-contrast examination less contrast agent is injected along with variable amounts of air. After the injection, the needle is withdrawn and the joint is moved several times to disperse the medium throughout the synovial cavity. Radiographs should be taken without delay because absorption and

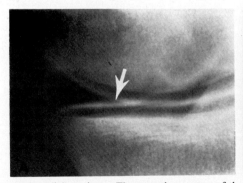 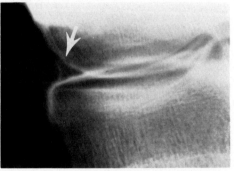

Fig. 1A. Normal medial meniscus. The smooth contours of the triangular cartilage are surrounded by contrast medium. Arrow points to inner edge of meniscus. **B.** Vertical tear of medial meniscus. Contrast medium has entered medial portion of triangular cartilage (arrow). (Courtesy of Dr. Richard A. McLeod.)

dilution cause a rapid decrease in contrast density after 10–20 minutes.

APPLICATIONS IN DIAGNOSIS AND EVALUATION

Arthrography has been used extensively to evaluate patients with internal derangement of the knee (Fig. 1A and B). Accuracy of 70–90 percent has been reported in the diagnosis of medial meniscus lesions. Lateral meniscus alterations, however, are more difficult to identify. Disruption of the medial and lateral collateral ligaments and the joint capsule are detected by extravasation of the medium outside of the confines of the joint. Stress maneuvers can be performed to improve visualization of abnormal structures. The cruciate ligaments and irregularities of the articular cartilage may be demonstrated but are difficult to assess. Cartilaginous loose bodies may be outlined. Hypertrophied synovial membranes producing nodular filling defects can be seen in villonodular synovitis and rheumatoid arthritis but are sometimes difficult to distinguish from fibrin clots.

The differential diagnosis of popliteal masses is aided by arthrography. This test may help separate popliteal cysts from popliteal artery aneurysms, neoplasms, or simply adipose tissue. Popliteal cysts are extensions or enlargements of normal knee bursae, particularly the gastrocnemius-semimembranosus bursa, or posterior herniations of the joint capsule (Fig. 2). Often the connection from the knee to the cyst is narrow and operates as a one-way flap valve into the cyst allowing synovial fluid to enter the cyst only during active flexion of the knee. Popliteal cysts may rupture into the calf, simulating thrombophlebitis. When an arthrogram is being performed to investigate a popliteal mass, the contrast agent is usually injected into the knee joint anteriorly. the knee

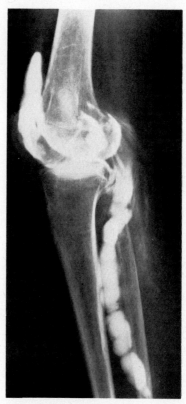

Fig. 2. Large popliteal cyst that has dissected nearly the entire length of the calf. (Courtesy of Dr. Richard A. McLeod.)

is then wrapped with an elastic bandage from the top of the suprapatellar pouch to the joint line and the patient is asked to walk a short distance. Extravasation of the contrast agent into the soft tissues of the calf indicates

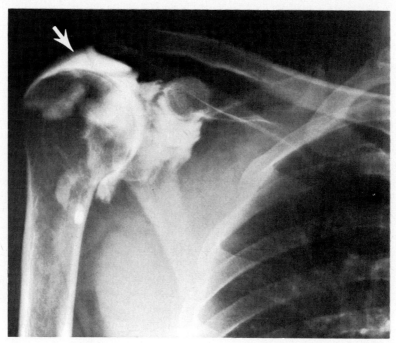

Fig. 3. Torn rotator cuff of shoulder. Contrast medium has entered subacromial bursa (arrow) from glenohumeral joint. (Courtesy of Dr. Richard A. McLeod.)

rupture of the popliteal cyst. Normal bursae may be distended by the injection of large amounts of contrast medium and confuse the diagnosis.

Arthrography is helpful in evaluating patients with shoulder pain, particularly those suspected to have injuries of the rotator cuff. The rotator cuff is a portion of the shoulder capsule and separates the joint cavity from the subacromial bursa. When this structure is torn, contrast medium injected into the glenohumeral joint can enter the subacromial bursa (Fig. 3). In adhesive capsulitis of the shoulder the joint space is contracted, and in recurrent dislocations of the humerus the degree of laxity of the anterior capsule and ligaments and enlargement of the axillary recess can be determined.

In the hip, arthrograms may help assess epiphyseal dysplasia, dislocations, adhesive capsulitis, and synovial chondromatosis. A more recent use has been to evaluate hip pain after total hip prosthesis surgery. Seepage of the contrast material between the methyl methacrylate and bone, whether in the acetabular or femoral components, indicates loosening. Abscess cavities and fistulous tracts may also be demonstrated.

Although experience with other peripheral joints is less extensive than for those discussed above, arthrograms have been used to evaluate synovial linings, the integrity of ligaments and capsules, and fistulous tracts related to nearly every joint.

REFERENCES

Carpenter JR, Hattery RR, Hunder GG, Bryan RS, McLeod RA: Ultrasound evaluation of the popliteal space. Comparison with arthrography and physical examination. Mayo Clin Proc 51:498, 1976

Desmet AA, Ting YM: Shoulder arthrography in rheumatoid arthritis. Radiology 116:601, 1975

Nicholas JA, Freiberger RA, Killoran PJ: Double-contrast arthrography of the knee. Its value in the management of two hundred twenty-five knee derangements. J Bone Joint Surg 52-A:203, 1970

Arthroscopy

Joseph J. Combs, Jr., and Gene G. Hunder

Arthroscopy is a precise and exacting endoscopic procedure employed to examine synovial joints. The procedure originated in Japan, and through the continued efforts of Watanabe, the arthroscope was finally developed as a practical diagnostic instrument. With the incorporation of perfected fiber optics and fiber light, the arthroscope has now achieved a technically superior design configuration over earlier models.

TYPES OF ARTHROSCOPES

Currently there are two basic types of arthroscopes in general use. The first is a needle scope having a diameter of 1.7–2.7 mm. The small size makes it ideal for use with local anesthesia; however, many arthroscopists feel this instrument is too small for examination of larger joints such as the knee. This debatable limitation can be precluded by making multiple insertions into the larger joints requiring arthroscopic examination. The second type is the diagnostic–operating arthroscope, which is 3.8–5 mm in diameter and has the advantage of a larger visual field (65°). This scope provides greater flexibility in angle of vision, varying from straight ahead direct vision (180°–170°) through various intermediate angles to a complete right angle. A special operative arthroscope is also available. With these, 90 percent of the knee joint can be accurately assessed from a single anterior approach, and when the needle scope is also used to examine the posterior compartment practically the entire joint is visualized.

APPLICATIONS IN DIAGNOSIS AND EVALUATION

Arthroscopy is most often used for the diagnostic evaluation of the knee; however, other joints, such as the shoulder, elbow, hip, and ankle, have also been examined. Arthroscopic findings greatly enhance the data derived from clinical, radiographic, and arthrographic examinations (Fig. 1). A recent prospective study of 100 patients with internal derangements of the knee compared and correlated clinical diagnosis, results of arthrography, and findings at arthroscopy and arthrotomy. The clinical diagnosis was correct in 72 patients, correct but incomplete in 10, and incorrect in 18. Arthroscopy was accurate in 94 patients and influenced subsequent surgical therapy in 55. Unexpected lesions were documented in 25 patients and arthroscopy was deemed critical for the diagnosis in 16. Unnecessary surgery was avoided in 21 of 23 additional patients analyzed who also underwent arthroscopy, but not arthrotomy. Diagnostic accuracy of arthroscopy varies directly with the experience and expertise of the examiner, and in all reported series the accuracy figure is 85–95 percent. Arthrographic accuracy in the series cited above was 78 percent overall (84 percent for medial meniscus and 72 percent for lateral meniscus). Arthroscopy and arthrography are complimentary procedures, each requiring comparable expertise not only in technique, but also in interpretation of findings.

The primary application for arthroscopy is in evaluation of the patient with recurrent or chronic knee pain, locking, giving way, or swelling for which no etiology has been established by all usual diagnostic procedures. This has been called by some the "problem knee." There are a number of other clinical situations in which arthroscopy should be considered: (1) examination of patients with medical–legal problems or compensation pending in whom it is desirable to avoid arthrotomy; (2) verification

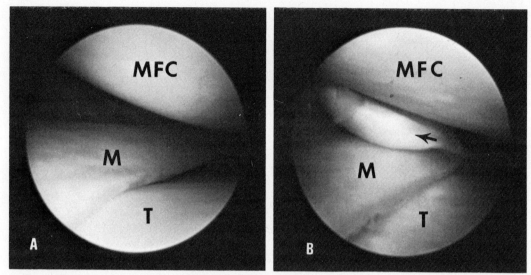

Fig. 1. Arthroscopic views of the medial compartment, left knee (lateral infrapatellar approach) in two patients. **A.** Medial femoral condyle (MFC), anterior-midsegment of the meniscus (M), and tibial plateau (T) are normal. **B.** Medial femoral condyle (MFC) and tibial plateau (T) are normal. Arrow indicates the disrupted segment of the posterior meniscus which is folded over the intact anterior meniscal segment (M). The arthrogram was reported as negative in this patient.

of the correct side of the meniscal lesion, since pain from one compartment is often referred to the opposite side; (3) examination of the adolescent girl with chondromalacia patella whose symptoms also suggest an additional problem; (4) removal of loose bodies or torn free edges of the menisci; and (5) detection of meniscal mimes. Obviously, identification and removal of minor lesions within the knee joint can preclude more extensive and possibly unnecessary surgery.

Meniscal mimes reported by Jackson comprise a variety of lesions simulating meniscal disruption or tear which may easily be identified by arthroscopy: (1) loose bodies; (2) chondromalacia (patellofemoral joint, femoral condyles); (3) osteochondral fractures; (4) anterior cruciate ligament lesions (isolated tears, chronic stubs); (5) hypermobile or dislocating menisci; (6) popliteal tendon (rupture or complete avulsion); (7) crystalline synovitis (gout or pseudogout); and (8) synovial impingement. A fibrous plica arising usually from the medial synovial wall, coursing over the femoral condyle, and inserting into the medial fat pad and synovium can also result in medial joint line pain, clicking, swelling, and rarely hemarthrosis (medial plica syndrome). Photographic documentation of intraarticular structures and pathologic findings provides further unique pictorial data to enhance the clinical record.

Direct vision synovial biopsy through the arthroscope can provide useful diagnostic data in various forms of arthritis such as rheumatoid arthritis, degenerative arthritis, crystalline-induced synovitis, and pigmented villonodular synovitis. Synovial membrane alterations may be localized, especially early in the disease, and therefore missed on a "blind" biopsy. Synovial hypertro-

phy occurs commonly in the intercondylar notch area surrounding the cruciate ligaments in milder early rheumatoid arthritis when the remainder of the synovial membrane appears normal. Radiographs in degenerative arthritis frequently appear normal; however, when the articular cartilage is viewed arthroscopically extensive chondromalacia of the femoral condyles and tibial plateau is encountered. A recent finding of interest is the presence of cartilage erosions of the non-weight-bearing areas of the femoral condyles in degenerative arthritis.

Clinical improvement in the course of degenerative arthritis has been reported by several observers following arthroscopy. This observation is probably not attributable to a placebo effect since in one series the clinical improvement lasted up to 5 years. Although reasons for this observation are as yet unknown, several tentative theories prevail. One possible reason is the effect of distension of the joint space itself and another is the extensive irrigation of the joint while the arthroscopic procedure is being carried out. The fluid evacuated from the knee of a patient with degenerative arthritis at the end of the arthroscopic procedure commonly contains considerable amounts of fibrinous and cartilaginous debris. Content of various enzymes in the synovial fluid, cartilage, and synovial membrane could conceivably be altered, but this theory warrants further investigation before any definitive conclusion is reached.

A stiff knee and a septic joint are the two important contraindications to arthroscopy. Hemarthrosis, if not cleared by adequate irrigation during the procedure, may decrease visual clarity but is not a contraindication.

Complications following this procedure are infrequent. The infection rate in all reported series has been less than 1 percent. Hemarthrosis is very unusual and usually no significant pain is experienced by the patient following arthroscopy.

In addition to diagnosis and therapy, arthroscopy appears to be a valuable tool for research in the various forms of arthritis, although it has not been used extensively as an investigative procedure in the past. The impact of the arthroscopic findings as they relate to diagnosis and surgical management cannot be overemphasized.

REFERENCES

DeHaven KE, Collins HR: Diagnosis of internal derangements of the knee (the role of arthroscopy). J Bone Joint Surg 57A:802, 1975

Jackson RW, Dandy DJ: Arthroscopy of the Knee. New York, Grune & Stratton, 1976

O'Connor RL: The arthroscope in the management of crystal-induced synovitis of the knee. J Bone Joint Surg 55A:1443, 1973

O'Connor RL: Arthroscopy. Philadelphia, Lippincott, 1977

DIFFERENTIAL APPROACH TO MAJOR RHEUMATIC SYNDROMES

Acute Monarticular Arthritis

Don L. Goldenberg

DIFFERENTIAL DIAGNOSIS OF ARTHRITIS AND NONARTICULAR RHEUMATISM

Acute pain and inflammation in a joint may be due to acute arthritis (synovial inflammation) or to pathology in an anatomic structure adjacent to the articular capsule (periarthritis or nonarticular rheumatism). Tendon sheaths, bursa, ganglia, vascular structures, and subcutaneous nodules may all become inflamed and enlarged, thereby simulating an acute arthritis of a contiguous joint.

The presence of a joint effusion is the most reliable sign of acute arthritis (Table 1). Although moderate amounts of excess synovial fluid are demonstrable by careful palpation of involved joints, small amounts of fluid may be confirmed only following an arthrocentesis. Massive synovial effusions are virtual proof of primary joint pathology. However, scant effusions may be due to a "sympathetic" reaction from an adjacent periarthritis or bone infection. For example, a prepatella bursitis or a quadriceps insertion tendinitis may cause small, noninflammatory knee effusions, merely as a reaction to the nearby inflammation.

The swelling associated with periarthritis is generally not extensive nor does it usually distend the articular capsule. It is often more discrete and firmer than that caused by acute synovitis. Periarthritis causes tenderness on palpation localized to one part of a joint such as a bursa or tendon insertion. This tenderness and inflammation often is not confirmed to the anatomic structure of the articular capsule. Arthritis usually causes diffuse tenderness over the whole joint. Although the range of motion may be limited by arthritis or periarthritis, the active range of motion is often much less than the passive range of motion in periarticular disorders such as bursitis and tendinitis. Arthritis generally results in an equal loss of active and passive ranges of motion.

Not only may it be difficult to differentiate arthritis from periarthritis, but many rheumatic diseases including rheumatoid arthritis, gout, gonococcal arthritis, and hepatitis cause simultaneous joint as well as surrounding soft tissue inflammation.

DIFFERENTIAL DIAGNOSIS OF ACUTE MONARTHRITIS

Certain rheumatic diseases typically cause an acute monarthritis (Table 2). Any patient who presents with an acute monarthritis should undergo immediate arthrocentesis. Even if a specific diagnosis cannot be made following a careful synovial fluid analysis, certain illnesses can be ruled out, and the synovial fluid analysis will be diagnostically helpful.

Fortunately, the most common types of acute arthritis as well as those rheumatic diseases that can be specifically treated are the same conditions associated with characteristic synovial fluid changes (Table 2).

Bacterial Arthritis

The most important cause of acute arthritis specifically diagnosed by synovial fluid analysis is septic arthritis (see the section on Infectious Arthritis in the fascicle on Specific Articular and Connective Tissue Diseases). In a recent 1-year review of patients admitted to Boston City Hospital with acute monarthritis, acute bacterial arthritis was the most common etiology. While disseminated gonococcemia often causes polyarthritis and tenosynovitis, most other types of bacterial arthritis cause an acute monarthritis (Table 3).

If gram stain smear demonstrates the microorganism, definitive therapy should be immediately begun. Although gram-positive cocci will be identified on a gram stain smear of the synovial fluid in the majority of cases of staphylococcal arthritis, most other organisms, especially *Neisseria gonorrhoeae,* will usually not be identified in this fashion. Helpful synovial fluid features while awaiting culture results include the following: leukocyte count greater than 50,000 cells/mm^3, greater than 90 percent polymorphonuclear leukocytes, a poor mucin clot, and a depressed synovial fluid glucose.

It is critical to be aware always of the possibility of septic arthritis. Special consideration of this diagnosis should be entertained in immunosuppressed hosts, patients with recent joint trauma, and patients with obvious bacteremia. It is especially important to consider superimposed septic arthritis in patients with chronic joint

Table 1
Differential Signs of Synovitis versus Nonarticular Rheumatism

Sign	Synovitis	Nonarticular Rheumatism
Swelling	Confined to articular capsule; may be massive	Localized; may be firm; usually small
Tenderness	Usually involves the whole joint	Usually a focal area which may extend beyond articular capsule
Restricted range of motion	Active = passive range of motion	Passive > active range of motion

disease such as rheumatoid arthritis. Therefore, if the etiology of a new joint effusion in a patient with previous arthritis is not perfectly clear, that joint must be aspirated and the fluid cultured and analyzed.

Gout. The most common etiology of acute monarthritis in an ambulatory care setting is gout. Usually small joints of the feet, especially the first metatarsophalangeal, are initially affected. However, large joints such as the knee and sometimes more than one joint are often acutely symptomatic. Clues to the diagnosis include the following: recurrent attacks of acute arthritis with no pain between attacks, precipitation of an attack by physical stress such as surgery, marked periarticular swelling and inflammation, and an abrupt explosive onset, which often begins in the early morning hours. Gout should not be a serious diagnostic consideration in premenopausal females. Radiographs are usually normal unless recurrent attacks have occurred over years and chronic tophaceous arthritis is present. The most helpful laboratory finding is hyperuricemia. However, nearly 20 percent of patients will not have an elevated serum uric acid during the attack of acute gouty arthritis, and hyperuricemia frequently is present in asymptomatic patients.

If possible, the diagnosis of gout should be confirmed by the demonstration of monosodium urate crystals by polarized microscopy (needlelike crystals demonstrating strong negative birefringence). However, it may be extremely difficult to obtain synovial fluid from small joints of the feet, and therefore a definitive diagnosis sometimes cannot be made. If gout is suspected but not confirmed by visualizing crystals, a therapeutic trial of colchicine is warranted. Adequate colchicine treatment (0.5 mg orally hourly for four to eight doses or 2 mg intravenously) generally produces remarkable relief of symptoms within 12–24 hours and helps to confirm the diagnosis (see section on Crystal-induced Arthritis: Gout in fascicle on Specific Articular and Connective Tissue Diseases).

Pseudogout. Calcium pyrophosphate dihydrate deposition disease may cause a chronic polyarthritis simulating rheumatoid arthritis or osteoarthritis, but most often it causes an acute or subacute monarthritis resembling gout (i.e., pseudogout, see section on Crystal-induced Arthritis: Pseudogout and Hydroxyapatite in fascicle on Specific Articular and Connective Tissue Diseases). Clues to the diagnosis of pseudogout include the following: large joint mon- or oligarthritis, middle-aged or elderly patients, x-ray evidence of chondrocalci-

nosis, and associated endocrine–metabolic diseases such as hyperparathyroidism, Charcot's joint, acromegaly, hemochromatosis, Wilson's disease, and ochronosis.

The definite diagnosis of pseudogout is confirmed by the demonstration of calcium pyrophosphate dihydrate crystals by polarizing microscopy. These crystals are weakly positively birefringent and are often small and pleomorphic; they may be missed unless a careful search is made. The acute attack of pseudogout frequently responds to joint aspiration without specific therapy, although antiinflammatory medications may hasten the recovery.

Patients may develop recurrent acute mon- or oligarthritis that simulates gout but crystals may not be initially identified by light and polarizing microscopy. In certain cases, the crystals are not visualized during the first few hours of the attack but are seen with subsequent synovial fluid analysis. In addition, calcium pyrophosphate, monosodium urate, and hydroxyapatite crystals have all been identified by electron microscopy even when not visualized by light and polarizing microscopy. These microcrystals are all capable of initiating a pathologic synovitis in man and animals.

Neoplasms

Other than septic arthritis and crystal-induced arthritis, only a few types of acute monarthritis are associated with specific synovial fluid characteristics. Solid tumors or lymphoproliferative disorders that involve joints may be diagnosed by the demonstration of malignant cells in a Wright's stain smear of the synovial fluid. However, in most other rheumatic diseases synovial fluid or synovial membrane pathologic changes are not of diagnostic significance unless research techniques not generally available in routine laboratories are employed.

Hemorrhagic Arthritis

Hemorrhagic synovial fluid associated with acute monarthritis is most often secondary to trauma, which can vary in severity from an osteochondral fracture to a minor event not even perceived by the patient (Table 2). If no history of trauma is obtained, the diagnosis may be obscure. Localized tenderness should alert the physician to a mechanical etiology of the hemorrhagic synovial fluid and arthrography or arthroscopy should be considered. Acute hemorrhagic arthritis secondary to hemophilia almost always begins in childhood, and adults not only will have a previous history of hemarthrosis, but radiologic sequelae of joint damage is also evident. A number of

Table 2
Differential Diagnosis of Acute Monarthritis

Causes	Definitive Diagnostic Test	Other Helpful Features
Common causes		
Bacterial arthritis	Gram stain, culture	"Purulent" synovial fluid (WBC > 50,000/mm³), decreased synovial fluid glucose
Gout	Uric acid crystals in synovial fluid	Podagra, hyperuricemia
Pseudogout	Calcium pyrophosphate dihydrate crystals in synovial fluid	Radiologic chondrocalcinosis
Trauma	—	Hemorrhagic synovial fluid, positive arthroscopy or arthrogram
Less common causes		
Degenerative joint disease	—	Usually more indolent
Sickle cell	Positive sickle cell preparation on blood	Often associated with painful "crisis"
Pigmented villonodular synovitis	—	Brownish bloody synovial fluid
Rheumatoid arthritis	—	Development of polyarthritis; rheumatoid factors
Rheumatoid variants	—	Extraarticular features, HLA-B27 marker
Rare causes		
Cancer	Malignant cells in synovial fluid or membrane	Bone destruction on x-ray
Hemophilia	"Factor" deficiency	Hemorrhagic synovial fluid
Lyme arthritis	—	Skin lesion, recurrent acute arthritis, geographic cluster of cases
Whipple's disease	Bacillary bodies in synovium	Extraarticular features

Table 3
Variable Presentations of Septic Arthritis

Etiology	Usual No. of Joints	Onset	Synovial Fluid		Associated Clinical Findings
			Mean Leukocyte Count (cells/mm³)	Percentage of Polymorphonuclear Cells	
Gonococcal	1–6	Abrupt	50,000	85–90	Rash, fever, genitourinary infection
Gram-positive cocci	1	Explosive	90,000	95	Fever
Gram-negative bacilli	1	Abrupt	90,000	95	Fever, urinary tract infection
Tuberculosis	1	Insidious	20,000	75	Osteomyelitis
Fungus	1	Insidious	10,000	50	Osteomyelitis
Hepatitis	4–10	Abrupt	2,000–20,000	10–75	Rash, abnormal liver function tests, detectable hepatitis surface antigen
Rubella	2–10	Abrupt	5,000	50	Rash
Lyme	1–2	Abrupt Recurrent	24,000	80	Erythema chronicum migrans

recent reports suggest that anticoagulants may be associated with spontaneous or trauma-related acute hemarthrosis. Benign and malignant tumors may also cause hemarthrosis. Hemangiomas and synovial osteochondromatosis are often diagnosed by the x-ray finding of multiple calcific densities, but are usually asymptomatic unless they interfere with joint motion. Pigmented villonodular synovitis, typically associated with a brownish red synovial fluid, generally causes the insidious onset of joint swelling and restricted motion. Lymphoma, leukemia, and primary or metastatic cancer may all cause acute arthritis which may be hemorrhagic.

Degenerative Processes

In most other causes of acute monarthritis, the synovial fluid analysis is of limited diagnostic utility (Table 2). Noninflammatory synovial fluid is most often associated with degenerative or mechanical processes. The synovitis associated with osteochondritis dissecans, chondromalacia patella, and osteoarthritis is typically more chronic and indolent, although an acute monarthritis may occur with these disorders. A past history of joint swelling, pain on joint motion, joint "locking," and typical x-ray evidence of degenerative arthritis or calcified loose bodies suggest a noninflammatory, mechanical synovitis. A period of observation and articular rest should be initiated. Orthopedic consultation should help determine the need for further studies such as an arthrogram or arthroscopy. Analgesics, antiinflammatory agents, and occasionally intraarticular corticosteroids are effective therapy.

Endocrine and Metabolic Disorders

Endocrine and metabolic disorders may cause noninflammatory subacute arthritis. The diagnosis is almost always entertained because of the extraarticular features of the illness such as occurs in hemochromatosis, acromegaly, hypothyroidism, and Wilson's disease. Acute monarthritis is unusual, unless calcium pyrophosphate deposition disease is also present.

Rheumatoid Arthritis

It is most difficult to differentiate causes of acute monarthritis when the synovial fluid is inflammatory and no definitive synovial fluid characteristics are present. In some reports as many as one-third of patients with rheumatoid arthritis present initially with acute monarthritis. Although the rheumatoid factor may be positive and striking lymphocyte synovial membrane infiltrates may occur within only 1–2 months of the onset of monarthritis, the diagnosis of rheumatoid arthritis can only be made with certainty if the characteristic symmetric polyarthritis develops.

Reiter's Disease

Reiter's disease may begin with an explosive inflammatory mon- or oligarthritis. If urethritis, conjunctivitis, circinate balanitis, or keratoderma blennorrhaggicum and acute arthritis are present, the diagnosis is not difficult. However, patients may first develop inflammatory oligarthritis without the other typical extraarticular manifestations of Reiter's disease. The presence of HLA-B27 antigen is diagnostically helpful in these cases since it is present in greater than 90 percent of patients with Reiter's disease but less than 8 percent of control populations.

Gonococcal Arthritis

Reiter's disease may be especially difficult to differentiate from acute gonococcal arthritis. Both illnesses may cause an acute monarthritis or polyarthritis in young, sexually active patients, and both may cause urethritis, conjunctivitis, and skin lesions. Since *Neisseria gonorrhoeae* are recovered in only about 50 percent of the synovial fluids from patients with suspected gonococcal arthritis, the differential diagnosis may necessarily be determined by a therapeutic trial of antibiotics. Patients with gonococcal arthritis generally respond dramatically after only 24–48 hours of antimicrobial therapy. Psoriatic arthritis similarly may cause an acute monoarticular arthritis. The diagnosis cannot be specific without the typical skin lesions.

Tuberculosis and Fungal Infections

Although acute bacterial arthritis is the most common example of an infection associated with oligarthritis, other infectious agents also cause acute monarthritis. Tuberculosis and fungal infections occasionally spread to joints, causing an insidious monarthritis of large peripheral joints, Rarely, the onset of the arthritis is abrupt. The chest x-ray may fail to reveal acute infiltrates. Positive skin tests and serologic evidence of recent infection are helpful. The diagnosis of tuberculous or fungal arthritis is best achieved with synovial membrane histopathology and culture (see chapter on Applications of Synovial Membrane Biopsy in the fascicle on Diagnostic Procedures).

Viral Arthritis

Viruses may cause acute arthritis, although the association of an arthritis with a specific virus is usually somewhat tenuous. The synovial fluid examined in patients with suspected viral arthritis has often been mildly inflammatory with a predominance of mononuclear cells.

Lyme Arthritis

Lyme arthritis causes an oligarthritis in children or adults heralded by an expanding, annular skin lesion. The monarthritis remits in a few weeks without specific therapy but is usually recurrent. Until the etiologic agent is identified, the diagnosis must rest on clinical and epidemiologic criteria. Two important causes of acute polyarthritis, acute rheumatic fever and hepatitis, rarely present with a monarthritis.

Acute Arthritis of Unknown Etiology

If there are no specific synovial fluid or serum findings and no evidence of infection nor characteristic extraarticular manifestations, the etiology of acute arthritis is usually not initially identified. Frequently, the monarthritis spontaneously subsides and acute arthritis may not recur. Occasionally an unusual clinical course of recurrent attacks of monarthritis such as described in recurrent hydrarthroses and palindromic rheumatism may continue for many years. Although infectious arthritis and gout are the most frequent causes of acute monarthritis seen at our medical center, monarthritis of unknown etiology has been the next most prevalent diagnosis. Fortunately, those cases that have been followed for a few years after the initial attack have not been recurrent and have required no specific treatment.

REFERENCES

Arnett FC, McClusky OE, Schecter BZ, et al: Incomplete Reiter's syndrome: Discriminating features and HLA-W27 in diagnosis. Ann Intern Med 84:8, 1976

Brandt KD, Cathcart ES, Cohen AS: Gonococcal arthritis. Arthritis Rheum 17:503, 1974

Cohen AS (ed): Laboratory Diagnostic Procedures in the Rheumatic Diseases (ed 2). Boston, Little, Brown, 1975

Espinoza LR, Spilberg I, Osterland CK: Joint manifestations of sickle cell disease. Medicine (Baltimore) 53:295, 1974

Goldenberg DL, Cohen AS: Acute infectious arthritis. A review of patients with non-gonococcal joint infections. Am J Med 60:369, 1976

Goldenberg DL, Kelley W, Gibbons RB: Metastatic adenocarcinoma of synovium presenting as an acute arthritis. Arthritis Rheum 18:107, 1975

Honig S, Gorevic P, Hoffstein S, et al: Crystal deposition disease; Diagnosis by electron microscopy. Am J Med 63:161, 1977

Resnick D, Niwayoma G, Goergon T, et al: Clinical, radiographic and pathologic abnormalities in calcium pyrophosphate dihydrate deposition disease. Radiology 122:1, 1977

Chronic Monarticular Arthritis

Robert H. Persellin and Richard M. Pope

FOREIGN BODY SYNOVITIS AND CHRONIC INFECTION

Persistent synovitis of greater than 2 months' duration in a single joint suggests an intriguing list of differential diagnostic possibilities (Table 1). Consideration must be given to indolent infections, local tumors, degenerative processes, foreign bodies, and inflammatory arthritides with atypical modes of presentation. The relative frequency of each of these causes of chronic monarthritis has been described in several retrospective analyses. About one-quarter of cases was due to degenerative joint disease and 6–27 percent were ultimately diagnosed as rheumatoid arthritis. Joint tumors, infections, osteochondritis dissecans, and chondrocalcinosis were other frequent diagnoses. Synovitis of undetermined cause accounted for approximately 30 percent of the patients.

A systematic approach to the patient with chronic monarticular disease utilizing elements of the history and physical examination, study of the synovial fluid and membrane, and radiologic evaluation will usually uncover the pathogenetic mechanism. Once the correct etiology is established, a high proportion of these disorders can be effectively treated and the prognosis for most is favorable.

FOREIGN BODY SYNOVITIS

Penetrating injuries by sharp, spiculated objects can initiate a chronic inflammatory synovitis. The foreign bodies most often identified have been plant thorns, especially from shrubs and palms, the spines of sea urchins, and fragments of brick and stone.

Plant thorn synovitis presents as a transient episode of acute synovitis immediately after the initial trauma. This is followed by a relatively quiescent period and later by chronic monarthritis. The knee, as in most forms of chronic monarthritis, is usually involved. The sedimentation rate is mildly elevated and the synovial fluid is inflammatory with approximately 20,000 white blood cells/mm^3, 90 percent of which are neutrophils. Plant

thorns cannot be detected radiographically, hence the history is essential to suggest this diagnosis. If the nondegradable vegetable material is allowed to persist within the joint, a chronic granulomatous inflammation results which may lead to flexion contractures and ultimately to bony erosions. Surgical excision is advocated for treatment. A careful microscopic examination of the synovium will reveal foreign body giant cells and vegetable tissue, which is best identified with the aid of polarizing microscopy.

Sea urchin spine puncture wounds are usually followed by systemic manifestations in addition to a marked local inflammatory reaction. The systemic symptoms will subside after removal of the protruding spine, but persistence of small fragments is associated with the smoldering chronic local reaction. Synovial fluid white blood cell count ranges from 8500 to 15,500 cells/mm^3. In contrast to plant thorn synovitis, most of the cells are lymphocytes. Radiographs demonstrate the retained spine fragments; if left in the joint, they will lead to a giant cell granulomatous reaction. Excision will alleviate both local and systemic symptoms.

An iatrogenic form of detritic synovitis can result from fragmented joint prostheses. Silicone particles will initiate a chronic inflammatory synovitis. These refractile, radiolucent foreign bodies can be found extracellularly in the synovium or within multinucleated foreign body giant cells in the granulomatous reaction, both within the synovium and in the medullary spaces of cancellous bone. These silicone fragments, ranging from 10 to 100 μm in diameter, have also been detected in lymph nodes and can cause a regional lymphadenopathy. Diagnosis requires synovial membrane or lymph node biopsy.

Blood can act as a foreign body in initiating a chronic synovitis. The recurrent hemarthroses seen in classic hemophilia underscore the inflammatory nature of blood and the ability of recurrent hemarthroses to cause a chronic proliferative, destructive synovitis. Blood prod-

Table 1
Chronic Monarticular Arthritis

Foreign bodies	Tumors	Noninflammatory disorders
Plant thorns	Benign	Trauma
Sea urchin spines	Pigmented villonodular synovitis	Degenerative joint disease
Silicone fragments	Synovial chondromatosis	Aseptic necrosis
Blood	Other benign tumors	Charcot joint
	Malignant	
Infectious diseases	Synovial sarcoma	Inflammatory rheumatic disorders
Tuberculosis	Chondrosarcoma	Rheumatoid arthritis
Atypical mycobacteria	Metastatic tumors	Juvenile rheumatoid arthritis
Brucellosis		Seronegative spondyloarthropathies
Fungi		Sarcoidosis
Common bacterial pathogens		Crystal-induced arthritis
Osteomyelitis		Synovitis of unknown cause
Congential syphilis		

ucts are believed to stimulate synovial cells to release neutral proteinases, including collagenase, as well as acid hydrolases and prostaglandins. These contribute to the degradation of articular cartilage and bony destruction. Similar chemical and histologic changes have been observed in experimental hemarthrosis. The knee, elbow, and ankle, followed by the shoulder and hip, are the most commonly involved articulations in hemophiliac arthritis.

CHRONIC INFECTION

The incidence of tuberculous arthritis has greatly diminished over the past 40 years and now accounts for less than 10 percent of cases of chronic monarthritis. The manner of presentation also appears to have changed. Patients now present earlier in the course of their disorder, and joint destruction is not as advanced. The age group most affected ranges from 51 to 60 years of age and active pulmonary tuberculosis at the time of monarticular joint involvement is unusual. This contrasts with the preantibiotic era, in which younger patients were more often affected and active pulmonary tuberculosis and arthritis frequently coexisted. Tuberculous arthritis is predominantly a chronic monarticular disease and a weight-bearing joint, particularly the knee or hip, is involved. The incidence of spinal tuberculosis has diminished. Joints less frequently infected include the shoulder, the sternoclavicular joint, and the volar carpal tunnel at the wrist.

The primary symptoms are swelling and pain. Synovial fluid analysis may reveal over 100,000 white blood cells/mm³ or may be more moderately elevated. However, only rarely do polymorphonuclear cells account for greater than 90 percent of synovial fluid leukocytes, as is the usual finding in other forms of bacterial arthritis. Glucose is reduced in approximately two-thirds of synovial fluids. The organism may be identified by acid fast stain or by culture of the synovial fluid. However, histologic examination and culture of synovial tissue are more reliable. The tuberculin skin test is usually positive unless the patient is anergic. Roentgenographic findings are not characteristic and range from soft tissue swelling and osteopenia early in the disease to cartilaginous destruction and subchondral erosions. The necessity for surgical debridement in the treatment of tuberculous joint involvement is unclear. With extensive joint damage, surgery together with appropriate chemotherapy is probably indicated.

While the incidence of tuberculous arthritis has diminished greatly, it is still the most common cause of a chronic granulomatous infectious arthritis. The atypical mycobacteria may also cause chronic monarthritis. Trauma, occupational exposure, prior intraarticular injection, and immunosuppression are factors that have been associated with these infections. The tendon sheaths of the hand are often involved. Diagnosis is most reliably made by histology and culture of synovial tissue. Surgical resection together with antibacterial drugs as indicated by susceptibility testing are recommended.

Since the widespread pasteurization of milk, brucellosis has become an uncommon cause of chronic, granu-

lomatous monarthritis. Culture of involved tissue, usually from the prepatellar bursa, knee, or hip, is necessary for diagnosis since the *Brucella* agglutination titer is frequently normal in these patients.

Other granulomatous infections of joints are uncommon. Articular involvement by infectious fungal organisms is seen in males with outdoor occupations in endemic areas. Coccidioidomycosis, endemic in the southwestern United States, usually initiates an acute arthritis with systemic manifestations that spontaneously resolves within a month. A chronic granulomatous disease develops in less than 1 percent of these individuals, and in this group monarticular joint involvement can be seen. Often the synovium is infected by direct extension from adjacent bone. Synovial tissue histology and culture are diagnostically more useful than synovial fluid. Blastomycosis, endemic in the Mississippi and Ohio River valleys and the southeastern states, if disseminated, will involve bones and joints in about 30 percent of cases. Often patients present with monarticular arthritis, the ankle or knee being the most frequent joint. Smear and culture of the synovial fluid are usually diagnostic. Sporotrichosis arthritis occurs without skin and lung involvement. Usually infecting the knee or ankle, this form of fungal arthritis is best identified by concomitant culture of the synovial membrane and fluid. Disseminated candidiasis can also initiate a chronic monarthritis. Infection by this unusual organism should be suspected in the immunosuppressed patient or in one receiving parenteral hyperalimentation. Diagnosis is established by culture of the synovial fluid. Chronic monarticular infections due to either histoplasmosis or cryptococcosis have been reported but are rare.

The clinical presentation of patients with chronic fungal arthritis is similar to that of tuberculosis. Patients are usually febrile and local pain and soft tissue swelling are apparent. Ocassionally deep cutaneous abscesses or draining sinus tracts are apparent in the region of infection. The synovial fluid analysis and radiographic appearance are not distinctive from tuberculosis.

Chronic granulomatous arthritis due to sarcoidosis is well known but is almost always polyarticular in nature. If noncaseating granuloma are noted on synovial biopsy material from a patient with chronic monarticular arthritis, the diagnosis is more likely to be tuberculosis or even fungal arthritis rather than sarcoidosis.

Septic arthritis due to common bacterial organisms, if not appropriately treated with antibiotics, may become chronic. Untreated, smoldering staphylococcal or gonococcal arthritis may present a picture similar to tuberculosis. This is uncommon today since the diagnosis of bacterial arthritis is usually made in its acute form. Chronic infections of the sternoclavicular and glenohumoral joints with common pathogens have been reported. Gram-negative bacilli, especially in heroin abusers, may cause a chronic sternoclavicular pyarthrosis. The presentation can be one of a several-month history of pain, swelling, and decreased movement.

Clutton's joint is low-grade inflammation of the knee

of children and adolescents with congenital syphilis. Occasionally monarticular, this rare cause of synovitis is present in patients with a positive serologic test for syphilis together with other manifestations of congenital syphilis such as interstitial keratitis, Hutchinson's teeth, and eighth-nerve deafness.

Osteomyelitis often presents as joint pain. A juxtaarticular focus of bone infection can result in a sympathetic joint effusion in which the synovial fluid is only minimally inflammatory and usually sterile. A true septic arthritis can result from a primary osteomyelitis if either the shoulder, hip, or elbow joint is involved since in these areas the joint capsule attaches to the periosteal bone distal to the epiphyseal plate. Rupture through the cortical bone would introduce infected osteomyelitic debris directly into the joint space in these areas. Osteomyelitis should be considered if the patient is a young adult with fever and joint splinting. Heroin abusers, immunosuppressed patients, and those with bacteremia are likely subjects.

REFERENCES

Arnold WD, Hilgartner MW: Hemophilic arthropathy. Current concepts of pathogenesis and management. J Bone Joint Surg 59-A:287, 1977

Fletcher MR, Scott JT: Chronic monarticular synovitis. Diagnostic and prognostic features. Ann Rheum Dis 34:171, 1975

Kelly PJ, Karlson AG: Musculoskeletal tuberculosis. Mayo Clin Proc 44:73, 1969

Pritchard DJ: Granulomatous infections of bones and joints. Orthop Clin North Am 6:1029, 1975

TUMORS, TRAUMA, AND INFLAMMATORY SYNOVITIS

Foreign bodies and infectious agents, though readily identifiable, are not frequent causes of chronic monarticular disease. The most common causes of chronic polyarthritis, that is, degenerative joint disease and rheumatoid arthritis, are also responsible for most cases of chronic monarthritis. The largest single group of patients with persistent monarticular disease has an inflammatory synovitis, and in many of these patients, rheumatoid arthritis will ultimately be diagnosed. Tumors, whether benign or malignant, are not often encountered in a general rheumatology practice. Regardless of etiology, the most commonly involved articulation in chronic monarticular disease is the knee.

BENIGN AND MALIGNANT TUMORS

Both primary and metastatic neoplasms in joints are characteristically monarticular. Special procedures such as arthroscopy or arthrography and biopsy or surgical exploration are required for definitive diagnosis. In addition to the tumors listed in Table 1 of the preceding chapter, bone neoplasms located in close proximity to articular structures can cause symptoms resembling primary joint disease.

Pigmented villonodular synovitis is the most common joint tumor. This lesion can occur in synovial tissue, in bursae, in tendon sheaths, or in the fascia and ligaments adjacent to tendons. Lesions are either nodular or diffuse and all bear the similar histologic characteristics of a fibrous stroma, hemosiderin pigment deposits, histiocytic infiltration, and multinucleated giant cells.

The exact pathogenesis of pigmented villonodular synovitis is uncertain. Most of the evidence suggests that it represents an inflammatory granulomatous reaction, but the stimulus initiating these tumors has not yet been conclusively identified.

The local form of nodular tenosynovitis is often seen in middle-aged females and develops in tendon linings about the fingers near the metacarpophalangeal or proximal interphalangeal joints, usually on the palmar surfaces. Less frequently, they occur in the foot or ankle. These small, usually painless masses may cause bone erosions. The localized form, when intraarticular, often occurs in the knees and presents the picture of internal derangement.

The diffuse form is usually found in young adult males, and 80 percent are in the knee. The hip and ankle are less often involved. The patient has a chronically swollen and painful joint and these symptoms become progressively more severe. Physical examination reveals localized tenderness and an intraarticular mass. The sedimentation rate is usually normal. The synovial fluid is characteristically serosanguinous or dark brown with a mild leukocytosis (3000–6000 cells/mm^3, of which only 25 percent are neutrophils). Numerous red blood cells are usually present. Radiographic examination shows soft tissue swelling; occasionally subchondral bone erosions will be present in the more chronic cases.

The preferred treatment for the extraarticular localized form is complete excision, although recurrence rates (up to 40 percent) are relatively high. Complete excision of the intraarticular localized form is more successful and essentially all patients are cured. Extensive synovectomy for the diffuse intraarticular form is followed by a high recurrence rate, especially if significant bone erosion has occurred. Some have advocated radiation therapy following total synovectomy. The finding of multinucleated giant cells will differentiate pigmented villonodular synovitis from synovial sarcoma, and thereby help avoid unnecessary radical resection.

Synovial chondromatosis (or osteochondromatosis if the lesions have calcified and ossified) is a less common benign disorder. Over half the cases occur in the knee, with the hip, elbow, and shoulder less commonly involved. The patients, usually adult males, complain of painful swelling and locking of the involved joint, and loose bodies are apparent on physical examination. The radiologic picture of osteochondromatosis is distinctive, showing multiple discrete calcified lesions within the joint. These findings are imparted by the numerous islands of highly cellular cartilage imbedded within the synovial membrane. If allowed to persist, degenerative arthritis will develop. As with other tumors, surgical resection is the treatment of choice.

The knee is also the most frequent site of hemangiomas, lipomas, and fibromas, other uncommon benign tumors. Hemorrhagic synovial fluid from the joint of a young adult without a history of antecedent trauma should suggest the possibility of a neoplasm. The erythrocyte sedimentation rate is usually normal in benign joint tumors.

The main primary malignant tumor of the synovium, synovial sarcoma, is an uncommon tumor. It usually originates in the paraarticular tissues of large joints of the lower extremity, often in young adults. Rarely is there an associated synovial effusion, presumably because the lesion does not involve the synovial membrane. Radiologic examination might detail osteolytic defects since the tumors cause a localized periosteal reaction and can invade bone. Approximately one-third will calcify. Synovial sarcoma invades regional nodes and disseminates to distant visceral and skeletal sites, producing "cannon ball" lesions in the lungs. This is a highly malignant tumor with a 5-year survival in the range of 45 percent. Either irradiation or chemotherapy following wide excision has been suggested, but the preferred method of treatment has not yet been substantiated by comparative studies.

TRAUMA AND DEGENERATION

Trauma is one of the most common causes of chronic monarticular arthritis. Meniscal or ligamentous injury may result in chronic pain and swelling. The knee is most commonly involved. A history of trauma and symptoms of joint instability or locking are helpful. Synovial fluid is usually noninflammatory but may be bloody if a ligamentous tear or fracture through the joint has occured. Degeneration of the joint may ultimately develop if there has been structural damage to the menisci, ligaments, or articular cartilage, or if a fracture has led to incongruity of the joint surface. Obviously, degenerative arthritis is also a consequence if the integrity of the joint has been disrupted by prior inflammatory disease, aseptic necrosis, congenital hip dysplasia, slipped capital femoral epiphysis, osteochondritis dissecans, or infection. These causes should be considered when chronic degenerative monarthritis occurs in a young adult, especially in the knee or hip. Generalized osteoarthritis without an identifiable underlying cause frequently presents as chronic monarticular disease. Radiographic examination will usually reveal the involvement of other joints.

The main symptom of traumatic or degenerative arthritis is pain made worse with activity. Synovial fluid is usually noninflammatory and the erythrocyte sedimentation rate is normal. In contrast to some other forms of chronic monarthritis, radiographic changes are of new bone formation with subchondral sclerosis, osteophyte formation, and joint space narrowing.

Aseptic necrosis, which may result in osteoarthritis, can produce a chronic monarthritis, usually of the hip. This ischemic degeneration of bone has been related to trauma, to gas or fat microembolism, and to the administration of corticosteroids. It has been frequently associated with disorders such as diabetes mellitus, alcoholism, systemic lupus erythematosus, and hemoglobinopathies.

Early in the course of aseptic necrosis of the hip, the radiographic appearance is normal. Sequential changes include an increased density of the femoral head followed by a faint line of radiolucency beneath subchondral bone. Later changes are those of collapse of the femoral head and degeneration.

Neuropathic arthropathy, most often a consequence of diabetic neuropathy or tabes dorsalis, is an extreme form of degenerative monarthritis. The involved joint, usually in the lower extremity, is initially painful, but there is little evidence of inflammation. Roentgenograms reveal fragmentation of subchondral bone, subluxation, and enthusiastic osteophyte formation. A neurologic examination will suggest the appropriate diagnosis.

INFLAMMATORY SYNOVITIS

A number of rheumatic disorders commonly presenting as polyarthritis should also be considered in the patient with chronic monarthritis. Included are adult or juvenile rheumatoid arthritis, Reiter's syndrome, psoriatic arthropathy, and ankylosing spondylitis. Even crystal deposition diseases, (gout and pseudogout), may produce a chronic monarthritis. The synovial fluid in these disorders is inflammatory, with cell counts usually exceeding 3000/mm³; and the erythrocyte sedimentation rate is often greater than 35 mm/hr.

Only a minority of all patients with definite or classic rheumatoid arthritis will have their disease start as monarthritis of more than 3 months' duration. Nevertheless, this disorder is so prevalent that it accounts for approximately 25 percent of all cases of monarticular disease. In one prospective analysis, 12 of 13 patients with chronic monarthritis considered to have rheumatoid arthritis ultimately developed the polyarticular form. In most of these patients, the wrist was the initial site of inflammation. The features suggestive of rheumatoid arthritis were an elevated erythrocyte sedimentation rate and a positive test for rheumatoid factor.

True monarticular arthritis as a presentation of juvenile rheumatoid arthritis is uncommon, accounting for less than 3 percent of all cases. In most patients with pauci- or oligoarthritis, more than one joint is inflamed. When a single joint is involved, it is usually the knee or, less commonly, the ankle. The association of iridocyclitis with this form of juvenile rheumatoid arthritis has been emphasized and periodic slit lamp examinations of the eyes are indicated. The outcome of monarticular juvenile rheumatoid arthritis is considered excellent.

The history and physical findings will usually suggest the appropriate diagnosis in patients with other inflammatory joint disorders. Thus, the history of urethritis or the finding of an asymptomatic penile or palatal ulcer will signal Reiter's syndrome. Pitting of the nails and localized patches of pustular psoriasis may be the only findings to suggest that a chronic synovitis is due to psoriatic arthritis. Spinal involvement in ankylosing spondylitis can develop without prominent back symptoms and the patient may present only when a peripheral large joint becomes inflamed.

Patients with calcium pyrophosphate deposition disease may present with chronic synovitis confined to a single joint. Most often this is the wrist, and radiographic findings are those of chondrocalcinosis and destructive arthritis. Usually other joints, especially the knees and hips, also demonstrate chondrocalcinosis. Synovial fluid analysis will show intracellular crystals of calcium pyrophosphate dihydrate. The other common crystal-induced disorder, gout, results in a chronic monarthritis only very rarely since urate crystals characteristically induce such a vigorous local reaction.

The single largest group of patients with chronic monarticular arthritis remains undiagnosed. In previous studies, "benign synovitis" accounted for 30 percent of all cases. Most often the knee was involved and there were no historical or physical features to indicate the underlying cause. When analyzed, synovial fluids from these patients revealed mild leukocytosis without other distinctive findings. Membrane histology was not diagnostic and the characteristic changes of rheumatoid arthritis were not observed. Analysis of the synovial fluids from these patients for rheumatoid factors was not car-

ried out but this test is probably of little diagnostic value. This form of chronic monarticular disease was considered benign since the course was usually favorable, the arthritis subsiding in most patients. However, in one prospective analysis, 3 of 21 cases initially diagnosed as synovitis of unknown cause ultimately developed typical changes of rheumatoid arthritis.

In most cases of chronic monarticular arthritis, a careful evaluation of the patient together with analysis of laboratory tests, including study of the synovial fluid and synovial membrane, will lead to the appropriate diagnosis. The prognosis for most forms, once the correct cause has been identified, is favorable.

REFERENCES

Fletcher MR, Scott JT: Chronic monarticular synovitis. Diagnostic and prognostic features. Ann Rheum Dis 34:171, 1975

Granowitz SP, D'Antonio J, Mankin HL: The pathogenesis and long-term end results of pigmented villonodular synovitis. Clin Orthop 114:335, 1976

Jaffee HL: Tumors and Tumorous Conditions of the Bones and Joints. Philadelphia, Lea & Febiger, 1958

Polyarthritis

John T. Sharp

CLINICAL FEATURES

The accurate diagnosis of polyarthritis requires a comprehensive knowledge of the diverse manifestations of rheumatic disease, an appreciation of the distinctive features of each condition, and a knowledge of those procedures and tests which provide critical diagnostic information in each condition.

Duration of Symptoms

Helpful distinctions are made by dividing patients according to the duration of polyarthritis (Table 1). Chronic arthritis in this discussion is arbitrarily taken as 6 weeks or longer following the diagnostic criteria for rheumatoid arthritis adopted by the American Rheumatism Association. In fact, many patients with rheumatoid arthritis are not seen by a physician until symptoms have been present for several weeks, perhaps because of the insidious onset. In contrast, patients with most acute forms of arthritis seek treatment soon after onset because of the severity of symptoms. Severity and duration often appear to be related, but exceptions are sufficiently frequent so that the two variables should be considered independently.

Many of the articular diseases occur either as acute or chronic processes and may be seen initially at any stage of illness. For example, a majority of patients with Reiter's syndrome have abrupt onset of symptoms and seek medical advice soon after the first manifestation of illness, but the occasional patient will not be seen until arthritis has been present for several months. Although

the majority of patients with Reiter's syndrome recover from the initial attack within a period of 2–4 months, some develop persistent arthritis from the beginning of illness.

In some diseases arthritis is characteristically episodic. This is particularly true of gout, which in most instances is characterized by complete recovery from acute attacks and totally symptom-free intervals, at least in the first few years after onset of attacks. Episodic arthritis should be distinguished from chronic arthritis characterized by a fluctuating course with periods of lesser disease intermingled with periods of exacerbation. Some articular diseases are characterized by recurrences. This is characteristic of gout, pseudogout, and Reiter's syndrome and may occur with any of the connective tissue diseases that go into remission. Some illnesses are a single event that are rarely or never recurrent. The acute polyarthritis associated with hepatitis B infection is not likely ever to recur, presumably because immunity to this virus is solid and long lasting, and thus after recovery a new infection will rarely occur. A few instances of second or third episodes of infectious arthritis due to gonococci or other bacteria have been described, but the likelihood of second infections is low.

In contrast to the acute form of polyarthritis from which there is complete recovery, there are some rheumatic diseases characterized by chronicity and persistence. Once degenerative arthritis in a weight-bearing joint becomes sufficiently severe to be symptomatic, the

Table 1

Articular Manifestations of Polyarthritis

Disease	Acute	Chronic (>6 wk)	Episodic	Small Joints	Large Joints	Spinal Involvement	Pauciarticular	Multiarticular	Limited to Arthralgia	Synovitis	Migratory	Additive
Acute rheumatic fever	+		+	±	+		+			+	+	
Hepatitis B Antigen polyarthritis	+			±	+		+			+		+
Infectious arthritis												
Gonococcal	+	±	+	±	+		+			+	±	+
Other	+	+	+	±	+		+			+		+
Gout	+	+	+	+	+		+			+	±	+
Pseudogout	+	+	+	±	+		+			+		+
Syphilis	+			±	+		+			+		
Systemic lupus Erythematosus	+	+	+	+	+		+	+	+	+	±	+
Periarteritis	+	+	+	+	+		+	+		+		+
Reiter's syndrome	+	+	+	±	+	+	+	±		+		+
Polychondritis	+	+	+	±	+		+			+		+
Hypertrophic osteoarthropathy	+	±			+		+		+	+		
Scleroderma	±	+	+	±	+		+		+	+		+
Dermatomyositis	±	+	+	±	+		+		+	+		+
Mixed connective tissue disease	±	+	+	±	+		+		+	+		+
Rheumatoid arthritis		+	±	+	+	C	±	+		+		+
Ankylosing spondylitis		+	±	±	+	+	+	±		+		+
Psoriatic arthritis		+	+	+	+	+	±	+		+		+
Enteropathic arthritis		+	+	+	+	+	+		±	+		+
Sarcoidosis		+		+	+		+		+	+		
Degenerative joint disease		+		+	+	+	+		+			+
Ochronosis		+			+	+			+			
Neuroarthropathy	+	+			+		+		+			+

Symbols: +, common manifestation; ±, feature is less frequent; C, cervical spine involvement.

disease is present for the duration of life unless there is surgical intervention, although symptoms may improve, sometimes to a remarkable extent. Similarly, many patients with rheumatoid arthritis have a chronic, persistent course that spans one or more decades.

Articular Involvement

In many instances the pattern of articular involvement is quite characteristic of a given condition (Table 1). As one example, this pattern is particularly striking in those cases of rheumatoid arthritis that some observers have called "typical." Such patients have arthritis involving the small joints in the wrists, fingers, and feet as well as several large joints. Often there is considerable symmetry, with the same joints involved on each side of the body. In the hands, metacarpophalangeal joints are involved more often than proximal interphalangeal joints, and the distal finger joints are involved the least frequently. Small joint involvement is less regular in most other forms of polyarthritis.

Rheumatoid arthritis is also characterized by the large number of joints involved in the majority of patients. Among the approximately 70 synovial joints that are located in the extremities or superficially on the trunk a few patients with rheumatoid arthritis have virtually every one of these joints involved, and many have 10–40 joints involved. Such widespread multiarticular involvement occurs at times in other forms of polyarthritis, but in most instances involvement is more limited. For example, nearly 75 percent of patients with gonococcal arthritis have two or more joints involved, but only the occasional patient has more than five. Acute rheumatic fever may eventually involve a large number of joints but usually is diagnosed after the arthritis has involved only a few joints. The connective tissue disorders are more variable in the number of joints manifesting arthritis, some patients having only a few joints involved and others mimicking rheumatoid arthritis in the extent of involvement.

Spinal involvement varies among the articular diseases. Characteristic forms of spondylitis occur regularly in Reiter's syndrome, ankylosing spondylitis, psoriatic arthropathy, enteropathic arthritis, degenerative joint disease, and ochronosis. Rheumatoid arthritis is frequently associated with arthritis in the cervical region and less frequently with involvement elsewhere in the spine.

The distinction between migratory arthritis and additive arthritis is often helpful. In the former, arthritis occurs for a limited time in a specific joint and then spontaneously remits completely. The second and subsequent joints to be involved develop symptoms later, usually with a period of overlap of variable duration. When involvement is additive, the second and subsequent joints are involved while the first joint still manifests arthritis, and each joint continues to manifest arthritis. Arthritis in rheumatic fever usually is migratory. In other forms of acute polyarthritis initial articular involvement is usually additive, but patients with systemic lupus erythematosus, polyarticular gout, gonococcal arthritis, and hepatitis B–

associated arthritis may mimic rheumatic fever in mode of onset.

In some patients articular manifestations may be limited to arthralgia for part or all of the course of illness even though the same disease in other patients may produce a frank synovitis with readily demonstrable signs of inflammation.

Extraarticular Manifestations

Extraarticular manifestations are often quite characteristic of a specific disease process. The presence of these features in various polyarticular diseases is summarized in Table 2.

Skin. Skin involvement is characteristic of a large number of the polyarticular diseases. In many, the skin lesions are quite distinctive, and in some instances the skin lesions are virtually diagnostic. Erythema marginatum in rheumatic fever, keratodermia blennorrhagica in Reiter's syndrome, psoriatic lesions, and scleroderma are all highly characteristic, distinctive lesions of diagnostic importance. In addition, a diffuse erythema is seen in some patients with systemic lupus erythematosus; nonthrombopenic purpuric lesions are seen in polyarteritis nodosa; urticarial lesions are found in hepatitis B polyarthritis; macular lesions on the palms and soles are found in secondary syphilis; violaceous lesions are found on the eyelids, knuckles, and elbows of patients with dermatomyositis; and vesiculopustular lesions are seen in gonococcal arthritis. All these findings are distinctive and contribute toward an accurate diagnosis.

Subcutaneous nodules are common in rheumatoid arthritis, acute rheumatic fever, polyarteritis, and gout, and are sometimes seen in scleroderma, dermatomyositis, sarcoid, and systemic lupus erythematosus. Firm, nontender nodules, usually several millimeters in diameter, in the olecranon bursa or 2–4 cm distal to the olecranon in a patient with chronic polyarthritis involving multiple small and large joints are helpful features in the positive diagnosis of rheumatoid arthritis.

Muscles. Muscle involvement with girdle weakness is most characteristic of polymyositis, mixed connective tissue disease, and scleroderma, but myositis can also be seen in rheumatoid arthritis, systemic lupus erythematosus, periarteritis, and sarcoid.

Serositis. Pleural and pericardial involvement are frequent in patients with systemic lupus erythematosus and are seen less frequently in rheumatoid arthritis, acute rheumatic fever, periarteritis nodosa, Reiter's syndrome, scleroderma, and dermatomyositis.

Lungs. Involvement of the parenchyma of the lung is particularly prominent in scleroderma and sarcoid and also occurs in dermatomyositis and mixed connective tissue disease. It is less frequently seen in several of the other rheumatic diseases, including rheumatoid arthritis, systemic lupus erythematosus, and periarteritis.

Cardiac involvement. Cardiac involvement is an important feature in distinguishing acute rheumatic fever from other forms of acute arthritis. Although Jones' criteria for the diagnosis of acute rheumatic fever can be met

Table 2

Extraarticular Manifestations of Polyarthritis

Disease	Fever	Skin Rash	Nodules	Muscle	Tendon and Bursa	Cartilage	Pleura	Peri cardium	Lung	Heart Muscle	Heart Valve	Kidney	Peripheral Nerve	Central Nervous System	Eye	Sjögren's Syndrome	Gastro intestinal	Liver
Acute rheumatic fever	+	D	+				+	+	±	+	+							
Hepatitis B Antigen polyarthritis	+	D																+
Infectious arthritis																		
Gonococcal	+	D				+	±	±			±							
Other	±		+			+												
Gout	±				+	+						+						
Pseudogout	±					+												
Syphilis	±	D										±						
Systemic lupus erythematosus	+	D	±	+		±	+	+	+	+	+	+		+	+		+	+
Periarteritis	+	D	+	+		+	+	+	+	+		+	+	+	+		+	+
Reiter's syndrome	+	D				+	±	±	±	+		+			+		+	
Polychondritis	+				+	+			+	+	+				+			
Hypertrophic osteoarthropathy									+									
Scleroderma	±	D	±	+	+	+	+	+	+	+		+			+	+	+	+
Dermatomyositis	±	D	±	+	+	+	+	+	±	+								
Mixed connective tissue disease	±			+		+	+	±	±	+	±	±	±					
Rheumatoid arthritis	±		+	+		+	±	±	+	±			±		+	+		
Ankylosing spondylitis	±								+	+					+		+	
Psoriatic arthritis	±	D				±									+			
Enteropathic arthritis	±	D				+			+								+	+
Sarcoid	+	D	+	+					+				±		+		+	+
Degenerative joint disease						+												
Ochronosis						+												
Neuroarthropathy													±	+				

Symbols: +, common manifestation; ±, feature is less frequent; D, distinctive skin lesions are seen.

without involvement of the heart, the certainty of the diagnosis is enhanced by the occurrence of pericarditis, congestive failure, or changing murmurs in a patient with migratory polyarthritis and serologic evidence of a recent streptococcal infection. Aortic insufficiency is seen in ankylosing spondylitis, Reiter's syndrome, and polychondritis, as well as in acute rheumatic fever. Myocarditis may be seen in scleroderma, dermatomyositis, and systemic lupus erythematosus; myocardial infarction occurs in periarteritis nodosa.

Kidneys. Involvement of the kidneys is frequently a prominent feature in patients with systemic lupus erythematosus and periarteritis. Rapid renal failure occurs in a minority of patients with scleroderma. Untreated, severe gout after several years' duration may be accompanied by renal disease.

Nervous system. The nervous system is affected by several of the connective tissue disorders. Central nervous system involvement occurs in many patients with systemic lupus erythematosus and periarteritis, and chorea may be a manifestation of acute rheumatic fever. Peripheral neuropathy may be a prominent feature of periarteritis nodosa and occurs in a few patients with rheumatoid arthritis.

Eyes. Iritis is particularly prominent in patients with ankylosing spondylitis, Reiter's syndrome, polychondritis, periarteritis nodosa, and sarcoid. In addition to iritis, the eye may be involved as a consequence of inflammation and fibrosis of the lacrimal gland in Sjögren's syndrome associated with rheumatoid arthritis, scleroderma, and systemic lupus erythematosus.

Digestive system. The esophagus, duodenum, and colon all may be involved in scleroderma. Disturbance in motility often leads to poor emptying of the esophagus and gastric reflux. The duodenum may be widely dilated, and wide-mouthed diverticula are commonly seen in the colon. In periarteritis nodosa infarction of the bowel may occur and may be a life-threatening manifestation. Reiter's syndrome may be heralded by the onset of diarrhea. Enteropathic arthritis is characterized by the association of arthritis with regional ileitis or ulcerative colitis. Arthritis is also a feature in Whipple's disease, an enteric infection that causes a wasting illness with malabsorption and diarrhea.

Liver. Involvement of the liver is seen in some patients with periarteritis, in hepatitis B induced polyarthritis, and in sarcoidosis. Some patients with scleroderma develop biliary cirrhosis.

Genitourinary system. Urethritis is a regular feature of Reiter's syndrome. In patients with gonococcal arthritis primary infection may occur by way of the genitourinary tract, but often such infection is inapparent, and in some instances other routes of entry occur. Thus, in actual practice, in recent years urethritis has not been common in patients with gonococcal arthritis. In the female salpingitis, vaginitis, and cervicitis may be present at the time of bacterial dissemination and arthritis.

LABORATORY STUDIES AND RADIOLOGIC FINDINGS
Laboratory Studies

Crystals. Laboratory studies provide definitive diagnostic information in only a few instances. The presence of monosodium urate or calcium pyrophosphate dihydrate crystals in joint fluid leukocytes is sufficient to establish a diagnosis of gout or pseudogout.

Bacteria. In patients with infectious arthritis, the presence of a pathogenic bacterium in joint fluid or blood cultures establishes the correct diagnosis.

Antibodies to ribonucleoprotein. In some instances the absence of a particular laboratory finding may be more helpful in the differential diagnosis than its presence. For example, in considering the possibility of mixed connective tissue disease, absence of antibodies to ribonucleoprotein (extractable nuclear antigen) essentially rules out the condition as it is now defined.

Rheumatoid factors. The presence of rheumatoid factor in the serum is not a particularly strong indication of rheumatoid arthritis, since a majority of persons with anti-IgG have no disease or a condition other than rheumatoid arthritis. On the other hand, in the differential diagnosis of a patient with subcutaneous nodules the absence of rheumatoid factor or anti-IgG antibodies in the serum is strong evidence against rheumatoid arthritis. In such instances biopsy of a nodule is mandatory for definitive diagnosis and the nodule should be fixed in absolute alcohol to prevent removal of urate so that a positive diagnosis can be made in those instances in which the nodule is a tophus.

Antinuclear antibodies. In considering the diagnosis of systemic lupus erythematosus the persistent absence of antinuclear antibodies argues against that diagnosis, since an extremely high percentage of patients with systemic lupus erythematosus have antinuclear antibodies soon after onset of illness. In contrast, the presence of antinuclear antibodies has little diagnostic specificity since many patients with other connective tissue diseases, including rheumatoid arthritis, scleroderma, dermatomyositis, and mixed connective tissue disease also have these antibodies. Antibodies to double-stranded or native DNA, however, have been observed infrequently in patients who have diseases other than systemic lupus erythematosus.

HLA-B27. The human lymphocyte antigen HLA-B27 is present in more than 90 percent of patients with ankylosing spondylitis and is found almost as frequently in patients with Reiter's syndrome, psoriatic arthritis with spondylitis, and enteropathic arthritis with spondylitis. However 4–6 percent of patients with other rheumatic conditions have the antigen, which is the same frequency as in the general population. Therefore, the presence of HLA-B27 on the lymphocytes of a patient undergoing diagnostic studies is supporting evidence for spondylitis or a related condition only if the clinical picture is consistent with such a diagnosis.

Table 3
Distinctive Features of Common Forms of Polyarthritis

Rheumatoid arthritis
  Clinical pattern of chronic arthritis, subcutaneous nodules
  Bony erosions and cartilage destruction by radiologic examination

Systemic lupus erythematosus
  Multisystem disease with prominent skin, articular, renal, central nervous system, hematologic, and serosal involvement
  Anti-nDNA antibodies present in many

Rheumatic fever
  Acute migratory arthritis
  Cardiac involvement in many
  Antistreptococcal antibodies present
  Responds to aspirin.

Periarteritis
  Multisystem disease with prominent arthritis, cardiac, gastrointestinal, renal, peripheral or central nervous system, and hepatic involvement
  Persistent hepatitis B antigen in many
  Angiograms characteristic
  Biopsy of involved vessel diagnostic

Hepatitis B antigen associated polyarthritis
  Acute arthritis
  Skin rash in many (usually urticarial)
  Abnormal liver function tests
  Hepatitis B antigen present transiently
  Responds to aspirin

Ankylosing spondylitis
  Thoracolumbar spine stiffness clinically
  Spinal and sacroiliac ankylosis radiologically
  HLA-B27 in most

Reiter's syndrome
  Triad of urethritis, conjunctivitis, and arthritis
  Recent or concomitant dysentery in many
  Characteristic skin lesions in some
  HLA-B27 in most

Psoriatic arthritis
  Chronic arthritis, terminal finger joints commonly involved
  Skin and nail lesions present
  HLA-B27 usually present when spine involved

Enteropathic arthritis
  Chronic arthritis associated with ulcerative colitis or regional ileitis
  HLA-B27 usually present when spine involved

Syphilitic arthritis
  Rash of secondary sphilis
  Serologic test positive
  Spirochetes in mucosal lesions

Hypertrophic osteoarthropathy
  Clubbing usually present
  Periosteitis demonstrated by x-ray examination

Neuroarthropathy
  Sensory defect
  Disorganized destruction of joint seen on radiologic examination

Sarcoid arthritis
  Associated with skin, lung, or liver lesions with characteristic histologic findings

Polychondritis
  Cartilage destruction in ears, nose, trachea
  Often associated with iritis and aortic insufficiency

Ochronosis
  Homogentisic acid in urine

Degenerative joint disease
  Heberden's nodes
  Persistent pain in a few large joints for months or years
  Loss of cartilage seen on radiologic examination

Infectious arthritis, gonococcal
  Acute arthritis associated with skin lesions in many
  Cultures of blood or synovial fluid frequently positive

Infectious arthritis, other septic
  Acute arthritis
  Cultures of blood or synovial fluid positive

Gout
  Acute, episodic arthritis
  Monosodium urate crystals in synovial fluid and tophi

Pseudogout
  Acute or chronic, episodic arthritis
  Calcium pyrophosphate dihydrate crystals in synovial fluid
  Knee cartilage calcified in most

Scleroderma
  Characteristic skin changes
  Lung involvement
  Raynaud's phenomenon
  Gastrointestinal and renal involvement

Dermatomyositis
  Muscle weakness
  Enzyme elevations
  Muscle biopsy frequently diagnostic
  Skin lesions in many

Mixed connective tissue disease
  Arthralgia
  Muscle weakness
  Skin lesions
  Dysphagia
  Lung involvement
  High-titer antibodies to ribonucleoprotein

Table 4
Methods of Diagnosing Polyarticular Diseases

I. History and physical examination provide the essential diagnostic information in:
  Rheumatoid arthritis—active synovitis in multiple small and large joints
  Ankylosing spondylitis—limited movement of spine
  Reiter's syndrome—triad of urethritis, conjunctivitis, and arthritis
  Psoriatic arthritis—typical skin lesions with arthritis
  Scleroderma—typical skin lesions
  Enteropathic arthritis—ulcerative colitis or regional ileitis with arthritis

II. Clinical laboratory tests along with history and physical examination provide the essential diagnostic information in:
  Gout—monosodium urate crystals in synovial fluid or tophi
  Pseudogout—calcium pyrophosphate dihydrate crystals in synovial fluid
  Infectious arthritis—bacteria cultured from synovial fluid or blood
  Systemic lupus erythematosus—antinuclear antibodies in most, anti-nDNA in many; leukopenia, anemia, or thrombocytopenia in many; proteinuria or hematuria in many
  Hepatitis B virus arthritis—HBsAg in serum, abnormal liver function tests
  Mixed connective tissue disease—anti-RNP in high titer
  Rheumatic fever—antibodies to streptococcal antigens
  Syphilitic arthritis—positive serologic test, identification of spirochetes in mucocutaneous lesions by dark-field microscopy
  Ochronosis—homogentisic acid in urine

IIIA. Radiologic examination along with history and physical examination provides essential diagnostic information in:
  Degenerative joint disease—loss of cartilage, osteosclerosis, juxtaarticular cysts, osteophytes

Pseudogout—calcification of fibrocartilage and/or hyaline cartilage of knees and other joints
Neuroarthropathy—disorganization and destruction of joint with fractures, fragmentation, aberrant calcification
Hypertrophic osteoarthropathy—periostitis of long bones

IIIB. Radiologic examination provides confirmatory diagnostic information in:
  Rheumatoid arthritis—juxtaarticular erosions and joint space narrowing of multiple small joints in the fingers and wrists
  Ankylosing spondylitis—ankylosis of sacroiliac and spinal apophyseal joints, calcification of spinal ligaments
  Periarteritis—aneurysms and segmental narrowing of small and medium-sized arteries demonstrated by angiograms of renal, mesenteric, or bronchial arteries
  Scleroderma—abnormal motility in esophagus and intestine, widely dilated duodenum, wide-mouth diverticula in colon
  Polymyositis—myositis ossificans

IV. Histologic examination along with history and physical examination provides essential diagnostic information in:
  Periarteritis—necrosis of arterial wall with inflammatory reaction
  Dermatomyositis—skeletal muscle fiber necrosis with inflammatory reaction
  Polychondritis—inflammation and necrosis of cartilage
  Sarcoidosis—noncaseating granuloma

Synovial fluid cell count. The synovial fluid reflects an inflammatory reaction when the white cell count is above 2000 or 3000/mm³, and often leukocyte counts are much higher in patients with rheumatoid arthritis, acute rheumatic fever, periarteritis, ankylosing spondylitis, Reiter's syndrome, gout, pseudogout, and infectious arthritis. In patients with systemic lupus erythematosus the white blood cell count in the joint fluid is usually less than 5000 and the majority of the cells are mononuclear.

Thrombocytopenic purpura. Thrombocytopenic purpura is seen most frequently in patients with systemic lupus erythematosus but occasionally is observed in scleroderma.

Muscle enzymes. Muscle enzyme activity is increased in the sera of patients with polymyositis, mixed connective tissue disease, and occasionally in scleroderma.

Serum complement. Serum complement is frequently decreased in patients with systemic lupus erythematosus, particularly at a time when renal disease is present and active. However, complement may be decreased in the absence of active renal disease in some patients with florid dermatitis and other manifestations of active lupus erythematosus. Serum complement is also occasionally reduced in patients with periarteritis and active nephritis.

Radiologic Findings

Radiologic examination of the joints provides helpful diagnostic information in degenerative joint disease, chondrocalcinosis, rheumatoid arthritis, ankylosing spondylitis, and neuroarthropathy. Characteristic findings in degenerative joint disease include loss of cartilage, osteosclerosis, and the presence of osteophytes.

In chondrocalcinosis the fibrocartilages in the knees,

wrists, and symphysis pubis often are calcified, and the hyaline cartilage of any joint may show a thin line of calcification outlining the articular surface. Chondrocalcinosis is most often found in the knees and is usually present when the patient is first seen for an attack of acute arthritis, even though another joint may be the site of the acute attack.

Rheumatoid arthritis is distinguished radiologically by the pattern of involvement of multiple small joints in the fingers and wrists. The characteristic lesions are erosions and loss of cartilage. Although no single lesion is diagnostic, the multiplicity and distribution of lesions in many instances constitutes a diagnostic pattern.

Ankylosing spondylitis is characterized radiologically by loss of joint space and ankylosis in the apophyseal joints and the development of calcification in the ligaments of the spine. In addition, usually there is marked involvement of the sacroiliac joints with erosions and partial or complete ankylosis. Neuroarthropathy is characterized by the disorganization and destruction seen in the bone adjacent to the articulation

Diagnostic information may be obtained by special radiologic procedures, including angiograms in periarteritis nodosa and examination of the gastrointestinal tract in enteropathic arthritis and scleroderma.

Tissue Biopsy

Tissue biopsies provide diagnostic information in periarteritis nodosa, polychondritis, and sarcoidosis, and biopsy of a nodule is essential in differentiating rheumatoid arthritis from gout in a few instances.

Summary

Table 3 is a summary of the features that are particularly useful in diagnosis of the various rheumatic diseases.

Table 4 presents diagnostic features of rheumatic diseases in the sequence in which a workup usually proceeds. From Table 2 the physician can design a workup to develop the data base necessary to establish a specific diagnosis taking into account all the important conditions in the differential diagnosis of polyarthritis.

REFERENCES

Duffy J, Lidsky MD, Sharp JT, Davis JS, Person DA, Hollinger FB, Min K-W: Polyarthritis, polyarteritis and hepatitis B. Medicine (Baltimore) 55:19, 1976

Gocke DJ, Hsu K, Morgan C, Bombardieri S, Lockshin M, Christian C: Vasculitis in association with Australia antigen. J Exp Med 134:330s, 1971

Goldenberg DL, Cohen AS: Acute infectious arthritis. Am J Med 60:369, 1976

McCarty DJ, Hollander JL: Identification of urate crystals in gouty synovial fluid. Ann Intern Med 54:452, 1961

Schlosstein L, Terasaki PI, Bluestone R, Pearson CM: High association of an HL-A antigen, W27, with ankylosing spondylitis. N Engl J Med 288:704, 1973

Sharp JT, Calkins E, Cohen AS, Schubert AF, Calabro J: Observations on the clinical, chemical, and serological manifestations of rheumatoid arthritis, based on the course of 154 cases. Medicine (Baltimore) 43:41, 1964

Zachariae H, Hjortshoj A, Kissmeyer-Nielsen F: Reiter's disease and HL-A 27. Lancet 2:565, 1973

Shoulder and Neck Pain

William P. Beetham, Jr.

Shoulder and neck pain may represent local or systemic disease. Pain in these areas may arise from the cervical spine, compression syndromes in the thoracic outlet, or disorders of the shoulder. Often symptoms in the shoulder and neck are diffuse and may extend into the upper extremity. Pain involving the shoulder and neck may also be referred from more distant sites due to disease affecting intrathoracic or diaphragmatic areas. A variety of articular or periarticular disorders can cause pain and disability in the neck and shoulder (Table 1). These disorders will be the primary concern of this section. The basic anatomy, normal function, and physical examination of the shoulder and neck are outlined in the chapter on the Shoulders and Neck in the fascicle on Regional Structures and Function: Basic Principles in Rheumatology.

DISORDERS OF THE NECK

Muscular Spasm of the Neck

Muscle spasm is a common cause of aching in the neck. In the upright position, the cervical spine normally has a lordotic curvature maintained with a minimum of muscular effort. Deviation of this position from poor posture or forward protrusion of the head may be associated with increased muscular tension. Anxiety and depression are often associated with muscular aching. Underlying disease of the spine can also cause painful muscle spasm with decreased neck motion and straightening of the normal lordotic curvature.

Cervical Sprain

A cervical sprain can be defined as injury to the supportive muscles and ligaments of the cervical spine. It is often caused by trauma, such as a car collision, which results in acute hyperflexion or hyperextension of the neck. The usual injury involves muscles primarily, and symptoms last only a few days to a few weeks. A more severe sprain can cause disruption of ligaments with severe pain and prolonged symptoms. The patient may be unable to hold the head upright when bending forward, and motion of the neck imposes painful tension on sprained ligaments. The use of the dramatic term *whiplash* injury may increase the likelihood of litigation. Its widespread use to describe minor injuries should be avoided. Roentgenograms of the neck usually reveal neg-

Table 1
Differential Diagnosis of Neck and Shoulder Pain

Neck Disorders	Shoulder Disorders
Chronic muscular strain (muscle spasm)	Calcific tendinitis and bursitis
Acute cervical sprain (whiplash)	Biceps tendon lesions
Torticollis (wryneck)	Bicipital tenosynovitis
Cervical spondylosis and osteoarthritis	Rupture of biceps tendon
Ruptured cervical disc	Rotator cuff tears
Ankylosing hyperostosis (Forestier's	Adhesive capsulitis (frozen shoulder)
disease)	Shoulder–hand syndrome (reflex neurovascular
Atlantoaxial and vertebral subluxation	dystrophy)
Other diseases of cervical spine	Articular disease
Infections	Infections
Inflammatory (rheumatoid arthritis,	Inflammatory (rheumatoid arthritis,
ankylosing spondylitis)	ankylosing spondylitis
Neoplastic	Degenerative
Metabolic (ochronosis, osteoporosis,	Neuropathic (Charcot's joint)
Paget's disease)	Crystal-induced arthritis (gout, pseudogout)
	Traumatic
Thoracic outlet syndrome (compression syndromes	Metabolic bone disease (osteoporosis,
of neurovascular bundle)	hyperparathyroidism, Paget's disease)
Cervical rib	Tumors (bone and soft tissue)
Scalenus anticus muscle	Muscular involvement
Costoclavicular syndrome	Fibrositis syndrome and myalgia
Hyperabduction of arm	Polymyalgia rheumatica
	Polymyositis and scleroderma
	Neurologic disorders
	Central nervous system
	Myelopathy
	Radiculopathy
	Brachial plexus
	Peripheral neuropathy
	Vascular disease
	Phlebitis
	Arteritis
	Occlusive
	Vasospastic
	Emboli
	Aneurysm
	Lymphedema
	Referred pain
	Intrathoracic
	Intraabdominal

ative findings except for straightening of the cervical spine from muscle spasm.

Cervical Spondylosis

Degenerative joint disease of the cervical spine may involve the intervertebral discs and adjacent vertebral bodies, the posterior apophyseal articulations, or the uncovertebral joints of von Lushka, which are located adjacent to the intervertebral foramina. The term *cervical spondylosis* is sometimes limited to degeneration of the intervertebral discs and changes in adjacent vertebral bodies. In this chapter spondylosis is used to describe derangement in any of the articulations already mentioned because all of these structures are interrelated and clinically produce similar symptoms when abnormal. Since degenerative changes in the intervertebral discs,

posterior apophyseal joints, and joints of von Lushka frequently occur together, the terms *osteoarthritis of the spine* and *spondylosis* are commonly used synonymously. However, only the posterior apophyseal articulations are true synovial joints.

Roentgenographic changes of cervical spondylosis commonly occur in patients who are asymptomatic. Nevertheless, patients with extensive radiologic abnormalities are more likely to have clinical symptoms than patients with only mild abnormalities. Cervical spondylosis increases with aging. Pain arising from the cervical spine is usually felt in the neck and back of the head but may extend into the shoulder and upper extremity if associated with nerve root compression. Pain from cervical disc disease can also be referred to the shoulder and

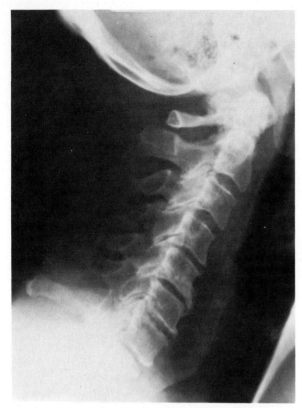

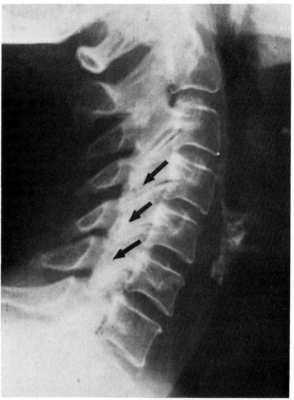

Fig. 1. This lateral view of the cervical spine reveals degenerative disc disease. The intervertebral spaces are narrow at C_{4-5}, C_{5-6}, C_{6-7}, and C_7–T_1. Osteophytes are present at the margins of C_5, C_6, and C_7 vertebral bodies. There is straightening of the normal cervical lordosis due to muscle spasm.

Fig. 2. This lateral view of the cervical spine demonstrates narrowing and sclerosis of apophyseal articulations (arrows). The intervertebral spaces and bodies are normal. (Reproduced from the Clinical Slide Collection on the Rheumatic Diseases produced by the Arthritis Foundation, New York, copyright 1972.)

upper arm without objective evidence of nerve root compression. Stiffness and pain on motion of the neck are often present.

Pathogenesis of disc disease. A basic knowledge of cervical spine anatomy is essential to an understanding of disease processes in this area. The intervertebral disc is composed of a central gelatinous core (nucleus pulposus) surrounded by an outer layer of fibrous material. The elasticity of the normal disc helps distribute stress exerted on the spine. Degeneration and aging are associated with dehydration and loss of proteoglycans within the nucleus, whose collagen content increases. When the disc loses its elasticity, it becomes more rigid and susceptible to herniation of the nucleus through defects in the outer layer if stress is exerted on the disc. Extrusion of the disc posteriorly or laterally may cause nerve root or cord compression.

Roentgenographic findings. Spondylosis is often associated with narrowing of the intervertebral disc spaces due to disc degeneration and the development of bony spurs on the margins of vertebral bodies (Fig. 1). Vertebral bodies adjacent to degenerative discs may have varying degrees of osteophyte formation and sclerosis of bone. Osteophytes that project anteriorly may nearly touch each other or even fuse. Bony spurs that project

posteriorly are usually less visible but, unlike spurs that project anteriorly, can cause significant nerve root or spinal cord compression. Degenerative changes may also involve the posterior apophyseal joints, which show sclerosis, irregularity, and narrowing of the joint space (Fig. 2). Apophyseal joint changes and degenerative disc disease can be visualized well on lateral roentgenograms of the cervical spine. The uncovertebral joints of von Lushka, which lie anterior to the intervertebral foramen, frequently participate in the degenerative process. Bony spurs that develop along the lateral aspect of the vertebral body may extend backward where they may compress the nerve root as it emerges from the intervertebral foramen. Encroachment of the intervertebral foramen is best visualized on an oblique roentgenogram of the cervical spine (Fig. 3). Anteroposterior views of the neck with the tube angled 12° caudocephalad are also helpful for evaluating bony impingement upon uncovertebral joints.

Compression Syndromes of the Cervical Spine

Mechanical lesions of the nerve roots and spinal cord in the cervical area can be divided into two types: nerve root compression causing radicular symptoms and spinal cord compression causing myelopathy. Because the nerve roots and spinal cord lie close together within the

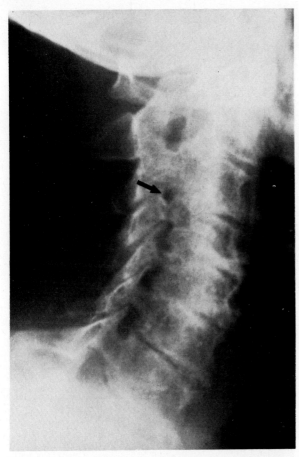

Fig. 3. Oblique view of the cervical spine showing bony impingement of intervertebral foramen most evident at level of 3–4 (arrow). Impingement can also be seen on the anterior aspect of the foramen at level of 4–5. (Reproduced from the Clinical Slide Collection on the Rheumatic Diseases produced by the Arthritis Foundation, New York, copyright 1972.)

spinal canal, both structures can occasionally be compressed together producing a combination of nerve root and spinal cord involvement.

Cervical nerve root compression (radiculopathy). Cervical nerve root compression may be due to bony spur formation, a soft lateral disc extrusion, or both. Compression of a cervical nerve root causes characteristic clinical features that are consistent in their pattern. The diagnosis is frequently missed, however, when the patient is seen initially, and often the patient must endure pain for weeks or months until the pain either subsides spontaneously or further evaluation reveals the correct cause of the distress. The diagnosis is missed because radicular pain is often most severe in the scapular region, shoulder, or arm and is rarely localized to the neck. Radiculopathy involving the upper limbs is characterized by muscular weakness and atrophy, diminution or loss of deep tendon reflexes, and paresthesias. The neurologic findings associated with compression of specific nerve roots of the cervical spine are summarized in Table 2. Neck motion, especially hyperextension, often aggravates the symptoms of nerve root compression. The majority of disc lesions develop at the site of maximum mobility of the cervical spine between C_{5-6} and C_{6-7} interspaces involving C_6 and C_7 nerve roots respectively.

Cervical myelopathy. Spinal cord compression in the cervical region is usually caused by bony spurs or intervertebral disc protrusion, but subluxation of the atlantoaxial joint and tumors may also occur. The most important factors in the development of clinical manifestations are extent of the lesion, rate of onset of the compression, and size of the spinal canal. The spinal cord is able to accommodate gradual forms of compression relatively well, such as that which occurs in spondylosis; acute compression, such as that which occurs in disc protrusion, however, may produce more severe impair-

Table 2
Findings in Compression of Specific Nerve Roots

Root	Motor Weakness	Sensory Loss	Distribution of Pain	Reflex Loss
C_5	Deltoid, supraspinatus	Uppermost outer arm	Neck, shoulder, upper arm	Biceps may be diminished
C_6	Biceps, brachioradialis, wrist extensors and flexors	Radial aspect of forearm; thumb and index fingers	Neck, scapular, lateral aspect of arm and forearm	Biceps and/or brachioradialis may be diminished or absent
C_7	Triceps, wrist, and sometimes finger flexors and extensors	Dorsum of forearm; index, middle, and fourth fingers	Neck, scapular, posterolateral arm, dorsum of forearm	Triceps may be diminished or absent
C_8	Finger extensors, interossei	Fourth and fifth fingers	Neck, posterior shoulder, medial aspect of arm, ulnar aspect of forearm	Triceps and/or wrist extensors may be diminished or normal

ment. A congenitally narrow spinal canal may produce cord or nerve root compression with relatively mild spondylitic changes whereas a wide canal can tolerate more extensive changes without signs of compression. If the anteroposterior diameter of the cervical canal is less than 12 mm, as measured radiographically, cord compression is likely. The cervical canal is widest at its upper end. Spinal injury at this level is unusual.

Spinal cord compression in the cervical region often causes radicular symptoms in the upper extremities and long tract signs in the lower extremities. Muscle weakness, atrophy, and loss of tendon reflexes in the arms with sensory impairment extending into the fingers may be noted. However, hyperreflexia may also occur in the upper extremities if the lesion is above C_5. In the lower limbs, spastic weakness, clonus, hyperreflexia, and extensor plantar reflexes may be present. Vibratory and, less often, position sense may be diminished in the legs. Loss of bladder and bowel control is relatively uncommon in cervical myelopathy.

Roentgenographic examination. Routine views of the cervical spine should be taken in the anteroposterior, lateral, and left and right oblique projections. Lateral views obtained with the neck in flexion and extension help reveal vertebral instability and subluxation. Open-mouth views may be necessary to demonstrate fractures of the odontoid process and should be obtained after cervical injury. In young patients the normal epiphysis at the base of the odontoid should not be confused with fracture.

The roentgenographic findings of cervical spondylosis have already been discussed. Cervical spine roentgenograms are helpful in revealing degenerative changes but are not reliable for determining the level of nerve root compression, which is best determined by the neurologic examination. Extensive radiologic abnormalities can be seen in the cervical spine of a patient who is asymptomatic. On the other hand, the roentgenogram may reveal normal findings in patients with ruptured cervical discs. Oblique views may reveal encroachment on a neural foramen by a bony spur, but these changes do not necessarily correlate with the actual site of compression, which may be at another level or may be caused by a soft, herniated disc that is not visible radiographically. Nevertheless, patients who exhibit extensive radiologic abnormalities are more vulnerable to nerve root compression than patients who have only mild changes.

Myelography. Myelography is used to detect mechanical impingement on nerve roots, spinal cord, and posterior fossa structures. Contrast material is introduced into the subarachnoid space. A filling defect in the column of contrast material or obliteration of the shadow, which forms the nerve root sleeve, occurs at the site of compression. Myelography also provides information regarding the size and location of the lesion. It is performed only when surgical treatment is being considered or when the cause of the compression is obscure. A normal cervical myelogram rules out cord compression at this level and makes nerve root impingement very unlikely.

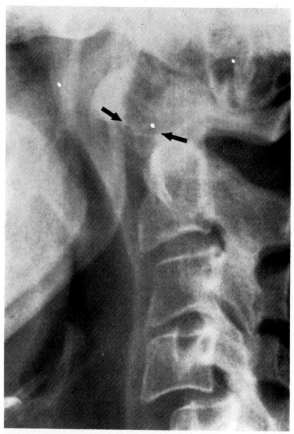

Fig. 4. Lateral view of cervical spine with neck in flexion showing atlantoaxial subluxation. The odontoid process is posteriorly displaced. The preodontoid space measures 8 mm (arrows) and should not exceed 3 mm in the normal adult. (Reproduced from the Clinical Slide Collection on the Rheumatic Diseases produced by the Arthritis Foundation, New York, copyright 1972.)

Cervical discography. The internal structure of the disc can be visualized by injection of radiopaque material. This may demonstrate small disc herniations not visible by myelography, but usually myelography is the preferable procedure.

Vertebral artery insufficiency. Compression of the vertebral artery by bony encroachment may reduce blood flow to the brain causing vertigo, nystagmus, diplopia, ataxia, deafness, and drop attacks without loss of consciousness. Rotation and hyperextension of the neck usually aggravate these symptoms. Significant vertebral artery compression by osteophytes is rare.

Rheumatoid arthritis (adult and juvenile). The cervical spine is commonly involved in children or adults with rheumatoid arthritis. Inflammatory erosion of bone and supporting ligaments may allow forward displacement of the atlas on the axis whose odontoid process may become eroded. Lateral roentgenograms obtained with the neck in flexion and extension are necessary to evaluate atlantoaxial subluxation. The atlantoodontoid space should not exceed 3 mm in adults (Fig. 4). If clinical symptoms of neurologic compression are present, flexion views

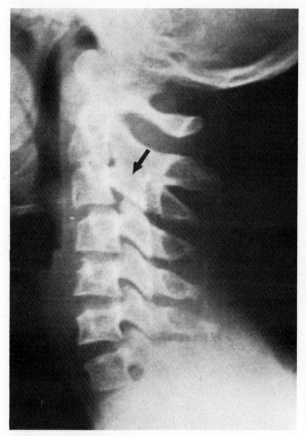

Fig. 5. Lateral view of the cervical spine showing fusion and obliteration of the apophyseal articulation between the second and third vertebrae (arrow) due to juvenile rheumatoid arthritis. (Reproduced from the Clinical Slide Collection on the Rheumatic Diseases produced by the Arthritis Foundation, New York, copyright 1972.)

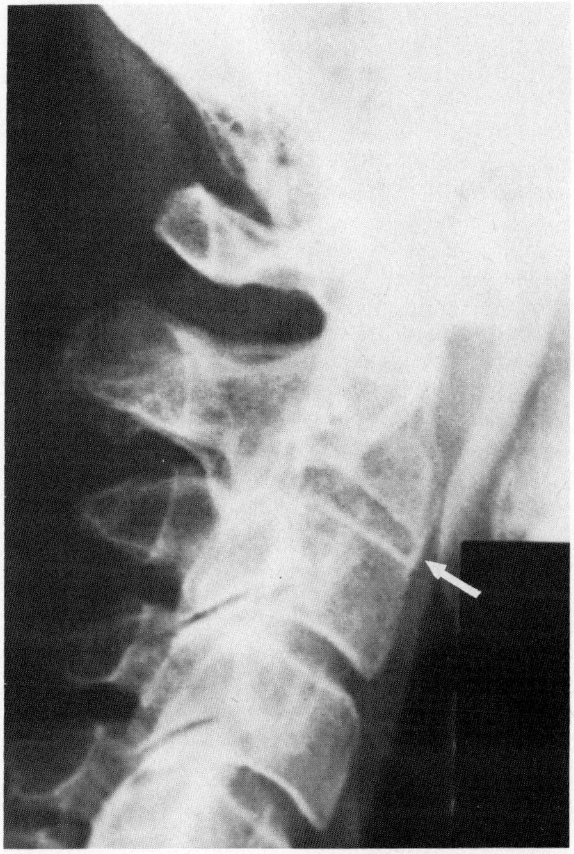

Fig. 6. Lateral view of the cervical spine showing a syndesmophyte bridging the space between the second and third vertebral bodies (arrow) due to ankylosing spondylitis. (Reproduced from the Clinical Slide Collection on the Rheumatic Diseases produced by the Arthritis Foundation, New York, copyright 1972.)

should be obtained with great caution to prevent aggravation of the compression. Ankylosis or fusion of the upper apophyseal joints is also common in juvenile rheumatoid arthritis (Fig. 5).

Ankylosing spondylitis. Typically, ankylosing spondylitis begins in the sacroiliac joints and lower spine but may extend into the neck in later stages causing pain and limitation of motion. Syndesmophytes may form extending from the margin of one vertebral body to the margin of the adjacent vertebral body (Fig. 6). The marginal syndesmophyte represents ossification of the outer portion of the intervertebral disc. The osteophytes associated with degenerative joint disease are thick bony spurs that project horizontally. They differ from the more delicate syndesmophytes associated with ankylosing spondylitis, which project vertically following the contour of the spine.

Ankylosing hyperostosis. Ankylosing hyperostosis (Forestier's disease) may involve the cervical spine, producing flowing calcification and ossification along the anterolateral aspect of several contiguous vertebral bodies with relative presentation of disc spaces.

Other destructive cervical disorders. Metastatic malignant tumors may involve the spine producing destructive radiologic lesions in the vertebral body that tend to spare the disc space. Compression fractures or posterior extension of the tumor may cause quadriplegia. A bone scan is often helpful in revealing "hot spots" associated with neoplastic invasion. The pain of malignancy is chronic and often worse at night while resting.

Roentgenograms may reveal a paravertebral soft tissue abscess or a disc space infection due to pyogenic organisms or tuberculosis. A disc space infection is characterized by narrowing of the disc space with destruction of adjacent vertebrae. Osteoporosis, osteomalacia, and Paget's disease can also involve the upper spine.

Thoracic Outlet Syndrome

Compression of the brachial plexus and subclavian artery or vein as these structures leave the neck and enter the region of the shoulder may cause pain, numbness, and tingling of the upper extremity. Vascular occlusion can also cause Raynaud's phenomenon on the involved side and predispose to thrombosis and embolization of the subclavian artery or vein. The compression may occur between the scalenus anticus muscle, clavicle, or pectoralis minor muscle and a cervical rib or the upper portion of the rib cage (see Fig. 6, page 133). Symptoms can be reproduced in certain positions, depending on the anatomic location of the compression, and are aggravated by strain and poor posture. Specific maneuvers, such as Adson's maneuver, hyperabduction of the arm, or downward pressure on the shoulder, can be performed to localize the site of compression (see the chapter on the Shoulders and Neck in the fascicle on Regional Structure and Function: Basic Principles in Rheumatology). A diminution or loss of radial pulse suggests vascular occlusion, especially when associated with a bruit above or below the clavicle. Pain, numbness, and tingling during these maneuvers suggest nerve compression. Care should be taken to distinguish this syndrome from cervical nerve root compression and the carpal tunnel syndrome. It can usually be treated in a conservative manner with appropriate exercises and is not significant clinically if the radial pulse is diminished during stress maneuvers in an asymptomatic patient.

DISORDERS OF THE SHOULDER

The shoulder is capable of a wide range of motion. It sacrifices some stability to achieve this remarkable mobility and is subject to strain, dislocation, and a variety of inflammatory and degenerative disorders that result in pain and limitation of motion. Both articular and periarticular soft tissues may be involved.

The technique of physical examination of the shoulder is reviewed in the chapter on Shoulders and Neck in the fascicle on Regional Structure and Function: Basic Principles in Rheumatology.

Calcific Tendinitis and Bursitis

Degenerative tendinitis is the commonest cause of shoulder pain and often occurs in the middle years of life. It usually involves the supraspinatus and infraspinatus tendons. Calcific deposits of hydroxyapatite are likely to form within or near these rotator tendons at sites of degeneration. About 3 percent of the middle-aged population have such calcific deposits, which are often asymptomatic. In many of these patients, however, pain develops as the result of inflammation of the tendon or overlying subacromial bursa.

Pathogenesis. Calcific deposits in the tendon are subject to repetitive pressure from daily use or strain and may absorb fluid when irritated, producing engorgement of the tendon. In the dry state the calcium is in powder form and the deposit usually is asymptomatic. When the calcified tendon is engorged, the calcium becomes liquid and chalky, causing pressure within the tendon. This chalky material may rupture into the subbursal space or into the overlying subacromial bursa, thereby producing an acute inflammatory reaction (Fig. 7). Bursitis rarely occurs as a primary condition and usually is secondary to degenerative lesions in rotator tendons.

Clinical manifestations. Symptoms resulting from inflammation of the tendon or bursa may be acute, subacute, or chronic. The acute syndrome is characterized by the relatively sudden onset of pain in the shoulder over the region of the deltoid muscle and upper arm. The pain is usually severe and is aggravated by any motion of the shoulder girdle or elevation of the arm. The typical patient comes in holding the arm at the side and removing the arm from a coat sleeve is likely to be extremely painful. Examination during the acute stage usually reveals exquisite tenderness over the anterolateral aspect of the shoulder. Pain at night is common because lying on the involved side aggravates the symptoms. In most cases the acute symptoms subside after a few days, but less often subacute distress may persist for weeks.

Roentgenographic findings. Roentgenographic studies frequently demonstrate a calcific mass in the subdeltoid area, but such deposits are not always present in symptomatic patients (see Fig. 1, page 332, in the chapter on Pseudogout in the fascicle on Specific Articular and Connective Tissue Diseases). Tendinitis can occur with-

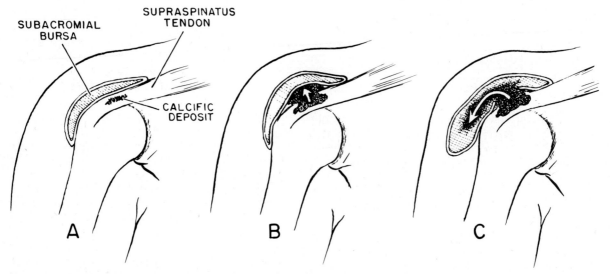

Fig. 7. Pathogenesis of acute calcific bursitis. **A.** Calcific deposit in tendon. **B.** Rupture of calcific bulge into subbursal space. **C.** Rupture of calcific deposit from tendon into subacromial bursa. (Modified from Cailliet R: Neck and Shoulder Pain. Philadelphia, Davis, 1964.)

out radiographic evidence of calcification. The calcific deposit may have a discrete linear pattern if localized to a tendon or a more diffuse lacy pattern if rupture has occurred into the subacromial bursa. The shoulder should be examined by anteroposterior views with the arm in both internal and external rotation to prevent nonvisualization of a calcific deposit by superimposing the calcium deposit over bony structures. Chronic involvement of rotator cuff tendons may result in bony changes that can be seen in the greater tuberosity of the humerus. The tuberosity appears cystic, sclerotic, and irregular and tends to decrease in size.

Biceps Tendon Lesions

Bicipital tenosynovitis.   The tendon of the long head of the biceps muscle emerges from the glenohumeral synovial sac to lie in the bicipital groove along the anterolateral aspect of the upper humerus (see Figure 2 in the chapter on Shoulders and Neck in the fascicle on Regional Structure and Function: Basic Principles in Rheumatology). It is covered by a synovial sheath as it lies in this groove. Tenosynovitis of the biceps tendon causes pain in the shoulder that radiates along the biceps to the forearm. The pain is accentuated by internal rotation or abduction of the shoulder. Bicipital tenosynovitis is characterized by tenderness over the bicipital groove. The pain is aggravated by resisted supination of the forearm with the elbow flexed at 90° (Yergason's sign). Roentgenographic studies usually reveal normal findings.

Rupture of biceps tendon.   Degenerative changes may occur in the biceps tendon with advancing age. Friction of the tendon against roughed margins of the bicipital groove causes fraying and weakening of the tendon, which elongates. When the tendon of the biceps is elongated, the biceps muscle becomes inefficient and no longer feels firm when the forearm is flexed against resistance. Spontaneous rupture of the tendon is associated with a sharp pain and immediate weakness in flexing the forearm. The biceps muscle is displaced distally in the upper arm where it forms an abnormal bulge.

Rotator Cuff Tears

Degenerative changes involving the supraspinatus, infraspinatus, and teres minor tendons can weaken the rotator cuff and predispose to rupture. Rotator cuff tears are frequently associated with trauma or strenuous use of the arm. A severe acute pain and sudden snap are often felt in the shoulder, followed by difficulty in abducting the arm. A complete tear results in inability to abduct the arm from the side, but it can be held in abduction if elevated to 90° or more by the action of the deltoid muscle. Partial tears cause milder pain and moderate weakness and may be difficult to differentiate from tendinitis or bursitis.

A contrast arthrogram may demonstrate a communication between the joint cavity and the subacromial bursa if a tear of the rotator cuff is present. It is important to realize, however, that the joint communicates with the bursa in some apparently normal, asymptomatic patients, especially with advancing age.

Adhesive Capsulitis (Frozen Shoulder)

The end result of chronic pain in the shoulder, regardless of cause, is often adhesive capsulitis or a frozen shoulder. It is characterized by chronic limitation of both active and passive motion in the shoulder. Patients with adhesive capsulitis may substitute scapular swing with elevation and depression of the shoulder girdle for true range of motion in the glenohumeral joint. This condition is caused by fibrosis and tightening of the joint capsule and periarticular ligaments and soft tissues. It is frequently associated with a variety of systemic or localized disorders, including coronary artery disease, cerebrovascular accidents, injury to the upper extremity, rotator cuff tears, calcific tendinitis, or postthoracotomy syndromes. It may also occur gradually without any obvious underlying disease and may be difficult to distinguish from rheumatoid arthritis involving the shoulders.

Shoulder–Hand Syndrome
(Reflex Neurovascular Dystrophy)

This syndrome is characterized by pain and limitation of motion in the shoulder, together with abnormalities in the hand. In the early stages, the hand abnormalities are due to stiffness, aching, swelling, and edema. In the later stages, trophic skin changes, vasomotor instability, and flexion contractures of the fingers may occur. The hand changes may resemble those seen in Dupuytren's contracture. The cause of this syndrome remains obscure but is presumed to result from a reflex sympathetic dystrophy similar to causalgia. The shoulder–hand syndrome is often associated with a variety of systemic or localized disorders including those already listed under adhesive capsulitis of the shoulder. The condition is bilateral in about 25 percent of patients.

Rheumatic Disease

Any of the diseases associated with synovitis may be responsible for pain and limitation of motion in the shoulder. Rheumatoid arthritis or ankylosing spondylitis may affect one or both shoulders. In the early stages of rheumatoid arthritis, roentgenograms may reveal only osteoporosis, but in later stages they may show bony erosion, loss of articular cartilage, or bony resorption of the distal clavicle. Septic arthritis due to pyogenic organisms or tuberculosis may cause permanent disability if inadequately treated. Pseudogout may affect the shoulder, but gout tends to spare the shoulder except in advanced stages. Hemophilia, sickle cell anemia, psoriasis, and inflammatory bowel disease are other systemic diseases that may involve the shoulder.

Degenerative joint disease of the glenohumeral joint is relatively uncommon, and when extensive it is often secondary to aseptic necrosis, ochronosis, infection, or trauma (Fig. 8). Neuropathic arthropathy (Charcot's joint) of the shoulder is usually due to syringomyelia. It occurs when loss of pain sensation deprives the joint of normal protective reactions. Joint discomfort remains mild relative to the severity of the joint destruction. Roentgenograms reveal severe disorganization of the joint with both destruction and proliferation of adjacent bone.

Polymyositis is a systemic form of muscle disease that causes aching and weakness of proximal muscles, including the muscles of the neck and shoulder girdle. Polymyalgia rheumatica should be suspected in elderly

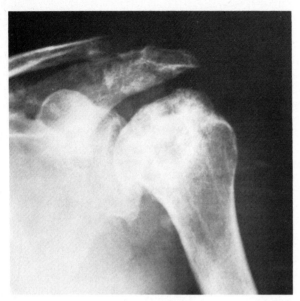

Fig. 8. Anteroposterior view of the shoulder showing marked sclerosis, deformity, and fragmentation of the humeral head due to aseptic necrosis. (Reproduced from the Clinical Slide Collection on the Rheumatic Diseases produced by the Arthritis Foundation, New York, copyright 1972.)

study and is associated with elevation of the serum alkaline phosphatase level.

Referred Pain

Intrathoracic or intraabdominal disease may produce pain in the neck and shoulder region. The pain of coronary artery disease is often felt in the left pectoral region and the ulnar surface of the left arm. Esophageal spasm and hiatus hernia may cause discomfort in the chest, shoulder, or arm. Pancoast's tumor, pulmonary infarction, or pericardial disease may produce pain in the region of the trapezius muscles. An intraabdominal perforated viscus or subdiaphragmatic abscess may also cause pain over the trapezius muscles. The pain of gallbladder disease is apt to be transmitted to the region of the right scapula. Aneurysms of the ascending aorta may produce pain over the right side of the neck and shoulder, whereas aneurysms of the transverse or descending aorta may cause referred pain over the left side of the back and shoulder. Lesions of the cervical spine frequently produce pain in the region of the shoulder or arm. Pain that is primarily localized over the deltoid muscle, however, is usually due to intrinsic disease of the shoulder and is not referred from other sites. When pain is referred into the region of the shoulder or neck from more distant sites, motion of the shoulder is usually normal and painless unless secondary adhesive capsulitis is present.

patients with generalized aching, especially in the region of the shoulder girdle. It is associated with marked elevation of the sedimentation rate, and, unlike in polymyositis, electromyographic studies, serum creatinine phosphokinase levels, and results of muscle biopsies are normal. The fibrositis syndrome is poorly defined. It is characterized by diffuse muscular aching and stiffness that may affect the neck and shoulder girdle. It is often worse with inactivity and improves with moderate activity; it is frequently associated with underlying systemic disease.

Nonrheumatic Disease

Leukemia and multiple myeloma in the region of the shoulder are best evaluated by roentgenographic studies, appropriate blood tests, and bone marrow examination. Metastatic malignancy produces destructive radiologic bone lesions and ''hot spots'' on the bone scan. Paget's disease of the shoulder is characterized by areas of increased and decreased bone density on roentgenographic

REFERENCES

Beetham WP Jr, Polley HF, Slocumb CH, et al: Physical Examination of the Joints. Philadelphia, Saunders, 1965
Cailliet R: Neck and Arm Pain. Philadelphia, Davis, 1964
Cailliet R: Shoulder Pain. Philadelphia, Davis, 1966
Fager CA: Diagnosis of cervical nerve root compression. Med Clin North Am 47:463, 1963
Jackson R: The Cervical Syndrome. Springfield, Ill, Thomas, 1971
Katz WA: Cervical spondylosis, in Katz WA (ed): Rheumatic Diseases: Diagnosis and Management. Philadelphia, Lippincott, 1977, pp 629–641
Katz WA: The shoulders and neck in the diagnosis of rheumatic diseases, in Katz WA (ed): Rheumatic Diseases: Diagnosis and Management. Philadelphia, Lippincott, 1977, pp 90–113
Steinbrocker O: The painful shoulder, in Hollander JL, McCarty DJ Jr (eds): Arthritis and Allied Conditions (ed 8). Philadelphia, Saunders, 1972, pp 1461–1502
Turek SL: Orthopaedics: Principles and Their Application (ed 3). Philadelphia, Lippincott, 1977, pp 739–789, 790–820, 821–865

Low Back and Hip Pain

Raymond E. H. Partridge

LOW BACK PAIN

Pain is the presenting symptom of disease affecting the spine, pelvis, and hips in the majority of patients. A few may present with swelling, weakness, or painless deformity, and in some physical abnormalities are discovered on routine physical examination. Anatomically the spine and pelvic girdle are closely interrelated, sharing certain mus-

cles and nervous pathways which allow symptoms to be referred from spine to pelvic girdle. Pain may also be referred to a point distant from the site of origin, as in knee pain from hip disease or sciatica from lumbar disc protrusion, but a large number of conditions involve local structures and the site of origin is usually not in doubt. The hip and spine may also be the site of referred pain from intraabdominal and pelvic pathology. Systemic disease of an inflammatory nature often causes musculoskeletal and spinal pain, although the major pathology may be located elsewhere.

The initial evaluation of the patient, consisting of a detailed history and physical examination, will usually provide sufficient data to enable first-stage or anatomic diagnosis to be made and is essential for planning a logical sequence of investigations for a more definitive pathologic and etiologic diagnosis. Age and sex provide helpful clues as the frequency of different diseases varies considerably in different decades and in some diseases there is a sexual bias.

Discitis is probably the commonest cause of back pain under the age of 3; ankylosing spondylitis has its highest frequency in men in the third and fourth decades. Prolapsed intervertebral disc is most common in men 20–50 years old, and postural pain is frequent in women of similar age. Osteoarthritis and degenerative disc disease are by far the most usual cause of back pain in individuals over 60; osteoporosis and vertebral collapse are also common in this age group. The onset of severe back pain for the first time over the age of 50 should be considered as indicative of tumor or infection until shown otherwise. A history of trauma is often given as an initiating event in many back syndromes, either as a direct cause of back pain or by unmasking existing disease. A positive family history may be present in some hereditary malformations or in ankylosing spondylitis and its variants.

SYMPTOMATOLOGY

The site, duration, character, severity, constancy, and radiation of the pain show some differences according to the type of pathology and the anatomic structures involved. Factors that alter pain significantly, such as rest, movement, or cough exacerbation, should be noted. Quite often, symptoms are difficult to interpret accurately because of the patient's reaction to pain and poor memory for past events. In all cases of back pain, a social and occupational history is important. Conscious or unconscious secondary gain or depressive reactions may cause persistence of symptoms.

Pain syndromes of the spine fall into two major categories, local pain and radicular pain, although often both are present. Local disease of vertebral bodies, intervertebral discs, apophyseal joints, and ligaments causes a deep, aching pain associated with varying degrees of muscle spasm and tenderness to palpation. The presence of morning stiffness is suggestive of an arthritic disorder; relief of pain by rest occurs with arthritis and disc disease, whereas constant pain, worsening at night, is characteristic of tumor, either of the vertebral body or spinal cord, and tuberculosis.

Radicular pain along the course of the lower lumbar of sciatic nerves is commonly due to root compression by a prolapsed intervertebral disc, but similar symptoms can be produced by spinal tumors, mechanical deformities, lumbar canal stenosis, epidural abscess, or, rarely, herpes zoster. Root compression may cause muscle weakness and tripping gait secondary to foot drop and peripheral paresthesia in the foot may be present. Symptoms of bilateral leg weakness, sensory loss, and urinary retention with overflow incontinence inply spinal cord involvement or a cauda equina lesion.

Examination of the patient should proceed as described in the chapter on Lower Back and Hip in the fascicle on Regional Structure and Function. The presence of spinal deformity, pelvic tilt, range of motion, local tenderness, gait, and neurologic abnormalities should be noted. A full physical evaluation, including examination of the rectum, pelvis, and breasts, is essential. After this stage of the evaluation it should be possible to estimate the probability that the back pain is caused by local problems (with or without nerve root involvement) associated with systemic disease or referred from extraspinal sites. Further evaluation requires routine radiologic and laboratory investigations, and in some cases special diagnostic studies are necessary to confirm the diagnosis.

DIAGNOSTIC STUDIES
Roentgenography

A routine x-ray examination includes anteroposterior, oblique, and lateral views of the lumbar spine and an anteroposterior view of the pelvis in order to visualize disc spaces, vertebral bodies, osseous structure, sacroiliac joints, hip joints, and soft tissues. The vertebral lamina and apophyseal joints are seen best in the oblique view. If sacroiliac disease is suspected, a 30° Ferguson view or oblique views of the sacroiliac joints are obtained. A lead shield for the genital area must be used in children. Stress films to evaluate the flexibility of the scoliotic curves may be useful. Tomography of the spine is helpful in delineating disease of the vertebral bodies and pedicles if these structures are poorly visualized in the standard x-rays.

Radioisotope Scanning

An increased uptake of technetium-99 polyphosphate is seen in bone lesions where there is primary or secondary osteoblastic activity; therefore, this technique is useful in detecting early inflammatory, neoplastic, or traumatic lesions before changes have occurred in the standard x-rays, although a distinction cannot be made between the types of lesion based on the scan alone. Inflammatory lesions of the discs and adjacent soft tissues can also be visualized by the use of gallium-51, which is helpful in the diagnosis of posterior abdominal wall tumor or abscess.

Computerized Axial Tomography (CAT)

A total-body scan that uses x-ray techniques that transect the spinal canal and intervertebral foramina is a new and useful technique in defining anatomic spinal lesions that are not appreciated by routine x-ray techniques. Spinal stenosis and spondylotic osteophytes encroaching on the intervertebral foramina may be seen by this method and soft tissue masses of the posterior abdominal wall are clearly outlined.

Laboratory Studies

Complete blood count, Westergren sedimentation rate, and urinalysis are done routinely. An elevated sedimentation rate is the most valuable indicator of an inflammatory or neoplastic lesion, although both false positives and false negatives can occur. The alkaline phosphatase is elevated in metabolic bone disease (osteomalacia), Paget's disease, and osteoblastic metastases; if necessary, fractionation should be done to distinguish bone from liver fractions. Increased acid phosphatase activity is seen in osteoblastic metastases from prostatic carcinoma. In cases of unexplained back pain with a high sedimentation rate, serum protein electrophoresis and immunoelectrophoresis may show an M spike, and free light chains (Bence Jones protein) may be found in the urine. Serum calcium is increased in malignant disease and reduced in osteomalacia.

The HLA-B27 antigen is present in 6–8 percent of whites and in a much smaller percentage of the black population. The aggregation of seronegative spondyloarthropathies in the B27-positive population has made this a useful additional test in some patients with backache. B27 antigen is present in 90 percent of patients with ankylosing spondylitis and in 70–80 percent of patients with Reiter's syndrome, reactive spondylitis, and the spondylitis associated with inflammatory bowel disease and psoriasis. A positive B27 antigen does not make the diagnosis of spondylitis or Reiter's syndrome but it is helpful in patients with early disease in whom radiologic changes of the lumbar spine and sacroiliac joints are equivocal or difficult to interpret. Other causes of back pain, however, such as lumbar disc disease, may occur as frequently in the B27-positive population as in the B27-negative. More recently, HLA-B7 has been shown to be associated with the development of ankylosing spondylitis in the B27-negative black population.

Electromyogram

Electromyographic abnormalities may be produced by lesions along a motor pathway from an anterior horn cell to a muscle fiber or along the course of sensory fibers. The technique is valuable in evaluating herniated discs with root pressure and distinguishing this from other neurologic syndromes. Myopathy produces a characteristic electrical pattern.

Further evaluation of back pain requires the use of invasive techniques that are generally only used if a lesion has been demonstrated by other methods.

Myelography

Myelography is not a routine procedure in the investigation of back pain. It is used to confirm the diagnosis of spinal canal block from tumor or other causes. It is also used in patients who exhibit neurologic defects on examination. It is done preoperatively before disc surgery to determine the level and site of disc protrusion.

Needle Aspiration and Biopsy

Aspiration of a disc space or vertebra under fluoroscopy is performed to obtain culture material in cases of discitis, vertebral osteomyelitis, or tuberculous abscess. A similar technique can be used for needle biopsy of bone to establish a pathologic diagnosis in destructive lesions of the spine.

DISEASE CLASSIFICATION

A classification based on pathology is shown in Table 1. No classification is completely satisfactory and it should be remembered that structural changes in the

---

Table 1
Differential Diagnosis of Low Back Pain

Infection	Structural
Discitis	Kyphoscoliosis
Osteomyelitis	Scheuermann's disease
Tuberculosis	Idiopathic scoliosis
Fungal infections	Spondylolisthesis
	Herniated lumbar disc
Nonspecific inflammation	Neuropathic Charcot spine
Spondyloarthropathies (HLA-B27 positive)	
Ankylosing spondylitis	
Reiter's syndrome	Paget's disease
Psoriatic arthropathy	
Reactive spondylitis	
Discitis (aseptic)	Neoplasia
	Spinal cord tumor
Trauma	Benign neoplasms
Vertebral fracture	Primary and metastatic tumors
Lumbosacral strain	
Degenerative	Osteitis condensans ilii
Osteoarthritis of the spine	
Lumbar spondylosis	
Diffuse idiopathic skeletal hyperostosis	Referred pain
Lumbar canal stenosis	Renal
	Pancreatic
Metabolic	Vascular
Osteoporosis	Tumor
Osteomalacia	
Hemachromatosis	
Ochronosis	Psychogenic pain

spine with kyphosis and scoliosis may accompany many other conditions. Structural abnormalities of the lumbar spine, herniation of lumbar discs, and lumbosacral strain are discussed in the chapter on Lower Back and Hip in the fascicle on Regional Structure and Function. These conditions and degenerative joint disease are the commonest causes of back pain but the possibility of other less common conditions must always be evaluated.

Infection

Discitis and vertebral osteomyelitis. Inflammation of the disc is the commonest cause of back pain in children under age 3 but may also occur in adults. The lumbar discs are often involved and the lumbar spine in children becomes flattened and even kyphotic. Vertebral osteomyelitis occurs mainly in children under the age of 12 or in individuals aged 50–70; the sex incidence is equal. The clinical features of discitis and osteomyelitis are similar: severe localized back pain, fever, chills, paravertebral muscle spasm, and restricted spinal motion occur in both. Young children present with fever and an inability to walk. *Staphylococcus aureus* and *Escherichia coli* are the common causative organisms; they spread from a focus by the hematogenous route and blood cultures may be positive during fever spikes (the source is seldom found in children). No invading organism is found in some cases of discitis in children and the etiology of the disease under these circumstances is uncertain.

In the early stage of discitis and osteomyelitis radiologic findings are negative, but bone scanning is positive early in over 90 percent of cases. Subsequently, discitis causes narrowing of the disc space and vertebral end plate irregularity. Destruction and collapse of the vertebral body occurs in osteomyelitis; a paravertebral abscess may be seen as a soft tissue shadow. The diagnosis can be confirmed by needle aspiration of pus under direct fluoroscopy and culture. Epidural abscess and cord compression may accompany both conditions.

A subacute, but severely painful back syndrome appears in brucellosis with symptoms similar to those described above. Splenomegaly is usually present.

Tuberculosis. Tuberculosis involves the vertebral body (often the first lumbar) most frequently in children or young adults, although the disease is now rare. The inflammation spreads across the discs into adjacent vertebrae (unlike malignant disease, which is usually limited by the disc) and into paraspinous tissues (tuberculous abscess). Collapse of the vertebrae occurs in untreated cases, causing an angulated spinal deformity and occasionally cord compression. Chronic pain, worse at night, and weight loss, anorexia, and low-grade fever are early symptoms. Examination presents a picture similar to that of other spinal infections with local pain, tenderness, and muscle spasm. Investigations may show an active tuberculous pulmonary focus on chest x-ray and a positive tuberculin test (a negative test virtually excludes the diagnosis). Routine x-rays of the spine are negative in the first few weeks of the disease but a bone scan is positive and tomography is helpful in demonstrating early lesions. Later bony rarefaction and destructive changes are seen.

Aspiration of a paravertebral abscess and needle biopsy for histology and culture confirm the diagnosis.

Inflammatory Disease: Seronegative B27 Spondyloarthropathies

Ankylosing spondylitis. Ankylosing spondylitis is an inflammatory synovitis of the spine and proximal joints with a male:female ratio of 10:1; it develops mainly between the ages of 18 and 40. A family history of spondylitis or back complaints is obtained in some cases. Early involvement of the sacroiliac joints occurs in over 90 percent of cases along with ascending inflammation of the apophyseal joints. Hip, shoulder, and knee synovitis occurs in more than one-third of cases and a small number have peripheral joint involvement. In addition to synovitis, inflammation of ligamentous attachments to bone (enthesopathy) leads to postinflammatory ossification of the annulus (syndesmophytes) and paraspinal ligament ossification, resulting in spinal fusion after a number of years. Early ankylosing spondylitis presents with pain and stiffness in the lumbar region, sacroiliac joints, buttocks, and posterior thighs. Occasionally pain is unilateral, causing confusion with disc protrusion. The pain awakens the patient from sleep in the early morning, and there is usually 1–2 hours of morning stiffness. Examination shows severe limitation of extension, lateral flexion, and forward flexion with a Schober test result of 1–3 cm. The sternomanubrial joint may be painful and heel pain is common. Twenty-five percent of patients have episodes of acute iridocyclitis that fluctuate independently of the spinal disease. Aortic ring dilation (incompetence) occurs late in 1–2 percent of patients. Male children from age 7 onward may present with oligoarticular arthritis of knees and hips and later develop typical spinal changes of ankylosing spondylitis.

Investigations show an elevated erythrocyte sedimentation rate, negative rheumatoid factor, and mild anemia. The B27 antigen is positive in 90 percent of cases. Early radiologic changes include symmetric irregular erosion and juxtaarticular sclerosis of the sacroiliac joints. Erosion of the anterior vertebral body margins causes vertebral squaring that can be seen on a lateral view. Tomography may demonstrate the vertebral body erosion. Early syndesmophyte formation is seen on the lower lumbar vertebrae and at T_{12}. A bone scan shows increased uptake around the sacroiliac joints early in the disease, but this does not appear to be a more sensitive test than careful x-rays of the sacroiliac joints. Later, joint space narrowing, ankylosis of sacroiliac joints, and progressive ossification of vertebral ligaments (bamboo spine) occur.

An arachnoiditis causing a cauda equina syndrome with lower limb neurologic deficit and bladder dysfunction is a rare complication of the disease.

Typical ankylosing spondylitis appears during the course of ulcerative colitis and Crohn's disease, predominantly in the HLA-B27 positive group. Unlike the peripheral arthropathy of inflammatory bowel disease, spondylitis may be progressive in spite of remission of bowel disease. A mild form of sacroiliitis that does not progress to the full clinical picture of ankylosing spondylitis appears to be a relatively common cause of chronic back pain in B27-positive individuals.

Reactive spondyloarthropathy. A reactive spondylitis with a somewhat different radiologic appearance occurs in Reiter's syndrome and psoriatic arthropathy. Twenty percent of patients with Reiter's syndrome have back pain, sometimes severe. Other features of the disease may also be present, including conjunctivitis, balanitis, urethritis, painless oropharyngeal ulceration, keratodermia blenorrhagica, and asymmetric involvement of ankles, knees, first metatarsophalangeal joints, and heels. The B27 antigen is positive in 70–80 percent of patients with Reiter's syndrome whether the spine is involved or not. Chronic back pain and stiffness occurs in 10–15 percent of patients with psoriatic arthropathy, but typical radiologic changes can also be seen in asymptomatic patients. Radiologically, sacroiliitis and syndesmophyte formation are often asymmetric. Periosteal pelvic "whiskering" is more frequent than in ankylosing spondylitis. Thick, paravertebral ossification from midbody to midbody of the vertebrae may be present.

Routine x-rays of the lumbosacral spine should be taken in all patients with seronegative inflammatory arthritis in order to screen for sacroiliitis—a helpful marker of this group of diseases.

Following infection with *Shigella, Salmonella,* or *Yersinia,* a transient polyarthritis may develop, mostly in B27-positive individuals with back pain and, in some, sacroiliitis. Postshigella arthritis occurring 1 month after dysentery has all the characteristics of Reiter's syndrome; postyersinia arthropathy is more like rheumatic fever. The diagnosis is made by positive stool culture and, in the case of *Yersinia,* by a rise in specific antibody titers.

Degenerative Joint Disease

Osteoarthritis. Osteoarthritis of the spine is a common disorder of the middle-aged and elderly, often in association with osteoarthritis of other joints. Heberden's and Bouchard's nodes and first carpometacarpal prominence are often present. It also develops after spinal injury and chronic deformity from any cause. The usual symptom is chronic back pain of gradual onset which is made worse by exercise and prolonged standing and relieved by rest. Stiffness occurs after sitting and short duration morning stiffness is present. There are no systemic symptoms. Variable deformity (usually mild lumbar scoliosis or flattening of lordosis) is present and the Schober test result (see the chapter on Lower Back and Hip in the fascicle on Regional Structure and Function) is reduced to 3–4 cm. The term *osteoarthritis of the spine* includes lumbar spondylosis with narrowing of the intervertebral discs, foraminal narrowing, and large osteophyte formation. Therefore, episodes of radicular pain are common. The lower apophyseal joints may show juxtaarticular sclerosis and joint space narrowing typical of diarthrodial joint osteoarthritis elsewhere, sometimes associated with pseudospondylolisthesis. The radiologic appearance of the spine reflects the process described but

does not correlate well with severity of the symptoms. Bone scans are negative or show only mildly increased uptake.

Lumbar canal stenosis. Progressive encroachment of the spinal canal by degeneration of the discs and hypertrophic ridging causes intermittent cauda equina dysfunction. Stenosis can also be congenital in origin, and a similar syndrome may be produced by massive central herniation of a disc. Chronic lumbar canal stenosis is commonest in men and causes limping and lumbar pain radiating to both legs on walking. Weakness and peripheral paresthesias occur in legs and feet. The pain resembles intermittent claudication of vascular origin but does not completely subside on rest. Physical examination may show saddle paresthesias and sometimes diminution or loss of reflexes, but often reflexes are normal. Straight leg raising and spinal motion may be diminished. The diagnosis when suspected can be made by measurement of the canal diameter (normal 22–25 mm) on standard x-rays and confirmed by CAT scan or myelogram.

Diffuse idiopathic skeletal hyperostosis. DISH, or Forrestier's disease, occurs predominantly in men over the age of 50 and clinically resembles ankylosing spondylitis in an older person. Severe diffuse spinal stiffness, central pain, and loss of motion occur gradually. Radiologically, ossification of the anterior and lateral ligaments is seen causing an effect like "candle wax" dripping down the spine, often best appreciated in the cervical or lower thoracic region. Disc spaces, sacroiliac joints, and apophyseal joints are preserved and there is no vertebral squaring. Large juxtaarticular osteophytes may limit hip motion. The diagnosis is made by standard x-rays of the spine: The B27 antigen is positive in 45 percent of cases.

Metabolic Bone Disease

Osteoporosis. Maximum skeletal mass is reached by age 20; thereafter a progressive diminution occurs in both sexes with an abrupt drop in mass (osteoporosis) in postmenopausal females. Postmenopausal osteoporosis in (usually thin) women is the most common type seen clinically. However, there are several causes of osteoporosis that may need to be excluded by appropriate studies, including endogenous or exogenous hypercortisonism, hyperthyroidism, and alcoholism. Multiple myeloma may also present as apparent osteoporosis, and severe osteoporosis may accompany rheumatoid arthritis. Osteoporosis is not painful, but pain is caused by microfractures or vertebral body collapse, usually in the lower thoracic and lumbar region.

Osteomalacia. Loss of mineral from bone results in osteomalacia. There are many causes, including malabsorption syndrome, poor nutrition, and pancreatic and renal disease, that should be evaluated. Chronic low back, hip, and thigh pain on movement gradually worsen if the disease is untreated. The rib cage, spine, and pelvis are tender to pressure. The bones become translucent and incomplete fractures (Looser's lines) may be seen late in the pelvis and femora. Serum calcium and phosphorous are normal or low and alkaline phosphatase is elevated.

Tumors

Metastatic carcinoma is a frequent cause of back pain in older age groups. Pain is characteristically severe and worse at night from collapse of a vertebral body. Radiographically, the vertebral end plate may be broken (unlike osteoporotic wedging) but the disc space is preserved. The pain of myeloma is insidious and aching at first, becoming severe when lytic lesions cause vertebral collapse. In the older age groups an elevated sedimentation rate and electrophoretic abnormalities should make one suspicious of malignancy. A bone scan is positive in metastatic carcinoma but only in one-half of the cases of myeloma.

Back pain can be caused by several benign and primary malignant neoplasms of bone at all age groups. Pathologic fracture and severe pain are characteristic of these lesions. Osteoid osteoma in the second or third decade typically causes night pain relieved by aspirin; a secondary scoliosis may develop.

Tumors of the spinal cord present with back pain that is often severe and usually worse at night. Early development of neurologic abnormalities in the lower limbs is characteristic of these disorders. A myelogram is essential for diagnosis.

Referred Pain

Back pain that clearly does not originate from the musculoskeletal system may be referred from posterior abdominal wall structures. Musculoskeletal examination is usually normal. Aortic aneurysm, pancreatic disease, and retroperitoneal tumors may all cause low back pain. Appropriate investigations, including pyelography, barium studies, echography, and abdominal CAT scan, are very useful.

Psychogenic Pain

After careful history and examination and thorough investigation a proportion of cases of back pain will remain undiagnosed. In some of these the pain is of psychogenic origin, most commonly a manifestation of depression or anxiety. Secondary gain, particularly if there is a history of trauma for which compensation is being sought, is another important factor. A long history of constant pain with a failure to respond to any standard therapy should arouse suspicion of a psychogenic origin.

HIP PAIN

SYMPTOMATOLOGY

Hip disease presents with pain in the groin, buttock, anterior thigh, or knee and a limp (antalgic gait). Stiffness is usually a predominant feature of hip arthritis. The symptoms of hip disease can be mimicked by bursitis, bone diseases of the upper end of the femur and pelvis, femoral hernia, inflammation of the inguinal lymph nodes, psoas abscess, and muscle disorders. Referred pain from prolapsed intervertebral discs often causes confusion with hip disease and the groin may be the site of referred pain along the course of T_{12} or L_1. Ureteric pain is also referred to the groin but the diagnosis is not usually difficult. A painless gait abnormality may occur with structural abnormalities, including uncorrected congenital dislocation of the hip and coxa vara, as a result of syphilitic neuropathic joint or myopathy. Swelling in the groin is rarely due to hip disease and if present is more likely to arise from structures in Scarpa's triangle or psoas abscess. Pelvic tilt from any cause will cause apparent swelling (unilateral prominence) of the greater trochanter.

The duration, site, radiation, and severity of pain and factors that exacerbate or ease the symptoms must be noted along with constitutional symptoms and the presence of arthritis elsewhere. The hip is frequently involved in different types of polyarthritis, the character of which is usually helpful in diagnosis. The examiner must be aware, however, of complications of polyarthritis, particularly joint sepsis, avascular necrosis, and fracture, that may occur during the course of the illness and be responsible for hip pain. Severe pain and inability to walk usually indicates infection (particularly if fever is present), fracture, or acute inflammatory synovitis. Milder pain and stiffness is characteristic of early degenerative joint disease in the middle-aged and elderly.

Age and sex are important considerations in diagnosis. In younger children the irritable hip syndromes of unilateral pain and limp are usually indicative of traumatic synovitis, "toxic synovitis," or Legg-Perthes disease. Hip pain can be the earliest sign of juvenile ankylosing spondylitis in male adolescents or of slipped femoral epiphysis. The most common hip pain in young and middle-aged adults is pain referred from a prolapsed intervertebral disc. Secondary osteoarthritis resulting from structural femoral head and acetabular abnormalities also presents in this age group. Primary osteoarthritis of the hip is the commonest cause of hip pain in older persons, but severe pain with inability to bear weight may be due to an unrecognized fracture of the femoral neck or pubic ramus, often without a history of injury. Polymyalgia rheumatica is associated with bilateral hip pain in patients over 50 years of age.

Examination of the patient should proceed as described in the chapter on Lower Back and Hip in the fascicle on Regional Structure and Function. A painless full range of hip motion is a strong indication of pain arising elsewhere and the spine and pelvis must be carefully examined. The contributions of combined hip and knee arthritis to limb dysfunction must be evaluated. A flexion contracture of the hip may result from muscle spasm secondary to psoas abscess or psoas irritation from appendicular or pelvic inflammation.

Appropriate diagnostic studies are helpful in evaluating the cause of hip pain and confirming the clinical impression.

DIAGNOSTIC STUDIES
Roentgenography

Routine roentgenography should include an anteroposterior and frog leg view of both hips and a lateral view of the involved hip. Appropriate views of sacroiliac joints and the lumbar spine should be taken if indicated. Tomography of the femoral head is very useful in detecting early changes of ischemic necrosis.

Radioisotope Scanning

Technetium-99 polyphosphate scanning will detect inflammatory and neoplastic lesions of the hip joint and adjacent bone. It is a useful technique for the assessment of hip pain if standard radiographs are normal, and it is also used to evaluate the nature of radiologically visible lesions.

Laboratory Studies

A complete blood count, erythrocyte sedimentation rate, urinalysis, and serum biochemistry should be done routinely. Rheumatoid factor, antinuclear antibody, and serum protein electrophoresis are helpful if an inflammatory lesion is suspected. The B27 antigen test is used to evaluate hip disease of adolescents and young males. The place of CAT scans in the diagnosis of hip disease has not yet been established. Arthrography is usually not helpful in diagnosis but may be used to establish the integrity of the cartilage and outline the synovial membrane. Aspiration of the hip is done under fluoroscopy if joint space infection is suspected.

DISEASE CLASSIFICATION

The classification (as shown in Table 1) is based on pathology.

Infection

Pyogenic arthritis and osteomyelitis. Essentially this is a disease of infancy and childhood caused by hematogenous spread of *Staphylococcus aureus*. There is usually associated osteomyelitis of the adjacent metaphysis. The child presents with extreme irritability, high fever, and painful muscle spasm causing flexion, abduction, and external rotation of the hip. There is a polymorphonuclear leukocytosis and high erythrocyte sedimentation rate. Radiographically, the earliest signs are bulging of the hip capsule and joint space widening; bone changes are not seen for 2 weeks. The organism is isolated by blood and synovial fluid culture. Osteomyelitis of the upper end of the femur presents with similar signs and symptoms.

Tuberculosis. The onset of tuberculosis is more insidious than that of pyogenic infection, with milder hip pain, limp, and deformity accompanying weight loss, anorexia, and fatigue. Night pain and muscle wasting are often present. The lesion may be in the synovial membrane or adjacent bone. The erythrocyte sedimentation rate is high and there may be chronic anemia. Radiographs will show distension of the hip capsule and osteoporosis followed by destruction of bone on both sides of the joint. The diagnosis is made by aspiration and culture or by open biopsy of the synovium. A search must be

Table 1
Differential Diagnosis of Hip Pain

Infection	Slipped femoral capital epiphysis
Pyogenic arthritis	
Tuberculosis	Paget's disease
Osteomyelitis	
? Viral arthritis	Regional (transient) osteoporosis
Psoas abscess	
	Villonodular synovitis
Nonspecific inflammation	
Spondyloarthropathies (HLA-B27 positive)	Neoplasia
Juvenile rheumatoid arthritis	Osteoid osteoma
Polymyalgia rheumatica	Leukemia
Toxic synovitis	Primary or metastatic tumor
	Multiple myeloma
Trauma	
Traumatic synovitis	Vascular
Fracture of femoral neck or pelvis	Intermittent claudication
Crystal-induced arthropathy	Myopathy
Gout	Myositis
CPPD disease	Muscular dystrophy
Degenerative	Hematologic
Osteoarthritis of the hip	Blood dyscrasias
	Hemophilia
Metabolic	
Osteoporosis with fracture	Meralgia paresthetica
Osteomalacia	
	Bursitis
Avascular necrosis	Trochanteric
Legg-Perthe's disease	Ischiogluteal
Steroid-induced	Iliofemoral
Alcoholism	
Blood dyscrasias	Referred pain
	Herniated lumbar disc
Neuropathic	Renal disease
Charcot's hip (syphilis)	Pelvic disease

made for active tuberculosis elsewhere, particularly in the genitourinary tract.

Inflammatory Diseases

B27 spondyloarthropathies. Ankylosing spondylitis may present with arthritis of the hip in adolescent males. Radiographs of the hip may be negative in the early stages and sacroiliac x-rays in adolescents can be difficult to interpret. A B27 antigen test is useful in this age group. Late in the disease one-third of patients with ankylosing spondylitis will develop hip disease which may progress to bony ankylosis. The hip joint is frequently involved in Reiter's syndrome. Severe, transient, painful synovitis of the hip is seen in psoriatic arthropathy, and progression to chronic arthritis may occur.

Juvenile rheumatoid arthritis (JRA). Hip involvement in JRA is most commonly seen during the course of acute febrile JRA (Still's disease) or the adult polyarticular form of the disease but is rarely the presenting feature of pauciarticular arthritis in patients under 4 years old. The antinuclear antibody (homogeneous pattern) is positive in 30 percent of these cases. Ischemic necrosis of the femoral head is often seen in association with hip arthritis if steroids have been used in treatment.

Adult rheumatoid arthritis. Hip joint involvement occurs late in rheumatoid arthritis and may be unilateral or bilateral. An adduction/flexion contraction with pelvic tilt often occurs, which causes the patient to flex the opposite knee on walking. The chronic stress on this knee will cause the so-called "long-leg arthropathy." If recognized early, correction of the hip lesion will prevent further contralateral knee damage. Narrowing of the joint space is the earliest radiologic sign of the rheumatoid hip. Gradual destruction of the femoral head, protrusio acetabuli, and acetabular fractures are later complications. Osteoporosis that causes fractures of the pelvic bones and severe hip pain can be seen in steroid-treated cases. Osteomalacia from poor nutrition must be excluded.

Crystal-induced arthropathy. Gout and pseudogout are very rare causes of acute hip arthritis in adults. Deposits of calcium pyrophosphate dihydrate (CPPD) can be seen radiographically in patients with CPPD disease as a thin radiopaque line in the articular cartilage adjacent to the femoral head.

Polymyalgia rheumatica. Severe shoulder and hip girdle pain with 2–3 hours of morning stiffness in individuals over the age of 50 are characteristic of polymyalgia rheumatica. Shoulder girdle pain is usually more severe than that in the hip. The sedimentation rate is high and temporal artery biopsy is positive for giant cell arteritis in 30 percent of cases.

Degenerative Joint Disease

Osteoarthritis is the commonest cause of hip pain in the middle-aged and elderly. Primary osteoarthritis is associated with arthritis of other joints and Heberden's nodes may be present. Secondary osteoarthritis develops at an earlier age as a result of femoral head–acetabular incongruity following femoral head abnormalities (see the chapter on Lower Back and Hip in the fascicle on Regional Structure and Function), infection, or trauma. Pain

is localized to the groin, buttock, or trochanter or is referred to the knee. Pain and stiffness are worse on exercise and relieved by rest, but late in the disease sleep may be disturbed. Stiffness after sitting is a common symptom and morning stiffness may last up to 1 hour. Loss of hip motion causes difficulty in putting on shoes and stockings. An antalgic gait is usually present on examination with loss of full extension and rotation of the hip joint in the early stages. Later, restriction of motion may be severe with adduction, flexion, and external rotation provoking contractures, causing pelvic tilt. Loss of cartilage and eburnation of bone results in severe crepitus on hip movement. Hip x-rays show narrowing of joint space from cartilage loss, subchondral sclerosis, and pseudocyst formation with osteophytes on the joint margin. There are no constitutional symptoms and laboratory tests are usually normal.

Tumors

Benign and malignant tumors can present with hip pain. Osteoid osteoma of the femoral neck or acetabulum is not uncommon in children and can be demonstrated radiographically as an area of lucency with a sclerotic rim. Tomography of the hip is helpful in the early stages. The pain is very responsive to aspirin. Acute leukemia in childhood can present with musculoskeletal symptoms that often include prominent hip and pelvic pain. The condition simulates infection or JRA. The blood count may be relatively normal in the early stages before blast cells appear. The platelet count is often depressed early, whereas in infections and JRA thrombocytosis is seen with active disease. Metastases to the upper end of the femur and pelvis present with hip pain. Radiographs may be normal in the early stages. A bone scan is essential in these cases, particularly if the sedimentation rate is raised.

Paget's Disease

The presentation of Paget's disease is similar to that of osteoarthritis of the hip. Pain is increased on exercise and is often present at rest. The diagnosis can usually be made radiographically before the characteristic deformities occur. Alkaline phosphatase is elevated during the active phase of the disease.

REFERENCES

Boston HC, Bianco AJ, Rhodes KH: Disc space infections in children. Orthop Clin North Am 6:953, 1975

Brewerton DA: HLA-B27 and the inheritance of susceptibility to rheumatic disease. Arthritis Rheum 19:656, 1976

Finneson BE: Diagnosis and Management of Pain Syndromes (ed 2). Philadelphia, Saunders, 1969

Howell DS, Sapolski AJ, Pita JC, Woessner JF: The pathogenesis of osteoarthritis. Semin Arthritis Rheum 5:384, 1976

Jacobs BW: Synovitis of the hip in children and its significance. Pediatrics 47:558, 1971

Paine KWE: Clinical features of lumbar and stenosis. Clin Orthop 115:77, 1976

Resnick D, Shaul SR, Robins JM: Diffuse idiopathic skeletal hyperostosis (DISH). Forrestier's disease with extra spinal manifestations. Radiology 115:513, 1975

Foot Pain

John J. Calabro

STATIC DISABILITIES OF THE FOOT

The foot is a very complex structure comprising one-fourth of the body's total bones and joints (see the chapter on Knees, Ankles, and Feet in the fascicle on Regional Structure and Function: Basic Principles in Rheumatology). As a moving appendage, it is rivaled in lifetime work only by the heart and lungs. In fact, it has been estimated that the average person walks 250,000 miles in a lifetime.

Foot disorders affect as many as 9 of 10 people at some time during their lives. Mostly static, these disorders may be traced primarily to the dictates of fashion or the use of shoes that lend a minimum of support, promote poor posture, and produce an imbalance between foot and body mechanics.

The major causes of foot pain are static disabilities, injuries, rheumatic diseases, and vascular disorders; of these, by far the most common are static disabilities.

Static disabilities are due to weak muscles or ligaments and to structural deformities of the foot that may be either congenital or acquired. They are commonly multiple (Fig. 1), since faulty mechanics from one disability often lead to another, thereby adding to the complexity of diagnosis and management.

FOREFOOT DEFORMITIES

The most common forefoot deformities are metatarsalgia, hammer toes, cockup toes, hallux valgus, hallux rigidus, bunions, warts, corns, and calluses. Metatarsalgia, or pain at the ball of the foot, may be due to a number of causes, including pes cavus (high longitudinal arch), a shortened Achilles tendon, Morton's neuroma, and inflammation of the metatarsophalangeal joints. Hammer and cockup toes may be caused by altered foot mechanics, tight shoes, or rheumatic disorders. Foot pain may also be caused by hallux valgus, or outward turning of the great toe, and by hallux rigidus, or stiffness of the big toe joint. Both hallux valgus and hallux rigidus are often accompanied by a painful bunion, due to adjacent bursal enlargement and inflammation. A painful bunionette may also form on the outside of the foot, adjacent to the little toe. Other painful soft tissue lesions include warts, corns, and calluses. These may occur singly or in combination and are usually secondary to irritation from confining shoes in the presence of other deformities, particularly hammer or cockup toes and metatarsal subluxation.

MIDFOOT DISABILITIES

The most common midfoot disabilities are foot strain and flat feet. Foot strain results from excessive body weight, occupational stress, or congenital or other

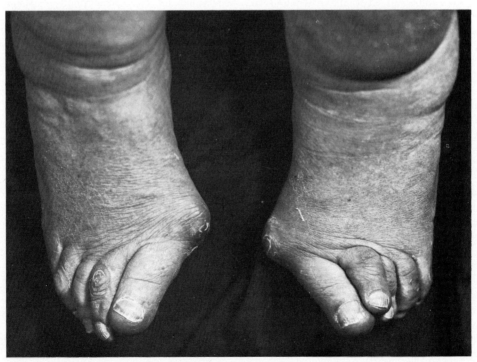

Fig. 1. Obesity-induced pes planus and striking forefoot deformities, including hallux valgus, bunions, hammer toes, corns, and spreadfoot.

causes. Overstretching of muscles and ligaments leads to varying degrees of foot pronation and valgus of the heel, abnormalities usually noted only with weight bearing. The major causes of flat feet (pes planus) are developmental (faulty posture or obesity), occupational (prolonged standing on hard surfaces), traumatic, neurologic, and rheumatic (rheumatoid arthritis). Flat feet may be flaccid (static), spastic, or rigid. In the flaccid type, which is the most common, the longitudinal arch is depressed only on weight bearing. If untreated, peroneal muscle spasm may result, producing the spastic flat foot, characterized by tender peroneal tendons and painful limitation of inversion. The end stage is a rigid flat foot in which the foot is fixed in abduction by contractures and adhesions.

HEEL PAIN

Heel pain is frequently caused by soft tissue inflammation from bursitis, tendinitis, and plantar fasciitis, or by calcaneal periostitis and spurs. Common causes are trauma and various rheumatic disease, including acute gout, rheumatoid arthritis, Reiter's syndrome, psoriatic arthritis, and ankylosing spondylitis. Heel pain may also result from soft tissue infection, osteomyelitis, fracture, local lipodystrophy, Sudeck's atrophy, Paget's disease, xanthoma of the Achilles tendon, bone tumor, osteochondritis, callus, or pump bumps.

Pain in back of the heel may be due to achillotendinitis, bursitis of the Achilles tendon (bursal inflammation between the skin and Achilles tendon), retrocalcaneal bursitis (bursal inflammation between the Achilles tendon and calcaneus), or a bony spur at the insertion of the Achilles tendon. In children, pain at the back of the heel may also be due to calcaneal apophysitis (osteochondritis); in young women, pain may be from shoe-induced achillotendinitis, callus, and pump bumps. The latter are painful soft tissue enlargements caused by irritation of prominent posterior calcanei from high-heel or pump shoes.

Pain at the bottom of the heel may be due to subcalcaneal bursitis or plantar fasciitis. These may be traumatic, secondary to rheumatic diseases, or idiopathic. Plantar fasciitis frequently leads to calcaneal periostitis and spur formation (Fig. 2). It may also result in diffuse plantar fascial thickening simulating Dupuytren's contracture at the palm.

There can be tenderness along the medial aspect of the heel from tenosynovitis of the posterior tibial tendon. This is especially common in adults with severely pronated feet. Less common is tenderness and swelling of the lateral aspect of the heel as a result of tenosnyovitis of the peroneal tendons.

REFERENCES

Calabro JJ: A critical evaluation of the diagnostic features of the feet in rheumatoid arthritis. Arthritis Rheum 5:19, 1962

Locke RK, Mennell J McM, Sgarlato TE: Foot complaints. Patient Care 6:20, 1975

Moseley HF: Static disorders of the ankle and foot. Ciba Clin Symposia 9:83, 1957

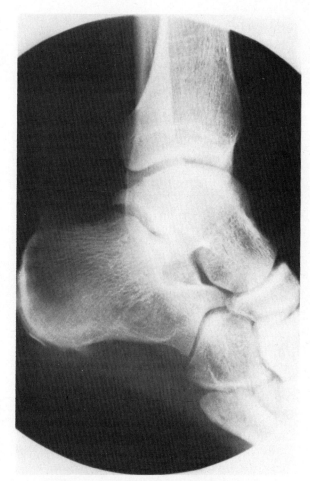

Fig. 2. Calcaneal spur due to plantar periostitis.

RHEUMATIC DISEASES AND OTHER DISORDERS OF THE FOOT

Of the 31 million or more Americans who suffer from musculoskeletal disorders, almost two-thirds have conditions that generally produce foot pain. Foot pain may also be caused by additional disorders, notably cutaneous, neurologic, and peripheral vascular diseases, or it may be due to injury, and in children, to osteochondritis.

RHEUMATIC DISEASES

Rheumatoid Arthritis

In terms of frequency of initial joint symptoms, foot problems outrank those of the hand, and are second only to those of the knee. Eventually, the feet become affected in up to 90 percent of rheumatoid arthritis patients, often constituting the major source of disability.

The metatarsophalangeal (MTP) joints are usually the first to become swollen and painful. Tenderness is elicited simply by applying light pressure to each of the MTP joints. Heel pain may also occur, occasionally as the initial complaint. In the back of the heel, pain results from achillotendinitis, bursitis of the Achilles tendon, retrocalcaneal bursitis, or rarely from subcutaneous nod-

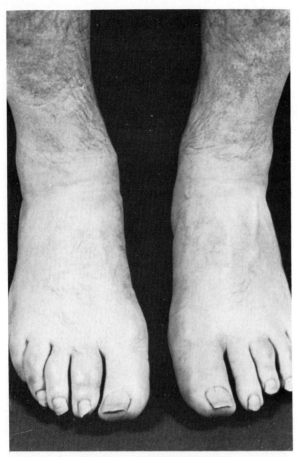

Fig. 1. Sausage toes in a patient with Reiter's syndrome. The right second and left first toes are diffusely swollen as a result of synovitis of the distal and proximal interphalangeal joints and intervening periostitis.

ules, which are usually painless. At the bottom of the heel, pain is most often caused by subcalcaneal bursitis or plantar fasciitis, and rarely by a subcutaneous nodule in the plantar fat pad.

Continuing MTP imflammation promotes contractures of ligaments and supporting structures. These, in turn, lead to progressive hallux valgus, hammer or cockup toes, subluxation of MTP joints, spreadfoot, and spastic flat foot. Secondary discomfort arises from shoe-induced microtrauma producing bunions, corns, and calluses. All of these foot problems call for aggressive therapy. Otherwise, the weight-bearing leg falls out of alignment, resulting in a valgus deformity of the knee. As a consequence of rheumatoid vasculitis, painful ulcerations and foot drop may also occur.

Gout

Initial or recurrent attacks of acute gout most often affect the great toe (first MTP joint) but may also occur in other toes, midfoot, instep, and heel. Joint pain is exquisite, produced in part by joint effusion as well as by edema of surrounding soft tissue. In chronic tophaceous arthritis, deformities similar to those observed in rheumatoid arthritis may evolve as a result of diffuse urate

deposition in multiple joints and soft tissues of the foot. The characteristic punched-out or erosive lesions noted on x-ray are prominent in the forefoot, uncommon in the midfoot, and rare in the heel.

Osteoarthritis

Foot pain and deformities due to osteoarthritis are primarily secondary to injury and to altered foot alignment from knee, hip, or back involvement. However, direct involvement of the first MTP joint may occur. Clinically, it is manifest as pain and progressive limitation (hallux rigidus), and on x-ray, as marginal sclerosis, osteophytes, and joint space narrowing.

An accelerated form of secondary osteoarthritis may occur in neuropathic (Charcot's) joints of the feet, most commonly from diabetes. The onset is often painless and insidious, hence early recognition is difficult. Typical deformities include soft tissue and bony proliferation of the midfoot, flattening of the longitudinal arch, and external rotation of the forefoot.

Spondyloarthropathies

Ankylosing spondylitis is the prototype of this group of disorders, which also includes Reiter's syndrome, psoriatic arthritis, enteropathic arthritis, and reactive arthritis following *Yersinia, Salmonella,* and *Shigella* infections. Each may be associated with foot pain from synovitis or heel pain from tendinitis, bursitis, plantar fasciitis, and periostitis, the latter being especially prominent in Reiter's syndrome (see Fig. 2, preceding chapter). Sausage toes, from diffuse swelling of an entire digit, occur with unusual frequency in Reiter's syndrome and psoriatic arthritis (Fig. 1). In both disorders, associated skin and nail changes are fairly distinctive. Occasionally, however, they may be similar, except that nail pitting does not occur in Reiter's syndrome.

Connective Tissue Disorders

Foot pain from synovitis may occur in these disorders, the most common of which are systemic lupus erythematosus, polymyositis, scleroderma, and polyarteritis. Foot pain and typical color changes following cold exposure from Raynaud's phenomenon may also occur, particularly in scleroderma. Vasculitis is also prominent, especially in polyarteritis and scleroderma; it is characterized by ischemic foot lesions, such as purple toes, soft tissue ulcerations, gangrene, and foot drop.

ADDITIONAL DISORDERS

Cutaneous Diseases

Common signs of aging skin are dryness, scaling, and atrophy. Breaks or fissures of the skin provide an easy avenue for bacterial, fungal, or contact dermatitis, the latter mostly from shoe dyes. At all ages, pressure from poor shoes may lead to painful subungual heloma, onychocryptosis (ingrown toe nail), plantar warts, corns, calluses, and bunions.

Neurologic Diseases

Problems of the foot and ambulation are common in neurologic disorders. For example, paresis of the lower extremity from a cerebral vascular accident may cause foot drop, trophic changes, and new weight-bearing areas for which the individual cannot compensate; these, in turn, can produce major foot problems. Tremor, rigidity, incoordination of movement, and peripheral neuropathies are other problems.

Foot pain, often severe, may be due to Morton's neuroma, Sudeck's atrophy (reflex sympathetic dystrophy), and nerve entrapment syndromes, such as the tarsal tunnel. The latter is due to compression neuropathy of the posterior tibial nerve within the tarsal tunnel, causing intermittent burning pain and parasthesias of the toes and sole which are worse at night. Point tenderness occurs at the medial side of the ankle, especially with tapping or direct pressure (Tinel's sign). There may be corresponding motor or sensory deficit and local fusiform swelling.

Peripheral Vascular Diseases

These diseases occur most commonly in the elderly, primarily from arteriosclerosis, varicose veins, and diabetes. The most prominent symptom is foot pain, especially with exercise, that may be associated with calf pain (intermittent claudication), weakness of foot muscles, edema, and numbness, tingling, or burning of the feet. The pulsations are diminished or absent. The overlying skin is usually thin, cool, and atrophic; the toe nails may be thickened. Severe circulatory impairment results in foot ulcers, which, in turn, predispose to infection and gangrene.

Injuries

Injuries that cause foot pain are usually obvious, except for march (stress) fracture. There is usually but not always a history of preceding injury or excessive walking. Fracture of a metatarsal shaft, usually the second or third, produces local pain, notably on walking, as well as tenderness and swelling. X-rays may be normal initially until callus forms several weeks later.

Osteochondritis

Of the various forms of osteochondritis, Freiberg's disease affects the metatarsal heads, usually the second. It is most common in teenagers, causing forefoot pain and swelling. On x-ray, there is widening and increased density of the affected metatarsal, followed later by fragmentation. Kohler's disease affects the navicular bone. It is common in children, producing medial midfoot pain and a limp. On x-ray, the navicular appears dense and flattened. Sever's disease, most common in teenage boys, involves the calcaneal apophysis, causing pain in back of the heel.

REFERENCES

Calabro JJ: A critical evaluation of the diagnostic features of the feet in rheumatoid arthritis. Arthritis Rheum 5:19, 1962

Calabro JJ, Garg SL: Neuropathic joint disease. Am Family Physician 7:90, 1973

Calabro JJ, Garg SL, Khoury MI, et al: Reiter's syndrome. Am Family Physician 9:80, 1974

Dickinson PH, Coutts MB, Woodward EP, Handler D: Tendoachillis bursitis. Report of twenty-one cases. J Bone Joint Surg 48-A:77, 1966

Edwards EG, Lincoln CR, Bassett RH III, Goldner JL: The tarsal tunnel syndrome: Diagnosis and treatment. JAMA 207:716, 1969

Hamilton EBD: Painful feet. Br Med J 3:342, 1969

Moskowitz RW: The painful foot. Gen Practitioner 27:100, 1963

Gastrointestinal Disease and Arthritis

Michael J. Reza and Carl M. Pearson

INFLAMMATORY BOWEL DISEASES ASSOCIATED WITH ARTHRITIS

Arthritis occurs in a significant number of patients with either ulcerative colitis or granulomatous ileitis (regional enteritis, Crohn's disease). Although estimates of its frequency vary from 10 to 40 percent, a recent large study documented the presence of arthritis in 23 percent of patients attending an inflammatory bowel disease (IBD) clinic. There are at least four major types of arthritis occurring in IBD: (1) colitic arthropathy, which is generally pauciarticular, occurs especially in the knees and ankles, and tends to flare concomitantly with flares in intestinal disease; (2) polyarthritis (rheumatoid factor negative); (3) spondylitis (HLA-B27 positive); and (4) combinations of the preceding.

PERIPHERAL ARTHRITIS

The peripheral arthritis of both ulcerative colitis and Crohn's disease are quite similar (each is discussed in detail in the chapters on Ulcerative Colitis and Arthritis and Granulomatous Ileocolitis and Arthritis in the next fascicle), and several general points should be kept in mind by the clinician. The arthritis is generally nondeforming, nonerosive, and sudden in onset. The synovitis is painful, migratory, usually oligoarticular, and usually of short duration. Peripheral arthritis is most common in the knees and ankles and tends to reflect underlying bowel activity. There is no sex predilection and recurrences or residual deformities are rare. Arthritis may occur prior to, during, or after the discovery of colitis.

As a general rule, patients with pancolitis, granulomatous colitis, perianal ulcers, pseudopolyps, uveitis, erythema nodosum, and pyoderma gangrenosum are more likely to develop arthritis. The peripheral arthritis usually responds to medication or surgical measures aimed at treating the underlying bowel disease.

SPONDYLITIS

Ankylosing spondylitis, which occurs in 5–20 percent of patients with IBD, carries a more serious prognosis than peripheral arthritis. It tends to occur before bowel disease is apparent, does not correlate with activity of bowel disease, and tends to progress despite adequate therapy or even cure of the bowel disease.

The vast majority of patients with ankylosing spondylitis and IBD are *positive* for HLA-B27 antigen. However, patients with colitis and enteropathic peripheral arthritis have *no increased* incidence of HLA-B27. Thus, there appear to be two major groups of patients with colitic arthropathy: those with a peripheral, inflammatory, rheumatoid-negative, HLA-B27–negative, arthritis that is self-limited; and those with sacroiliitis and/or ankylosing spondylitis who are positive for HLA-B27, but rheumatoid factor negative, and share many features similar to those of idiopathic ankylosing spondylitis.

WHIPPLE'S DISEASE

Arthritis or arthralgias occur in as many as 90 percent of patients with this rare disorder, which afflicts predominantly middle-aged white males. This disease should be suspected in an older male who presents with fever, abdominal pain, lymphadenopathy, hypotension, diarrhea or steatorrhea, and joint symptoms.

Diagnosis is made by demonstration of PAS-positive macrophages and, on electron microscopy, rod-shaped bacilli in the lamina propria in a biopsy of the small intestine. Joint symptoms may precede intestinal disease by as much as 20 years. The arthritis is characteristically fleeting, polyarticular, and migratory, and it may be quite subtle. The pathogenesis of Whipple's arthritis is poorly understood, but recent investigations have demonstrated rod-shaped bacilli in the synovium of involved joints. Spondylitis also occurs in approximately 15 percent of patients. The arthritis may respond to appropriate antibiotic therapy for Whipple's disease.

BEHÇET'S DISEASE

This chronic, inflammatory disease of unknown etiology is characterized by oral, ocular, and genital ulcerations as well as arthritis and widespread vasculitis. Esophagitis and colitis may also develop, and thus mimic granulomatous colitis. Sacroiliitis and spondylitis may also occur in Behçet's disease, but there is no increased incidence of HLA-B27.

REITER'S SYNDROME AND
INFECTIOUS DIARRHEA

Although in the United States, Reiter's syndrome most commonly occurs after an episode of nongonococcal urethritis, the original case reported by Hans Reiter occurred following an episode of dysentery. However, the presence of gonorrhea or even gonococcal arthritis does not exclude the possibility of Reiter's syndrome in those individuals who happen to be HLA-B27 positive. Thus, typical Reiter's syndrome may be associated with episodes of infectious diarrhea caused by *Salmonella, Shigella,* and *Yersinia enterocolitica.* It has been shown that postdiarrheal Reiter's syndrome is more likely to develop in those individuals who are HLA-B27 positive. When arthritis does occur it it is usually in those patients with acute, fulminent episodes of dysentery. Some authors feel that *Yersinia* infections cause a "reactive" arthritis as opposed to a classic Reiter's syndrome.

ARTHRITIS AFTER INTESTINAL
BYPASS SURGERY

A symmetric, erosive, but usually nondeforming polyarthritis that mimics rheumatoid arthritis may occur, in as many as 21 percent of patients after intestinal bypass surgery for morbid obesity. The arthritis is most common after jejunocolic bypass but also occurs after jejunoileal bypass. In several cases circulating cryoglobulins and immune complexes have been demonstrated and implicated in the pathogenesis of this disease. Bacterial overgrowth secondary to stasis in the blind loop may be a causative factor since antibiotic therapy occasionally alleviates this form of arthritis.

REFERENCES

Greenstein AJ, Janowitz HD, Sachar DB: The extraintestinal complications of Crohn's disease and ulcerative colitis: A study of 700 patients. Medicine (Baltimore) 55:401, 1976

Hawkins, DF, Farr M, Morris CH, et al: Detection by electron microscope of rod-shaped organisms in synovial membrane from a patient with the arthritis of Whipple's disease. Ann Rheum Dis 35:502, 1976

VARIOUS GASTROINTESTINAL DISEASES ASSOCIATED WITH ARTHRITIS

It has become increasingly apparent that certain gastrointestinal diseases may be associated with or complicated by arthritis or other rheumatic symptoms. On occasion the presence of arthritis may be the first clue to occult or incipient colitis, enteritis, or hepatitis. Much light has been shed upon the seemingly peculiar association of inflammatory bowel disease and arthritis or spondylitis by the recent discovery of a remarkable association between the histocompatibility antigen HLA-B27 and ankylosing spondylitis, Reiter's syndrome, ulcerative colitis, and granulomatous ileitis.

The gastrointestinal disturbances discussed in this chapter have been associated with arthritis or other rheumatic complaints.

LIVER DISEASES
Viral Hepatitis

Arthralgias and low back pain are common in viral hepatitis. It also has recently become apparent that an acute symmetric small joint polyarthritis associated with an urticarial skin rash may be a significant early clinical feature of viral hepatitis [hepatitis B antigen (HBsAg) positive]. The arthritis, in fact, precedes clinical signs of hepatitis and resolves when jaundice or liver function abnormalities occur. Elegant work by several investigators has demonstrated circulating immune complexes consisting of HBsAg (HAA) and antibody to it. Several patients with the prodromal arthritis of viral hepatitis had marked hypocomplementemia, especially of total hemolytic complement (CH_{50}) and C4, and to a lesser extent of C3. Hypocomplementemia abates, as does the arthritis, when jaundice appears. This illness is thus quite similar to classic serum sickness.

Chronic Active Hepatitis

Patients with chronic active hepatitis may develop a severe necrotizing vasculitis indistinguishable from classic polyarteritis nodosa. They usually have persistence of the HBsAg, and in some HBsAg has been localized by immunofluorescent techniques in the synovial membrane. The disease has a significant mortality rate but may respond to corticosteroid and cytotoxic therapy. Thus, it appears to be a chronic immune complex disease and ranks as an important discovery in that it comprises one of the first demonstrations of a chronic rheumatic disease presumably caused by a virus in humans.

Alcoholic (Laennec's) Cirrhosis

Patients with moderately severe alcoholic cirrhosis may develop a self-limited rheumatoidlike polyarthritis which develops as their liver function studies improve. The pathogenesis of this disorder is not understood.

Other Liver Diseases Associated with Arthritis

Arthritis or rheumatic symptoms may occur in association with a variety of other hepatic conditions, although the relationship between these conditions is not clearly understood. Some of these are listed below:

1. Wilson's disease, in which osteoporosis and a premature osteoarthritis occur
2. Hemochromatosis, in which a peculiar arthritis with features of osteoarthritis, rheumatoid arthritis, and chondrocalcinosis occurs
3. Fitz-Hugh-Curtiss syndrome, in which perihepatitis occurs and may be associated with the disseminated gonococcal dermatitis–arthritis syndrome
4. Amyloidosis
5. Temporal arteritis and/or polymyalgia rheumatica and liver function abnormalities
6. Primary biliary cirrhosis and the CREST syndrome
7. Granulomatous liver disease and arthritis (e.g., sarcoid, coccidioidomycosis, etc.)
8. Mixed essential cryoglobulinemia and chronic active liver disease
9. Mucopolysaccharidoses
10. Tuberculosis
11. Syphilis
12. Drug sensitivities

CONNECTIVE TISSUE DISEASES

Almost all the major connective tissue diseases may affect the gastrointestinal tract, as well as the joints, in a variety of ways. A discussion of these diseases is beyond the scope of this chapter but some major pertinent examples are listed below:

1. Hepatic and intestinal vasculitis and perforation associated with systemic lupus erythematosus
2. Esophageal dysfunction and, rarely, intestinal hypomotility associated with typical poly- or dermatomyositis
3. Esophageal dysfunction and Raynaud's disease
4. Esophageal dysfunction and intestinal vasculitis with mixed connective tissue disease
5. Esophageal dysfunction, reflux esophagitis, bacterial overgrowth in the small bowel, megoduodenum, duodenal and colonic diverticulum, and pneumatosis cystoides intestinalis in progressive systemic sclerosis
6. Gastrointestinal hemorrhage in Henoch-Schonlein purpura
7. Gastrointestinal vasculitis and hemorrhage as well

as pancreatitis and chronic hepatitis in mixed essential cryoglobulinemia
8. Nodular regenerative hyperplasia of the liver
9. Felty's syndrome in rheumatoid arthritis
10. Granulomatous hepatitis in Wegener's granulomatosus
11. Intestinal lymphoma and achlorohydria in Sjögren's syndrome

PANCREATIC DISEASE

Subcutaneous nodules, panniculitis, arthritis, and bone lesions, especially medullary fat necrosis, may be associated with both pancreatic carcinoma and pancreatitis.

MISCELLANEOUS DISEASES

The following is a list of additional diseases:

1. Ehlers-Danlos syndrome
2. Familial Mediterranean fever
3. Weber-Christian disease
4. Coeliac sprue
5. Pseudoxanthoma elasticum
6. Serum sickness
7. Osteogenesis imperfecta
8. Type II hyperlipoproteinemia
9. Hemophilia

DRUG TOXICITY

Gastrointestinal hemorrhage, peptic ulcer disease, colitis, hepatic dysfunction, and pancreatitis are common side effects of many of the standard drugs used in treating the connective tissue disorders, most of which also have articular symptoms. Physicians should familiarize themselves with these toxic effects associated with drugs such as aspirin, steroids, indocin, gold, azathioprine, allopurinol, methotrexate, etc. Furthermore, arthritis has been reported in antibiotic (ampicillin, clindamycin) induced colitis.

SUMMARY

Physicians should be aware of the frequent association of gastrointestinal and rheumatic diseases. Patients with arthritis, back pain, uveitis, or spondylitis in whom no connective tissue disease can be readily diagnosed may, in fact, have their diagnosis established by such tests as simple as a barium enema or UGI x-ray. The UGI x-ray should include a small bowel follow-through, as terminal ileitis may be the only manifestation of Crohn's disease. On the other hand, in the patient with IBD in whom back pain or peripheral arthritis develops, determination of the HLA-B27 may prove quite useful. Arthritis in young persons may also be a prodrome to viral hepatitis.

REFERENCES

Alpert E, Isselbacher KJ, Schur PH: The pathogenesis of arthritis associated with viral hepatitis. N Engl J Med 285:185, 1971

Duffy J, Lidsky MD, Sharp JT, et al: Polyarthritis, polyarteritis and hepatitis B. Medicine (Baltimore) 55:19, 1976

Sergent JS, Lockshin MD, Christian CL, et al: Vasculitis with hepatitis B antigenemia. Medicine (Baltimore) 55:1, 1976

Shagrin JW, Frame B, Duncan H: Polyarthritis in obese patients with intestinal bypass. Ann Intern Med 75:377, 1971

Skin Disease and Arthritis

Evelyn V. Hess and Baher S. Foad

ERYTHEMA, PURPURA, URTICARIA, AND NODULES ASSOCIATED WITH ARTHRITIS

Many rheumatic diseases have associated skin and mucosal manifestations which may be invaluable in making a diagnosis, for example the skin changes of scleroderma, psoriasis, and gonococcemia. Occasionally, the skin lesions do not provide specific diagnostic information; for example, erythema multiforme can be caused by numerous drugs or can occur in association with rheumatic or other diseases.

In this chapter erythema, purpura, urticaria, and nodules will be discussed and their relationship to rheumatic diseases will be highlighted.

ERYTHEMA
Facial Erythema

Among the rheumatic diseases, facial erythema occurs in systemic lupus erythematosus (SLE) and dermatomyositis. Facial erythema also occurs in photosensitivity reactions, rosacea, seborrheic dermatitis, and erysipelas.

SLE. Erythema occurs in the butterfly area of the face (Fig. 1), often following sun exposure (photosensitivity), and consists of diffuse erythema, sometimes with mild scaling and fine telangectasia. Erythema also occurs on the neck, the "V" area of the chest or back, in periungual and palmar sites. Alopecia and Raynaud's phenomenon are also common in SLE. Other skin signs include purpura, urticaria, discoid lesions, leg ulcers, facial and periorbital edema, hyperpigmentation, and digital gangrene. Mucosal ulcers can develop in the mouth or nose. Immunofluorescence studies of the skin lesions in SLE have demonstrated immunoglobulin and complement deposition not only at the dermal–epidermal junction, but also in blood vessels and epidermal cell nuclei. Activation of both the classic and alternative complement pathway has been reported. Immune deposits in the skin are due to immune complexes rather than antibodies to basement membrane. Such deposits have also been demonstrated in 60 percent of clinically uninvolved skin (lupus band test).

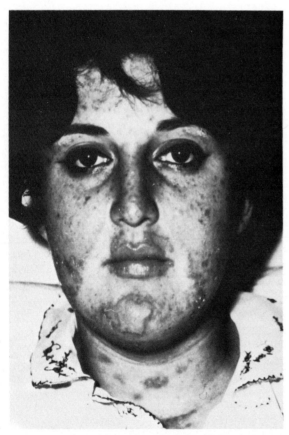

Fig. 1. Butterfly rash. (Reproduced from the Clinical Slide Collection on the Rheumatic Diseases produced by the Arthritis Foundation, New York, copyright 1972.)

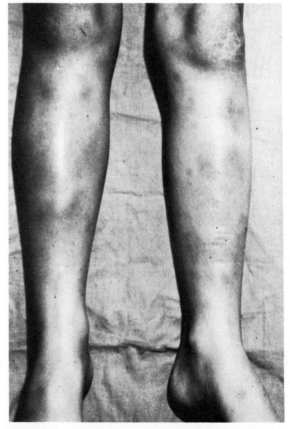

Fig. 2. Erythema nodosum. (Reproduced from the Clinical Slide Collection on the Rheumatic Diseases produced by the Arthritis Foundation, New York, copyright 1972.)

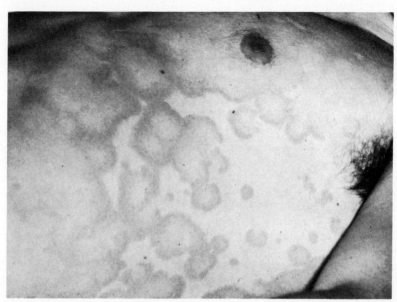

Fig. 3. Erythema marginatum. (Reproduced from the Clinical Slide Collection on the Rheumatic Diseases produced by the Arthritis Foundation, New York, copyright 1972.)

Dermatomyositis. Dusky butterfly erythema is common with purplish red (heliotrope) erythema of the upper eyelids with edema. Scaly erythema occurs on the extensor surfaces of elbows and knees.

Erythema Nodosum

Erythema nodosum consists of painful, tender, raised erythematous nodules, usually in young adult females (Fig. 2). It occurs most commonly on the anterior aspect of the legs. The lesions vary in size from one to several centimeters and may occur in crops. They develop over a few weeks, then regress. Arthralgias and/or arthritis may precede or occur with the nodules and usually involve the ankles and knees. The erythrocyte sedimentation rate is usually elevated. Common causes of erythema nodosum include sarcoidosis, drug reactions, streptococcal infections, and inflammatory bowel diseases. In many cases no cause can be established. The polyarthritis and erythema nodosum are self-limiting, but arthralgias may last for a few to several months.

Erythema Multiforme

Erythema multiforme consists of symmetric, erythematous, maculopapules on feet, legs, and forearms which may become generalized. The lesions may enlarge, become confluent, and form concentric rings (iris lesion). It is common in children and is self-limiting. Severe cases develop bullae and involve mucosal surfaces with associated fever and arthralgias (Stevens-Johnson syndrome). Causes of erythema multiforme include the following: reaction to drugs; viral, fungal, and bacterial infections; rheumatic diseases (acute rheumatic fever, SLE, dermatomyositis, vasculitis); and internal malignancy.

Erythema Marginatum

Erythema marginatum consists of erythematous ring macules with a pink outer margin and clear center (Fig. 3); it usually occurrs on the trunk and extremities. Individual lesions appear and disappear within a few hours.

Erythema marginatum occurs in acute rheumatic fever, usually with carditis.

PURPURA

The common causes of purpura in the rheumatic diseases are discussed below (see Table 1).

SLE

Purpura can be due to thrombocytopenia or vasculitis.

Rheumatoid Vasculitis

The purpura in rheumatoid vasculitis is usually associated with peripheral neuropathy, ischemic nail fold lesions, and leg ulcers. It usually occurs in patients with high-titer rheumatoid factors and subcutaneous nodules. A correlation with IgG rheumatoid factor and low molecular weight IgM has been described, suggesting that rheumatoid vasculitis is mediated by immune complexes. Sural nerve biopsy is useful in confirming the vasculitis; if done early it may show immune deposits of IgG, IgM and C3.

Cutaneous Vasculitis

Cutaneous vasculitis may present as palpable purpura or urticaria. It usually involves the lower extremities and occurs in crops lasting 1–4 weeks with residual hyperpigmentation or atropic scars. Fever, arthralgias, or myalgias may precede the purpuric lesions. If the vasculi-

Table 1
Purpura in Rheumatic Diseases

Systemic lupus erythematosus
Rheumatoid vasculitis
Cutaneous vasculitis
Cryoglobulinemia
Henöch-Schonlein purpura
Hyperglobulinemic purpura
Reaction to drugs

tis is widespread, there may be involvement of the lungs, kidneys, and nerves. Some patients have low serum complement. Complement components have been demonstrated in the skin by immunofluorescence studies. The blood vessels in the dermis are infiltrated with polymorphonuclear leukocytes (leukocytoclastic angiitis).

Cryoglobulinemia

The skin manifestations of cryoglobulinemia include Raynaud's phenomenon, purpura, and cold urticaria. Arthralgias, peripheral neuropathy, and renal disease may also occur. In the rheumatic diseases, cryoglobulins have been described in rheumatoid arthritis, SLE, Sjögren's syndrome, and vasculitis. In some cases no underlying disease can be found (essential cryoglobulinemia). The cryoglobulins are often immune complexes and exhibit rheumatoid factor activity (for example, hepatitis B antigen host IgG and IgM rheumatoid factor cryoglobulin).

Henöch-Schonlein Purpura

This is a type of hypersensitivity angiitis characterized by a tetrad of purpura, arthralgias, abdominal pain, and glomerulonephritis. Initially the skin lesions are erythematous macules or urticarial, usually in the lower extremities, and become purpuric. Skin biopsy shows a picture of leukocytoclastic angiitis; IgG and C3 deposits are found on immunofluorescence studies.

Hyperglobulinemic Purpura

Recurrent episodes of purpura develop on the legs associated with hyperglobulinemia. Rheumatoid factor is often present due to IgG anti-gamma globulin, which may be monoclonal in nature.

Drug Reactions

Gold, corticosteroids, salicylates, and phenylbutazone can cause purpura.

URTICARIA

Lesions are pruritic, sharply circumscribed, elevated areas of skin edema that may involve subcutaneous tissues (angioedema). The urticaria may be due to the release of histamine or other chemical mediators by immunologic or nonimmunologic mechanisms. There are many causes for chronic urticaria among the rheumatic diseases. Urticaria occurs in SLE, serum sickness, vasculitis, cryoglobulinemia, acute rheumatic fever, and juvenile rheumatoid arthritis. In familial angioneurotic edema due to deficiency of C1 esterase inhibitor, edema occurs in the skin, gastrointestinal tract, and larynx.

NODULES

Rheumatoid Nodules

Rheumatoid arthritis.   In rheumatoid arthritis, subcutaneous and subperiosteal nodules occur in 20 percent of adult patients (Table 2). The nodules, which are firm and nontender, occur over pressure points. Histologically, the nodules consist of three regions: a necrotic center surrounded by palisading macrophages, which in turn are surrounded by chronic inflammatory cells and fibroblasts. In some patients, the nodules are numerous (rheumatoid nodulosis) and result in cystic areas on x-ray.

Rheumatic fever.   Nodules in rheumatic fever usually occur with severe carditis. They are smaller than rheumatoid nodules and usually last for less than 1 month.

SLE.   Nodules in SLE occur in 5–10 percent of patients and histologically may resemble rheumatoid nodules.

Erythema Nodosum

Nodules in erythema nodosum are discussed above.

Panniculitis

The term *panniculitis* refers to a degeneration of fat cells and an infiltration with macrophages and chronic inflammatory cells. The common causes include the following: (1) Panniculitis may be seen in erythema nodosum. (2) Weber-Christian panniculitis consists of episodic, tender, subcutaneous nodules in the subcutaneous fat of the buttocks and thighs, mostly in women. Atrophic scars develop with healing. Fever, malaise, and weakness may precede the onset of the nodules. When the mesenteric and mediastinal fat is involved, gastrointestinal or cardiac symptoms develop and then the term *Weber-Christian disease* is used. (3) SLE may present with panniculitis. (4) In pancreatitis and pancreatic carcinoma, subcutaneous and periarticular fat necrosis leads to the development of subcutaneous nodules and polyarthritis.

Vasculitis

Nodules along the course of peripheral arteries occasionally occur in polyarteritis nodosa. These nodules are usually painful and tender and may pulsate.

Sarcoidosis

The skin lesions in sarcoidosis may be papules, nodules, or plaques. Histologically, sarcoid granulomas are seen. The lesions involve the face and extremities. In acute sarcoidosis hilar adenopathy, fever, erythema nodosum, arthralgias or arthritis may occur (Lofgren's syndrome). The ankles and knees are commonly involved and swelling can be both periarticular and synovial. In chronic sarcoidosis, chronic skin and joint symptoms may be associated with granulomatous involvement in the viscera.

Amyloidosis

The skin is commonly involved in primary amyloidosis as papules, purpura, or nodules that usually occur in the groin, axilla, face, or neck. Carpal tunnel syndrome is common. Amyloid arthritis differs from rheumatoid arthritis in the absence of significant morning stiffness, noninflammatory synovial effusion, and the absence of

Table 2
Nodules in Rheumatic Diseases

Rheumatoid nodules
Erythema nodosum
Panniculitis
Vasculitis
Sarcoidosis
Amyloidosis
Calcinosis
Xanthomas
Gouty tophi
Multicentric reticulohistiocytosis
Sweet's syndrome

destructive changes on x-ray. Nodules similar to those in rheumatoid arthritis may occur in the elbow region.

Calcinosis

Calcinosis occurs in scleroderma and dermatomyositis (dystrophic calcification). In scleroderma the calcific deposits are circumscribed and occur on fingers, elbows, knees, and pelvis. Ulceration and extrusion may occur. In dermatomyositis, calcification involving the muscles and subcutaneous tissues form widespread sheets. Calcinosis is more common in childhood dermatomyositis.

Xanthomas

Xanthomas occur in hyperlipidemic states. Tuberous xanthomas occur on extensor surfaces of elbows and knees. Tendon xanthomas occur in the Achilles, prepatellar, and extensor tendons of hands and feet. Both tuberous and tendon xanthomas occur in types II and III hyperlipoproteinemias and may be associated with migratory polyarthritis and Achilles tendonitis. Eruptive xanthomas consist of numerous small yellow-red papules over the buttocks, thighs, back, and elbows occurring in types I, IV, and V hyperlipoproteinemia; they may be associated with joint pain, stiffness, tenderness, and hyperthesia.

Gouty Tophi

Gouty tophi should be considered in the differential diagnosis of nodules in the elbow region.

Multicentric Reticulohistiocytosis (Lipoid Dermatoarthritis)

This is due to infiltration of the dermis and synovium by histiocytes and giant cells containing lipid. Painless, firm, reddish brown or yellow papules and nodules occur on the face and hands and may involve mucosal surfaces. A destructive polyarthritis similar to rheumatoid arthritis may develop.

Sweet's Syndrome (Acute Febrile Neutrophilic Dermatosis)

Recurrent episodes of raised painful nodules, plaques, or pustules associated with fever, leukocytosis and nondeforming peripheral arthritis may occur.

DISCOLORATION AND OTHER SKIN CHANGES ASSOCIATED WITH ARTHRITIS

In this chapter other skin changes, including discoloration, induration, plaques, ulcers, papules, and nail changes, will be discussed.

DISCOLORATION OF THE SKIN

Raynaud's Phenomenon

Raynaud's phenomenon is cyclical discoloration of the fingers on cold exposure. Vasoconstriction of digital blood vessels produces blanching or pallor, associated with pain, numbness, and tingling. Relaxation of the vasospasm results in cyanosis, and, on rewarming, redness may occur due to reactive hyperemia. A two- or three-color change (pallor, cyanosis, erythema) is required to confirm the presence of Raynaud's phenomenon. Pathologically there is vasospasm and/or occulsion of digital blood vessels triggered by cold exposure. Re-

current episodes result in atrophy of soft tissues at the tips of the fingers and occasionally ulceration. Bone resorption of the terminal tufts may occur. Underlying rheumatic diseases include scleroderma, SLE, dermatomyositis, rheumatoid arthritis, and cryoglobulinemia. Raynaud's phenomenon may precede other manifestations of scleroderma or SLE by several years.

Hyperpigmentation

Hyperpigmentation may be seen in scleroderma, dermatomyositis, and ochronosis, or it may be secondary to medications such as gold and antimalarials.

OTHER SKIN CHANGES

Scleroderma

The skin changes in scleroderma pass through three stages: edematous swelling, replaced by induration, followed by atrophy. The skin is tight, shiny, and indurated. Raynaud's phenomenon is common. Telangectasia and calcinosis may occur. The face is commonly involved. Histologically there is an increase of dermal collagen. X-rays of the hands may show soft tissue atrophy at the finger tips, resorption of terminal phalanges, and calcinosis. Joint capsules, tendons, and ligaments are involved by the fibrotic process, leading to stiffness, pain, and limitation of movement; occasionally synovitis is seen.

Two syndromes similar to scleroderma have been described recently: mixed connective tissue disease syndrome and eosinophilic fasciitis. In mixed connective tissue disease, swollen fingers, acrosclerosis, and Raynaud's phenomenon are associated with arthritis and myositis. Esophageal and pulmonary involvement can occur. The antinuclear antibody test is positive in a speckled pattern and the hallmark of the syndrome is the presence of antibodies to an extractable nuclear antigen. Eosinophilic fasciitis is due to inflammation and eosinophilic infiltration of the fascia between the subcutaneous tissue and muscle. The skin of arms and legs becomes erythematous and indurated with relative sparing of the hands and face. Eosinophilia and hyperglobulinemia are present.

Papules, Plaques, and Ulcers

Psoriatic arthritis. Erythematous scaling plaques are common on the elbows, knees, scalp, and trunk. The nails are commonly involved in patients who develop arthritis. Psoriatic arthritis may involve peripheral joints or the spine. The peripheral arthritis usually occurs a few years after skin involvement but may occur simultaneously or precede the skin psoriasis. Flare-ups of the skin are usually accompanied by flare-ups of arthritis.

Reiter's syndrome. This syndrome is a tetrad of urethritis, conjunctivitis or iritis, arthritis, and skin and mucosal lesions. Superficial ulcers are common on the penis, oral mucosa, and tongue. Coalescence of ulcers on the glans penis produces circinate balanitis. The palms and soles are commonly involved by maculopapular lesions that become keratotic. Large areas of the soles may be affected, producing keratodermia blenorrhagica; keratotic lesions of the fingernails are common. The arthritis in Reiter's syndrome can be similar to that of psoriasis.

Ulcerative colitis and Crohn's disease. The arthritis of inflammatory bowel disease may be associated with erythema nodosum, oral ulcerations, uveitis, and flares with exacerbations of colitis. Pyoderma gangrenosum occurs in some patients with colitis.

Behçet's syndrome. This is a multisystem disease characterized by oral and genital ulcers, iritis, and frequently involvement of skin. The skin lesions are varied and include papules, vesicles, pustules, pyoderma, and erythema nodosum. Pustules commonly occur following punctures of the skin.

Gonorrhea

In gonococcemia with fever and arthrits, distinctive skin lesions may occur. Initially a small erythematous macule occurs and it may become vesiculopustular with a dark necrotic center.

NAIL CHANGES

Keratosis and pitting of the nails occur in psoriasis and in Reiter's syndrome. Telengectasia may occur in scleroderma, SLE, and vasculitis. Vascular lesions in nail folds occur in SLE, dermatomyositis, and vasculitis. Clubbing, such as occurs in hypertrophic pulmonary osteoarthropathy, may be associated with periostitis and arthritis.

REFERENCES

Duffy J, Lidsky MD, Sharp JT, et al: Polyarthritis, polyarteritis and hepatitis B. Medicine (Baltimore) 55:19, 1976

Farström L, Winkelmann RK: Acute panniculitis. Arch Dermatol 113:909, 1977

Krauser RE, Schumacher HR: The arthritis of Sweet's syndrome. Arthritis Rheum 18:35, 1975

Moore PC, Willkens RF: The subcutaneous nodule: Its significance in the diagnosis of rheumatic disease. Semin Arthritis Rheum 7:63, 1977

Soter NA: Clinical presentations and mechanisms of necrotizing angiitis of the skin. J Invest Dermatol 17:354, 1976

Tan EM: Immunopathology and pathogenesis of cutaneous involvement in systemic lupus erythematosus. J Invest Dermatol 67:360, 1976

Braverman IM: Skin Signs of Systemic Disease. Philadelphia, Saunders, 1970

Connective Tissue Disease: Overlap Syndromes

Charles L. Christian

The diagnosis of connective tissue syndromes is based more on descriptive phenomena than on precise knowledge of pathogenesis or recognition of etiologic factors. The definitions of systemic lupus erythematosus, rheumatoid arthritis, and progressive systemic sclerosis require clinicopathologic patterns of organ involvement; to a lesser degree diagnosis depends on serologic tests that have varying degrees of association with different syndromes but lack absolute specificity. For each of the several syndromes there is a "classic" pattern of disease, upon which all observers agree in diagnosis. However, the clinical and laboratory components of each individual syndrome may be shared by one or more of the others.

Synovitis can be a significant feature of all of the connective tissue diseases. Myositis, characteristic of polymyositis, is present in a significant number of patients with systemic lupus erythematosus, progressive systemic sclerosis, rheumatoid arthritis, and a syndrome that is called *mixed connective tissue disease*. Interstitial pneumonitis, most frequently encountered in progressive systemic sclerosis, is also a significant feature of other connective tissue syndromes. Thus, by present criteria for diagnosis, groups of patients with systemic lupus erythematosus, progressive systemic sclerosis, or rheumatoid arthritis manifest varying combinations of several features. The permutations are such that each syndrome can be divided into multiple subsets on the basis of organ patterns of involvement, natural history, and laboratory data. Frequently individual patients with multisystemic disease exhibit abnormalities that are consistent with arbitrary criteria of more than one connective tissue syndrome. The nosologic frustration that ensues is expressed in phrases such as "overlap syndromes," "mixed connective tissue disease," "undifferentiated connective tissue disease," or in conjunctive terms such as "sclerodermatomyositis," "lupoderma," "rupus," rheumatoid arthritis/systemic lupus erythematosus, systemic lupus erythematosus/progressive systemic sclerosis, and so on.

The American Rheumatism Association has proposed arbitrary criteria for classification of rheumatoid arthritis and systemic lupus erythematosus: these criteria are not "diagnostic criteria;" rather they provide uniformity in the classification of disease for the purpose of clinical, therapeutic, and epidemiologic studies.

As we gain new information regarding the pathogenesis and etiology of the connective tissue syndromes, the nomenclature will probably become less confusing and our current terms may have no more than historical significance. Some examples of new concepts are HLA-B27 associations with rheumatic disease, demonstration of the role of hepatitis B virus in the induction of acute polyarthritis and vasculitis syndromes, and the recognition that "mixed cryoglobulins" and paraproteins are involved in the pathogenesis of vasculitis in some patients.

SHARED CLINICAL AND LABORATORY FEATURES OF THE CONNECTIVE TISSUE SYNDROMES

For each of the rheumatic disease syndromes there are typical or classic forms, defined by combinations of clinical manifestations and laboratory data. Even the typical patterns of an individual syndrome share features

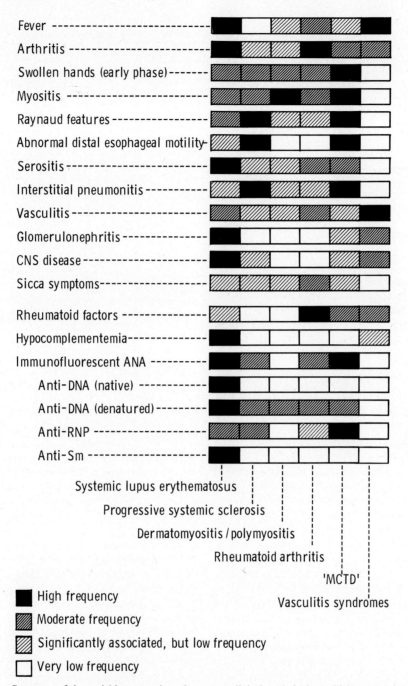

Fig. 1. Summary of the variable expression of common clinical, pathologic, and laboratory abnormalities in individual connective tissue disease syndromes. MCTD, mixed connective tissue disease.

with the other connective tissue diseases (Fig. 1). Arthritis, myositis, serositis, interstitial pneumonitis, Raynaud's phenomena, and sicca features are observed with varying frequency in systemic lupus erythematosus, progressive systemic sclerosis, dermatomyositis/polymyositis, rheumatoid arthritis, and a pattern of disease that has been termed "mixed connective tissue disease." Deforming polyarthritis was once considered unique to rheumatoid arthritis, but such changes are observed with significant frequency in otherwise typical cases of systemic lupus erythematosus, systemic sclerosis, myositis syndromes, and mixed patterns of disease.

Laboratory phenomena help define individual syndromes; e.g., hypocomplementemia, anti-native DNA antibodies, and anti-Sm antibodies are characteristic of systemic lupus erythematosus, but, with the possible exception of anti-Sm antibodies, none of these is specific for the disease.

Table 1
Representation of the Heterogeneity Manifest in Patients with Systemic Lupus Erythematosus

Features	Clinical Variants*								
	I	II	III	IV	V	VI	VII	VIII	IX
Clinical									
Fever	+	+	+	+	0	+	0	0	0
Arthritis	+	+	+	+	+	+	+	+	0
Photosensitive dermatitis	+	0	0	0	+	+	0	+	0
Serositis	+	+	0	0	0	0	0	0	0
Glomerulonephritis	+	0	+	+	0	+	0	0	0
CNS disease	+	0	0	0	0	0	0	0	0
Myositis	0	0	0	+	0	0	+	0	0
Raynaud's phenomena	0	0	0	+	0	0	+	+	0
Sicca features	0	0	0	0	+	0	0	0	0
Interstitial pneumonitis	0	0	0	0	+	0	+	0	0
"Rheumatoid" nodules	0	0	0	0	+	0	0	0	0
Laboratory									
Antinuclear antibodies	+	+	+	+	+	0	+	+	+
Anti-DNA (native)	+	+	+	+	+	0	0	+	+
Hypocomplementemia	+	+	+	+	0	+	0	+	+
Rheumatoid factors	0	0	0	0	+	0	0	0	0
Leukopenia	+	0	+	0	0	+	0	0	0
Hemolytic anemia	0	0	0	0	0	0	0	0	0
Thrombocytopenia	0	0	+	0	0	0	0	0	+
BFP Wassermann	+	0	0	0	0	+	0	0	0
Anticoagulant	+	0	0	0	+	0	0	0	0

*The "clinical variants" are designated types I–IX only for the purpose of discussion (see text).

VARIABLE PATTERNS WITHIN INDIVIDUAL SYNDROMES

For a particular syndrome such as systemic lupus erythematosus, the dozen or more clinical and laboratory manifestations that characterize the syndrome are variably expressed in individual patients. This variability is most striking when comparing patients at single points in time. A patient may exhibit predominantly rheumatic disease at the onset, later have hematologic and cutaneous abnormalities, and still later manifest chronic renal or central nervous system illness. Even with summation of features, the clinical heterogeneity is such that one can recognize and analyze subsets of systemic lupus erythematosus. The "clinical variants," arbitrarily designated types I–IX in Table 1, refer to this heterogeneity.

In this classification (proposed only for the purpose of discussion), type I represents "classic" systemic lupus erythematosus. Cases that show the characteristic serologic features of systemic lupus erythematosus but do not manifest clinical abnormalities (type IX) are conceptually considered a part of the spectrum of systemic lupus erythematosus. (This situation, discovered by accident or in epidemiologic or family studies, is probably more frequent than is recognized.) Cases that exhibit typical clinical features of systemic lupus erythematosus but lack antinuclear factors are represented by type VI disease. Type V refers to cases with clinical abnormalities characteristic of rheumatoid arthritis and serologic phenomena ordinarily associated with systemic lupus erythematosus. The pattern of illness designated type VII in Table 1 can

be viewed as a "variant" of systemic lupus erythematosus or as mixed connective tissue disease (see below).

The heterogeneity in syndromes other than systemic lupus erythematosus can also be analyzed in terms of subsets. Variations in patterns of rheumatoid arthritis relate to factors such as seropositivity, polyarticular versus oligoarticular, sustained versus intermittent course, presence or absence of antinuclear antibodies, extraarticular manifestations, etc. The group of patients with rheumatoid arthritis and high titers of antinuclear antibodies is not homogeneous: it includes those with severe "classic" rheumatoid disease that do not manifest clinical features of systemic lupus erythematosus and others that exhibit various admixtures of the two syndromes. The spectrum of progressive systemic sclerosis includes patients with typical "hidebound" cutaneous disease and little or no visceral abnormalities, individuals with severe gastrointestinal, renal, or cardiovascular manifestations of the syndrome who lack cutaneous abnormalities, patients with the CREST* syndrome, and those with chronic Raynaud's features who exhibit equivocal cutaneous or visceral abnormalities.

OVERLAP PATTERNS OF CONNECTIVE TISSUE DISEASE

Inevitably, controversies arise in the arbitrary classification of patients who exhibit features of more than one syndrome. A patient with Raynaud's symptoms, diffuse

*Calcinosis, Raynaud's manifestations, altered esophageal motility, sclerodactyly, and telangectasia.

scleroderma, and myositis could be viewed as having two syndromes (progressive systemic sclerosis and polymyositis) or as having only progressive systemic sclerosis if inflammatory myopathy is considered part of the spectrum of that syndrome. In the absence of specific markers for systemic lupus erythematosus and rheumatoid arthritis, patients with features of both diseases could be considered to have either one or the other or both diseases. The variety of "overlap" or undifferentiated syndromes is large: one pattern, which includes features of systemic lupus erythematosus, polymyositis, and progressive systemic sclerosis, has been identified and termed *mixed connective tissue disease.*

MIXED CONNECTIVE TISSUE DISEASE

Sharp and his colleagues proposed this term in 1972 to describe an "overlap" pattern of disease that was observed in 25 patients. The most prominent clinical features were rheumatic symptoms, diffusely swollen hands, Raynaud's features, abnormal esophageal motility, and myositis. None of the initial group of patients manifested evidence of renal disease, a minority had serologic features associated with systemic lupus erythematosus, and all had high titers of antibodies reacting with what was initially termed an "extractable nuclear antigen," subsequently characterized as nuclear ribonucleoprotein (RNP). (Both anti-RNP and anti-Sm specificities result in speckled immunofluorescent antinuclear patterns; the former is not reactive with ribonuclease-treated nuclear substrate.)

Arbitrarily, definition of mixed connective tissue disease *requires* the presence of anti-RNP antibodies in high titer; on clinical grounds alone a significant number of the patients could have been classified as having systemic lupus erythematosus or progressive systemic sclerosis.

A larger multiinstitutional study of 100 patients with high titers of anti-RNP hemagglutinating antibodies confirmed the initial observations regarding clinical correlations (Table 2). Renal disease, relative to its incidence in systemic lupus erythematosus, was infrequent. It should be noted that there is very little information on the natural history of mixed connective tissue disease; most reports have recorded observations at one point in time. A follow-up study of the first 25 patients reported disclosed that 7 patients had died: 1 from sclerodermalike malignant hypertensive disease, 1 from nephrotic syndrome, 2 from suicide, 2 from cardiovascular problems (probably incidental to their underlying illness), and 1 from gastric hemorrhage. Ten of the living patients who were examined included some with persistent features of scleroderma, some with myositis, some with chronic arthritis, and others who had experienced complete remission of their disease.

A significant percentage of patients with rheumatoid arthritis, systemic lupus erythematosus, and progressive systemic sclerosis have anti-RNP antibodies, although usually lower in titer than in mixed connective tissue disease. In a prospective study of 50 patients with systemic lupus erythematosus, the frequency of anti-RNP

Table 2

Clinical and Laboratory Characteristics of 100 Patients with anti-RNP Antibodies

Characteristic	Percent
Raynaud's features	85
Swollen hands	66
Sclerodermatous changes	33
Myositis	63
Skin rash	38
Fever	33
Neurologic abnormalities	10
Renal disease, definite	5
Renal disease, possible	5
Serositis	27
Arthritis/arthralgia	95
Abnormal esophageal motility	67 (75)
Decreased pulmonary diffusing capacity	67 (63)
Lymphadenopathy	39
Splenomegaly	19
Hepatomegaly	15
Sicca features	7
Hashimoto's thyroiditis	6
Anti-RNP	100
Anti-Sm	0 (67)
Anti-native DNA	12
LE cell positive	14
Hypocomplementemia	4 (70)
Rheumatoid factor	55 (62)
Hypergammaglobulinemia	73
Leukopenia (WBC <4500/mm³)	35

Figures in parentheses indicate the number of patients examined for individual characteristics when fewer than 100 were studied.

Adapted by permission from Sharp et al. and the *New England Journal of Medicine* 295:1149, 1976.

antibodies was 16 percent; titers did not fluctuate significantly over a 4-year period. The presence of anti-RNP antibody did not appear to identify a subgroup of lupus patients with individual clinical characteristics but other observations have suggested that systemic lupus erythematosus patients with anti-RNP antibodies exhibit a low incidence of major renal disease.

VALUE OF DIAGNOSTIC CLASSIFICATION

This discussion reflects the author's prejudice regarding arbitrary categorization and subclassification of connective tissue syndromes. Nevertheless, there is a rationale in the analysis of subsets and hybrid syndromes when such efforts yield information on prognosis and management of individual groups of patients or when a special research focus on such groups provides clues regarding etiology and pathogenesis.

Regarding prognosis and management, disease nomenclature has no more than statistical relevance. The pattern of organ involvement gives a more accurate guide. As a group, patients with mixed connective tissue disease who have high titers of anti-RNP antibodies and lack serologic markers of lupus are less likely to manifest life-compromising renal or nervous system complications than are patients with typical systemic lupus erythematosus; but in individual patients with the mixed syndrome, glomerulonephritis and other visceral complications may be prominent, and the prognosis is therefore altered.

The strongest argument for subclassification of connective tissue syndromes and the analysis of overlap patterns relates to the search for new information regarding etiology and pathogenesis. The recognition of shared manifestations between the several syndromes and mixed patterns in individual patients lends support to the hypothesis that the clinical variety reflects variable host responses to common etiologic factors. Anti-RNP antibodies are maximally expressed in a mixed pattern of disease, yet they are significantly associated with the other rheumatic disease syndromes. There may be a unique opportunity to characterize the genesis of anti-RNP antibodies by detailed studies of patients with mixed connective tissue disease, and this information could elucidate pathogenetic events in systemic lupus erythematosus, progressive systemic sclerosis, and rheumatoid arthritis.

SUMMARY

All of the connective tissue syndromes have in common a variable set of clinical, pathologic, and laboratory features, and the heterogeneity within a given syndrome (by current definitions) is large. Several overlap syndromes have been described: one, which includes features of systemic lupus erythematosus, progressive systemic sclerosis, and myositis and high titers of anti-RNP antibodies, has been termed *mixed connective tissue disease.*

Only in a statistical sense are prognosis and management influenced by diagnosis, whether typical, atypical, or overlap. The natural history and the treatment of patients with connective tissue diseases are determined more by organ patterns of involvement than by syndrome labeling.

The atypical and overlap syndromes may provide a special opportunity for characterizing etiologic and pathogenetic factors that are common to all of the connective tissue diseases.

REFERENCES

Bresnihan B, Grigor R, Hughes GRV: Prospective analysis of antiribonucleoprotein antibodies in systemic lupus erythematosus. Ann Rheum Dis 36:557, 1977

Fries JF: Mixed connective tissue disease. Current concepts (discussion). Arthritis Rheum S181:186, 1977

Notman DD, Kurata N, Tan EM: Profiles of antinuclear antibodies in systemic rheumatic diseases. Ann Intern Med 83:464, 1975

Reichlin M: Problems in differentiating SLE and mixed connective-tissue disease. N Engl J Med 18:1194, 1976

Sharp GC, Irvin WS, May CM, Holman HR, McDuffie FC, Hess EV, Schmid FR: Association of antibodies to ribonucleoprotein and Sm antigens with mixed connective-tissue disease, systemic lupus erythematosus and other rheumatic diseases. N Engl J Med 295:1149, 1976

Sharp GC, Irvin WS, Tan EM, Gould RG, Holman HR: Mixed connective tissue disease—An apparently distinct rheumatic disease syndrome associated with a specific antibody to extractable nuclear antigen (ENA). Am J Med 52:148, 1972

The Eye and Connective Tissue Diseases

Wallace V. Epstein

Of all the organ systems affected by the rheumatic diseases, none has provided a greater diagnostic and therapeutic challenge than the eye. Ocular disease may be the presenting manifestation of a rheumatic disorder, may develop into the most disabling expression of the disease even when the musculoskeletal manifestations are fully developed, and may provide unique insights into the etiology and pathogenesis of the entire disease complex. The eye may be involved in forms of synovitis associated with lymphocytic infiltration, as in the Sjögren–sicca syndrome, as well as in those rheumatic conditions associated with immune complex formation such as the nodular scleritis of rheumatoid arthritis.

The eye is subject to the same forms of immunologic attack as the skin and other target organs of the body. The eye may be irreversibly injured by such an attack. The interaction between the ophthalmologist and those treating rheumatic diseases calls for a common vocabulary and mutual appreciation of diagnostic and therapeutic problems. As the eye does not allow biopsy examina-

tion of involved tissues in most cases, so the musculoskeletal system does not afford repeated direct observation of the level of inflammation. Daily slit lamp examination of the anterior chamber of the eye with recording of flare (i.e., light scattering due to increased protein) and cells may provide a highly responsive expression of the underlying inflammatory process and, as such, can be a guide to the institution and continuation of drug therapy. Internists are well advised to remember the striking incidence of ocular manifestations of rheumatic diseases and to inquire of and examine the patient for these; most importantly, they should make appropriate referrals to an ophthalmologist when eye disease is overt or is a distinct possibility.

ANATOMIC CONSIDERATIONS

To make the highly diverse manifestations of ocular rheumatic conditions comprehensible, it will be necessary to review anatomic relationships and a few specialized terms so that the ophthalmologist's report is most helpful and the diagnostic possibilities can be narrowed.

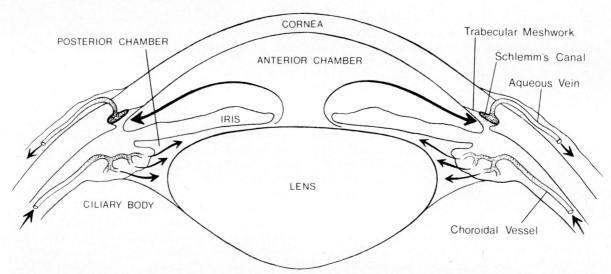

Fig. 1. Cross-section of anterior segment of eye showing aqueous circulation from the area of formation in ciliary body of outflow through canal system of the anterior chamber angle. (The author gratefully acknowledges the assistance of Ms. J. Weddell, who prepared this figure.)

Disorders located in or anterior to the ciliary body are designated anterior segment disease; disorders posterior to the ciliary body are designated posterior segment disease. The anterior segment is divided by the iris into the anterior and posterior chambers (Fig. 1). These anatomic boundaries are of importance because, for reasons that are not entirely clear, ocular inflammation associated with particular rheumatic diseases tends to occur in either the anterior or posterior segment.

Two circulations within the eye determine not only the distribution of infections or other etiologic modalities but also the localization of the inflammatory response. Aqueous humor, which is synthesized in the ciliary body, flows through the posterior aqueous chamber anteriorly past the pupillary margin of the iris into the anterior aqueous chamber. The trabecular meshwork, and ultimately Schlemm's canal at the angle of the anterior chamber, filters and then returns the aqueous to the vascular system. It may not be too fanciful to see similarities between this system and the process of manufacture of synovial fluid. Indeed, an aspiration of the aqueous for examination, although technically a good deal more difficult than joint fluid aspiration, may provide some of the same types of information as does synovial fluid analysis. Obstruction to the flow of aqueous from the posterior to anterior chamber by fibrous bands at the iris pupillary margin (synechiae) may cause segments of the iris to adhere posteriorly to the lens epithelium. In most forms of anterior uveitis, such posterior synechiae are sought out and treated promptly. Both obstruction to flow and obstruction to effective drainage of aqueous lead to glaucoma and elevated chamber pressure. Diminished production of aqueous due to chronic cyclitis (ciliary body inflammation) can lead to an even more ominous finding than the hard eye of glaucoma: a soft or hypotonous eye.

Two essentially nonanastomotic vascular circulatory systems coexist in the eye, both derived from the ophthalmic branch of the internal carotid artery. The central retinal artery supplies the circulation of the inner portion of the retina, while the long and short ciliary arteries provide the uveal tract with its nutrition. The uveal tract itself consists of the iris, ciliary body, and choroid. Nutrients to the outer portion of the retina diffuse from choroidal vessels, but direct vascular anastomoses do not exist between most of the retinal and uveal circulation. Thus, choroiditis may occur without associated retinitis.

The common circulation of the anterior and posterior portions of the uveal tract provide an explanation of the progression of posterior uveitis to anterior uveitis and the reverse. Despite this, anterior uveitis without posterior manifestations remains characteristic of ankylosing spondylitis.

Inflammation of the iris, ciliary body, or choroid, i.e., "uveitis," may present initially as iritis (iris alone) or iridocyclitis (iris and ciliary body), or it may be manifest by cells, fibrin, and inflammatory debris in the anterior chamber (anterior uveitis) or the vitreous (posterior uveitis). Iridocyclitis, as seen in juvenile rheumatoid arthritis, may follow the continuity of the uveal circulation with the sequential appearance of iritis and cyclitis.

Diseases of the outer coats of the eye can involve the uveal tract by contiguous spread. For example, the nodular scleritis of rheumatoid arthritis may lead to an anterior uveitis; posteriorly, a serous retinal detachment may result from involvement of the choroid or other structures. External ocular tissues such as the conjunctiva, episclera, and sclera are each associated with characteristic rheumatic afflictions to be discussed.

Corneal disease also follows anatomic planes; e.g., the keratitis of juvenile rheumatoid arthritis and the Sjögren–sicca syndrome appears in the subepithelial and epithelial layers, whereas the keratopathy of syphilis begins deep in the corneal stroma close to the corneal endothelium. Adequate examination of the cornea and the anterior chamber is not possible with the ophthalmoscope alone. Evaluation of the cornea, anterior chamber, and lens all demand slit lamp examination.

One further distinction concerning the ocular inflammation associated with rheumatic diseases involves the appearance of the aqueous and vitreous on slit lamp examination. Granulomatous uveitis refers to the presence of large cells, usually macrophages and monocytes, together with fibrin strands. Nongranulomatous uveitis is characterized by small cells, usually lymphocytes or polymorphonuclear leukocytes, fibrin, and inflammatory debris. Nongranulomatous uveitis is characteristic of ankylosing spondylitis and juvenile rheumatoid arthritis, but it should be noted that this distinction is not one always made with ease and a patient's uveitis may be classified as granulomatous at one time and nongranulomatous at another.

OCULAR MANIFESTATIONS OF RHEUMATIC CONDITIONS

The incidence of sites of ocular inflammation in particular rheumatic diseases is shown in Table 1.

Adult Rheumatoid Arthritis

Approximately 10 percent of nodule-forming, serum rheumatoid factor–positive adult rheumatoid arthritics develop an overt ocular manifestation of their rheumatic disease. Whatever process results in the formation of subcutaneous rheumatoid nodules can occur in the scleral layers of the eye. Conjunctivitis, episcleritis, and scleritis can all develop; their distinction is essential but not always simple, since combinations of these manifestations is the rule rather than the exception. Conjunctivitis is best identified by diffuse fine vessel engorgement and our ability to move such vessels with a cotton applicator. Episcleritis has a rather sudden onset and the vessels are discrete, purplish pink, and frequently perpendicular to the limbus (periphery of the cornea). These vessels cannot easily be shifted by applicator pressure, although, as in the case of conjunctival vessel engorgement, topical 10 percent phenylephrine will constrict the vessels.

Scleritis, involving the deepest layers, is associated with the more gradual onset of pain and manifests a deep purple-redness. Usually distinct vessels cannot be seen and topical vasoconstrictors have no effect. Scleritis always has some associated episcleritis and can occur both anteriorly, where it can be easily appreciated, or posteriorly, where it cannot. The scleritis can be diffuse, nodular, or necrotizing and can, by mechanisms already described, lead to anterior, posterior, or panuveitis, choroiditis, and keratitis. These in turn can lead to glaucoma, retinal detachment, thinning of the sclera, and rarely to spontaneous rupture of the globe. The histology of nodular scleritis in patients with rheumatoid arthritis is similar to that of subcutaneous nodules found elsewhere, and patients who have such ocular nodules have a greater than usual number of nodules elsewhere as well as pericarditis, pleurisy, and vasculitis. Ophthalmologists who treat patients with scleritis find, on consultation, that almost one-third of such patients have rheumatoid arthritis, and almost 60 percent have positive serologic tests for rheumatoid factor. When nodular scleritis is progressive and vision threatening, therapy is best undertaken by administration of immunosuppressive drugs. Reports of the use of either cyclophosphamide or chlorambucil suggest a far better response than previous attempts with either local or parenteral adrenocorticosteroids. Other conditions to be considered as causes of scleritis include syphilis, sarcoidosis, tuberculosis, and disseminated vasculitis.

Juvenile Rheumatoid Arthritis

In contrast to the painful red eye that is typical of the nodular scleritis of adult rheumatoid arthritis and the anterior uveitis of ankylosing spondylitis, the ocular lesion of juvenile rheumatoid arthritis may progress in the

Table 1
Incidence of Ophthalmic Manifestations of Rheumatic diseases

Diagnoses	Conj.	Episclera	Sclera	Cornea	Iris	Ciliary Body	Choroid	Retina
Adult RA	0	3	3	1	1	1	1	2
Juvenile RA	0	0	0	3	3	3	1	1
Sjögren's syndrome	4	0	0	4	0	0	0	0
Ankylosing spondylitis	0	0	0	0	4	2	0	0
Reiter's syndrome	4	0	0	0	2	0	0	0
Arthritis with colitis	0	0	0	2	3	3	0	0
SLE	2	0	0	0	0	0	0	4
Temp. arteritis	1	1	2	0	0	0	0	3
Behçet's syndrome	0	1	1	0	4	3	0	4
Periarteritis	2	3	3	2	1	1	1	3
Wegener's granulomatosis	0	0	3	2	0	0	0	2
Polychondritis	2	4	2	1	3	0	0	2

Scale of 0–4 refers to incidence not severity.

absence of pain or redness. Juvenile rheumatoid arthritis associated with ocular disease probably represents a 20 percent subset characterized by involvement of females more than by males (5:1) and a pauciarticular onset of disease. A minimally symptomatic iritis may lead to a nongranulomatous anterior uveitis with posterior synechiae resulting in pupillary irregularity. Two sequelae of chronic anterior chamber inflammation that can lead to vision loss are glaucoma and cataract formation.

The formation of calcium plates in the subepithelial region of the cornea (band keratopathy) is characteristic but not diagnostic of juvenile rheumatoid arthritis. If the band is in the optical axis, even with optimal medical management, significant vision loss occurs in one-half of such children. Whereas corneal band formation can be treated by chelation, the fibrous scar that sometimes accompanies the calcific deposits is not affected by chelation. Rather than wait to observe or have the child's parents report changes in pupil shape or opacity of the eye (cataract), it is wise to perform regular slit lamp examinations to detect anterior chamber inflammation. In 20–40 percent of such youngsters, the anterior uveitis may be manifest as red, painful iridocyclitis in which photophobia due to contraction of an inflamed ciliary body may result and in which pain may be the presenting manifestation. Rarely, posterior segment disease including papilledema and loss of central visual acuity, may develop. Primary inflammation of the posterior segment is not characteristic of juvenile rheumatoid arthritis. One-half of the patients with iridocyclitis have positive serum antinuclear antibody (ANA) tests, whereas one-third of the group with juvenile rheumatoid arthritis is ANA positive in the absence of ocular manifestations. Early detection, aggressive therapy with mydriatic-cycloplegic drugs and local corticosteroids, and meticulous follow-up are mandatory in this as they are in all ocular complications of rheumatic disease.

Sjögren's Syndrome

Keratoconjunctivitis sicca may occur in the absence of any rheumatic condition or it may be associated with typical rheumatoid arthritis, scleroderma, systemic lupus erythematosus (SLE), or other rheumatic conditions. It is difficult to be certain how to classify the ocular manifestations of such combinations. For example, many of the ocular manifestations attributed to scleroderma devolve from the sicca syndrome rather than from the sclerodermatous process per se. The ocular involvement in the Sjögren–sicca syndrome is a consequence of two processes: (1) infiltrative damage to the major and accessory lacrimal glands resulting in a keratopathy due to loss of the protective action of tears; and (2) less commonly, conjunctivitis and/or anterior uveitis. The well-known gritty or burning sensation associated with the early phases of the disease can be studied by measurement of the total lacrimal flow rate, quantitation of lysozyme in tears, and staining of the damaged epithelium (rose bengal test). Occasionally, patients may complain of the opposite symptom, i.e., excessive tearing; but upon examination, the lacrimal output is found deficient in protein and lysozymal enzyme.

The classic Schirmer test measuring tear production by paper wetting is a gross test and requires care in placement of the paper strips. Remember that normal elderly persons manifest less than 15 mm wetting in 5 minutes. There is no very close correlation of ocular symptoms with the magnitude of the decrease in tear formation until there is almost no tear production. As the corneal surface suffers loss of normal lubrication, the superficial epithelium is damaged and an inflammatory process develops in both the superficial corneal layers and in the bulbar conjunctiva. In its latter stages, a hazy keratitis develops, epithelium is denuded, and Bowman's membrane may be exposed. *Keratitis filiformis* refers to strands of corneal epithelium hanging free from their attachment to the corneal surface. This is the usual reason for the complaint that patients with this condition have difficulty opening their eyes after sleeping. Rarely corneal ulcerations ensue.

The use of artificial tears and the avoidance of topical corticosteroids best describe the local management. Some feel that an increase in tear production may be seen if the infiltrative process that affects the lacrimal glands responds to systemic therapy, but remissions rarely occur, even when other tissues affected by the infiltrative process appear to respond to treatment.

Scleroderma

Scleroderma is frequently associated with ocular manifestations, but most of these occur when a clinical mixture of keratoconjunctivitis sicca or a full Sjögren's syndrome coexists. Most of the external ocular manifestations such as lid tightness, keratitis, decreased tearing, and, rarely, episcleritis relate to an associated rheumatic condition. Retinal lesions are most frequently those associated with hypertension, a not uncommon sequela of scleroderma per se.

Wegener's Granulomatosis

Approximately one-half of the patients with Wegener's granulomatosis develop ocular manifestations. Proptosis, the most frequent complication (22 percent) is usually a consequence of sinusitis or a cavernous sinus thrombosis, but may occur in the absence of definite sinus involvement. Ten to 15 percent of patients have conjunctivitis, episcleritis, scleritis, or vision loss due to optic nerve effects—all thought to be secondary to small vessel vasculitis. A central scotoma and retrobulbar pain may both be manifestations of granulomatous infiltration of the optic nerve. Vasculitis of the posterior ciliary artery may lead to an ischemic optic neuropathy, while a similar process involving the anterior ciliary artery may result in a corneoscleral ulcer. These manifestations of anterior and posterior ciliary artery vasculitis may be seen in patients with SLE, rheumatoid arthritis, and polyarteritis. Wegener's granulomatosis may also be associated with vasculitis of the central retinal artery, resulting in ischemia of the retina and optic nerve atrophy. Inflammation of the uveal tract has also been reported, and in contrast to most other forms of uveitis associated with rheumatic diseases, this one tends to be granulomatous uveitis and has been reported in association with retinal phlebitis, vitreous hemorrhage, and neovascular glaucoma.

Ankylosing Spondylitis

The ocular complications of ankylosing spondylitis may become the dominant clinical problem in some patients. In approximately 25 percent of patients, a nongranulomatous iritis or more typically an iridocyclitis is seen. Occasionally a spillover of inflammatory cells into the anterior vitreous may be seen on slit lamp examination. In contrast to the anterior uveitis of juvenile rheumatoid arthritis, this condition results in a red, painful eye. The inflammatory process leads to cellular and protein deposits on the endothelial surface of the cornea (keratitic precipitates) and at the iris margin (Koeppe nodules). Adhesion of the iris margin to the lens results in posterior synechiae with the potential for obstruction to aqueous flow and thereby for developing glaucoma. This chronic inflammatory process, together with the side effects of corticosteroid therapy, may contribute to the formation of posterior subcapsular cataracts.

Topical corticosteroids are usually used together with mydriatics if synechia formation is threatened, but, unfortunately, these do not always completely control the inflammation. Institution of local therapy early in the course of an attack of iridocyclitis is essential. Periodic slit lamp examination is mandatory in patients with ankylosing spondylitis who have developed this complication. It is of interest that ophthalmology has its own method of diagnosing spondylitis: Verhoeff's test for spondylitis is declared positive when the patient is unable to extend the cervical vertebrae well enough to put his chin on the slit lamp apparatus.

Whether uveitis represents a subset of ankylosing spondylitis based on HLA-B27 characteristics is uncertain, since 80–90 percent of all ankylosing spondylitics are HLA-B27 positive and over one-half of all patients with acute uveitis of other origins are found to be HLA-B27 positive.

It is of interest that of the eight most common conditions affecting the sacroiliac joints, all but osteoarthritis and osteitis condensans ilii have an associated ocular complication (Table 2). Since the ocular event only develops in a subset of patients with each condition, a common genetic susceptibility in the several subgroups will probably be found.

Table 2
Conditions Leading to Sacroiliitis

Ulcerative colitis	Psoriasis
Reiter's disease	Whipple's disease
Ankylosing spondylitis	Osteoarthritis
Regional enteritis	Osteitis condensans ilii

Systemic Lupus Erythematosus

Most of the ocular manifestations of SLE develop as a result of small blood vessel inflammation. The most common manifestations are discrete infarctions of the nerve fiber layer of the retina resulting in fluffy white lesions in or around the posterior pole called *cytoid bodies*. Retinal hemorrhages and edema are also seen. Patients with SLE and hypertension may provide a challenge on examination of the fundus, since both hypertensive exudates and cytoid bodies may be present simultaneously. Retinal hemorrhages are seen in approximately 10 percent of patients with or without hypertension. Retinal vasculitis with arteriolar narrowing, especially of peripheral vessels with retinal degenerative changes, is also seen. Disturbances of extraocular eye muscle function resulting in diplopia may result from ischemic lesions associated with nutrient vessel vasculitis, while visual defects may be caused by lesions in any part of the visual pathway from the retina to the visual cortex. As indicated in the section on Wegener's granulomatosis, specific lesions may result from vasculitis of the anterior and/or posterior ciliary arteries. Hallucinations, scotomas, homonymous field defects, and cortical blindness have all been reported in SLE resulting from posterior cerebral artery involvement.

Reiter's Syndrome

Although the conjunctivitis of Reiter's syndrome is part of the clinical triad that defines the disorder, it may be both transient and of minimal clinical significance. Attempts to associate the conjunctivitis with a specific infectious agent have been unsuccessful. It is in the small minority of patients with Reiter's syndrome that we may see a severe anterior nongranulomatous uveitis not unlike that seen with ankylosing spondylitis. Recurrent iritis in both conditions may lead to synechiae that could result in glaucoma. Rarely, papillitis, retrobulbar neuritis, retinitis, intraocular hemorrhage, and keratitis occur. Although specific infectious agents such as those of the chlamydial group have been considered as possible etiologic agents for both articular and extraarticular manifestations, there is no evidence that the active eye lesions regularly harbor this agent.

Temporal Arteritis

The threat of vision loss in the granulomatous arteritis of temporal arteritis results primarily from ischemic effects on the two ciliary branches of the ophthalmic artery. A retinal lesion due to choroidal ischemia (posterior ciliary artery) may lead to peripapillary "cotton-wool spots." It is a matter of controversy whether some involvement of the central retinal artery in its extraocular course may also contribute to the loss of vision. Transient episodes of retinal ischemia due to involvement of either vessel must be treated immediately with parenteral corticosteroids. The exact initial dose remains subject to debate; but at least in this condition, one generally errs on the high side for the initial dose. Self-medication by the knowledgeable patient if sudden changes in vision develop appears to be highly desirable. It is extraordinarily rare to see initiation or progression of the ocular lesions of temporal arteritis when the patient is receiving oral adrenocorticosteroids or when the erythrocyte sedimentation rate has been brought down to the normal range.

Relapsing Polychondritis

Although relapsing polychondritis is infrequently seen, there is a surprisingly high incidence of ocular involvement (65 percent) in patients with this disease. Although episcleritis is the most common finding, scleritis, iritis, and keratitis may also be found. Although less common, chorioretinitis, extraocular muscle palsies, and optic neuritis may occur. In addition to a lesion of cartilage, and presumably of antigenically similar elements in the sclera, polychondritis is also characterized by a vasculitis. The lesions just described are also seen in temporal arteritis and in Takayasu's disease. Ischemic optic neuropathy related to posterior ciliary artery vasculitis has been reported in this condition, and, indeed, is one of the most common forms of optic nerve disease seen in the older age group usually prone to arteriosclerotic disease of these vessels.

Behçet's Syndrome

This syndrome, with its triad of recurrent oral, genital, and ocular lesions, may also manifest arthritis and both central nervous system and skin manifestations. The ocular lesions include conjunctivitis, episcleritis, iritis, choroiditis, and retinal vascular lesions. The dominant clinical picture is that of an anterior uveitis with profuse outpouring of inflammatory cells in the anterior chamber that, together with fibrin, settle to the bottom of the chamber (hypopyon). The initial retinal lesions usually appear as a periarteritis or periphlebitis, sometimes with thrombosis and hemorrhage. The rapidity with which this ocular lesion can cause blindness, frequently by simultaneous anterior and posterior segment disease, is remarkable. The introduction of alkylating agents (chlorambucil) to the treatment of this ocular catastrophy appears to have added a significant therapeutic modality, while large amounts of corticosteroids add little and should not be considered a necessary first step before chlorambucil is prescribed.

Bowel Disease

Both ulcerative colitis and terminal ileitis can be associated with episcleritis and uveitis, especially iritis; and both appear to correlate with the activity of the bowel lesions. Anterior nongranulomatous uveitis and corneal ulcers may occur in 2–4 percent of patients. Approximately one half of the patients with ocular disease associated with bowel disease also manifest arthritis, usually sacroiliitis. One third of the patients with bowel and joint lesions also manifest ocular pathology.

Polyarteritis

Polyarteritis, like the ocular arteritis associated with rheumatoid arthritis, SLE, and Wegener's granulomatosis, may involve both external and internal ocular structures. Involvement of the various coats of the eye leads to conjunctivitis, episcleritis, and both nodular and diffuse scleritis. Occasionally, in all of these conditions associated with intense vasculitis, limbal corneal ulcers may develop (necrotizing sclerokeratitis). This intensely painful, necrotizing condition can lead to perforation. The combination of interstitial keratitis and vestibuloauditory disease (vertigo and eighth nerve deafness) due to vasculitis (Cogan's syndrome) may also be seen. A wide range of retinal vascular lesions, including choroidal and retinal ischemia with hemorrhage, edema, and exudates, is not uncommon.

In addition to the highly variable intraocular manifestations, consequences of vasculitis involving cranial nerves and the visual pathway can produce diplopia, palsies (cranial nerves III and IV), hemianopia, and nystagmus.

Antirheumatic Medications

The complexity of the interrelations between ocular and articular diseases is increased by the ability of several commonly used antirheumatic medications to cause ocular disease. Topical and parenteral glucocorticoids can cause glaucoma in those with a genetically determined susceptibility to the disease. Posterior subcapsular cataracts may be associated with adrenocorticosteroid administration. Synthetic antimalarials have been responsible for corneal deposits, diminished corneal sensitivity, and retinopathy. The symptoms can include night blindness, ring scotomata, and visual loss. Since this appears to be dose related, it can be avoided by not exceeding 100–200 mg of hydroxychloroquine daily, although even at this level regular ophthalmologic examination is advisable. Gold therapy has been associated with conjunctivitis, corneal deposits, and, rarely, keratitis. Indomethacin administration has also been associated with corneal deposits. Clearly, an inventory of the patient's current and previous antirheumatic medications is necessary in the evaluation of ocular manifestations of the rheumatic diseases.

REFERENCES:

Brandt K, Lessel S, Cohen AS: Cerebral disorders of vision in systemic lupus erythematosus. Ann Intern Med 83:163, 1975

Chajek T, Fainaru M: Behcet's disease report of 41 cases and a review of the literature. Medicine (Baltimore) 54:179, 1975

Chylack LT: The ocular manifestations of juvenile rheumatoid arthritis. Arthritis Rheum [Suppl] 20:217, 1977

Epstein WV: Ocular complications of rheumatic diseases. Calif Med 118:17, 1973

Gold DH, Morris DA, Henkind P: Ocular findings in systemic lupus erythematosus. Br J Ophthalmol 56:800, 1972

Haynes BF, Fishman ML, Fauci AS, Wolff SM: The ocular manifestations of Wegener's granulomatosis: Fifteen years experience and review of the literature. Am J Med 63:131, 1977

Hogan MJ, Alvarado JA, Weddel JE: Histology of the Human Eye. Philadelphia, Saunders, 1971

Hogan MJ, Kimura SJ, Thygeson P: Signs and symptoms of uveitis: I. Anterior uveitis. Am J Ophthalmol 47:155, 1959

Hurd ER, Snyder WB, Ziff M: Choroidal nodules and retinal detachments in rheumatoid arthritis. Am J Med 48:273, 1970

Kimura SJ, Hogan MJ, O'Connor GR, Epstein WV: Uveitis and joint diseases: Clinical findings in 191 cases. Arch Ophthalmol 77:309, 1967

Kimura SJ, Thygeson P, Hogan MJ: Signs and symptoms of uveitis: II. Classification of the posterior manifestations of uveitis. Am J Ophthalmol 47:171, 1959

Mamo JG, Azzam SA: Treatment of Behcet's disease with chlorambucil. Arch Ophthalmol 84:446, 1970

Ostler HB, Dawson CR, Schachter J, Engleman EP: Reiter's syndrome. Am J Ophthalmol 71:986, 1971

Watson PG, Hayreh SS: Scleritis and episcleritis. Br J Ophthalmol 60:163, 1976

Wirostko E, Johnson LA: Cytology of inflamed acqueous humor in patients with rheumatoid arthritis. Am J Clin Pathol 54:369, 1970

Pulmonary Manifestations of Connective Tissue Diseases

Gary R. Epler

PULMONARY RESPONSE TO CONNECTIVE TISSUE DISEASES

Virtually all connective tissue diseases affect the lungs, which may respond in several ways (Table 1). Interstitial pneumonia is one of the most important responses. It is a progressive, dynamic process, and for this reason, the terms *acute* and *chronic pneumonia* and *fibrosing alveolitis* are preferable to the older term *fibrosis* since the latter refers merely to the scar or end product of some previously active lesion. Different types of pneumonias occurring in the connective tissue diseases include (1) usual interstitial pneumonia (UIP), (2) acute interstitial pneumonia, and possibly (3) desquamative interstitial pneumonia (DIP).

UIP is characterized by an entire spectrum of lesions ranging from normal alveolar walls to fibrotic, end-stage lesions. The interstitium contains polymorphus cellular infiltrates and the epithelial lining in small air spaces ranges from large, rounded cells on less damaged alveolar walls to cuboidal and squamous cells on more scarred alveolar walls. Acute interstitial pneumonia is characterized by epithelial necrosis, massive edema, the presence of hyaline membranes, and sparse cellular infiltrates. DIP is occasionally seen, but it is not yet certain whether this is caused by connective tissue disease or is a chance association. It is characterized by a lesser interstitial infiltrate and large mononuclear cells filling alveolar spaces. Histologic classification of these pneumonias is important in the connective tissue diseases since this can be used to forecast prognosis and response to therapy.

Since serosal membranes are a major target of the connective tissue diseases, the pleura is often involved. This involvement begins as an inflammatory response

Table 1
Frequency of Pulmonary Manifestations in Connective Tissue Disorders

Disease	Acute Interstitial Pneumonia	Chronic Interstitial Pneumonia	Pleural Effusion	Pulmonary Angiitis	Aspiration	Comments
Rheumatoid arthritis	0	+	++	+	0	Rheumatoid nodule; low glucose in effusion
SLE	+	+	+++	+	0	
Scleroderma	0	++	+	++	+	Poor prognosis
Polymyositis and dermatomyositis	+	+	0	+	+	Hypoventilation syndrome
Ankylosing spondylitis	0	0	+	0	0	Upper lobe infiltrates and bullae
Sjögren's syndrome	+	+	0	0	0	Lymphocytic interstitial pneumonia pseudolymphoma; lymphoma
Wegener's granulomatosis	0	+	+	+++	0	Multiple nodules, cavities
Behçet's syndrome	0	+	0	0	0	Hemoptysis
Polyarteritis nodosa	0	0	0	+	0	
Reiter's syndrome	0	0	0	0	0	Upper lobe infiltration
Mixed connective tissue disease	0	+	0	0	0	

Notation: 0, rare or questionable; +, occasional (< 10 percent); ++, frequent (10–20 percent); +++, common (> 20 percent).

with pleural effusion and subsequent pleural fibrosis or adhesions. In addition, the vascular system is often involved in these diseases and arteritis or fibrinoid necrosis may develop in small pulmonary vessels.

PULMONARY MANIFESTATIONS OF SPECIFIC CONNECTIVE TISSUE DISEASES

RHEUMATOID ARTHRITIS

Although pleural involvement occurs in 20 percent of patients with rheumatoid arthritis, effusions are seen in only 3–5 percent, probably because effusions go undetected in patients without symptoms. Pleural effusions may develop at any time and may precede or occur at the onset of joint symptoms. They are unilateral or bilateral, their glucose content is often less than 20 mg/dl, and some have a low complement. Pleural biopsy shows nonspecific fibrosis in half of the cases, but is diagnostic in others if rheumatoid nodules are seen. Most effusions are transient and resolve in several months, and systemic or intrapleural steroid therapy does not alter the final outcome. Occasionally, serious complications such as fibrothorax or empyema with pneumothorax may develop. Surgical decortication may improve dyspnea and physiologic impairment caused by fibrothorax in some patients.

Chronic interstitial pneumonia is more common in patients with rheumatoid arthritis than in the general population. Radiographic evidence of this lesion is seen in less than 5 percent of chest roentgenograms but physiologic abnormalities may be more common. As in pleural disease, interstitial involvement occurs at any time during the course of rheumatoid arthritis. These patients often have progressive dyspnea and end-inspiratory crackles. Physiologic studies indicate abnormally low vital capacity or diffusing capacity with increased alveolar–arterial oxygen tension difference. Exercise measurements show further deterioration of gas exchange. The radiographs may be normal or they may have linear opacities at the bases or honeycombing in severe cases. Lung biopsy reveals UIP and immunoflorescence may demonstrate IgM in alveolar walls in some specimens. As suggested by these histologic findings the clinical course may be indolent with minimal symptomatic, radiographic, or physiologic changes over a period of years; it may show a rapidly progressive process of fibrosis, end-stage honeycombing, or cor pulmonale; or it may be at an inbetween stage. Steroid therapy may accelerate the natural course of this disease and is often harmful. Insufficient information is available to be able to determine the efficacy of immunosuppressive agents for the treatment of this pulmonary complication.

The necrobiotic (rheumatoid) nodule of the lung is occasionally seen; it is called *Caplan's syndrome* when associated with the pneumoconioses. Nodules generally are subpleural, 1–2 cm in diameter, and occur bilaterally.

They develop during active rheumatoid arthritis but may precede the disease. Cavity formation occurs in one-third of the cases and can rupture into the pleural surface causing pneumothorax, but often the patients have no symptoms, signs, or pulmonary function abnormalities. Histologically the nodule has a characteristic structure: a central zone of fibrinoid necrosis, an intermediate zone of histiocytes and fibroblasts radiating in pallisade fashion, and a peripheral zone of connective tissue. These lesions are identical to those seen in the subcutaneous tissue and other organs. The nodules often regress spontaneously but may persist or in some cases enlarge. Therapy is not indicated, but since rheumatoid nodules mimic tuberculosis, neoplasm, or necrotizing granulomatoses, biopsy may be needed for verification.

Pulmonary vascular disease may occur as a result of advanced interstitial pneumonia and cor pulmonale, or less frequently as rheumatoid vasculitis. Fibrinoid necrosis and acute arteritis are seen histologically in this form of vasculitis, and immunofluorescence may demonstrate IgM in pulmonary arterioles.

Bronchiolitis obliterans has been reported in patients with rheumatoid arthritis. In contrast to interstitial pneumonia, in which there is no large airway involvement, physiologic evidence of severe airflow obstruction is seen in these patients, and several deaths have been reported as a result of this complication. In addition, patients with rheumatoid arthritis have a higher prevalence of bronchiectasis, bronchitis, and bilateral pneumonia. Finally, rheumatoid arthritis may involve the cricoarytenoid, causing chronic laryngitis, altered phonation, and dysphasia. Although laryngoscopic examination may show abnormalities in these patients, acute laryngeal obstruction is unusual. This lesion should be considered in patients receiving anesthesia or endotracheal intubation.

SYSTEMIC LUPUS ERYTHEMATOSUS

Clinical manifestations of pleural and pulmonary involvement occur in 30–50 percent of patients with systemic lupus erythematosus (SLE) and may even be the initial complaint. Pleuritic pain is the most common symptom and a pleural effusion is seen in half of such patients. The effusion may be massive and bilateral and may contain LE cells or have a low complement. These effects are usually transient, but residual fibrosis may develop, resulting in a pleura three to four times the usual thickness.

Although chronic interstitial pneumonia is seen in most histologic specimens at autopsy and physiologic evidence of this lesion is quite common, the chest roentgenogram is abnormal in only 5–10 percent of patients. Dyspnea and productive cough are frequent symptoms and basilar crackles are heard in two-thirds of such patients. Functional studies indicate decreased vital capacity and single-breath diffusing capacity. Histologically, these lesions resemble UIP. The disease is generally slowly progressive but in some long-term survivors honeycombing and cor pulmonale may develop.

Acute interstitial pneumonia has also been described

in SLE. This disease is characterized by the sudden onset of dyspnea, cough, and fever. Diffuse alveolar densities are seen radiographically and effusions are common. In contrast to the chronic form of pneumonia, these patients may show a dramatic response to high-dose corticosteroid therapy. Therefore, in patients with SLE, classification of the lung biopsy may help to differentiate patients with acute interstitial pneumonia in whom therapy may be beneficial from those with UIP in whom therapy may not be effective.

Lesions are not as common in the pulmonary circulation as they are in the systemic vasculature, but an inflammatory infiltrate of small arteries with fibrinoid change or onionskin lesions may occur in some cases. Symptoms are not commonly associated with these vascular changes, but physiologic changes may be detected, especially during exercise studies.

Pulmonary infections are only slightly more common in patients with SLE, but infections with agents such as *Pneumocystis carinii* are often associated with long-term steroid or immunosuppressive therapy.

SCLERODERMA

Among the visceral organs involved in scleroderma, the lung is second only to the esophagus, and pulmonary complications are a major cause of death. More than half of these patients may develop symptoms, abnormal physiologic studies, or radiographic abnormalities during the course of illness.

Chronic interstitial pneumonia is the most common pulmonary manifestation. Findings include progressive dyspnea, crackles, and an abnormal diffusing capacity. Radiographically, a diffuse reticular–nodular pattern is seen at the lung bases. Biopsy reveals histologic features of UIP and small airway involvement has been described. The interstitial processes are more active in these patients; therefore, prognosis tends to be unfavorable and end-stage honeycombing with cyst formation may develop. Occasionally, pneumothorax results from these cystic spaces. Steroid therapy has no effect on this type of histologic lesion and may cause harm by increasing susceptibility to infection. Even though the skin surrounding the chest may be extensively involved, this finding ususally does not decrease the vital capacity or lung volumes.

Pulmonary vascular disease is an important feature of scleroderma and may be found in over one-third of these patients. Clinical findings include dyspnea and abnormal exercise gas exchange studies. Radiographic evidence of enlarged pulmonary vasculature may be seen in some patients. Histologically, the large arteries are spared but the small and medium arteries show thickening of the intimal layer. The most consistent lesion is concentric fibrosis of the arteriolar intima, and the lumen is frequently narrowed or at times completely occluded. Although the CREST syndrome (calcinosis, Raynaud's phenomenon, esophageal dysfunction, sclerodactyly, telangiectasia) tends to have a slowly progressive course,

pulmonary vascular disease may develop in these patients.

The pleural membranes are also involved in scleroderma. Adhesions are commonly found at autopsy and, as expected, effusions develop in some of these patients. Aspiration resulting from esophageal dysfunction may cause acute or recurrent pneumonitis. Other manifestations include bronchiectasis, chest soft tissue calcification (calcinosis), and bronchiolitis obliterans.

POLYMYOSITIS AND DERMATOMYOSITIS

Interstitial pneumonia has been reported in less than 5 percent of patients with polymyositis or dermatomyositis. If the lesion is acute, there is histologic evidence of active cellular alveolitis with minimal scarring, and it is responsive to steroid therapy, but in the chronic UIP form, there may be extensive fibrosis with no steroid response and a poor prognosis. Small pulmonary arteries and arterioles may have medial or intimal thickening but vasculitis is rare.

Neuromuscular involvement may cause aspiration pneumonia, a poor prognostic sign, or hypoventilation syndrome, which causes hypercapnia.

MISCELLANEOUS DISORDERS

Pulmonary involvement is seen in less than 5 percent of patients with ankylosing spondylitis. The most common abnormality is bilateral upper lobe fibrosis. Bullae, sometimes containing aspergilloma, are often associated with these fibrotic changes. Other manifestations include pleural thickening, effusions, pneumothorax, and, very rarely, cor pulmonale.

Approximately 9 percent of patients with Sjögren's syndrome have pulmonary involvement. UIP is the most commonly seen lesion. It is associated with cough and dyspnea but no hemoptysis. Effusions may develop in some of these patients. The lymphoreticular system is involved in this connective tissue disease, which in some cases results in lymphocytic interstitial pneumonia, pseudolymphoma, and malignant lymphoma. Results of therapy with corticosteroids and immunosuppressive agents have been variable but, if clinically appropriate, a short trial of therapy should be given.

Pulmonary involvement in Wegener's granulomatosis is characterized by destructive inflammatory angiitis and areas of liquefactive necrosis and fibrosis. Cough, hemoptysis, and pleuritic pain are common symptoms. The roentgenogram shows single or multiple pulmonary nodules with diameters of 1–10 cm and frequent cavitation. Pneumothorax and effusion may develop but are uncommon. Steroid therapy or immunosuppressive agents are beneficial in some patients.

Pulmonary involvement in Behçet's syndrome is rare but life-threatening hemoptysis may develop as well as chronic interstitial pneumonia.

The bronchial arteries in patients with polyarteritis nodosa may show fibrinoid necrosis and perivascular infiltration. Upper lobe pulmonary fibrosis may develop as a late manifestation in Reiter's syndrome. UIP may be seen in patients with mixed connective tissue diseases.

The pulmonary lesions of sarcoidosis are discussed in the section on Sarcoidosis in the fascicle on Specific Articular and Connective Tissue Diseases.

REFERENCES

Carrington CB, Gaensler EA, Coutu RE, FitzGerald MX, Gupta RG: Natural history and treated course of usual and desquamative interstitial pneumonia. N Engl J Med 298:801, 1978

Epler GR, McLoud TC, Gaensler EA, Mikus JP, Carrington CB: Normal chest roentgenograms in chronic diffuse infiltrative lung disease. N Engl J Med 298:934, 1978

Gross M, Esterly JR, Earle RH: Pulmonary alterations in systemic lupus erythematosus. Am Rev Respir Dis 105:572, 1972

Israel HL, Patchefsky AS, Saldana MJ: Wegener's granulomatosis, lymphomatoid granulomatosis and benign lymphocytic angiitis and granulomatosis of lung. Ann Intern Med 87:691, 1977

Matthay, RA, Schwartz MI, Petty TL, Stanford RE, Gupta RC, Sahn SA, Steigerwald JC: Pulmonary manifestations of systemic lupus erythematosus: Review of twelve cases of acute lupus pneumonitis. Medicine (Baltimore) 54:397, 1975

Rosenow EC, Strimlan CV, Muhm JR, Ferguson RH: Pleuropulmonary manifestations of ankylosing spondylitis. Mayo Clin Proc 52:641, 1977

Schwarz MI, Matthay RA, Sahn SA, Stanford RE, Marmorstein BL, Scheinhorn DJ: Interstitial lung disease in polymyositis and dermatomyositis: Analysis of 6 cases and review of the literature. Medicine (Baltimore) 55:89, 1976

Strimlan CV, Rosenow EC, Divertie MB, Harrison EG: Pulmonary manifestations of Sjogren's syndrome. Chest 70:354, 1976

Walker WC, Wright V: Pulmonary lesions and rheumatoid arthritis. Medicine (Baltimore) 47:501, 1968

Weaver AL, Divertie MB, Titus JL: Pulmonary scleroderma. Chest 54:490, 1968

SPECIFIC ARTICULAR AND CONNECTIVE TISSUE DISEASES

Rheumatoid Arthritis

EPIDEMIOLOGY, ETIOLOGY, PATHOGENESIS, AND PATHOLOGY

Edward D. Harris, Jr.

Rheumatoid arthritis is a chronic disease of joints. Beginning with inflammation in the synovium, it may go into remission, run an intermittent course, or progress to a proliferative synovitis capable of erosion of bone and destruction of cartilage and tendons. Evidence for systemic disease frequently accompanies joint symptoms, and organs other than the synovium can be involved in a chronic proliferative and inflammatory tissue reaction.

The cause of rheumatoid arthritis remains unidentified. In contrast, multiple factors which doubtlessly are responsible for amplifying and perpetuating the initial pathology are now recognized. It may well be that there is no single etiologic factor and that many similar or diverse stimuli brought to bear upon the susceptible host may trigger reactions leading to the clinical syndrome which we recognize as rheumatoid arthritis.

EPIDEMIOLOGY

Studies designed to determine the prevalence and distribution of rheumatoid arthritis are difficult to carry out and interpret because no specific criteria exist for diagnosis. The American Rheumatism Association (ARA) criteria (Table 1) were the first developed for any connective tissue disease and have served to classify populations with reasonable sensitivity and specificity (see the section of Epidemiology in the fascicle on Regional Structure and Function). However, the ARA criteria are not diagnostic in an absolute sense. Only more detailed clinical and laboratory correlations will enable us to refine them to the point where specific disease etiologies are known.

The occurrence and distribution of rheumatoid arthritis can be summarized as follows:

1. "Definite" or "probable" rheumatoid arthritis exists in 1–3 percent of the adult population. Certain studies have suggested a higher prevalence in certain groups (e.g., Finns, Jamaicans, New Zealanders, and the Blackfeet and Pima Native American tribes).

2. Rheumatoid arthritis is two to three times more common in females than in males, and the altered physiology of pregnancy often is associated with remission of the disease.

3. Onset of classic rheumatoid arthritis can occur at any age, but the peak incidence is between ages 25 and 55.

4. Prevalence of rheumatoid arthritis has been found to be increased (approximately twofold) in first-degree relatives of patients with rheumatoid arthritis. However, a lack of concordance in twin studies and the failure of family studies to suggest a specific inheritance pattern have blocked attempts to establish a firm a genetic basis for rheumatoid arthritis. Recent work, however, has shown a high degree of association of rheumatoid arthritis and the histocompatibility antigen Dw4. The D locus within the major histocompatibility complex (MHC) on the sixth chromosome in man, tested for by the mixed lymphocyte culture technique, may be a reasonable functional expression of immune response genes.

5. Socioeconomic class, work exposure, specific nutritional deficiency, personality disorders or personality patterns, and autonomic nervous system dysfunction have not been demonstrated to be associated with either an increased or decreased incidence of rheumatoid arthritis.

ETIOLOGY

An exogenous infection or molecular components of an infectious agent are likely candidates for the primary etiologic agent(s) in rheumatoid arthritis. Specific data have not conclusively linked infection to rheumatoid arthritis and Koch's postulates to prove infectious etiology have not been met; however, increasing knowledge about the life cycles of certain forms of infectious agents and their chemical and immunologic features has made it apparent that infectious agents of different types are versatile, can persist in tissues, can share identity of molecular fragments with host cell components, and can trigger inflammation in such a way that it may become self-perpetuating. The appreciation of the variations in the immune response from individual to individual also highlights the possibility that small alterations in the structure of host components in connective tissue may lead to an acute and then chronic immune response.

Table 1
Criteria for Rheumatoid Arthritis

Criteria	Classification
Morning stiffness	Classical rheumatoid arthritis: 7 criteria
Pain on motion or tenderness in at least one joint	
Swelling (soft tissue or fluid) of at least one joint	Definite rheumatoid arthritis: 5 criteria; joint signs or symptoms continuous for at least 6 weeks
Swelling of at least one other joint	
Symmetric joint swelling, same joint on both sides of body (excluding terminal phalangeal joint)	Probable rheumatoid arthritis: 3 criteria; joint signs or symptoms continuous for at least 6 weeks
Subcutaneous nodules	Possible rheumatoid arthritis: 2 criteria; joint signs or symptoms continuous for at least 3 weeks
Roentgenographic changes (at least bony decalcification)	
"Rheumatoid factor" (any method)	
"Poor" mucin precipitate	
Characteristic histologic changes—synovium	
Characteristic histologic changes—nodules	

From Kellgren et al (eds): The Epidemiology of Chronic Rheumatism, vol 1, 1963. Courtesy of Blackwell Scientific.

Infectious Agents

Bacteria. Streptococcal infections were linked to rheumatoid arthritis in the 1920s, and recent studies have provided more than an epidemiologic association between these organisms and rheumatoid arthritis. The administration of cell wall fragments of group A streptococci to Sprague-Dawley rats induces a chronic peripheral polyarthritis not unlike rheumatoid arthritis. In associated studies, great interest has centered on the role of bacterial cell wall peptidoglycans in the pathogenesis of chronic inflammation. Rabbits hyperimmunized with streptococcal vaccine synthesize rheumatoid factors (7S) which can bind to group A peptidoglycan. Similar peptidoglycans are found in Freund's complete adjuvant, an emulsion of killed mycobacteria in oil; this material produces chronic arthritis after injection into rats. It is possible that, as in the experimental arthritis, arthritogenic cell wall components may be relatively indigestible and may persist within macrophages; in the genetically susceptible host they may activate an immune response.

Diphtheroid organisms and *Corynebacterium acnes* were once isolated from rheumatoid synovial tissues and fluid, but these studies have not been confirmed. *Erysipelothrix* organisms produce an arthritis in swine; the organism can be recovered during the acute onset of disease, but not after the synovitis becomes chronic. The reason for this may be that a component of the organism (e.g., peptidoglycans of cell wall or another molecular species) is all that persists to make the lesion chronic, or that the initial inflammation itself leads to chronicity.

Mycoplasma. An appreciation of the versatility of *Mycoplasma* species is just emerging in numerous sophisticated studies. In addition to being hard to detect in tissues, *Mycoplasma* have been shown to absorb host cell membrane antigens and/or immunoglobulins. This transfer of molecular species may be sufficient to render certain *Mycoplasma* in susceptible hosts resistant to immune clearance, yet arthritogenic. Absorption of host 7S gamma globulin by the *Mycoplasma* might alter the immunoglobulin sufficiently to make it immunogenic, resulting in production of rheumatoid factor. Although the experimental *Mycoplasma*-induced chronic synovitis in pigs has many similarities to rheumatoid arthritis, no data in humans have confirmed reports that *Mycoplasma* species could be isolated from synovial tissue and fluid from patients with rheumatoid arthritis.

Viruses. There are multiple ways in which a virus could serve as the initial antigenic challenge in rheumatoid arthritis yet remain virtually undetectable. Viruses can induce host cells to form a protective membrane for the viral core. Slow viruses can replicate within cells without killing them and can alter the composition of the host cell membrane; these hybrid membranes could be an effective stimulus for a host immune response. Viruses may, through infection of cells in synovium or other tissues, induce sufficient change in one or more connective tissue components to make them antigenic and arthritogenic.

Early reports that rheumatoid synovial cells could resist infection by viruses and therefore presumably were already infected by a virus capable of inducing interferon synthesis have not been confirmed. The possibility that viral antigens could be recovered from cyroprecipitates in serum or synovial fluid has a precedent in the recovery of hepatitis B virus from cyroprecipitates. Relatively large amounts of cryoprecipitate are found in serum of patients with Lyme arthritis (see the chapter on Lyme Arthritis in the section on Infectious Arthritis), which, for strong epidemiologic reasons, seems related to an as yet unproved viral infection. Attempts to devise sensitive assays to detect the presence in rheumatoid tissue of the enzyme reverse transcriptase (RNA-directed DNA polymerase) associated with latent C animal RNA tumor viruses have to date been unsuccessful.

Patients with rheumatoid arthritis frequently have a circulating antibody referred to as *rheumatoid arthritis precipitin* which reacts with a nuclear antigen present in B lymphoblast cells grown in tissue culture. This antigen is not rheumatoid factor. Peripheral blood lymphocytes can be induced to form this antigen after infection and transformation by Epstein-Barr virus.

Autoimmunity: An Immune Response Directed against Host Components

Rheumatoid factor—antibody to altered IgG. The puzzle of whether antibodies to host components have a causal relationship to a disease or whether they are simply another manifestation of it remains unsolved. This is particularly true for rheumatoid factor. Although many data support the observation that the presence of high-titer rheumatoid factor is associated with greater morbidity (joint erosions, extraarticular manifestations of rheumatoid arthritis, etc.) than is found in seronegative disease, it is known that many patients with a clinical diagnosis of rheumatoid arthritis have no detectable rheumatoid factor. Once formed, however, it is apparent that anti-IgG antibodies (e.g., rheumatoid factor) have a pathogenic potential, particularly when formed in an immune complex with IgG itself. The Fab region of rheumatoid factor recognizes altered antigenic sites in the Fc region of IgG. Thus a molecule of rheumatoid factor could link with another molecule of rheumatoid factor and these "self-associated" rheumatoid factor complexes may have the capacity to generate inflammation. If this sequence were proven to occur, then the chronicity of rheumatoid inflammation could be understood once it was known how the first anti-IgG was generated.

Connective tissue components—collagen and proteoglycans.   Antibodies to collagen and its denatured form (gelatin) are found more often in the serum and synovial fluid of rheumatoid than nonrheumatoid patients. The antibodies may be generated in response to immunologically altered collagen molecules created by inflammation in connective tissues. In experimental animals intraperitoneal injection of type II collagen (that found in articular cartilage) has the capacity to evoke chronic polyarthritis. Whether this occurs in man as cartilage (normally avascular and slowly metabolized) is infiltrated with new blood vessels and is destroyed by granulation tissue (perhaps releasing previously sequestered antigens into the circulation) is not known.

The emerging theories that bacterial cell wall peptidoglycans that are both arthritogenic and poorly degradable might serve as a chronic and persistent stimulus to arthritis in the properly prepared host (see above) complement older data and hypotheses suggesting that altered host proteoglycan molecules could initiate and sustain an immune response by the host. It was shown that short-chain glycopeptides from bacterial cell walls could (perhaps in response to stimuli ranging from a viral infection to trauma) be taken up by synovial cells or chondrocytes, incorporated into proteoglycans and/or hyaluronic acid by these cells, and released and included in the extracellular matrix. The altered matrix component might function as an immunogen; its location in the matrix would make it difficult to eradicate by phagocytic defense mechanisms. Antibodies to cartilage proteoglycan subunits have been found in both rheumatoid and in nonrheumatoid synovial fluids.

PATHOGENESIS AND PATHOLOGY

To explain rheumatoid arthritis fully, one must address the following question: Why does the inflammation initially occur in joints? Hypotheses are offered in lieu of proof. First, joints are moving parts. Experimentally induced arthritis in animals is more severe and more inflammatory in moving than in paralyzed limbs. Patients with paralysis from stroke who develop rheumatoid arthritis have more active erosive disease in the movable

extremities. Second, connective tissue matrices appear to attract and trap complexes that include IgG. In avascular tissue, such as articular cartilage, antigen–antibody complexes may be sequestered and serve as a chronic stimulus to the immune system as well as to activation of complement and other mechanisms which could lead to a proliferative (and potentially destructive) synovitis. Third, a factor inherent in the structure of joints may predispose them to synovitis. There is no epithelium lining the joint space; normal synovium is formed of mesenchymal cells loosely collected into a pseudolining which provides no substantial barrier between synovium and synovial fluid. A large network of capillaries provides access to cells for protein, low molecular weight biologically active substances, and solute from the circulation whenever an inflammatory stimulus is present. It may be that the very loose organization of the cells in normal synovium facilitates the enormous (100-fold or more) increase in cell number in rheumatoid synovium.

Early Synovitis: Inflammation and Cellular Proliferation

The earliest abnormality in rheumatoid arthritis is an increase in blood flow to the synovium. This leads to edema within the synovial lining. Increased permeability of vessels leads to increased accumulations of synovial fluid. Superficial synovial lining cells proliferate. Lymphocytes and monocytes from the circulation accumulate in the subsynovial areas around blood vessels (Fig. 1). Fibrin is precipitated on and within synovium. Polymorphonuclear leukocytes (PMN) are attracted by chemotaxis to the joint space, rarely remaining within synovial tissue itself.

Early in the rheumatoid process a dissociation of the acute inflammatory reaction (represented by the findings in synovial fluid) and the chronic inflammatory response (represented by the synovial proliferation) can be seen. The reactions in synovial fluid are characteristic of responses to antigen–antibody complex formation, whereas within the synovium the pathophysiology is what one would expect from lymphokine-mediated disease. The degree of inflammation manifested in synovial fluid can be gauged by the pain, redness, and swelling of the joints. The proliferative synovitis, however, can be silent and destroy joints without outward signs of inflammation. It is the interaction among the cellular elements of the synovium (synovial cells, endothelium, macrophages, lymphocytes, and plasma cells) and soluble mediators of inflammation that makes rheumatoid arthritis a complex as well as self-sustaining process.

One poorly understood characteristic of rheumatoid arthritis is its *polarization*. Why does rheumatoid synovium not invade in a centrifugal manner out through capsule and skin? Instead, the synovial pathology has a centripetal organization and destroys cartilage from the periphery to the center. The periphery (the subsynovial and capsular parts of the joint), in contrast, are characterized by proliferation, not destruction. The capsule becomes thickened and less pliable.

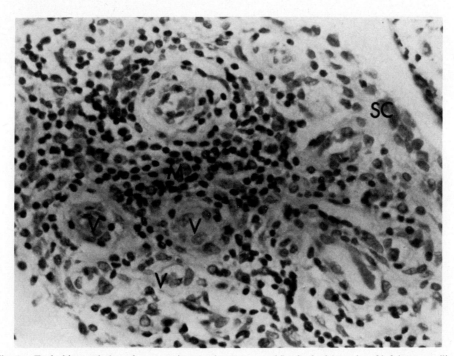

Fig. 1. Early histopathology from a patient (male, 41 years old) who had 2 weeks of left knee swelling and subsequently developed classic seropositive rheumatoid arthritis. The synovial cells (SC) have not proliferated greatly. There are many new small blood vessels (some are marked V), and mononuclear cells (M) have begun to appear in the extravascular space around the new capillaries. Later these may form small follicles beneath the synovial cells which may proliferate to many cell layers in depth.

The initial focus of polarization within the joint is at the junction between the synovium and perichondrial periosteum. Here connective tissue cells appear to be recruited by the vascular, highly cellular synovium and combine to form the cellular "pannus," which replaces both cartilage and bone by direct extension as does a localized malignancy.

In areas not at the invasion front, such as the supra-patellar inflection or pouch, the free synovium becomes grossly villous and arborized in appearance as it develops an enormous surface area. It takes on a characteristic tan color and is intricately laced with fine small blood vessels.

With progression and chronicity, bone mass near the joints is depleted, the cartilage is progressively eroded, ligaments and joint capsule are stretched by cellular and fluid proliferation within the joint, and the incongruity of damaged joint surfaces articulating with one another leads to progressive degenerative joint disease superimposed upon the inflammatory process.

Underlying the pathology sketched above are multiple pathologic mechanisms that have been described chemically and physiologically. Just as it may be inappropriate to search for a single cause of rheumatoid arthritis, it is inappropriate to attempt to arrange the known pathogenic mechanisms in a series, as if one led to the other. Instead, they will be discussed in parallel and interactions among them will be recognized.

Vascular proliferation. Essential to any tissue growth is the presence of new blood vessels. Inflammation attracts capillaries which branch off from thin-walled terminal arterioles in the subsynovial regions and leave via thin-walled venules. Factors involved in the genesis of new blood vessel formation are being searched for using many techniques. Culture medium from activated macrophages *in vitro* is capable of stimulating new vessel formation in experimental animals. Endothelial cells spearhead the invasion of new vessels. These cells are metabolically active and, by unknown mechanisms, form into a tubular structure as connective tissue is penetrated.

Endothelial cells, the primary cells in the establishment of new vasculature and inflammation, have secretory as well as structural functions. They have been shown to synthesize a precoagulant, clotting factor VIII, type III and IV α chains of collagen (for subendothelial connective tissue and basement membrane, respectively), elastin microfibrils, sulfated mucopolysaccharides, a reninlike enzyme capable of generating angiotensin from synthetic renin substrates, and both angiotensins I and II. Vessels mature, flow increases, the temperature within joints increases, a factor which may in turn increase the velocity of reactions involving joint destruction in the inflammatory process.

As inflammation and synovial blood flow increases, capillaries become permeable to molecules that they normally would retain within their lumen. Endothelial cells

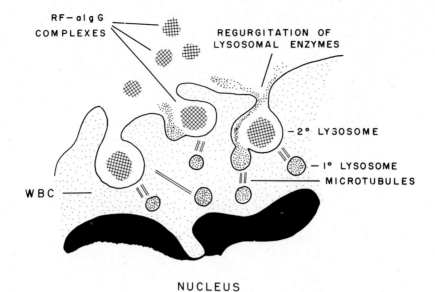

Fig. 2. Release of lysosomal enzymes through the mechanism "regurgitation during feeding." A PMN (WBC) has come into contact with rheumatoid factor—aggregated IgG-antiIgG complexes and has begun to phagocytose these immune complexes. Primary lysosomes (azurophil and specific granules) fuse with the secondary lysosomes and enzymes escape from the cell. (Courtesy of Dr. G. Weissmann.)

hypertrophy; small thrombi plug vessels and stasis develops. Erythrocytes extravasate between endothelial cells, and high molecular weight proteins as well as solute escape into the synovial fluid. Fibrinogen and enzymes of the clotting system appear extravascularly and, in response to many possible stimuli for activation of Hageman factor, the clotting cascade is activated. Fibrin covers the surface of synovium and cartilage, perhaps interfering with normal nutrition of the avascular cartilage. Within pools of edema in synovial villous fronds fibrin clots form, leading to a separation of vessels and subsynovial cells; the tips of the villi are infarcted. In severe cases these infarcted synovial fragments may break off, organize, and become "rice bodies"—egg shaped, homogeneous, and compacted aggregates of fibrin and dead cells. Paralleling terminal microvascular obstruction is a decrease in oxygen tension and pH in synovium and synovial fluid.

Cellular infiltrates in synovial fluid and tissues: functional morphology. Polymorphonuclear (PMN) leukocytes. In rheumatoid arthritis, effusions in joints are chronic; the pathology of the synovial membrane is one of chronic inflammation, yet the synovial fluid has an abundance of PMN leukocytes. These cells are drawn into the joint by multiple chemotactic factors. It is likely that the joint space is a trap for these cells and that during a 24-hour period most PMN leukocytes die, are lysed, and are replaced by cells influxing from the subsynovial vasculature. The half-life of granulocytes within synovial effusions is not more than 6 hours, which suggests that within a moderately inflammatory rheumatoid effusion the daily breakdown within the synovial cavity might exceed one billion cells. In active rheumatoid patients, chemotoxis for neutrophils as well as the phagocytic

capabilities of these cells are impaired, perhaps because the rheumatoid cells have been exposed to much debris and products of inflammation.

Lysosomal enzymes from PMN leukocytes are capable of degrading virtually all components of tissues (including nucleic acids, collagen, elastin, proteoglycans, vascular basement membranes, fats, and cell membranes). In addition to using normal connective tissue components as substrates, the contents of lysosomes are arthritogenic in and of themselves by either nonspecific irritating effects or more specific induction of inflammation. PMN leukocytes from the blood of rheumatoid patients may have greater total proteinase activity per cell than do cells from normal patients. Lysosomal enzymes have kinin-generating activity. A family of cationic proteins released with enzymes from lysosomes have antibacterial activity and produce vascular permeability and fever.

Death and lysis of the PMN leukocytes is not the only way that lysosomal enzymes can be released. Regurgitation during feeding and reverse endocytosis are additional mechanisms pertinent to rheumatoid arthritis (Fig. 2). The first is seen as lysosomal material is extruded from phagosomes during active phagocytosis by the cells. The second is initiated when the PMN leukocytes encounter immune complexes or other stimuli to phagocytosis adherent to or a part of nonphagocytosable surfaces such as collagen fibrils within cartilage matrix or basement membranes; this induces a prompt selective release of lysosomal enzymes directly outside the cell during this unsuccessful attempt at phagocytosis.

When large quantities of proteinases accumulate within joint fluid the normal inhibitory proteins that regulate proteinase activity extracellularly (α_2 macroglobulin,

α_1 proteinase inhibitor, and β_1 anticollagenase) may become saturated, and enzyme activity normally masked in synovial fluid may be demonstrated. This probably occurs at PMN leukocyte concentrations of over 50,000/ mm^3.

The PMN leukocyte has the capacity to generate superoxide ion radicals during phagocytosis. Unless promptly scavenged by regulatory substances such as superoxide dismutase, these free radicals can be toxic to cells as well as to components of the extracellular matrix.

Platelets. Platelets and PMN cells have the same phylogenetic ancestry and have similar functions as effectors of inflammation. The platelet's function is limited to vessels, however, unlike the PMN leukocyte which functions primarily in extracellular tissues. Platelets may be mobilized more quickly in inflammation than are the PMN cells. Similar to the PMN cells, the granules of platelets contain biologically active cationic proteins that increase vascular permeability and may generate chemotactic factor formation. Platelets accumulate in vessels adjacent to inflammation or tissue necrosis, and this may facilitate thrombosis and tissue infarction in synovial villi.

Macrophages. It has been demonstrated in experimentally produced arthritis in animals that blood monocytes migrate into synovium and reside there permanently as macrophages. No direct evidence for the origin of macrophagelike cells is available in rheumatoid arthritis but it is likely that the same sequence occurs. Unlike the short-lived PMN cells macrophages survive and function actively in tissues for long periods, although after activation they divide very infrequently.

Many factors serve to activate macrophages, transforming them into actively phagocytic and secretory cells. Activation factors include complex lipid compounds, endotoxins, products of activated lymphocytes, endotoxins, immune complexes, substances from PMN leukocytes and the C3b component of complement. Receptors for the Fc component of IgG (both monomeric and aggregated forms) and C3b-coated particles have been found on macrophage plasma membranes. The receptors endow macrophages with many functions within the rheumatoid synovial lining: (1) active phagocytosis of tissue debris, including effete white and red blood cells and iron granules; (2) trapping, transporting, and processing of antigens for lymphocytes; and (3) secretion of enzymes utilized in cartilage and bone destruction. Parenthetically, the same receptors of Fc components of IgG on macrophages make these cells specific targets in experimental systems for IgG-coated liposomes carrying drugs or enzymes.

Products produced by the macrophage for export from the cells include enzymes (lysozyme, plasminogen activator, elastase, collagenase), complement components (C2, C3, C4), leukocyte pyrogen, interferon, and a substance(s) that stimulates colony formation of PMN cells in vitro.

The function of the macrophage in the immune response is a significant one. Activation of T lymphocytes responding to thymus-dependent antigens requires that the antigen be processed and presented by macrophages which share with the T cell similar gene products of the MHC.

Experimental data suggest that multinucleate giant cells may originate from macrophages. Giant cells are often found in rheumatoid synovium and form spontaneously in cultures of rheumatoid synovial and synovial fluid cells. They divide infrequently and may have a greater capacity to produce and release proteinases than do mononuclear cells.

Synovial cells. There are three morphologic types of normal synovial cells to which certain functions have been ascribed. Type A cells are macrophagelike with abundant cell processes, intracellular vacuoles, and mitochondria. Type B cells are dominated intracellularly by endoplasmic reticulum; they have few filopodia and are thought to be involved in the synthesis of protein and/or glycoproteins for export from the cells. Type C cells (often present in large numbers) have morphologic features of both A and B cells (see the chapter on Synovial Membrane in the fascicle on Regional Structure and Function). Synovial cells are programmed to produce hyaluronic acid and glycoproteins involved in cartilage/ cartilage lubrication. These cell products join with the ultrafiltrate of plasma from subsynovial vessels to form synovial fluid.

Evidence is accumulating that demonstrates that high molecular weight hyaluronic acid found in normal noninflamed joints has suppressive effects on inflammation and the immune response. Rheumatoid synovial fibroblasts, isolated by outgrowth from primary explants, have characteristics different from normal synovial cells: they have higher rates of glycolysis, produce more lactate, have an increased doubling time, produce more hyaluronate which is less viscous than normal, and synthesize less collagen than do normal cells. In rheumatoid synovium an increase in the relative proportion of type B cells has been demonstrated; it is possible that the biochemical changes reported merely reflect a shift in function toward that of B cells as they normally function.

The cells in rheumatoid synovium removed at surgery can be dissociated from one another and cultured in vitro. About half the dissociated cells do not adhere to culture dishes; these represent lymphocytes and dead cells. The adherent cells are of different morphologic types. Some are flat spindle-shaped cells which appear as undifferentiated fibroblasts. Others are round with many inclusions and a ruffled border. A third type appears as a dendritic cell with many radially directed arborized extensions. The percentage of dendritic cells has a relationship to the amount of neutral proteinases (collagenase and plasminogen activator) produced by the adherent cells. Many of the dendritic cells and some macrophagelike cells contain more than one nucleus. Roughly half of the adherent cells are phagocytic early in culture. Many stain for membrane-associated collagen.

These nonimmunocytes of rheumatoid synovium appear to have multiple functions, all of which contribute to a proliferative inflammatory lesion. They apparently can synthesize collagen and hyaluronic acid, release large amounts of collagenase, neutral proteinases, cathepsins, and prostaglandins, and continue as active scavengers of cellular debris. They function while being continually exposed to soluble mediators of inflammation and mitogenesis.

Lymphocytes and the synovial immune response. Below the proliferating synovial lining cells and macrophages are infiltrates of lymphoid cells. The cells are arranged around the postcapillary venules through which they have migrated. Blast cells are found in the center of these clusters or follicles and may comprise up to 5 percent of the total lymphocyte population. More thymus-dependent (T) lymphocytes than thymus-independent (B) cells are present in rheumatoid synovial lymphocyte collections, although the presence of many plasma cells and the detection of rheumatoid factor synthesized by rheumatoid synovial lymphocytes attests to significant numbers of antibody-producing cells. The rate of immunoglobulin synthesis by rheumatoid synovial lymphocytes is similar to that of spleen or lymph nodes, but there is evidence that these plasma cells and their presursor B lymphocytes are committed to formation of antibody directed against different antigens than are cells within central lymphoid organs. It is possible that these local antigenic stimuli reside on altered IgG. The antigen-combining sites of the immunoglobulins match combining sites of the surface receptors of the B lymphocytes which produced the antibody. Because the number of types of chemical structure against which antibodies can be made is enormous, so must be the variability in B cell receptors.

The functional characteristics of T lymphocytes and studies of their receptor specificity are discussed in the section on Cellular Immunology in the fascicle on Immunology. T lymphocytes recognize antigens on cell surfaces and thus distinguish self from nonself on *live* cells. Antigens can be divided into two broad classes, thymus dependent or thymus independent. The latter stimulate B cells without helper T lymphocyte intervention; thymus-dependent antigens need help from T cells to stimulate B lymphocytes. The regulatory influence of T lymphocytes on the immune response is mediated by subclasses of these cells, *helper* and *suppressor* cells.

The fine regulation of T lymphocytes upon B lymphocyte differentiation and function is probably mediated through surface antigens coded for by the MHC. The functions of this regulation include determination of relative amounts of IgG and IgM antibody produced to a given antigen, and the affinity of that antibody for its antigen. Altered IgG, the immunogen which generates rheumatoid factor, is probably a thymus-dependent antigen.

All the cell types necessary for immunologic function described above—macrophages and T and B lymphocytes—are found within the deep synovial infiltrate of chronic inflammatory cells. The complex interactions among MHC gene products, thymus-dependent antigens, and the immunocytes are potentially different enough

from individual to individual to explain the presence of severe arthritis in one person, mild arthritis in another, and transient arthritis in a third, all of whom have had exposure to the same antigen.

Soluble mediators of inflammation. Soluble mediators of inflammation can effect changes within synovial tissue as well as within synovial fluid. There are multiple pathways through which one system of mediators can interact with another (Fig. 3).

Prostaglandins. Prostaglandins are a family of 20-carbon unsaturated fatty acids widely distributed in vertebrate tissues (see the chapter on Prostaglandins in the fascicle on Regional Structure and Function). A microsomal enzyme complex, prostaglandin synthetase, regulates production of these compounds. The finding that certain drugs (salicylates and indomethacin) inhibited prostaglandin synthesis was a major impetus in sorting out the role of prostaglandins in many biologic systems. Prostaglandin concentration in exudates parallels the intensity of the exudate. PGE_2 is produced in large quantities by rheumatoid synovial cells in culture. Production in vitro is inhibited by low concentrations of indomethacin and corticosteroids. PGE_2 and endoperoxide metabolites of metabolism are potent stimulators of bone resorption, and release of these compounds from chronic proliferative synovitis may be responsible for the justaarticular bone resorption seen in this disease. Rheumatoid synovial cells have been shown to become refractory to stimulation by prostaglandins: after exposure to prostaglandins and the expected rise in cAMP content and fall to normal, rechallenge by prostaglandins produces no increase in cAMP. It is possible that in the presence of chronically elevated prostaglandin concentrations (as in rheumatoid arthritis) the synovial cells may become refractory to prostaglandins, and that this refractory state may alter the cell growth cycle, membrane transport, and/or protein synthesis. Synovial cells fixed in a chronic refractory state by prostaglandins may be especially sensitive to lymphokines or other factors which could stimulate cell proliferation or proteinase production.

Kinin system. The end result of activation of the kinin system is bradykinin, a nanopeptide (NH_2 Arg–Pro–Pro–Gly–Phe–Ser–Pro–Phe–Arg OH) which can cause (1) slow concentration of blood vessels, (2) an increase in capillary permeability and arteriolar dilatation, and (3) pain when applied at certain nerve endings. The kinin system, complement, and the clotting system are the major endogeneous mediators of inflammation. Activation of kinins is a cascade and amplification system, initiated by activated Hageman factor. Activation of Hageman factor—probably the initial step for each of these systems—may be triggered by exposure to basement membrane collagen, endotoxins, plasmin, kallikrein, and perhaps to immune complexes in the presence of high molecular weight kininogen. Activated Hageman factor or Hageman factor fragments cleave prekallikrein to kallikrein. Prekallikrein is closely related, if not identical, to plasma plasminogen activator. Kallikrein, a serine proteinase, also is chemotactic for PMN cells. Kallikrein

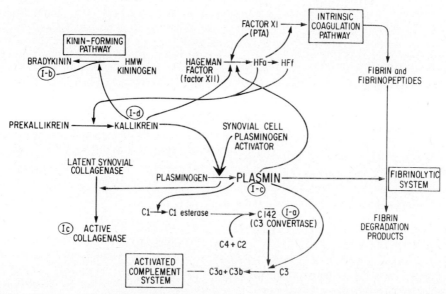

Fig. 3. Functional interrelationships of plasmin with the clotting, fibrolytic, kinin-forming, and complement systems. Abbreviations: HFa, activated Hageman Factor; HFf, activated Hageman factor fragment; PTA, plasma thromboplastin antecedent; C1, first component of complement. Inhibitors of components in this system include: I-a, C1 esterase inhibitor; I-b, kininase (C3a or C5a inactivator); I-c α_2 macroglobulin, α_1 trypsin inhibitor, tissue-specific inhibitors of neutral proteinases; I-d, kallikrein inhibitors. (Schema constructed with concepts of Dr. Kirk Wheupper, Dr. Allan Kaplan, and others.)

cleaves both a high (170,000) and/or a low (80,000) molecular weight kininogen, releasing bradykinin from the interior of the molecular. C1 inhibitor serves as a circulating regulator of this system, inhibiting Hageman factor and both kinin-generating and chemotactic functions of kallikrein. α_2 Macroglobulin inhibits kallikrein as well, but α_1 proteinase inhibitor (α_1 antitrypsin) does not. Bradykinin itself is inactivated by kininases which are carboxypeptidases.

Complement activation. Intact rheumatoid synovial tissue explants as well as macrophages have the capacity to synthesize complement components C2, C3, C4, and C5 and properdin factor B. Despite this, the concentrations of C4, C2, and C3 in rheumatoid synovial fluids are lower than in synovial fluids from patients with other joint diseases, indicating that significant complement consumption during aggregation with immune complexes takes place within the joint space.

There are two principal effects of complement activation in rheumatoid arthritis. One is production of a complex which binds to membranes of cells, targeting them for destruction; the other is production of multiple biologically active fragments. Initiating factors in complement activation can be the binding of C1q to the Fc portion of aggregated IgG or IgG–anti-IgG. C3 convertase activity has been demonstrated in rheumatoid synovial fluid, especially in patients with seropositive active disease and vasculitis. Plasmin and the activated C42 complex are probably the principal components of C3 convertase activity.

Biologically active components of complement activation are produced through the entire cascade. C3a, a small fragment released as C3 is cleaved, is an anaphylotoxin. C3b promotes immune adherence. C5a and other fragments produced by cleavage of C5 are the most active chemotactic factors produced during complement activation. Modulating these activities are multiple inhibitors in plasma and tissues: C3b inactivator, anaphylatoxin inactivator, and a serum component named chemotactic factor inactivator are particularly effective inhibitors of specific inflammogenic proteins.

Although the initial activating process of the alternative (properdin) system is unknown, it is clear that activated factor B of this system complexed with C3b and properdin acts as an effective C3 convertase. The role of the alternative pathway in rheumatoid arthritis has not been defined.

C-reactive protein. One factor not newly discovered but recently appreciated as being biologically active is C-reactive protein (CRP). This glycoprotein has five identical subunits with a molecular weight of about 120,000. It is opsonic, is synthesized by hepatocytes, and not uncommonly rises 1000-fold in concentration in response to tissue necrosis or inflammation. CRP has a striking amino acid homology with amyloid P component, but has no sequence homology with IgG or HLA antigens. The following functions have been demonstrated for CRP and some may be effective at concentrations achieved in vivo:

1. C1q binding
2. Activation of the alternative pathway of complement

3. Stimulation of macrophage phagocytic mechanisms
4. Suppression of T cell function in vitro
5. Binding with choline phosphatides—a mechanism for its binding to cells

Clotting and fibrinolytic system. Initiation of clot formation by activation of Hageman factor sets in motion a complex system involving platelets as well as plasma components. Once the firm clot is formed, processes begin to clear away fibrin which was deposited. Activation of plasmin provides such a mechanism. Plasminogen, the zymogen of plasmin, is present in high concentrations in inflammatory exudates and is cleaved to active plasmin by plasminogen activator(s). Rheumatoid synovial cells in culture release plasminogen activator, and circulating prekallikrein may be identical to plasma plasminogen activator. Active plasmin can digest fibrinogen and fibrin, activate Hageman factor, and activate collagenase from its latent forms generated by rheumatoid synovial cells and PMN. Despite plasmin activation, fibrin accumulation exceeds its removal within the rheumatoid joint. Its presence coating cartilage may interfere with chondrocyte metabolism; these cells are dependent upon a free flow (during compression and release of cartilage) of solute from synovial fluid. It is believed that excessive fibrin deposition within and on synovium leads to a hypoxic state and to conditions predisposing to tissue necrosis and establishment of potential sites for sequestration and growth of bacteria. Some evidence indicates that fibrin itself may act as an antigen that stimulates humoral and cell-mediated immune responses within joints.

Transfer factor. Transfer factor is a dialyzable, nonantigenic, nonimmunoglobulin composed of polynucleotides and/or polypeptides which may initiate cellular immunity by converting lymphocytes to an antigen-responsive state. This quality separates its presumed function from that of lymphokines, which can be considered effectors of cellular immunity produced by antigen-stimulated lymphocytes. Transfer factor exists as a basic constituent of lymphocytes and can be extracted after cellular disruption. When given to a recipient animal it appears to induce a new clone of antigen-responsive lymphocytes which, in the presence of appropriate antigen, express all the capacities of natively sensitized lymphocytes. The role of transfer factor, if any, in the pathogenesis of rheumatoid arthritis has not been defined. Its lack of antigenicity, combined with its capacity to make dormant clones of lymphocytes antigen-responsive, has led to early trials of transfer factor in the treatment of rheumatoid arthritis.

Lymphokines. As stated above, very little is known about the nature of receptors on T lymphocytes. In vitro systems do, however, enable us to characterize the lymphocyte mediators produced after the interaction of certain sensitized lymphocytes and antigen. In addition to the specific biologic activity demonstrated in various assay systems, it is likely that the most important role for these lymphocyte mediators (lymphokines) is one of am-

plification. A few sensitized lymphocytes may produce enough mediators to involve a large number of cells. For example, antigen may stimulate just a few T lymphocytes, and the T lymphocytes will produce a B cell mitogen.

In general, lymphokines are glycoproteins with molecular weights of less than 60,000 daltons. There are many types of lymphokine activity:

1. Lymphokines affecting inflammatory cells:
   a. factors affecting adhesion, motility, chemotaxis
   b. mitogenic factor
   c. factors amplifying response of cells to antigen
   d. macrophage activation factor
   e. lymphocytotoxins
2. Lymphokines causing cellular proliferation and excess production of gene products:
   a. mitogenic factor and cell growth inhibitor
   b. factors stimulating collagen and collagenase synthesis by fibroblasts and synovial cells
   c. angiogenesis factor
   d. osteoclast activation factor

The broad effects of lymphokines are illustrated by reports of multiple effects upon macrophage function. These soluble factors affect macrophage metabolism (increased glucose oxidation, protein synthesis, and glucosamine uptake), the cell surface (altered cell membrane composition and electrophoretic mobility), cell migration (inhibit macrophage migration and are chemotactic for macrophages), activation (stimulation of phagocytosis and secretion of proteinases), and cell-mediated cytotoxicity.

"Activation" peptides. Lymphocytes, platelets, and exudative leukocytes in culture produce similar but not chemically identical connective tissue activating peptides (CTAP). CTAP induce metabolic and growth changes in normal synovial cells in culture that are similar to those described in rheumatoid synovium: glucose utilization and lactate formation increase, synthesis of low molecular weight hyaluronic acid accelerates, and glycosaminoglycan synthesis and (with CTAP III from platelets) mitogenesis increase. CTAP may be an important component of the reparative response to chronic inflammation. This characteristic is manifested by increased connective tissue turnover and enzymatic remodeling of tissues. The similarities of CTAP to other stimulatory factors is striking and emphasizes the fact that many such mediators are produced by cells in response to inflammation, including nonsuppressible insulinlike activity from serum, somatomedin, fibroblast growth factor, and primate platelet factor. These factors as well as CTAP may be involved in the proliferative response which transforms a thin synovial membrane into a bulky, inflamed, highly vascularized, and locally destructive mass of cells.

Rheumatoid factor. Circulating antibodies with specificity for IgG immunoglobulins are a constant finding in the sera and synovial fluid of 70–80 percent of patients with a clinical diagnosis of rheumatoid arthritis.

These antibodies are of the 19S IgM class, but 7S IgM and IgG rheumatoid factors are found as well. IgM rheumatoid factor is produced by lymph nodes, by the spleen, and by immunocytes within rheumatoid synovium.

A number of lines of evidence do *not* support a primary role for rheumatoid factor in the pathogenesis of this disease. For example, rheumatoid factor is not found only in patients with rheumatoid arthritis (see the chapter on Biologic Functions and Clinical Significance of Rheumatoid Factors in the fascicle on Diagnostic Procedures). It is also of great interest that children with juvenile rheumatoid arthritis rarely have circulating rheumatoid factor even though the disease pathologically and clinically resembles adult rheumatoid arthritis. Similarly, a rheumatoidlike illness (but without significant joint destruction) often occurs in patients with agammaglobulinemia.

Nevertheless, the following observations support the hypothesis that rheumatoid factor is deeply involved in the pathogenesis of this disease.

1. IgG, IgM, rheumatoid factor, and complement are found in complexes in rheumatoid synovium and synovial fluid as well as in intracytoplasmic complexes within PMN leukocytes.

2. Polyclonal rheumatoid factors do fix and activate complement via the classic pathway.

3. Numbers of rheumatoid factor plaque-forming cells in the peripheral blood of seropositive patients correlate with disease activity as reflected by acute synovitis, the erythrocyte sedimentation rate, and the presence of extraarticular manifestations such as vasculitis.

4. Injection of autologous IgG into affected joints of rheumatoid patients produces an inflammatory response which has been attributed to complement activation, phagocytosis of immune complexes by PMN, and subsequent release of lysosomal enzymes.

5. Certain patients with seronegative arthritis (including some with juvenile rheumatoid arthritis) have rheumatoid factor masked by other proteins during in vitro tests; rheumatoid factor can be detected in IgM factions after serum has been passed through gel filtration columns.

6. Recently, self-associating rheumatoid factor has been observed in the sera of several patients with rheumatoid arthritis. Each IgG molecule serves as both antigen and antibody. Intermediate-sized complexes, ranging from dimers of IgG to large complexes (19S) have been isolated. If such self-association of rheumatoid factors were a general rather than an isolated phenomenon, immune complexes of IgG could form in the synovial fluid without the presence of another antigen.

How and why IgG becomes immunogenic has not been satisfactorily explained. The molecule must be altered in some fashion. Perhaps formation of an immune complex with certain antigens would be sufficient to make the IgG immunogenic. Structural or conformational alterations of IgG induced by viral infections or by nonspecific effects of inflammation could trigger antiglobulin formation, particularly if helper T cells were sensitized to such changes or if suppressor T lymphocytes were inadequate or deleted. Noninfectious, metabolic causes of altered IgG have been suggested (e.g., a diminished concentration in serum of endogenous sulfhydryl inhibitors that normally protect synovial fluid gamma globulin from denaturation by sulfhydryl–disulfide interchange).

Progression of Established Rheumatoid Synovitis: Destruction of Articular Tissue

Pathology of established rheumatoid synovitis. Once chronicity and proliferation have become established within the rheumatoid joint, the pathophysiology of the disease can be viewed from two aspects. One way is to consider the abnormal function of the synovium, which becomes thickened into many villous folds, and as a result, surface area is enormously increased. Blood vessels (capillaries, arterioles, and venules) are a major component of this tissue and the increased blood flow in perpheral joints (normally at temperatures in the range of 31°–34°C) may rise to intraarticular temperatures of 35°–38°C. Microhemorrhages, induced by trauma and/or inflammation, result in deposits of fibrin within and on the surface of synovium and "rice bodies" may develop as infarction of terminal villi occurs. Concurrent with the production of proteinases, their release along with lysosomal enzymes, and the synthesis of rheumatoid factor and lymphokines by the sublining plasma cells and lymphocytes, there is proliferation of extracellular connective tissue. Collagen deposition within the joint capsule and subsynovial tissue increases the bulk of the tissue and is associated with an increased blood flow. The increased cellularity and blood flow in the presence of inflammation results in a large amount of synovial fluid filling the low resistance reservoir of the joint space. Multiple chemotactic factors within the fluid lead to a massive influx of PMN, most of which do not escape but are degraded within the joint space. All these factors produce a significant change in the physiology of the rheumatoid joint.

Abnormal physiologic function in the rheumatoid joint. The following list summarizes the functional abnormalities induced in joint structures by the rheumatoid process before destruction begins:

1. Cartilage
   a. loss of ability to rebound from a deforming force
   b. decreased lubrication
2. Capsule and synovium
   a. increased blood flow and temperature
   b. decreased compliance
   c. alteration in synthetic capacity
   d. increased metabolic demands
3. Synovial fluid
   a. decreased oxygen tension and pH
   b. diminished lubricating capacity
   c. increased hydrolytic enzyme capacity
   d. increased intraarticular pressure

Early effects on cartilage are cause by depletion of normal proteoglycans from the matrix. The proteoglycans probably are replaced by water; the volume of cartilage does not change. Normally these polyanions, after release of compression of normal cartilage during weight bearing or muscle contraction, act as an electronegative spring, due to repulsion of like charges, to restore the cartilage to normal volume. Very early in the rheumatoid lesion, enzymes from PMN leukocytes, synovial cells, and possibly chondrocytes are responsible for proteoglycan depletion. Elastase (extracellularly) and cathepsin D (within phagolysosomes) are the principal enzymes effecting this destruction of proteoglycans. The cartilage may appear the same grossly, but it has lost the normal capacity to rebound from a deforming load. This interferes with chondrocyte function because normal chondrocyte nutrition is dependent on the dynamics of squeeze-film lubrication: the force of weight bearing squeezes out interstitial fluids in cartilage, and release of pressure results in fluid with higher pO_2, pH, and glucose being pulled into the matrix through a sponge effect. Lubrication of cartilage surfaces is accomplished through this squeeze-film phenomenon at high loads only. At lower loads a form of boundary lubrication by glycoproteins is operative. The chondrocyte and synovial cell may synthesize this lubricant component; it is likely that tissues in the rheumatoid joint synthesize less of this lubricating glycoprotein and that the lubricating fractions are susceptible to the multiple proteinases free in synovial fluid.

Hyaluronic acid contributes more to soft tissue lubrication (e.g., synovium on synovium) than to cartilage on cartilage lubrication. Inflamed joint fluid contains shortened hyaluronic acid chains with low viscosity. Loss of normal lubricant as well as the enormous bulk of articular structures in arthritis may contribute to subjective stiffness as the soft tissue folds move against each other and generate friction.

Some studies have reported increased sympathetic nervous tone within peripheral tissues of rheumatoid patients. Induced by inflammation, this effect might lead to localized pain as the many nerve endings in the joint capsule become ischemic.

Rheumatoid synovial tissue explants in vitro are known to metabolize glucose more rapidly than normal and to produce an excess of lactate. The increased metabolic rate of the synovial tissue is reflected in the abnormal respiratory gases and lactate in rheumatoid synovial fluid. Although the effective regional blood flow to joints is increased in rheumatoid arthritis, this increase is insufficient to meet the increased metabolic demands of the synovium. As a result, in the synovial fluid pH is depressed, pO_2 falls, and lactate increases—all roughly in proportion to each other and to the severity of joint disease as manifested by proliferation of synovial cells, focal necrosis, and focal obliterative microangiopathy.

Another aspect of altered synovial membrane physiology is the intraarticular pressure changes produced by the increased volume of synovial fluid. Although small joint effusions accumulate at almost no resistance, the thickened joint capsule is not elastic; after it becomes distended the intraarticular pressure increases greatly when the effective volume of the joint increases, such as when the patient performs a deep knee bend. This pressure (as high as 1000 mm Hg) may be sufficient to cause rupture of a joint.

Rheumatoid pannus.   A second aspect of the established rheumatoid process is the activity beginning at the synovial–osteochondral junction which progresses to pannus development and ends with destruction of cartilage and pseudorepair by ankylosing fibrosis.

The reasons for this centripetal polarization of the obliterative process are not known but they may be related to sequestration of antibody–antigen complexes within collagenous and relatively cellular cartilage interstices. Studies of early lesions have indicated that in addition to synovial cells there is a recruitment of periosteal and perichondrial fibroblasts, which proliferate and replace cartilage. Chondrocytes that are near the advancing edge of pannus replicate within their lacunae (Fig. 4); these may be activated to produce enzymes capable of degrading both collagen and proteoglycans. In general, early destruction of subchondral bone is greater than that of the cartilage itself, which may lead to cartilage lipping. Erosion of bone may be facilitated by both soluble mediators (e.g., prostaglandins) released by synovium and periosteocytic resorption of mineral. The adjacent sites of periosteal demineralization are then invaded by the rheumatoid pannus. Collapse after such resorption of bony support systems produces fragments of cartilage which either are engulfed and included within the invasive synovial tissue or float free in synovial fluid, where they die and become mineralized or degraded or else remain viable and actually grow in size by obtaining nutrition from synovial fluid.

Although cellular replacement of cartilage begins at the periphery of joints, surface damage is seen as well, probably caused by hydrolytic enzymes from PMN cells in the joint fluid. Precipitation of fibrin intertwined with cellular debris on the surface of the cartilage may smother it by preventing normal flux of synovial fluid solutes in and out.

The junction of the cartilage and pannus is the focus of degradative activity within the rheumatoid joint. Immunofluorescent studies have revealed deposits of collagenase and cathepsin D at this junction but not elsewhere. Different patterns are observed depending on the virulence of resorption at the particular tissue in each patient. Election microscopic studies have shown that in very invasive disease the first line of pannus cells (which appear either as macrophages or fibroblasts) penetrate deep within the cartilage matrix with fine cellular processes (Fig. 5); occasionally cartilage collagen fragments are seen within phagolysosomes of the cells at the invasive front. In less aggressive disease, an amorphous zone several micrometers in width may separate cartilage from pannus cells; it appears that here there is progressive destruction of cartilage extracellularly by enzymes released from the cells. Inactive lesions are characterized principally by hypovascular and relatively acellular fibrosis at this invasion front. Occasionally areas are de-

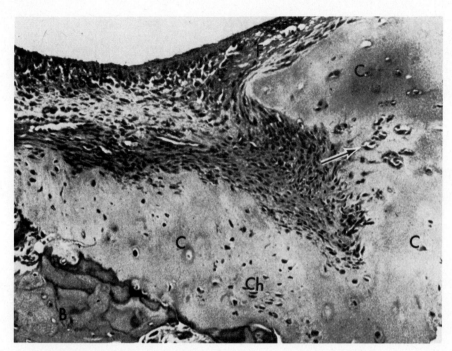

Fig. 4. Early destruction by invasive synovial cells at joint margin. The synovial cells are most actively progressing with fingerlike extensions into the cartilage (C) in the direction of the arrow. Chondrocytes (Ch) in proximity to invasive pannus often replicate within enlarged lacunae. Erosion at the left of bone (B) is seen also. A thin layer of amorphous material, probably fibrin (F), overlies the synovial cells (SC). (Courtesy of Dr. Kingsley Mills.)

scribed where the invasive tissue is composed almost entirely of small new blood vessels with perivascular clusters of mononuclear cells.

Deep in the invasive layers there is exuberant scar formation. Thick and thin bands of collagen with moderate numbers of new blood vessels and relatively little inflammation produce thickened joint capsules. The cap-

sule contains relatively little elastin and its rigidity contributes to joint stiffness.

Synovial proliferation occurs within tendon sheaths as well as within joints. These tendons are at a high risk of spontaneous rupture by hydrolytic enzymes and ragged bony prominences created by the same processes.

The loss of normal congruity of joints produces al-

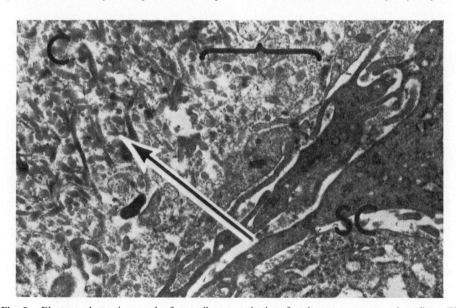

Fig. 5. Electron photomicrograph of a small area at the interface between pannus and cartilage. The erosive process is moving in the direction of the arrow. Thin cell processes of a synovial cell (SC) run parallel to the invasion.

tered mechanical stress very early. Whether cartilage is depleted of its normal proteoglycans by enzymes from chondrocytes (as proposed for degenerative arthritis) or by hydrolytic enzymes from inflammatory cells and a proliferative synovium (as in rheumatoid arthritis), the degenerative process begins. Small trauma is magnified by articular incongruity. Motion exaggerates the inflammatory response. Muscle contraction, tendon slippage due to stretching or erosion of tendon sheaths and ligaments, or other joint constraints produce abnormal stress, subluxation, and inefficient, sometimes painful function.

It is the combination of aggressive rheumatoid synovitis and physical acitivity that leads to the production of subchondral pseudocysts: invagination of pannus through cartilage and subchondral bone produces a pear-shaped accumulation of granulation tissue. Scarring of the superficial pannus tends to "wall off" the subchondral pseudocyst.

Pathology of Extraarticular Manifestations of Rheumatoid Arthritis

A common factor in the genesis of extraarticular manifestations of rheumatoid arthritis is an increased reactivity of mesenchymal tissue. This is exemplified particularly by the rheumatoid nodule. Vasculitis underlies the pathologic sequence. Beginning as a small focus of proliferating cells surrounding inflammatory changes in small arteries, this lesion expands centrifugally. Concentric scarring and perivascular cuffing by lymphocytes surrounds a very cellular medial portion with radial orientation of cells and connective tissue bundles. Within the center, necrosis is found. The necrotic material is composed of immature collagen fibrils, filamentous material (probably fibrin), cells, and cellular debris. Necrosis may develop because the center of the original lesion becomes insufficiently vascularized as the lesion expands and the activated histiocytes in radial orientation produce proteinases and collagenase sufficient to degrade the supporting scaffold of connective tissue on which they rest. Continuing obliterative terminal arteriolitis contributes to the progression of the necrosis as well. The occurrence of nodules on body parts exposed to pressure (including the occiput in bedridden patients) accentuates the excess cellular reactivity that rheumatoid patients manifest. In other organs (e.g., the pericardium or the eye) the reactive inflammation may not be manifest as a classic nodule, but in the lung it may.

REFERENCES

Castor CW, Lewis RB: Connective tissue activation. Scand J Rheumatol 5:41, 1975

Cooke TD, Hurd ER, Ziff M, Jasin HE: The pathogenesis of chronic inflammation in experimental antigen-induced arthritis. J Exp Med 135:323, 1972

Dayer J-M, Krane SM, Graham R, Russell G, Robinson DR: Production of collagenase and prostaglandins by isolated adherent rheumatoid synovial cells. Proc Nat Acad Sci USA 73:945, 1976

Falchuk MD, Goetzl EJ, Kulka JP: Respiratory gases of synovial fluids. Am J Med 49:223, 1970

Fries JF, Mitchell DM: Joint pain of arthritis. JAMA 235:199, 1976

Hadler NM: A pathogentic model for erosive synovitis: Lessons from animal arthritides. Arthritis Rheum 18:256, 1976

Hamerman D: New thoughts on the pathogenesis of rheumatoid arthritis. Am J Med 40:1, 1966

Haselwood DM, Castles JJ: The biology of the rheumatoid synovial cell. West J Med 127:204, 1977

Harris ED Jr. (ed): Rheumatoid Arthritis, New York, Medcom Press, 1974

Hollander JL, Fudenberg HH, Rawson AJ, Abelson NM, Torralba TP: Further studies on the pathogenesis of rheumatoid joint inflammation. Arthritis Rheum 9:675, 1966

Hollingsworth JW, Siegel ER, Creasey WA: Granulocyte survival in synovial exudate of patients with rheumatoid arthritis and other inflammatory joint diseases. Yale J Biol Med 39:289, 1967

Johnson PM, Faulk WP: Rheumatoid factor: Its nature, specificity, and production in rheumatoid arthritis. Clin Immunol Immunopathol 6:414, 1976

Paul WE, Benacerraf B: Functional specificity of thymus-dependent lymphocytes. Science 195:1293, 1977

Pelus LM, Strausser HR: Minireview—Prostaglandins and the immune response. Life Sci 20:903, 1977

Ryan GB, Majno G: Inflammation. Kalamazoo, Mich, Upjohn, 1977

Werb Z, Mainardi CL, Vater CA, Harris ED Jr: Endogenous activation of latent collagenase by rheumatoid synovial cells. N Engl J Med 296:1017, 1977

Ziff M: Relation of cellular infiltration of rheumatoid synovial membrane to its immune response. Arthritis Rheum 17:313, 1974

CLINICAL PRESENTATION AND COURSE OF RHEUMATOID ARTHRITIS

James L. McGuire and Edward D. Harris, Jr.

Patients with rheumatoid arthritis may first present themselves to physicians at any stage of disease. They may be crippled, with joints already destroyed and with extraarticular manifestations of rheumatoid vasculitis. Some may have proliferative synovitis which has not yet led to joint destruction and may shown few signs of extraarticular disease. Still others may present early with synovitis and with insufficient criteria to make a diagnosis. What ever the stage of the process, the keystone of successful management of patients with rheumatoid arthritis is an adequate understanding of the pathogenisis of the disease, the clinical patterns in which it presents, and the course of established disease manifested in the joints as well as in extraarticular sites.

EARLY DISEASE
Common Patterns of Onset

The usual mode of onset of rheumatoid arthritis is insidious. First symptoms may be nonarticular and may be manifested by fatigue, diffuse aching, or bursitis. Joint symptoms involving the hands, ankles, shoulders, feet, or neck are usually morning stiffness, weakness, or pain. Rheumatoid arthritis beginning in the knees is frequently painless; the chief symptom is stiffness related to synovial effusions. Disease in the elbow may be completely asymptomatic and may be discovered as a painless loss of full extension on examination. Symmetry of joint involvement is found frequently, and this criterion applies to certain joints within one group (e.g., proximal interphalangeal or metacarpophalangeal joints) as well as to those groups themselves. It is these patients with symmetric, progressive, insidious onset of pain and swelling in many joints that most easily fulfill diagnostic criteria (see Table 1 in preceding chapter).

Approximately 80 percent of patients eventually have rheumatoid factor in serum, but it may take months to appear and does so coincident with findings of justaarticular osteopenia on roentgenograms and development of subcutaneous nodules.

Unusual Patterns of Onset

Acute onset of symmetric polyarthritis. These patients may be acutely ill and may be completely immobilized with aggressive inflammatory synovitis in many joints. High fever, malaise, and exquisitely painful joints necessitate exclusion of sepsis as a cause of disease. The acute form of presentation, however, has no special prognostic connotations. Some patients may respond to antiinflammatory drugs rapidly, improve rapidly, and stay in a prolonged remission; others, in contrast, may progress to chronic progressive and destructive synovitis with a course similar to that occurring with insidious onset of disease.

Presentations similar to juvenile rheumatoid arthritis. A symptom complex similar to Still's disease is seen occasionally, particularly in young men. Initial symptoms are fever of unknown origin with or without evanescent maculopapular skin eruptions, lymphadenopathy, or splenomegaly. Prognosis is generally good, and after 1 year 50 percent of patients are likely to be well while the remainder may have some degree of recurrent disease controlled by a conservative drug regime.

Seronegative polyarthritis. These patients, usually less than 45 years of age, have a presentation indistinguishable from those who have rheumatoid factor present in the serum. HLA-B27 is common in this group (25 percent), and in a subset of young males with an associated sacroiliitis the diagnosis of HLA-B27–associated spondyloarthropathy becomes more appropriate.

Palindromic rheumatism. This is a puzzling syndrome. These patients have irregular, 3–5-day attacks of acute pain and swelling of joints (particularly knees and wrists) which subside completely. A certain percentage, probably less than 25 percent, develop persistent synovitis which evolves gradually into a pattern consistent with rheumatoid arthritis.

Age-associated modes of onset. Young women in the late teens or early twenties may present with bilateral knee effusions and stiffness without any other signs of disease. Symptoms and signs are directly related to use: exercise exacerbates symptoms; rest alleviates them. The long-term prognosis generally is good. One group of elderly patients presents with diffuse shoulder pain, and these patients are often considered to have polymyalgia rheumatica. Another older group, particularly males, presents with hand and wrist disease marked by extraordinary diffuse swelling of the entire hand and stiffness to the point of rigidity. All of these symptoms can evolve into definite or classic rheumatoid arthritis.

Factors Affecting the Course and Progression of Disease

Most patients with rheumatoid arthritis receive treatment, so that it is difficult to talk of the "natural history" of the disease. However, the degree of chronicity of persistent active synovitis is perhaps the most important determinant of the rapidity and extent of joint destruction. Patients with remissions—either spontaneous or induced by therapy—invariably do better than those with continuous active disease. Patients with intermittent inflammation in joints seem to have fewer stimuli for the development of synovial proliferation. These patients are unlikely to develop erosive disease and joint destruction. Those with chronic proliferative disease will very likely have progression of both symptoms and signs; the degree of progression will depend on the virulence of the process at the cartilage–bone–pannus junction.

Many associated circumstances in patients with rheumatoid arthritis may alter the course of disease. A few factors are associated with remission of disease. One is pregnancy, although arthritis may flare to its original severity or worse after parturition. A second is a marked change in life style which produces an effective decrease in stress on the mind and joints. A third, usually an unwelcome event, is paralysis; a paretic limb invariably has less inflammation and proliferative synovitis. In contrast, a patient with the tremor of Parkinson's disease is given no rest from motion and articular destruction may be rapid. The obese patient submits each weight-bearing joint to excessive stress and the mechanical contribution to joint destruction is accentuated in these patients. In diabetes, abnormal carbohydrate metabolism may interfere with proteoglycan metabolism in connective tissue and inadequate or altered matrix components may develop, leading to excessively rapid joint destruction. One subgroup of patients has a predilection to develop tendon/muscle contractures early in disease. This interferes with function as well as with physical therapy to improve joint function. Patients with positive tests for rheumatoid factor are likely to have more joint erosions and more extraarticular manifestations of disease. Eosinophilia, persistently high erythrocyte sedimentation rate, and rheumatoid factors in high concentration are associated with erosive disease.

Although a sudden flare of symptoms in one joint may reflect increased activity of the synovitis, the possibility of superimposed sepsis upon the rheumatoid process is a real one. Aspiration of acutely flaming joints is essential to rule out infection.

ARTICULAR MANIFESTATIONS OF ESTABLISHED DISEASE

In the preceding chapter the manner in which rheumatoid synovitis affects joints in general was outlined. The patterns of progression of arthritis in specific joints,

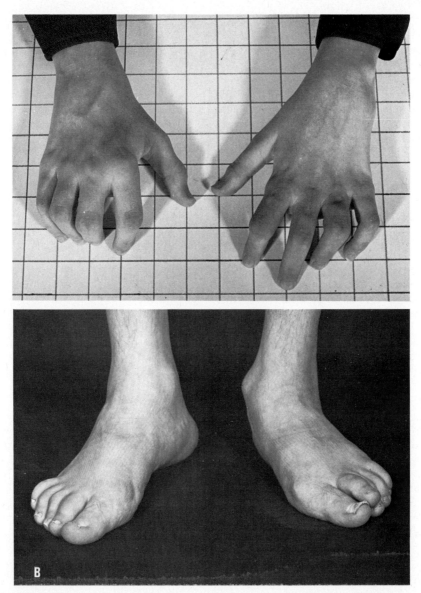

Fig. 1.   Hands and feet of a young man with rheumatoid arthritis. **A.** The hands are shown in a position of maximal finger extension. These flexion contractures resulted both from destruction of cartilage and bone at the PIP and loss of gliding function within flexor tendon sheaths from fibrosis secondary to chronic inflammation. **B.** The toes are relatively spared. There is a moderate hallux valgus on the left, however dorsal subluxation of the phalanges on the metatarsals is only slight. Progressive synovitis of the left ankle has resulted in an eversion deformity and loss of the plantar arch. In this patient, the same deformity was avoided on the right by spontaneous functional fusion of the tibiotarsal joint.

however, are programmed by both the structure and function of those joints.

Hand

Distal interphalangeal joints (DIP) are rarely affected in rheumatoid arthritis. This fact is helpful in diagnosis, but the reasons for it are unknown, other than the fact that there is little synovium to be affected in those joints.

Proximal interphalangeal joint (PIP) disease is associated with tense soft tissue swelling unlike the bony enlargement of erosive osteoarthritis. Chronic extension of the joint leads to stretching of joint capsule and liga-

ments. The relationship of flexor and extensor tendons to the joint is distorted. Altered forces across the PIP, in combination with contraction of inflamed intrinsic muscles of the hands and elongation of tendons, leads to "boutonniere" (DIP extension and PIP flexion) and "swan neck" (DIP flexion and PIP hyperextension) deformities (Fig. 1A).

The second and third metacarpophalangeal joints (MCP) are often the earliest MCP to be diseased. Effusions here are often large enough to aspirate. The pattern of joint deformity in the MCP is classically one of progressive volar and ulnar subluxation. Theories abound to explain the dynamics of this deformity, but they all have tendon–joint incongruity as a common denominator. It is likely that with progressive disease the metacarpal head becomes eroded so that it no longer effectively supports the base of the proximal phalanx. Similarly, the accessory collateral ligaments and the membranous portion of the volar plate become stretched and destroyed by direct extension of the invasive synovium. Flexor tendons, which tend to "bowstring" at the MCP during grip and pinch, further stretch the suspensory ligaments; as a result, during grip stress is applied not to the metacarpal head, but to the proximal phalanx. Contractures of interosseous muscles may lead to volar subluxation with permanent flexion contracture of the proximal phalanx. Finally, destruction of the wrist compartments producing radial rotation may produce a "zig-zag" phenomenon by resulting in exertion of a greater ulnar–volar force upon the long flexor tendons than is usual.

Wrist

In the wrist, tenosynovitis in the extensor carpi ulnaris sheath manifests itself early as an asymptomatic swelling over the ulnar styloid. Low-grade but chronic disease stretches the ligaments restraining the ulnar styloid and it may become lax and sublux dorsally. Later in the disease synovial proliferation can lead to firm cystlike structures surrounding the long tendons on the dorsum of the wrist. Spontaneous rupture of extensor tendons may occur. Carpal arthritis is usually quite painful and causes marked limitation of motion on flexion and extension of the wrist. Chronic rheumatoid synovitis affects all compartments of the wrist joint, destroying cartilage and bone, which leads to ulnar drift, ligamentous stretching, and volar subluxation. The carpal tunnel syndrome— e.g., median nerve compression with pain in the hand and forearm (particularly at night), tingling in the thumb, second, and third fingers, and alterations in normal pain sensation and regulation of sweating and temperature— in one or both hands may be a presenting symptom of rheumatoid arthritis. If unrecognized and untreated, this can progress to permanent weakness of intrinsic muscles of the hand. It is caused by swelling of synovial tissue within the volar tendon compartments of the wrist; pressure around the median produces a delay in nerve conduction. Definitive diagnosis can be made by nerve conduction studies.

Shoulder

Arthritis involving the shoulder, especially the glenohumeral joint and the acromioclavicular joint, is common in rheumatoid arthritis. The arthritis is usually bilateral and must be distinguished from other common problems such as peritendonitis, bursitis, and rotator cuff injuries. Joint effusions are best palpated anteriorly, with the arm in a position of external rotation.

Head and Neck

Cricoarytenoid arthritis can present as hoarseness, dyspnea, dysphagia, or even aspiration during swallowing. Rarely, stridor develops. Involvement here is more common than is generally appreciated. The temporomandibular joint can be affected in rheumatoid arthritis, which usually causes pain, swelling, and difficulty with mastication, all of which are more symptomatic in the morning. The clavicle may be involved at either of its ends. Distal erosions leading to a "sharpened-pencil" deformity at the acromioclavicular joint develop in severe disease. Proximally, the sternoclavicular joint may be swollen and tender. Cervical spine disease causes pain on rotation and flexion of the neck. Multiple foci of proliferative granulomatous synovitis lead to shortening and ankylosis. Narrowed intervertebral disc spaces and osteopenia are seen together in the cervical spine in rheumatoid arthritis but in few other conditions.

At the atlantooccipital joint, erosion and attenuation of the ligament holding the odontoid process against the transverse process of C_1 leads to posterior subluxation of the odontoid during flexion of the neck. This can result in symptomatic spinal cord compression with occipital pain or shooting pains in the arms. Vertical subluxation of C_2 occurs as well. Roentgenograms are diagnostic of subluxation if there is more than 3 mm between the odontoid and the arch of C_1 with the patient's head held in flexion and if more than 4.5 mm of the odontoid projects above a line drawn from the posterior hard palate to the anterior occiput.

Hip

The hip is frequently involved early. One of the first signs of disease may be a loss of full hip rotation in extension. Decreased flexion and/or flexion contracture may not evolve until later. Severe, progressive inflammatory disease may lead to adductor and abductor contractures which prevent the patient from carrying out normal bladder, bowel, and sexual function. Degenerative changes are shown in Figure 2.

Lower Extremity

The knees, ankles, and small joints of the feet are usually involved in a symmetric fashion. In the knee, synovial proliferation is more profuse than in any other joint. Involvement in the suprapatellar pouch leads to bulky swelling and accumulations of large volumes of synovial fluid. Meniscal cartilages may be destroyed, and loss of the cruciate ligaments to the proliferative pannus leads to instability in an anteroposterior direction. Preexisting deformity (genu varus or valgus) becomes accentuated as preferential destruction of the femoral–condyle and tibial plateau develop on the side bearing the greatest stress.

The eponym *Baker's cyst* is given to synovial outpouching in the popliteal fossa. With synovial tissue acting as a ball valve, fluid may be forced into the posterior pouch without means for decompression. A popliteal cyst may retard venous and lymphatic flow. The appearance of signs of thrombophlebitis in a rheumatoid patient may, in fact, be caused by a large popliteal cyst. With sudden rises in pressure within the knee, the cyst may herniate along muscle planes in the calf or even rupture into the calf. An ecchymotic area around the lateral malleolus called the "crescent sign" may be seen shortly after rupture. Diagnosis of rupture can be confirmed by arthro-

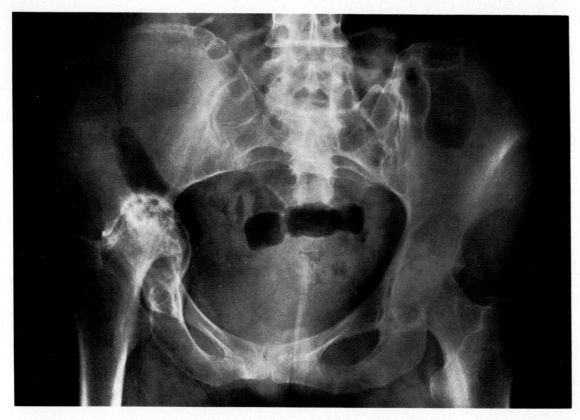

Fig. 2. Pelvic x-rays of a patient with severe rheumatoid arthritis. Both hips are involved, the right more than the left. Sacroiliac joints are normal. The right femoral head shows remodeling and flattening. Loss of the apparent joint space signifies loss of articular cartilage. At this point secondary degenerative changes have developed, producing sclerosis and cysts on both sides of the joint. The acetabulum has responded by remodeling away from pressure; the result is protrusion of the acetabulum into the pelvic cavity. The left hip is less destroyed but the osteopenia around the joint, irregular femoral head, loss of joint space and subchondral cystic areas suggest that degenerative changes may develop soon. (Courtesy of Dr. Gary S. Hoffman.)

gram, which will reveal extravasation of the dye from the joint. Intact popliteal cysts can be outlined by ultrasound examination.

Nonspecific mild ankle edema is an early manifestation of rheumatoid arthritis and may make minimal swelling of the ankle joint itself difficult to detect. Longstanding ankle arthritis results in limitation of dorsiflexion and plantar flexion; subtalar arthritis limits inversion and eversion of the ankle, making walking on uneven ground very painful. It is common for rheumatoid patients with foot and ankle involvement to develop progressive eversion and valgus deformities (Fig. 1B). Painful synovitis of metatarsophalangeal joints leads to pain during stepping off in a normal gait, which leads to early plantar subluxation of these joints. The metatarsal heads may be palpated on the ball of the foot as phalanges sublux vertically; callous formation and collections of submetatarsal bursal fluid are common. The "cocked-up toe" deformity may be found on examination before the patient complains of foot symptoms. A pre-Achilles tendon bursitis or subcutaneous nodules along the tendon often present as heel pain.

Rheumatoid Nodules

Subcutaneous nodules develop in multiple areas with a special propensity for skin over pressure points, including extensor surfaces of the ulna, the ischial tuberosities, the Achilles tendons, and the occiput. Gliding function with tendon sheaths can serve as a stimulus to nodule formation. In active disease, small nodules can be palpated within the palm and flexor tendon sheaths over proximal and middle phalanges. Occasionally they cause painful impairment of finger motion. It is extremely unusual for the rheumatoid nodules to develop without both arthritis and a positive test for rheumatoid factor in blood. Tophi and xanthomas can mimic nodules on clinical examination, but only granuloma annulare has both clinical and histologic similarities to the rheumatoid nodule.

EXTRAARTICULAR
MANIFESTATIONS

Abnormalities in rheumatoid arthritis in systems other than joints and muscles can be classified by their chronologic appearance. Early extraarticular manifestations are important for diagnosis and prognosis, while the late complications of rheumatoid disease may be life-threatening.

Anemia and Thrombocytosis

Anemia in rheumatoid arthritis is mild: the hemoglobin is 10–11 g/dl with normochromic, normocytic indices. As in other forms of anemia of chronic disease, there is a functional failure of iron utilization by the precursors of erythrocytes in the bone marrow. The result is hypoproliferative anemia. The presence of a microcytic hypochromic anemia and hemoglobin of 8–9 g/dl should prompt a thorough review of the antiinflammatory agents being used and a search for a bleeding source in the gastrointestinal tract. Hemolysis is not a component of the anemia of rheumatoid arthritis. The platelet count rarely increases to levels which would produce increased thrombotic complications of disease.

Felty's Syndrome

Felty's syndrome is defined as neutropenia and splenomegaly in a patient with rheumatoid arthritis. Platelets may be decreased and anemia is usually present. Infection (pneumonia, cellulitis, or urinary tract infections) can herald the appearance of the syndrome. Physical examination usually reveals mild to moderate splenomegaly, advanced deforming arthritis, and subcutaneous nodules. Neutrophil counts of less than 500/mm^3 can be found. The etiology of the neutropenia may reflect several interacting problems. Increased margination of the white blood cells accounts for part of the neutropenia. Antibodies directed against both the nuclei and the cell membrane of PMN have been described. The enlarged spleen may trap cells within sinusoids, accounting for thrombocytopenia and part of the anemia. Antibodies to the neutrophil have been found in cryoprecipitates in serum.

Sjögren's Syndrome

Sjögren's syndrome may be present, by strict criteria (see the section on Sjögren's Syndrome), in as many as 50 percent of patients with classic or definite rheumatoid arthritis. It is generally believed to represent a late extraarticular manifestation, particularly in women with high titers of rheumatoid factor, although symptoms of eye irritation and dry mouth may present early in the disease.

Rheumatoid Vasculitis

Vasculitis is almost always associated with severe disease. It is postulated that deposition of immune complexes within blood vessels precipitates the clinical events. In some cases, IgG, IgM, and components of complement have been demonstrated by immunofluorescent studies within vessel walls. Clinical manifestations are a function of the size of the vessels involved. One form involves small arterioles; histologic sections reveal obliterative vasculitis with intimal proliferation and occasionally fibrinoid necrosis of vessel walls. Polyarteritis classically affects larger caliber vessels than does the vasculitis of rheumatoid arthritis.

The potential sites of involvement of rheumatoid vasculitis are many. Males with rheumatoid factor are most likely to have this form. Skin ulcers with necrotic centers and heaped-up proliferative edges resemble pyoderma gangrenosum and occur on the lower legs. Involvement of the vasa vasorum supplying large peripheral nerves produces a mononeuritis multiplex as all functions of one peripheral nerve are impaired. Distal functions disappear first; the result is foot drop or paresthesias in the hands. Rare patients with rheumatoid vasculitis develop necrotizing involvement of medium size vessels of the central nervous system. At the other end of the spectrum is a mild peripheral sensory neuropathy with fluctuating symptoms and an inadequately studied pathologic basis. Vasculitis resembling polyarteritis may strike the gastrointestinal tract, causing bowel dysfunction and/or hemorrhage. The linkage of vasculitis to corticosteroid therapy is tenuous, but it must be appreciated that any abrupt change in the milieu surrounding a rheumatoid patient—whether it be personal emotional trauma, withdrawal of suppressive treatment, or intercurrent illness—may precipitate a flare of arthritis and/or vasculitis.

When comparing organ systems involved in rheumatoid vasculitis with those of another connective tissue disease, systemic lupus erythematosus (SLE), it is striking that there are organ systems affected by the deposition of immune complexes in SLE that are not affected by immune complexes of rheumatoid factor and IgG in rheumatoid arthritis. In particular, glomerulonephritis is rare in rheumatoid arthritis.

Rare patients may develop digital obliterative endarteritis. This proliferative arterial lesion, not dissimilar to the pathology of Raynaud's disease, may present with fingertip ulceration and nail abnormalities. Progression to frank necrosis and gangrene is rare.

A small vessel vasculitis with the pathology of leukocytoclastic angiitis has been described in patients with rheumatoid arthritis. This is "palpable purpura." It presents with crops of erythematous macules and urticarial papules which may evolve to a palpable purpuric rash, particularly on dependent parts such as the legs. When biopsied, all lesions seem to be at the same stage of development. Cryoglobulinemia has been associated with the clinical findings and histopathology of leukocytoclastic vasculitis and should be looked for in all rheumatoid arthritics who develop this small vessel vasculitis.

Pulmonary Complications

The underlying pulmonary disease in rheumatoid arthritis is a vasculitis; however, the various syndromes of pulmonary complications have been described thoroughly enough to warrant consideration of them as organ-specific complications.

Pleurisy with effusion is the most common rheumatoid manifestation in the lung. More common in males, the pleurisy may be painless and occasionally precedes joint symptoms. The effusions generally have low glucose concentrations because the rheumatoid inflammation inhibits glucose transport into the pleural cavity. White blood cell counts show inflammation, but cell counts greater than 25,000/mm^3 are rare. Thoracentesis is important for differential diagnosis; tuberculosis, empyema, and pulmonary embolism must be ruled out.

Rheumatoid nodules in the lung are usually asymptomatic and are first noticed on routine chest roentgenograms. The patient characteristically has multiple subcutaneous nodules and advanced arthritis. Pulmonary nodules may erode through bronchioles to produce a bronchopleural fistula. Single rheumatoid nodules must be differentiated from the many etiologies of coin lesions, of which carcinoma is the most serious. Multiple nodules appear as metastatic disease or tuberculosis. Diagnosis by bronchoscopy or percutaneous needle biopsies may be necessary in difficult cases. In no instance is the excessive mesenchymal reactivity of rheumatoid patients demonstrated better than in Caplan's syndrome: rheumatoid patients who also had exposure to mineral dusts from coal mining developed rapidly progressive, coalescing rheumatoid nodules. Pulmonary insufficiency may be a sequel to this lesion.

Variable degrees of pulmonary interstitial fibrosis may be seen in rheumatoid arthritis; like the pulmonary nodules, this develops without prominent symptoms. Physical exam may reveal fine, crisp rales at the bases posteriorly, while the chest roentgenograms are usually normal. Using sophisticated techniques, such as postexercise arterial oxygen tension determinations and pulmonary function tests, some abnormalities of pulmonary function can be demonstrated in approximately 50 percent of patients with rheumatoid arthritis. Lung biopsies confirm the presence of interstitial fibrosis. The pathology may vary from an exudative appearance with edema, cellular infiltrate, and little fibrosis to dense fibrosis with few cells. At the other end of the spectrum is far advanced fibrosis, which leads to severe respiratory symptoms and an abnormal chest x-ray with diffuse fibrosis. Pulmonary fibrosis is a late complication of rheumatoid arthritis seen more frequently in females than males. Rarely, a patient has obliterative pneumonitis with both exudative and fibrotic lesions.

Cardiac Involvement

The recent utilization of ultrasound techniques has revealed pericardial effusions in as many as one-half of patients with active rheumatoid arthritis. Only a small percentage of this group is symptomatic, however, The pericarditis can precede arthritis but usually follows the onset of joint symptoms and may accompany a flare of disease activity. Tamponade is rare. Pericardial fluid, as do pleural and joint fluids in rheumatoid arthritis, may have a low glucose concentration and contain "ragocytes," PMN with large inclusions.

Involvement of the endocardium and myocardium is associated with severe active disease. The pathology, depending on the virulence of a particular case, will range from well-structured rheumatoid granuloma formation on valve leaflets or within the myocardium to diffuse coronary arteritis. Similarly, clinical manifestations range from murmurs and mild conduction abnormalities to valve perforation and papillary muscle dysfunction.

Ocular Complications

The eye is involved in rheumatoid arthritis in several ways. Sjögren's syndrome and keratoconjunctivitis sicca were discussed in the section of Sjögren's syndrome in this fascicle. Scleritis is a deep penetrating inflammation of the scleral coat of the eye and has pathology resembling rheumatoid granulation tissue elsewhere. Patients may be asymptomatic or complain of severe pain and blurring of vision, as would patients with acute iritis. The inflammation in the sclera heals with atrophy. The scleral coat may be thinned sufficiently to see the dark choroid beneath. If the damaged sclera becomes infarcted, the softened tissue may fall apart, producing rupture of the globe; this is the dreaded scleromalacia perforans. Scleritis occurs in adult rheumatoid patients, whereas anterior uveitis (both acute and chronic) is seen in chronic juvenile arthritis.

Complications of treatment of rheumatoid arthritis include posterior subcapsular cataracts induced by corticosteroid therapy and retinopathy due to antimalarial drugs.

Muscle Involvement

Nonarticular pain in the extremities in rheumatoid arthritis may be a manifestation of a focal myositis not associated with muscle enzyme elevations. Weakness is not usual and when present it commonly represents disuse atrophy around a chronically inflamed joint rather than a primary myositis. During acute flares of rheumatoid disease, excruciating pain in muscle bundles may reflect reversible ischemia generated by the pressure of inflammation and edema. Myopathy associated with corticosteroid therapy usually develops in patients treated with fluorinated compounds (e.g., triamcinolone) and is reported to be associated with an elevated urinary creatine excretion in comparison with patients who have a primary myositis.

Bone Involvement

The other component of the musculoskeletal system that is involved in multiple ways in rheumatoid arthritis is the osseous system. The first finding is that of decreased bone mass around involved joints. Prostaglandins released by the proliferative synovial tissue resorb bone, and soluble products of activated lymphocytes can generate osteoclasts in the subchondral bone. Adding to the stimuli to local osteopenia is disuse of inflamed, painful limbs. Poor nutrition, decreased absorption of calcium secondary to interference with gastrointestinal absorption by corticosteroid therapy, and the antianabolic effects of these drugs produce axial osteoporosis. Superimposed on these causes of decreased bone mass is the unfortunate fact that persons at the highest risk for rheumatoid arthritis—women in middle age and older—are also at high risk for developing osteoporosis as normal menses cease.

Amyloidosis

Amyloidosis of the amyloid A (AA) protein type may be a complication of the chronic inflammatory process in rheumatoid disease. The presumed serum precursor of protein AA (SAA) has been found to be elevated in rheumatoid arthritis. Clinically, infiltrations of the liver, spleen, and kidney are most characteristic of this secondary amyloidosis (see the section on Amyloidosis).

REFERENCES

Benedek TG: Rheumatoid pneumoconiosis—Documentation of onset and pathogenic considerations. Am J Med 55:515, 1973

Bluestone R, Bacon PA: Extra-articular manifestations of rheumatoid arthritis. Clin Rheum Dis 3:385, 1977

Bujak JS, Aptekar RG, Decker JI, et al: Juvenile rheumatoid arthritis presenting in the adult as fever of unknown origin. Medicine (Baltimore) 52:431, 1973

Chamberlain MA, Bruckner FE: Rheumatoid neuropathy. Ann Rheum Dis 29:609, 1970

Fleming A, Dodman S, Crown JM, Corbett M: Extra-articular features in early rheumatoid disease. Br Med J 1:1241, 1973

Franco AE, Levine HD, Hall AP: Rheumatoid pericarditis. Ann Intern Med 77:837, 1972

Ganda PO, Caplan H: Rheumatoid disease without joint involvement. JAMA 228:338, 1974

Jayson MI, Jones DEP: Scleritis and rheumatoid arthritis. Ann Rheum Dis 30:343, 1971

Nasrallab NS, Masi AT, Chander RW, Fergenbaum SL, Kaplan SB: HLA-B27 antigen and rheumatoid factor negative peripheral arthritis. Am J Med 83:379, 1977

Ropes MW, Bauer W: Rheumatoid arthritis: Its varied clinical manifestations. N Engl J Med 233:592,618, 1945

Short CL: Rheumatoid arthritis: Types of course and prognosis. Med Clin North Am 52:549, 1968

Wayed MA, Brown DL, Currey HLF: Palindromic rheumatism, clinical and complement study. Ann Rheum Dis 36:56, 1977

LABORATORY TESTS FOR DIAGNOSIS OF RHEUMATOID ARTHRITIS

Edward D. Harris, Jr.

SYNOVIAL FLUID ANALYSIS

Aspiration of fluid from inflamed joints is an essential component of proper diagnosis (see the chapter on Synovial Fluid Analysis in the fascicle on Diagnostic Procedures). All specimens should be cultured for bacteria as outlined in an earlier section and for fungus and *Mycobacterium* if joint involvement is monarticular. The tests of synovial fluid relevant to rheumatoid arthritis are summarized in Table 1.

Other tests on synovial fluid, some of which are more costly but are sometimes important for correct diagnosis include the following:

1. *Search for "ragocytes."* A "ragocyte" is a PMN that has phagocytosed immune complexes (IgG, rheumatoid factor, and complement) which are apparent as homogeneous inclusions. Immunofluorescent studies of the inclusions confirm this. Smears of rheumatoid synovial fluid stained for immunoglobulins may reveal large amounts of extracellular immunoglobulin aggregates. Many other inclusion-containing cells exist in synovial fluid and may be confused with "ragocytes."

2. *Complement (CH_{50}, C3, C4) tests.* These tests are often below normal in rheumatoid effusions because the complement system is activated by IgG–rheumatoid factor immune complexes. For accurate determinations, complement activity should be expressed in a ratio to total globulin.

3. *Protein electrophoresis of IgG.* Plasma cells within the rheumatoid synovial membrane may synthesize sufficient IgG to raise levels in synovial fluid to greater than normal; rarely the synovial fluid IgG concentration may approach that of serum.

4. *Proteinase tests.* At PMN counts of over 50,000/mm^3 the natural inhibitors of proteinases may be saturated, permitting enzyme activity normally inhibited in body fluids to be active and directly measurable. These enzymes include elastase, collagenase, and cathepsins.

BLOOD AND URINE TESTS

The diagnosis of rheumatoid arthritis can be made in many patients without multiple and expensive laboratory tests. Some patients with a typical presentation of rheumatoid arthritis may need additional tests to rule out other diseases, but the following tests are sufficient to confirm the diagnosis and start appropriate therapy in most patients with active synovitis:

1. complete blood count (hemoglobin, white blood cell count, and differential smear with platelet estimate)
2. erythrocyte sedimentation rate (Westergren technique)
3. rheumatoid factor test
4. antinuclear antibody determination
5. urinalysis

The white blood cell count in rheumatoid arthritis is normal or elevated (usually < 12,000 WBC/mm^3). Hemoglobin is variably decreased in proportion to activity and chronicity of the inflammation. Values less than 10 g/dl caused only by rheumatoid arthritis are unusual, and lower values should prompt a search for additional causes of anemia. Examination of the blood smear is essential for evaluation of red cell morphology, white cell differential count, and platelet estimate. Thrombocytosis is not unusual in active rheumatoid arthritis. Eosinophilia has been correlated with active systemic rheumatoid disease. Tests for rheumatoid factor in serum, measured by standard latex or other particle agglutination procedures, detect IgM anti-IgG and are positive in over 85 percent of patients with classic or definite rheumatoid arthritis. Very high titers are found in patients with clinical manifestations of rheumatoid vasculitis.

Antinuclear antibodies (ANA) are present in titers of over 1:32 in the sera of over 30 percent of patients with active rheumatoid arthritis. The pattern is usually a homogeneous one. A rising ANA titer with evolution of a peripheral nodular or specked pattern may be associated with a change from rheumatoid disease into a clinical picture more consistent with SLE or the mixed connective tissue disease syndrome.

Urinalysis is usually normal in rheumatoid arthritis

Table 1
Synovial Fluid Analysis in Rheumatoid Arthritis

Parameter	Normal	Rheumatoid Arthritis	Comments
Appearance	Faint yellow and clear	Yellow to white; mild turbidity to creamy; fibrin flecks are common; significant hemorrhage is rare in early disease	Turbidity reflects increased leukocyte concentration; fibrin precipitate indicates chronicity sufficient to allow larger molecules (e.g., α_2 macroglobulin and fibrinogen) to pass into the effusion
Mucin clot	Normal: sodium hyaluronate precipitates as a ropy clump	Normal ("good mucin"), "fair mucin" (many flecks and strands loose from the main tight precipitate), or "poor mucin" (no major precipitate; many diffuse flecks and strands in the solution)	Mucin clot reflects the fact that sodium hyaluronate is a polyanion and precipitates in weak acids; this clot is *not* fibrin and its loss of integrity is believed to result from enzymatic breakdown of long chains of hyaluronate to shorter ones, as well as from production of lower molecular weight hyaluronate by rheumatoid synovial cells
String test	Long thread connects a drop falling from a needle	Normal, short, or absent threads	Semiquantitative index of viscosity, reflecting integrity of hyaluronate chains, similar to the mucin clot
WBC	<1000/mm³	1000 to >100,000 mm³	Good index of the degree of inflammation in the joint; findings in RA span the range from mild inflammatory fluids (seen in SLE, vasculitis, and scleroderma) to severe inflammation (seen in sepsis or acute gout)
Differential WBC	< 50% PMN	80%–95% PMN	As the WBC increases, the percentage of PMN increases; very early in RA, the percentage of lymphocytes may be higher than expected
Glucose	30% difference from fasting blood glucose	Normal, low, or very low	Rheumatoid process interferes with normal transport of glucose into the joint fluid; very low values in synovial fluid (< 10 mg/dl) are seen only in tuberculous, acute bacterial infection and rheumatoid arthritis
Crystal	None	None	Polarized light microscopy is essential for adequate crystal detection

unless it is complicated by amyloidosis, and evidence for renal disease should prompt a search for an additional or different diagnosis.

ADDITIONAL DIAGNOSTIC TECHIQUES

In most situations, clinical examination, blood tests, and synovial fluid analysis are sufficient for the diagnosis of rheumatoid arthritis. Exceptions usually occur when involvement is monarticular. Some of the following techniques may help in diagnosis. None are available routinely.

1. *Synovial needle biopsy.* Although simple to perform with appropriate needles and stylet, the small tissue samples obtained only occasionally provide specific diagnoses. The synovium is limited in the ways it can respond to inflammation. Only the presence of dense lymphoid follicles amidst proliferative synovial cells can approach specificity for rheumatoid arthritis and the heterogeneity of synovium from different locations in one joint is great.

2. *Arthoscopy.* This procedure is expensive because it must be done in the operating room, but it does not require inpatient hospitalization in most cases. It can demonstrate different pathologies and derangements of structure. Biopsy can be a selective instead of a random process as with needle biopsy.

3. *Joint imaging with nucleotides.* Technetium-99 pyrophosphate isotopic scans are nonspecific. Indication for their use is generally restricted to determination of sacroiliac involvement.

4. *Thermography.* This techique is noninvasive. Increased blood flow produces higher joint temperatures, which are reflected in the overlying skin. Correlation with effective therapy is excellent and its use as a parameter for drug studies is well established.

5. *Arthrography.* In rheumatoid arthritis this technique is used to define effects secondary to destructive synovitis (such as meniscal cartilage damage and the loss of articular cartilage thickness) and to determine the size of popliteal cysts.

As noted above, it is important not to miss the diagnosis of another disease which presents as rheumatoid arthritis, but laboratory tests to rule out other causes of arthritis should be obtained for specific clinical indications and not as screening procedures.

Assessment of a rheumatoid patient is a different process than diagnosis. It involves an initial determination of function in activities of daily living and a comparison of these data with objective musculoskeletal examination and laboratory tests by the physician. It is this assessment that forms the basis for initial and continued therapy.

REFERENCES

Cohen AS (ed): Laboratory Diagnostic Procedures in the Rheumatic Diseases (ed 2). Boston, Little, Brown, 1975

DIFFERENTIAL DIAGNOSIS

Gary S. Hoffman and Edward D. Harris, Jr.

SEPTIC ARTHRITIS

In the differential diagnosis of arthritis it is important not to label a patient's problem prematurely. An erroneous diagnosis, formulated too soon from too few data, is of more potential harm to the patient than an error on the side of restraint in providing a definite diagnosis. The clear exception to this is septic arthritis. Of all the diagnoses listed in Table 1, this is one which must always be ruled out on clinical grounds and results of arthrocentesis. This specter of possible infection underlies the rheumatologists' desire to aspirate joint effusions as a major aid in making a diagnosis in any patient with arthritis. Compounding this problem are the statistics indicating that septic arthritis has a higher occurrence rate in joints involved with a rheumatoid process than in normal joints. For this reason, the patient with rheumatoid arthritis who has an acute or subacute "flare" in one or several joints should have these joints aspirated and cultured.

CRYSTAL-INDUCED ARTHRITIS

Gout may mimic sepsis in a joint, but it may also present as polyarthritis in approximately 5 percent of cases. Acute polyarthritis has been the first manifestation of gout in a very few patients. Usually, polyarticular gout is asymmetric and most involved joints are in the lower extremities. Diagnosis may be difficult because serum uric acid, even in cases of documented microcrystalline synovitis, may be less than 7 mg/dl. It also has been observed that acute gouty arthritis can rarely occur in rheumatoid joints. Erosions in rheumatoid arthritis do not occur beyond the confines of the joint capsule because this marks the limits of the synovium. Microcrystalline disease, in contrast, can produce a granulomatous response to crystals with subsequent erosions of bone outside the joint capsule.

Calcium pyrophosphate dihydrate (CPPD) microcrystalline disease incites less of an inflammatory response in most patients than does gout, and 5 percent of affected patients have subacute or chronic polyarticular disease that may be associated with synovial proliferation and erosions of subchondral bone. CPPD crystals may be difficult to find in joint fluid, even during acute attacks, so that other clues for differential diagnosis from rheumatoid

Table 1
Differential Diagnosis of Polyarthritis and Joint Pain

Chronic Synovitis with Potential for Articular Erosion	Synovitis, Usually Without Articular Erosions	Rarely Significant Synovitis
Ankylosing spondylitis	Amyloidsis	Hemochromatosis
Psoriatic arthritis	Arthritis of inflammatory bowel disease	Hemoglobinopathies
Reiter's syndrome	Behçet's syndrome*	Hyperparathyroidism**
Rheumatoid arthritis	Cryoglobulinemia	Hypothyroidism
Hemophilic arthritis	Degenerative joint disease—reactive synovitis	Osteoarthritis
Microcrystalline diseases	Hepatitis without vasculitis	Pancreatitis and periarticular fat necrosis
Mixed connective tissue disease and other "overlap" syndromes	Hypertrophic osteoarthropathy, primary or secondary	Polymyalgia rheumatica/giant cell arteritis
Sarcoid arthritis*	Leukemic arthritis*	Reflex sympathetic dystrophy†
Septic arthritis, acute or insidious (fungal or mycobacterial)	Postinfectious arthritis (*Yersinia, Shigella, Salmonella*)	Subacute bacterial endocarditis
Lyme arthritis*	*Rubella,* spontaneous and postvaccination	
	Other viruses	
	SLE, systemic sclerosis, dermato- or polymyositis	
	Vasculitis, polyarteritis, Wegener's granulomatosis, hepatitis B virus arthritis with vasculitis and/or cryoglobulinemia	
	Rheumatic fever	

*Erosions rarely occur.
†Special studies may reveal synovitis.
**In the absence of calcium pyrophosphate dihydrate arthropathy.

arthritis must be used. Roentgenographic evidence of chondrocalcinosis, subchondral cysts, sclerosis, and osteophyte formation in carpal and MCP joints may help in the diagnosis of CPPD (see the section on Crystal-induced Arthritis).

PSORIATIC ARTHRITIS

About 5 percent of psoriasis patients have some form of arthritis. There may be a generalized reactivity in mesenchymal tissue in joints below involved skin; the result can be pain and inflammation from skin down through bone resulting in rapidly progressive, destructive arthritis. This is particularly notable in DIP joints when there is severe skin and nail involvement. In contrast, some patients with psoriasis may have very few skin lesions restricted to rarely examined areas such as the peri-anal or scalp. In these patients arthritis may be clinically indistinguishable from rheumatoid arthritis (see the chapter on Psoriatic Arthritis in the section on Sero-negative Polyarthritis).

HLA-B27–POSITIVE SPONDYLOARTHROPATHIES

Patients with asymmetric seronegative polyarthritis present an interesting differential diagnosis which includes seronegative rheumatoid arthritis. Roentgenograms of the spine and sacroiliac joints may be helpful. Twenty to 25 percent of young males with ankylosing spondylitis first present with peripheral arthritis. The presence of sacroiliitis and the absence of mucocutaneous lesions, onycholysis, urethritis, and a preceding acute diarrhea help to rule out Reiter's syndrome. Patients with psoriasis who have HLA-B27 antigen on cell membranes are more likely to develop spondylitis than are those without HLA-B27. The same applies to patients with inflammatory bowel disease (ulcerative colitis and granulomatous colitis). Patients with inflammatory bowel disease with peripheral arthritis do not have an increased incidence of HLA-B27.

Determination of the presence or absence of HLA-B27 is an available but expensive test. When is it indicated? The answer must reflect the fact that the presence of HLA-B27 on a given patient's cells does not make a specific diagnosis in the absence of appropriate historical, physical, and radiographic evidence. The importance of the data accumulated on HLA-B27 is that it has brought together a number of disorders which have in common a high risk of developing spondyloarthropathy. The inference drawn is that diverse stimuli in patients with this genetic marker may lead to a common pathologic response, i.e., sacroiliitis and/or spondylitis. A practical setting in which HLA typing may be useful would be a patient with back or neck pain but without roentgeno-graphic evidence of spondylitis (e.g., vertebral squaring or syndesmophytes) and without firm evidence of psoriasis, Reiter's syndrome, or inflammatory bowel disease. If the B27 antigen is present in such a case, a diagnosis of "B27-related" disease might be more appropriate than "seronegative rheumatoid arthritis."

PATTERNS OF JOINT INVOLVEMENT

Differential diagnosis of arthritis by joint patterning is helpful (see the section on Radiology of Joints in the fascicle on Diagnostic Procedures). Rheumatoid arthritis frequently involves the neck (but not the back), temporo-mandibular joints, and sternoclavicular joints. DIP joint disease is common in osteoarthritis and psoriasis, but is rare in rheumatoid arthritis. Symmetric involvement of MCP joints (particularly the second and third) with bony thickening suggestive more of osteoarthritis than the soft tissue proliferation of rheumatoid arthritis is an indication to rule out hemochromatosis and other calcium pyrophosphate dihydrate associated conditions. Extremely painful small joints of the hands without synovial thickening are often found in virus-associated arthritides, such as in spontaneous rubella infection, the postvaccination rubella syndrome and the arthritis which may precede the icteric phase of viral hepatitis. Lyme arthritis, with its unknown cause and vector but a distinctive prodromal skin eruption and systemic symptoms, may in contrast rarely progress to a proliferative and erosive synovitis.

Large joint involvement should lead one to consider other disorders in the differential diagnosis. Villonodular synovitis occurs most frequently in the knee. It may or may not be painful. Large effusions and soft tissue (synovial) proliferation are usually apparent. Subchondral cysts may form, and because of repeated hemorrhage from microtrauma to the very vascular tissue, synovial fluid is often dark in color with a high lipid (cholesterol from cell membranes) content.

RHEUMATIC FEVER

Revisions of the Jones criteria for guidance in the diagnosis of rheumatic fever have emphasized the importance of establishing antecedent streptococcal infection. The criteria are listed in the section on Rheumatic Fever. Arthritis is a major criterion, and arthralgia remains a minor one. In the case of monarticular arthritis, arthralgia in other joints strengthens the case for rheumatic fever if adequate numbers of other major and minor criteria are present. In the adult, of course, no stronger suggestion of rheumatic fever exists than a previous history of a definite acute attack. Recurrent episodes of rheumatic fever are often mimetic (i.e., presenting with the same constellation of original symptoms as the initial attacks). Recurrent attacks occur almost exclusively among patients not receiving regular chemoprophylaxis, but may occur as long as 20 years after initial attacks.

OTHER CONNECTIVE TISSUE DISEASES

The connective tissue diseases, often considered along with rheumatoid arthritis in most classifications include SLE, scleroderma (systemic sclerosis), polymyositis, and mixed connective tissue disease. Early specific diagnosis may be impossible in these processes. In none is persistent proliferative synovitis as common as in rheumatoid arthritis. Reliance for diagnosis on specific tests such as anti-DNA titers is unwise; such antibodies may be present in undetectable titer early in SLE, and rheumatoid patients occasionally have significant titers of antibodies to nuclei and their components. Frequent follow-up examination in patients with undiagnosed polyarthritis is essential to search for telltale skin lesions and nonarticular symptoms compatible with one of these diagnoses.

PERIARTHRITIS

An important component of physical examination is determination of whether a painful joint reflects true arthritis or periarthritis. The latter may be associated with intense erythema of the skin, but full slow passive range of motion can be accomplished. In contrast, passive range of motion of a joint involved with true acute synovitis is very painful. Periarthritis is seen in sarcoidosis (often accompanied by erythema nodosum), microcrystalline disease, deep lesions of fat necrosis of panniculitis, and occasionally in amyloidosis, leukemia, and hypertrophic osteoarthropathy.

POLYMYALGIA RHEUMATICA

The decision as to whether or not true synovitis is present is crucial in a patient presenting with proximal joint pain, fever, anemia, and an elevated erythrocyte sedimentation rate. If true synovitis with an inflammatory joint fluid is present in any joint in such a syndrome, the diagnosis of polymyalgia rheumatica becomes less tenable. In this syndrome, probably a manifestation or variant of giant cell arteritis, symptoms usually can be localized to muscle groups around shoulders or hips rather than to the joints themselves. A similar problem may rarely occur in differential diagnosis between rheumatoid arthritis and reflex sympathetic dystrophy. The latter may present with swollen joints; periarticular demineralization and, rarely, some erosions of bone occur.

DEGENERATIVE JOINT DISEASE

The most common form of degenerative joint disease or osteoarthritis to be confused with rheumatoid arthritis is the form involving PIP joints and the first carpometacarpal joints, called *erosive osteoarthritis*. Patients are usually middle-aged and have hard bony swelling at the joints accompanying striking loss of motion. Acute attacks of pain with erythema of the skin can resemble gout. Roentgenograms show marked joint destruction without bony demineralization and with new bone proliferation. Heberden's nodes are usually seen at DIP joints. All forms of degenerative joint disease may have a reactive synovitis associated with the degenerative processes in joints. The synovitis may contribute to joint destruction. Indeed, the end stages of rheumatoid arthritis and degenerative joint disease may resemble each other clinically and pathologically.

REFERENCES

Bland JH, Frymoyer JW: Rheumatic syndromes of myxedema. N Engl J Med 282:1171, 1970
Bluestone R: Rheumatologic complications of some endocrinopathies. Clin Rheum Dis 1:95, 1975
Budiman-Mak E, Weitzner R, Lertratanakul Y: Arthropathy of hemochromatosis. Arthritis Rheum 20:1430, 1977
Gordon DA, Pruzanski W, Ogryzlo MA, et al: Amyloid arthritis simulating rheumatoid disease in five patients with multiple myeloma. Am J Med 55:142, 1973
Hadler NM, Franck WA, Bress NM, et al: Acute polyarticular gout. Am J Med 56:715, 1974
Schumacher HR, Andrews R, McLaughlin G: Arthropathy in sickle cell disease. Ann Intern Med 78:203, 1973
Silverstein MN, Kelly P: Leukemia with osteoarticular symptoms and signs. Ann Intern Med 59:637, 1963
Spruance SL, Metcalf R, Smith CB, et al: Chronic arthropathy associated with rubella vaccination. Arthritis Rheum 20:741, 1977

TREATMENT

John R. Ward and
C. O. Samuelson

Rheumatoid arthritis (RA) is a syndrome of unknown cause and unpredictable course. Pathophysiologic mechanisms are being identified and emphasize the complex nature of this inflammatory response. However, it has been impossible to design therapeutic agents which specifically interrupt the rheumatoid process. Because treatment is essentially nonspecific and certainly not curative, management of this disease is based on control of specific manifestations and preservation of function. The treatment program for the patient must be individualized. In all cases it should include objectives agreed upon by patient and physician, methods for measuring and following disease activity, definitions of possible risk as well as expected benefit of each treatment modality, and alternative plans should additional interventions be necessary.

GENERAL MANAGEMENT

Effective patient education is essential for proper management. The physician should adopt an optimistic approach but must be frank about the lack of knowledge of the etiology of RA and the absence of any absolute cure. The patient must be cautioned about those who claim to have developed specific "cures" and the major emphasis should be placed on the management and control of the disease over the long term. Patient education should include an estimate of what might be expected in the future. The possibility of complete remission and the improbability of eventual complete crippling should be emphasized, but the probability of continuing disease should be acknowledged.

Family members and other significant individuals should be involved in the educational and therapeutic processes. Compliance in a long-term program is dependent in part on the acceptance of the program by patient and family, knowledge of the disease process, and active support for the patient by the family, close friends, employers, and others. Repeated review and discussion are important factors not only in enhancing compliance with the medical program, but also in successfully persisting with physical therapy, making necessary alterations in life style, and coping with disability in the new role forced upon the patient by the disease. It must be clear to the patient that the illness potentially affects all facets of life. Opportunity for discussion of potential as well as actual problems should be provided and sexual activity as well as other sensitive areas should be frankly and openly considered with the patient.

Rest and exercise are extremely critical in the management of RA and emphasis must be placed on their becoming an integral part of the daily routine. An inflamed joint may be made worse by excessive or inappropriate activity and usually improves with rest. Complete long-term bed rest is difficult to justify and if protracted may lead to muscle atrophy, contractures, and osteoporosis. Therefore, an individualized rest program should be developed. This might include an initial period of total bed rest or merely daily rest periods. In addition, protective splints for specific joints may be useful in selected patients.

A daily physical therapy program is implemented with emphasis on active or active–assisted range of motion exercises. The exercises are designed to obtain optimal joint mobility and to maintain and/or improve muscle strength. Instructions should be specific and objectives set. An objective may be to merely maintain the current status or may include modest improvement goals which can be measured. Close cooperation between physical therapist and physician is essential. The use of heat or cold for temporary relief of pain and stiffness should be a matter of patient preference. There is no unique attribute of any different form of heat, such as paraffin or diathermy. Whatever works should be used and should be simple and safe so that it is practical for home use.

For selected patients, much can be done by modification of the home or work environment. It is best to enocurage the patient and the family to use their ingenuity with the assistance of the occupational and/or physical therapist. Simple appliances and minor behavior changes may do much to improve the quality of life.

RA produces mechanical deformities which should be identified and managed appropriately as they usually are not responsive to drug therapy. An example of such a mechanical deformity is the dorsal subluxation of the toes at the metatarsophalangeal joint. The prominent metatarsal heads are associated with atrophy of the plantar fat pads and the development of callosities which cause pain with weight bearing. Metatarsal appliances may alleviate the problem. Other patients may benefit from surgical intervention.

DRUG THERAPY

Inflammation is a normal, protective, complex, and homeostatic response to injury of any type and is associated with tissue repair. In RA, persistent uncontrolled inflammation becomes dysfunctional, leading to pain and in some patients eventual joint destruction. Suppression of inflammation results in symptomatic improvement in RA, but unless the inciting factor is eliminated, drug effects are only suppressive and temporary. In RA, agents which are termed "quick-acting antiinflammatory drugs" have not been shown to alter the underlying disease process and merely tend to relieve symptoms. They do perhaps modify or suppress to some degree the inflammatory response. Another group, the slow-acting drugs, such as gold, D-penicillamine, and immunoeffective agents, may have the potential to alter the actual progression of the disease.

The proper use of drugs requires a knowledge of available agents, including their properties, and a plan for deciding which medication to give for what purpose, and for how long. It is useful to remember that individual variation is the rule in response to most drugs. If a patient is a "nonresponder" one should ask: Was the dose adequate? Did the patient take the drug as prescribed? Did the patient take it for a sufficient length of time? Was the diagnosis correct? Was the drug given for the appropriate indication? For "responders" one should ask: Is continued drug therapy necessary? Could the dose be reduced? Are there any safer, better tolerated, and/or less expensive alternative drugs? In any case, the majority of patients with RA will require antiinflammatory drugs and convention recommends a quick-acting nonsteroidal antiinflammatory agent as the first choice.

Nonsteroidal Antiinflammatory Drugs (NSAID)

There are a number of nonsteroidal antiinflammatory drugs (NSAIDs) currently available and many more are likely to be developed in the future. While this spectrum of choice has advantages, it also requires appropriate decisions on such issues as which agent to try first, what dose to use and for how long, and what drug to select next if necessary. In addition, one must consider if intolerance to one drug predicts intolerance to another and if the agent of choice will create new or additional problems for the patient. For convenience, drugs of similar chemical classes will be grouped for discussion.

Salicylates. *Efficacy and indications.* Salicylates are analgesics, and at high doses they are antiinflammatory. They do not prevent cartilage or bone destruction, but it is generally agreed that they are the most effective and widely used simple analgesics for RA. For patients who tolerate adequate doses, they are the preferred NSAID for beginning drug treatment of active RA.

Pharmacokinetics. Aspirin absorption from the stomach and small bowel is rapid and complete. While food may retard and diminish the rate of absorption, it does not reduce total bioavailabiilty. After absorption acetylsalicylic acid is rapidly hydrolyzed. The half-life of salicylates in man increases with increasing doses. Probable mechanisms include saturation of hepatic pathways such as those involved in glycine conjugation, which convert salicylate to salicylurate, and the salicylphenolic glucuronide pathway. At plasma concentrations associated with optimal antiinflammatory effect, the limited capacities of the salicylurate and salicylphenolic glucuronide pathways are exceeded and salicylic acid becomes the predominant excretory product. Salicylate conjugates are excreted at a more rapid rate than salicylate ion, which is excreted by a pH-dependent mechanism. Salicylate excretion is slow at the usual acid pH of urine and is increased by raising urinary pH. Thus, after a dose of 300 mg aspirin, the plasma half-life is about 2.5 hours but approaches 20 hours with high-dose aspirin treatment.

Mechanism of action. It is beyond the scope of this chapter to enumerate the multiple actions of salicylates. They probably not only inhibit the production of mediators of inflammation but may also interfere with the peripheral effects. They have widespread cellular actions, including partial suppression of the leukocyte chemotactic response and altered lymphocyte function. The mechanisms of these multiple effects are unclear and have not completely explained their antiinflammatory properties.

Contraindications and precautions. The only certain contraindication to the use of salicylates is a confirmed history of aspirin hypersensitivity. Relative contraindications include recent or active peptic ulcer disease and/or gastroduodenal hemorrhage, hemorrhagic states such as hemophilia, severe renal impairment and/or analgesic nephropathy, pregnancy, and breast feeding.

Appropriate precautions include monitoring of liver function in children, watching for anemia and occult gastrointestinal blood loss, avoidance of low doses in patients with hyperuricemia, and awareness of possible drug interactions such as the enhancement of oral anticoagulant activity, possible enhancement of oral hypoglycemic drug effects, and blocking of the uricosuric effect of probenecid.

Toxicity. Aspirin frequently induces dyspepsia and there is little doubt that it can cause gastritis, gastric erosions, and occult gastric bleeding. Salicylates cause gastric injury in part by damaging the mucosal cells and thus promoting hydrogen ion back diffusion with further cell damage. There is no convincing evidence that aspirin leads to duodenal ulcers.

Salicylism with tinnitus and/or hearing loss usually occurs at salicylate levels of around 20 mg/dl. In the very young and very old, auditory changes do not always occur. Frank salicylate intoxication with respiratory alkalosis progressing to metabolic acidosis and coma occurs at higher levels. This usually results from excess dose, failure to appreciate the long serum half-life at high doses, or alterations in the excretion pattern. Serious toxicity is particularly found in youngsters with intercurrent diseases such as diarrheal syndromes with dehydration and acidosis.

Anemia may result from salicylate-induced gastric mucosal bleeding. Aspirin increases bleeding time, decreases platelet adhesiveness and aggregation, and in large doses may cause hypoprothrombinemia. The syndrome of rhinorrhea, nasal polyps, and asthma may be due to chemoreceptor or biochemical idiosyncrasy, rather than a simple allergic response.

Hepatotoxicity, observed especially in juvenile patients on high doses, is usually mild, acute, and reversible with discontinuation of therapy. In some the drug can be continued at a reduced dose without recurrence.

Analgesic nephropathy from aspirin alone cannot be confirmed in humans, but when taken concurrently with large doses of phenacetin, salicylates may contribute. Low-dose salicylates impair uric acid excretion by the kidney and can contribute to hyperuricemia. Institution of salicylate therapy may reduce the creatinine clearance by as much as 25 percent through mechanisms not related to impairment of glomerular function.

Aspirin may prolong gestation slightly. Aspirin also enters the fetal circulation and may increase perinatal mortality.

Preparations and regimen. Numerous salicylate preparations are available and range from plain, buffered, and enteric-coated aspirin to time-released preparations. There are sodium and magnesium salts, choline conjugates, salicylsalicylic acid, and mixtures of these. Plain aspirin tablets are inexpensive and often are preferred. In some patients buffered or enteric-coated preparations apparently cause less gastric distress. Other forms may also be better tolerated.

The total daily dose should be that which achieves the desired effect. If an antiinflammatory effect is sought, doses of 3500–6000 mg/day are required.

The therapeutic goal is to achieve a serum salicylate level of 15–30 mg/dl. Because salicylate has a longer half-life at high doses, small dosage increases produce proportionately greater serum salicylate levels and it may take 5–7 days to reach this new equilibrium. Likewise, at high doses, aspirin need not be given every 4 hours.

Phenylalkanoic acids. Three of the recent NSAID's are phenylalkanoic acid derivatives and many more are in the offing. Those approved at the present time for use in the United States are ibuprofen (Motrin) naproxen (Naprosyn), and fenoprofen (Nalfon). Each has a proprionic acid substitution. Each is analgesic, antipyretic, and antiinflammatory in the appropriate dose.

Efficacy and indications. These drugs are equivalent to full doses of aspirin in the treatment of RA. They also appear to be essentially equivalent to each other in efficacy. As is aspirin, they are indicated for active disease, either as single agents or in combination with steroids or "slow-acting drugs." They are not to be used with each other or with therapeutic doses of aspirin as no enhancement of efficacy has been demonstrated.

There may be subsets of responders and nonresponders and these may be different for each drug. Therefore, some patients will not respond at all and others will obtain varying benefit. Thus it may be useful to try more than one drug in any given patient.

Table 1

Preparations, Mean and Maximum Dosages, and Frequency of Administration of Nonsteroidal Antiinflammatory Drugs (Phenylalkanoic Acids)

Drug	Dosage Form (mg)	Mean Daily Dosage (mg)	Maximum Daily Dosage (mg)	Schedule
Ibuprofen (Motrin)	300 & 400	1800	2400	qid
Fenoprofen (Nalfon)	300 & 600	2400	3200	qid
Naproxen (Naprosyn)	250	500	750	bid

Many believe that new NSAID such as these should replace aspirin as the drug of first choice primarily because these drugs are better tolerated than aspirin. Certainly, these drugs should be considered for patients who are intolerant of aspirin or have failed to respond.

Pharmacokinetics. All are readily absorbed after oral administration and peak plasma levels are achieved by 90–120 minutes. The approximate half-life for each drug is as follows: ibuprofen, 2 hours; fenprofen, 3 hours; and naproxen, 13 hours. The major route of excretion is renal. Ibuprofen and fenoprofen are primarily metabolized in the liver and then excreted by the kidney, whereas naproxen is excreted in the urine, either unchanged or as the glucuronide conjugate.

Mechanism of action. None of the many effects of these drugs on biochemical systems explain their mode of action in RA. Thus the reader is referred to the extensive reviews for further information.

Contraindications and precautions. The only absolute contraindication to the use of these drugs is established hypersensitivity to that drug. However, cross sensitization has been observed between these drugs and other NSAID, including aspirin, and thus caution should be exercised in using the agents in sensitized persons.

Patients who have been intolerant to one drug may experience similar adverse effects with others of this group. Although these drugs have been successfully employed in patients with peptic ulcer disease, they should be used with caution and care. Similarly, prudence should be exercised when these drugs are given to patients who have bleeding disorders, hypertension, or congestive heart failure or are taking highly protein-bound drugs such as warfarin.

Toxicity. Side effects are similar for all of these agents. Nausea and epigastric distress are the most common but are seldom severe. Occasional mild and usually transient elevations of hepatic enzyme levels are observed but definite hepatotoxicity is not seen. Other common effects include skin rashes, edema, and interference with platelet adhesiveness, which may occasionally prolong the bleeding time. Uncommon side effects include headache, lightheadedness, and other central nervous system disturbances. Toxic amblyopia is a rare complication of ibuprofen and is rapidly reversible when the drug is stopped.

Preparations and regimen. Although Table 1 lists recommended doses, it is always necessary to tailor the dose to the needs and tolerance of individual patients. In general, higher doses are advised to achieve observable benefits which should be evident within 1–2 weeks. If helpful, the dose can then be adjusted to maintain these benefits. If no antirheumatic effect is seen, then alternative therapy is undertaken.

Interactions. Under certain circumstances, such as concurrent administration of aspirin and fenoprofen, there may be reduction in serum levels of each drug, but the clinical importance of this effect is doubtful. Similarly, the potential for displacement of other strongly protein-bound drugs exists, but again the clinical relevance has not been established.

Indoles, indenes, and pyroles. Despite early controversy, indomethacin (Indocin) is an effective antirheumatic drug. More recently, sulindac (Clinoril), an indene, and tolmetin (Tolectin), a pyrole, have also been shown to be effective. Because these drugs have chemical and clinical similarities they will be discussed together.

Efficacy and indications. Indomethacin, sulindac, and tolmetin seem as effective in RA as aspirin and the phenylalkanoic acids. In addition, 50–100 mg of indomethacin at bedtime has been shown to reduce night pain, sleep disturbance, and morning stiffness in RA patients.

Pharmacokinetics. Each drug is rapidly absorbed after oral administration. Tolmetin has a plasma half-life of approximately 45 minutes, indomethacin has a half-life of about 2 hours, and sulindac has a half-life of 8 hours, while the mean half-life of the sulfide metabolite is about 16 hours. Tolmetin is excreted mainly in urine either unchanged, conjugated, or as an inactive dicarboxylic acid metabolite. Urinary excretion accounts for 60 percent of indomethacin, either as indomethacin, glucuronides, or metabolites. The remainder is excreted in feces as metabolites.

Following absorption, sulindac undergoes reversible reduction to the active sulfide metabolite and irreversible oxidation to a sulfone metabolite. There is enterohepatic circulation which may contribute to the sustained plasma levels. The major route of excretion is renal, although approximately 25 percent of the drug, primarily as sulfone and sulfide metabolites, is found in the feces.

Mechanism of action. Multiple actions have been described but no specific mechanism of action for effect in RA is known.

Contraindications and precautions. The only absolute contraindication is hypersensitivity to the specific drug. Relative contraindications are definite peptic ulcer disease, severe hepatic disease, or bleeding diathesis. Patients who have been intolerant to indomethacin may be able to tolerate tolmetin or sulindac.

Toxicity. The major problems with indomethacin are gastrointestinal and central nervous system effects, which are partly dose-dependent. Nausea and epigastric pain are frequent and have been associated with gastric ulcers. Some patients develop diarrhea, headaches, and, less commonly, lightheadedness, vertigo, confusion, and frank psychosis. Hypersensitivity reactions are very rare but are more likely in patients who have experienced such reactions to aspirin. Retinopathy is questionable and toxic hepatitis is rare.

Tolmetin and sulindac have similar toxicity but to a lesser degree.

Preparations and regimen. Indomethacin is supplied in capsules containing either 25 or 50 mg. An initial dosage of 25 mg three times daily can be increased to 150 mg/day if response is not adequate. An occasional patient may require *and* tolerate doses as high as 200 mg/day. In some patients who have significant night pain, 50–100 mg of indomethacin at bedtime will be well tolerated and reduce night pain, improve sleep, and reduce morning stiffness. Tolmetin is available in 200-mg tablets. The usual starting dose for tolmetin is 300–400 mg four times daily with a maximum daily dosage of 1800 mg or as little as 800 mg. As with other NSAID agents, the dosage must be individualized to achieve maximum benefit and the drug effect should be evident within 1–2 weeks.

Sulindac is supplied as tablets containing either 150 or 200 mg. The usual starting dose is 150 mg morning and evening, with a maximum daily dosage of 400 mg.

Pyrazolon Derivatives

Phenylbutazone (Butazolidin), a congener of antipyrine and aminopyrine, has been used in the treatment of RA since 1949. Oxyphenbutazone (Tandearil) is a hydroxy analogue of phenylbutazone.

Efficacy and indications. In adequate doses, phenylbutazone and oxyphenbutazone appear to be essentially equal to aspirin and other NSAID in treating RA. However, their toxicity precludes their selection as frequently used drugs or for long-term therapy of RA.

Pharmacokinetics. Phenylbutazone is rapidly absorbed from the gastrointestinal tract and peak plasma levels are reached in 2 hours. Phenylbutazone undergoes glucuronidation at C-4 of the central ring and, to a lesser extent, hydroxylation at one of the phenyl rings, or at the butyl side chain. C-glucuronidation appears to be the important biotransformation reaction for removal of oxyphenbutazone. The plasma half-life of phenylbutazone when given in multiple doses ranges from 47–142 hours with a mean of 70–80 hours. An increased dose does not produce a proportional increase in plasma concentration. About 60 percent of the drug (as metabolites) is excreted in the urine and most of the remainder is excreted in the feces.

Contraindications and precautions. These drugs are contraindicated in patients who have an established history of drug sensitivity, definite peptic ulcer disease, or significant hematologic problems, or who are concomitantly using another highly protein-bound drug (such as warfarin) or hematotoxic drug (such as gold). The drugs should rarely be considered for use in patients with congestive heart failure, hypertension, or significant liver or renal disease. If employed, careful monitoring is required (see below).

Toxicity. These drugs are generally poorly tolerated; side effects occur in perhaps one-third of patients. Unwanted reactions are in part dependent on dose, duration of therapy, and age of patient. About 20 percent occur during the first several weeks of therapy and about 50 percent within the first 3 months. The most common is gastric intolerance with heartburn, nausea, and vomiting. There may be associated gastritis and acute peptic ulceration with consequent complications. Salt and water retention may occur.

The most serious reactions are hematologic. Agranulocytosis usually occurs early in the course of therapy and is often preceded by a rash. Thrombocytopenia also occurs. Aplastic anemia is most frequently seen in patients over 60 years of age who have been treated for at least 6 months; it has a mortality of approximately 50 percent.

Other side effects include a variety of skin rashes and severe reactions include Stevens-Johnson and Lyell's syndromes. Salivary gland enlargement may develop early in therapy and clears when phenylbutazone is stopped. Toxic and cholangitic hepatitis have been reported.

Preparations and regimens. Phenylbutazone (Butazolidin) and oxyphenbutazone (Tandearil) are supplied as 100-mg tablets. Enteric-coated preparations, buffered preparations, and combinations including steroid are available. These combinations should not be used. In most instances 100-mg three or four times a day is sufficient, but in acute flares 200 mg three or four times a day for several days may be helpful. Long-term therapy should rarely be employed and, if used, careful and regular monitoring for side effects—including complete blood count, platelet count, blood pressure determination, and surveillance for other side effects—is necessary. There is no advantage of oxyphenbutazone over phenylbutazone.

Interactions. These drugs potentially could have significant interactions with other protein-bound drugs. Thus phenylbutazone can enhance effects of warfarin. It can reduce plasma digoxin levels and enhance the hypoglycemic effects of acetohexamide and tolbutamide, perhaps by displacement from protein-binding sites as well as effects on enzymes. Desipramine and other tricyclic antidepressants inhibit the absorption of phenylbutazone, as may cholestyramine.

Gold

Efficacy and indications. Gold compounds have been used in the treatment of RA for 50 years. Controlled studies have repeatedly demonstrated that they produce symptomatic improvement and significant decrease in joint swelling. The proportion of patients reported to experience benefit is variable and only estimates can be developed. In general, about 20–40 percent of patients who successfully complete a course of gold treatment experience a "remission" and 40–60 percent have major improvement; 10–20 percent experience no benefit. Approximately one-third of patients may be considered as treatment failures, including those who are unresponsive to chrysotherapy, those who eventually escape its effect, and those who develop toxic effects. Remission occurs in less than 10 percent and major improvement occurs in less than 20 percent of untreated patients over comparable periods of observation. A recent double-blind study of RA patients treated with gold compounds for 2 years showed that the progression of rheumatoid joint disease as evaluated by x-rays was significantly reduced or arrested.

It is generally agreed that patients with active rheumatoid synovitis not controlled by more conservative therapy should be considered for gold treatment. Disease should have been persistently active for at least 4–6 months and reversible arthritis (i.e., soft tissue inflammation) should be evident. The arthritis must be of sufficient severity to justify potential risks. In later stages, when cartilage and bone damage have occurred, gold can only offer hope of retarding further progression in joints with active synovitis. Thus, gold treatment is not indicated for mild disease, pauciarticular disease, or inactive RA. Chrysotherapy is also beneficial in juvenile rheumatoid arthritis.

It is essential that no contraindications are present (see below). Mild neutropenia and Felty's syndrome, however, are not absolute contraindications and may improve with gold therapy. Gold toxicity may be more frequent in patients with psoriasis, and gold compounds may exacerbate psoriasis. Nonetheless, the mere presence of psoriasis does not contraindicate gold treatment. Gold may be given to the RA patient with Sjögren's syndrome as well as the occasional patient with RA-associated eosinophilia.

Pharmacokinetics. Within hours after intramuscular injection of gold compounds, serum gold levels reach a peak and the serum half-life is 5–6 days. The gold is largely bound to albumin for transport and the bulk is deposited in tissues, particularly in the reticuloendothelial system and renal cortex. Gold is excreted principally in the urine and less in feces. From 20 to 50 percent of a single dose is retained in the body after 180 days and gold excretion may continue for over 1 year. Thus there is a relatively short serum and a long whole-body half-life.

Most investigators have found no correlation between serum gold concentration and either therapeutic effect or toxicity. Tissue levels likewise have not been found useful in monitoring therapy.

Mechanism of action. The exact mechanism(s) of action in RA remain unknown. Gold compounds are antimicrobial (including mycoplasmas). Gold compounds

react with sulfhydryl groups and bind avidly to plasma proteins and all cell constituents. They can measureably affect the function of enzymes (including lysosomal), the first component of complement, phagocytic cells, and lymphocytes. They are not "immunosuppressive" in patients. Unfortunately, these observations do not provide an understanding of their action in RA, and particularly we have no insight into the slow response to gold treatment.

Contraindications and precautions. Chrysotherapy is contraindicated in the following circumstances: (1) previous failure to respond to an adequate course of gold therapy; (2) confirmed history of gold sensitivity and/or toxicity, especially hematologic and renal; (3) significant renal disease and/or proteinuria; (4) blood dyscrasia; (5) pregnancy or breast feeding; and (6) concomitant administration of D-penicillamine. Relative contraindications are as follows: (1) active hepatitis and/or serious liver disease; (2) concomitant use of drugs known to produce bone marrow depression, neutropenia, and/or thrombocytopenia; (3) presence of significant dermatologic disease; and (4) presence of significant allergic disease.

During therapy, careful inquiry for pruritis, rash, metallic taste, stomatitis, facial flushing, light-headedness, fainting, or diarrhea is done before each injection. A complete blood count, including platelet and differential cell counts, and a complete urinalysis should be done within 24 hours preceding each injection. If any of the above symptoms are elicited or if evidence of toxicity appears on laboratory testing, treatment is discontinued until the problem is resolved. Gold toxicity will not be prevented, but early cessation of treatment can usually avoid serious reactions.

Toxicity. Chrysotherapy would clearly be more useful if it were free of the frequent unwanted and potentially serious reactions. Adverse reactions occur in about one-third of patients; they are in part dependent on dose of administered gold and usually are not serious. Perhaps 15 percent of patients will not be able to complete a course of gold therapy because of toxic reactions. Serious reactions are reported in less than 5 percent. Death is an infrequent complication and occurs in probably less than 0.25 percent.

Mucocutaneous side effects are the most frequent. Rashes, which may occur in as many as 30 percent of patients, are almost always pruritic and are often similar to lichen planus or pityriasis rosea. They most frequently are difficult to classify and may be generalized, patchy, or localized. Gold dermatitis generally worsens with continued gold administration and may rarely progress to generalized exfoliative dermatitis. Most rashes, however, respond to cessation of gold treatment and, if severe, they can be suppressed with topical and/or systemic corticosteroids. Gold can often be reinstituted without recurrence of a rash. A small challenge dose of 5–10 mg is used as a preamble to cautious reimplementation of gold in either reduced or full-dose schedules. There are no definite predictors for gold rashes.

Stomatitis is frequently painless and often is preceded and/or accompanied by a metallic taste; it can be localized to gingival or buccal and sublingual mucosa. It usually recurs if the patient is rechallenged with gold.

Proteinuria occurs in 2–10 percent of patients and is expected to clear in weeks after stopping gold, although an occasional patient has persistent proteinuria which lasts for months. Serious renal disease as manifested primarily by nephrotic syndrome is rare. The predominant lesion is membranous glomerulonephritis with deposits of IgG, IgM, and beta-1C globulins. More than two-thirds of affected patients recover and treatment with corticosteroids in the range of 60 mg prednisone daily is often advised in severe renal disease.

Hematologic complications include eosinophilia, leukopenia, agranulocytosis, thrombocytopenia, and aplastic anemia. Eosinophilia is most common and is considered to be a predictor of toxicity by some. Granulocytopenia may appear abruptly and is usually reversible with cessation of gold treatment. Severe granulocytopenia and agranulocytosis are rare, thus prognosis and treatment are difficult to assess. Treatment considerations would include high-dose corticosteroids and anabolic steroids.

Thrombocytopenia is another uncommon but potentially fatal complication of gold treatment. It is probably not the result of isolated bone marrow toxicity. As with agranulocytosis, prognosis and treatment are anecdotal. Treatment would clearly dictate discontinuation of gold and possible corticosteroid treatment with or without splenectomy.

"Nitritoid" reactions resemble the pharmacologic effects of nitrites and include facial flushing, nausea, light-headedness, and impending syncope. They tend to occur more frequently with aurothiomalate and may be managed by switching to another gold compound, decreasing the dosage, administering the injection with the patient supine, and keeping the patient at rest for varying periods of time.

Unusual manifestations of gold toxicity include diffuse interstitial pneumonia, intrahepatic cholestasis, enterocolitis, and peripheral neuropathy. Predictable effects are gold deposits in the cornea (chryseosis) of patients who have received over 1500 mg of gold compound, and skin deposits, often with pigmentary changes (chrysiasis), in patients who have received even larger doses of gold. Neither of these require treatment.

Preparations and regimen. Gold compounds that are commonly used are the aqueous solutions sodium aurothiomalate (50 percent gold) and sodium thiosulfate (37 percent gold) and an oil suspension, aurothioglucose (50 percent gold). All of these preparations are given by intramuscular injection. An oral gold preparation and intraarticular administration of gold and/or radioactive

gold colloid have been suggested but are not advised because of lack of availability and/or proven efficacy.

The recommended schedule consists of an initial dose of 10 mg of the gold *compound* followed in 1 week by 25 mg, and then weekly injections of 50 mg until 1000 mg has been given. If major clinical improvement occurs before or by the time the schedule is completed, maintenance therapy is implemented. Gold compounds are then given every 2 weeks for 2–20 weeks, then every third week, and finally every fourth week for an indefinite period of time. While maintenance gold therapy is frequently required, the specifics remain to be studied.

Controlled studies have shown that higher doses of gold are more toxic and no more effective. Recent studies suggest that lower doses might be employed. Gold is also useful in the carefully selected juvenile rheumatoid arthritis patient in a dose of 1 mg/kg/week with a maximum dose of 50 mg/week.

Antimalarials

Aminoquinoline antimalarial drugs have been used in the treatment of RA since the early 1950s. Original enthusiasm for these compounds has waned with the demonstration that they may lead to serious retinal toxicity which frequently is progressive even after the drug is stopped. Although several drugs of this group have been proposed for use in RA, the major controlled studies have been restricted to chloroquine and hydroxychloroquine.

Efficacy and indications. Several double-blind studies on chloroquine and hydroxychloroquine have been similar in design and results. Antimalarial drug–placebo comparisons at 3 months tend to favor the drug but usually not at statistically significant levels. The most impressive differences were seen in studies with the drug administered for 1 year. Thus, while all studies suggest that these drugs are more effective than placebo, the differences were usually slight; however, they improved in extended periods of study.

Antimalarials may be useful in carefully selected patients in combination with NSAID or low-dose corticosteroids. Historically, these drugs have been suggested for early and mild disease, but because of their possible serious toxicity and only modest benefit, they should be reserved for patients who need additional therapy beyond NSAID but are not candidates for gold or D-penicillamine.

Pharmacokinetics. The aminoquinolines are almost completely absorbed from the gastrointestinal tract. Approximately 50 percent is bound to plasma proteins and there is prolonged retention in the tissues. They are largely degraded in the body by mechanisms that are still unclear and only about 10 percent is found in the urine unchanged. Small amounts of drug or metabolite may be found in the urine for weeks or months after cessation of therapy. Animal studies show extremely high tissue concentrations in the liver, spleen, kidney, lung, and heart. In addition, there is selective accumulation in the pigmented tissues of the eye. It is likely that the drug has special avidity for melanin pigments since the selective ocular deposition is not found in albino animals.

Mechanism of action. The known pharmacologic effects of the 4-aminoquinolines do not adequately explain the antirheumatic action of these drugs. Chloroquine is concentrated in nuclear material and lysosomes and is able to bind to nucleic acids and stabilize lysosomal membranes. Chloroquine may also impair leukocyte chemotaxis, suppress lymphocyte responsiveness, and interfere with sulfhydryl binding in proteins.

Contraindications and precautions. These agents are contraindicated in the presence of retinal and visual field changes, especially those attributable to 4-aminoquinolines, and in patients with known hypersensitivity to these compounds. These agents should be used very cautiously in the presence of hepatic disease or glucose-6-phosphate dehydrogenase deficiency. Aminoquinolines may exacerbate psoriasis or cutaneous porphyria and should not be used in pregnancy.

Toxicity. Long-term therapy, such as that required in RA, may lead to retinal toxicity, which appears to be dose and duration of administration related. Retinopathy has been reported in as few as 0.1 percent to as many as 15 percent of treated patients. The retinopathy appears to correlate with the selective deposition of the drug in the pigmented retinal layers.

Additional minor toxic reactions include transient headache, gastrointestinal upset, and pruritis. These rarely require termination of treatment.

Preparations and regimen. Hydroxychloroquine (Plaquenil) is supplied as a 200-mg tablet and the usual starting dose is one tablet two to three times a day. While superior antirheumatic effect is achieved with higher doses, the incidence of toxicity is unacceptable. With response the dose is reduced to one tablet one to two times a day. Treatment for less than 6 months at these levels carries little risk but regular ophthalmologic examination at 3–6-month intervals is mandatory during the course of treatment.

Interactions. While specific interactions with other drugs have not been reported, the use of these agents concomitantly with gold or pyrazoline drugs should be avoided because of the frequency of skin rashes with these compounds.

D-Penicillamine

D-penicillamine, recently approved for use in RA by the U.S. Food and Drug Administration, has received widespread acceptance, particularly in Great Britain. In the United States it is being used more frequently and represents a useful "slow-acting drug."

Efficacy and indications. D-penicillamine has been shown repeatedly to be a slow-acting drug in RA, and is apparently as effective as gold. It may also be useful for treating extraarticular manifestations such as vasculitis, rheumatoid lung disease, Felty's syndrome, and excessive nodule formation. Its use is reserved for patients who have persistent disease which is unresponsive or progressive despite optimal use of conventional drugs. It should be used before deformities and irreversible structural changes have developed and can be considered an alternative to gold therapy.

Pharmacokinetics. Absorption from the gut is rapid, with a peak blood level in 1 hour. There is protein binding and the drug is still detectable in plasma after 48 hours. It is largely oxidized to penicillamine disulfide and 80 percent is excreted within 24 hours.

Mechanism of action. A number of actions, such as sulfydryl reduction, chelation, blocking of viral RNA replication, and lathyrogenic effect, have been described but cannot be related to an effect in RA.

Contraindications and precautions. Contraindications are hypersensitivity to D-penicillamine, the presence of proteinuria, thrombocytopenia, leukopenia, or pregnancy, and the uncooperative patient. A history of penicillin allergy is *not* a contraindication, but the initial doses of D-penicillamine should be given cautiously and in a setting prepared to treat anaphylaxis. Prior toxic reactions to gold do *not* indicate similar reactions to D-penicillamine.

Toxicity. Side effects of D-penicillamine therapy are frequent and are, in part, dependent on dose and duration of treatment. Renal and hematologic toxicity are serious and potentially fatal. Loss, impairment, or alteration of taste occurs in 25–30 percent of patients. It appears at about 6 weeks of therapy and gradually disappears over another several months. Gastrointestinal disturbances, most commonly nausea and anorexia, also occur most frequently in the first several months. D-penicillamine is *not* ulcerogenic.

Rashes occur in up to 20 percent of patients. They may occur at any time, but a generalized maculopapular or morbilliform rash occurs in the first months of treatment. Cessation of D-penicillamine treatment leads to prompt recovery and it is frequently possible to resume therapy at low doses without recurrence of the rash. A late pruritic rash with irregular scaly plaques often requires withdrawal from treatment. Pemphigus demands discontinuation and *no* rechallenge. Elastosis perforans serpiginosa is thought to be induced by many years of treatment.

Hematologic adverse reactions include leukopenia, thrombocytopenia, and aplastic anemia. The incidence of these reactions is impossible to determine. Leukopenia of 3000 WBC/mm^3 or less or an absolute PMN count below 1500/mm^3 requires stopping D-penicillamine and no subsequent rechallenge is permitted. If the platelet count falls below 100,000/mm^3, the drug is stopped and not restarted. Thrombocytopenia may herald aplastic anemia but is most commonly an isolated and self-limited event. Hematologic toxicity can appear suddenly and at any time.

Proteinuria develops in 10–15 percent of patients, usually after several months of treatment. Proteinuria may clear with only modest reduction in the daily maintenance dose. If proteinuria exceeds 1–2 g/day the drug should be discontinued. In uncomplicated patients the proteinuria slowly clears, although it may take as long as 1 year to do so. Nephrotic syndrome is uncommon but demands cessation of therapy and no rechallenge. Persisting hematuria also necessitates stopping D-penicillamine as the renal lesion has the characteristics of an immune complex nephritis.

Other adverse effects include drug fever, stomatitis, mammary gigantism, Goodpasture's syndrome, myasthenia gravis, polymyositis, lupus syndrome, and obliterative bronchiolitis.

Preparations and regimen. D-penicillamine is marketed as 125- and 250-mg capsules in the United States. The optimal dose and duration of therapy have not been fully established. It appears, however, that response is slow and may occur on low doses. Furthermore, toxicity and side effects seem to be decreased on low as opposed to high doses. Thus treatment is initiated at 250 mg/day, taken on an empty stomach. A complete blood count including platelet count and urinalysis is done every 2 weeks to check for toxicity. If no response is evident after 3 months, the dose is increased to 500 mg, which can be given as a single daily dose. In successive 3-month intervals the dose can be increased to 1.0 g/day. Rarely, a patient will require larger doses. Once a good response is obtained and maintained, attempts to reduce the dose by reversing the above schedule seem appropriate.

Interactions. D-penicillamine is not to be given with gold.

Corticosteroids

Few clinical observations in the history of medicine rival the discovery by Hench and his co-workers that cortisone could suppress the inflammation of RA. Following the initial burst of enthusiasm for corticosteroid therapy came the realization that it is not curative and that side effects and toxicity are significant. While some disagreement still exists, corticosteroids continue to be used frequently and offer important benefits to the carefully selected patient.

Efficacy and indications. Corticosteroids are at least temporarily effective in suppressing the inflammation of RA. There is a lack of evidence, however, that these agents alter the natural course of the disease. Whenever these drugs are used, there must be a conscious assessment that the expected beneficial results from corticosteroid therapy will outweigh the risk of serious adverse effects. For example, the needs of a breadwinner to remain active may be different than those of other patients. Finally, the aim in corticosteroid treatment should be to ameliorate symptoms rather than to suppress them completely.

Steroids should be neither the initial agent used in RA nor the only drug employed. They should be administered only after conscientious trials with more conservative medications have been unsuccessful. There are con-

ditions associated with RA, however, that are either potentially so devastating or life-threatening that corticosteroids should be given in high enough doses to be suppressive. It is generally agreed that these drugs should be used in severe vasculitis, disabling pericarditis, and pleuritis associated with RA, life-threatening Felty's syndrome, RA leg ulcers not responsive to other modes of therapy, and currently or previously steroid-dependent patients undergoing surgery or other major stress. Steroids are not indicated in patients responsive to other agents nor in those without active inflammation.

Pharmacokinetics. Cortisol and most synthetic analogs are readily absorbed after oral administration. Parenteral administration is used to obtain high concentrations rapidly in body fluids or to maximize local effects. Corticosteroids exist in plasma, and approximately 90 percent are reversibly bound to protein, either "corticosteroid-binding globulin" or albumin. When radioactively labeled steroids are intravenously injected, most of the radioisotope is recovered in the urine in 72 hours, and fecal, biliary, or pulmonary excretion is trivial. Serum half-life is short for most preparations and ranges from 0.5 to 5 hours.

Mechanism of action. There is evidence that implicates both antibody-mediated and cell-mediated processes in rheumatoid inflammation. For corticosteroids to influence the rheumatoid inflammatory process significantly, they need to suppress both components; that implies suppression of the ability of circulating sensitized lymphocytes to transform into activated immune lymphocytes or of the ability of the latter to synthesize the soluble mediators of cellular hypersensitivity, or both (see the section on Mechanisms of Inflammation in the fascicle on Immunology).

Contraindications and precautions. While absolute contraindications are few, relative contraindications are many and thus must be carefully weighed in each patient. In addition, side effects tend to be dose related; therefore, the smallest possible dose consistent with the necessary pharmacologic effect should be used. Corticosteroids should be avoided in patients with systemic infections, especially those not readily controlled by antibiotic therapy—in particular, disseminated fungal and tuberculous infections, but also some viral and bacterial infections. Other contraindications include generalized osteopenia, selected psychiatric problems, thromboembolic disease, diabetes mellitus, congestive heart failure, hypertension, glaucoma, and cataracts. Corticosteroids should be used cautiously with ocular herpes infections to avoid corneal perforation and with ulcerative colitis if there is a possibility of abscess or perforation.

Exogenous corticosteroid administration may lead to suppression of hypophyseal pituitary adrenal axis function and thus the dosage must be gradually reduced before withdrawing completely and supplemental steroid must be given during stress such as surgery or severe infection. Furthermore, there is an enhanced effect of

Table 2
Comparison of Antiinflammatory Corticosteroids

Corticosteroid	Relative Antiinflammatory Potency	Equivalent Dosage (mg)	Plasma Half-Life (min)	Sodium-retaining Effect
Cortisone	0.8	25	30	++
Hydrocortisone	1	20	90	++
Prednisolone	4	5	200	+
Prednisone	4	5	60	+
Methylprednisolone	5	4	180	0
Triamcinolone	5	4	300	0
Dexamethasone	25	0.75	200	0

these agents in patients with cirrhosis and hypothyroidism.

Finally, the use of steroids in the presence of peptic ulcer is disputed but the agents should be avoided if possible in this setting.

Toxicity. Two categories of toxic effects are observed with adrenocorticosteroids which are related to continued use of large doses and to withdrawal of the drugs. A Cushing-like syndrome follows long-term use of moderate to high-dose therapy, and a secondary adrenal insufficiency syndrome develops when these drugs are stopped or tapered too rapidly. The toxicity of corticosteroids is dose and time dependent.

The following abnormalities have been reported in conjunction with long-term exogenous steroid administration: Fluid and electrolyte disturbances include sodium and fluid retention, congestive heart failure, hypokalemia with or without alkalosis, and hypertension. Musculoskeletal manifestations are muscle weakness and myopathy, osteoporosis, vertebral compression fractures, aseptic necrosis of femoral and humeral heads, and pathologic fractures of long bones. Gastrointestinal toxicity includes peptic ulceration with possible perforation and/or hemorrhage, pancreatitis, abdominal distention, and ulcerative esophagitis. Dermatologic problems reported are impaired wound healing, thin and fragile skin, petechiae and ecchymoses, facial erythema, increased sweating, and suppression of skin test reactions. Possible neurologic complications mentioned are pseudotumor cerebri, seizures, vertigo, and headache. Metabolic and endocrine toxicity may include negative nitrogen balance, menstrual irregularities, development of a Cushingoid state, secondary adrenocortical and pituitary unresponsiveness, growth suppression in children, decreased carbohydrate tolerance, and exacerbation of diabetes mellitus. Ophthalmologic problems include posterior subcapsular cataracts, increased intraocular pressure, glaucoma, and exophthalmos.

Preparations and regimen. A large number of synthetic adrenocorticosteroids have been synthesized. Those commonly used in RA are listed in Table 2. Most of these compounds share the same pharmacologic properties, apart from mineralocorticoid effect, and differ only with respect to absolute dosage. It should be empha-

sized that no drug in this group is unique with respect to a separation of therapeutic and toxic effects.

Corticosteroids are administered orally, parenterally (intravenous, intramuscular, intraarticular, and intralesional routes), and topically. Some absorption into the systemic circulation occurs with all forms of topical administration.

Oral administration is most frequent in the treatment of RA. For carefully selected patients, intrasynovial injection may be appropriate. Other routes of administration are usually not recommended. Hypophyseal pituitary adrenal (HPA) axis suppression is likely if greater than physiologic doses are used. To minimize the side effects associated with corticosteroid therapy, many regimens have been recommended. In general, it is best to use the lowest possible dosage, such as prednisone 5–10 mg/day, given in two to four divided doses, consistent with the desired level of suppression of RA activity. For equivalent total doses, a single morning dose causes less HPA axis suppression than multiple doses, and alternate day administration results in even better HPA axis function. Unfortunately, in RA, larger doses are usually required to achieve acceptable benefit with less frequent administration.

Intraarticular injections, while frequently helpful, are only adjunctive therapy to a general program. Special care must be taken in injection technique to avoid infection.

Cytotoxic (Immunosuppressive) Drugs

These agents are discussed in detail elsewhere (see the section on Immunosuppressive Drugs in the fascicle on Immunology). They will be briefly reviewed here as they are used in patients with rapidly progressive RA who have not responded to other drugs. Two drugs, azathioprine and cyclophosphamide, are employed in the treatment of RA.

Efficacy and indications. Controlled studies have shown that both azathioprine and cyclophosphamide are useful in suppressing rheumatoid synovitis and are comparable to gold in efficacy. Their immediate toxicity and particularly their potential oncogenic effects make them only rarely indicated. The following guidelines are suggested for the use of these drugs in rheumatic disease; (1) life-threatening or potentially seriously crippling disease must be present; (2) reversible lesions must be present; (3) there must be a failure to respond to, intolerable side effects from, or contraindication to the use of conventional drugs, including gold and D-penicillamine; (4) there must be no contraindications, including infection, hematologic abnormalities, and prior history of malignancy; (5) informed consent must be obtained; (6) there must be meticulous follow-up for signs of toxicity, both immediate and delayed, and for evaluation of benefit to justify continued use; and (7) there should be peer review.

Pharmacokinetics and mechanism of action. This information is presented in the section on Immunosuppressive Drugs in the fascicle on Immunology.

Contraindications and precautions. Some contraindications and precautions have been described above and elsewhere (see the section on Immunosuppressive Drugs in the fascicle on Immunology). Additional contraindications are pregnancy, breast feeding, concurrent use of other drugs which could produce bone marrow suppression, and unreliability of patients. In patients with significant renal impairment, the clearance of azathioprine and cyclophosphamide is reduced. In patients receiving allopurinol, the metabolism of azathioprine is inhibited and a reduction in dose of one-third to one-fourth the usual dose of azathioprine is advised. Cyclophosphamide is "activated" by liver microsomes; thus drugs such as phenobarbital can increase the rate of metabolism and enhance its effects. Conversely, drugs that decrease microsomal enzyme activity such as phenothiazines should also be avoided when cyclophosphamide is administered.

Toxicity. These drugs are cytotoxic and immunosuppressive. Side effects include gastrointestinal intolerance, infection, and bone marrow depression. Cyclophosphamide also causes hair loss, hemorrhagic cystitis, azoospermia, and anovulation. Azathioprine may cause fever, rash, and hepatic injury. Thus the use of these agents demands full knowledge of their immediate and delayed toxicity (discussed further in the section on Immunosuppressive Drugs in the fascicle on Immunology).

Preparations and regimen. Both azathioprine and cyclophosphamide are supplied as 50-mg tablets. There is increasing evidence that lower doses of these drugs may be effective. Thus either drug in doses of around 1.0 mg/kg/day might be tried in selected patients. Response is slow and may not be maximal for 4–6 months. For unresponsive patients, doses of 1.5–3.0 mg/kg/day may be required.

Complete blood counts are done every 2 weeks. For patients on cyclophosphamide, urinalysis and tests for blood in the urine are done biweekly.

These agents have also been reported to be helpful in treating rheumatoid lung disease and vasculitis.

MISCELLANEOUS TREATMENTS

A number of other drugs have been reported to be helpful in RA. Either uncertain toxicity or unconfirmed benefit prevent any from being recommended for use at the present time.

Zinc sulfate has been reported to be a slow-acting antirheumatic drug. If it has an effect it is apparently mild and confirmation of efficacy is needed. L-Histidine has also been advocated but efficacy has not been established.

Levamisole is an antihelminthic agent with immunostimulatory properties. While optimal dosages have not been developed, a levamisole regimen of 100–150 mg/day for 3–4 days each week has shown it to be an effective slow–acting antirheumatic drug. A major drawback to its use is sudden unpredictable agranulocytosis.

Thoracic duct lymph drainage results in dramatic improvement in RA. However, when drainage of lymphocytes is discontinued the arthritis returns. Leukophoresis and extracorporeal irradiation of leukocytes have not been refined as therapeutic approaches.

SURGERY

Surgical intervention to relieve pain and improve function is a dramatic and rewarding approach for selected patients. Operative procedures on joints include synovectomy, arthrodesis, and arthroplasty. In some circumstances osteotomy and bone resection can be done. Tenosynovectomy, tendon repair, and release of "trapped" nerves are examples of nonarticular surgery.

Surgical synovectomy may be considered for persistent painful synovitis before radiologic changes of joint damage have developed. In some instances, synovectomy may retard progression and provide pain relief. It is most successful in metacarpophalangeal joints and knees.

Arthrodesis is rarely performed except in isolated finger joints to provide improved function. Likewise, osteotomy, such as proximal tibial osteotomy to correct valgus or varus deformity of the knee, is not commonly advocated in RA.

Total joint replacement has been a major advance in abolishing pain and restoring motion and function in severely damaged joints. Virtually any joint can be replaced. Total hip replacement is predictably successful and durable despite some late effects such as loosening of the prosthesis, infection, and fractures. Total knee replacement is also immediately satisfactory, although long-term success is less certain; it should be reserved for carefully selected patients. For other joints, consultation with an experienced orthopedic surgeon will be required to identify the rare candidate for surgery.

Surgery of the hand is often successful in correcting deformities or retarding their progression; it is mainly performed to improve function. Soft tissue procedures for swan neck and boutonniere deformities, synovectomy, resection arthroplasty, joint replacement, and selective arthrodeses are all options. Selection of patients for surgery requires consultation with a surgeon experienced in rheumatoid hand surgery. Tenosynovectomy for "trigger fingers" is often helpful. Immediate repair of ruptured tendons and, if diagnosis is delayed, tendon transfers are successful in restoring function.

Forefoot deformities in RA can be severe and disabling and surgical correction is indicated when more conservative measures such as metatarsal appliances are unsuccessful in relieving pain.

Nerve entrapment syndromes, such as median nerve compression in the carpal tunnel, may require surgical decompression for relief.

REFERENCES

Bluhm GB: The treatment of rheumatoid arthritis with gold. Semin Arthritis Rheum 5:147, 1975

Champion GD, Day RO, Graham GG, Paul PD: Salicylates in rheumatoid arthritis.Clin Rheum Dis 1:245, 1975

Famaey JP, Lee P: More recent nonsteroidal anti-rheumatic drugs. Clin Rheum Dis 1:285, 1975

Fauci AS, Dale DC, Balow JE: Glucocorticoid therapy: Mechanisms of action and clinical considerations. Ann Intern Med 84:304, 1976

Fowler P: Phenylbutazone and indomethacin. Clin Rheum Dis 1:267, 1975

Gerber RC, Paulus HE: Gold therapy. Clin Rheum Dis 1:307, 1975

Gottlieb NL: Chrysotherapy. Bull Rheum Dis 27:912, 1976–1977

Hamilton LDB, Scott JT: Hydroxychloroquine sulfate (Plaquenil) in treatment of rheumatoid arthritis. Arthritis Rheum 5:502, 1962

Hill HFH: Treatment of rheumatoid arthritis with penicillamine. Semin Arthritis Rheum 6:361, 1977

Huskisson EC: Antiinflammatory drugs. Semin Arthritis Rheum 1:1, 1977

Jaffe IA: D-Penicillamine. Bull Rheum Dis 28:948, 1977–1978

Jasani MK: The importance of ACTH and glucocorticoids in rheumatoid arthritis. Clin Rheum Dis 1:335, 1975

Mills JA: Drug therapy: Nonsteroidal anti-inflammatory drugs. N Engl J Med 290:781, 1002, 1974

Mowat AG, Huskisson EC: D-penicillamine in rheumatoid arthritis. Clin Rheum Dis 1:319, 1975

Paulus HE, Whitehouse MW: Nonsteroid anti-inflammatory agents. Ann Rev Pharmacol 13:107, 1973

Rheumatology Workship: A modern review of Geigy pyrazoles. J Intern Med Rev 5 [Suppl 2]:1, 1977

Smith MJH, Smith PK: The Salicylates. New York, Interscience, 1966

Zvaifler NA: Antimalarial treatment of rheumatoid arthritis. Med Clin North Am 52:759, 1968

Rheumatic Fever

John Baum

DEFINITION AND EPIDEMIOLOGY

Rheumatic fever is an inflammatory state principally involving the heart, the large peripheral joints of the body, the brain, and the skin and its supporting structures. The development of rheumatic fever follows a prior infection of the pharynx with group A streptococci.

DEFINITION

There had been difficulty in defining rheumatic fever in the past because of its numerous modes of presentation but it has been easier since the appearance of Jones' criteria. Certainly, as the name implies, fever is a prominent symptom; however, the most important manifestation is the inflammatory carditis, which can result in permanent damage to the heart. Other manifestations such as arthritis, chorea, subcutaneous nodules, and skin rashes are of a temporary nature and are only of minor importance aside from their value in diagnosis. Since the work of Coburn in the early 1930s the relationship of rheumatic fever to a prior pharyngeal infection with group A streptococci has been extended and confirmed. It must be noted, however, that today streptococci play a more important role in the United States as causal agents in skin infections and nephritis.

In a recent review of the literature it was pointed out that streptococcal infection is a frequent cause of erythema nodosum. Although arthritis and fever can appear with erythema nodosum and with the finding of β-hemolytic streptococcus in the throat (as well as a raised antistreptolysin titer), erythema nodosum is *not* a feature in those patients who develop rheumatic fever. Indeed, the appearance of erythema nodosum virtually rules out the development of cardiac lesions, even in the presence of arthritis and fever.

Pharyngitis, the only type of streptococcal infection that leads to rheumatic fever, has been demonstrated to occur in epidemics and, again, as one would expect, these infections will occur during periods when there is more contact between persons; that is, during the cooler times of the year. Not only must there be prior pharyngeal infection with the organism, but it is evident that the streptococcus must be present long enough to induce an immune response. This response, measured in terms of antibody level, is stronger in those patients developing rheumatic fever. Because there is individual variation in response, the level in an individual patient is not diagnostic.

Although most physicians will recognize a full-blown hemolytic streptococcal sore throat, many of the cases are of much less intensity and often are clinically unrecognized. In the classic case, a patient will present with a sudden onset of sore throat which is sometimes associated with abdominal pain and nausea (especially in children) and accompanied by constitutional symptoms such as malaise, headache, and fever.

The signs of this condition are redness and edema of the throat, the presence of an exudate on the tonsils, enlargement and tenderness of the anterior cervical nodes, a fever of 101°F or greater, leukocytosis of greater than 12,000 leukocytes/mm³, and an elevated erythrocyte sedimentation rate. These signs will be helpful, but only the growth of the organism from a throat culture is diagnostic.

EPIDEMIOLOGY

Rheumatic fever has shown a remarkable decrease in incidence in the past 30 years. The attack rate, which has been estimated in the past as being from 0.14 to 1.70 percent of children with streptococcal pharyngitis, is probably even lower today. This has been noted in a number of countries around the world, especially in the industrialized countries whose inhabitants have enjoyed a general improvement in living status and nutrition. In addition to the decline in the total number of cases there has been a decline in the frequency of carditis in those patients who do get the disease. Chorea has also become less frequent and a greater proportion of those patients who develop the disease present with arthritis. In addition to the improved living standards and a more knowledgeable detection of the presence of β-hemolytic streptococcal pharyngitis leading to early therapy, other factors may also have played a role in decreasing the number of cases of rheumatic fever. The suggestion has been made that an increasing proportion of the streptococcal organisms recovered from pharyngeal infections contain little or no M protein, that factor which has been chiefly associated with virulence.

As with many diseases in which there has been a decrease in the total number of cases, interest has fallen and this alone has probably led to poorer follow-up and possibly less case reporting. The use of antibiotics alone has not accounted for the decrease in rheumatic fever in the United States. Although there may be no real difference in the numbers of streptococcal sore throats in children in the United States, there has been a significant drop in the number of patients with acute rheumatic fever. The circumstances that have helped produce this improvement may be related to improvements in nutrition and housing but the precise answer remains in doubt. Some investigators believe that the continuing deterioration of inner city areas may cause a change in the frequency of rheumatic fever. There is some credence to this point of view since rheumatic fever does appear to be increasing in blacks (the major inhabitants of crowded urban areas in recent years). A recent study in the southern part of the United States found that the incidence of acute rheumatic fever in blacks was two times that in whites. When these patients were followed up the incidence of rheumatic heart disease was three times as high in blacks. Carditis with the initial attack of rheumatic fever was a significant indicator for the subsequent development of heart disease; the carditis occurred more frequently in blacks.

The fall in the death rate from rheumatic fever and rheumatic heart disease has been most striking in the younger age groups. This correlates well with decreased frequency of diagnosis.

Several groups have looked at HLA phenotypes in patients with rheumatic fever. In a study of 109 patients with rheumatic fever a significantly increased frequency of BW35 was found as compared to the controls, while B18 was more common in patients with acute carditis. In another study of 86 patients with chronic rheumatic heart disease, however, the HLA frequencies were not found to differ significantly from those found in the control group.

Other studies have found still different frequencies of transplantation antigens. In one, a decreased frequency of A3 was found. Another group compared frequencies in patients from different geographic areas: New Zealanders of European origin, Maori, and Europeans. In the Maoris a slight but significant increase in the frequency of A3 and A8 and a decrease in A10 was observed. In the patients of European descent there was a significant relationship of the transplantation antigens to the development of rheumatic fever.

REFERENCES

Leirisalo M: Rheumatic Fever. Am J Clin Res [Suppl] 9:1, 1977
Leirisalo M, Laitinen O, Tiilikainena: HLA phenotypes in patients with rheumatic fever, rheumatic heart disease and Yersinia arthritis. J Rheumatol [Suppl] 3:78, 1977
Markowitz M: The changing picture of rheumatic fever. Arthritis Rheum [Suppl] 20:369, 1977

PATHOGENESIS AND CLINICAL FEATURES

Although much is known of the etiologic factors in rheumatic fever, the mechanisms of tissue damage are still unclear. Diagnosis and the clinical appearance of the disease have been extensively studied and represent what is best known about this condition. The therapy of streptococcal infection has been well established and its application has been one of the more important reasons for the diminishing importance of rheumatic fever, with its crippling sequelae, as an important disease in the United States.

IMMUNOPATHOLOGY

The characteristic rheumatic lesions found in the heart are termed *Aschoff bodies;* they represent focal breakdown of muscle. The lesions contain fragments of muscle fibers and what may be regeneration or an attempt at regeneration. Aschoff bodies are found in the atrial appendages of many patients with mitral stenosis at the time of surgery, however, in most cases there is no clinical or laboratory evidence of rheumatic fever at the time. The fact that Aschoff bodies can be found in the ventricular myocardium at the same time is some indication that their presence represents persistant inflammatory activity so localized that peripheral evidence of inflammation is not found.

In a recent review of Aschoff bodies reported in patients operated on for mitral stenosis, 38 percent had them in the excised atrial appendages. This was confirmed in patients operated on for mitral lesions at the

National Institutes of Health over a period of 21 years (1954–1974); 25 percent had Aschoff bodies.

The cause of the damage to myocardial tissue is still not clear. There is some evidence, however, that anti-streptococcal antibodies react to cardiac tissue or at least bind to it. This would speak for a direct effect on heart tissue of a humoral component induced by the presence of streptococcal antigen. Other evidence suggests that circulating immune complexes consisting of cardiac antigen plus antiheart antibodies could localize in cardiac tissue and induce damage. Antiheart antibody has been found in a number of diseases but seems to be most prominent in active rheumatic fever, bacterial heart disease, and myocardial infarction. When antiheart antibodies in patients with rheumatic fever were specifically compared to those in patients with rheumatic heart disease there was a strikingly higher frequency in rheumatic fever. Although it is difficult to determine the importance of these antibodies in the development of the cardiac lesions, it is of interest that when immunofluorescent staining is done on cardiac tissue there is marked staining of the sarcolemmal membranes of myofibrils. This type of staining has a higher frequency and is of greatest intensity in patients with acute rheumatic fever and lends credence to the belief that this humoral factor has some relationship to the development of the cardiac lesions.

Further evidence for immunologic activity in the development of the lesion has been the identification of complement components in myocardium of valves in postmortem studies of rheumatic hearts. The least well characterized mechanism appears to be the role of cell-mediated immunity in the destruction and damage of cardiac tissue. However, in tissue culture studies using lymphocytes from patients with rheumatic fever and cultured cardiac tissue there appears to be some deleterious effects of these lymphoid cells on the cardiac muscle fibers.

Although the precise mechanism for the appearance of rheumatic fever following streptococcal infection has not been proven there are a number of immunologic cross reactions that have been found between some of the cellular components of the streptococcus and a number of different body tissues. The M protein found in the cell wall is a large molecule consisting of protein, lipid, and carbohydrate that has been found to show cross-reactivity with heart muscle. In addition, a cell wall polysaccharide appears to cross-react with a mucoprotein found in the heart valves. An assumption would then be made that antibodies produced to these substances might have an effect on heart tissue. This rather simplistic observation may hold because the rheumatic fever develops long enough after the infection so that high titers of antibody to these streptococcal antigens are present. Although not generally used clinically, levels of antibody to streptococcal polysaccharide may have some value in the diagnosis of rheumatic fever. A higher level of this antibody can be observed in patients with rheumatic fever, especially when cardiac involvement is present. Thus the presence of this antibody may have value in the diagnosis of rheumatic valvular heart disease and carditis.

Hypersensitivity has not been definitely proven to be a mechanism in the development of rheumatic fever after streptococcal infection, but some studies of blood lymphocytes have shown a decrease in the number of T cells in this group of patients. In addition, it was found that there is decreased phytohemagglutinin stimulation of lymphocytes, but, as would be expected, when streptococcal antigens were used there was an increase in lymphocyte stimulation. This again may not indicate a direct relationship to the development of the tissue lesion in rheumatic fever but may be seen as a paraphenomenon.

Examination of the synovial tissue from an involved joint shows dilitation of blood vessels with small focal infiltrates of polymorphonuclear leukocytes and lymphocytes. There is edema of the synovial tissue. There is no exuberant overgrowth of the synovial tissue (pannus) or collections of lymphocytes as in rheumatoid arthritis.

The nodule of rheumatic fever has a central necrotic zone surrounded by fibroblasts and histiocytes. Small vessels may be surrounded by lymphocytes and polymorphonuclear cells. There is no palisading or zoning such as that seen in the nodule of rheumatoid arthritis.

CLINICAL FEATURES

The diagnosis of rheumatic fever is still best made using the modified Jones criteria. The major criteria include carditis, polyarthritis, chorea, subcutaneous nodules, and erythema marginatum. The minor criteria are fever, arthralgia, prolonged P-R interval, increased erythrocyte sedimentation rate, presence of C-reactive protein or elevated white blood cell count, evidence of preceding β-hemolytic streptococcal infection, previous history of rheumatic fever, or the known presence of rheumatic heart disease.

It should be emphasized that these criteria rigidly applied can exclude patients who subsequently are found to have rheumatic fever. This group is most likely to include patients who may show several of the minor criteria and none or one of the major criteria. Another group who could be excluded are patients appearing with monarthritis as the only major manifestation of the disease.

With the current changes in the presentation of rheumatic fever suggestions have been made for altering the criteria. Since carditis and polyarthritis are the major problems in rheumatic fever and there is evidence that there has been a fall off in these manifestations, some investigators believe the presence of either one or both along with supporting information such as the presence of streptococcal antigens may be the most important means of making the diagnosis of rheumatic fever. After the streptococcal infection occurs there is a latent period before the appearance of rheumatic fever; it averages about 19 days but varies from 7 to 37 days.

Any one of the major or minor manifestations can appear at the onset of the rheumatic fever. Of the major criteria, chorea usually appears late in the course of rheumatic fever. In addition to the neurologic changes there may be emotional instability. The patient is unable to maintain a tight hand grip and shows repetitive irregular milkinglike motions. Other notable features are the involuntary motion of the extremities, the face, and the tongue. This can best be described as jerky movements. Chorea has been seen much less frequently in recent years, and probably occurs in no more than 10–15 percent of patients with rheumatic fever today. The chorea of systemic lupus erythematosus, also caused by involvement of the central nervous system, is similar in its appearance.

Erythema marginatum, although characteristic of rheumatic fever, is also rare. The lesions are characterized by a somewhat pink central area with a sharply outlined periphery. They are occasionally mistaken for the rash of systemic onset juvenile rheumatoid arthritis. However, in the latter condition there is no well-outlined edge and the lesions are usually smaller and lighter in color and have a pale center. These coalesce, rather than spread from a single area, with serpiginous moving borders as is seen in erythema marginatum.

The subcutaneous nodules usually appear over bony prominences. They most often appear with carditis and, as in erythema marginatum, are an uncommon manifestation occuring in about 5 percent of the patients.

Carditis presents in several ways. Murmurs are the most prominent reflection of cardiac involvement. A significant apical systolic murmur is the most common since the mitral valve is frequently involved. It is heard best at the apex and is a pansystolic, loud, high-pitched, blowing murmur. The next most important is the low-pitched apical middiastolic murmur. A basal or aortic diastolic murmur is less frequent. Since bivalvular disease can occur it can be heard along with the murmurs showing involvement of the mitral valve. Pericarditis may present with a pericardiac friction rub, chest pain, or pericardial effusion. Pericarditis is seen as part of the rheumatic carditis in the child and is rare in the adult. The most rare manifestation of acute rheumatic fever is congestive heart failure. It occurs in 5–10 percent of patients with rheumatic fever who have cardiac involvement.

Other indications of cardiac involvement are tachycardia (especially during sleep), changes in the heart sounds (as an accompaniment of rheumatic myocarditis), and the appearance of a gallop rhythm.

The most common manifestation of acute rheumatic fever is arthritis, which occurs in most patients. Arthralgia or joint pain without objective signs of joint inflammation is a minor criterion for diagnosis. As pointed out earlier, monarthritis, though not part of Jones' criteria, can be seen, and in one series was found in 25 percent of the patients who developed arthritis. The joints that are involved are usually the large ones; the knee is involved most often, and there may also be involvement of the hips, ankles, and elbows. Occasionally there is small joint involvement and the diagnosis of rheumatic fever should not be ruled out if small joints of the fingers or toes are involved. It has long been stated and is apparently true that cardiac damage is less likely in patients who have active joint involvement.

Classically, the arthritis is migratory, involving one or several joints; after other joints are involved, the arthritis remits in the original ones. Redness and marked tenderness is a more distinctive feature of the arthritis of rheumatic fever than of rheumatoid arthritis. This aspect of the disease, like the others, is self-limiting; the joints are involved for about 1 week, and the total course lasts about 3 weeks.

Jaccoud's syndrome or joint deformity secondary to repeated attacks of rheumatic fever is a medical curiosity that has been reported only twice in the United States. With repeated attacks of inflammatory synovitis the metacarpophalanageal joint capsules become enlarged and thickened by fibrosis. The fingers show ulnar deviation due to the pull of the intrinsic muscles. However, normal alignment can be restored by holding the hand on a flat surface. X-ray films do not show any evidence of bony erosions.

Although it was stated in the past that a rapid response of joint inflammation to aspirin is characteristic of rheumatic fever, this type of response can occasionally be seen in acute rheumatoid arthritis and cannot be depended upon as a diagnostic test.

Examination of synovial fluid obtained from the joints of patients with rheumatic fever shows an elevated total white blood cell count consisting mostly of polymorphonuclear leukocytes at the onset of the arthritis. The mean count in 12 fluids in one series was 13,600 cells/mm³. If the synovitis is present longer than 4–7 days the fluid shows predominently mononuclear cells. The proteins in the fluid are elevated and the sugar content is normal. There is nothing diagnostic in the synovial fluid of these patients.

DIAGNOSIS

The antibody response to the streptococcal antigens takes time to appear. The initial rise in antibody levels can be seen within the first 7 days after the streptococcal infection, and the maximum level occurs at 20–40 days following infection. The titers then gradually fall over the next several weeks but the rate of fall varies with the individual. There is variation in the response to individual streptococcal antigens; testing should therefore be done for more than one antigen. Occasionally the antibody levels are measured at the period of peak levels so that subsequent measurements are lower, and an antibody rise, which would be a positive indication of streptococcal infection, cannot be demonstrated. A two-tube dilution change in titer, however, is usually significant. One can compare the value of throat cultures to tests showing the presence of antibodies to various antigens of the streptococcus. A positive culture, if it is due to streptococcus, can often be obtained within 12 hours, with cultures becoming less positive over the next few days. Then the antibodies such as antistreptolysin O, anti-DNAse, antihyaluronidase, anti-NADase, or antistreptokinase appear. The most efficient method is to use the recently described streptozyme test, which measures a number of streptococcal antibodies and is more sensitive than any of the previously mentioned antigens.

The prior presence of a β-hemolytic streptococcal sore throat is, as has been proven, a necessity for the development of rheumatic fever. This requirement presents occasional dilemmas. Many patients do not report having had a sore throat before the development of rheumatic fever. Once rheumatic fever has developed an attempt to culture streptococcus from the throat produces a low yield. Elevated levels of antistreptolysin O titer are usually found four to five times as frequently as isolation of the organism. It may be helpful to obtain throat cultures of contacts of the patient.

The streptozyme test was devised using a standardized suspension of aldehyde-fixed sheep blood cells sensitized with the following five antigens: antistreptolysin O, antistreptokinase, antihyaluronidase, anti-DNAse, and anti-NADase. It has been reported that there is a good correlation between antistreptolysin O and the antistreptozyme test. However, the streptozyme test using multiple antigens increases the frequency of the serologic diagnosis of streptococcal infection.

Another valuable though not specific test to detect inflammation is the erythrocyte sedimentation rate. With the occurrence of an inflammatory disease such as rheumatic fever, acute-phase reactants are produced; these are proteins (e.g., fibrinogen; alpha globulins) produced nonspecifically. The proteins are present in the circulation and because of their inherent stickiness adhere to red cells, which then act to form rouleaux. These packets of red cells (like a roll of coins) have an increase in volume compared to their surface area, making them fall more rapidly in the sedimentation tube. The signs and symptoms of rheumatic fever (except for "pure" chorea) are accompanied by an elevation in the erythrocyte sedimentation rate. There is no difference in the degree of elevation of the sedimentation rate if either polyarthritis or carditis is present. With treatment, especially with corticosteroids, the sedimentation rate will fall. However, if therapy is stopped and the signs and symptoms of rheumatic fever rebound the sedimentation rate will also rebound.

Although after treatment of streptococcal infection with penicillin, the fall in the white blood count follows the clinical response to therapy by several days, the erythrocyte sedimentation rate is slower to respond, sometimes taking 2–3 weeks before falling to normal levels.

C-reactive protein is another acute phase reactant produced in the liver. There is a generally held opinion that it is more responsive to the acute stage of rheumatic fever and will return to normal levels before the erythrocyte sedimentation rate. In any event it is exceedingly difficult to make the diagnosis of acute rheumatic fever in the absence of either an elevated sedimentation rate or the presence of C-reactive protein.

Stollerman has pointed out the usefulness of fluoroscopic examination of the heart in detecting the dilatation of the "inflow tract" of the left ventricle and the posterior wall of the left atrium. However, since standardized criteria could not be established because of the marked variation in normals, a simple anteroposterior view of the heart is the most reliable method of detecting cardiac enlargement. Congestive heart failure is now a rare accompaniment of rheumatic carditis but should be suspected if vascular congestion and patchy edema is seen on the chest x-ray films. This can be observed before other signs or symptoms of congestive heart failure are readily apparent. In addition to the presence of a significant murmur and pericarditis, cardiac enlargement by roentgenography fulfills the criterion for acute carditis. However, if only cardiac enlargement and failure are present, that is sufficient to make the diagnosis of carditis.

Too much reliance should not be placed on the electrocardiogram in the diagnosis of rheumatic fever. There is no characteristic pattern that can unequivocally indicate the presence of carditis. The prolongation of atrioventricular conduction as measured by a prolonged P-R interval occurs in 40 percent of patients with acute rheumatic fever. It is related to the overall disease process and is not specifically indicative of cardiac involvement since it can also be seen with polyarthritis alone. Even more suggestive of this limited role is the fact that there is no relationship between the appearance of a prolonged P-R interval and the subsequent development of rheumatic heart disease. The persistence of this finding after the subsidence of the acute attack again is no indication of future cardiac damage.

Flattened or inverted T waves are seen with myocarditis but also have no clear relationship to the degree of involvement since they can come and go in the presence of definite myocarditis. The same holds true for the corrected QT interval. Pericarditis has a recognizable association with electrocardiogram changes but again this is not consistent. Deviation of the ST segment with T wave inversion in some of the precordial leads may occur. The ST elevation is also seen to a lesser degree in the limb leads.

COURSE

Recurrent attacks of rheumatic fever are frequent. Although there is some evidence that there is a period of relative resistance in adults during the first few months after an attack, the attack rate is highest within a few years after the initial attack. Myocarditis and endocarditis can recur without any other manifestation of rheumatic fever. As time goes on the chance of recurrence decreases for unknown reasons. Does the high frequency of recurrences point to a susceptible population or to alterations in the immune system with the first attack that increase susceptibility?

Rheumatic fever is uncommon in the adult. When it does occur in the adult age group it appears to be more benign and cardiac involvement is rare. It is harder to diagnose in the adult because some of the features seen in children, such as subcutaneous nodules and chorea, are rarely observed. Erythema marginatum is also very unusual in adults. Adult patients are usually in their 20s; rheumatic fever is rare in the elderly. For unknown reasons arthritis has always been the most common manifestation of rheumatic fever in adults. Carditis is found in about 20 percent of the patients. As in the children, the recurrence rate of rheumatic fever is higher in those patients who have developed rheumatic heart disease compared to patients who had rheumatic fever without any evidence of valvular disease in their initial attack. It is important to follow the adult patient as closely as one follows children. If rheumatic heart disease is present one must be watchful, because with the minimal disease so often seen in the adult recurrent attacks of carditis could be missed.

TREATMENT

The treatment of rheumatic fever starts with prevention of the disease. The American Heart Disease Committee report entitled *Prevention of Rheumatic Fever* contains detailed recommendations for therapy. In general, streptococcal infection should be treated as soon as the infection is diagnosed. Penicillin continues to be the recommended drug. Either intramuscular administration of benzathine penicillin G or 10 days of oral therapy is recommended. In patients who are allergic to penicillin, erythromycin is the recommended drug for the acute attack. However, for long-term treatment after the development of proven rheumatic fever, intramuscular benzathine penicillin is the best agent. Compliance is the greatest problem in long-term therapy of any type. The use of intramuscular penicillin on a monthly basis is the way to be sure that the patient is actually taking the medication. A good rule of thumb is that any patient who shows fairly good evidence of taking the medication regularly and faithfully for at least 1 year will be a good risk for long-term oral therapy. In a study from the southern part of the United States it was pointed out that there were no recurrences of rheumatic fever in those individuals who received regular prophylaxis with intramuscular penicillin G benzathine. The investigators felt that recurrences in patients taking oral prophylaxis occurred because there was poorer compliance in this group. Compliance is often worse in the individuals who require it most. Patients who develop carditis in the initial attack of rheumatic fever or develop it subsequently are best served by prophylaxis by injection. If penicillin allergy develops in the patient then the sulfonamide drugs are recommended.

The requirements for drug therapy with penicillin, or other agents if allergy is present, have not changed from earlier reports. It was reemphasized that the tetracyclines are not useful because many of the streptococcal strains are highly resistant. It was stated that patients who continue to have positive cultures for group A streptococcus and in whom reinfection has not been proven should not continue to be treated after several courses of therapy. It was noted, but again was left more or less to the physi-

cian's discretion, that family contacts of a high-risk patient may be cultured when they develop upper respiratory symptoms. It probably is of advantage to culture all of the family contacts, including those who are asymptomatic, because of the possibility that a carrier state has developed in one of the family members.

In a Public Health Service Hospital Study, it was found that in an epidemic situation it is most effective and least costly to treat all patients at risk with penicillin. Different strategies were effective in the endemic situation. It was felt that all patients should be treated with penicillin when the positive throat culture yield is at least 20 percent. If the yield of positive group A streptococcus cultures is 5–20 percent only those patients with positive cultures should be treated. If the yield is below 5 percent then no treatment is most cost effective.

In addition, this group made the point that early penicillin treatment for the typical clinical findings that go along with hemolytic streptococcal sore throat show not only more effectiveness in preventing acute rheumatic fever but also a decreased length of illness. Early treatment also will cut down the spread of the organism, and certainly early treatment has the advantage of producing less medical expense to the patient. These features, they felt, outweigh the occasional danger of allergic reactions to penicillin.

It should be reemphasized that we may be more indebted to some unknown factors for the present-day rarity of rheumatic fever in the United States. However, these unknowns will not help the individual patient who might contact the proper strain of streptococcus and develop disabling cardiac disease. We must continue to watch for the organism and provide the appropriate treatment.

REFERENCES

Kaplan EL, Bisno A, Derrick W, Facklam R, Gordis L, Houser HB, Jackson WH, Millard HD, Shulman ST, Taranta AV, Wannamaker LW: Prevention of Rheumatic Fever. American Heart Association Committee Report. Circulation 55:51, 1977

Kaplan MH: Autoimmunity in rheumatic fever: Relationship to streptococcal antigens cross-reactive with valve fibroblasts, myofibres and smooth muscle, in Dumonde DC (ed): Infection and Immunology in the Rheumatic Diseases. Philadelphia, Lippincott, 1976

Otaka Y (ed):Immunopathology of Rheumatic Fever and Rheumatoid Arthritis. Tokyo, Igaku Shoin, 1976

Stollerman GH: Rheumatic Fever and Streptococcal Infection. New York, Grune & Stratton, 1975

Tompkins RK, Burnes DC, Cable WE: An analysis of the cost-effectiveness of pharyngitis management and acute rheumatic fever prevention. Ann Intern Med 86:481, 1971

Zabriskie JB: Rheumatic fever: A streptococcal-induced autoimmune disease, in Dumonde DC (ed): Infection and Immunology in the Rheumatic Diseases. Philadelphia, Lippincott, 1976

Seronegative Polyarthritis

INTRODUCTION

Rodney Bluestone

Recent scientific advances and distinctive clinical profiles have led to subcategorization within the previously amorphous group of rheumatic diseases labelled *seronegative polyarthritis*. *Polyarthritis* means inflammation of multiple joints, usually manifest locally as a visably and palpably swollen, painful, and tender articulation. When the inflammatory process affects many joints throughout the skeleton, the afflicted individual usually suffers from widespread pain, stiffness, and disability. The acuteness, extent, and distribution of a polyarthritis will largely determine the clinical severity of the disease. The term *seronegative polyarthritis* refers to a pathologic process of this kind which is not associated with readily detectable serum rheumatoid factor. Conventionally, this implies an absence of IgM agglutinating antibody against human or rabbit IgG, as detected in a latex or bentonite flocculation test or a sheep cell agglutination test. Rheumatoid arthritis is usually, and perhaps nearly always, eventually associated with serum rheumatoid factor. Thus, the classic clinical appearance of established rheumatoid arthritis is as a seropositive polyarthritis particularly common in young or middle-aged women. The distribution of a rheumatoid polyarthritis is usually widespread and symmetric in its extent and most notably affects the peripheral synovial joints.

Hence, the diagnostic use of the term *seronegative polyarthritis* emphasizes the fact that there are many forms of polyarthritis that are not due to rheumatoid disease but still may be characterized by acute or chronic inflammation of several or many synovial and cartilaginous joints. Regardless of their chronicity or pattern of skeletal distribution they are, by definition, seronegative for conventionally detected rheumatoid factor. However, the recognition of a seronegative polyarthritis does not imply a diagnostic "wastebasket" in which to place every young arthritic patient who does not have clear-cut rheumatoid arthritis. The diagnosis encompasses some well-defined rheumatic diseases that may or may not clinically resemble rheumatoid arthritis but do not appear to be associated with the immunologic aberrations of true rheumatoid disease. The seronegative polyarthritides fall into three main diagnostic groups: First, there is the group of closely related (and probably genetically determined) diseases best referred to as the *seronegative spondyloarthropathies*. Second, there are many systemic disorders in which transient or significant polyarthritis may be but one localized manifestation of the underlying disease process. Third, true rheumatoid arthritis may present in an atypical and incomplete form that may initially be seronegative.

SERONEGATIVE SPONDYLOARTHROPATHIES

This is a group of rheumatic diseases that probably share similar pathogenetic factors and display many pathologic, radiographic, and clinical features in common. The usual differences between the individual clinical syndromes are mainly related to acuteness, extent, and symmetry, which, together with certain extraarticular features, characterize the clinical profiles. The primary pathologic process within the musculoskeletal tissues is common to all of the seronegative spondyloarthropathies and appears to consist of a mononuclear cell inflammation of cartilage, subchrondral articular bone, joint capsule, ligamentous–bony junctions, periarticular periosteum, and, to a lesser extent, joint synovium. The typical distribution of this chronic inflammatory process includes the large central cartilaginous joints of the body—especially the sacroiliac joints, sternomanubrial junction, symphysis pubis, and intervertebral joints (discs) of the spine. Even when synovial joints are primarily involved, the inflammation of extrasynovial articular structures is important, particularly in the small synovial joints of the spine (apophyseal and costovertebral articulations) and in the large proximal synovial joints (hips and shoulder). Involvement of more peripheral synovial joints is seen but it is rarely as widespread or symmetric as in patients with rheumatoid arthritis.

The inflammatory process possesses some intrinsic properties that explain many of the radiographic and clinical findings. The chronic inflammatory exudate resolves by fibrosis, and this scar tissue has a remarkable tendency to ossify. Thus, inflammation in or around a joint capsule may heal, with secondary ossification resulting in complete immobilization and fusion of that joint in the relative absence of significant intraarticular pathology. Similarly, the periarticular osteitis and periostitis leads to the formation of bony spurs that may bridge adjacent vertebral bodies (syndesmophytes) or protrude as sensitive bone spurs (e.g., around the hindfoot or margins of the pelvis). Thus, the radiographic changes of the seronegative spondyloarthropathies are rather distinct and include blurring of the cartilaginous–bony interface with irregular loss of joint space, fluffy looking central and marginal articular erosions, subchrondral osteitis with healing sclerosis, periarticular new bone formation with bony bridging, and intraarticular ossification with eventual complete fusion of joints. Once the intervertebral joints of the spine become fused by such a process, profound vertebral body osteoporosis is inevitable.

The seronegative spondyloarthropathies are all strongly associated with the histocompatibility antigen HLA-B27. At present the significance of this association is unclear, but it raises several pathogenetic possibilities: a direct role for the B27 antigen on the cell surface in host susceptibility to infectious agents; an antigenic minicry between B27 and invading microbes which might generate a damaging immune response to autoantigens; or a close association between the gene coding for B27 and other genetic material within the major histocompatibility complex on the sixth chromosome, comparable to HLA-linked immune response genes widely identified in other species. In the case of the seronegative spondyloarthropathies, the putative immune response genes would indeed be disease susceptibility genes and govern either a hypo- or hyperresponsiveness to environmental agents or to altered host tissues in the propagation of chronic inflammatory rheumatic disease.

Clinical examples of the seronegative spondyloarthropathies include the following: ankylosing spondylitis in adults, in children, and in association with chronic inflammatory bowel disease; Reiter's syndrome, whether following bacillary dysentery or sexual intercourse; other postinfectious "reactive" arthropathies such as post-*Salmonella* and post-*Yersinia* arthritis; and psoriatic arthritis. Although many individuals may be identified with these "pure" clinical syndromes, it is becoming increasingly clear that patients may present with one type of clinical picture and then evolve to resemble better another distinct form of seronegative spondyloarthropathy. Moreover, because susceptibility to these rheumatic diseases appears to be closely associated with genetic material coding for HLA-B27, they naturally show a strong familial incidence. Patients with each or any of the B27-related arthropathies usually have relatives with similar afflictions. The risk for an asymptomatic, B27-positive, first-degree relative of a patient with ankylosing spondylitis to develop a related seronegative spondyloarthropathy appears to be greatly increased, although precise epidemiologic data are still awaited. Moreover, many patients appear to have an incomplete or subclinical form of a seronegative spondyloarthropathy. These patients may present with a clinically incomplete syndrome so that conventional diagnostic criteria are not met; and yet the clinical features, family history, and presence of HLA-B27 strongly suggest a "forme fruste" spondyloarthropathy.

SERONEGATIVE POLYARTHRITIS AS A LOCALIZED MANIFESTATION OF UNDERLYING SYSTEMIC DISEASE

There are many diseases in internal medicine that may result in transient but troublesome polyarthritis. Even though this polyarthritis may be quite widespread and may symmetrically involve many small peripheral joints, the clinical resemblance to rheumatoid arthritis is only superficial. As one might expect, as the underlying systemic disease waxes and wanes, so may the arthritis become more or less obvious. The pathologic process in many of these diseases appears to be a subacute inflammation of the synovium, and recent studies suggest that this synovitis may be associated with the presence of circulating immune complexes.

Examples of this type of seronegative polyarthritis might include the following: the transient large joint involvement of chronic inflammatory bowel disease frequently accompanied by erythema nodosum and pyoderma gangrenosum; the widespread arthralgias and occasional destructive arthritis of Whipple's disease; the transient symmetric small joint polyarthritis of acute sarcoidosis; the occasional and transient pauciarticular arthritis of Behçet's syndrome and familial Mediterranean fever; the transient knee joint effusions of subacute bacterial endocarditis; the small joint upper limb polyarthritis of preicteric Australia antigen hepatitis; the sympathetic effusions associated with periarticular erythema nodosum; and the occasional large joint arthritis accompanying erythema multiforme due to any provoking cause. Not uncommonly, systemic lupus erythematosus can present as a rheumatoid factor–negative arthritis. However, the rich serologic stigmata of the disease are soon apparent. In all of these disorders the systemic disease may present as or feature a seronegative polyarthritis. Nevertheless, careful clinical scrutiny usually suggests the unlikelihood of a primary rheumatic disease, and suggests the peripheral manifestation of a more systemic relapsing disorder.

Finally, patients with polyarticular gout may present in this fashion. Thus, although acute gouty arthritis is usually monoarticular and clinically distinct, a few patients may present with recurrent polyarticular synovitis resembling a chronic seronegative inflammatory syndrome. Under these circumstances, however, appropriate synovial analysis with crystal identification and recognition of the typical radiographic changes should dispel all such diagnostic confusion.

SERONEGATIVE RHEUMATOID ARTHRITIS

The vast majority of patients with rheumatoid arthritis eventually exhibit a positive test for serum rheumatoid factor. However, early in the course of the disease the conventional laboratory tests for antiglobulins may be negative or only weakly positive. Moreover, occasional patients with rheumatoid arthritis may produce high-avidity antiglobulins that remain locally trapped in the synovial cavity for many months, and the testing of synovial fluid for rheumatoid factor presents technical problems, with a tendency to false-negative results. In addition, the production of circulating IgG (7 S) antiglobulins would escape detection using conventional laboratory techniques.

Conceivably, every patient with rheumatoid disease makes antiglobulins from the onset of their illness, but the autoantibody may remain confined within synovial plasma cells. In clinical practice it is only those patients with circulating IgM agglutinating antibody directed against IgG that we refer to as being seropositive. Thus, true and apparent seronegative rheumatoid arthritis probably does occur and necessitates diagnostic consideration of some of the disorders discussed above. The natural history and course of the rheumatic disease, the distribution of the arthropathy, the distribution and nature of the radiographic changes, and the recognition of other extraarticular features all serve to solve the diagnostic dilemma eventually. The recent recognition of forme fruste seronegative spondyloarthropathy, notably in middle-aged males presenting with large joint arthritis, undoubtedly accounts for some patients previously regarded as having seronegative rheumatoid arthritis. In the juvenile forms of the disease, however, a well-characterized rheumatoid arthritis is usually seronegative. Most children with juvenile rheumatoid arthritis, regardless of the nature of its onset or course, are seronegative for conventional rheumatoid factor.

Clinical descriptions of the various rheumatic diseases that may present to the clinician as a seronegative polyarthritis are presented in the next eight chapters. They encompass a diagnostically convenient group of patients, since the concept of widespread articular inflammation in the absence of rheumatoid factor raises certain diagnostic possibilities. Many of the diseases in this section are typical and readily diagnosed. Others may present as incomplete or atypical syndromes, and still others almost certainly represent a heterogeneous collection of various rheumatic diseases awaiting further categorization. Pathogenetically, pathologically, and clinically most are quite distinct from rheumatoid arthritis.

REFERENCES

Bluestone R: HLA W27 and the "rheumatoid varients." Hosp Practice 10:131, 1975

Bluestone R: The seronegative spondyloarthropathies, in Vaughn JH (ed): Immunological Diseases. Boston, Little, Brown, (in press)

Brewerton D, James DCO: The histocompatibility antigen (HL-A27) and disease. Arthritis Rheum 4:191, 1975

Kohler P: Clinical immune complex disease. Manifestations in systemic lupus erythematosus and hepatitis B virus infection. Medicine (Baltimore) 52:419, 1973

Schaller JG, Hanson V (eds): Proceedings of the First ARA Conference on the Rheumatic Diseases of Childhood. Arthritis Rheum [Suppl] 20:145 1977

Wright V, Moll JMH: Seronegative Polyarthritis. New York, North-Holland, 1976

ANKYLOSING SPONDYLITIS

Rodney Bluestone

Ankylosing spondylitis (AS) is an ancient rheumatic disease characterized by inflammatory stiffening of the spine. Adult AS probably represents the purest clinical phenotype of the group of disorders referred to as the seronegative spondyloarthropathies; an understanding of its pathogenesis, pathology, radiology, and clinical characteristics is important for the recognition of all the other rheumatic diseases in this group. Recently a strong association between AS and the histocompatibility antigen HLA-B27 has been confirmed throughout the world. The further exploration of this association has led to a dramatic broadening of our clinical horizons for this disease. Thus, it is now clear that AS exists as a spectrum of clinical presentations ranging from the fully expressed profile of progressive spinal inflammation and total fusion to various forme fruste syndromes in which the pathologic process may be relatively inconspicuous or atypical. Moreover, since AS shares many of its clinical and radiographic features with the other seronegative spondyloarthropathies (such as chronic Reiter's syndrome and psoriatic arthritis), certain patients may at sometime during their illness display features of any or all of these related rheumatic disorders.

PATHOGENESIS

The etiology of AS is unknown but recent studies may provide valuable pathogenetic clues. Approximately 90 percent of all whites with AS are HLA-B27 positive compared to an 8 percent frequency in normal individuals. The incidence of B27 in U.S. blacks with the disease appears to be somewhat lower at about 50 percent, but this is still significantly greater than the 4 percent incidence of the antigen in normal U.S. blacks. This association holds for patients suffering from AS complicating chronic inflammatory bowel disease, as well as in the juvenile form of AS, which may mimic pauciarticular juvenile rheumatoid arthritis in its initial presentation.

The association of human disease with HLA antigens has raised many new pathogenetic considerations. As far as AS is concerned, it has been postulated that the presence of the B27 antigen on the cell surface might render the connective tissues more susceptible to an infectious agent. However, not all patients with AS are B27 positive, so the antigen does not appear to be mandatory for developing the disease. A second possibility is one of antigenic modulation or mimicry. If an infectious agent could in some way modify B27-positive cell surfaces so as to render them autoantigenic, an autoimmune inflammatory state might be induced. Alternatively, an appropriate immune response to an exogenous agent might cross-react with B27-positive host tissues, thereby initiating an autoaggressive immune reaction. The third and most widely considered hypothesis is the possibility that the gene coding for HLA-B27 is linked to an immune response or disease susceptibility gene closely situated within the major histocompatibility complex on the sixth chromosome, in a fashion analogous to the HLA-linked immune response genes documented in many animal species. Expression of a B27-linked disease susceptibility gene could explain the development of AS in B27-negative individuals, as well as the very occasional B27-negative family member of a proband with established AS who, in turn, later develops a seronegative spondyloarthropathy. Moreover, the expression of such a disease susceptibility gene might depend on interaction with other environmental and/or genetic factors as yet unrecognized.

There is as yet no absolute evidence that immune response genes exist in humans, but this hypothesis has led to reconsideration of the potential role of infectious agents as a precipitating cause of AS. Such data include an increased incidence of chronic prostatitis in patients with AS, and the recognized development of spondylitic features in patients recovering from postdysenteric Reiter's syndrome. However, most of the animal models in which a putative immune response gene appears to govern the development of experimental or naturally occurring autoimmune disease are characterized by detectable immune aberrations. Traditionally, AS is thought of as an immunologically quiet disorder when compared to the other serologically rich rheumatic diseases such as rheumatoid arthritis and systemic lupus erythematosus. Although minor and inconstant immune aberrations have been reported in patients with AS, it is hard to identify any single abnormality of humoral or cellular immunity that might reflect the presence of a pathogenic immune response gene linked to HLA-B27.

DIAGNOSTIC CRITERIA AND PREVALENCE

The accepted diagnostic criteria for AS are those declared in Rome and later modified in New York. The Rome criteria reflect the typical symptoms and signs of established disease, and are weighted heavily toward the detection of radiographic sacroiliitis. Unfortunately, mild or even moderate degrees of sacroiliitis may not be radiographically distinct. Moreover, many other diseases may undoubtedly affect the sacroiliac articulation. In practice, a single posteroanterior radiograph centered on the pelvis is most suitable for detecting sacroiliitis, and only if a doubtful abnormality is observed are special views of the sacroiliac joints desirable. However, it may be wrong to interpret asymptomatic radiographic sacroiliitis routinely as indicating AS, and this error may account for some of the confusion surrounding the true prevalence and incidence of this disease.

Most original prevalence data for AS were based on the detection of radiographic sacroiliitis, with or without clinical examination of the patients. These data revealed a prevalence of 1.5–2 persons/1000 in predominantly white populations, with a male to female preponderance of about 7:3. Such studies suggested the role of genetic factors influencing the development of AS, with a strong familial aggregation of the disease expressed either as a full clinical syndrome or as asymptomatic radiographic sacroiliitis. More recent surveys have confirmed the widespread geographic incidence of AS together with some racial variability.

Review of the epidemiologic data in light of the disease association with HLA-B27 suggests that AS is far more prevalent in our society than was hitherto suspected. Preliminary studies suggest that up to 25 percent of "normal" B27-positive individuals reveal the symptoms or radiographic signs of the disease. Moreover, this subclinical AS is equally distributed between the sexes. If confirmed, these data would indicate a true prevalence figure approaching 2 percent, with a nearly equal sex distribution. The familial aggregation of the disease may be explained since the putative gene coding for suscepti-

bility to AS appears to be largely transmitted with the gene coding for HLA-B27. Similarly, the distinctive racial distribution of the disease can also be correlated with the prevalence of the gene coding for HLA-B27 in any ethnic group. Thus, AS is far commoner in whites than in black Afroamericans or pure Africans. In addition, the very high prevalence of AS in Haida Indians correlates with the high incidence of HLA-B27 in that tribe with about one-quarter of the gene carriers developing radiographic sacroiliitis or frank AS. Clearly, the diagnostic criteria for AS as they now stand may not include a large population of subjects with subclinical disease who nevertheless carry the putative disease susceptibility gene and are capable of transmitting AS to their future generations.

PATHOLOGY

The chronic inflammatory lesion of AS consists of lymphocytes and macrophages. This inflammatory infiltrate primarily affects cartilage (especially fibrocartilage), subchondral bone, periarticular periosteum, the ligamentous–bony junctions, joint capsules, and, to a lesser extent, the synovial membrane of some synovial joints. Although no skeletal structure may be immune from the inflammatory process, there is a characteristic distribution of the disease. The major target organs are the joints of the axial skeleton, which include the following: the cartilaginous nonsynovial synchondroses of the intervertebral spaces; the diarthrodial (synovial) apophyseal, costovertebral, and neurocentral joints; the largely cartilaginous sacroiliac joints; the central cartilaginous joints of the anterior chest wall; and the symphysis pubis (Fig. 1). Proximal synovial joints are frequently involved, notably the shoulders, hips, and knees. More distal joints may become inflamed and swollen at any time during the course of AS, but severe and widespread involvement of small peripheral joints is unusual.

The inflammatory process within the component tissues of these joints generates extensive fibroblastic scar tissue. This organizing fibrous tissue possesses a remarkable tendency to calcify and eventually ossify. It is this ossifying fibrosis that leads to fusion of articular tissues and irreversible loss of skeletal mobility. Even when proliferative synovitis is present, it is rarely as extensive as that seen in rheumatoid arthritis and the concomitant inflammation within the joint capsule and subchondral bone contributes as much to the erosion and fusion of the joint as does the synovial process. Thus, the inflammatory process of AS may lead to bony fusion of spinal, central, or peripheral joints in the relative absence of synovitis.

The inflammatory process of AS may also involve certain selected extraarticular tissues as described below:

1. A recurrent nongranulomatous acute iritis is said to occur in up to 25 percent of all patients with AS at sometime during the entire course of their disease. Unusually severe scarring and secondary glaucoma can occur. Of great interest is the occurrence of "idiopathic" iritis in B27-positive individuals in the absence of other

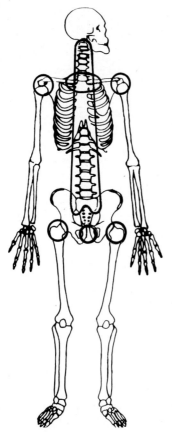

Fig. 1. Joints of the axial skeleton typically affected by ankylosing spondylitis.

features of AS. It remains to be seen whether these patients represent a forme fruste of a seronegative spondyloarthropathy or will eventually develop other rheumatic manifestations.

2. A perivascular lymphocytic infiltration of the aortic vasa vasorum has been detected in the aorta of some patients with early AS. This process may be followed by necrosis of the medial coat with replacement of the normal arterial wall by fibrous tissue. This is associated with overlying thickening and atrophy of the intima. Although the process can occur throughout the entire aorta, the important long-term sequelae are restricted to the proximal part of the vessel, where medial coat destruction near the valve ring may result in a structurally intact but incompetent aortic valve. Thus, chronic aortic regurgitation is thought to occur in approximately 1–2 percent of all patients with longstanding AS, but is nearly always associated with other advanced stigmata of the disease. Occasionally, the subaortic scarring becomes extensive enough to involve the cardiac conduction tissue, thereby causing all degrees of heart block in addition to aortic regurgitation.

3. Rarely, patients with AS may develop a bilateral pulmonary apical fibrosis, probably secondary to a low-grade interstitial pneumonitis that has resolved by fibrosis

and cavitation. The pulmonary changes are nearly always seen in the presence of obvious skeletal disease and, although nontuberculosis in origin, any such cavitation may become colonized by opportunistic bacteria or fungi.

4. A few patients with AS appear to develop a low-grade spinal arachnoiditis early in their disease course. This probably explains the observation of moderate and transient elevations of cerebrospinal fluid protein concentrations detected in some patients. This may be one possible mechanism of dural cyst development which then presents in later life as a cauda equina syndrome due to the formation of posterior lumbosacral arachnoidal diverticulae.

RADIOLOGY

The nature and distribution of the pathologic process within the skeletal system results in certain characteristic radiographic changes. The sacroiliac joints are usually the most conspicuous areas of radiographic involvement. The inflammatory process results in the progressive destruction of the sacroiliac cartilage, with erosive destruction of the subchondral bone most apparent on the iliac side of the joint. The erosions appear as punched-out areas extending deep into the subchondral trabeculae initially leading to "pseudowidening" of the joint space. The adjacent bone initially undergoes a brisk osteoblastosis, resulting in radiographic sclerosis, and this juxtaarticular sclerosis is often the most obvious radiographic sign of the disease when the discrete erosions are no longer evident. Since there is no cartilege in the upper third of the sacroiliac joint, the early inflammatory changes are not well visualized there. However, the intraarticular ligamentous inflammation in the upper part of the joint quickly leads to bony bridging, with mature osteoid tissue totally replacing the original joint space. Once the sacroiliac joint is completely fused by new bone, radiographic periarticular osteopenia is usual. The inflammatory process at the ligamentous-bony junctions of the pelvis may manifest as fluffy periostitis which eventually matures into irregular new bone formation, noted particularly at the insertions of the sacrotuberous and sacrospinous ligaments, as well as along the inferior rami of the ischiopubis and along the superior iliac crests.

Chondritis of the intervertebral discs usually begins at their perimeter, underlying the attachment of the vascular annulus fibrosus. The inflammatory process may destroy any amount of disc substance, but usually undergoes early healing so that radiographic loss of disc spaces is unusual. However, an adjacent subchondral vertebral body osteitis may be detected as a lytic lesion surrounded by sclerotic bone. As any chondritis and osteitis heals, calcification and new bone formation attacks to and replaces the annulus fibrosus, resulting in syndesmophytes which may thereby bridge the adjacent margins of one vertebral body to another (see Fig. 3B, page 96). The osteitis and destruction of the peripheral portions of the subchondral vertebral bodies followed by syndesmophyte formation is frequently accompanied by a low-grade periostitis of the anterior margins of the vertebral bodies. This combined process serves to blunt the vertebral corners and to fill in the normally concave anterior vertebral margin, resulting in radiographic squaring of the bodies. Thus, thoracic vertebral squaring is often one of the earliest radiographic signs of AS and may be detectable before any other radiographic abnormality develops. The uniform development of widespread annulus fibrosus ossification and syndesmophyte formation, together with a similar process within the perispinal ligaments, and the subsequent enchondral ossification of completely immobilized intervertebral cartilages all contribute to the classic end-stage radiographic "bamboo spine" of AS.

Occasionally the vertebral chondritis and osteitis may be locally severe with erosion of the end plate and gross vertebral body destruction. The radiographic appearance then mimics that of a septic discitis with osteomyelitis, but the other typical features of the rheumatic disease are usually obvious. The synovial apophyseal and costovertebral joints of the spine may similarly be involved in the pathologic process. Here, joint capsular inflammation may quickly result in bony fusion in the absence of significant intraarticular joint pathology. Radiographically, this is most apparent in the cervical apophyseal joints as progressive loss of joint space and an irreversible kyphosis of the whole cervical spine. However, atlantoaxial subluxation can paradoxically occur in the presence of an otherwise completely fused neck. Radiographic involvement of the manubriosternal and symphysis pubis articulations may be detected as subchondral erosions, with eventual disruption of the joint often accompanied by adjacent sclerosis and periostitis.

A synovitis within proximal limb joints may result in marginal erosions similar to those seen in rheumatoid arthritis. However, the early metaplasia of the inflammatory synovial tissue to fibrocartilage and bone, together with the associated chronic inflammation within the periarticular tissues, leads to a radiographic appearance of joint destruction paralleled by intra- and extraarticular new bone formation and eventual bony fusion. The smaller synovial joints can radiographically resemble those of rheumatoid disease but are more asymmetric and reveal a greater tendency to "whiskery" marginal and central articular erosions with proliferative new bone formation around the disrupted cortices.

The active skeletal inflammation anywhere tends to promote osteoblastosis so that a positive scintigraphic bone scan may be obtained, even before radiographic changes are apparent. This principle can be applied to the detection of preradiographic sacroiliitis mainly using ^{99m}Tc-polyphosphate as the localizing radionuclide. It should be remembered that multiple areas of active osteitis or postinflammatory osteoblastosis may be detected as "hot spots" in many patients with AS and usually do not indicate metastatic disease.

CLINICAL FEATURES

Ankylosing spondylitis usually presents clinically in a late adolescent or young adult male with symptoms of persistent low and midback pain and stiffness. Although symptoms may be felt in any part of the spine (including the neck), most are localized to the lumbosacral region

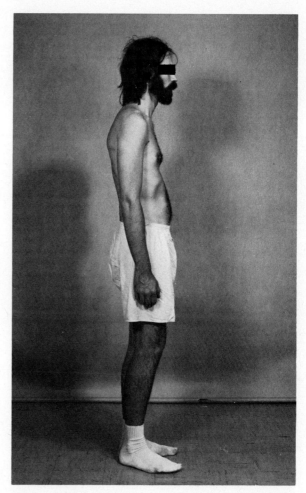

Fig. 2. Position of increased stoop resulting from ankylosing spondylitis.

and posterior pelvis, with exacerbation after prolonged sitting or lying and relative relief following active physical movement. Radiation of the pain down the back of the leg is not uncommon, but is rarely as severe or extensive as in true sciatica. Physical signs may include point tenderness localized directly over the posterior aspects of the sacroiliac joints and a variable degree of tender paraspinal muscle spasm at any level on the posterior torso.

There is very early loss of motion of the entire spine and its articulations, and a variety of clinical maneuvers may be used to detect and measure this. If the inflammatory disease continues and is untreated, a typical sequence of deforming events may slowly develop over the years. This is noted as an early loss of the normal lumbar lordosis, an increase in the thoracic and cervical kyphosis, restriction of chest wall expansion, and a position of increasing stoop with flexion contractions of the hips and knees (Fig. 2). Eventually, complete axial fusion may lead to the appearance of a cachectic man imprisoned in a fixed position of total body flexion, walking with a shuffling gait with his vision involuntarily transfixed to the floor.

Acute iritis may be apparent at the time of initial presentation. More usually, however, past episodes of iritis will result in chronic scarring and depigmentation of the iris, with irregularity of the pupil. Aortic regurgitation may be detected in 1–2 percent of patients with advanced disease. A variable number of patients with longstanding AS may develop secondary systemic amyloidosis.

The disease can present in childhood, when the usual clinical picture is of a little boy with pauciarticular arthritis affecting lower limb large joints and mimicking one form of juvenile rheumatoid arthritis. However, the predominant symptom of backache eventually becomes noticeable, and the child may develop the typical clinical features of adult AS by adolescence. Usually, recurrent episodes of acute iritis or detection of the B27 antigen have clarified the diagnosis by then. Ankylosing spondylitis associated with chronic inflammatory bowel disease appears to be pathologically, radiographically, and clinically identical to the idiopathic form of the disease. In a majority of patients the rheumatic disease follows the overt intestinal disorder, but the presence of colitis may be latent, asymptomatic, or unnoticed until later years.

LABORATORY TESTS

Laboratory tests may reveal a low-grade normocytic anemia of the type associated with any chronic inflammatory disease. An elevated blood sedimentation rate is usual in the early stage of the disease but becomes less reliable as an indicator of disease activity once the pathologic process is well established. A moderate elevation of the serum alkaline phophatase concentration may be noted, and it is probably due to the release of the enzyme from inflamed subchondral bone. Any degree of prolonged immobilization aggravates the osteopenia and may induce hypercalcuria. The vast majority of patients with AS are HLA-B27 positive. In patients who show involvement of peripheral synovial joints, synovial fluid examination reveals no distinctive features. A moderately inflammatory fluid is usually evident, rarely with any evidence of local complement consumption.

DIFFERENTIAL DIAGNOSIS

The diseases discussed here will not include other clinical forms of the seronegative spondyloarthropathies. It may become merely a semantic exercise to distinguish clinically between chronic Reiter's disease, chronic psoriatic arthritis, and AS. Rather, the physician's clinical skills must be focused on recognizing the other types of articular disease that may superficially resemble the spondyloarthropathies.

Low back pain is an extremely common symptom among all segments of the population and may be due to a large variety of pathologic and psychologic factors. The diagnosis of lumbosacral disc disease, fibromyalgia, lumbago, lumbar strain, chronic pelvic disease, or psychosomatic backache in a young individual should only be considered after excluding the possibility of inflammatory spondylitis. Under certain circumstances, it may be necessary to maintain a high index of suspicion for AS while keeping the clinical, radiographic, and scintigraphic features of the illness under observation.

Osteoarthrosis affecting the apophyseal and intervertebral joints of the lumbosacral spine is very common. The clinical setting of an older individual with characteristic radiographic changes usually leads to the correct diagnosis. However, the sacroiliac joint may be involved in the degenerative process, especially in its lower portion where the radiographic loss of joint space and bridging osteophytes may mimic AS. Nevertheless, the upper ligamentous part of the degenerative joint is usually normal. The proliferative degenerative condition of the spine referred to as "benign senile hyperostotic spondylosis" (Forrestier's disease) may result in extensive perispinal hypertrophic new bone formation (see Fig. 6, page 100). Careful inspection of the radiographs, however, reveals intact and discrete vertebral bodies beneath the struts of new bone, and the sacroiliac joints should appear normal.

Postinflammatory fusion of the apophyseal joints in the cervical spine, which can resemble the radiographic appearance of AS, can be seen in two extreme forms of rheumatoid arthritis. First, the apophyseal joints of children with polyarticular rheumatoid arthritis may fuse following persistent synovitis at the site (see Fig. 2A, page 95). Furthermore, radiographic changes in the sacroiliac joints of these children may well reflect the abnormal stresses of altered weight bearing secondary to hip joint disease, as well as a low-grade erosive synovitis arising from the small amount of synovium lining the anterior capsule of the joint. Second, postinflammatory fusion of the cervical spine has been described in elderly chronic rheumatoid arthritics as a terminal radiographic feature of their disease. In both of these situations, the recognition of the underlying rheumatoid arthritis is usually apparent. Although hip and shoulder joint involvement is a common manifestation of AS, it is unusual to detect persistent and deforming synovitis of the smaller peripheral joints in patients with the disease. Occasionally, however, a peripheral joint erosive arthritis dominates the clinical presentation but is rarely as widespread and symmetric as that seen in rheumatoid arthritis. Nevertheless, the axial skeletal changes eventually develop and a careful radiographic and scintigraphic examination of such individuals nearly always reveals subtle degrees of sacroiliitis and spondylitis. Indeed, there is an increasing recognition of middle-aged males who present with seronegative, B27-positive, large peripheral joint polyarthritis, some of whom appear to be suffering from incomplete AS. AS and rheumatoid arthritis can occasionally occur together in the same patient. Under those circumstances, the presence of high-titer rheumatoid factor, rheumatoid nodules, and widespread erosive peripheral joint arthropathy in a patient with obvious AS should suggest the diagnosis of two unrelated rheumatic diseases.

Various conditions affecting the vertebral bodies may superficially resemble the radiographic changes of AS. These include intrabody disc herniations (Schmorl's nodes), reactive vertebral sclerosis following fracture of the end plates, and septic discitis with associated osteomyelitis of adjacent vertebral bodies. Similarly, metabolic bone diseases may manifest in the spine and lead to some diagnostic confusion. One example of this is seen when Paget's disease crosses the sacroiliac joint. Finally, any adult presenting with pain and tenderness in the spine should be scrutinized for the presence of metastatic disease or myelomatosis.

There are several forms of vertebral or paravertebral ossification that occasionally may resemble AS. They include the idiopathic calcification in the posterior longitudinal ligament of the upper cervical spine reported in normal elderly Japanese subjects, and the very florid paravertebral ossification and sacroiliac joint fusion seen in some patients with spinal cord injuries and paraplegia. None of these changes, however, appear to be postinflammatory in nature. A nonspecific and almost certainly noninflammatory sclerosis of the iliac subchondral bone is seen in parous women and is known as *osteitis condensans ilii*. It is a completely innocent condition but may occasionally resemble the sacroiliac sclerosis of AS. Similarly, a painful erosive destruction of the symphysis pubis, osteitis pubis, may be seen in women who have undergone pelvic or urologic surgery (presumably complicated by sepsis). In such individuals, however, the destructive process is sharply localized and the previous genitourinary infective episodes are suspected or proven. Rarely, the arthropathies of familial Mediterranean fever and Behçet's disease may damage large joints, including the sacroiliac articulations. By the time this happens, the systemic nature of the episodic syndrome is obvious.

TREATMENT

At present there is no specific therapy for this disease. The main theme for the management of patients with AS is to maintain the maximum degree of skeletal mobility and to prevent the natural progression toward immobilizing flexion contractures. In the vast majority of patients with AS these objectives are readily achieved, but they require a life-long and regular active exercise program aided by the judicious use of a few carefully selected antiinflammatory drugs.

This exercise program may have to be temporarily modified during very active phases of the inflammatory process. However, complete immobilization and bed rest should always be discouraged because of the risks of accelerated bony fusion, osteopenia, hypercalcuria, and renal stone formation. The importance of maintaining a good posture is crucial and the patients should be trained to hold themselves erect when sitting or standing, and to sleep at night on a firm mattress or board with only one pillow so as to minimize cervical spine flexion. Appropriate active exercises are designed to maintain chest expansion, full extension of all the spine, and a complete range of motion in the proximal joints. The ability to perform these exercises may be facilitated by the prior use of hot showers or cold compresses applied to local areas of painful muscle spasm. Natural sports activities that facilitate spinal extension and joint motion such as walking and swimming should likewise be encouraged.

The principle role of antiinflammatory and analgesic drugs in this disease is to suppress some of the pain and subjective stiffness, thereby facilitating pursuit of the exercise program. There is no evidence that any currently available drug can favorably modify the natural history of AS, although many can evoke a significant degree of symptomatic relief. The most popular and useful antiinflammatory drugs for patients with the disease include phenylbutazone (at a maximum dosage of 400 mg/day), indomethacin (at a maximum dosage of 200 mg/day), and any or all of the newer propionic acid derivatives. For reasons that are unclear, salicylates are less useful in treating this type of arthritis. Nevertheless, a small percentage of patients with AS do benefit from aspirin treatment and it should be considered as one therapeutic option. There is no evidence that corticosteroids or gold are beneficial in controlling the symptoms or modifying the outcome of AS. However, topical corticosteroids may be used in the management of acute iritis and occasionally in the suppression of a persistent peripheral joint synovitis. Very rarely, low-dose radiotherapy directed at the entire spine and sacroiliac joints is necessary to induce a temporary remission in patients with severe disease who are totally unable to tolerate or absorb oral agents. This form of treatment is generally to be avoided due to the demonstrated long-term association with hematologic malignancies.

Some surgical procedures are of great potential benefit to patients with end-stage disease. In particular, total joint replacement has been used even for young patients with completely immobilized hips. Similarly, ankylosed temporomandibular joints can be treated by condylar resection; and heroic cervical or lumbar osteotomies have helped patients with devastatingly severe spinal kyphosis. Severe aortic regurgitation is amenable to valve replacement with little fear of undue postoperative complications.

Although not curable, AS is one of the most rehabilitatible of all the chronic rheumatic diseases. Given the appropriate effort in patient education, a well-designed exercise program, and the use of carefully selected antiinflammatory drugs, it is possible to restore the vast majority of patients to their normal lifestyles.

REFERENCES

Ball J: Heberden Oration, 1970: Enthesopathy of rheumatoid and ankylosing spondylitis. Ann Rheum Dis 30:213, 1971

Bluestone R, Pearson CM: Ankylosing spondylitis and Reiter's syndrome: Their interrelationship and association with HLA B27, in Stollerman G (ed): Advances in Internal Medicine. Chicago, Year Book, 1977

Brewerton DA, Hart FD, Nicholls A, Caffrey M, James DCO, Sturrock RD: Ankylosing spondylitis and HL-A 27. Lancet 1:904, 1973

Calin A, Fries JF: Striking prevalence of ankylosing spondylitis in healthy W27 positive males and females. N Engl J Med 293:835, 1975

Mason RM, Murray RS, Oates JK, Young AC: Prostatitis and ankylosing spondylitis. Br Med J 1:748, 1958

Paronen I: Reiter's disease. A study of 344 cases observed in Finland. Acta Med Scand [Suppl] 131, 1948

Patton D, Woolfenden J: Radionuclide bone scanning in diseases of the spine. Radiogr Clin North Am 15:177, 1977

Ramer S, Bluestone R: Colitic arthropathies. Postgrad Med 61:141, 1977

Resnick D, Niwayama G: On the nature and significance of bony proliferation in "rheumatoid variant" disorders. Am J Roentgenol 129:275, 1977

Resnick D, Niwayama G, Goergen TG: Comparison of radiographic abnormalities of the sacroiliac joint in degenerative disease and ankylosing spondylitis. Am J Roentgenol 128:189, 1977

Romanus R, Ydén S: Destructive and ossifying spondylitic changes in rheumatoid ankylosing spondylitis (pelvo-spondylitis ossificans). Acta Orthop Scand 22:88, 1952

Schaller JG, Hanson V (ed): Proceedings of the First ARA Conference on the Rheumatic Diseases of Childhood. Arthritis Rheum [Suppl] 20:145, 1977

Schlosstein L, Terasaki PI, Bluestone R, Pearson CM: High association of an HL-A antigen, W27, with ankylosing spondylitis. N Engl J Med 288:704, 1973

Wright V, Moll JMH: Seronegative Polyarthritis. New York, North-Holland, 1976

JUVENILE RHEUMATOID ARTHRITIS

John Baum

Juvenile rheumatoid arthritis (JRA) is persistent (longer than 6 weeks) arthritis of unknown etiology appearing in a child. It is no longer considered a single disease, and today we recognize three types. All eventually show arthritis as the major manifestation but differ in type of onset (the first 6 months of disease), course, prognosis, and some laboratory features. An arbitrary upper age limit of 16 years is often used to separate childhood-onset from adult-onset arthritis. This distinction is clearly artificial since there are a number of reports of the juvenile form with systemic onset starting in the late teens and twenties. Puberty has no relationship to or effect on the onset (or course) of JRA.

EPIDEMIOLOGY

The epidemiology of JRA has not been well defined. There are a number of estimates based on surveys of diseases in children and surveys of the relative frequency of JRA as compared to adult rheumatiod arthritis. In the United States the frequency of JRA is approximately 1/1000 children under age 16. Allowing for undiscovered cases, the total U.S. population of JRA is estimated to be about 100,000–150,000.

Although adult rheumatoid arthritis seems to have the same frequency in many parts of the world, there are relatively fewer cases of JRA among oriental populations in the United States and among children in Japan. Studies in Hawaii and Vancouver, B.C., Canada, have also confirmed the rarity of JRA in oriental populations.

CLINICAL TYPES
Systemic

In the first type of JRA, systemic features precede the onset of arthritis. Although there is a peak onset at about age 2, patients with this systemic type continue to be seen throughout childhood, with girls and boys affected equally. The most striking presenting feature of the systemic type is fever. Although the fever may occasionally be as high as 105°F, as a rule the elevations are about 102°–103°F. There is usually a daily spike in the late afternoon, returning to normal by morning. Less often the spikes are bimodal, occurring both in the morning and afternoon. The characteristic feature of the fever is a daily return to normal levels.

A rash often described by parents as reminiscent of measles frequently accompanies the fever. The individual lesions are usually nonpruritic, frequently have a pale center, and often are coalescent. Most commonly, the rash appears on the chest and on the back of the neck, thighs, and upper arms. Involvement of the skin of the hands and feet is rare. The rash may be further elicited by scratching near the affected area or is brought out by a hot bath.

Lymphadenopathy, especially markedly enlarged axillary nodes, is another important sign. Splenomegaly and, less commonly, hepatomegaly are other features of the systemic illness. This phase of the disease can sometimes antedate any joint manifestation by months and occasionally years. Generally, as the joint involvement becomes more prominent the systemic features diminish. As in the adult, morning stiffness can be as prominent and disabling as the joint disease.

Pauciarticular (Oligoarticular)

Pauciarticular (or oligoarticular) arthritis refers to that subtype of JRA in which four or fewer joints are involved. This is the most frequent in our experience and constitutes 40–50 percent of all JRA cases. The pauciarticular type, which also seems to have its peak onset at about 2 years of age, has a female predominance, especially at this age of onset. The knee is the most common site when a single joint is involved. There may also be involvement of one knee and ankle or both knees and ankles. Although small joints are infrequently involved, unusual combinations (e.g., a knee and one proximal interphalangeal joint in the hand) can be seen. Asymmetry is characteristic; for example, often a knee and the opposite ankle are symptomatic. Fever and rash are not considered part of this subtype. Although the pauciarticular form has a greater frequency of remission than the other forms, there may be physical residua.

An important feature of pauciarticular athritis is the frequent appearance of chronic uveitis, most often in females with onset under 4 years of age. In one study, up to one-quarter of the patients with pauciarticular disease had uveitis, particularly those with antinuclear antibody present in their blood. Because of this association it is customary to recommend ophthalmologic examinations in this group of children three to four times a year. A routine ophthalmoscopic examination will not pick up the early appearance of cells in the anterior chamber, for this requires slit lamp examination.

Children with monarticular arthritis of the knee can develop two types of complication. With inflammation involving a single joint, almost always the knee, there is an increased blood supply to this area, causing over-growth of the leg. In most cases a lift on the opposite shoe is useful and surgery has rarely been required. The second problem is the development of demineralization in the bones around an involved joint. Children so afflicted may during play or athletics fall and fracture either the femur or the tibia on the side with the monarticular arthritis.

Polyarticular

Polyarticular disease is the form closest to that seen in adults. The older the child at onset the more this subtype of disease resembles the adult form, although the joint manifestations are still not identical to those seen in the adult.

Regardless of the type of onset, when the hand is involved in JRA the most marked changes are usually in the proximal interphalangeal joint. These produce a ''spindling'' or fusiform swelling of the fingers. The distal interphalangeal joints are more rarely involved. The metacarpophalangeal joints are involved about as often as in the adult. With progression of disease in the hands, the fingers of adult patients tend to go into ulnar deviation. In children, however, the fingers usually are straight with a tendency to develop some degree of flexion contracture so that there is a clawlike appearance of the hand. Wrist involvement in the child tends to destroy the growth centers and cause fusion of the carpal bones. As in the adult, minor degrees of flexion contracture of the elbow can be present even with minimal inflammatory involvement noted in the elbow joint.

Hip involvement is often a major problem with children. The involvement itself may be of two types: In some, the major type is similar to that seen in ankylosing spondylitis, where stiffness and decreased mobility is the most disabling feature of the disease. In most, however, the disease is similar to that seen in the adults, with joint destruction, movement of the hips restricted by pain, and destruction and flattening of the femoral head. There is also more often involvement of the cervical spine, usually presenting first as neck pain and restriction of motion. About 50 percent of these children will eventually have some cervical spine involvement.

Micrognathia due to interference with growth of the ramus of the jaw may be another prominent feature seen in polyarticular JRA, especially in children in whom the disease starts before 6 years of age. It is most frequently seen in those children whose illness started as systemic then became polyarticular disease. Restriction in growth and subsequent lack of height appears to be related to the degree of inflammatory activity. As originally reported by Still, this is most commonly seen in those children with systemic onset.

Unlike adult rheumatoid arthritis, in which rheumatoid factors are usually present, there is no single laboratory test that can be used to confirm the presence of JRA if rheumatoid factor is not present. Thus, differential diagnosis largely rests on careful attention to history and the elimination of all other possible causes of arthritis in children.

LABORATORY AND X-RAY CHANGES

The major laboratory and clinical findings in the three types of JRA are listed in Table 1. The white blood cell count is frequently elevated and indeed can be extremely high, with values as high as 50,000–60,000/mm^3 in children with systemic onset. Chronic anemia, a frequent accompaniment of JRA and more marked in the systemic and polyarticular forms, is usually normochromic, normocytic accompanied by a low serum iron and iron-binding capacity. Sometimes part of the anemia is due to bleeding secondary to aspirin therapy. In making the differential diagnosis between inflammatory arthritis and trauma—which must always be considered in the differential diagnosis of monarticular arthritis—the erythrocyte sedimentation rate is of particular value. Even with pauciarticular disease, the sedimentation rate is frequently elevated, often markedly so, with only slight evidence of joint activity. The sedimentation rate is, however, occasionally normal in the face of active joint involvement.

Tests for autoantibodies are rarely of value. Rheumatoid factors are rarely present except in children with polyarticular disease onset, and even then they are likely to be present only in the older child. Antinuclear antibody, rarely found in systemic and polyarticular disease, is more frequent in the pauciarticular form and may correlate with the development of chronic uveitis.

Immunoglobulin levels and serum complement were studied in a group of children with JRA and compared to normal controls. When the comparison was made, dividing the children according to the mode of onset of disease as well as the course, higher IgA levels were found in children whose onset was polyarticular. If children with systemic or monarticular onset went on to polyarticular involvement elevated IgA levels were again seen in those children. When the entire group was divided into those children who had active disease and those whose disease was inactive, active disease was characterized by higher levels of IgA but there were also elevations of IgG. It

Table 1
Laboratory Features of Juvenile Rheumatoid Arthritis

Type of JRA	ESR	WBC	Hb	RF	ANA
Systemic	↑ ↑ ↑	↑ ↑ ↑	↓ ↓ ↓	0̄	0̄
Pauciarticular	↑	→	↓	±	+(≈25%)
Polyarticular	↑ ↑	↑	↓ ↓	+(≈30%)	±

Abbreviations: ESR, erythrocyte sedimentation rate; WBC, white blood count; Hb, hemoglobin; RF, rheumatoid factors; ANA, antinuclear antibodies.

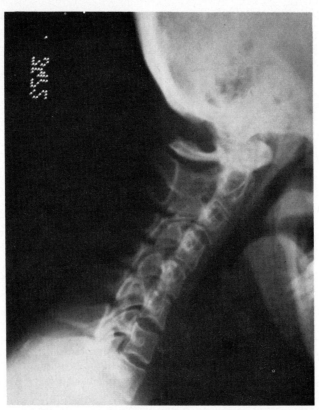

Fig. 1.   Typical x-ray film of the cervical spine in JRA. There is loss of the normal curve in flexion
(straightening of cervical spine) and fusion of C2 and C3.

appears from such data that elevated levels of IgA in children reflect increased disease activity.

Early in the course of arthritis, no specific joint changes are seen. Soft tissue swelling and osteoporosis appear within weeks of the onset of joint activity. Although periosteal new bone formation adjacent to involved joints is an early finding, it is not seen with monarticular arthritis but only with polyarticular involvement. With progress of the disease, cartilage destruction as measured by narrowing of joint space appears, then bone destruction and, subsequently, ankylosis. Bony ankylosis is a late manifestation. Another problem that can be detected on the x-ray film is subluxation, which can be seen in the hips, knees, and cervical spine.

Findings on roentgenologic examination of the cervical spine range from early straightening of the normal curvature through complete fusion of all cervical vertebrae. The earliest radiologic change seen is demineralization. Subluxation of vertebrae, especially at the atlantoaxial joint, may also occur. The most common roentgenographic manifestation, virtually pathognomonic for juvenile arthritis, is the fusion of the bodies of C₂ and C₃ (Fig. 1).

PATHOLOGY

Synovial tissue obtained by biopsy generally shows nonspecific synovitis. IgG has been demonstrated in the plasma cells of the infiltrate.

Bywaters has reported that there is no great difference in the appearance of the synovitis in the juvenile form of the disease, as compared to the adult. However, the much thicker hyaline cartilage in children protects the destruction of the bone to a greater degree than is possible in adults. The erosions are also more likely to be marginal. Periostitis close to the joint is secondary in inflammation raising the periostium and is more common in children. Fibrous ankylosis is more likely to occur in the child than in the adult and is most frequently seen in the hips and knees. The synovitis appears to be less severe in patients with monarticular disease than in those with polyarticular disease.

PROGNOSIS

In one analysis of the literature it was found that at any given time of examination between 5 and 15 years after onset, 30–50 percent of children have grossly active disease and 70–90 percent of patients are in class I–II functional status. Thus, in comparison to studies that have been reported on the prognosis of adult rheumatoid arthritis, children seem to fare better.

As in many chronic diseases, there is a somewhat increased frequency of death in JRA as compared to normals. What is of interest is that the death rate in JRA is four times as high in Europe as it is in the United States and the major cause of death there is renal failure secondary to amyloidosis, while in the United States the most frequent cause of death is infection. The infections are often related to the use of high-dose corticosteroid therapy.

The reason for this discrepancy and for the high frequency of secondary amyloidosis in several European areas (Poland, England, Germany, and Scandinavia) is unknown.

DIFFERENTIAL DIAGNOSIS

Differential diagnosis in the early stages of JRA is often difficult. The involvement of the joints in rheumatic fever follows a typical migratory pattern, more frequently involving larger rather than the smaller joints. In addition, redness and pain of the involved joints is more striking than in rheumatoid arthritis. The fever is typically persistently elevated, whereas in the systemic form of JRA a daily return to baseline levels after fever spikes is usually seen. Erythema marginatum, which occurs in rheumatic fever, is readily distinguished from the rash of JRA. The most frequent age of onset of JRA is about 2 years whereas rheumatic fever is rare before age 4.

Cardiac involvement in rheumatic fever is usually a prominent feature of that disease, whereas cardiac involvement is a more unusual feature in children with JRA. Acute cardiac enlargement with dilatation and pericarditis can occur in JRA. Endocarditis is not seen. Both can show an elevation of the anti-streptolysin O titer.

The other connective tissue diseases may present problems in the differential diagnosis. Systemic lupus erythematosus in the adolescent, although most strikingly manifested by renal involvement, does occasionally present with joint disease. Laboratory examination may be of assistance. If the fluorescent test for nuclear antibody is available and can be titrated, a high titer (or positive LE preparation) will almost always confirm the presence of systemic lupus erythematosus. Although a positive antinuclear antibody test is seen in pauciarticular disease in about 25 percent of patients, the titer is usually low and the LE preparation is not positive.

Dermatomyositis has as its major manifestation weakness, swelling, and muscle pain. Arthritis can appear but the muscle signs are decidedly more prominent. Children often show as the sole skin manifestation a heliotrope rash on the upper eyelids.

Henoch-Schonlein purpura occasionally includes arthritis involving the lower extremities. This is overshadowed by the typically purpuric rash over the buttocks and lower legs with edema. Hematuria may also be seen, and it is not present in JRA.

Ankylosing spondylitis may present in adolescence and is initially indistinguishable from JRA. The spinal involvement appears after the peripheral manifestations and may not present until the late teens or early twenties. Adolescent boys presenting with pauciarticular disease of the lower extremities or with the presentation of "sausage toes" should be studied for the presence of HLA-B27. "Sausage toes" is a diffuse swelling of the involved toe with purplish appearance.

Monarticular arthritis may be a medical emergency since it can represent acute septic arthritis. In more than 90 percent of cases in a child septic arthritis occurs in a single joint. Although fever is often present, the child may be afebrile. The white blood cell count and differential also may not be helpful diagnostically since there may be an elevation and a shift to the left with monarticular JRA. A history of trauma is often elicited in the presence of monarticular disease but should not be too quickly accepted as a cause of an acute effusion. Because septic arthritis is rapidly destructive, joint aspiration and examination of the fluid should be accomplished promptly. Although grossly purulent synovial fluid usually indicates septic arthritis, a high white cell count may also be found in JRA. Therefore, a gram stain and culture should be done immediately.

Traumatic synovitis, by definition, is inflammation of a joint due to direct trauma. Although the physician is often given a history of trauma, it is sometimes difficult to be sure of the relationship to the appearance of the effusion. We have frequently seen monarticular arthritis supposedly brought on by trauma. The absence of any systemic signs of disease, e.g., a normal sedimentation rate, and evidence as well as history of local trauma will be of great help in making the correct diagnosis. If there is any doubt, the joint should be aspirated. A traumatic joint may be grossly bloodly but usually will show viscous fluid with a white cell count of not more than several hundred cells, most of which are mononuclear.

Although there are several syndromes of nonspecific extremity and joint pain the only one that may be a problem in the differential diagnosis of JRA is one involving the hip. Nonspecific synovitis of the hip is seen in equal numbers in males and females and is characterized by pain in one hip with painful limitation of motion, occasionally a slight fever, occasionally a slight increase in the sedimentation rate, negative x-ray films, and a total course of about 1 week.

Nonspecific pain in the legs, sometimes called "growing pains," thought by some to be a distinct entity, presents as a complaint of night pain without any evidence of arthritis.

THERAPY

The basic therapy of JRA is aspirin. Since JRA is an inflammatory disease, the first objective is to decrease inflammation and the second to relieve pain. Pain is not a major complaint in children. The antiinflammatory effects of aspirin are probably only reached when maximum tolerated dosages are given. In children, this maximal dose ranges between 80 and 120 mg/kg. Side effects may occur before an antiinflammatory dose can be reached. Tinnitus is the most common side effect, although gastrointestinal upset is also frequent. Hepatotoxicity has recently been reported as a rare side effect of aspirin therapy. The symptoms are nausea, vomiting and anorexia. However, mild elevations of the SGOT and SGPT, seen more frequently, do not require discontinuance of aspirin. The appearance of nasal polyps or mild bleeding is rare. To avoid gastric irritation parents must be warned

(Ⓧ) Prednisone

that aspirin should never be given on an empty stomach but preferably with meals or, if a nighttime dose is used, with milk or an antacid. For convenience, it is best given four times a day; that is, with meals and at bedtime. If taken consistently, a satisfactory and persistent level can be achieved. If the patient appears to be fully compliant, taking a maximum dose with a minimal therapeutic response, a salicylate level should be drawn. If the level is not 20–25 mg/dl, it is clear that a satisfactory antiinflammatory effect cannot be achieved in that particular child. In this event, there are a limited number of other nonsteroidal antiinflammatory drugs that can be used.

Apart from exacerbations requiring increases in aspirin or the use of another antiinflammatory drug, another difficult decision involves when to discontinue therapy after a period of quiescence of the disease. No controlled studies have been done to establish whether aspirin has a prophylactic effect and thereby diminishes the frequency of recurrences. Nevertheless, when it appears that the disease has been inactive for 3 months or longer, the full dose should be gradually reduced and eventually discontinued over a period of approximately 1–2 months.

Tolmetin, one of the newer analgesic antiinflammatory drugs, is the only one of the newer drugs that has thus far been approved by the FDA for use in children in the treatment of JRA. It has been tested in double-blind and long-term studies of children with JRA at doses up to 30 mg/kg and its effectiveness seems to be about that of aspirin. Its side effects are probably slightly less and it is apparently better tolerated at higher doses than is aspirin. One interesting point noted with the use of this drug is the absence of any hepatotoxicity.

Indomethacin has been used extensively in Europe and to a limited degree in the United States. Its present limitation to adult use is due to problems reported early in its use for JRA, some of which may not have been related to the drug or may have been due to excessive dosage.

Phenylbutazone may be effective but is also not recommended because of its possible effects on bone marrow. When pain is an important feature of the disease, either due to deformities or severe erosive changes, pure analgesics such as codeine may on rare occasions be added to the medication regimen. A drug such as acetaminophen should *not* be used as the basic treatment for JRA, for while this drug is an analgesic it is not antiinflammatory.

If morning stiffness is a problem it can be treated either by adding a nonsteroidal antiinflammatory agent at night, or, if this does not succeed, by administering 2.5–5 mg of prednisone. These should be given in the form of a single bedtime dose. Another method of reducing morning stiffness recently described is to have the child sleep on his bed in a sleeping bag.

Corticosteroids can also be used in the treatment of JRA, but only in those few children in whom nonsteroidal antiinflammatory drugs have not been effective and who are not responding well to the long-term therapy discussed below. Prednisone is almost exclusively preferred since it can be used more easily in small children when low doses are desired. Dosages above 2 mg/m³ are said to inhibit growth. Alternate day steroids will not inhibit growth but are unlikely to control the disease.

Steroid

If steroids are needed for control of disease, the child should be started on 2.5 mg of prednisone twice a day. The dose can be slowly raised but should be kept below a total of 10 mg/day if possible. Once a child is started on a steroid one must attempt to reduce and eventually eliminate it; 1-mg prednisone tablets can be used to reduce the dose. For example, to reduce from 7.5 mg/day it is probably better to change from the 5-mg tablets to 1-mg tablets, and the next reduction would be to 6 mg (2 mg tid), i.e., about a 1-mg reduction from the daily dose at weekly or 2-week intervals.

Intraarticular steroids are occasionally used in the treatment of pauciarticular or monarticular arthritis. If frequent injections are needed (i.e., as often as once every 2–3 weeks), steroids should probably not be used.

For long-term therapy several drugs are available. Gold is effective in JRA. The drug is given by intramuscular injection, 25 mg/week, for a total course of about 500 mg. If the child responds to this therapy, subsequent injections can be given at longer intervals (every 2–4 weeks). Treatment with gold should be followed by blood counts and urinalysis twice monthly. The appearance of a drop in the white cell count or of protein in the urine is reason to stop therapy. If a pruritic rash appears the gold should also be discontinued, but once the rash disappears the gold can be restarted. If the rash reappears again, therapy should not be continued.

Antimalarials such as chloroquine or hydroxychloroquin continue to be used by some rheumatologists in place of gold. The long-term effect, however, with deposition of the drug in pigmented tissue of the retina, is a drawback since this can eventually lead to loss of vision. If this drug is to be used on a regular basis, the child must be followed with regular ophthalmologic examination since early changes are reversible.

Penicillamine is a relatively new drug proposed for the treatment of JRA. It has been used in Europe in place of gold in the treatment of children, and good results have been reported. An advantage is that this drug can be given orally. In adults its side effects are reported to be not as severe as those seen with gold. However, the side effects of penicillamine that have been reported to date include severe depression of the bone marrow as well as Goodpasture's syndrome, both of which are severe enough to mitigate against its use except in special circumstances.

Immunosuppressive drugs have occasionally been given in the treatment of patients with severe JRA; however, the risks entailed with these drugs restrict their use to the very rare patient with severe, unremitting disease.

In adults, synovectomy has been a popular operation for rheumatoid arthritis. The long-range results, however, have not been good and it is doubtful that synovectomy will have any major role in the treatment of this disease in children. The replacement joint protheses that have recently come into extensive use in the treatment of adult arthritis have been shown to be of some benefit in certain children. Those with severe hip disease in whom maximum growth potential has been achieved are candidates for this type of therapy.

Physical therapy plays a major role in the treatment of children with JRA and should be begun from the time they are first seen. A formal program performed exclusively by physical therapists is usually not necessary since most parents can be taught appropriate exercises. Parents acquire proper techniques more readily, however, when this instruction is first given by a therapist who shows them step by step what is to be done. The exercises are directed mostly at maintaining muscle strength and preventing contractures. Periodic assessment by a physical therapist is appropriate to reinforce and to correct therapy and to revise therapeutic goals and procedures. In addition to maintaining a normal pattern of regular activity—walking, stair climbing, and some athletics—these children should be encouraged to swim as much as possible.

REFERENCES

Ansell BM (ed): Rheumatic Diseases in Childhood. Clinics in Rheumatic Diseases. 2. Philadelphia, Saunders, 1976

Brewer EJ Jr: Juvenile Rheumatoid Arthritis. Philadelphia, Saunders, 1970

Schaller JG, Hanson V (eds): Proceedings on the First ARA Conference in Rheumatic Diseases of Childhood. Arthritis Rheum [Suppl] 20:145, 1977

PSORIATIC ARTHRITIS

Evelyn V. Hess
and Beverly A. Carpenter

The association between psoriasis and arthritis was first noted over 100 years ago. Since then, there has been controversy whether this is a coincidental association of arthrits with psoriasis or a distinct entity of psoriatic arthritis. Data from epidemiologic, radiographic, familial, and genetic studies substantiate psoriatic arthritis as a distinct clinical entity. Psoriasis affects 1–2 percent of the general population. Psoriatic arthritis occurs in approximately 7 percent of psoriatics. The male to female ratio is 1:1.04, similar to psoriasis, but different from the 1:3 ratio in rheumatoid arthritis. In 75 percent of men and 68 percent of women the onset of psoriasis precedes the manifestations of arthritis. In 15–25 percent joint manifestations may precede skin involvement. The age of onset of joint symptoms ranges from 20 to 50 years (mean 27 ± 11 years for females and 29 ± 12 years for males). A few cases of psoriatic arthritis have been reported in childhood.

CLINICAL GROUPS

Psoriatic arthritis has a number of clinical presentations. The following five groups have been defined:

1. Predominantly distal interphalangeal (DIP) joint involvement with almost all DIP joints involved. Dystrophic psoriatic nail changes commonly occur with DIP involvement. Although considered the "classic" presentation of psoriatic arthritis, this group represents only 5 percent of cases of psoriatic arthritis.

2. Arthritis mutilans, a severe deforming arthritis involving multiple small joints of the hands and feet. This is a progressive arthritis characterized by periarticular erosions, osteolysis, and ankylosis often resulting in marked functional impairment. Sacroiliac and spinal joint involvement occurs frequently. It is associated with more severe psoriasis and the males have a higher incidence of genital skin involvement. Arthritis mutilans occurs in 5 percent of psoriatic arthritis cases (Fig. 1).

3. Peripheral joint involvement simulating rheumatoid arthritis. This is a symmetric polyarthritis, commoner in females, with negative rheumatoid factor tests. It accounts for approximately 15 percent of cases of psoriatic arthritis.

4. An asymmetric monoarticular or oligoarticular arthritis. Single joints or a few DIP, proximal interphalangeal (PIP), metacarpal, and metatarsophalangeal joints are involved. This group accounts for approximately 70 percent of cases of psoriatic arthritis.

5. Predominantly spinal involvement with sacroiliitis and spondylitis. These patients, in contrast to those with idiopathic ankylosing spondylitis, may have few or absent low back symptoms. Sacroiliitis or spondylitis may be noted only on routine x-rays. Peripheral joints may or may not be involved. This group represents 5 percent of psoriatic arthritis cases.

It should be noted that the occurrence of spondylitis in psoriatic arthritis has been observed to be as high as 57 percent in screening x-ray studies. It is becoming increasingly evident that spondylitis is commoner in psoriatic arthritis and in psoriasis than previously noted.

SYMPTOMS AND SIGNS

Psoriatic arthritis is inflammatory in type and can be acute or insidious in onset. The most frequent initial sites of involvement are the DIP and PIP joints of the hands. The symptoms are pain and swelling with or without erythema involving the small joints of the hands and feet, wrists, knees, and ankles. Synovial proliferation does occur but is not as striking as the boggy synovitis in rheumatoid arthritis. "Sausage-shaped" fingers and toes may be present (Fig. 2). Dystrophic psoriatic nail changes occur in 80 percent of cases of psoriatic arthritis as opposed to 30 percent of cases of uncomplicated psoriasis. The nail changes, characterized by pitting and splitting, occur more commonly with extensive DIP joint involvement. In many cases, the skin changes may be occult and patients are unaware that they even have psoriasis. Therefore, in asymmetric polyarthritis, the clinician should search carefully for classic psoriasis of elbows, knees, and other sites such as the intergluteal, submammary, axillary, umbilical, genital, and perineal areas. A careful family history for psoriasis and arthritis should be obtained, as many cases are familial.

Other less well-known features observed in psoriatic arthritis include the following: (1) Temporomandibular joint involvement similar to that in rheumatoid arthritis

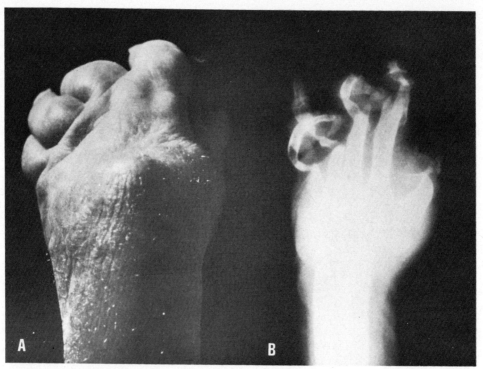

Fig. 1.   **A.** Arthritis mutilans of the hand with multiple deformities. **B.** X-ray of the hand with extensive destruction of all joints.

may be seen. There is stiffness and pain with radiographic changes. (2) There may be cervical spine involvement, which is also present in rheumatoid arthritis and ankylosing spondylitis. In one series of patients with deforming psoriatic arthritis, 30 percent had cervical spine disease. Narrowing and marginal sclerosis of the apophyseal joints, subluxation of atlantoaxial joints accompanied by neck pain, and neurologic deficits have

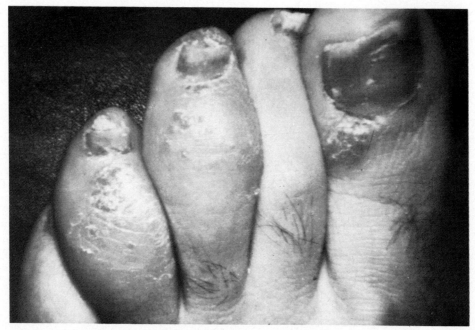

Fig. 2.   Psoriatic lesions of the first, third, and fourth toes with psoriatic arthritis of the interphalangeal joints and "sausage-shaped" swelling. (Reproduced from the Dermatologic Teaching Slide Series by permission of the American Academy of Dermatology.)

been reported in severe cases. Careful cervical spine and neurologic examinations must be performed in all patients with psoriatic arthritis. (3) In one series ocular involvement was noted in 32 percent of patients with psoriatic arthritis. Conjunctivitis was the commonest lesion, occuring in 19.6 percent, and was twice as frequent as in uncomplicated psoriasis. Iritis, episcleritis, and keratoconjunctivitis sicca were also observed.

LABORATORY FINDINGS

There are no pathognomonic diagnostic tests for psoriatic arthritis. The most important parameters for diagnosis are the absence of rheumatoid nodules and rheumatoid factor coupled with the appropriate clinical and radiologic manifestations (Table 1).

RADIOLOGY

The radiologic features of peripheral psoriatic arthritis reflect the clinical manifestations in that they are asymmetric and involve mainly the small joints of the hands and feet. The progressive radiologic changes are indicative of an inflammatory arthritis accompanied by erosions, bone resorption, destruction, and eventual ankyloses. Early in the course of disease, there may be only juxtaarticular soft tissue swelling, as in rheumatoid arthritis. Osteoporosis is not a feature of psoriatic arthritis. The radiologic changes most often seen in the five groups of psoriatic arthritis are as follows:

1. ''whittling'' of the phalanges, metacarpals, and metatarsals
2. the classic ''pencil-in-cup'' deformity, with the proximal ends of the phalanges and metacarpals ''cupped,'' and the opposing phalange, metacarpal, or metatarsal whittled (Fig. 1B)
3. asymmetric erosions of the DIP and PIP joints with relative sparing of the metacarpal, phalangeal, and metatarsophalangeal joints
4. ankylosis of phalanges, metacarpals, and metatarsals
5. acroosteolysis of the terminal phalanges
6. sacroiliitis and spondylitis

The radiologic changes of psoriatic sacroiliitis and spondylitis are similar to those of ankylosing spondylitis. A straight spine and squared vertebrae are less common in psoriatic spondylitis. Destruction of adjacent intervertebral surfaces with disc calcification can occur. Psoriatic sacroiliitis shares many features with Reiter's syndrome: (1) the asymmetry of sacroiliac changes; (2) the erosions, destruction, and sclerosis of sacroiliac joint margins but less frequent involvement of symphysis pubis, iliac crest, ischial tuberosities, spinous and transverse processes and apophyseal joints; and (3) less commonly, the progression from sacroiliac joints upward to the cervical spine.

DIFFERENTIAL DIAGNOSIS

Reiter's syndrome may have similar cutaneous lesions and nail changes. It occurs predominantly in men. Large joints are more often affected than small joints, and the lower limb is more often involved than the upper. Reiter's syndrome and psoriasis may have ocular manifestations. The incidence of HLA-B27 positivity is higher

Table 1
Laboratory Profile in Psoriatic Arthritis

Blood
  Negative rheumatoid factor
  Negative antinuclear factor
  Normal complement
  Anemia; normocytic
  Leukocytosis
  Elevated sedimentation rate
  Hyperuricemia (10–20%)
Synovial fluid
  Inflammatory exudate; type II fluid
Synovial pathology
  Nonspecific inflammatory changes with increased fibrous
   tissue

in Reiter's than in psoriatic arthritis. It may be very difficult to differentiate radiographic findings in the sacroiliac joints and spine in these two diseases. Heel spurs are often present in Reiter's syndrome.

Ankylosing spondylitis lacks cutaneous manifestations. The sex distribution is similar; the joint distribution is as in Reiter's syndrome.

The arthritis associated with inflammatory bowel disease is similar, but the skin manifestations of psoriasis and the bowel manifestations of inflammatory bowel disease are helpful distinguishing factors.

Rheumatoid arthritis at times is difficult to distinguish from psoriatic arthritis. The latter, however, lacks nodules and rheumatoid factor, has typical psoriatic skin lesions, and shows a tendency to more asymmetric involvement of other joints. Typical radiologic changes of psoriatic arthritis should help to differentiate the two diseases.

Erosive osteoarthritis may mimic peripheral asymmetric psoriatic polyarthritis involving the DIP and PIP joints. The onset occurs mostly after 50 years of age and Heberden's and Bouchard's nodes are usually present in erosive osteoarthritis.

The hyperuricemia associated with severe psoriasis may suggest gout when a patient develops acute monarthritis, especially of the big toe. The skin lesions of psoriasis and the clinical course should distinguish these two entities.

Behçet's syndrome can be distinguished by mucous membrane manifestations.

ETIOLOGY AND PATHOGENESIS

Psoriasis is a disease of epidermal hyperplasia, the etiology of which is not known. A genetic predisposition to psoriasis is supported by familial aggregation of psoriasis in the absence of spouse aggregation. The mode of inheritance of psoriasis is multifactorial, involving both genetic and environmental factors.

Psoriasis is associated with histocompatibility antigens HLA-B13 and HLA-BW17. Individuals bearing either of these antigens are at four to five times higher risk of developing psoriasis than other individuals. The incidence of psoriasis in the general population is 2 percent and rises to approximately 6 percent in people with either

HLA-B13 or HLA-BW17. In some studies from France and the United States, HLA-BW38 (part of w16) is associated with psoriasis significantly above the control population; this was not so in a Scandanavian study. One gene linked with the HLA-B locus cannot entirely explain the inheritance of psoriasis. Other gene relationships as well as environmental factors may be necessary to support the theory of a multifactorial mode of inheritance.

In an extensive study to determine the familial occurrence of psoriatic arthritis, 12.5 percent of 88 probands had at least 1 relative with confirmed psoriatic arthritis. The overall prevalence of psoriatic arthritis in first-degree relatives of probands with psoriatic arthritis was 5.5 percent. In first-degree relatives of patients with psoriatic arthritis, the prevalence of sacroiliitis and spondylitis, not necesarily associated with psoriasis, increased to 7.4 percent and 6.3 percent, respectively. In these first-degree relatives and those of other probands with psoriasis uncomplicated by arthritis, the incidence of psoriasis was also increased.

These findings suggest that familial aggregation of peripheral psoriatic arthritis and of psoriasis are due to genetic and environmental factors and that of sacroiliitis is predominately genetic.

The association between psoriatic arthritis and HLA-B27 supports this conclusion. The overall prevalence of HLA-B27 in psoriatic arthritis is 25–30 percent. The presence of sacroiliitis and/or spondylitis accounts for an increased frequency of HLA-B27 positivity. The incidence of HLA-B27 positivity in patients with peripheral psoriatic arthritis without sacroiliitis is insignificant but rises to 64.3 percent in the presence of psoriatic spondylitis and to 50 percent in psoriatic sacroiliitis. The association between HLA-B27 and peripheral psoriatic arthritis is less clear. Some studies have shown that in patients with predominately DIP psoriatic arthritis, there is a significant increase in HLA-B27 positivity. Others have shown either no increase in positivity or a 23 percent positivity in psoriatic arthritis including all peripheral joints. These discrepancies may represent the differences in types of patient populations investigated and the clinical and radiologic criteria used to define psoriatic arthritis.

The Koebner phenomenon is of interest. This reaction is characterized by the capacity to reproduce skin lesions at sites of local injury in approximately one-half the patients with psoriasis. It is speculated that there is a specific enzyme deficiency resulting in a low level of joint fluid hyaluronic acid which increases the vulnerability of the joint to trauma. It is possible that in genetically predisposed individuals trauma and/or other factors may be a stimulus in the expression of psoriasis and/or psoriatic arthritis.

There is scintigraphic evidence that psoriasis and psoriatic arthritis may represent a systemic inflammatory disorder. Using highly sensitive ^{99m}Tc-labeled media, 95 percent of patients with psoriasis but lacking clinical or radiographic evidence of psoriatic arthritis were found to have an abnormal uptake in the joints, usually associated with psoriatic arthritis. This represents an inflammatory process in the involved joints.

It is known that collagen metabolism in psoriatic skin is deranged and that the level of prolyl hydroxylase is four times greater in psoriatic skin than in normal or uninvolved psoriatic skin. There is also evidence that DNA synthesis may be increased in psoriatic skin. ^{99m}Tc-labeled medium preferentially binds to immature collagen. This supports the concept that psoriasis and psoriatic arthritis may represent a spectrum of a generalized collagen disease with varying degrees of clinical expression.

COURSE AND THERAPY

The severity of the arthritis usually parallels the severity of the skin disease. Consequently, conventional therapy of psoriasis with coal tar, ultraviolet light, steroid creams, and ointments is indicated. Mild psoriatic arthritis can adjunctively be controlled with therapeutic doses of aspirin. In cases unresponsive to aspirin, indomethacin, 75–150 mg/day in divided doses, can be given. Gold therapy has given inconsistant results. Antimalarial drugs which may aggravate psoriasis and cause exfoliative dermatitis are contraindicated.

Psoriatic arthritis may have a progressive, severe, and destructive course even with controlled psoriasis. If conventional and antiinflammatory drugs do not control the arthritis, systemic steroids may be tried.

Methotrexate is of value in severe, uncontrolled psoriasis. Methotrexate, azathioprine, and 6-mercaptopurine have been found of benefit in some cases of severe, progressive psoriatic arthritis. These drugs should be used with caution because of their toxic side effects.

Preliminary results suggest that azaribine, an oral antipyrimidine agent, may be of benefit in refractory psoriatic arthritis, but further studies are needed. Azapropazine, a new antiinflammatory agent undergoing clinical trials in Europe and Japan, has been shown to have beneficial effects in psoriatic arthritis.

Physical therapy programs are important supportive measures in the total management of chronic psoriatic arthritis, as they are in any other chronic arthropathy.

Surgical treatment of the chronic deformities may be necessary in some patients.

REFERENCES

Baum J, Hurd E, Lewis D, Ferguson JL, Ziff, M: Treatment of psoriatic arthritis with 6-mercaptopurine. Arthritis Rheum 16:139, 1973

Eastmond CJ, Woodrow JC: The HLA system and the arthropathies associated with psoriasis. Ann Rheum Dis 36:112, 1977

Lassus A, Karvonen J: Reactive arthritis, Reiter's disease and Psoriatic arthritis. Clin Rheum 3:281, 1977

Metzger AL, Morris RI, Bluestone R, Terasaki PI: HL-A W 27 in psoriatic arthropathy. Arthritis Rheum 18:111, 1975

Moll JMH, Wright V: Familial occurrence of psoriatic arthritis. Ann Rheum Dis 32:181, 1973

Moll JMH, Wright V: Psoriatic arthritis. Semin Arthritis Rheum 3:55, 1973

Roberts MET, Wright V, Hill AGS, Mehra AC: Psoriatic arthritis follow-up study. Ann Rheum Dis 3.5:206, 1976

Roux H, Mercier P, Maestracci D, Serratrice G, Sany J, Seignalet J, Serre H: Psoriatic arthritis and HLA antigens. J Rheumatol [Suppl] 3.4:64, 1977

REITER'S SYNDROME

John L. Decker

The most persistent feature of this disease, which predominantly affects young men, is a nonsuppurative polyarthritis that is classically associated with urethritis and conjunctivitis. The cause is unknown and the course varies from mild and transient to an abrupt prostrating illness accompanied by high fever with many joints involved. Relapses after complete recovery are common, whereas other patients evince a chronic course with protracted, mild disease activity.

The syndrome bears the name of Hans Reiter, a German physician who ascribed a case seen in a cavalry officer to a spirochete not found in subsequent cases. The first recognition of the syndrome in the United States (1942) referred to Reiter's report and applied his name to the syndrome although searches of older literature make it clear that, among others, Brodie in England and Launois in France had described it much earlier. In France the disease is called the Fiessinger-Leroy syndrome.

The illness continues to arouse great interest for several reasons. Exogenous, self-replicating agents are regularly invoked to account for the initiation of illnesses such as rheumatoid arthritis and systemic lupus erythematosus; if any of the sterile polyarthritides are caused by an infectious agent, Reiter's syndrome preeminently must be of such origin and yet its cause continues to be a puzzle. The diversity of its manifestations and the unfortunate physician tendency to apply "gun-barrel vision" to his special area of interest—be it inflammed oral mucous membranes, conjunctivitis, nonspecific urethritis, or low back pain—often delay diagnosis and fragment treatment. Finally, Reiter's syndrome appears to be capable of "evolving" into ankylosing spondylitis or psoriatic arthritis, a fact which widens speculations on their unknown causes and makes more piquant the recently recognized high prevalence of the HLA-B27 lymphocyte surface genetic marker in all three.

CLINICAL FEATURES

There is no identifying or specific tag for the syndrome. Current concepts are built upon descriptions of past patients, some of whom exhibited only fragments of the picture. Its manifestations seem to vary both geographically and by patient selection from, for example, venereal disease, rheumatic disease, or ophthalmologic clinics. Thus, as with most diseases, it is not possible to describe its manifestations with unbiased precision.

The illness is a disease of young men, with the male to female ratio in the range of 10–15:1. Juvenile cases, sometimes in families, are being described with increasing frequency. It is uncommon for the disease to appear for the first time beyond 45 years of age.

Typically, the manifestations develop over 1–4 weeks, starting with diarrhea or urethritis, then ocular inflammation, and finally culminating in an asymmetric polyarthritis sometimes accompanied by a dermal eruption. These features may be compressed into a few days, the patient presenting with large joints involved, continuing urethritis, the beginnings of a skin rash, and high fever. Such patients often have a hectic, severe course, resistant to treatment and resulting in weight loss, debilitation, and juxtaarticular osteoporosis. Much more commonly the manifestations are milder and outpatient management is possible.

In Europe, the syndrome often begins with watery diarrhea associated with cramps, usually without blood. This may be of a specific nature, particularly in epidemic situations. The syndrome has been recognized, for example, with wartime epidemics of shigella dysentery; the diarrhea is then followed by a urethritis.

The urinary symptoms are usually those of frequency and burning on micturition with minimal, clear to mucoid penile discharge. Cystitis, often the only finding in the female, is common in men as well. The picture is one of nonspecific urethritis but the presence of gonorrhea does not exclude the diagnosis of Reiter's syndrome; when gonorrhea is present, the purulent discharge responds readily to penicillin and the patient is left with the clear, watery discharge of nonspecific urethritis, a symptom complex which may respond to broad-spectrum antibiotics such as tetracycline. The urethritis is often accompanied by limited perimeatal erosion of the glans penis.

The conjunctivitis is characterized by sensations of ocular irritation and burning, bulbar and palpebral conjunctival injection, and discharge which may be purulent and voluminous but is usually scant. The mildest and most transient of the features, it is the one most often overlooked and most likely to be missing from the triad. Iridocyclitis of the acute, anterior type may be seen but probably in less than one-third of those with ocular inflammation.

Arthritis is asymmetric and tends to involve the large joints of the lower extremity, the ankles and knees. Monarticular presentation is common but not persistent. Usually four to seven joints are asynchronously involved in an attack. Any joint may be involved, including the synarthrodial sacroiliac joints. Peripheral joints swell, are painful whether in motion or at rest, and may show redness and heat. Synovial fluid is of an inflammatory nature, exhibiting primarily polymorphonuclear leukocytes up to roughly 50,000/mm³ and a poor mucin clot. Glucose levels are often substantially lower than those of the blood, and hemolytic complement is increased, a notable finding which is often useful in differential diagnosis.

Much of what is commonly referred to as "arthritis"

is, in fact, not synovitis at all but inflammation of ligamentous and tendinous insertions into bone—enthesopathy of tendons themselves or of the periosteum. These features are so prominent as to encourage experienced clinicians to suggest a diagnosis of Reiter's syndrome in a young man who presents with *none* of the other features. Local findings often noted are tendonitis of the extensor hallucis longus extending well up on the dorsum of the foot, painful enlargement of the insertion of the Achilles tendon into the calcaneus, periostitis of the shaft of the phalanges of one or two toes with the production of a "sausage digit" (see Fig. 1 in the chapter on Static Disabilities of the Foot in the preceding fascicle), focal tenderness in a dime-sized area on the anterior surface of the patella, and throbbing pain and bony tenderness about the lower shins. These features, characteristic but not pathognomonic, raise other possibilities such as gout, gonococcal arthritis, hypertrophyic pulmonary osteoarthropathy, and ankylosing spondylitis.

The musculoskeletal manifestations, coming on 2–3 weeks after the onset of diarrhea or urethritis, may be of limited duration but usually persist for several months before slowly receding. The illness is self-limited and only rarely leaves residua of any significance.

As Reiter's syndrome has become more clearly separated from Neisserian infection, it has become apparent that it is also characterized by a group of mucocutaneous manifestations which together can be considered a fourth feature, converting the triad to a tetrad. The oral mucous membrane of the tongue, cheeks, or palate shows erosions, rarely deep enough to be called an ulcer, and strikingly asymptomatic even upon ingestion of acidic fluids. Histologically these correspond closely to lesions that can be identified in the male urethra by urethroscopy. Similarly, multiple erosions may develop and coalesce on the glans or foreskin of uncircumcized males, again virtually without symptoms. In the circumcized male the lesions are discrete and usually separate from the meatus; they have a central, yellowish papule and a red scaly border. The lesions are referred to as *balanitis circinata*.

Very similar painless lesions, appearing particularly on the weight-bearing aspect of the soles or the palmar skin of the hand, are referred to as *keratoderma blennorrhagica*, a complete misnomer since parakeratosis is more common than hyperkeratosis and blennorrhagica is derived from *blennorrhea*, an antique designation for gonorrhea. The almost waxy, cone-shaped papule of dark yellow or brown with desquamation at its margins looks like a volcanic island, lapped around by white sand and waves as seen from the air. They may coalesce and desquamate into much more impressive lesions measuring centimeters in diameter and they may spread to virtually any place on the body; in intertriginous areas, erosions are more likely than papules. The nails may be involved, either at the base, looking like a mycotic paronychia, or under the leading edge of the nail, where cornified tissue can build up resulting in lifting and sometimes loss of the nail.

Histologically the oral, urethral, and dermal lesions all show microabscesses—focal collections of neutrophilic leukocytes in vacuoles. In the skin, the rete pegs are elongated and hypertrophied and parakeratosis and acanthosis are found. The histologic picture is indistinguishable from that of pustular psoriasis and, clinically, some patients with keratoderma blennorrhagica will, at later times, have unequivocal psoriasis. It is impressive to watch the healing of keratoderma blennorrhagica; even the most severely involved areas, usually the soles and nails, do return to complete normality in time.

Rarely, cardiac lesions, simulating those of ankylosing spondylitis and particularly including conduction defects and nonvalvular, aortic insufficiency, result from Reiter's disease. Even more rarely, a variety of neurologic lesions, both peripheral and central, have been observed.

The laboratory findings are no more diagnostically specific than are the individual clinical features. The sedimentation rate is elevated, some increase in circulating complement activity is often found, and leukocytosis beyond 15,000/mm^3 is rare. Urinalysis may reveal evidence of lower urinary tract disease but smears of urethral discharge or of fluids expressed by prostatic massage will be more telling. These are bacteriologically sterile although coincidental bacterial infection does not exclude Reiter's syndrome.

Radiologic abnormalities are absent in the early course but become more frequent if the illness persists or if films are made during a second or a third relapse. Juxtaarticular osteoporosis and periostitis are the major findings. The latter may be of the whiskery type seen about the iliac crests, the inferior ramus of the pubis, and the ischial tuberosities, or of the circumferential type as laid down about pedal phalanges or the distal tibia. Plantar heel spurs, often soft and feathery in outline and accompanied by erosions in active disease, may be prominent. Sacroiliac joint involvement, usually symmetric but more frequently asymmetric than in early ankylosing spondylitis, is common in relapsing disease; ankylosis may result and some patients go on to vertebral squaring, apophyseal joint disease, and classic ankylosing spondylitis. A few chronic cases have shown extraordinary lateral bridging between vertebral bodies, bridges which began as spurs in midbody.

The disease may be no more than a single 3–6-week episode with no recurrence in as many as one third of patients. The first attack may be much more prolonged, however, with articular and cutaneous manifestations persisting for 4–6 months. In most instances initial attacks do clear but relapses are common, probably occuring in two-thirds of all patients. The relapses often differ from the original attack and may be confined, for example, to iritis or balanitis; they may be characterized by recurrent back pain or heel pain without preceding diarrhea or urethritis. Indeed, these limited patterns or forme fruste may antedate as well as follow the fully expressed syndrome. Recurrences have been observed after prostatic massage or diarrhea induced by antibiotics. After 5–

10 years of such attacks or of persistent problems not clearly discerned as "attacks," examinations done without benefit of historical information would find ankylosing spondylitis in 10–15 percent of patients and psoriatic arthritis in another 5 percent. Follow-up studies suggest that the outlook is less favorable in the epidemic type than in the endemic.

ETIOLOGY

Infectious and genetic factors appear to be intertwined in the cause of Reiter's syndrome. The epidemic form seems to be related to lack of hygienic facilities and bacillary dysentery. In one remarkable outbreak 9 cases appeared aboard a U.S. Naval vessel. Roughly one-half of the large crew developed bacillary dysentery after eating a specific meal; the 9 who developed Reiter's syndrome had all had dysentery. The endemic disease appears to be of venereal origin, commonly follows venereal exposure, is more frequent in port cities, and seems to be associated with promiscuity. Historically difficult to distinguish from gonococcal arthritis, in more recent years it has been ascribed to mycoplasma or pleuropneumonialike organisms and to organisms of the Bedsonia group, the cause of trachoma, lymphogranuloma venereum, and psittacosis, Neither type of organism, however, has been regularly isolated from fresh cases and all efforts to identify a viral cause have failed. It has been suggested that viral penetration with resultant disease might be facilitated by antecedent mucous membrane bacterial infection due, for example, to *Shigella* or gonococcus.

The virtual restriction of a venereal disease to males is based upon unknown factors, perhaps anatomic considerations or, less likely, upon sex hormone regulation of the response to an exogenous agent. Cases may appear in several men after contact with the same, apparently healthy female.

Systematic studies of the families of persons with the disease show no overt Reiter's syndrome but, notably, do show an increased prevalence of ankylosing spondylitis and of psoriasis as compared to similarly ascertained disease in the general population. Such findings are very much in accord with the more recent and most striking demonstration that 75 percent or more of patients with Reiter's syndrome carry the HLA-B27 antigen on their lymphocyte surfaces; this antigen has been identified in only 6–8 percent of comparable normal populations but in 95 percent of patients with ankylosing spondylitis. As expected, the sacroiliitis, ankylosing spondylitis, and anterior uveitis seen in Reiter's syndrome are virtually confined to that portion of patients who are B27 positive. Indeed, it is surprising that, given this genetic feature, such a relatively small proportion of the Reiter's patients develop full-blown spondylitis. It has been suggested that the presence of the antigen makes the patient susceptible to "reactive arthritis" in the wake of bacterial infections not actually invading the articular tissues. In this view, reactive arthritis seen after *Salmonella* or *Yersinia* infection would be comparable to Reiter's syndrome following bacillary dysentery.

The pathogenetic contribution of the lymphocyte antigen to the disease is, in fact, uncertain but it emphasizes the relationship to ankylosing spondylitis and, as indicated earlier (see chapter on Seronegative Spondyloarthropathies), has the effect of expanding our view of Reiter's syndrome by encouraging the study cf HLA-B27–positive individuals who clinically exhibit only portions of the tetrad.

TREATMENT

Since some patients may be seen initially with high fever, purulent urethritis, and a few large joints showing acute synovitis, one must take great pains to exclude septic arthritis and gonoccocal disease. Even when bacterial organisms are not found on smears of the urethral discharge and synovial fluid it may be wise to proceed promptly with penicillin therapy. If fever persists and new joints are involved within the next several days on the drug, a diagnosis of Reiter's syndrome becomes increasingly likely and the antibiotic may be stopped as the results of cultures become available. Some feel that tetracycline will shorten the course of nonspecific urethritis but such drugs have no effect on the musculoskeletal disease.

As a rule, neither the urethritis nor the conjunctivitis require treatment. However, local corticosteroids may be useful in the latter, and if keratitis or uveitis develop systemic steroid therapy should be added.

The arthritis and musculoskeletal features may be intensely symptomatic and are treated with full doses of a nonsteroidal antiinflammatory drug. Traditionally, phenylbutazone or indomethacin have been widely used, but salicylate derivatives or other short-acting antiinflammatory agents are also effective. Corticosteroids appear to have remarkably little effect in some individuals, even at substantial dose levels, and are usually avoided in management. When possible, simple arthrocentesis may result in notable relief of symptoms in the tightly distended joint.

In severe attacks with keratoderma blennorrhagica continuing to produce new lesions and pyrexia persisting over weeks, the administration of methotrexate may be followed by prompt and dramatic relief. Using doses below levels often complicated by mucosal ulceration or leukopenia, one can often achieve improvement which will persist after only 1–2 weeks of medication, thus avoiding the hepatic injury which is a major concern in chronic methotrexate administration. The folic acid antagonist, however, is not an approved drug for use in Reiter's syndrome.

Prophylaxis against subsequent episodes, a worthy objective, has not been subjected to detailed study. Low-dose, chronic tetracycline therapy has been advised. Patients in whom recurrences could be prevented by the use of a condom in sexual intercourse have been described.

REFERENCES

Brewerton DA, Caffrey M, Nicholls A, Walters D, Oates JK, James DCO: Reiter's disease and HL-A27. Lancet 2:996, 1973

Calin A, Fries JF: An "experimental" epidemic of Reiter's syndrome revisited: Follow-up evidence on genetic and environmental factors. Ann Intern Med 84:564, 1976

Hancock JAH: Surface manifestations of Reiter's disease in the male. Br J Vener Dis 36:36, 1960

Lawrence JS: Family survey of Reiter's disease. Br J Vener Dis 50:140, 1974

Sairanen E, Paronen I, Mahonen H: Reiter's syndrome: A follow-up study. Acta Med Scand 185:57, 1969

Weinberger HW, Ropes MW, Kulka JP, Bauer W: Reiter's syndrome, clinical and pathological observations; A long term study of 16 cases. Medicine (Baltimore) 41:35, 1962

Wright V, Moll JMH: Seronegative Polyarthritis. New York, North-Holland, 1976, pp 237–291

ULCERATIVE COLITIS AND ARTHRITIS

Michael J. Reza
and Carl M. Pearson

Ulcerative colitis is a chronic, intermittent inflammatory disease of unknown etiology affecting the large intestinal mucosa and submucosa. As with Crohn's disease, many extraintestinal manifestations may occur, including arthritis, uveitis, a variety of liver disturbances, stomatitis, cutaneous lesions, thromboemboli, and other complications. The arthritis that may accompany ulcerative colitis is of two major types: peripheral and spinal.

PERIPHERAL ARTHRITIS

Peripheral arthritis is an important extraintestinal manifestation of ulcerative colitis occurring in up to 26 percent of patients. The arthritis was first described in detail by Wright and Watkinson, who found evidence of rheumatic symptoms in even a somewhat greater percentage of 269 patients. Although polyarthritis may occur, typical "colitic" arthropathy is an acute, monarticular, and asymmetric lower limb disease.

The arthritis most commonly occurs after bowel disease is evident but occasionally may precede symptomatic colitis. It tends to be acute, episodic, and temporally related to flares in the bowel disease. It generally becomes apparent a short time after the colitis develops, but colitis may be present for as long as 10 years before the first attack of synovitis.

The joints most commonly involved are the ankles and the knees. Asymmetry is the rule, but on occasion a symmetric synovitis mimicking rheumatoid arthritis may occur. When polyarticular, the pattern of spread is often migratory as in rheumatic fever. Attacks occur abruptly, reaching maximum intensity within 24 hours. The duration of arthritis is usually quite short, rarely lasting more than several months. Attacks occur relatively infrequently and permanent joint damage is exceedingly uncommon. Rheumatoid nodules are absent, and serologic tests for rheumatoid factor and antinuclear antibodies are generally negative; when present they are of low titer. Joint erosions are not seen on x-ray examination. Syno-vial biopsy during acute attacks reveals nonspecific signs of inflammation. Joint fluid is usually inflammatory.

Peripheral arthritis tends to occur in those patients with extensive disease and is related to both local and systemic complications of the colitis. It tends to be more common in those patients with perianal disease, pseudopolyps, skin lesions such as pyoderma gangrenosum and erythema nodosum, uveitis, and oral ulcerations. Both sexes are affected equally.

The incidence of the HLA-B27 tissue type in patients with ulcerative colitis with or without peripheral arthritis is not increased.

Thus, peripheral arthritis is an extraintestinal complication of ulcerative colitis, not a genetic accompaniment as is ankylosing spondylitis. Its causation is not clear but is presumably related to the increased permeability of the diseased colon, thus allowing entry of foreign materials into the circulation. Conceivably, these materials could include bacteria, bacterial cell wall components, bacterial breakdown products, viruses, and other infectious or noninfectious agents. Subsequently, these agents could directly irritate synovial tissue or, more probably, initiate an immunologically mediated process similar perhaps to serum sickness in which joints become target organs.

Alternatively, it is possible that ulcerative colitis itself is an immunologically mediated disease, and the synovium is affected by the same process that inflames the bowel. Some immunologic abnormalities that have been demonstrated in ulcerative colitis include: antibodies to colonic epithelial cells; antibodies directed against fecal bacteria in the colonic mucosa of some patients; circulating lymphocytotoxic antibodies in 40 percent of patients; circulating immune complexes; anergy to dinitrochlorobenzene; infiltration of the colon with plasma cells and lymphocytes; and other possible mechanisms. Further support for an immunologic basis is that the disease frequently responds to therapy with corticosteroids, which are known to inhibit certain aspects of immune response.

Treatment is aimed at the underlying bowel disease. Surgical removal of diseased bowel almost always is curative of the peripheral arthritis. This is in contradistinction to the peripheral arthritis of Crohn's disease, which is often ameliorated but not cured by bowel surgery. Presumably, this ineffectiveness is related to the fact that it is often not possible to remove all the diseased bowel in Crohn's disease.

The arthritis can usually be managed by standard conservative therapy including rest, joint aspiration, joint protection, and carefully monitored therapy with standard antiinflammatory medications such as aspirin, indomethacin, or phenylbutazone in full therapeutic doses. Gold is contraindicated. Corticosteroids are rarely needed for arthritis alone, but when used provide dramatic relief. Thus, when oral, intravenous, or even colonic infusions of corticosteroids are employed to treat the colitis, the arthritis frequently abates as well. We have seen some patients in whom rectal steroid enemas failed to completely ameliorate the colitis but relieved the arthritis. In general, antiinflammatory medications are necessary only for short periods of time, unless the colitis is severe and unremitting.

ANKYLOSING SPONDYLITIS

Ankylosing spondylitis is seen in 4–6 percent of patients with ulcerative colitis. This is a much higher incidence than would be expected in the general population. Thus, it had been thought that ulcerative colitis might in some way predispose to or cause ankylosing spondylitis. As opposed to the peripheral arthritis, however, ankylosing spondylitis often precedes the onset of ulcerative colitis and is not affected by flares or remissions in the bowel disease. In fact, the spondylitis typically progresses in spite of total colectomy. It thus does not behave as an extraintestinal manifestation of ulcerative colitis.

An explanation for this curious association between ankylosing spondylitis and ulcerative colitis became apparent with the discovery of the high frequency of the HLA-B27 histocompatibility antigen in those patients with both colitis and spondylitis. Thus, the majority of patients with ankylosing spondylitis and inflammatory bowel disease will be HLA-B27 positive, as opposed to a normal frequency of this antigen in those with colitis and peripheral arthritis. It has been calculated that the risk for developing ankylosing spondylitis in a patient with ulcerative colitis who is HLA-B27 positive is 47 percent, which may be a conservative estimate.

The spondylitis that occurs in ulcerative colitis is virtually indistinguishable from idiopathic ankylosing spondylitis. Radiographically, typical sacroiliitis and syndesmophytosis occur and may progress to the rigid, so-called "bamboo" spine in advanced cases. Although males with spondylitis still predominate, the male to female ratio is much lower in colitis associated with spondylitis than it is in idiopathic ankylosing spondylitis (Marie-Strümpell disease). Sacroiliitis may occur without spondylitis and both may be associated with uveitis. An increased incidence of sacroiliitis and spondylitis is seen in family members of patients with ulcerative colitis (even in those without signs of rheumatic disease), and these persons may be either HLA-B27 positive or negative.

The management of spondylitis in ulcerative colitis patients is similar to that of idiopathic ankylosing spondylitis. Attention must be paid, however, to the gastrointestinal toxicity of antiinflammatory medications such as indomethacin. Exercise, heat, deep-breathing exercises, and maintenance of an erect posture are paramount.

SUMMARY

There are two major types of arthritis that occur in ulcerative colitis: Peripheral arthritis, which occurs in about one-quarter of patients, is an extraintestinal complication that tends to parallel activity of intestinal disease. Spondylitis, on the other hand, occurs in about 5 percent of patients and is genetically determined. The HLA-B27 antigen is found only in those patients with spondylitis. Whereas men born with the HLA-B27 antigen have a predisposition to developing ankylosing spondylitis, those with both ulcerative colitis *and* the HLA-B27 antigen have an even higher likelihood of developing spondylitis.

Patients with colitis may have both spondylitis and peripheral arthritis but only if the HLA-B27 antigen is present. Sacroiliitis may occur (with or without the HLA-B27 antigen) without necessarily progressing to spondylitis. Peripheral arthritis usually occurs after colitis becomes apparent, whereas spondylitis not uncommonly may antedate the bowel disease. Thus, the possibility of occult inflammatory bowel disease should be kept in mind in a patient (particularly a female) who develops spondylitis. Because of its strong predictive value, those patients with ulcerative colitis who develop rheumatic complaints, especially back pain and/or uveitis, should be tested for the histocompatibility antigen HLA-B27.

REFERENCES

Brewerton DA, Caffrey M, Nicholls A, et al: HLA-B27 and arthropathies associated with ulcerative colitis and psoriasis. Lancet 1:956, 1974

Greenstein AJ, Janowitz HD, Sachar DB: The extra-intestinal complications of Crohn's disease and ulcerative colitis: A study of 700 patients. Medicine (Baltimore) 55:401, 1976

Morris RI, Metzger AL, Bluestone R, et al: HL-A-W27—A useful discriminator in the arthropathies of inflammatory bowel disease. N Engl J Med 290:1117, 1974

Wright V, Watkinson G: The arthritis of ulcerative colitis. Br Med J 2:670, 1965

GRANULOMATOUS ILEOCOLITIS AND ARTHRITIS

Michael J. Reza
and Carl M. Pearson

Granulomatous ileocolitis, also known as regional enteritis or Crohn's disease, is a chronic inflammatory disease that may involve any portion of the gastrointestinal tract; however, the terminal ileum is most commonly involved. When disease is confined to the large intestine only (as it is in 10 percent of patients) it is known as granulomatous colitis. Its cause remains unknown, but a viral etiology is strongly suspect. Diagnosis is made most definitively by gastrointestinal radiographs. The course of this disease is chronic, intermittent, and highly variable.

Crohn's disease is particularly common in young adults and teenagers, has no sex predilection, is probably more common in Jews than non-Jews, and appears to be increasing in incidence. As opposed to ulcerative colitis, inflammation in Crohn's disease involves all layers of the intestinal wall and even adjacent lymph nodes and mesentery.

It has long been recognized that rheumatic symptoms and complaints occur with some frequency in Crohn's disease. In fact, 2.3 percent of Crohn's personal series of patients were noted to have arthritis. Recently, however, careful investigations of large groups of patients with Crohn's disease, both in the United States and abroad, has revealed that as many as 20 percent have arthritis. The arthritis is of two major types: peripheral and spinal. When it occurs in peripheral joints it is considered to be a specific extraintestinal complication of Crohn's disease.

PERIPHERAL ARTHRITIS
(INTESTINAL SYNOVITIS)

This complication is the most common musculoskeletal manifestation of Crohn's disease; it occurs in 18–20 percent of patients. When monarticular it has been referred to as the "colitic" pattern, when polyarticular, as the "polyarthritic" pattern. Peripheral arthritis in Crohn's disease may thus be mon-, olig-, or polyarticular. In general, it tends to be an episodic, acute polyarthritis involving larger joints more than small joints, especially in the lower extremities. Although any joint may be involved, the knee is most commonly afflicted, followed in frequency by the ankle, shoulder, and wrist.

Although peripheral arthritis may precede intestinal symptoms, it most commonly occurs concomitantly with or after the onset of Crohn's disease. The synovitis generally parallels the activity of the intestinal disease as opposed to spondylitis (see below). Thus, flares in the intestinal disease are commonly accompanied by flares in the peripheral arthritis. Surgery frequently improves the arthritis, but not completely, as it may do in ulcerative colitis.

Peripheral arthritis tends to occur more often in those patients with active, extensive, severe disease and other extraintestinal manifestations such as erythema nodosum, iritis, and oral ulcerations. The arthritis may occur regardless of the location of involved bowel but is most common in granulomatous colitis. The incidence is lowest in those patients with small intestinal disease only, and intermediate in those with granulomatous ileocolitis.

The arthritis itself is almost invariably nondeforming and nonerosive and usually is of short duration. It rarely lasts more than several months, and joint function is usually well maintained. Rheumatoid nodules are not seen and tests for rheumatoid factor, antinuclear antibodies, and anti-DNA antibodies are negative. There is *no* increased incidence of the histocompatibility antigen HLA-B27 in these patients with peripheral arthritis only. Knee effusions may be large and synovial fluid is usually inflammatory. Synovial histology is that of a nonspecific inflammatory response.

Treatment of the arthritis is best accomplished by treating the underlying bowel disease. In addition, traditional conservative therapy with salicylates, nonsteroidal antiinflammatory agents, rest, and joint aspirations may be effective. If the bowel disease prevents the use of aspirin, phenylbutasone, indomethacin, or similar drugs, then a short course of systemic corticosteroids is almost always effective. Gold therapy is *not* indicated and should not be used. Although surgery is generally

avoided in this disease, it may partially improve peripheral arthritis but not spondylitis.

ANKYLOSING SPONDYLITIS

Ankylosing spondylitis (spondylitic pattern) occurs in 7 percent of patients with Crohn's disease and often precedes intestinal disease. As opposed to peripheral arthritis, it is *not* an extraintestinal manifestation of Crohn's disease, but rather a genetic accompaniment. Its course is not affected by that of the bowel disease. The is clinically and radiologically identical to idiopathic ankylosing spondylitis. The majority of patients with Crohn's disease and ankylosing spondylitis have the histocompatibility antigen HLA-B27. In contrast, patients with Crohn's disease and peripheral arthritis or Crohn's disease alone have no increased incidence of HLA-B27. Sacroiliitis alone may occur in 9.5 percent of patients and may not necessarily always progress to ankylosing spondylitis. Thus, approximately 17 percent of patients will have sacroiliitis with or without spondylitis. As opposed to idiopathic ankylosing spondylitis, the male predominance is much less in patients with Crohn's disease and ankylosing spondylitis.

The significance of the HLA-B27 antigen in the spondylitic arthropathy of Crohn's disease is important in that it implies a different pathogenesis than the peripheral arthritis of Crohn's disease. In addition, it has been calculated that the risk of developing iritis or ankylosing spondylitis in an HLA-B27–positive patient with Crohn's disease is at least 14 percent.

The treatment of ankylosing spondylitis in Crohn's disease is basically no different from that of primary ankylosing spondylitis. However, gastrointestinal toxicity of the antiinflammatory medications must be carefully watched for. Bowel surgery rarely, if ever, has any bearing on the spondylitis. Peripheral arthritis and spondylitis may both occur in an HLA-B27–positive patient.

ETIOLOGY AND PATHOGENESIS

The etiology of Crohn's disease, although unknown, has long been suspected to be infectious. Other suggested factors include genetic, immunologic, environmental, or some combinations of these. Viral agents have been cultivated from intestinal tissue, and appear to be picornaviruses. Filtrates of Crohn's disease tissue have induced the disease in laboratory animals. Thus, it is also possible that the peripheral arthritis is related to the virus. More probably, inflammation of the bowel allows increased permeability to a variety of agents, including bacteria. Thus, it is conceivable that "foreign" antigens (perhaps bacterial wall components) are absorbed into the circulation, inducing antibodies. Subsequent antigen–antibody complexes (immune complexes) might be filtered out in joint tissues and induce synovial inflammation. It is also possible that the synovium shares common antigens with intestinal mucosa as well.

This mechanism would fit with the observed high incidence of peripheral arthritis in those patients with large colon involvement where the concentration of bacteria is highest. On the other hand, ankylosing spondylitis, which is probably genetically determined, can be seen in any patient with Crohn's disease (and the HLA-B27 antigen) regardless of location of bowel disease.

Although an immunologic basis for peripheral arthritis in Crohn's disease has not been proven, there is much to support this theory. First, the peripheral arthritis bears some clinical resemblance to serum sickness. Second, many immunologic abnormalities have been shown to exist in Crohn's disease, including anticolonic epithelial cell antibodies, immune complexes, antibodies to cross-reacting enterobacterial antigens, decreased numbers of T cells, decreased responsiveness of lymphocytes to mitogenic stimuli, and anergy to dinitrochlorobenzene. Furthermore, both Crohn's disease and the peripheral arthritis of Crohn's disease may respond to immunoregulatory drugs such as corticosteroids, azathioprine, and levamisole, as do many rheumatic diseases known to be immunologically mediated.

MISCELLANEOUS MUSCULOSKELETAL COMPLICATIONS

Less common musculoskeletal manifestations of Crohn's disease incude clubbing of the fingers and/or toes (in 11 percent), periarthritis, cervicobrachial pain, granulomatous myopathy, granulomatous bone disease, osteomyelitis of the right iliac wing, and cutaneous vasculitis (erythema nodosum).

REFERENCES

Goldin RH, Bluestone R: Tissue typing in the rheumatic diseases. Clin Rheum Dis 2:231, 1976

Greenstein AJ, Janowitz HD, Sachar DB: The extra-intestinal complications of Crohn's disease and ulcerative colitis: A study of 700 patients. Medicine (Baltimore) 55:401, 1976

Haslock I, Wright V: The musculo-skeletal complications of Crohn's disease. Medicine (Baltimore) 52:217, 1973

Morris RI, Metzger AL, Bluestone R, et al: HL-A-W27—A useful discriminator in the arthropathies of inflammatory bowel disease. N Engl J Med 290:1117, 1974

WHIPPLE'S DISEASE

Alan Rubinow

Whipple's disease is a rare disorder described by George Whipple in 1907. His patient, a 36-year-old man, had suffered gradual weight loss, low-grade fever, persistent cough, steatorrhea, anemia, and polyarthritis. At autopsy deposits of neutral fat and fatty acids were seen in the dilated enteric lacteals and mesenteric lymph nodes and large mononuclear cells were found in the lamina propia and submucosa of the small bowel.

Since the first description, over 150 cases have been reported. The disorder is most common in whites 40–60 years of age with a male predominance of 9:1. It occurs less commonly in women and has been recorded during childhood. The disease is usually sporadic but has been noted in siblings. Although the environmental or genetic

setting for this disorder has not been defined, many patients have been farmers and prolonged exposure to animals or birds may have etiologic significance.

Initially, Whipple's disease was considered to be a primary disturbance of fat metabolism; however, in 1949 it was demonstrated that the foamy mononuclear cells in the affected areas of the intestine were not lipid but glycoprotein that stained intensely with a periodic acid–Schiff (PAS) stain. These PAS-positive granules in the macrophages constitute the hallmark of the disease and are composed of sickle-shaped particles averaging 2–3 μm in diameter. The particles are comprised of closely packed membranes, vesicles, and granules derived from remnants of phagocytosed rod-shaped bacteria that have been incompletely digested. They have been found in virtually every organ studied, including the liver, lymph nodes, spleen, pancreas, heart, lung, synovium, serosal membranes, and central nervous system.

ETIOLOGY

Bacteria have been implicated as the etiologic agents, but a specific organism has not been isolated and Koch's postulates have not been filled. Electron microscopic studies have identified clusters of rod-shaped bacterialike bodies in the lamina propia of the jejunal mucosa. They appear to be most heavily concentrated just below the epithelium and in the mesenteric lymph nodes. The reversibility of the clinical and pathologic features of Whipple's disease with the institution of antimicrobial therapy is further evidence for an infective and probably bacterial cause. A cell wall–deficient streptococcus has been grown from a prolonged monolayer cell culture of a lymph node taken from a patient with Whipple's disease, but the disease has not been reproduced in experimental animals.

Despite the overwhelming circumstantial evidence for an infectious etiology, the male predominance, the inability to isolate specific organisms, and the unique cellular response point to the impairment of host factors as an important factor in the pathogenesis. The incomplete lysis of phagocytosed bacteria may be due to defective macrophage function, but substantive evidence for this hypothesis is also lacking. Some patients with active disease may have impaired cell-mediated immunity that usually persists but occasionally disappears upon successful antibiotic therapy. The role played by these alterations in immune function in the etiology and pathogenesis of Whipple's disease has not been determined.

CLINICAL FEATURES

Clinical manifestations attributable to virtually every organ system may occur in Whipple's disease and frequently may appear years or decades prior to the onset of classic gastrointestinal symptoms (Table 1); rarely are they recognized as prodromata. Polyarthritis is the most common prodromal feature. Low-grade fever, weight loss (independent of diarrhea and malabsorption), lymphadenopathy, arterial hypotension, hyperpigmentation, polyserositis, and pleural effusions are seen with varying frequency. In the preantibiotic era, sudden death in pa-

Table 1
Extraintestinal Manifestations of Whipple's Disease

General
  Fever
  Weight loss

Musculoskeletal
  Polyarthritis
  Sacroiliitis
  Ankylosing spondylitis
  Myopathy

Central nervous system
  Personality changes
  Dementia (presenile)
  Myoclonic seizures
  Spastic paralysis
  Acute encephalopathy
  Hypersomnia
  Ophthalmoplegia (supranuclear)

Ophthalmologic: decreased vision
  Retrobulbar neuritis
  Bilateral central scotoma
  Papilledema
  Vitreous inflammation

Auditory
  Hearing loss

Serosal
  Pericarditis
  Ascitis
  Pleural effusion

Cutaneous
  Hyperpigmentation
  Nonthrombocytopenic purpura

Hematologic
  Lymphadenopathy
  Anemia
  Leukocytes (neutrophilia)

Cardiovascular
  Arterial hypotension
  Myocarditis
  Endocarditis
  Sudden death

Endocrine
  Panhypopituitarism
  Hypothyroidism
  Impotence

tients with Whipple's disease was attributed to cardiac involvement, and indeed myocardial and endocardial lesions are commonly seen at autopsy.

Central nervous system abnormalities usually occur in late, untreated cases but may appear early in the course of the disease. The spectrum of neurologic involvement includes personality changes, memory loss, ataxia, presenile dementia, myoclonus, spastic paresis, hyperreflexia, hypersomnia, and seizures. In addition, papilledema, ophthalmoplegia (often transient), retrobulbar neuritis, bilateral deafness, and impotence appear to be secondary to brain disease. PAS-positive macrophages have also been identified in the thoracic duct lymph, alveolar wall capillaries, bone marrow, and endocardial vegetation, suggesting their deposition from circulating blood. Anemia and leukocytosis with neutrophilia are common hematologic manifestations of active disease but eosinophilia is rare. In the late phase, the patients are usually febrile and emaciated with weight loss, diarrhea, and malabsorption dominating the clinical picture. From 1 to over 30 years may lapse from the prodromal phase to the development of gastrointestinal symptoms. Advanced disease, almost invariably fatal in the past, responds dramatically to antibiotic therapy.

Peripheral arthritis is a common accompaniment, and 60–90 percent of patients experience articular involvement. Joint symptoms usually precede the more typical features by 1 to as many as 35 years (usually 4–5 years). In over 50 percent of patients, articular symptoms are the sole initial manifestation of the disease. Characteristically, the attacks of arthritis are acute in onset and often transient and intermittent. They occur at infrequent intervals and typically last from only a few hours to a few days, usually remitting spontaneously. In some cases, the attacks may be of longer duration and on rare occasions may continue relentlessly for several years.

The pattern of joint involvement is usually polyarticular and often migratory, involving at least three or more joints in the majority of patients. Less frequently, the joints may be involved in a symmetric fashion, and sometimes only one joint is affected. In some instances, the patient only complains of mild recurrent aches in the joints with no objective signs of inflammation, while in others, a mild to florid synovitis with a severely hot, swollen, and painful joint may be observed. The joints affected in order of frequency are the knees, ankles, wrists, elbows, small joints of the hands and shoulders. Other infrequently encountered articular features include subcutaneous nodules and fingernail clubbing; residual joint deformity is usually absent or mild. Roentgenologic changes in the joints are rare but ankylosis, juxtaarticular osteoporosis, and even subchondral erosions have been observed.

Interestingly, the arthritis has been known to subside a number of months to 2 years prior to the onset of weight loss and diarrhea. The arthritis usually resolves within 2 months after the institution of antibiotic therapy. A relapse precipitated by the premature discontinuation of therapy may be heralded by the reappearance of joint symptoms.

The frequency of axial joint involvement in association with Whipple's disease is controversial. Although in one review 18 of 95 patients with Whipple's disease were considered to have spondylitis, only 1 could be classified as definitely having ankylosing spondylitis and 2 as probably having ankylosing spondylitis when current criteria were applied. According to these criteria the frequency of sacroiliitis and ankylosing spondylitis in association with Whipple's disease is similar to that observed in patients with ulcerative colitis or regional enteritis and is fourfold greater than the expected rate in a white population. Two patients have been examined for the presence of HLA-B27 histocompatibility antigens. One was positive, and one negative.

The ability to recognize the early arthritic features as attributable to Whipple's disease requires a high index of suspicion and clinical acumen. In most such patients the articular symptoms resemble the periodic syndromes such as gout and palindromic rheumatism and respond equivocally to colchicine or antiinflammatory agents. Many cases are treated for years as atypical rheumatoid arthritis. With the development of multisystem features, the disease is most often confused with sarcoidosis, lymphoma, Addison's disease, and systemic lupus erythematosus. Patients who enter into the malabsorptive stages of the disease become easily recognizable. However, some may die of intercurrent disease, and in others a milder form of the disease may never lead to malabsorption or other significant organ dysfunction. In some instances, the disease process is entirely asymptomatic and is identified during diagnostic procedures (small bowel roentgenographs, lymph node biopsy, or laparotomy) that are performed for other reasons.

LABORATORY FINDINGS

The synovial fluid findings vary with the clinical severity of the arthritis. Arthrocentesis performed during an attack shows a moderately inflammatory synovial fluid in which the white cell count ranges from a few thousand to about 36,000 cells/mm^3, with 95 percent polymorphonuclear leukocytes. A mucin clot is fair to poor and no PAS-positive cells have been observed in suitably stained smears of synovial fluid. On the other hand, a high percentage of mononuclear cells are observed in synovial fluids demonstrating less inflammatory changes.

On light microscopy, the synovial membrane pathology parallels the acuteness of the arthritis and the synovial fluid leukocyte count. At the peak of an attack, a heavy, dense polymorphonuclear infiltrate is present within the membrane. In addition, hypervascularity, thickened vessel walls, and some synovial lining cell hyperplasia may be observed. The changes in the synovial membrane during the intercritical period or in relatively mild bouts of arthritis show a nonspecific chronic inflammation of normal membrane. Large foamy vacuolated cells containing discrete PAS-positive granules may be seen during the more acute attacks. They are either more difficult to discern or absent in patients with less florid synovitis.

Rod-shaped bacteria in various stages of degradation identical to those present in the small bowel have been observed in the synovial membrane on two occasions. It appears that direct bacterial infiltration of the synovium, possibly from hematogenous spread, is responsible for

the arthropathy of Whipple's disease and not a "hypersensitivity" reaction as previously postulated. The factors that precipitate the episodic arthritis or activate bacteria that have been dormant in other organ systems for many years remain unknown. On the institution of therapy, the above changes resolve completely.

The disorder should be suspected in male patients with arthritis and gastrointestinal disease, especially if malabsorption is present. The diagnosis lies in the recognition of PAS-positive macrophages in the small bowel, as obtained by peroral jejunal biopsy, or in extraintestinal sites. Electron microscopy demonstrates classic inclusions. Laboratory tests for rheumatoid factors or antinuclear antibody are negative and the erythrocyte sedimentation rate is often moderately elevated.

TREATMENT

The treatment of Whipple's disease includes a combination of penicillin, 1.2 million units, and streptomycin, 1 g, for 10–14 days followed by maintenance therapy with tetracycline, 1 g/day. The disease, in some cases, has proved to be refractory to long-term tetracycline and prolonged penicillin treatment has been advocated. Therapy should be continued for at least 1 year as some patients have relapsed due to premature discontinuation.

The bacteria disappear rapidly from the small intestine, while PAS-positive macrophages either remain or regress at a slower rate. Relapse may be heralded by fever, arthritis, or neurologic symptoms and antibiotic therapy should be reinstituted. Corticosteroids were used with variable success prior to the proven effectiveness of antibiotics, but are not currently employed.

REFERENCES

Caughey DE, Bywaters EGL: The arthritis of Whipple's syndrome. Ann Rheum Dis 22:327, 1963

Cohen AS: An electron microscopic study of the structure of the small intestine in Whipple's disease. J Ultrastruct Res 10:124, 1964

Hawkins CF, Farr M, Morris CJ, Hoare AM, Williamson N: Detection by electron microscope of rod-shaped organisms in synovial membrane from a patient with the arthritis of Whipple's disease. Ann Rheum Dis 35:502, 1976

Kelly JJ, Weiseger BB: The arthritis of Whipple's disease. Arthritis Rheum 6:615, 1963

Maizel H, Ruffin JM, Dobbins WO III: Whipple's disease: A review of 19 patients from one hospital and a review of the literature since 1950. Medicine (Baltimore) 49:175, 1970

BEHÇET'S DISEASE

Thomas A. Medsger, Jr.

Behçet's disease is a multisystem disorder sharing clinical features with Reiter's syndrome and several connective tissue diseases, particularly systemic lupus erythematosus and the vasculitides. The eponym honors the Turkish dermatologist whose 1937 description of the disease, although not the first, was both timely and comprehensive. Often called the "mucocutaneous-ocular syndrome" or the "tri-symptom complex," Behçet's three cardinal features are recurrent oral and genital ulcerations and ocular inflammation. In recent years, the recognition of many other organ system involvements has served to broaden the spectrum of the disease considerably.

EPIDEMIOLOGY

The first reports of Behçet's disease emanated primarily from countries bordering the Mediterranean Sea, but current series indicate its world-wide occurrence, including Japan, other parts of Europe and the Middle East, and the United States. In one district in Japan, the incidence was estimated at 1 patient per 10,000 population. In most areas, however, it is suspected that Behçet's patients are both misclassified and under-diagnosed. Age of onset ranges from 6 to 70 years with a median in the third decade. Males predominate in most series in a ratio of 2–4:1, but, as in the connective tissue diseases, rates among females are highest during the childbearing ages of 15–45. Familial clustering has been observed.

Because of the rarity of Behçet's disease and the need for diagnostic consistency and reliability in reporting its occurrence and manifestations, several sets of criteria have been proposed. All emphasize the major features noted above and also include a group of less common and less specific findings as minor criteria. Authors differ somewhat in terms of which criteria they consider major or minor.

CLINICAL FEATURES

Oral ulcerations, always painful, occur in 90–95 percent of patients. They typically begin as raised erythematous spots that rapidly ulcerate within 24 hours and acquire a gray-yellow base. Ulcers may be located anywhere within the mouth or pharynx. These lesions are usually discrete, but may be either single or multiple (crops); their size ranges from a few millimeters to several centimeters in diameter. Oral ulcerations often resolve in 1–2 weeks but tend to be recurrent. Biopsy reveals focal ulceration of the oral mucosa with a mononuclear infiltrate at the base but without vasculitis. The appearance, natural history, and histopathology of these lesions are indistinguishable from those of aphthous stomatitis, although the latter lesions are usually somewhat smaller. The oral ulcers in Reiter's syndrome are shallow and most commonly asymptomatic, a helpful differential point.

In males, the genital lesions take the form of punched-out, painful ulcers on the scrotum or penile shaft. In contrast, the vulvar and vaginal ulcerations in women may go entirely unnoticed, and thus a thorough pelvic examination is necessary. The overall frequency of these lesions in reported case series is 60–70 percent.

The eyes are affected at some time in the course of Behçet's disease in 80–85 percent of patients. The classic finding is iritis with a purulent collection in the anterior chamber (hypopyon). Conjunctivitis, episcleritis, keratitis, iridocyclitis, and optic neuritis have also been observed. The late complications of cataracts, glaucoma,

and blindness appear to be sequelae restricted to patients with previous posterior segment inflammation.

Cutaneous involvement (70–85 percent) occurs as an erythema nodosumlike nodular vasculitis of the lower extremities, as "pathergic" erythema and induration at sites of trauma (e.g., needle puncture), or as papulopustular lesions. These changes tend to remit spontaneously within 7–14 days but to be recurrent after variable periods of time (days to months). Vasculitis is the typical microscopic finding.

The subcutaneous tissue may show migratory or superficial thrombophlebitis (20 percent) or deep venous thrombosis (5 percent), rarely including the renal veins or venae cava. Especially in patients with phlebitis, there is decreased plasma fibrinolytic activity and a tendency to excessive fibrin deposition in vessels.

Arthralgias or, less often, arthritis, are noted in over one-half of patients. An asymmetric polyarticular involvement is most common, usually affecting the knees or ankles and sparing small joints of the extremities. Recurrent bouts of arthritis are frequent; the duration of episodes is variable, ranging from several weeks to a few years. Synovial fluid leukocytes may be less than 2000 cells/mm^3 in the transient arthritis associated with erythema nodosum or greater than 20,000/mm^3. As in Reiter's disease, the serum and synovial fluid complement values are normal or high. The histologic picture is that of chronic, nonspecific synovitis, but permanent deformity or roentgenographic changes are rare.

Gastrointestinal involvement (30 percent) consists chiefly of episodes of diarrhea and abdominal pain, tenderness, or distention. The clinical and roentgenographic picture usually fits best with either ulcerative colitis or regional enteritis, but a malabsorption syndrome may supervene.

Central nervous system manifestations (20 percent) are varied and may take the form of meningitis, transverse myelitis, or a brain stem syndrome. Benign intracranial hypertension with papilledema, organic confusional states, and psychiatric disorders have also been noted. Increased numbers of cells (chiefly mononuclear) and elevated protein levels in the cerebrospinal fluid may be found. This complication may carry a somewhat higher survival risk, but its poor prognostic outlook appears to have been exaggerated.

The sequence of clinical involvement is indeed variable, and "incomplete" cases are now accepted even though the accumulation of criteria is insufficient for a definite diagnosis. Oral ulcerations usually appear first, while joint, eye, and especially central nervous system lesions tend to be delayed in onset. Typically, 1–5 years may elapse in "complete" cases before all of the major features make their appearance. Exacerbations and remissions of unpredictable duration characterize the subsequent course.

LABORATORY FINDINGS

There is no single laboratory test available to confirm the diagnosis of Behçet's disease. During exacerbations, the sedimentation rate is usually elevated, and diffuse hypergammaglobulinemia is often found. Low-grade anemia may be present, as well as a mild leukocytosis. Serologic abnormalities are unusual. A high proportion (60 percent) of individuals have high titers of serum antibodies directed against human oral mucosa and some have peripheral lymphocytes that are stimulated by mucosal antigen. These findings are not specific since aphthous stomatitis patients have similar responses. Biopsy specimens show no deposition of immune reactants in affected areas by immunofluorescence techniques.

In Japan, a strikingly increased frequency of the tissue typing antigen HLA-B5 has been found in Behçet's patients compared with controls. This work is not yet confirmed and a large series from the United States found no such association and no increase in HLA-B27 which might link Behçet's disease more closely to Reiter's syndrome.

TREATMENT

No specific therapy exists for this disorder. Nonsteroidal antiinflammatory agents may be useful for the symptomatic treatment of arthralgias and/or arthritis. Corticosteroids have been administered with variable, inconsistent results, as have fibrinolytic compounds. In large doses, the former may be of benefit for the control of acute central nervous system Behçet's disease. In some patients, blood transfusions were felt to induce a clinical remission. Because of recurrent, potentially debilitating (ocular, gastrointestinal) or fatal (central nervous system) complications, immunosuppressive drugs have been used and hold some promise for controlling resistant cases.

ETIOLOGY

Speculation about an infectious agent etiology was entertained for many years after Behçet's original description of "elementary bodies" in smears of hypopyon fluid and oral ulcerations and the observation of inclusion bodies in synovial fluid leukocytes. Several claims of virus isolation from patients with Behçet's disease have been made but were never convincingly or repeatedly confirmed. Considering the recognized geographic concentrations of cases, familial clustering, and the HLA-B5 association in Japan, host factors appear to play an important role. Whether or not autoimmune mechanisms are prominently involved has not been determined. It is most likely, as in Reiter's syndrome, that the pathogenesis of Behçet's disease is multifactorial.

REFERENCES

Chajek T, Fairnaru M: Behçet's disease. Report of 41 cases and review of the literature. Medicine (Baltimore) 54:179, 1975

Monacelli M, Nazzaro P (eds): Behçet's Disease. New York, Karger, 1966

O'Duffy JD, Carney JA: Behçet's disease: Report of 10 cases, 3 with new manifestations. Ann Intern Med 75:561, 1971

O'Duffy JD, Goldstein NP: Neurologic involvement in seven patients with Behçet's disease. Am J Med 61:170, 1976

Ohno S, Aoki K, Sugiura S: HL-A5 and Behçet's disease. Lancet 2:1383, 1973

Oshima Y, Shimizu T, Yokohari R, Matsumoto T, Kano K, Kagami T, Nagaya H: Clinical studies on Behçet's syndrome. Ann Rheum Dis 22:36, 1963

Systemic Lupus Erythematosus

Edgar Cathcart

DIFFERENTIAL DIAGNOSIS AND EPIDEMIOLOGY

Systemic lupus erythematosus (SLE) is a chronic inflammatory disease that usually involves the skin (classically with a butterfly rash over the cheeks and nose) and often is associated with arthritis, glomerulonephritis, serositis, and central nervous system (CNS) disease. Many abnormalities of the immune system have been described and the presence of antinuclear antibodies and the lupus erythematosus (LE) cell is characteristic of the disease.

DIAGNOSTIC CRITERIA AND DIFFERENTIAL DIAGNOSIS

As in many other chronic multisystem disorders of unknown etiology, precise diagnostic criteria for SLE are not available. The American Rheumatism Association criteria for SLE were designed for classification rather than bedside diagnosis and they have been most helpful in studies of the natural history of the disease, in epidemiologic surveys, and in drug trials. A clinical diagnosis of SLE is generally based on the finding of multisystem disease, e.g., diffuse erythematous rash plus arthritis, serositis, or CNS involvement. The laboratory diagnosis of SLE depends on the demonstration of LE cells or antinuclear antibodies (ANA) at some point in the disease. Certain immunopathologic features, particularly the demonstration of immunoglobulin and complement components in skin or renal biopsies, are of great diagnostic significance. SLE is frequently characterized by exacerbations and remissions, and disease activity should be evaluated periodically by attempting to quantify major clinical manifestations and pertinent laboratory findings such as the erythrocyte sedimentation rate (ESR), serum complement levels and antibody titers to native ("double-stranded" or undenatured) DNA.

Discoid lupus and drug-induced lupus syndromes probably deserve separate classification criteria, although the diagnostic workup of both of these conditions is often identical to that of SLE. Sometimes a diagnosis of two or more connective tissue diseases is made in a patient with SLE. The most common "overlap syndrome" concerns patients who have typical features of rheumatoid arthritis

Table 1
American Rheumatism Association Criteria for SLE

Arthritis without deformity	Psychosis/seizures
Facial erythema	LE cells
Discoid lupus	False-positive serologic test for
Pleurisy/pericarditis	syphilis
Alopecia	Hemolytic anemia/leukopenia/
Photosensitivity	thrombocytopenia
Raynaud's phenomenon	Proteinuria (>3.5 g/24 hr)
Oral/nasal ulcers	Cellular casts

and SLE, but others have been described in which SLE is associated with classic findings of polymyositis, scleroderma, or periarteritis nodosa. The relationship of "mixed connective tissue disease" to SLE is unclear. Although there may be a number of distinguishing features, particularly the results of antibody tests for extractable nuclear antigens, it is possible that they share the same etiology and pathogenesis.

The differential diagnosis of SLE is fraught with many problems and often requires a keen clinical acumen regarding various types and patterns of inflammatory joint diseases, mucocutaneous syndromes, seizure disorders, coagulopathies, and the like. The American Rheumatism Association criteria for SLE have helped greatly to bring some order to a very confusing area of clinical mecidine, but it must be noted that the 14 features listed in Table 1 are but a sample of the symptoms, signs, and laboratory abnormalities that are encountered in patients with SLE and lupuslike syndromes.

A symmetric polyarthritis is the most frequent manifestation of SLE, but many other systemic diseases, including rheumatoid arthritis and the other connective tissue disorders, infectious and chronic active hepatitis, acute bacterial endocarditis, and sarcoidosis, may present with an identical clinical picture. The synovitis of SLE does not cause pannus formation and seldom results in joint contractures. Thus, because of its greater discriminatory powers, several authorities recommend that the term "arthritis without deformity" might be replaced by "arthritis without bone erosions."

A butterfly rash is evident in over 60 percent of patients, but equally specific though less spectacular skin

Table 2
Additional Clinical and Laboratory Criteria for Use in
Differential Diagnosis of SLE

Fever	Antinuclear antibodies
Joint deformities without erosions	Hypocomplementemia
Periungual erythema/	Cryoproteins/immune
telangiectases	complexes
Pupura	Fibrin-split products
Livido reticularis	Lymphocytotoxins
Cytoid bodies	Circulating anticoagulants
Migraine/visual hallucinations	Free urinary L-chains
Splenomegaly	Proteinuria (<3.5 g/24 hr)
Lymph node enlargement	Hyperglobulinemia
Aseptic necrosis	Elevated ESR

changes in SLE include periungual erythema and scattered telangiectases on the fingers, palms, and upper eyelids. Approximately 10 percent of patients with SLE manifest livido reticularis, and although the causes of purpura are manifold, hemorrhagic lesions in the skin may be the first indication that a bleeding or clotting disorder is present.

"Cotton-wool" exudates (cytoid bodies) in the absence of hypertension or diabetes frequently signal the onset of widespread vasculitis, and complaints of headache and visual hallucinations, either formed or unformed, should alert the physician to the possible diagnosis of SLE. Fever, splenomegaly, and lymph node enlargement are also common manifestations of many systemic disorders, including infectious and lymphoproliferative diseases, but one or all of these findings can be the initial manifestation of SLE. Likewise, aseptic necrosis of the bone may have multiple causes, but an increasing awareness of its clinical and radiologic features renders it a valuable diagnostic sign in SLE.

Of the myriad of abnormal laboratory tests that occur in SLE, the findings of LE cells, chronic false-positive serologic tests for syphilis, and hemolytic anemic, leukopenia, and thrombocytopenia, have received the most attention. The sensitivity and specificity of the various ANA tests for SLE have been thoroughly evaluated and there is general agreement that higher titer fluorescent ANA tests of "homogeneous" pattern may be a more sensitive indicator of SLE than a positive LE cell preparation, that "peripheral" or "rimmed" patterns usually herald the onset of active renal disease, and that the "speckled" patterns are more characteristic of rheumatoid arthritis, scleroderma, and mixed connective tissue disease.

Apart from the additional findings of massive proteinuria and cellular casts, the criteria based on laboratory tests in SLE are limited and might well be expanded to recognize the more frequent occurrence of mild or minimal glomerulonephritis in SLE (proteinuria less than 3.5/24 hr), the marked association between hypocomplementemia and immune complex deposition, and the highly specific finding of circulating anticoagulants in subsets of the SLE population. Other nonspecific but diagnostically useful laboratory abnormalities in SLE are listed in Table 2 and include an elevated ESR, hyperglobulinemia, cryoproteinemia, and the frequent finding of lymphocytotoxins and fibrin-split products in the peripheral blood.

One of the most controversial aspects of the diagnostic workup of patients with SLE concerns the indications for and interpretation of a renal biopsy. Although the finding of casts or proteinuria serves to alert the physician to the presence of renal disease, it usually does so only in advanced cases of lupus nephritis, missing the early lesions that lack these flagrant signs; moreover, occasionally SLE patients have been found with advanced nephritis but negative urinalysis. For these reasons, definitive diagnosis still requires the renal biopsy and light or electromicroscopic examinations of the specimens. As stated elsewhere, the role of newer noninvasive techniques in the differential diagnosis of SLE needs further investigation. Fortunately, these techniques may be of greatest value in clinical situations such as endocarditis and "cerebritis" in which more traditional laboratory procedures seem to be least helpful.

EPIDEMIOLOGY

It now appears that SLE has a greater incidence and, in the majority of cases, a more benign outcome than previous studies indicated. The overall incidence of SLE is approximately 7.6 cases per 100,000: in women aged 15–64 years, who are at higher risk, the prevalence is about 1 in 700. Blacks have SLE, whether systemic or chronic discoid, three times more frequently than their representation in the general population, and the condition may be as common as rheumatoid arthritis in black women aged 15–64 years. A striking increase in the incidence of SLE in females as compared to males is evident in the second to fourth decades, but data to support linkage to genetic factors, including the X chromosome, HLA antigens, and immune response genes, are inconclusive to date. Apart from scattered reports of SLE occurring in families, there is no clear-cut evidence of familial aggregation. Extremely high concordances of clinical SLE and serologic abnormalities between monozygotic twins have recently been reported.

REFERENCES

Cohen AS, Reynolds WE, Franklin EC, Kulka JP, Ropes MW, Shulman LE, Wallace SL: Preliminary criteria for the classification of systemic lupus erythematosus. Bull Rheum Dis 21:643, 1971

IMMUNOPATHOLOGY

Although histologic examinations may reveal no specific abnormalities in certain tissues, the most characteristic light microscopic finding in SLE is the hematoxylin body. This is an oval, smudgy, eosinophilic body, larger than a cell nucleus; it usually occurrs in clusters in synovial membrane, heart, kidney, and almost any tissue of the body. It is the tissue equivalent of the LE cell and is pathognomonic of SLE. Another well-known lesion is "fibrinoid," a homogeneous eosinophilic material in the ground substance which has been shown by immunochemical techniques to contain a variety of substances, including fibrinogen and immunoglobulins; it is nonspecific in nature. Vasculitis involving capillaries and small arterioles is readily identified in the skin or glomeruli of most patients with active SLE. Sometimes vasculitis is widespread, but in other cases the vascular changes are confined to one or a few organs, including testes, ovary, brain, spinal chord, lungs, liver, gall bladder, stomach, intestines, breast, and uterus. Inflammatory changes may vary from small foci in cross sections of the vessel to complete involvement of all three layers. Necrotizing

arteritis, indistinguishable from that seen in periarteritis nodosa, is sometimes found in SLE.

Electron microscopic studies have disclosed microtubular particles, resembling myxoviruses, in circulating white blood cells and within the microvascular lining of multiple organs from patients with SLE. Several reports have confirmed the high incidence of viruslike inclusions in glomeruli from patients with lupus nephritis, while their occurrence in other renal biopsies has been rare. The nature of these tubular structures and their relation to the etiology of SLE is unknown.

KIDNEY INVOLVEMENT

Pathologic abnormalities in lupus nephritis may be separated into at least three main categories: mild (focal) proliferative glomerulitis, severe (diffuse) proliferative glomerulonephritis, and membranous glomerulonephropathy (Table 1). In the first type, microscopically evident disease activity is confined to portions of only a few of the glomeruli sampled (for an accurate diagnosis, renal biopsy specimens must contain no fewer than 5 glomeruli, preferably about 10). Typically, the basement membrane is only minimally thickened, if at all. The focal lessions show a proliferation of endothelial and mesangial cells, usually at the periphery of the glomerular tufts involved, together with swelling, focal necrosis, and infiltration by polymorphonuclear leukocytes. By immunofluorescence all glomeruli show prominent mesangial staining, and by electron microscopy dense deposits are confined mainly to mesangial cells and segmental lesions.

In diffuse proliferative disease, the microscopic findings are basically those found in focal disease, but they are much more extensive: all or almost all of the glomeruli are swollen and necrotic, and the proliferation of endothelial and mesangial cells is often so severe that many capillairies are obliterated. In addition, inflammation commonly extends to the tubules and the interstitium. So-called "wire-loop lesions" (segmental thickening of the glomerular tufts' basement membrane) are frequent, and immunofluorescence shows a thickened, irregular outline ("granular" or "lumpy-bumpy pattern") with specific staining for immunoglobulins, complement

Table 1
Kidney Involvement

Clinical Features*	Histologic Classification
Normal	Mesangial (minimal)
Proteinuria (<3.5 g/24 hr), hematuria, and/or cellular casts	Focal proliferative (mild) and/or interstitial
Renal insufficiency	Diffuse proliferative (severe) and interstitial and ?sclerosing
Nephrotic syndrome	Membranous
End-stage and/or malignant hypertension	Sclerosing and/or arteriolitis (fibrinoid)

*It has been clearly demonstrated that some patients with normal renal function or with minor clinical abnormalities may have diffuse proliferative changes on renal biopsy.

components, DNA, and anti-DNA antibodies. Properdin B has also been identified in these lesions. Electron microscopy reveals thick, granular material deposited along the endothelial side of the basement membrane, in the membrane itself, or (rarely) along the epithelial side of the membrane.

In severe diffuse proliferative nephritis, mesangial and endothelial cell proliferation is prominent and epithelial crescents involving 30 percent or more glomeruli have been noted. Staining for IgG and C3 is usually heavy, and stains for IgA and IgM are often positive, but usually in lesser amounts. Fibrin is commonly seen in crescents and focally in scattered lobules adjacent to the crescents. Electron micrographs demonstrate diffuse dense deposits in all sites. In some patients, the principal glomerular abnormality is irregular sclerosis. This type of lesion has been designated *sclerosing lupus nephritis* and should probably be considered as a variant of severe proliferative glomerulonephritis. The presence of deposits of immunoglobulin and complement in such cases suggest that the basic pathogenetic mechanism, the accumulation of immune complexes, continues to operate.

In membranous glomerulonephropathy, the characteristic histologic appearance is an almost uniform thickening of the glomerular capillary walls caused primarily at the electron microscopic level by diffuse basement membrane thickening. These deposits, present in all types of lupus nephritis, but more numerous and more evenly distributed in this type, contain immunoglobulin and complement. On immunofluorescence the characteristic pattern is "finely granular." This helps to distinguish membranous lupus nephritis from anti-basement membrane nephritis (Goodpasture's syndrome), in which the fluorescent pattern is typically smooth and linear. In contrast to the proliferative types of lupus nephritis, the membranous form rarely shows any necrosis or leukocyte infiltration.

The classification of lupus nephritis into three basic categories (there may be overlap of the three individual cases) dates from about 1970. Recent findings indicate, however, that there may be two more basic types: an early form of glomerular disease that is confined to mesangial cells (minimal glomerulitis), and an extraglomerular lesion in which disease activity is mainly, sometimes totally, confined to the interstitium. In the latter, most glomeruli, if not all, appear to be normal or show only a slight increase in populations of mesangial cells by light microscopy. Among the glomeruli and surrounding renal tubules, however, there is widespread mononuclear cell infiltration with varying degrees of interstitial edema and fibrosis, tubular atrophy, and thickening of tubular basement membranes. Immunofluorescence reveals bright, granular deposits of immunoglobulin and complement along tubular basement membranes or in the interstitium. Electron microscopy shows numerous interstitial lymphocytes and mast cells, and, again, electron-dense deposits in the thickened tubular basement membrane. These lesions may have important pathogenetic and clinical implications since similar interstitial abnormalities,

with comparitive sparing of the glomeruli, have been described in acutely rejecting kidney transplants.

The mesangial lesion is characterized by a proliferation of the scavengerlike mesangial cells in the glomerulus and by deposits of immunoglobulin and complement in thickened mesangial matrix and glomerular capillaries. The precise significance of mesangial lesions is difficult to define, since some mesangial abnormality is probably present in all patients with SLE, and no clinical correlation can be found between the extent of mesangial abnormalities and the presence or absence of clinical renal disease. Progression from the mesangial lesion to the diffuse proliferative form has been documented, and on occasion, regression of diffuse proliferative glomerulonephritis to the mesangial form has been reported in association with clinical remission. Necrotizing vasculitis in the kidney, associated with severe hypertension and rapidly progressive renal failure occurs in about 20 percent of patients with diffuse proliferative glomerulonephritis. The vascular lesions that involve arterioles and interlobular arteries are characterized by acellular necrosis of the vessel walls, frequently with proteinaceous thrombi occluding the lumens. Intimal proliferation and mural hemorrhage of the interlobular arteries may be seen in association with the necrotic lesions in about one-half of cases. Fluorescence microscopy demonstrates IgG and C3 in some of the lesions and nonspecific accumulation of plasma proteins in others.

SKIN LESIONS

Histologic examination of the acute lupus skin eruption reveals hyperkeratosis of the epidermis with plugging of the hair follicles. There may be either atrophy (acantholysis) or hypertrophy (acanthosis) of the prickly cell layer of the skin; the capillaries and lympatics are dilated and mononuclear cells surround the blood vessels and infiltrate the dermal appendages. The histologic findings in chronic SLE skin lesions reflect their macroscopic "discoid" appearance with marked atrophy of the epidermis in the center of each lesion and hypertrophy in the periphery. Inflammatory cell infiltration is more pronounced in the dermal layers of the discoid lesions and there is little or no edema in the epidermis.

Immunofluorescent "band" tests have revealed immunoglobulin, properdin B, and complement components not only in the walls of dermal blood vessels, but more specifically along the derm–epidermal junction in both acute and chronic lesions. Noninvolved skin from patients with SLE yields positive results in over 50 percent of cases, and a positive band test is said to correlate with biopsy-proven glomerulonephritis, diminished serum complement levels, and increased titers of antibodies to native DNA, although not all observers accept this association. Lupus profundus is a rare manifestation of SLE in which acute and chronic inflammation of the subcutaneous fat causes palpable painful subcutaneous nodules. Histologically, the lesions are characterized by acute and chronic vasculitis; the overlying skin may be normal, but sometimes sclerotic plaques with central ulcerations or skin atrophy may occur.

INVOLVEMENT OF LYMPH NODES, SPLEEN, AND THYMUS

The lymph nodes are enlarged in the majority of patients with SLE. Distortion of the architecture by engorgement of sinuses and infiltration with many plasma cells, monocytes, polymorphonuclear cells, and macrophages are changes that frequently occur and are quite characteristic of SLE. Areas of necrobiosis with surrounding granulomatous tissue may replace follicles and germinal centers. There is marked reticular hyperplasia and phagocytosis of erythrocytes.

The spleen is grossly enlarged in 10–45 percent of cases. The most characteristic finding in that organ is the "onion skin" lesion consisting of concentric rings of collagen laid down around the arterioles. Histologic examinations of the thymus have been unremarkable in most autopsy series.

NEUROLOGIC FINDINGS

When neuropsychopathic problems develop, they tend to be multiple and to occur when the SLE is otherwise active. This activity is apt to be in the form of thrombocytopenia or vasculitis. These observations seem to suggest bases for the neurologic lesions, but the neuropathologic record shows that the majority of cases are not inflammatory or hemorrhagic. In more than one-third of autopsied cases, small brain infarcts or single areas of nerve cell loss (encephalomalacia) are observed. These changes, which are not grossly visible, tend to occur in the cerebral cortex and brain stem and are related to changes in the capillaires and small arterioles. There is good correlation between the clinical signs and the encephalopathic changes but poor correlation with the site of damage. One-third of SLE patients show no pathologic changes on postmortem examination, but the remainder usually have evidence of choriomeningitis or vasculitis with or without subarachnoid and intracerebral hemorrage. There have also been cases in which there is a necrotic myelopathy not directly related to vascular lesions or demyelination.

The fluffy white exudates that are frequently observed by funduscopic examination may be defined histologically as "cytoid bodies." They occur in the superficial nerve fiber layer of the retina and appear to be foci of microinfarcts with surrounding edema. Other nonpathognomonic changes in the fundus associated with SLE include small, superficial retinal hemorrhages, round cell infiltration, and edema of the choroid and papilledema. Demyelination and loss of axons have been described in several patients with SLE, but ischemic optic atrophy is rare.

CARDIAC INVOLVEMENT

At postmortem, pericardial abnormalities have been reported in over 80 percent of cases of SLE. Microscopic inflammatory changes vary in type and degree. In some cases there are only rare foci of fibrinoid degeneration or minimal infiltration of inflammatory cells. In others, extensive areas of fibrinoid and/or heavy infiltration with mononuclear cells have been described. A superficial layer of fibrin is occasionally present and adhesions have been noted in one-half of the cases. Myocardial involvement is less commonly seen, varying from small areas of perivascular inflammation to widespread diffuse interstitial inflammation. Myocardial infarction, with and without atherosclerosis of the coronary vessels, is being reported with increasing frequency.

Evidence of endocarditis or valvular lesions undiagnosed during life are found at autopsy in about 40 percent of cases. The classic findings were first described by Libman and Sacks, who noted small verrucous vegetations, chiefly on the ventricular side of the mitral valve. They consist of dense connective tissue, inflammatory cell infiltrates, and sometimes hematoxylin bodies. Immune complex deposition as evidenced by positive fluorescent staining for IgG and complement has been reported in a typical Libman-Sacks lesion.

PULMONARY INVOLVEMENT

Despite the frequency on chest x-ray, pulmonary infiltrates are often poorly defined and appear nonspecific by histologic examination. At postmortem, many small branches of the pulmonary arteries show extensive subintimal proliferation.

SYNOVIAL MEMBRANE CHANGES

Synovial membrane changes both in joints and tendons vary from none to marked inflammation in SLE. As in the pleura and pericardium, abundant fibrin deposits on or just below the surface lining cells, with apparent atrophy or loss of synoviocytes and relatively little exudation of inflammatory cells, have been described in some cases.

MUSCLE INVOLVEMENT

Focal areas of perivascular and interstitial inflammation have been noted on histologic examination of muscle biopsy specimens from patients with SLE and a peculiar type of vacuolar myopathy has been described.

CLINICAL FEATURES

Emotional and physical stress, pregnancy, infections, drug ingestion, and photosensitivity have all been implicated as precipitating factors either at the onset or prior to an exacerbation of SLE. In approximately 30 percent of SLE patients, the onset is acute and there is evidence of multisystem involvement within 2 months. Patients who present with a typical skin eruption usually have a gradual onset; when only one system is initially involved (whether it be skin, joints, or other), it may remain the sole manifestation of the disease for many months, or even years.

Proteinuria, in the absence of urinary tract infection, is the commonest and most reliable sign of clinical renal involvement in SLE. It usually precedes hematuria, the finding of red cell casts, and a rise in the serum creatinine level. Proteinuria is the initial manifestation in about 5 percent of patients, but by the end of the first year over 50 percent of cases with four or more American Rheumatism Association criteria for SLE have evidence of renal

Table 1
Prevalence of the Major Clinical Manifestations of SLE

Manifestations	1954	1965	1966	1971	1975
Arthritis	90	92	91	95	62
Fever	86	84	61	77	—*
Skin lesions	85	72	89	81	86
Nephritis	65	46	86	53	49
Adenopathy	58	59	78	36	40
Pleurisy	56	45	55	48	31
Pericarditis	45	31	29	38	25
Neuropsychiatric	37	26	65	59	40
Splenomegaly	15	9	46	18	10
Mouth ulcers	14	9	41	7	29
Photosensitivity	11	33	34	—	50
Raynaud's phenomenon	10	18	12	21	45
Alopecia	3	25	46	37	38
Aseptic necrosis	—	5	2	7	8
Subcutaneous nodules	—	5	22	11	11

Reports from Johns Hopkins (1954), Los Angeles County Center (1965), Massachusetts General (1966), Columbia-Presbyterian (1971), and Wellesley (1975) Hospitals.
*Not reported.

involvement. The probability of new onset of nephritis decreases the longer a patient has SLE.

Although fever has been recorded in the majority of patients with SLE, it is a presenting sign in 5 percent or less. On the other hand, when a lupus "crisis" develops it is manifested by high fever, extreme generalized weakness and fatigue, severe headache, marked abdominal pain, and often chest pain. It may be accompanied by severe involvement of the CNS or cardiovascular system and is frequently complicated by life-threatening infections. Unfortunately, a small but significant group of patients with SLE have a rapidly progressive downhill course in which one or more crisis may lead to death within 2 years despite all forms of treatment.

In the less serious and more chronic forms of SLE, there is no characterisitic pattern of the disease as it unfolds and very little can be done to predict the clinical course of an individual patient once the diagnosis has been made. The 5-year survival rate has increased from 54 percent, as reported in the series from John Hopkins Hospital in 1954, to 75 percent, as reported from the Wellesley Hospital in Toronto in 1975. The only study of survival based upon a population survey indicates that over 90 percent of patients will be alive 10 years after the diagnosis of SLE is made by standard criteria. At one time, damage to the CNS was a leading cause of death in SLE, but the situation has changed so that now it accounts for only about 10 percent of deaths. On the other hand, in one series patients with neuropsychiatric abnormalities had a high association with nephritis and a 5-year survival of less than 55 percent.

KIDNEY DISEASE

In patients with renal involvement, the overall prognosis varies with the type and severity of the renal lesions. Longer survival is more likely in patients showing only mesangial or focal glomerulitis in contrast to those

with glomerulonephritis. Median survival for patients with diffuse proliferative glomerulonephritis was originally calculated to be 2.5 years, but most recent estimations now exceed 5 years. The prognosis with patients with nephrotic syndrome (proteinuria greater than 3.5g/24 hr) is also not as bad as originally thought, although patients with a mixed picture of both proliferative and membranous glomerulonephritis usually fare the worst whether treated with steroids and immunosuppressive agents or not. The onset of impaired creatinine clearance and/or hypertension are considered bad prognostic signs.

Recently, attention has been focused on the vascular events of the later stages of SLE. Accelerated atherosclerosis, hypertension, and end-stage lupus nephropathy often dominate the late clinical course and finally lead to death.

JOINT DISEASE

Arthritis has been noted in 62–95 percent of patients with SLE and is the most prevalent clinical manifestation in most series (Table 1). Joint disease, as characterized by pain and/or soft tissue swelling in multiple joints, is typically intermittent in SLE and leaves few residual changs over the years (Table 2). Arthralgia is the first symptom in about two-thirds of the patients, but its migratory and transient nature plus a notable absence of objective physical signs often lead to a delay in establishing a definitive diagnosis. A true symmetric arthritis

Table 2
Joint and Bone Involvement in SLE

Arthralgias	Deforming (nonerosive) polyarthritis
Tenosynovitis	Subcutaneous (rheumatoid) nodules
Nondeforming polyarthritis	Aseptic necrosis of bone

mainly involving knees, interphalangeal, and metatarso-phalangeal joints favors a diagnosis of rheumatoid arthritis rather than SLE, but a relatively benign course and the absence of bone erosions is highly suggestive of the latter condition. Tenosynovitis is often described in SLE and it may be that periarticular inflammation, rather than intrinsic joint disease, produces the "flipper-hand" and "swan-neck" deformities that occur in about 5 percent of patients. Unfortunately, there is no one clinical criterion by which one may differentiate the arthritis of SLE from that of rheumatoid arthritis, and there are even occasions when the two diseases appear to "overlap" in the same patient.

Unusual symptoms of articular disease in SLE include hoarseness due to cricoarytenoiditis and nonpainful dislocation of the sternoclavicular joint. Subcutaneous nodules are sometimes found but the lupus nodules seem to occur in crops, tend to be smaller and more superficial than rheumatoid nodules, and seldom persist longer than 1–2 months. Joint pain in patients with SLE may be due to acute bone infarction rather than synovitis. There appears to be significant association with the administration of high-dose steroids, but there are patients who develop aseptic necrosis in the absence of steroids. Unfortunately, aseptic necrosis is a common and often highly symptomatic problem in the patients with advanced lupus and some of them require surgical treatment with replacement arthroplasties to prevent pain and disability.

SKIN LESIONS

A diffuse erythematous rash is present on one or both cheeks and/or the bridge of the nose in the majority of patients who are observed from the onset of their disease to the confirmation of the diagnosis of SLE (by the presence of four or more of the American Rheumatism Association criteria). The facial lesions may either be flat or raised and vary in degree from a faint blushlike appearance of the cheeks to discreet red maculopapular eruptions involving the entire face and including the perioral and periorbital regions. A butterfly rash usually blanches on pressure and is distinguished from the classic rash of discoid lupus, which forms in raised, erythematous patches with adherent keratotic scaling and follicular plugging. The acute facial rash is less likely to produce atrophy and scarring than chronic discoid lesions and has a far greater tendency to be associated with multisystem disease. A small but definite proportion of cases of discoid lupus evolve into the classic picture of disseminated disease, but there is abundant clincial and serologic evidence to prove that patients with chronic skin disease are at the benign end of the spectrum of SLE.

The frequent occurrence of skin lesions on the face is probably related to an increased prevalence of photosensitivity in patients with SLE (approximately 30 percent). On the other hand, despite a marked tendency to exacerbation of SLE by sun exposure, there is no higher incidence or onset of disease during the summer months. Skin lesions also occur frequently in nonexposed areas and vary from scattered erythematous macules to typical areas of atrophy, follicular plugging, and telangiectases, and rarely to vescicles and ulcers. Other skin lesions seen in patients with SLE include upper-eyelid telangiectases, periungual erythema, red spots on the hands, and palmar erythema.

Alopecia, usually estimated as loss of 50 percent or more of the hair, has been noted in about one-half of the patients with SLE. Scalp lesions with erythema, scaling, or residual areas of atrophy accompany most of the episodes of alopecia, but sometimes, a marked loss of hair may be the only sign of active disease. Oral or nasopharyngeal ulcerations are also exceedingly common in SLE. Mouth lesions range from small, red, painless "canker sores" on the hard palate to large ulcerating vesicles on the tongue and buccal mucosa which may be very painful. In general, the appearance of mouth lesions heralds more severe exacerbation of systemic disease activity.

HEART DISEASE

Pericarditis is the most common cardiac manifestation of SLE. It is usually transient, asymptomatic, and detectable only in about 30 percent of all lupus patients because of an audible rub. While the occurrence of pericarditis is not necessarily cause for alarm, cardiac tamponade sometimes intervenes. Rarely, constrictive pericarditis occurs in association with SLE. The presence of pericarditis, often in association with myocarditis, probably explains the frequent notation of abnormal T waves by electrocardiogram in patients with active SLE.

The clinical diagnosis of myocarditis is certainly a difficult one and often depends on the finding of tachycardia out of proportion to body temperature or a level of anemia. Clinical evidence of endocarditis is even less common than myocarditis. Though there have been reports of mitral and aortic valvular insufficiency in scattered cases of SLE, Libman-Sacks endocarditis remains, in general, an autopsy diagnosis. On the other hand, the increasing use of echocardiography and other noninvasive techniques may help to determine the physiopathologic significance of unexplained murmurs in patients with SLE and the other connective tissue diseases. In this regard, coronary angiographic studies have already confirmed the remarkable tendency of longstanding cases of SLE to develop premature atherosclerosis. In some instances, the atherosclerotic changes in the coronary vessels have been related to preexisting or concomitant vasculitis. There is no doubt that an increasing prevalence of myocardial infarction in SLE contributes to the second phase of the bimodal mortality pattern that has recently been described.

HYPERTENSION

Hypertension occurs with increased frequency in SLE and is probably secondary to renal involvement and the common use of prolonged steroid therapy. Rarely, the blood pressure is excessively high and very poorly responsive to antihypertensive therapy for unexplained reasons. Pulmonary hypertension, presumably secondary to vasculitis of the pulmonary vessels, may result in cor pulmonale.

VASOMOTOR ABNORMALITIES

Vasomotor abnormalities have been frequently described in patients with SLE. The usual symptoms are excessive coldness or sweating of hands and feet. A history of Raynaud's phenomenon with a characteristic two-phase color reaction is obtained in at least 20 percent of the patients. In some it represents the first sign of the disease and may be present for months or even years before systemic involvement is evident. In severe cases, Raynaud's phenomon is related to widespread vasculitis and may be accompanied by digital ulcers or gangrenous lesions in the finger tips, toes, upper arms, legs, buttocks, face, and ears. An increased incidence of thrombophlebitis in SLE has been reported by some observers but not by others.

LUNG DISEASE

Chest pain is very common in SLE and is usually related to an underlying pleurisy. When a rub is not present it is difficult to differentiate pleural from musculoskeletal pain, although the latter is usually found over the lower ribs anteriorly or in the axillae. Routine serial chest x-rays reveal pleural effusions in more than 50 percent of patients with SLE and in some autopsy series the incidence of pleural involvement approaches 100 percent. Areas of increased lung density, representing small areas of basal atelectasis or pneumonitis, are also frequently seen in SLE. It is sometimes difficult to decide whether the parenchymal lung infiltrates are aseptic or not and antibiotic therapy is often instituted despite negative bacterial cultures. Diffuse intersitital pulmonary fibrosis is occasionally seen in patients with SLE, but the association is less common than in other connective tissue diseases.

Unfortunately, patients with SLE are often compromised hosts and their lungs may be seeded by common or uncommon infectious agents. Thus, pneumonitis takes an added toll with respect to morbidity and mortality, and the medical literature on SLE is replete with case eports of patients with pneumonitis due to opportunistic organisms, e.g., *Pneumocystis carinii, Candida albicans,* etc.

NEUROPSYCHIATRIC ABNORMALITIES

In his original report, Kaposi first noted that stupor and coma may be terminal manifestations of SLE. Osler mentioned a patient "who imagines all sorts of things," and in 1904 there was an excellent description of delirium, aphasia, and hemiparesis in a patient with SLE. Although it is uncommon for the disease to present this way, neuropsychiatric manifestations appear at some time in the course of the illness in 25–75 percent of patients. Table 3 is a list of the neuropsychiatric abnormalities that have been described.

Approximately one-half of the patients with SLE appear to be psychologically intact with normal anxiety and depression in relation to their illness. Some patients are noted to be psychoneurotic with more severe episodes of anxiety and a tendency to chronic depression.

Table 3
Neuropsychiatric Abnormalities

Neurosis
Psychosis
  Acute brain syndrome
  Functional schizophrenia, depression
Seizures (convulsions)
  Generalized
  Partial (motor or sensory)
Upper motor neuron lesions (paresis/paraplegia)
Cranial nerve palsies (diplopia, etc.)
Visual pathway lesions
  Retinopathy (hemorrhages, exudates, papilledema)
  Optic and chiasmal neuropathy (visual field defects)
  Retrochiasmal dysfunction (hallucinations, migrainelike syndrome)
Aseptic meningitis
Chorea and other movement disorders
Transverse myelopathy
Peripheral neuropathy

Patients with profound emotional disturbances may present with an acute brain syndrome or with a functional psychosis. The former may be associated with hallucinations, disorientation in time, place, or person, gross memory defects, perseveration, confabulation, and visual and auditory hallucinations. The behavior of patients with functional psychosis may be either paranoid or catatonic (schizophrenia) or characterized by severe depression. Psychosis may first appear when a patient is given a higher dose of steroids than was previously required to control disease activity. On the other hand, a psychotic episode may be the first manifestation of SLE and is frequently observed in patients who are not receiving steroids.

CNS DISORDERS

Generalized seizures (convulsions) or partial seizures affecting focal motor or sensory areas of the brain represent the most common CNS manifestation of SLE. The majority of patients have a single seizure but some have recurrent attacks of generalized convulsions. Fortunately, hemiparesis and cranial nerve palsies tend to recover quickly in patients with SLE.

In addition to diplopia, which is frequently observed in many series, visual disturbances may arise due to retinopathy (hemorrhages and exudates in the fundus), increased intracranial pressure (papilledema), optic and chiasmal neuropathy (visual field defects), and retrochiasmal problems. The latter seems to account for the visual hallucinations and migrainelike syndromes that are often described by patients with active SLE.

Since all portions of the CNS may be affected in SLE it is not surprising that patients will also be encountered with symptoms and signs of aseptic meningitis, transverse myelopathy, and peripheral neuropathy (sensory and/or peripheral). Unusual complications of SLE include chorea and other types of tremor, vertigo, nystagmus, and a bizarre clinical picture simulating an intracranial mass lesion.

Attempts to pinpoint the anatomic site and nature of

CNS lesions in SLE are not always successful, even with the most modern and sophisticated techniques. Following a lumbar puncture and cerebrospinal fluid analysis, patients suspected of having lupus "cerebritis" may be studied using electroencephalograms (EEG), brain scans, or computerized tomography. Abnormal EEG patterns are common in patients with SLE with or without overt neurologic signs and there is often little correlation between the clinical findings and the brain wave changes. In general, diffuse slowing is seen in patients with encephalopathy and more localized changes following a cardiovascular accident. 99m/Tc scintigrams and computerized tomography scans are being used increasingly, but the verdict as to their diagnostic potential in SLE has not been reached. In the final analysis, a careful history and physical examination is still the most reliable way of making the diagnosis of CNS lupus.

GASTROINTESTINAL SYMPTOMS

Gastrointestinal symptoms may include nausea, vomiting, dysphagia, and abdominal pain. Dysphagia is quite rare, although esophageal motility studies have revealed a positive correlation between abnormal peristalsis and Raynaud's phenomenon. Abdominal pain may be due to gastric erosions, intestinal ulcers, or pancreatitis, but it is more often secondary to a sterile form of peritonitis. The clinical picture may be even more confused in patients receiving steroids or immunosuppressive drugs.

LIVER DISEASE

Hepatomegaly is said to occur in 20–50 percent of patients with SLE, but the clinical consequences are negligible. Chronic active hepatitis must be carefully differentiated from SLE since patients with the former condition may have prominent extrahepatic manifestations, especially rash and polyarthritis. Although certain laboratory abnormalities, including ANA, are found in both diseases, clinical and autopsy studies indicate that hepatic involvement is rarely a complication of SLE. Thus the term *lupoid hepatitis syndrome,* which originally was applied to a series of young women with jaundice, hypergammaglobulinemia complications, and positive LE cell preparations, has lost favor and is now considered obsolete.

SLE IN CHILDHOOD

Differences in the clinical manifestations of SLE between adults and children are not as great as those observed, for example, in rheumatoid arthritis. Infants born of mothers with active SLE frequently have evidence of ANA and other placentally transferred autoantibodies during the neonatal period, but direct inheritance of SLE is exceedingly rare. There is a 5:1 preponderance of females over males and the peak age of onset is evenly divided between childhood and adolescence. The higher proportion of males in the younger age group is significant, and some authors believe that there might even be a slight peak in male incidence in adolescents paralleling that of females.

Arthritis, arthralgias, rash, and fever are the cardinal presenting complaints. Although the disease does not differ markedly from SLE in adults, the incidence of hepatomegaly and lymphoadenopathy in children is higher. The most persistent problems are related to cardiac, neurologic, or renal involvement. Factors influencing prognosis do not appear to differ greatly from those in adults, but a greater ratio of male versus female deaths suggests that SLE may be more severe in boys. The cause of death in children, as in adults, remains primarily renal followed closely by sepsis; more than one-half of the deaths that occur in children with SLE are due to extrarenal causes.

SLE AND PREGNANCY

Because of its predilection for women of childbearing age, pregnancy is often a factor that must be considered in the management of patients with SLE. Although most patients appear to be unaffected during the normal 9-month gestional period, spontaneous abortion occurs twice as often in pregnant SLE patients as compared to normals. An increased incidence of premature births and toxemia of pregnancy has been noted in several series and exacerbations of disease activity occur in as many as 38 percent of pregnancies, including flares after miscarriages and caesarian section. The period of pregnancy during which an exacerbation occurs varies greatly, ranging from the first month to many weeks after delivery. On the other hand, exacerbations rarely occur in patients who have been in clinical remission for many years. Although the use of hormones for contraception may not be advisable, pregnancy should be avoided at least during the time the disease is active.

SLE AND INFECTION

The incidence of infection in SLE is said to be 10 times greater than in normal controls. The actual risk of infection is greatly magnified by the frequency with which SLE patients receive steriods and cytotoxic drugs and by progression to impaired renal function to certain cases. Unfortunately patients with lupus may also have exacerbations following infection(s) and their clinical problems may be compounded by flare of the underlying disease with its known effect on the immune system. Finally, for some patients it is most difficult to determine whether infection is present, whether signs and symptoms suggesting infection represent an exacerbation of SLE, or whether both infection and SLE are occurring together.

SLE AND OTHER SYSTEMIC DISEASES

There have been claims of a significant association between SLE and other systemic diseases including Sjögren's syndrome, Hashimoto's thyroiditis, thrombotic thrombocytopenic purpura, myasthenia gravis, and neoplasia. The prevalence of severe keratoconjunctivitis sicca and xerostomia ranges from 1 to 8 percent in most series, but a prospective study using a battery of tests (Schirmer's test, rose bengal staining, sialography, radionuclide excretion of technetium-99, scintiscans, and lip biopsy) revealed clinical or subclinical manifestations of Sjögren's syndrome in all but 1 of 50 unselected consecutive patients with SLE. While these striking results await confirmation by other investigators, they suggest that lacrimal and salivary gland dysfunction may have been overlooked in many patients with SLE. The association between Hashimoto's thyroiditis and SLE is more tentative and has been challenged by the negative results of one excellent postmortem study.

Thrombotic thrombocytopenic purpura—a rare febrile multisystem disease of young females with the typical pathologic changes of thrombi and esoinophilic deposits in arterioles, venules, and capillaries—has been described in several patients with classical SLE. The coexistence of myasthenia gravis and SLE, either before or following thymectomy, has been recorded in the literature. A postulated association between SLE and malignancy is intriguing because of the common deficits of cellular immune function in both conditions.

REFERENCES

Baldwin DS, Lowenstein J, Rothfield NF, Gallo G, McCluskey RT: The clinical course of the proliferative and membranous forms of lupus nephritis. Ann Intern Med 73:929, 1970

Dubois EL: Lupus Erythematosus (ed 2). Los Angeles, University of Southern Cormimia Press, 1976

Estes D, Christian CL: The natural history of systemic lupus erythematosus by prospective analysis. Medicine (Baltimore) 50:85, 1971

Gillian JN, Cheatum DE, Hurd ER, Stastny P, Ziff M: Immunoglobulin in clinically univoled skin in systemic lupus erythemoemotosus. J Clin Invest 53:1434, 1974

Harvey AM, Shulman LE, Tumulty PA, Conley CL, Schonreich EH: Systemic lupus erythematosus: Review of the literature and clinical analysis of 138 cases. Medicine (Baltimore) 33:291, 1954

Johnson RT, Richardson EP: The neurological manifestations of systemic lupus erythematosus. Medicine (Baltimore) 47:337, 1968

Lee P, Urowitz MB, Bookman AAM, Koehler BE, Smyth HA, Gordon DA, Ogryzlo MA: Systemic lupus erythematosus. Q J Med 46:1, 1977

Ropes MW: Systemic Lupus Erythematosus. Cambridge, Mass, Harvard University Press, 1976

Urowitz MB, Bookman, AA, Koehler BE, Gordon DA, Smythe HA, Ogryzlo MA: The bimodal mortality pattern of systemic lupus erythematosus. Am J Med 60:221, 1976

LABORATORY ABNORMALITIES

HEMATOLOGY
Plasma Proteins

Plasma protein abnormalities are remarkably common in SLE. They are so fundamental to the understanding of this disease that some investigators regard SLE as one of the major diseases in which autoimmune processes take place. Serum albumin is depressed in the chronically ill patient and often reflects the severity of excessive proteinuria in patients with nephrotic syndrome. Acute phase reactants, particularly α_1 antitrypsin, haptoglobin, and C-reactive protein may rise at the onset of SLE, but serial measurements of these proteins are much less helpful than the ESR determinations in assessing disease activity. Parallel measurements of the ESR and C-reactive protein may be useful in differentiating exacerbations

due to SLE from intercurrent infections, for it has recently been suggested that C-reactive protein levels rise during sepsis but tend to be low or unchanged during active lupus.

Serum Complement

There is increasing awareness that patients with classic SLE or lupuslike syndromes may have inheritable deficiences of specific complement components. The usual cause of low serum total hemolytic complement activity in SLE is increased consumption by circulating or fixed antigen–antibody complexes, but more than a score of patients with heterozygous or homozygous absence of C2 have been reported to date, and examples of deficient C1 inhibitor, C1r, C1s, C4, C5, and C8 have been well documented.

Immunoassays to quantify serum levels of C3 and C4 are probably the most convenient methods for screening for the presence of immune complexes, differentiating gross abnormalities of the classic and alternative pathways, and monitoring disease activity, particularly in patients with lupus nephritis. Over 90 percent of patients with depressed serum C3 levels have demonstrable cold-insoluble complexes (cryoproteins), and it has been shown that the major constituents of these cryoprecipitates are native DNA and anti-DNA antibodies. Immune complexes of varyious sizes and solubilities have also been detected in SLE serum using more sensitive but possibly less specific techniques—for example, Raji cell, C1q, and monoclonal IgM binding.

Serum Antibodies

ANA abound in the serum of patients with SLE (see the section on Antinuclear Antibodies in the fascicle on Diagnostic Procedures). Fluorescent antibody techniques and radioimmunoassays have virtually replaced the LE cell test in most laboratories, but it should be pointed out that in an unexpected lupus crisis the ability to recognize a positive LE cell preparation may provide a diagnosis long before results of the more sophisticated method are available. Typical LE cells have also been described in synovial, pericardial, and pleural effusions from patients with active SLE.

Increased titers of antibodies to native DNA as measured by immunofluorescence, complement fixation, or radioisotopic techniques have strong correlations with active lupus nephritis. Other autoantibodies occur with frequency in SLE and probably contribute to the marked increase in total IgG, IgA, and IgG which prevail in that disease. Rheumatiod factors are noted in approximately one-third of the patients, and when they are detected in unusually high titers the clinical association with Sjögren's syndrome should be borne in mind since the symptoms of a dry nose, dry mouth, and dry eyes are too often disregarded in patients with SLE. Occasionally patients will show the presence of antithyroid antibodies.

Test for Syphilis

Another abnormal finding is the chronic, biologic false-positive test for syphilis, as defined in a person with no clinical or epidemiologic evidence of syphilis who has a repeatedly positive serologic test for 6 months or more and negative treponemal antibody tests. Large numbers of these patients have been followed for years, and it has been ascertained that in a significant percentage of them SLE develops. Conversely, a small percentage of patients with proven lupus are found to have false-positive serologic tests for syphilis. These reactions have served as indices for determining the epidemiology and the natural history of this disorder and already have indicated that in many cases SLE is present for a much longer time than had been suspected.

Anemia

Anemia (less than 12 g hemoglobin/dl) occurs in 50 percent or more of patients with SLE. The causes of anemia are multiple and may be of immune or nonimmune pathogenesis (Table 1). As in many other chronic diseases, the total red cell mass may be reduced despite normal appearing bone marrow and adequate iron stores. This normochromic, normocytic anemia is associated with low serum iron levels and diminished iron-binding capacity.

Acquired hemolytic anemia may be the sole presenting sign of the disorder and is found in about 10 percent of patients with four or more American Rheumatism Association criteria. A much larger proportion of patients with SLE who lack positive signs of hemolytic anemia (elevated reticulocyte count, low serum haptoglobin level, or a sharp fall in blood hemoglobin in the absence of hemorrhage) give a positive direct Coombs' test either against immunoglobulin alone, immunoglobulin plus complement (usually C3 or C4), or complement alone. Erythrocyte-bound immunoglobulin not detected by the standard Coombs' reagents can also be demonstrated using the more sensitive complement-fixing antibody consumption test. Occasionally, hemolytic anemia in SLE has been attributed to increased titers of cold agglutinins.

A bizarre peripheral blood smear characterized by many distorted fragmented red cells (triangular, helmet, and burr cells) is not infrequently found in patients with lupus nephritis and suggests the diagnosis of microangiopathic anemia and uremia. Drug-induced anemias, either on an immune or nonimmune basis, have also been reported with increased frequency in SLE.

Leukocyte Differential

Leukopenia is one of the hallmarks of SLE. Reduced numbers of polymorphonuclear cells or mononuclear cells will not be appreciated unless frequent peripheral blood white cell and differential counts are performed. The neutropenia is probably autoimmune in origin, although recent studies have implied that at least part of the granulocytopenia in SLE may be due to marrow inhibition. Qualitative abnormalities of granulocyte function have also been noted and several studies have indicated abnormalities of chemotaxis in SLE. Lymphopenia in active SLE is even more prevalent than neutropenia and may be of pathogenic significance.

An analysis of the peripheral blood lymphocytes in SLE has shown that both the absolute number and proportion of T (thymus-derived) and B (bursa-equivalent) cells are reduced. Patients with active disease show the

Table 1
Pathogenesis of Anemia in SLE

Chronic disease
Iron deficiency
Hemolysis
  Hypersplenism
  "Warm" antibodies and complement (Coombs' test)
  Cold agglutinins
  Drug-induced
  Microangiopathy

greatest reduction, whereas inactive patients have values that are only slightly below normal controls. The magnitude of the T cell depression not only parallels disease activity but also correlates with impaired cellular immune function as measured by skin test delayed hypersensitivity, lymphocyte transformation to phytohemagglutinin stimulation in vitro, and macrophage-inhibition factor production. In contrast to T and B cells, the absolute number of null cells (lymphocytes lacking complement and immunoglobulin receptors and failing to rosette sheep red blood cells) is increased even though the total number of circulating lymphocytes is decreased.

Lymphocytopenia may be caused by IgM lymphocytotoxic antibodies, which have been identified in as many as 80 percent of patients with active SLE. The presence of these antibodies correlates inversely with the leukocyte count and serum C3 levels and directly with fever, skin, CNS, and hematologic abnormalities. IgM lymphocytotoxins not only react with T and B cells in vitro, but also destroy fetal thymus tissue and cross-react with antigens found in human brain. An examination of family members and close household contacts of patients with SLE showed that 73 percent of consanguinous and 50 percent of nonconsanguinous relatives had detectable levels of lymphocytotoxic antibodies.

Platelets

The following disorders of hemostatic function have been observed in SLE: thrombocytopenia, qualitative platelet disorder, circulating anticoagulant, hypoprothrombinemia, and acquired Von Willebrand's syndrome. Thrombocytopenia is the most common cause of impaired hemostasis in SLE and may be associated clinically with purpura, hematuria, gastrointestinal bleeding, or intracerebral hemorrhage. From 25 to 50 percent of patients have platelet counts of less than 100,000 cells/mm^3 at some time during the course of the disease, but only about 8 percent have bleeding manifestations. Antiplatelet antibodies of the IgG class have been demonstrated in the serum of almost 80 percent of patients with SLE.

Coagulation Defects

Approximately 10 percent of patients with SLE have abnormal factors in the serum that interfere with blood coagulation. An in vitro coagulation defect is associated with a prolonged clotting time accompanied by a normal or prolonged partial one-stage prothrombin time and an abnormal partial thromboplastin time. All other tests, including the thromboplastin generation test, are normal.

Anticoagulant activity invariably resides within the immunoglobulin fractions of circulating plasma, and its delaying effect on the recalcified clotting time and partial prothrombin time of normal plasma can be titered out as though it were an antibody.

The partial thromboplastin time and, rarely, the prothrombin time may also be prolonged in the presence of fibrin-split products, in which case the thrombin time is also prolonged. Fibrin-split products are commonly elevated in patients with SLE, but usually not enough to affect these tests. There is an increased incidence of fibrin-split products in patients with active lupus nephritis, and it has been postulated that intravascular coagulation may contribute to the renal pathologic changes and the presence of hemolytic anemia.

URINALYSIS

Other laboratory abnormalities pertain to specific organ or tissue involvement. Urine concentrations of polyclonal L chains (immunoglobulin light-chains) are elevated during and just prior to exacerbations of kidney disease in SLE. L chains are metabolized by enzymatic protolysis after glomerular filtration, and accurate quantitation of these proteins in the urine seems to be a sensitive assay of renal tubular function. Less common urinary abnormalities in SLE include impaired secretion of potassium ions (with an associated hyperkalemia) and latent renal tubular acidosis.

SYNOVIAL FLUID ANALYSIS

Synovial fluid analysis of painful or swollen joints often reveals a surprising absence of inflammatory changes, with relatively low leukocyte counts and a proportionate increase in the number of mononuclear cells. LE cells many be seen in the direct smear of synovial fluid. Mucin precipitates are almost always normal and the relative viscosity is correspondingly high. The low absolute numbers of neutrophils in synovial fluid are duplicated in pericardial, pleural, and asitic fluid of patients with SLE.

CEREBROSPINAL FLUID ANALYSIS

Apart from patients with aseptic meningitis, pleocytosis is not usually present in the cerebrospinal fluid of patients with SLE. Cerebrospinal fluid total protein is often elevated in patients with organic brain disease and may be correlated with increased concentrations of polyclonal IgG and anti-DNA antibodies. Serial determinations of C4 are said to be helpful in following the course of certain patients with CNS involvement, but C4 hemolytic titers must be performed on the day that the lumbar puncture has been carried unless the cerebrospinal fluid is stored at −70°C.

LIVER FUNCTION TESTS

Liver function abnormalities, particularly elevated serum bilirubin levels are rare in SLE, and elevations of SGOT and lactic acid dehydrogenase usually suggest hepatotoxicity due to aspirin or other therapeutic agents. Anti-smooth muscle antibodies are not associated with liver abnormalities in SLE and if present in high titer suggest a diagnosis of chronic active hepatitis.

REFERENCS

Budman DR, Steinberg AD: Hematologic effects of systemic lupus erythematosus. Ann Intern Med 86:220, 1977

DRUG-INDUCED LUPUSLIKE SYNDROMES

During the past 20 years a steady accumulation of reports has described a lupuslike syndrome induced by various drugs. At least 40 agents have been incriminated; the list includes 7 anticonvulsant agents, 6 phenothiazines, many antibiotics, and miscellaneous drugs, particularly sulfonamides, isoniazide, procainamide, hydralazine, α-methyldopa, propylthiouracil, penicillamine, P-amino salicylic acid, and oral contraceptives. The implication that drugs may activate an illness that resembles idiopathic SLE is most convincing for hydralazine and procainamide, and somewhat less strong for isoniazide, chloropromazine, and the various anticonvulsants. Most of the other drug associations have been reported sporadically, and many of the cases treated with these agents may have already had SLE prior to commencement of drug therapy.

PROCAINAMIDE

Genetic variations in the acetylation of procainamide, hydralazine, and other aromatic compounds are known to exist and it has been clearly demonstrated that "slow acetylators" are more prone to develop side effects, including the drug-induced lupuslike syndrome, after long-term therapy with these agents. While these observations may have an important bearing on the pathogenesis of drug-induced SLE, it should be pointed out that 90 percent of patients with idiopathic SLE also demonstrate slow acetylation of isoniazide when tested under appropriate conditions.

Antinuclear antibodies develop in approximately 75 percent of patients taking procainamide. Only a small proportion of these patients, however, develop a lupuslike clinical reaction, as characterized by polyarthralgia, myalgia, fever, pulmonary infiltrates, pleurisy, and pericarditis. As in other forms of drug-induced SLE, renal disease, CNS involvement, and a classic rash are notably absent, and the clinical abnormalities disappear after the drug is discontinued. On the other hand, since procainamide is usually prescribed for elderly patients with organic heart disease, the additional cardiopulmonary problems may result in death unless therapy is promptly discontinued.

The absence of antibody to native DNA in procainamide-induced SLE has been reported by several laboratories and, although antibody to denatured DNA is present, serum complement levels are normal. There are some experimental data to support the notion that drug–DNA complexes altering DNA immunogenicity may play a pathogenic role in procainamide-induced SLE. The persistence of slowly falling titers of antinuclear antibody for years after the administration of the drug has been stopped indicates that a significant alteration in tolerance to self has occurred in patients receiving procainamide for 6 months or longer. High titers of antibodies to ribonucleoprotein (RNP) have been noted in a large series of patients with myocardial infarction following short-term therapy with procainamide. The relationship of anti-RNP antibodies in the procainamide-treated patients to similar antibodies in SLE, mixed connective tissue disease, and other disorders remains to be defined.

HYDRALAZINE

Immune responses to hydralazine have been detected in patients with hydralazine-induced SLE, but not in patients taking hydralazine without developing toxicity. Although the clinical manifestations of hydralazine- and procainamide-induced lupuslike syndromes are similar, circulating antibodies to native DNA have been described only in the former condition. This suggest that hydralazine hypersensitivity more closely represents an induced or activated form of SLE, but differs pathogenetically with respect to renal, CNS, and possibly skin involvement. Interestingly, hydralazine can be used safely in hypertensive patients with SLE who are receiving concomitant immunosuppressive therapy.

ETIOLOGIC FACTORS AND POSSIBLE THERAPEUTIC INTERVENTION

The preceding chapters in this section are based mainly on clinical experience at Boston University Medical Center and the published accounts of large series of patients seen at Johns Hopkins, Los Angeles County Center, Massachusetts General, Columbia-Presbyterian, and Wellesley Hospitals. Although there may be sampling and classification differences between one series and another, a remarkable uniformity emerges with respect to mode of presentation, prevalence of major system involvement, pathologic findings, and autoimmune abnormalities in SLE. Unfortunately, there is not comparable agreement in the literature regarding etiologic factors in SLE. The pathogenesis is also speculative, although many of the clinical and pathologic findings seem to be related to immune complex deposition. The results of treatment are equally obscure, and it is still not known whether steriods alter the natural history of SLE, almost 30 years after their introduction as therapeutic agents in this disease. For these reasons, it seems appropriate to consider etiologic factors and possible therapeutic intervention in the same chapter. Only by sifting fact from theory will a true appreciation of the role of the various therapeutic agents in SLE become apparent.

ETIOLOGY

The notion that SLE may be an immune complex disease is not a new one. Some of the supporting evidence has already been mentioned—namely, immunofluorescent and electron microscopic findings of immunoglobulin and complement in renal and skin specimens. Similar findings have also been noted in lung and pleural biopsy specimens and in tissue obtained postmortem

from Libman-Sacks heart valve vegetations and brain meninges. In addition, it has been demonstrated that kidney tissue eluates from patients with advanced disease contain high concentrations of ANA, suggesting that the immunoglobulin there is in the form of a complex rather than as a result of nonspecific trapping in the damaged tissue.

Some patients with lupus nephritis have been shown to have circulating free DNA at one time and circulating anti-DNA antibodies at other times, suggesting that complexes are being formed repeatedly. In some instances it has been possible to demonstrate DNA within glomerular deposits or within cryoprecipitates of lupus serum, findings which are tantamount to direct evidence for the presence of the antigen portion of an immune complex. It has also been shown that the highest avidity anti-DNA antibodies are localized to IgG eluated from the glomerulonephritic kidney, and that the anti-DNA antibodies of lowest avidity prevail in the serum of patients with lupus nephritis.

Perhaps the most striking pathogenic abnormality in SLE is the patient's propensity to form autoantibodies not only to cell nuclei but to cell membranes, cytoplasmic ingredients, and plasma proteins. It can be argued that all the clinical and pathologic abnormalities in SLE are directly related to autoimmune phenomena. Anemia, leukopenia, and thrombocytopenia may be at least partially caused by cell membrane toxins. The false-positive biologic tests for syphilis and the factors that interfere with the clotting mechanism may share specific affinity for lipid or glycolipid cellular determinants, and it has been shown that anti-T cell antibodies cross-react with antigens in human brain tissue.

The etiologic events leading up to the autoantibodies and, *pari passu*, circulating immune complexes are unknown. Nevertheless, in formulating approaches to the management of the patient with SLE, certain assumptions about these events are commonly made and acted upon. Generally the assumptions involve an interplay of infectious, genetic, and immunologic factors. Although an etiologic agent has not been identified in patients with SLE, a naturally occurring experimental model is found in the NZB/NZW hybrid mouse; this condition is most interesting because of its close resemblance to the human disease. Chronic viral infection has been demonstrated in these animals and there is impressive though inconclusive evidence that the murine oncogenic type C virus is a causative agent of this lupuslike syndrome. A unique feature of the endogenous oncornaviruses is that the genes of these organisms are present in mice as normal constituents of cellular DNA, inherited by offspring from their parents. A remarkable concentration of oncornaviral envelope glycoprotein has been identified in the tissue and serum of NZB mice as compared to non-NZB-related strains.

A naturally occurring multisystemic disease resembling human SLE has also been recognized in several breeds of dogs, and there is preliminary evidence that

Table 1

Hypothetical Sequence of Events in SLE Etiology with Possible
Therapeutic Intervention

Sequence	Event	Possible Therapy
1.	Vertical transmission of type C virus	Antibiotics
2.	Virus replication in T cells	Genetic counseling
3.	T cell destruction	Soluble immune response suppressor
4.	Defective cellular immunity	Thymic hormones
5.	Enhanced expression of chronic virus infection	Prostaglandins
6.	Hyperactive antibody (B cell) response	High-dose steroids; immunosuppressive agents
7.	Immunologic reaction to viral and host antigens	DNA tolerogens
8.	Circulating immune complexes	Avoidance of UV light Intermediate-dose steroids
9.	Inflammatory response	Salicylates/antimalarials Low-dose steroids
10.	End-stage lupus nephritis	Chronic dialysis; kidney transplantation

type C RNA virus may be present in filtrates from affected tissues in these animals. Independent evidence obtained by different techniques in different laboratories shows that type C virus antigens are present on the peripheral blood lymphocytes of certain patients with SLE, and, as noted previously, cytoplasmic inclusions resembling the nucleocapsid of paramyxvirus have been seen in the kidney and skin of patients with SLE.

Type C virus replication in the thymus or an enhanced immunologic response to the viral antigens could possibly lead to a pathogenic sequence of events as depicted in Table 1. The thymic lesions alter and eventually destroy T cell function, either directly or through an autoimmune mechanism. Defective cellular immunity allows further viral replication and dissemination, inducing an escalating humoral response. Other etiologic events that may apply to both SLE and the autoimmune mouse model are a premature switch from IgM to IgG anti-DNA antibody synthesis, and the protective effect of androgenic hormones with respect to thymic function.

THERAPY

We now appear to be entering a new era in which therapeutic intervention in patients with SLE will make it possible to prevent some if not all of the steps leading to the deposition of immune complexes in renal tissue. The optimal approach would appear to be fourfold:(1) identify genetic markers for the disease such as specific HLA antigens or immune response (Ir) genes; (2) isolate and eradicate the causative exogeneous agent(s); (3) repair the primary immunologic (thymic?) lesion; and (4) prevent the formation of anti-DNA soluble immune complexes.

The most promising methods of preventing or arresting autoimmune phenomena are the result of a recent discovery that NZB/NZW mice lose precursors of "suppressor" T cells and the ability to produce soluble immune response suppressor (SIRS) factor after exposure to the mitogen concanavalin A. Restoration of suppressor cell function in aging NZB/NW mice has already been achieved by the administration of thrice-weekly injections of SIRS obtained from young non-NZB-related mouse spleen cell suspensions and 1-year survival has been favorably altered from 7 percent to 93 percent.

Hormones and Cytotopic Drugs

Other possible ways of lessening the autoimmune features of SLE include the administration of thymic hormones to thymic deficient subjects and modulation of "femaleness" of affected individuals by androgenic hormones. In a novel approach, several investigators have recently shown that treatment of lupus nephritis in adult NZB/NZW F1 mice by cortisone-facilitated tolerance to nucleic acid antigens leads to greatly improved survival. Other regimens which have been reported to lessen disease activity and improve survival in the lupus mouse model include azathioprine, cyclophosphamide, and prostagandin E_1 administration. Unfortunately, the results obtained in experimental animals do not always pertain to the human disease and it has already been proven, for example, that the use of cytotoxic drugs in patients with SLE has been less effective than in the animal model.

Steroids

The role of steroids in the day-to-day management of patients with SLE is still controversial. Steroids are indicated for acute hemolytic episodes, for severe leukopenia, and for thrombocytopenia. Steriods should not be used routinely in all patients, many of whom (with mild or moderate disease) can be maintained on salicylates and antimalarial drugs alone. Patients who have more severe and occasionally life-threatening complications (that is, pericardial effusion with tamponade, myocarditis, or severe inanition or "crisis") in addition to the hemotologic complications already mentioned may often benefit from steroids given for short periods. SLE, however, is not always life threatening, and since steroids are difficult to withdraw and have many severe side effects, these drugs should always be used with caution.

The role of corticosteroids in lupus nephritis is not clear-cut. It is generally agreed that low doses (that is, less than 30 mg prednisone/day or its equivalent) will not affect the course of severe diffuse proliferative glomerulonephritis. There are some who believe that intermediate doses (60–100 mg prednisone/day for periods of up to 6 months) will favorably influence renal disease. There are, however, no controlled studies to support this view, whereas data are accumulating indicating that a number of patients with apparently severe renal disease will do well even without steroids and that serious complications of steroid therapy often outweigh its possible beneficial effects.

The use of intermittent high-dose intravenous "pulse" steroids provides an alternative to the prolonged administration of low or intermediate doses of steroids, but its effectiveness and possible reduction of side effects needs testing in a controlled fashion.

Antimetabolites

Antimetabolites such as 6-mercaptopurine, azathioprine, and cytoxan have also been used in lupus nephritis, usually together with systemic steroids. Although this form of therapy has many advocates and may be beneficial in individal cases, the overall results have been disappointing, and there is mounting evidence that the prolonged use of immunosuppressive agents may lead to a more serious complication, namely, neoplasia.

Nondrug Management

Since there is no specific treatment for SLE, a number of nonspecific measures may be exceedingly helpful in attaining remissions, and some are occasionally lifesaving. In general, patients with active disease should have complete bed rest and an adequate diet, and should avoid stressful situations such as elective surgery, emotional stress, or nonessential drugs. The patients should also avoid direct sunlight and drugs known to sensitize (especially sulfa derivatives, procainamide, trimethadione, and other anticonvulsive agents). The patients with articular disease should have a conservative program of heat and exercises, as outlined in the chapter on treatment in the section on Rheumatoid Arthritis.

Antiinflammatory Agents

Patients with active SLE often feel better on antiinflammatory medication, starting with the most benign agents (salicylates). Aspirin should be prescribed to tolerance, but liver function tests should be performed at regular intervals since it has been shown that salicylates and other nonsteroidal antiinflammatory drugs used in the treatment of lupus may cause liver enzyme abnormalities and biopsy changes indistinguishable from those seen in chronic active hepatitis.

The patient who does not respond to salicylates may show a good response to antimalarial agents.The most commonly used is hydroxychloroquine sulfate (200-mg tablets), 1 tablet twice a day for 1 week, then 1 tablet per day thereafter. One must be cautious in utilizing antimalarial agents, however, because of potential ocular toxicity. Although minor side effects (transient leukopenia or gastrointestinal irritation) may be avoided by changing the dose schedule, the ocular toxicity may lead to scotomata and increasing loss of vision. This complication is probably related to dose and duration of treatment; patients receiving these agents should have a careful opthalmologic examination every 4–6 months.

Summary

In summary, the therapeutic armamentarium for SLE falls far short of desirable, particularly in treating the most severe manifestations such as CNS vasculitis and proliferative diffuse glomerulonephritis. Improved therapeutic intervention probably awaits better understanding of the etiologic and pathogenic events that often lead to end-stage renal disease, atherosclerosis, or permanent cerebrovascular injuries. Promising new avenues of research have been opened, and progress may depend on a better understanding of the murine model, which has already yielded much useful information on the immunobiology of immune complex disease.

REFERENCES

Cathcart ES, Scheinberg MA, Idelson BA, Couser NG: Beneficial effects of methylprednisolone "pulse" therapy in diffuse proliferative nephritis. Lancet 1:163, 1976

Decker JL, Klippel JH, Plotz PH, Steinberg AD: Cyclophosphamide or azothioprine in lupus glomerulonephritis. A controlled trial: Results at 28 months. Ann Intern Med 83: 606, 1975

Kaplan D: Treatment of systemic lupus erythematosus. Arthritis Rheum 20:S175, 1977

Phillips PE: The virus hypothesis in systemic lupus erythematosus. Ann Intern Med 83:709, 1975

Scleroderma (Systemic Sclerosis)

Joseph H. Korn and E. Carwile LeRoy

DEFINITION

Scleroderma (systemic sclerosis) is a multisystem disorder involving primarily the connective tissue and small blood vessels. As the name indicates, cutaneous involvement is the most prominent feature, manifested as swelling, induration, and thickening of skin. The most severe manifestations, however, result from the involvement of visceral organs by fibrotic, vascular, and inflammatory components of the disease. Although the etiology is obscure, there is evidence that metabolic, vascular, and immunologic abnormalities contribute to pathogenesis. Vascular abnormalities (such as Raynaud's syndrome) are usually the earliest clinical features and may precede classic fibrotic changes by years.

Scleroderma is often considered an indolent but inexorably progressive disease; the actual clinical spectrum is varied and broad. Early in the illness, vascular features (Raynaud's phenomenon, telangiectasia) alone may be present and definitive diagnosis may not be possible. This phase may last for weeks in some patients and years in others before fibrotic features become evident; some patients with Raynaud's syndrome never develop characteristic cutaneous scleroderma. At the opposite extreme are patients with widespread and often rapidly progressive fibrotic and vascular processes involving both skin and internal organs, hence the name *progressive systemic sclerosis*. In between are patients with variable proportions of vascular and fibrotic disease of the skin and viscera. The acronym CREST has been used to define a subgroup of patients with (cutaneous) *calcinosis, Raynaud's* syndrome, *esophageal* hypomotility, *sclerodactyly* (scleroderma limited to the digits), and *telangiectasia*. There are also patients with long-term, severe cutaneous disease without detectable visceral involvement. Others may have limited and stable visceral involvement for years. Finally, there are localized forms of scleroderma such as linear scleroderma and morphea that are not associated with either visceral disease or vascular abnormalities.

Whereas characteristic cutaneous features distinguish scleroderma, inflammatory and serologic abnormalities often lead to confusion with other rheumatic disease. Often, individual patients may present with or develop syndromes embodying features of several rheumatic diseases. Cutaneous and/or myositic features of dermatomyositis, cutaneous and/or serologic abnormalities of systemic lupus erythematosus, symmetric polyarthritis, Raynaud's syndrome, and cutaneous scleroderma may appear in various combinations either simultaneously or consecutively in a single patient. Thus, scleroderma not only has a vertical spectrum of severity or involvement, but is itself part of a horizontal spectrum of rheumatic disease that may appear in overlapping or mixed form.

EPIDEMIOLOGY

Scleroderma is the third most common rheumatic disease, following rheumatoid arthritis and systemic lupus erythematosus in prevalence. The disease occurs worldwide and in all races. The incidence in the United States is estimated at 12 cases per million population per year. There is a predilection for women, with a 3:1 female:male ratio. The disease may appear at any age and has been reported in infants as well as octogenerians. Age of onset peaks between the third and sixth decades. The incidence of Raynaud's phenomenon may be 50 times that of definite scleroderma.

Although the disease does not appear to be inherited, 12 families have been reported in which more than 1 member has scleroderma. In addition, scleroderma has been associated within the same family with Raynaud's disease or with other rheumatic diseases. The relative contribution of genetic and environmental factors in these associations is not clear.

CLINICAL AND PATHOLOGIC FINDINGS

Raynaud's Phenomenon

The most common initial symptom of scleroderma is the episodic vasomotor abnormality known as Raynaud's phenomenon. Episodes are characterized by a triphasic reaction involving fingers, toes, and occasionally the face. Initial vasoconstriction and pallor are followed by a dusky cyanosis. With return of flow, there is hyperemia and swelling. Raynaud's phenomenon is most commonly associated with exposure to cold but may also be triggered by stress. On examination, the fingers may be abnormally cool. If the process has been particularly severe or prolonged, there may be ulcerations at the tips of digits or scars of healed ulcerations. At times this may manifest as flattening or concavity of the distal finger pulp. There may also be loss of hair over the second phalanx and tautness of the skin over the distal fingers (sclerodactyly). The toes and occasionally the nose or ears may be similarly involved.

Patients with Raynaud's phenomenon have decreased capillary blood flow and decreased skin temperature, even at usual indoor temperatures. The difference between patients with Raynaud's and normals is exaggerated with cold exposure. A decrease in ambient temperature may result in cessation of cutaneous capillary blood flow in a significant proportion of patients with Raynaud's phenomenon. There is a decrease in the number of skin capillary loops which is most readily seen at the nailfold but is also present in the skin over the distal phalanges. In association with this, there is often marked dilatation and distortion of the remaining capillaries. Larger blood vessels are also abnormal; angiographic studies demonstrate luminal narrowing in the digital arteries. On section, arterioles show the distinctive vascular lesion of scleroderma: arteriolar intimal proliferation which may progress to total occlusion, medial thinning, and a perivascular cuff of connective tissue (Fig. 1).

Skin Manifestations

Cutaneous involvement in scleroderma ranges from subtle alterations in skin thickness and texture to a severe, deforming, hidebound appearance. Although involvement of the hands is usually prominent and most severe, any part of the body may be affected. In general, involvement is worse on the appendages and face than on the axial skeleton and more severe distally than proximally. In the earliest stages, the patient may complain of swelling and stiffness in the hands. Puffiness with nonpitting edema may be noted on examination. Initial sclerotic changes consist of a change in skin texture, apparent thickening of the dermis, and loss of hair over affected parts (Fig. 2A). There is a decrease in skin pliability and an inability to lift the skin from the underlying loose connective tissue. Subsequently, as fibrosis continues, there is marked thickening of dermis, tautness of skin with loss of normal skin creases, and thinning and fragility of epidermis which becomes atrophic with both hyper- and hypopigmentation. Eventually, there is a hidebound appearance with marked loss of skin mobility and contractures due to the fibrotic process. Ulcerations of skin may be prominent and persistent because of poor blood supply, epidermal fragility, and poor healing. Calcium deposition in the dermis may occur and become widespread with time; it is sometimes associated with overlying draining ulcerations.

When involved with scleroderma, the face may ap-

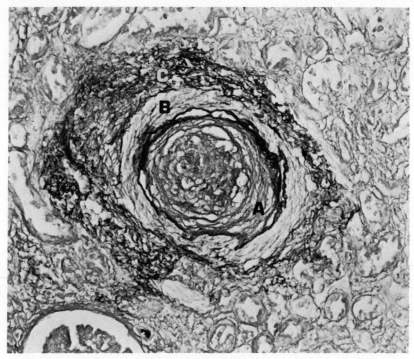

Fig. 1. Artery from kidney of a patient with scleroderma. There is marked intimal proliferation (A), medial thinning (B), and perivascular cuffing of connective tissue (C). The elastic membrane is intensely stained. Resorcin–fuchsin. ×250. (Courtesy of Dr. J. Upshur.)

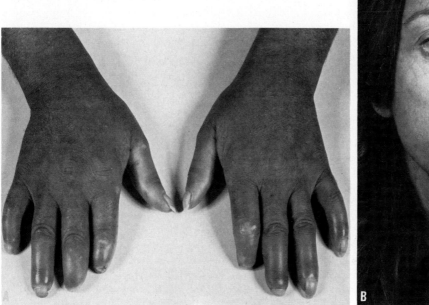
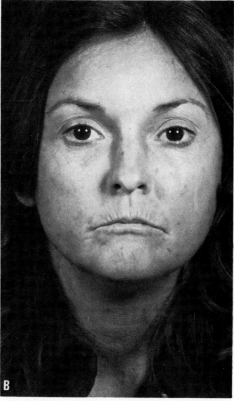

Fig. 2. Hands and face of a patient with scleroderma. **A.** The skin over the distal and middle phalanges is tightened and shiny. There is resorption of the distal phalanges of several digits. **B.** Circumoral constriction by sclerodermatous skin is evident. A few telangiectases are present on the nose, cheeks, and chin.

pear immobile and expressionless. There is inability to open the mouth widely because of constriction of sclerodermatous perioral skin; this may lead to a characteristic "mouselike" appearance or "mauskopf" (Fig. 2B). Telangiectases may be prominent, especially over the cheeks.

On histologic examination, scleroderma skin shows a widening of dermis with increased collagen deposition in the subcutaneous tissue. There is increased ground substance in the skin biopsies of some patients. Dermal mononuclear cell infiltrates are commonly seen; these are most prominent in early and intermediate stages of the disease, although they may be found in late fibrotic stages as well. In advanced scleroderma, atrophy is prominent, with epidermal thinning, loss of glandular structures, and increased melanin deposition. Subcutaneous fat is replaced by collagen fibers. Small arteries show the same changes noted previously: intimal proliferation which may progress to occlusion and an adventitial cuff of collagen.

Gastrointestinal Manifestations

The gastrointestinal tract is the most common visceral organ system involved in scleroderma. Almost any portion may be affected, including the teeth, salivary glands, oropharynx, esophagus, small intestine, large intestine, stomach, pancreas, liver, and gallbladder. Esophageal disease is most frequent, with symptoms present in approximately 40 percent of patients and subclinical involvement present in another 50 percent. There is hypomotility of the distal esophagus and incompetence of the lower esophageal sphincter. Esophageal disease is also present in a majority of patients with the CREST syndrome as well as in a significant proportion of patients with Raynaud's disease alone.

An early symptom is occasional sticking of food in the midchest with pain and fullness. Similar symptoms may be noted after drinking of ice water, suggesting an esophageal counterpart of Raynaud's phenomenon. Heartburn or regurgitation of food, especially in the recumbent position, may result from gastroesophageal reflux; chronic peptic esophagitis can lead to stricture and severe dysphagia.

On radiographic examination, the characteristic findings are hypomotility and dilatation of the distal two-thirds of the esophagus; gastroesophageal reflux of barium may be seen. Abnormal radiographs are found even in asymptomatic patients, particularly in cinéesophagrams taken in the recumbent position. Esophageal pressure determinations (manometrics) are even more sensitive and are abnormal in 90 percent of scleroderma patients.

Symptoms related to the remainder of the alimentary tract are also largely due to hypomotility. The stomach is infrequently involved clinically; poor emptying may lead to nausea and abdominal fullness. Involvement of the small intestine may manifest itself by abdominal distention, bloating, and pain. Stasis leads to bacterial overgrowth and a "blind loop" syndrome with deconjugation

of bile salts, vitamin deficiency, malabsorption, diarrhea, and weight loss. Intestinal telangiectases may be a source of chronic blood loss resulting in anemia.

X-ray contrast studies show gastric dilatation and poor emptying, small intestinal dilatation, especially of the duodenum, slow transit time throughout the bowel, and distinctive wide-mouthed sacculations of the colon. Laboratory evaluation may reveal the common abnormalities of malabsorption: steatorrhea, hypoalbuminemia, vitamin deficiency (especially vitamin B_{12} and the fat-soluble vitamins), and, less commonly, calcium and electrolyte inbalance.

Autopsy studies show smooth muscle atrophy and/or fibrosis of the distal esophagus in almost three-quarters of the patients. Similar involvement of the remainder of the intestinal tract is the cause of the dilatation and hypomotility that is seen. Fibrosis and atrophy may also be the etiology of the gastric achlorhydria that has been reported in some patients. Cellular infiltrates in the bowel wall are similar to those seen in sclerodermatous skin.

Pancreatic and biliary abnormalities are rarely of clinical significance but are more common than ordinarily appreciated. Over one-half of the patients have abnormal pancreatic secretory patterns in response to secretin infusion. Approximately one-third have pancreatic deficiency; some show hypersecretion. Decreased biliary flow and decreased gastric acid secretion are also common. Overt hepatic involvement is rare, but nonspecific ultrastructural abnormalities consisting of giant hepatic mitochondria have been reported in a high proportion of patients studied. A number of patients have been reported who have scleroderma in association with primary biliary cirrhosis and often Sjögren's syndrome as well. Reported salivary gland abnormalities in scleroderma may be due to associated Sjögren's syndrome. Dental involvement is present in approximately one-third of scleroderma patients, with marked widening of the periodontal membrane (Blackburn's sign); it is not usually of clinical significance.

Pulmonary Manifestations

Pulmonary involvement in scleroderma may include disease of the vascular tree and pleura as well as lung parenchyma. Pulmonary symptoms are common in both early and later phases of the disease. The most common complaint is mild dyspnea on exertion. An intermittent cough, occasionally productive of whitish sputum, is often present. The most frequent physical finding is the presence of dry, crackling rales at the lung bases. An increase in the intensity of the second heart sound suggests the development of pulmonary hypertension. With more advanced disease, this may be accompanied by widened splitting of the second heart sound and findings of right ventricular enlargement.

The classic roentgenographic finding is interstitial fibrosis, most prominent at the lung bases. In early stages, an alveolar pattern may also be present, suggesting an inflammatory component. Pleural effusions are seen occasionally. Pulmonary function tests are a more sensitive indicator of lung involvement and may be abnormal in the presence of a normal chest x-ray. Disease of the small airways occurs early and may be detected by an abnormal closing volume, an increase in residual volume, and an abnormal diffusion capacity. A somewhat later finding is the restrictive picture of interstitial fibrosis: decreased vital capacity and total lung capacity. Obstructive disease may be seen as well, but it is the least specific finding. On right heart catheterization there may be elevation of pulmonary artery pressures resulting from interstitial lung disease as well as from primary involvement of the pulmonary vasculature.

At autopsy, pulmonary arteries show medial hypertrophy and an intimal proliferation similar to that seen in other organs. There is smooth muscle atrophy of the bronchiolar wall with loss of elastic tissue and resultant bronchiolectasia. Parenchymal fibrosis leads to both airway narrowing and thickening of the alveolar–capillary membrane. Lung biopsies in some patients with pulmonary symptoms of recent onset have shown vasculitis, leading to the suggestion that this might be an early and perhaps causative pathologic lesion.

Cardiovascular Manifestations

All three layers of the heart may be involved in scleroderma. Pericardial disease is most common and may present as acute or chronic pericarditis. Chronic pericardial tamponade with peripheral edema may be mistaken for congestive heart failure. Pericardial effusions are found by echocardiography in about one-half of patients with scleroderma; a similar proportion of patients who come to autopsy have effusions and/or pericardial inflammation.

Myocardial involvement was thought to be a common cause of cardiac symptoms in scleroderma patients. Although myocardial fibrosis is seen in the majority of patients with scleroderma, this is a common pathologic finding in elderly nonscleroderma patients as well. Only in younger scleroderma patients studied at autopsy is there a significant increase in myocardial fibrosis compared to control populations. It should be remembered that pulmonary disease, pericardial effusions, and hypertensive heart disease may each lead to cardiac decompensation in the scleroderma patient. In addition, the scleroderma patient is not immune to the arteriosclerosis which afflicts the rest of the population. Thus, it is not clear that a fibrotic "scleroderma heart" plays a major role in the etiology of clinically evident cardiac disease. Right ventricular disease secondary to disease of the lungs and pulmonary vasculature has already been mentioned. Involvement of the endocardium and heart valves in scleroderma has been reported but is uncommon and is rarely a cause of functional abnormality.

Renal Manifestations

Renal disease in scleroderma is the single most important indicator of prognosis. Fortunately, only a minority of patients with scleroderma ever develop renal disease, for its appearance is almost invariably an omen of a rapidly progressive and fatal course. Renal involvement is manifested clinically by the appearance of hypertension (blood pressure greater than 140/90), proteinuria, or azotemia. The appearance of any one of these symptoms is associated with rapidly progressive oliguric renal failure. The presence of preexistent hypertension (i.e., documented hypertension prior to the development of scleroderma) may not have the same poor prognostic significance.

The basic lesion in the scleroderma kidney is found in the small blood vessels. Magnification angiography can demonstrate vascular abnormalities in intralobular renal arteries and loss and narrowing of cortical vessels. Hemodynamic studies show a reduction in renal cortical blood flow measured by labeled xenon infusion. In patients followed prospectively, abnormalities in renal blood flow and angiographic patterns may antedate the appearance of hypertension, proteinuria, or azotemia.

On pathologic examination, the characteristic triad of scleroderma vascular involvement is seen: intimal proliferation, medial thinning, and adventitial cuffing of collagen. This process involves interlobular arteries, intralobular arteries, and afferent arterioles. Fibrinoid necrosis of arteriolar walls may be present. The vascular lesion is distinguishable from that of malignant hypertension by the presence of medial thinning and an adventitial cuff of collagen. Such lesions may be seen even in the kidneys of patients who do not have clinical hypertension. In addition to arterial lesions, there may be associated cortical infarcts, sclerosis or necrosis of glomeruli, interstitial edema, inflammation or fibrosis, and nonspecific tubular changes such as swelling, atrophy, and epithelial degeneration. Indirect immunofluorescence of scleroderma kidneys has inconsistently demonstrated the deposition of fibrinogen, immunoglobulin, and complement.

The ureters and bladder may also be involved with the sclerodermatous process. Rarely, ureteral fibrosis may result in obstruction. Bladder atony resulting from muscular fibrosis has also been seen.

Musculoskeletal Manifestations

Arthralgia and joint stiffness are common in scleroderma and may be the presenting symptoms. True arthritis with warm or swollen joints is uncommon. In later stages of the disease, stiffness of the hands secondary to dermal involvement may be perceived as articular by the patient. Joint deformity usually results from fibrosis and contracture of skin rather than from articular disease per se. Sclerodermatous involvement of tendon sheaths can contribute to flexion contractures of joints. Examination may reveal audible or palpable crepitus over the tendon sheaths.

Radiographic studies rarely demonstrate erosive arthritis; indeed, bony erosions should suggest coexistent rheumatoid disease. A characteristic finding is resorption of the distal phalangeal tuft of fingers and toes. This is due to vascular disease and may be found in patients with severe Raynaud's phenomenon without scleroderma. Intraarticular calcium deposition with calcific effusion has been reported. Pathologically, the synovium may show changes similar to but less extensive than those seen in rheumatoid arthritis: synovial proliferation and mononuclear cell infiltration. A distinctive finding is the deposition of a fibrin coat over the synovium and occasionally within synovial tissue.

Disease of striated muscle is common in scleroderma and may account for the frequent complaints of myalgia and weakness. In general, however, muscle involvement is not severe. There may be muscle tenderness and objective weakness; more often, physical examination is unrevealing. Mild elevations of creatinine phosphokinase and aldolase are seen in the majority of scleroderma patients. Electromyographic and histologic findings are usually normal but sometimes support the diagnosis of inflammatory myositis. Occasionally, myositis may dominate the clinical picture and result in severe proximal muscle weakness and tenderness, marked elevations in muscle enzymes, and grossly abnormal electromyograms. The term "sclerodermatomyositis" has been used to describe patients with cutaneous scleroderma and severe myositis.

Neurologic Manifestations

Involvement of the nervous system in scleroderma is uncommon. Peripheral neuropathy has been reported but is rarely apparent clinically. Increased thickness of the perineural connective tissue sheaths seen on histologic section may play a pathogenetic role. A number of patients with scleroderma have developed trigeminal neuralgia in the course of their illness but involvement of the other cranial nerves rarely, if ever, occurs. Similarly, central nervous system disease due to scleroderma is rare, perhaps nonexistent.

Sjögren's Syndrome

Sjögren's syndrome (sicca complex) has been demonstrated in a high proportion of patients with scleroderma. In our experience, involvement is rarely of clinical significance.

Laboratory Findings

The diagnosis of scleroderma rests upon a constellation of clinical symptoms and signs. There are few specific or distinctive laboratory abnormalities. Radiographic or manometric evidence of disordered esophageal hypomotility is probably the most helpful finding. Other abnormalities include (1) serologic findings common to a number of rheumatologic and chronic inflammatory states and (2) indicators of specific organ involvement. A mild anemia is found in one-third to one-fourth of patients and is usually normochromic and normocytic. Elevation of the erythrocyte sedimentation rate is common and may relate to disease stage or activity. Serum globulins are often elevated, especially IgM, and there may be hypoalbuminemia. Circulating cryoglobulins have been detected in almost half the patients studied. Tests for rheumatoid factor are positive in one-third of patients and are often associated with cryoglobulinemia. Antinuclear antibodies are found frequently; in many patients there is a distinctive nucleolar pattern on indirect immunofluorescence. Antibodies directed againsted sin-

gle-stranded RNA, specifically uracil nucleotides, have been found in a high proportion of patients studied. Lupus erythematosus (LE) cells are seen rarely, except in those patients who also have clinical features of systemic lupus erythematosus.

Some laboratory tests may provide a clue to early or subclinical involvement of different organ systems. The finding of proteinuria or an elevated BUN almost invariably predicts the development of severe and fatal renal disease. Microangiopathic hemolytic anemia is often seen in patients with renal disease and hypertension. Elevations of creatinine phosphokinase and aldolase indicate the presence of myositis. Lactic acid dehydrogenase and glutamic oxaloacetic transaminase elevations may result from both muscle and pulmonary disease. As previously noted, pulmonary function tests, echocardiography, and tests for intestinal absorption may detect visceral involvement before it becomes clinically evident. Evaluation of renal blood flow by radioactive xenon infusion and renal arteriography are invasive procedures, but they may be useful in the early detection of renal disease. Similarly, cardiac catheterization may identify patients with pulmonary hypertension.

The usefulness of skin biopsies in the diagnosis of scleroderma has been limited. In general, the biopsy findings reflect what is already clinically apparent. In patients with early disease, full-thickness skin biopsies which include the subcutaneous tissues may reveal cellular infiltration that is suggestive but not diagnostic of scleroderma. In these early cases, the characteristic vascular lesions are usually not present or are not severe enough to allow diagnosis on histologic grounds.

ETIOLOGY AND PATHOGENESIS

Although the etiology of scleroderma is unknown, in recent years considerable information has accumulated about a number of possible pathogenetic mechanisms. Investigative approaches to scleroderma have been directed by the clinical findings of vasculopathy, vascular lesions, fibrosis, and immunologic abnormalities. The results of various studies have suggested that vascular, metabolic, and inflammatory events may play pathogenetic roles.

Vascular, Metabolic, and Immunologic Factors

The outstanding clinical vascular feature of scleroderma is the presence of Raynaud's syndrome. This temperature-dependent phenomenon results from abnormal vascular reactivity in the small to medium-sized arteries of the extremities. The abnormal response to cold extends to vessels supplying the visceral organs as well; renal blood flow in scleroderma patients has been shown to be temperature sensitive and, as previously noted, esophageal symptoms may be triggered by cold exposure. The cause of the pathologic vasospastic response is unclear. Raynaud's phenomenon may be reproduced in normal volunteers by the intraarterial injection of serotonin. Isolated blood vessels of patients with scleroderma and Raynaud's syndrome demonstrate increased sensitivity to serotonin. It is interesting that injection of serotonin can cause fibrosis of human skin and that patients with serotonin-producing (carcinoid) tumors develop fibrosis in visceral organs. Studies of scleroderma patients have failed to reveal a disorder of serotonin metabolism.

The role of the microvasculature in scleroderma was recognized over 50 years ago when the association was made between Raynaud's phenomenon and abnormalities of the capillary circulation at the nailfold. There was decreased capillary blood flow, a decrease in the number of capillary loops, and marked capillary dilatation and tortuosity. These distinctive capillary findings have been confirmed and are seen only in patients with scleroderma, dermatomyositis, and Raynaud's disease. The visceral counterpart of this abnormality is best displayed by the loss of vessels and an abnormal vascular pattern in sclerodermatous kidneys. A correlation has been demonstrated between the severity of capillary abnormalities observed at the nailfold and the extent of visceral disease. Peripheral microvascular abnormalities may prove a useful means of early detection of visceral involvement; such early detection is critical in view of the rapidly progressive nature of some forms of visceral disease.

Two findings suggest that microvascular abnormalities in scleroderma may be a consequence of vascular injury. A factor has been reported in the serum of scleroderma patients with cytotoxic activity specific for endothelial cells. In another study, evidence was found for increased endothelial cell proliferation in the dermal blood vessels of some scleroderma patients. Thus, the intimal proliferation and vessel occlusion seen on histologic examination could represent an endothelial response to injury.

Several abnormalities in connective tissue metabolism have been observed in scleroderma. The most interesting of these is the demonstration that scleroderma skin fibroblasts synthesize more collagen in vitro than do normal fibroblasts. Furthermore, this abnormality persists after multiple passages in tissue culture. The expression of this defect in vivo is evidenced by the accumulation of excessive collagen in sclerodermatous skin. Additional evidence for excess collagen synthesis in vivo is the presence of increased protocollagen proline hydroxylase in the skin of some scleroderma patients. This enzyme converts proline to hydroxyproline in the precursor molecule of collagen. Thus, a primary defect in the regulation of collagen synthesis may play a role in the pathogenesis of scleroderma.

The frequent finding of immunologic abnormalities in scleroderma and the occasional appearance of clinical features of lupus erythematosus, polymyositis, and rheumatoid arthritis in scleroderma patients suggest that scleroderma may be, at least in part, an autoimmune disease. In addition to antibodies directed against IgG and nuclear antigens, antibodies to mitochondrial, smooth muscle, gastric parietal cell, and thyroid antigens have been found in scleroderma patients. The depression of cellular immune function common in patients with systemic lupus erythematosus is not seen in scleroderma. Delayed hypersensitivity skin responses to common antigens are normal. The proportions of T and B lymphocytes, as well as the response of scleroderma lymphocytes to mitogens, have been variously reported as normal or moderately depressed.

The above findings are commonly seen in a number of immunologic and chronic inflammatory states and probably have little direct bearing on disease pathogenesis. Other abnormalities of immune function may have more specificity or relevance for scleroderma. Scleroderma lymphocytes have been shown to be cytotoxic in vitro to both fibroblasts and smooth muscle cells. Cell-mediated immunity to collagen has been demonstrated in some patients with scleroderma but in some patients with rheumatoid arthritis and systemic lupus erythematosus as well. Recent studies have demonstrated the production of migration inhibition factor by scleroderma lymphocytes when they are exposed to extracts of skin. The frequent finding of cellular infiltrates in sclerodermatous skin suggests that cellular immune mechanisms directed against connective tissue antigens may operate in vivo.

Model of Pathogenesis

A hypothetical model of the pathogenesis of scleroderma can be constructed that considers the immunologic, metabolic, and vascular abnormalities. Immunologically mediated injury to the microvasculature, humoral and/or cell mediated, leads to vascular occlusion and decreased blood flow. One consequence of the vascular lesion is injury to the surrounding connective tissue. Such injury results in fibroblast proliferation and excessive collagen deposition. Hypoxia and other metabolic consequences of vascular injury, as well as factors released by inflammatory cells, may select fibroblast populations that synthesize excessive collagen. Perivascular accumulation of collagen alters blood vessel distensibility and contractility, causing further derangement of blood flow and Raynaud's phenomenon. A secondary result of injury to connective tissue could be an immunologic response to (altered) connective tissue or cellular antigens with perpetuation of the whole process.

Support for such a model comes from the study of graft versus host reactions in both experimental animals and man. The transfer of nonhistocompatible bone marrow cells or spleen cells from normal mice to immunosuppressed mice results in an immune reaction of donor cells against the recipient host. Vascular lesions seen in such animals strongly resemble those of scleroderma. A similar pathology is seen in blood vessels of rejected human allografts. Furthermore, the appearance of scleroderma-like skin lesions has been reported in several patients who developed graft versus host reactions after receiving bone marrow transplants from nonidentical twins for the treatment of aplastic anemia. Thus, both vascular and fibrotic abnormalities of scleroderma can be reproduced in part by an immunologically mediated process.

Genetic Factors

The role of genetic factors in the pathogenesis of scleroderma is unclear. As already noted, several studies report familial aggregation of scleroderma and/or Raynaud's syndrome. In the vast majority of cases, however, there is no family history of rheumatic disease. Several recent reports, though, suggest that genetic factors may play a role; chromosomal abnormalities have been found in a high proportion of scleroderma patients. Furthermore, an abnormally high incidence of chromosomal abnormalities was found in over two-thirds of first-degree relatives of patients studied. Sera of scleroderma patients with chromosomal abnormalities contained a factor which could induce chromosome breaks in normal cells. The relationship of vascular, metabolic, and immunologic abnormalities in scleroderma is unknown.

Environmental Factors

Another clue to the pathogenesis of Raynaud's syndrome and scleroderma comes from reported occupational associations with these diseases. It has long been known that workers using vibrating instruments such as jackhammers and reciprocating saws have an abnormally high incidence of Raynaud's syndrome. More recently, it has been reported that polyvinyl chloride workers may develop not only Raynaud's syndrome, but also microvascular capillary abnormalities and acroosteolysis similar to that seen in scleroderma. An increased incidence of scleroderma has been reported in South African gold miners and French miners with silicosis. In these groups of patients, pulmonary and cutaneous findings predominated. Thus, environmental factors can predispose to the development of both the vascular and fibrotic aspects of scleroderma.

DIFFERENTIAL DIAGNOSIS
Raynaud's Phenomenon

The diagnosis of scleroderma presents no difficulty in the patient who presents with Raynaud's phenomenon and characteristic hidebound skin. When Raynaud's phenomenon alone is present, the diagnostic challenge is greater. Raynaud's phenomenon may be present in other rheumatic diseases (e.g., rheumatoid arthritis or systemic lupus erythematosus) as well as in association with occlusive or obliterative vascular disorders (e.g., arteriosclerosis and Buerger's disease), local trauma or structural lesions (e.g., thoracic outlet obstruction), occupational exposure to vibrating instruments, and serum hyperviscosity with circulating cryoproteins such as cold agglutinins and cryoglobulins. Each of these considerations should be evaluated systematically. In our experience, when the above causes are not present, the majority of patients with Raynaud's phenomenon go on to develop scleroderma. Patients with more severe symptoms and those who develop secondary skin changes such as digital ulcerations and sclerodactyly are at greatest risk. It is important, therefore, to search for evidence of visceral scleroderma in patients with Raynaud's phenomenon by careful examination of the various organ systems. Evidence of esophageal hypomotility, abnormalities in pulmonary function tests, and elevations of the muscle enzymes are among the earliest findings seen in asymptomatic patients.

Rarely, a patient may present with Raynaud's phenomenon and widespread visceral scleroderma but without the characteristic cutaneous findings (so-called scleroderma sine scleroderma). In these patients the diagnosis can only be made on the basis of the characteristic visceral pathology described earlier. Distal esophageal hypomotility, duodenal dilatation, and colonic sacculations are lesions strongly suggestive of scleroderma.

Sclerodermalike Skin Changes

A number of disease entities have cutaneous features that may be confused with scleroderma. Scleredema (of Buschke) presents with an indurated, often hidebound, appearance of the skin that may be indistinguishable from scleroderma. A clue to diagnosis is the presence of predominantly truncal and proximal extremity involvement; there is absolute or relative sparing of the hands, forearms, and feet, which are most commonly involved in scleroderma. Eosinophilic fasciitis is an inflammatory disease of skin, subcutaneous tissue, and muscle that may resemble scleroderma. Peripheral eosinophilia, the absence of Raynaud's phenomenon, marked hyperglobulinemia, and occasionally eosinophilic infiltration on histologic section distinguish this entity from scleroderma. Sclerodermalike skin changes have also been reported in porphyria, Werner's syndrome, amyloidosis, progeria, acrodermatitis chronica atrophicans, lichen sclerosis and atrophicus, acromegaly, and infiltrating carcinomia. Shoulder–hand syndrome, especially when bilateral, may cause diagnostic confusion, particularly with the early, puffy phase of scleroderma.

CREST Syndrome

In our opinion, the importance of diagnostic differentiation between scleroderma and the CREST syndrome has been overemphasized. As mentioned earlier, scleroderma and CREST are both part of a broad spectrum of disease. The optimism based on initial reports of the benign course of the CREST syndrome has been tempered by the progression, with time, of significant numbers of patients to classic scleroderma with extensive visceral disease. In this respect, patients with CREST resemble those who have Raynaud's syndrome alone for long periods of time before the development of scleroderma.

Mixed Connective Tissue Disease

Similarly, the value of distinguishing "pure" scleroderma from scleroderma with overlapping features of other rheumatic diseases has been overly emphasized. The favorable response of patients with "mixed connective tissue disease" to steroid therapy reflects not so much the diagnosis as the systems involved and the stage of that involvement. Thus, myositis is generally steroid responsive whether it occurs in pure scleroderma, systemic lupus erythematosus, polymyositis, or mixed connective tissue disease. Although it was initially suggested that patients with mixed or overlapping disease have an almost invariably favorable course, more recent data do not support this conclusion. Some of these patients have developed severe renal disease unresponsive to conventional therapy. When followed long enough, many, if not most, patients with mixed features of two or more rheumatic diseases develop a more classic picture of a single connective tissue disorder—usually scleroderma, and less often systemic lupus erythematosus.

MANAGEMENT

No specific therapy is presently available that can prevent visceral disease in scleroderma. The absence of specific curative therapy should not, however, discourage the physician from employing useful therapeutic modalities that may benefit the patient. These measures are mainly directed at ameliorating symptoms and preventing complications resulting from involvement of various organ systems.

General Management

The psychologic aspects of chronic disease are often given inadequate attention by the physician. For the patient, the knowledge that he or she suffers from an incurable and progressive disease is often devastating. The importance of patient education with regard to available therapeutic modalities, as well as the patient's own role in maintaining optimal health, cannot be overemphasized. He or she must be encouraged to lead a normal life within the limitations created by the disease. Physical activity should be encouraged and, in some patients, physical therapy may be necessary. Such measures are helpful in combating the contractures and muscle wasting which accompany a passive and sedentary approach to the disease. Indeed, regular exercise is beneficial; patient fears to the contrary are common and should be dispelled.

Raynaud's Phenomenon

The first line of therapy against cold-induced vasoconstriction is the use of protective physical measures. Excessive cold exposure should be avoided. Gloves and extra pairs of socks should be worn to shield affected extremities, as well as extra layers of clothing to keep the trunk warm and induce peripheral vasodilatation. The patient should feel warm, even to the point of mild perspiration.

A pharmacologic approach to the treatment of Raynaud's phenomenon has been moderately successful. Drugs with direct vasodilating properties as well as sympatholytic agents have been used for many years. Sympathetic blocking agents such as guanethidine, methyldopa, phenoxybenzamine, and reserpine have generally been more effective in management than direct vasodilating drugs. Therapy should be initiated at low doses and gradually adjusted upward until the desired effect is obtained or side-effects supervene. The most troublesome side-effects are orthostatic hypotension with guanethidine and methyldopa, impotence with guanethidine, sinus and atrial tachycardias with phenoxybenzamine, and depression and nasal stuffiness with reserpine. Less commonly, methyldopa may cause hepatic dysfunction or autoimmune hemolytic anemia. Because guanethidine has few side effects and may be administered in a single daily dose, many clinicians prefer it to other agents. No one agent is clearly superior to any other; indeed, at least part of the therapeutic response results from a placebo

effect. Nonetheless, many patients report a decrease in the frequency of attacks of Raynaud's phenomenon and show objective signs of improvement such as the absence of new digital ulcerations and healing of existing ones.

Reserpine administered intraarterially has also been effective in treating Raynaud's phenomenon. The administration of 0.5 mg reserpine as a single dose into the brachial artery has resulted in improved blood flow with healing of digital ulcerations in some patients. Beneficial effects are of variable duration (from several weeks to 6 months). Interestingly, some patients also show improved esophageal motility after intraarterial reserpine. In patients with more severe vascular disease unresponsive to physical and pharmacologic treatment, surgical sympathectomy may be temporarily beneficial. A substantial proportion of patients respond to this more drastic measure; unfortunately, the benefits are often not permanent. Some studies suggest that patients with Raynaud's syndrome in association with scleroderma are less likely to have a permanent or long-lasting response to surgical sympathectomy than patients with idiopathic Raynaud's phenomenon (Raynaud's disease).

Skin Involvement

Although a variety of drugs has been advocated for the treatment of cutaneous scleroderma, none has, as yet, stood the test of time. The use of D-penicillamine and colchicine was prompted by knowledge of their capacity to inhibit collagen synthesis. D-penicillamine inhibits collagen cross-linking and is active in the dissolution of disulfide bonds. Colchicine inhibits microtubular function, thereby impairing movement of collagen out of the cell; it also stimulates collagenase activity, which should result in dissolution of collagen that has already formed. Although some reports suggest the effectiveness of both these agents in treating the dermal manifestations of scleroderma, more extensive trials are necessary before general use can be advocated. One should remember that, following initial reports, there was optimism about dimethylsulfoxide, para-aminobenzoic acid, and vitamin E for the treatment of scleroderma; early enthusiasm waned when subsequent studies showed little or no beneficial effect. It is also not generally appreciated that hidebound skin may soften spontaneously after several years. Wider cognizance of this feature of scleroderma might reduce the number of enthusiastic reports of therapy.

Nonspecific approaches such as local creams to prevent dryness are useful. Infected ulcerations should be treated aggressively with local debridement and antibiotic ointments. Finally, measures that improve vascular flow will generally also be successful in treating and preventing cutaneous ulcerations.

Gastrointestinal Involvement

Although esophageal hypomotility and incompetence of the lower esophageal sphincter are common in scleroderma, they are usually asymptomatic. When symptoms are present, they may be managed with the same measures used in treatment of gastroesophageal reflux of other causes. Avoidance of the recumbent position after meals helps reduce regurgitation of food. Elevation of the head of the bed on 6–12-inch blocks and antacid preparations are helpful in the treatment of peptic esophagitis. Metoclopramide has been reported effective in improving esophageal sphincter pressure and reducing symptoms. It has been suggested that antacids and bed elevation be used routinely in scleroderma patients as prophylaxis against esophageal stricture which might result from chronic reflux esophagitis.

Other gastrointestinal symptoms such as diarrhea, abdominal distention, steatorrhea, malabsorption, weight loss, and occasionally intestinal obstruction result from severely disordered motility of the alimentary tract, most critically the third and fourth segments of the duodenum and the proximal ileum. The nutritional consequences of stasis-induced bacterial overgrowth can be ameliorated with the cyclic use of broad-spectrum antibiotics such as tetracycline. Occasionally, low-residue diets and medium-chain triglycerides are necessary to enhance intestinal absorption and improve the general nutritional state. Episodes of adynamic ileus can generally be treated with conservative measures; surgical intervention is rarely necessary and may have catastrophic consequences.

Pulmonary Involvement

Once the fibrotic process is established in the lungs, there is little to offer other than supportive care. This consists of oxygen when necessary, respiratory exercises, and aggressive treatment of supervening infection. Although no agents that are currently available have been shown to suppress or arrest the fibrotic and vascular processes, the hope for future therapy lies in the early detection of pulmonary involvement. In some patients, early biopsies have shown a vasculitic and inflammatory process which may be responsive to glucocorticoid therapy.

The course of the pulmonary disease is usually an indolent one. Interstitial involvement may be present for some years before symptoms become evident. Even then, the patient may function in a restricted capacity for several years before the appearance of end-stage pulmonary disease, fatal infection, or fatal involvement of other organ systems.

Cardiac Involvement

Symptoms of dyspnea and dependent edema may result from cardiac as well as pulmonary disease. Right heart catheterization may be necessary to detect pulmonary hypertension and cor pulmonale. Even with relatively normal heart size on roentgenogram, a significant pericardial effusion may be present; echocardiography should be done on all patients with symptoms of congestive heart failure. In our experience, the development of congestive heart failure with pericardial effusion has been a poor prognostic sign, leading to oliguric renal failure within 6 months in some patients.

Patients with scleroderma who develop acute pericarditis usually respond well to antiinflammatory agents or short-term corticosteroids. Steroids are not effective in the treatment of established myocardial disease, with the possible exception of rarely occurring myocarditis. Congestive heart failure due to presumed myocardial involvement with scleroderma is best managed with digitalis, diuretics, and salt restriction. If the earliest lesions in cardiac scleroderma are vasculitic or inflammatory, one might presume that steroids would be effective. The inability to date to detect and treat such early myocardial disease precludes a definitive statement. Recently developed techniques such as combined gallium–xenon myocardial scans may be helpful in detecting early myocardial scleroderma.

Hypertension and Renal Failure

No effective therapy is available for the cure or prevention of renal disease in scleroderma. This is particularly distressing because renal involvement is the single most important predictor of an unfavorable course. Thus, at present, the detection of renal disease is of prognostic rather than therapeutic importance. Reliable indicators of renal involvement include the development of hypertension, proteinuria, and azotemia. Plasma renin activity is often, but not always, elevated.

Hypertension should be treated aggressively. Occasionally, control of blood pressure may be impossible with standard therapy, particularly in patients with rapidly progressive renal disease. Combinations of drugs should be used, including propranolol to suppress renin activity. Nephrectomy in combination with hemodialysis or transplantation has been used in a limited number of patients with rapidly progressive oliguric renal failure. The results to date suggest that such a program may be effective in some patients in avoiding what would otherwise be a fatal course. The use of newer, potent antihypertensive agents or combinations of antihypertensive agents such as minoxidil, propranalol, and methyldopa has not been adequately explored but may represent an alternative to nephrectomy. Corticosteroids and immunosuppressive agents have not been useful in this setting; indeed, it has been suggested that the use of corticosteroids may accelerate the disease process.

Musculoskeletal Involvement

Significant myositis with muscle weakness is frequently seen in scleroderma. Corticosteroids are the basic treatment and should be used at a dose of 1 mg/kg prednisone equivalent per day, in divided doses. As in other rheumatic diseases, the response is usually prompt, with improvement in both clinical and chemical parameters. There has not been adequate experience with the use of immunosuppressive agents and methotrexate in the treatment of those patients with scleroderma myositis who are either steroid unresponsive or require long-term steroids for control of their disease. In asymptomatic patients with mild elevations of muscle enzymes, steroid therapy has generally not been successful in improving the chemical parameters.

Articular disease in scleroderma is usually not severe. When carefully questioned, the patient may reveal

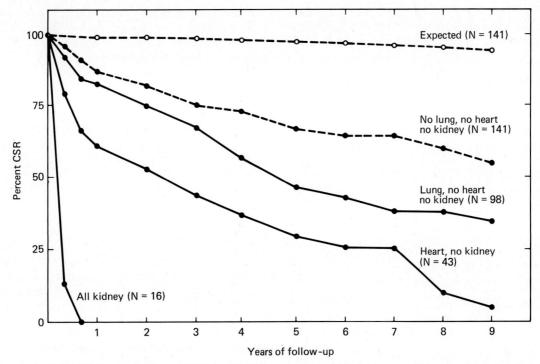

Fig. 3. Observed cumulative survival rates (CSR) for scleroderma patients with lung, heart, or kidney involvement and observed and expected CSR for patients with none of these involvements at entry to study. (Courtesy of Dr. T. Medsger.)

that his "joint pain" actually derives from stiffness, immobility, and contractures of the skin. Symptoms are best controlled with moderate doses of aspirin or, in the aspirin-intolerant patient, other nonsteroidal, antiinflammatory agents.

Future Therapy

As already noted, treatment of scleroderma as a whole has not met with any considerable success. Over the past two decades, a number of agents have been used in the general treatment of scleroderma. Corticosteroids were among the earliest drugs used; they have not been shown to have an effect on the natural course of the disease. In the early inflammatory phases of the illness, transient improvement from steroids may be seen, but benefits must be weighed against potential risks. The therapeutic value of immunosuppressive agents has not been demonstrated. Although some reports suggest improvement of cutaneous disease with D-penicillamine treatment, no effect on visceral involvement has been shown. Colchicine is currently under investigation as a therapeutic agent but the information to date is inadequate to make a definite judgment. The lack of efficacy of some of the drugs tested may be a result of our inability to detect scleroderma in the earliest and potentially most treatable stages. The future of scleroderma therapy may depend on both earlier diagnosis, especially of visceral disease, and a better understanding of underlying pathogenetic mechanisms.

COURSE AND PROGNOSIS

As already noted, the course of scleroderma is highly variable. In the individual patient, prognosis is determined by the site and extent of visceral disease (Fig. 3). In general, patients over the age of 50, males, and blacks have a poorer prognosis. Renal involvement is most serious; patients who develop hypertension, azotemia, or proteinuria follow a course that almost invariably leads to death within 6–12 months. The employment of dialysis and/or renal transplantation as life-supporting measures after renal failure has met with only limited success; patients often succumb to pulmonary infection or hemorrhage.

Cardiac and pulmonary scleroderma, in that order, follow renal involvement as predictors of mortality. Gastrointestinal disease is not an independent risk factor except when untimely death is precipitated by surgical intervention in severe adynamic ileus. Similarly, the severity, extent, and duration of cutaneous disease have no effect on survival. Nonetheless, even patients without clinical renal, cardiac, or pulmonary disease have a shorter life expectancy than normal, probably because of unrecognized visceral involvement.

Scleroderma represents a challenge to the physician in its early detection, in careful monitoring for the appearance of visceral involvement without inducing unnecessary anxiety, and in aggressive intervention when life-threatening involvement occurs. A greater understanding of this multistage, multisystem disease with widely vary-ing rate and sites of involvement will be required before more rational therapy can become available.

REFERENCES

Campbell PM, LeRoy EC: Pathogenesis of systemic sclerosis: A vascular hypothesis. Semin Arthritis Rheum 4:351, 1975

Cannon PJ, Hassar M, Case DB, Casarella WJ, Sommers SC, and LeRoy EC: The relationship of hypertension and renal failure in scleroderma (progressive systemic sclerosis) to structural and functional abnormalities of the renal cortical circulation. Medicine (Baltimore) 53:1, 1974

D'Angelo WA, Fries JF, Masi AT, Shulman LE: Pathologic observations in systemic sclerosis (scleroderma). A study of fifty-eight autopsy cases and fifty-eight matched controls. Amer J Med 46:428, 1969

Fleischmajer R, Perlish JS, Reeves JRT: Cellular infiltrates in scleroderma skin. Arthritis Rheum 20:975, 1977

Kondo H, Rabin BS, Rodnan GP: Cutaneous antigen-stimulating lymphokine production by lymphocytes of patients with progressive systemic sclerosis (scleroderma). J Clin Invest 58:1388, 1976

LeRoy EC: Increased collagen synthesis by scleroderma skin fibroblast *in vitro*. A possible defect in the regulation or activation of the scleroderma fibroblast. J Clin Invest 54:880, 1974

Medsger TA, Jr, Masi AT, Rodnan GP, Benedek TG, Robinson H: Survival with systemic sclerosis (scleroderma). A life table analysis of clinical and demographic factors in 309 patients. Ann Intern Med 75:369, 1971

Norton WL, Nardo JM: Vascular disease in progressive systemic sclerosis (scleroderma). Ann Intern Med 73:317, 1970

DIFFUSE EOSINOPHILIC FASCIITIS

Lawrence E. Shulman

This is a newly recognized connective tissue disease that initially appears to be either scleroderma or dermatomyositis but has distinguishing clinical, laboratory, and histopathologic features that allow it to be clearly separated from both diseases. In most patients the disease seems to follow (by hours, days, or weeks) physical exertion that is either unusual or excessive for that individual. Even though flexion contractures of the extremities may develop, the disorder seems reversible, often completely; prolonged corticosteroid therapy seems to afford gradual progressive and gratifying results in most patients. Spontaneous recovery has also been reported.

When first described in 1974, the disease was called "diffuse fasciitis with hypergammaglobulinemia and eosinophilia." In subsequent reports it has been designated as "eosinophilic fasciitis" or "diffuse eosinophilic fasciitis."

The disease may begin gradually or explosively. The patient first notes swelling and stiffness of one or more extremities. Even though these symptoms may begin in only one leg or arm, they usually proceed to involve all four extremities in a symmetric manner. The extremities then become tight and patients complain of pulling sensations in legs and arms. Subsequently, they develop flexion contractures of knees and elbows, and in extreme cases, of ankles and wrists. In some patients the trunk and neck also become involved; a few have restricted respiratory excursion or limited neck rotation.

DIAGNOSIS AND PATHOGENESIS

On superficial inspection, the skin appears to have the changes of scleroderma, principally because the skin is firmly bound down to underlying structures. However, the distribution of the involvement of the extremities is opposite to that found in scleroderma: it is nonacral (less or absent distally) in fasciitis, and acral (more distally) in scleroderma. On close inspection of the skin, the ability to make fine wrinkles is normal, and hair distribution and sweating are intact. Another helpful diagnostic feature is the irregularity of the process, causing the skin to have a "puckered" or "orange peel" appearance. Such changes may be seen over the trunk as well as over the extremities. Rarely, there is initially a slight blotchy erythema over an involved area. In the fully developed case, elbows or knees cannot be fully extended, abduction at the shoulders is limited, and ankle movement is so restricted that the patient must walk on his toes. There is no muscle weakness.

The most common laboratory abnormalities are peripheral blood eosinophilia, elevated erythrocyte sedimentation rate, and hypergammaglobulinemia. The eosinophilia may be modest or very high (over 50 percent). Sedimentation rate elevations are usually moderate. The hyperglobulinemia consists largely of IgG elevations even greater than 4.0 g/dl. Bone marrow examinations reveal eosinophilia and plasmacytosis. In most patients there is no anemia, and the platelet count is normal. Very recently, however, patients with fasciitis have been found to develop aplastic anemia or thrombocytopenic purpura.

A properly obtained biopsy provides the most definitive diagnostic information. The optimal surgical technique is to obtain a long, deep, eliptical, continuous, and through-and-through specimen, extending from skin through fat and fascia to include muscle, in an area of intense clinical involvement, usually on an extremity. Thickening of the fascia between muscle and subcutaneous fat can be seen even on gross examination in some cases. Under the microscope, the fascia is greatly thickened with collagenous hypertrophy and a scattered cellular infiltrate, at times in follicular form. The predominant cells in the infiltrate are lymphocytes and plasma cells. Occasionally, eosinophils and/or histocytes are also seen in the lesions. These changes (i.e., collagenous hypertrophy and cellular infiltration) may extend to involve the septa between muscle bundles and/or the connective tissue septa in the subcutaneous adipose tissue; in extreme cases, the dermis the may be involved. In such cases, however, the center of gravity of the lesions is in the fascia. Immunofluorescent studies of the lesions have not revealed any consistent abnormalities; occasionally, staining for IgG or complement has been observed. Electron microscopic studies of the lesions have not added new information.

In most patients, diffuse fasciitis can be readily distinguished from scleroderma by the normality of the skin on close inspection and histologic examination (in almost all cases), the nonacral central distribution of the disease, the irregularity of the lesions, the absence of Raynaud's phenomenon, and the lack of visceral involvement (gut, lung, heart, and kidney). In contrast to dermatomyositis, patients with fasciitis do not have muscle weakness, muscle enzymes are not elevated, and myocytes appear normal on muscle biopsy. Circulating autoantibodies, such as antinuclear antibodies and rheumatoid factors, and serum complement are normal.

Diffuse fasciitis seems to be an unusual, peculiar immunologic reaction to some type of antigen or stimulus engendered in most patients by heavy exercise or undue physical exertion. Jogging, weight-lifting, exercycling against resistance, swimming, marching, and furniture moving are examples of the types of physical activity in which patients have engaged before the onset of fasciitis. In a few patients there is no history of such unusual exertion. Fasciitis has been found in children, adolescents, and adults of all ages, and in both sexes. Cases have recently been discovered in Europe, Asia, and South America.

THERAPY

The response to corticosteroid therapy has been very gratifying. The starting dose is usually 30–40 mg prednisone daily. The sedimentation rate and eosinophil count are valuable guides for monitoring steroid dosage. Clinical improvement is gradual over weeks or months, leading in many patients to complete clinical remission, including the reappearance of normal "skin" and the disappearance of flexion contractures. Remissions persist in most patients after steroids have been discontinued. There also have been a few reports of spontaneous complete remission without any therapy.

REFERENCES

Caperton EM, Hathaway DE: Scleroderma with eosinophilia and hypergammaglobulinemia: The Shulman syndrome. Arthritis Rheum 18:391, 1975

Rodnan GP, DiBartolomeo AG, Medsger TA, Burnes EL Jr: Eosinophilic fasciitis: Report of seven cases of a newly recognized scleroderma-like syndrome. Arthritis Rheum 18:422, 1975

Schumacher HR: A scleroderma-like syndrome with fasciitis, myositis and eosinophilia. Ann Intern Med 84:49, 1976

Shulman LE: Diffuse fasciitis with hypergammaglobulinemia and eosinophilia. A new syndrome? J Rheumatol 1 [Suppl 1]: 46, 1974

Shulman LE: Diffuse fasciitis with eosinophilia: A new syndrome. Trans Assoc Am Physicians 88:70, 1975

SCLEREDEMA

Lawrence E. Shulman

This rare benign disorder was termed "scleredema adultorum of Buschke" in 1900 to distinguish it from sclerema neonatorum. This designation, however, is clearly a misnomer, in that the disease frequently begins in childhood or adolescence. In fact, a 1963 review of world literature, yielding 209 cases, found that 29 percent of patients were children under 10 years of age and an additional 22 percent were between 10 and 20 years of age. Approximately two-thirds of the cases were female.

CLINICAL FEATURES, ETIOLOGY, AND PATHOLOGY

The skin lesions begin as indurated, nonpitting, edema that initially occurs over the neck, face, and shoulders and then extends to involve the upper arms and trunk, down to the waist. The disease affects the hands very rarely, and the feet never. The involved skin appears diffusely thickened, feels leathery and firm, wrinkles poorly, and is immobile. There may be transient erythema at the onset. The face is smoothly thickened with fewer than normal wrinkles and may be devoid of expression. Mobility of the neck and shoulders may be limited, and mouth opening is impaired. In severe cases, chest expansion may be reduced. The evolution of the skin changes is rapid, usually within a few weeks.

Etiologically, there are at least two forms of the disease: (1) idiopathic, and (2) a recently described form associated with diabetes mellitus. The idiopathic form occurs mostly in young persons, often following a presumably infectious febrile illness, most commonly a streptococcal infection. In one review, 65 percent of patients with scleredema had a history of antecedent infectious disease (tonsillitis, pharyngitis, influenza, or scarlet fever) a few days to 6 months before the skin changes began. Evidence of streptococcal infection was present in half the cases. Several observers have reported a sharp decline in the incidence of scleredema since World War II, perhaps coincident with a decline in streptococcal infection or the use of antibiotics.

The standard description of the course of the idiopathic form is that the disease resolves, usually completely, leaving no sequelae, in 6 months to 2 years. More recent reports, however, differ: in one, 25 percent of cases had no improvement or only partial improvement 2 or more years after onset; in another report, the disease persisted for 20 years in one patient and 38 years in another. There have also been rare reports of relapses after 2 and 20 years.

The association of scleredema and diabetes mellitus was not generally recognized until the 1960s. It seems to be an unusual complication of diabetes, occurring in middle-aged or elderly persons who have had longstanding adult-onset diabetes, usually are obese, and require high doses of insulin. The limited information available to date indicates that the scleredema is persistent and may last for several years. The diabetic form otherwise resembles the idiopathic form very closely, both clinically and histopathologically.

The essential pathologic lesion is the accumulation of acid mucopolysaccharide in the dermis, and to a lesser degree in the subcutis. The collagen fibers of the dermis are pushed apart by a substance that stains metachromatically. The substance is largely hyaluronic acid, since the metachromasia can be blocked by pretreatment with hyaluronidase. These morphologic observations have been confirmed by histochemical studies of scleredematous skin, indicating an increased content of acid mucopolysaccharides, but a normal content of collagen and water.

The disease is usually benign and limited to the skin; most distress comes from the stiffnes and immobility. However, there have been reported changes in other organs—the tongue, muscles, heart (pericardium and myocardium), and esophagus, roughly in order of decreasing frequency. The importance and specificity of these observations remain to be determined.

THERAPY

There is no known treatment for the scleredema. Certain modalities of physical therapy may help to counteract the limited mobility.

REFERENCES

Curtis AC, Shulak BM: Scleredema adultorum: Not always a benign self-limited disease. Arch Dermatol 92:526, 1965
Fleischmajer R, Faludi G, Krol S: Scleredema and diabetes mellitus. Arch Dermatol 101:21, 1970
Greenberg LM, Geppert CX, Worthen HG, et al: Scleredema in children: 3 cases with histochemical study and review of world literature. Pediatrics 32:1044, 1963
Sowa JM, Woody EM, Shulman LE: Scleredema adultorum and diabetes mellitus. Arthritis Rheum 9:542, 1966

Polymyositis (Dermatomyositis)

Mary Betty Stevens

ETIOLOGY, PATHOGENESIS, AND PATHOLOGY

Polymyositis is a diffuse inflammatory disease involving primarily striated skeletal muscle. It may occur alone, in association with neoplastic lesions, or as one manifestation of other connective tissue disorders such as systemic lupus erythematosus (SLE), systemic sclerosis (PSS) or Sjögren's syndrome. In approximately 40 percent of patients with polymyositis, characteristic skin lesions accompany the myopathy (hence, the term, dermatomyositis); it is particularly within this subset that one finds childhood disease and the myositis of adults with neoplasms. Clinically, the hallmark of polymositis, regardless of type (adult polymyositis, childhood dermatomyositis, polymyositis with malignancy, or polymyositis with connective tissue disorders), is weakness of the proximal limb girdle muscle groups. The characteristic features of polymyositis are summarized in Table 1.

Polymyositis, or dermatomyositis, can occur at any age, but is most often seen in adults over the age of 40 years. Women are affected more frequently than men, especially when the myositis occurs in the setting of other multisystem connective tissue disease. There is no sex predominance in childhood, and racial and ethnic factors have not been identified.

ETIOLOGY AND PATHOGENESIS

The cause of polymyositis is unknown. In fact, when one considers the spectrum of clinical associations with this inflammatory myopathy, it becomes unlikely that polymyositis results from a single etiologic agent. Recently, high titers of antibodies to *Toxoplasma gondii* were reported with unusual frequency in patients with this disorder, but no other evidence of toxoplasmosis, either clinically or bacteriologically, could be found. Nor have other infectious agents been detectable. Pathogenetically, polymyositis is generally considered an immunologic, autoreactive disorder. The association of this inflammatory myopathy with autoantibodies to nuclear antigens and clinical features of such diseases as systemic lupus erythematosus (SLE) and Sjögren's syndrome lends support to this concept. Furthermore, the autoimmune hypothesis is reinforced by the recent evidence that muscle inflammation may result from cytotoxic lymphocytes specifically sensitized to striated muscle antigens.

PATHOLOGY

Histologically, the cardinal feature of polymyositis, regardless of clinical setting, is the inflammatory, cellular infiltration with associated necrosis of muscle fibers. Both type I and type II fibers are involved in the inflammatory process. Degeneration of muscle fibers may be remarkably focal or segmental in some patients, or may even be absent on biopsy of clinically involved sites. More often, however, extensive degeneration is found with interspersed regenerating fibers characterized by their altered basophilic staining, centralization of nuclei, and variation in cross-sectional fiber diameter. Similarly, the inflammatory infiltrates, composed of lymphocytes, other mononuclear cells, and occasionally plasma cells, may be scattered diffusely throughout entire muscle groups or clustered in focal aggregates in the interstitum, particularly in perivascular locations.

In children, a severe angiitis may be found not only in muscle but also in skin and subcutaneous tissue, in perineurium, and throughout the gastrointestinal tract. Such a necrotizing arteritis is rarely, if ever, associated

Table 1
Characteristic Features of Polymyositis

Type	Characteristics
Polymyositis	Adults, females (3:1), over 40 years of age Insidious onset and slow progression in those without skin lesions Facial rash and Gottron's lesions in less than half, arthralgias in 25 percent, Raynaud's phenomenon in 15 percent Antinuclear antibodies and rheumatoid factor uncommon
Childhood	No sex dominance Facial and extremity lesions present Usually an acute onset Steroid responsive Calcinosis and contractures common Vasculitis often prominent
Polymyositis with malignancy	Adults, males (3:1), over 40 years of age Onset usually acute Typical skin lesions in vast majority Responsive to removal of tumor, not steroids Malignancy may be occult
Polymyositis with connective tissue disorders	Features of SLE, systemic sclerosis, mixed connective tissue disease, and, less frequently, Sjögren's syndrome and rheumatoid arthritis Raynaud's syndrome and arthralgias in over half Antinuclear antibodies and rheumatoid factors common

with the polymyositis (or dermatomyositis) of adults. Later, a postinflammatory interstitial fibrosis can be marked, particularly in those children who have had extensive, severe muscle inflammation and necrosis. These are also the patients who may develop prominent subcutaneous calcinosis and contractures. Although clinically the skin lesions of dermatomyositis are characteristic and even diagnostic (Gottron's papule), histologically the inflammatory reaction in the dermis is quite nonspecific.

REFERENCES

Currie S, Saunders M, Knowles M, Brown AE: Immunologic aspects of polymyositis. The in vitro activity of lymphocytes on incubation with muscle antigen and with muscle cultures. Q J Med 157: 63, 1971

Dawkins RL, Mastalgia FL: Cell-mediated cytotoxicity in polymyositis. New Engl J Med 288: 434, 1974.

Johnson RL, Fink CW, Ziff M: Lymphotoxin formation by lymphocytes and muscle in polymyositis. J Clin Invest 51: 2435, 1972

Kagan LJ, Kimball AC, Christian CL: Serologic evidence of toxoplasmosis among patients with polymyositis. Amer J Med 56: 186, 1974

CLINICAL FEATURES

Polymyositis, with or without the skin lesions of dermatomyositis, varies broadly in onset and course of disease. Nonetheless, weakness of the proximal limb girdle muscle groups is the dominant manifestation. Any striated muscle site can be involved, and weakness of the neck flexors and the cricopharyngeal musculature is present in approximately one-half of patients. Pain on stretch and tenderness with pressure in involved muscle groups are less often present and occur most frequently in those cases with an acute, fulminant onset.

The onset of polymyositis is most often subtle and insidious. Patients may note the slow progression of difficulty in rising from a chair or climbing stairs, or, with shoulder girdle involvement, lifting objects of moderate weight or performing activities that require abduction or elevation of the arms. Even the transfer of a book from an overhead shelf or combing the hair becomes increasingly difficult. In the few patients with an acute onset, weakness in raising the head from the pillow or, in those with involvement of the pharyngeal muscles, problems in initiating the swallow of solid foods and dysphonia may accompany the early skeletal symptoms. Rarely, the respiratory muscles are involved, leading to complicating pulmonary infections and even death. Late in the course, if the disease is untreated or refractory to therapy, muscle atrophy and shortening can occur, with resultant limb contractures and such profound weakness that the patient becomes confined to a wheel chair or bedridden.

SKIN MANIFESTATIONS

A variety of skin lesions occur in patients with polymyositis, regardless of type. In those with true dermatomyositis, the typical rash is a common initial feature. Particularly characteristic are the dusky, violaceous, so-called "heliotrope" upper eyelids and the erythematous, scaling plaques (Gottron's sign) overlying the knuckles. Similar erythematous patches may overlie elbows, knees, and malleoli, and diffuse macular erythema may be present over the face, V-neck area, and upper trunk. Prominent periungual erythema is present in the majority of patients. Occasionally, particularly in children and those with an acute onset, edema of soft tissues, linear warmth, and erythema may overlie the involved proximal limb muscle groups. In these patients, myalgia and muscle tenderness are prominent. Of course, the characteristic cutaneous manifestations of SLE and scleroderma are seen when polymyositis occurs in association with these disorders.

OTHER CLINICAL MANIFESTATIONS

The other clinical manifestations, like the skin lesions, vary with the setting in which the inflammatory myopathy occurs. For example, Raynaud's phenomenon occurs in less than 20 percent of patients with uncomplicated polymyositis (or dermatomyositis) and almost never in those with malignancies; but it occurs in approximately half of the patients with other connective tissue disorders.

Like skeletal muscle, the myocardium may be involved by the inflammatory process, which leads to arrhythmias and congestive heart failure. Interstitial pneumonitis and pulmonary fibrosis can occur but rarely result in hypoxemia and cor pulmonale.

Several gastrointestinal problems may develop. Dysphagia with difficulty initiating the swallow occurs when the cricopharyngeal musculature is involved. Substernal discomfort after eating as well as reflux symptoms in recumbency are due to lower esophageal motor dysfunction, which is especially prominent in those with Raynaud's phenomenon or systemic sclerosis. In childhood dermatomyositis, severe abdominal pain, gastrointestinal ulceration and hemorrhage, and death may result from the severe vasculitis that rarely, if ever, occurs in adults.

In polymyositis of all types, constitutional symptoms are usually prominent early in the course. Fever is usually intermittent and low grade, and flulike symptoms with malaise, fatiguability, and diffuse musculoskeletal aching initially may mask the evolving muscle weakness in those with an insidious disease onset. Myalgia and stiffness related to involved muscle groups are frequent but seldom severe. Similarly, polyarthralgias are noted in at least 25 percent of patients but frank arthritis is uncommon in the uncomplicated myopathy.

NEOPLASMS

In the older adult, concern for a possible occult neoplasm should arise when polymyositis appears, especially in the presence of typical skin lesions (i.e., dermatomyositis) and in the absence of Raynaud's phenomenon and other features of connective tissue disease. Malignancies are not associated with the dermatomyositis of childhood. The true prevalence of tumors among those with polymyositis has not been established, but a search for a neoplastic lesion should be undertaken in all patients presenting at over 50 years of age, especially men. Any solid tumor, especially carcinoma of the breast, lung, stomach, colon, prostate, uterus, or ovary, may show such an association. Rarely, even lymphomas have been reported. It is important to realize that muscle weakness or skin lesions may be the initial expression of such neoplasms in a significant number of patients, if not the majority, with localizing tumor symptoms lagging behind by weeks or months. Consequently, in the older adult in whom a search for malignancy has been negative, close follow-up and often reevaluation are necessary if early diagnosis is to be made.

CONNECTIVE TISSUE DISORDERS

In approximately one-quarter of patients with polymyositis, features of other connective tissue disorders are so prominent that dual diagnoses have been made. In order of descending frequency, these disorders are systemic sclerosis, SLE, and, rarely, Sjögren's syndrome and rheumatoid arthritis. Usually the muscle inflammation is an early feature of active disease in patients with SLE or systemic sclerosis. In those patients with overlapping features of systemic sclerosis and SLE—the so-called mixed connective tissue disease syndrome—myositis is an especially prominent feature.

REFERENCES

Barnes BE: Dermatomyositis and malignancy: A review of the literature. Ann Intern Med 84:68, 1976

Bohan A, Peter JB, Bowman RL, Pearson CM: A computer-assisted analysis of 153 patients with polymyositis and dermatomyositis. Medicine (Baltimore) 56:255, 1977

Frazier AR, Miller RD: Interstitial pneumonitis in association with polymyositis and dermatomyositis. Chest 65:403, 1974

Medsger TA, Robinson H, Masi AT: Factors affecting survivorship in polymyositis: A life table study of 124 patients. Arthrtis Rheum 14:249, 1971

Sharp GC, Irvin WS, Tan EM, et al: Mixed connective tissue disease: An apparently distinct rheumatic disease syndrome associated with a specific antibody to an extractable nuclear antigen. Am J Med 52: 148, 1972

Williams RC Jr: Dermatomyositis and malignancy: A review of the literature. Ann Intern Med 50:1174, 1959

DIAGNOSIS

The diagnosis of polymyositis is generally based upon the presence of a proximal limb girdle weakness in association with (1) the elevation of one or more muscle enzymes in serum, (2) the characteristic changes of an inflammatory myopathy on electromyography and (3) a confirmatory histology on muscle biopsy. Since none of the ancillary studies is universally positive in patients with polymyositis, it becomes essential to rule out an array of diverse disorders which, by virtue of muscle weakness, can mimic polymyositis (see Differential Diagnosis). In those with cutaneous involvement (Gottron's sign), the clinical picture itself is diagnostic.

LABORATORY FEATURES

The basic hematology is usually normal in patients with active polymyositis except for the elevation in sedimentation rate. While nonspecific, the sedimentation rate occasionally correlates well with disease activity and may, serially followed, be a useful measure of therapeutic response. A significant degree of anemia, if present, should alert the physician to an underlying malignancy or, if hemolytic and Coombs positive, to associated autoimmune disease (especially SLE).

Chemically, the salient abnormality is the elevation of one or more of the muscle enzymes in serum. In our experience, the creatine phosphokinase (CPK) level is most sensitive in this regard; it is difficult to establish a diagnosis of polymyositis in the presence of a normal CPK. Usually, elevations in serum glutamic oxalic transaminase, serum glutamic pyruvic transaminase, lactic acid dehydrogenase, and aldolase also accompany active disease. It is the very rare patient who has biopsy evidence of muscle inflammation and completely normal serum enzyme levels, but in those with advanced disease, focal inflammation, or reduced muscle mass, such a discrepancy can be seen.

Hyperglobulinemia due to a polyclonal increase in the gamma fraction is noted particularly in patients with associated neoplastic or connective tissue disease. The prevalence of serologic abnormalities must similarly be considered in relation to the specific clinical setting. In general, children with dermatomyositis and adults with tumor syndromes are seronegative.

Antigammaglobulin ("rheumatoid") factors, determined by the latex-fixation test system, occur in approximately 10 percent of adults with uncomplicated polymyositis, with or without skin lesions. Antinuclear antibodies, determined by immunofluorescent assay, occur less frequently in this group (5 percent or less) and, as expected, vary in character and prevalence with respect to associated connective tissue disorders. Our preliminary observations suggest, however, a particular association between myositis and antibody to nuclear ribosenucleoprotein not only in the mixed connective tissue disease syndrome but also in SLE and systemic sclerosis. In one series, a low β-1-C was found in 67 percent of 21 patients, although the total hemolytic complement was reduced in only one individual.

ELECTROMYOGRAPHY

The majority of patients with polymyositis and dermatomyositis have characteristic, although not entirely specific, findings on electromyography. Three primary types of abnormalities occur: (1) fibrillations that occur spontaneously at rest; (2) potentials of short duration and less than normal amplitude that are evoked by voluntary muscle contraction; and (3) repetitive pseudomyotonic discharges of high frequency that follow such mechanical stimulation of muscle as an electrode insertion. In at least three-quarters of patients, all these changes are recorded from actively inflamed muscle bundles. Thus, electromyography not only is of direct diagnostic value, but also can provide a useful guide to the selection of a suitable site for muscle biopsy. Furthermore, serial studies provide one means of monitoring the response to suppressive therapy.

MUSCLE BIOPSY

If the site is well chosen, nearly all patients with active myositis will have myopathology on biopsy. Muscles most likely to yield positive results are those that are symptomatic but not markedly atrophic, usually proximal sites such as the deltoid or quadriceps femoris. Again, abnormal electrical activity may be helpful in identifying inflamed muscles appropriate for biopsy. However, it must be recognized that the needle insertion for electromyography is irritative and can evoke a local cellular infiltration, so that the biopsy should be taken at some distance from the actual testing sites.

The pathologic changes described earlier vary in character and intensity from one patient to another. Occasionally one is surprised by an apparent dissociation between the intensity of inflammation histologically and the degree of enzyme elevations in the serum; rarely, inflammatory changes on biopsy may be found in patients with normal serum enzyme levels. Thus the prime indication for biopsy comes from the clinical setting.

DIFFERENTIAL DIAGNOSIS

A multiplicity of disorders can present with dominant muscle pain and weakness and thus must be considered in the differential diagnosis of polymyositis. The presence of characteristic skin lesions (i.e., dermatomyositis) or features of associated connective tissue disorders may simplify the diagnostic problem; but even then, treatable disorders of metabolism, endocrinopathies, infectious disease, and toxicities must be considered and specifically ruled out.

A variety of infections, especially viral, may be characterized by acute, intense polymyalgias but rarely muscle weakness. On the other hand, trichinosis can be both an acute and chronic illness with severe muscle pain and periorbital edema as early manifestations. The presence of hyperpyrexia and digital splinter hemorrhages, and the laboratory demonstration of eosinophilia and skin test positivity to the *Trichinella* antigens are useful determinants. However, the major clue to diagnosis may be the history in the young adult with a dietary predilection for rare beef or pork. Biopsy demonstration of the trichinae establishes the diagnosis. Rarely, toxoplasmosis mimicking an acute viral infection may be confused with polymyositis.

Metabolic disorders and endocrinopathies are more frequent, occult problems which can present as a myopathy. Hyper- or hypofunction of the thyroid gland, especially in older adults, must be searched for by appropriate laboratory tests since muscle weakness may be the only clinical symptom of such disorders. Similarly, hyperparathyroidism, which is equally treatable, should be ruled out in those with an unexplained myopathy. Proximal limb girdle weakness is characteristic of Cushing's syndrome and is of major concern in patients receiving corticosteroids as well as in those presenting initially with the problem of a proximal myopathy. However, in neither primary Cushing's nor iatrogenic steroid-induced myopathy are the muscle enzymes or sedimentation rate elevated. Furthermore, on biopsy, inflammatory changes in muscle are uniformly lacking in these patients. Similarly, those with muscle weakness secondary to Addison's disease are "biopsy negative"; in addition, their muscle weakness is more diffuse and generally distributed and they show characteristic electrolyte abnormalities. Hypokalemia from any cause (most frequently diuretic induced) cannot only mimic polymyositis clinically but also may be accompanied by serum elevations in CPK and other muscle enzymes. The diagnosis may be determined by the lack of characteristic changes on electromyography and muscle biopsy as well as by improvement, clinically and chemically, after discontinuance of the offending agent.

Direct myotoxicity independent of potassium depletion can result from drugs and ethanol. The history of exposure is the key to diagnosis, as it is in the instance of an acute myolysis following unusual and intense physical exercise. Marked myoglobinemia, while not specific, may characteristically occur in these individuals.

In the older age groups, polymyositis may be particularly confused with any one of several processes. Polymyalgia rheumatica (PMR) in the elderly woman may be associated with conspicuous muscle weakness as well as the dominant aching pain in proximal limb muscle groups. Although the sedimentation rate is elevated in both PMR and active polymyositis, muscle enzymes and biopsy are uniformly normal in PMR and the electromyographic changes of inflamed muscle are lacking in this disorder. Noninflammatory carcinomatous myopathy and neuromyopathy are similarly ruled out by ancillary studies. Although structural changes in the axial skeleton (i.e., cervical and lumbar spondylosis, degenerative disc and joint disease) are commonplace with increasing age, one must attribute myopathic symptoms to them only after careful exclusion of alternative causes. The electromyogram and regional nerve conduction times are especially useful in this regard.

A careful history and physical examination should distinguish myasthenia gravis from polymyositis in most instances. The diurnal variation in weakness and the frequent involvement of ocular and palatal musculature in myasthenia contrast the more constant, progressive, and proximal muscle weakness of polymyositis. The positive Tensilon test of myasthenia is usually negative in inflammatory myopathies, although occasionally a pseudomyasthenic response can be observed in the patient with polymyositis. In myasthenia, however, the muscle enzymes are not elevated, the muscle biopsy is negative for inflammatory changes, and electromyography characteristically shows decreasing potentials with repetitive testing.

Features of many less common and less treatable disorders can occasionally mimic polymyositis: the muscle weakness and cramping pain of heritable type V glycogen storage (McArdle's) disease, the insidious weakness of muscular dystrophy, and the intermittent pain in the axial and proximal girdle musculature of the "stiff man syndrome." Differentiation can usually be readily established on clinical and laboratory grounds, except in muscular dystrophy, which may be associated with enzyme elevations, electromyographic abnormalities identical to those of polymyositis, and even inflammatory change on muscle biopsy.

TREATMENT

The approach in the therapy of polymyositis is to suppress the inflammatory tissue process and thereby minimize residual loss of muscle mass and strength. Early diagnosis with prompt institution of appropriate antiinflammatory drugs is the key to optimal recovery in those patients without underlying neoplasia; in those with malignancies, tumor ablation is also attempted. Corticosteroids are the drugs of choice and are usually initially administered in high (approximating 50 mg prednisone or its equivalent daily) divided doses. Response to therapy is closely monitored both clinically and in the laboratory; improvement in muscle strength a less sensitive indicator than the serum indices of muscle inflammation. The mus-

cle enzymes and sedimentation rate are serially followed, at first at least weekly; only when the enzyme battery has returned to normal is consideration given to corticosteroid tapering. In our experience, the sedimentation rate is a more variable and less reliable therapeutic guide. In the majority of patients who do respond, corticosteroid tapering should be done slowly over a period of weeks, or even months, with constant chemical monitoring and persistent control of enzymes within the normal range. Low-dose maintenance therapy (5–15 mg prednisone or its equivalent daily) may be required for years if not indefinitely.

Major therapeutic responses may occur promptly (within days), especially in the younger patient with an acute disease onset. Others may require weeks before significant return of muscle strength and normal levels of enzymes are observed. Still others cannot be adequately controlled at all by corticosteroids, either because the disease is refractory or they cannot tolerate steroids at the dosage required for disease suppression. In either instance, the addition of an immunosuppressive agent is indicated, and methotrexate seems to be the cytotoxic drug of choice. Intravenous administration on a weekly schedule is the optimal route, with 5 mg as the starting dose. If no adverse reactions are noted (i.e., membrane ulcerations, hepatotoxicity, or leukopenia), 10 mg is administered 1 week later, then 15 mg and so on until a 35–50-mg weekly dose is established. As with corticosteroids, only after clinical and chemical response is the minimum maintenance dosage defined through cautious tapering. It is imperative that patients be serially monitored chemically throughout the treatment period; every effort should be directed toward returning and then maintaining the serum enzymes within the normal range. Clinical evaluation alone (i.e., monitoring of proximal limb girdle strength) is insufficient; it is particularly difficult in those patients receiving corticosteroid therapy in view of the possibility of weakness from a steroid-induced myopathy.

In addition to antiinflammatory drug therapy, general supportive and physical measures may be the key to minimizing residual weakness and functional limitation. Initially, when myositis is acute, intensive exercise programs are not well tolerated. As inflammation subsides, progression from passive and isometric exercises to the active and resistive exercise of involved groups may aid in maintaining strength and function. Resting splints, especially in children, may help to minimize contractures.

REFERENCES

Arnett FC Jr, Whelton JC, Zizic TM, Stevens MB: Methotrexate therapy in polymyositis. Ann Rheum Dis 32:536, 1973

Metzger A, Bohan A, Goldberg L, et al: Polymyositis and dermatomyositis: Combined methotrexate and corticosteroid therapy. Ann Intern Med 81: 182, 1974

Pearson CM: Patterns of polymyositis and their response to treatment. Ann Intern Med 59:827, 1963

Mixed Connective Tissue Disease

Gordon C. Sharp

MANIFESTATIONS AND DIAGNOSIS

Clinicians have long been aware of patients with overlapping features of more than one rheumatic disease who do not fit into traditional classifications. Patients having a combination of clinical features similar to those of systemic lupus erythematosus (SLE), progressive systemic sclerosis (PSS), and polymyositis and unusually high titers of circulating antibody to a nuclear ribonucleoprotein (RNP) antigen have recently been described under the name *mixed connective tissue disease* (MCTD). MCTD patients frequently respond well to treatment with corticosteroids and appear to have a relatively favorable prognosis.

SEROLOGIC FINDINGS

Almost all patients with MCTD have high titers (usually greater than 1:50 and frequently over 1:1000) of fluorescent antinuclear antibodies (ANA), which produce a speckled pattern. With a very sensitive passive hemagglutination technique these patients have typically been found to have very high titers (frequently more than 1:100,000) of antibody to a nuclear antigen extractable in isotonic buffers (ENA). Treatment of ENA-coated red cells with ribonuclease (RNase) eliminates or greatly reduces the hemagglutination reaction with the patient's serum in MCTD.

Immunodiffusion studies have shown that ENA consists of at least two distinct antigens, one sensitive to RNase and trypsin, which appears to be a nuclear ribonucleoprotein (RNP), and the other resistant to RNase and trypsin, which has been termed the *Sm antigen*. Antibodies to RNP, Sm, and several other nuclear acidic protein antigens all produce speckled ANA patterns. Patients with MCTD characteristically have very high titers of antibody to RNase-sensitive ENA by hemagglutination and only antibody to RNP and not to the Sm antigen by immunodiffusion. These high titers of circulating RNP antibody usually persist during periods of both disease activity and remission. Rarely, patients with clinical features of MCTD are negative for RNP antibody or have both RNP and Sm antibodies.

The serologic pattern of RNP antibodies in high titer and no Sm antibodies is very frequently associated with MCTD; it is much less common in SLE or PSS, and occurs rarely, if at all, in patients with polymyositis, rheumatoid arthritis, and other rheumatic diseases. The fact that some patients with high titers of antibody to RNP may begin with more limited disease (usually suggesting SLE, PSS, or rheumatoid arthritis) and then develop additional clinical features resulting in a picture typical of MCTD is a further indication that this serologic pattern may have a very high specificity for MCTD.

LE cells and antibodies to native DNA are infrequent in MCTD. Serum complement levels are slightly to moderately reduced in only about 25 percent of patients. Rheumatoid agglutinins are positive—frequently with high titers—in over half of MCTD patients. The erythrocyte sedimentation rate is frequently elevated, and diffuse hypergammaglobulinemia, often ranging from 2–5 g/dl, occurs in about three-quarters of these patients.

CLINICAL FEATURES

The prevalence of MCTD is unknown, but it may be more common than polymyositis and less frequent than SLE. Approximately 80 percent of patients have been female, and the age range is 5–80 years with a mean of 37 years.

The typical clinical pattern of MCTD is characterized by Raynaud's phenomenon, polyarthralgia or arthritis, swelling of the hands leading to a sausage appearance of the fingers, esophageal hypomotility, pulmonary disease, and inflammatory myopathy. In some patients, all these disease manifestations appear simultaneously. However, since clinicians have become more aware of MCTD and testing for RNP antibody has become more readily available, larger numbers of patients have been identified in an early phase of the disease. During this phase they frequently have minimal symptoms such as Raynaud's phenomenon, arthralgias, myalgias, and fatigue, and laboratory studies may reveal hypergammaglobulinemia and a speckled ANA pattern—findings insufficient to make a definite diagnosis. As these patients continue under medical observation over a period of months or years they may develop other disease manifestations resulting in a diagnosis of MCTD.

The initial appearance of Raynaud's phenomenon and swollen hands may suggest PSS, while proximal muscle weakness at the onset may suggest polymyositis. When pleuritis and/or pericarditis occurs in conjunction with fever, arthralgias, and an erythematous rash, one suspects SLE. Adults may appear to have rheumatoid arthritis and children initially are often thought to have juvenile rheumatoid arthritis. Dyspnea on exertion related to pulmonary involvement or prominent lymphadenopathy suggesting a lymphoma are less frequent early presenting features. Whatever the initial presentation, there is a tendency for limited disease to progress slowly to become more widespread and for changes in the major clinical problem to occur over time.

Raynaud's phenomenon, noted in approximately 85 percent of patients with MCTD, may precede other disease manifestations by months or years. Ischemic necrosis or ulceration of the fingertips, common in PSS, are rarely seen in MCTD.

Skin Lesions

The most frequent skin manifestation, which occurs in over two-thirds of MCTD patients, is swelling of the fingers, leading to a sausage appearance. The skin may be taut and thick, with histologic changes of an increase in dermal collagen content as well as considerable edema. Sclerodermalike changes are sometimes more extensive, but diffuse involvement of the skin or tightly bound-down skin with contractures is rarely seen. Lupuslike rashes may occur, including the following: acute malar eruptions; diffuse, nonscarring, erythematous subacute lesions; and/or chronic scarring discoidlike lesions. Other frequent findings include violaceous discoloration of the eyelids, erythema over the knuckles, elbows, and/or knees, diffuse nonscarring alopecia, hyperpigmentation and hypopigmentation, periungual telangiectasia, and "squared" telangiectasia over the hands and face.

Arthritis

Polyarthralgias occur in most patients, and three-quarters have frank arthritis. Usually the arthritis is nondeforming. However, features may be typical of rheumatoid arthritis, including erosive changes on x-ray and subcutaneous nodules.

Muscle Symptoms

Proximal muscle weakness with or without tenderness is common. Serum levels of creatine phosphokinase and aldolase may be elevated, and electromyograms are typical of inflammatory myositis. Biopsies show muscle fiber degeneration and perivascular and interstitial infiltrates of lymphocytes and plasma cells. Even when clinical findings are minimal, immunofluorescent analysis of biopsies may reveal IgG or IgM deposition within blood vessels, within fibers, and along the sarcoplasmic membrane.

Esophageal Involvement

Systematic cine esophagram and manometric studies of 35 consecutive MCTD patients have revealed dysfunction in 80 percent, including 70 percent of asymptomatic patients. Abnormalities include decreased lower esophageal sphincter pressure, decreased amplitude of peristalsis in the distal two-thirds of the esophagus, and a decrease in upper sphincter pressure. Severity of esophageal dysfunction appears directly related to disease duration.

Pulmonary Involvement

Pulmonary dysfunction likewise may not be clinically apparent and thus may fail to be detected unless thorough pulmonary evaluations are carried out. Studies performed in 30 consecutive MCTD patients disclosed an 80 percent incidence of pulmonary disease, including 69 percent of asymptomatic patients. Abnormalities regularly included decreased diffusing capacity (30–70 percent of normal) and, less often, reduced lung volume. Chest x-rays showed diffuse interstitial infiltrates and, less frequently, volume loss or pleural disease. Occasionally, pulmonary involvement is the predominant clinical problem in MCTD, leading to exertional dyspnea and/or pulmonary hypertension.

Cardiac Involvement

Cardiac involvement appears to be less common than pulmonary disease in MCTD. However, in a recent report of MCTD in children, 64 percent had cardiac involvement, including pericarditis, myocarditis with congestive heart failure, and aortic insufficiency. On occasion, adults with MCTD have been thought to have a viral pericarditis until the sustained duration and subsequent recognition of other clinical features led to the correct diagnosis.

Renal Involvement

Renal disease indicated by proteinuria, hematuria, and/or an abnormal kidney biopsy occurs in only about 10 percent of patients with MCTD. Often it is mild, but on occasion it has been a major clinical problem and patients have died with progressive renal failure. Twenty renal biopsies performed in 300 patients with MCTD showed 5 that were normal, 5 had mesangial hypercellularity only, 5 had focal glomerulitis, 3 had membranous glomerulonephritis, 1 had diffuse membranoproliferative glomerulonephritis, and 1 demonstrated severe intimal proliferative vascular changes. Immunofluorescent analyses in some cases show granular deposits of IgG, C3, and C4 in the glomerular basement membrane. In a few cases, electron-dense deposits have been noted in subepithelial and deep mesangial regions on electron microscopy.

Neurologic Abnormalities

Serious neurologic abnormalities are noted in only 10 percent of MCTD patients. A trigeminal sensory neuropathy is the most frequent neurologic finding. Other neurologic problems have included organic mental syndrome, "vascular" headaches, aseptic meningitis, seizures, multiple peripheral neuropathies, and cerebral infarction or hemorrhage (probably related to hypertension and atherosclerosis).

Miscellaneous Manifestations

Moderate anemia and/or leukopenia occur in 30–40 percent of patients with MCTD. Clinically significant Coombs-positive hemolytic anemia and thrombocytopenia are rare. However, in a recent report of 14 children with MCTD, 6 had severe thrombocytopenia, including 2 who required splenectomy because of severe thrombocytopenia only partially responsive to corticosteroids.

Lymphadenopathy and fever are noted in about one-third of MCTD patients. Hepatomegaly and splenomegaly may occur, but serious disturbances of liver function have been very rare. Other less frequent findings include intestinal tract involvement similar to that seen in PSS, Hashimoto's thyroiditis, Sjögren's syndrome, and persistent hoarseness.

DIFFERENTIAL DIAGNOSIS

As noted in Table 1, the MCTD syndrome differs from SLE by virtue of its high incidence of Raynaud's phenomenon, swollen hands, esophageal hypomotility, pulmonary disease, and myositis, and low incidence of serious renal disease, antibodies to native DNA or Sm, LE cells, and hypocomplementemia. The higher incidence of myositis, polyarthritis, lymphadenopathy, leukopenia, and hypergammaglobulinemia and infrequency of diffuse sclerosis distinguishes MCTD from PSS. The incidence of Raynaud's phenomenon, swollen hands,

Table 1
Differential Diagnosis of Mixed Connective Tissue Disease

Finding	MCTD	SLE	PSS	PM
Raynaud's phenomenon	++++	+	++++	+
Swollen hands	+++	Rare	+++	Rare
Esophageal hypomotility	+++	+	+++	+
Pulmonary disease	+++	+	++	+
Myositis	+++	Rare	+	++++
Polyarthritis	++++	+++	+	+
Lymphadenopathy	++	++	Rare	Rare
Leukopenia	++	+++	Rare	Rare
Serious renal disease	+	+++	++	0
Diffuse sclerosis	+	Rare	++++	+
Hypergammaglobulinemia	++++	+++	+	+
High-titer antibody to RNP	++++	+	Rare	0
Antibody to native DNA	+	++++	+	Rare
Antibody to Sm	Rare	+++	0	0
LE cells	+	+++	+	Rare
Hypocomplementemia	+	+++	+	Rare

Abbreviations: MCTD, mixed connective tissue disease; SLE, systemic lupus erythematosus; PSS, progressive systemic sclerosis; PM, polymyositis.

esophageal hypomotility, pulmonary disease, arthritis, lymphadenopathy, leukopenia, and hypergammaglobulinemia is much higher in MCTD than in polymyositis.

The characteristic serologic finding of high titers of antibody to RNP is much more frequently associated with MCTD than with other rheumatic diseases. Therefore, detection of RNP antibody permits a presumptive diagnosis of MCTD at a time when disease manifestations are limited. In an early phase, when symptoms may simulate SLE, PSS, rheumatoid arthritis, or polymyositis, the finding of a high-titer speckled ANA should suggest the diagnosis of MCTD and lead to a test for RNP antibody. Because patients with MCTD (unlike patients with PSS and rheumatoid arthritis) frequently respond favorably to corticosteroids, it is important to pursue the diagnosis when clinical or serologic clues are present.

REFERENCES

Notman DD, Kurata N, Tan EM: Profiles of antinuclear antibodies in systemic rheumatic diseases. Ann Intern Med 83:464, 1975

Sharp GC, Irvin WS, LaRoque RL, Velez C, Daly V, Kaiser AD, Holman HR: Association of autoantibodies to different nuclear antigens with clinical patterns of rheumatic disease and responsiveness to therapy. J Clin Invest 50:350, 1971

Sharp GC, Irvin WS, May CM, Holman HR, McDuffie FC, Hess EV, Schmid FR: Association of antibodies to ribonucleoprotein and Sm antigens with mixed connective tissue disease, systemic lupus erythematosus and other rheumatic diseases. N Engl J Med 295:1149, 1976

Sharp GC, Irvin WS, Tan EM, Gould RG, Holman HR: Mixed connective tissue disease—An apparently distinct rheumatic disease syndrome associated with a specific antibody to an extractable nuclear antigen (ENA). Am J Med 52:148, 1972

Singsen BH, Bernstein BH, Kornreich HK, King KK, Hanson V, Tan EM: Mixed connective tissue disease in childhood. J Pediatr 90:893, 1977

ETIOLOGY AND TREATMENT

ETIOLOGY AND PATHOGENESIS

The etiology and pathogenesis of MCTD are unknown. The following clues suggest that immune aberrations may be involved: (1) persistence over years of extremely high titers of RNP antibody (which might suggest continuing antigenic stimulation or absence of normal cellular regulatory mechanisms); (2) marked hypergammaglobulinemia; (3) mild to moderate hypocomplementemia in 25 percent; (4) preliminary evidence of circulating immune complexes during active disease; (5) specific deposition of IgG, IgM, or complement within the walls of blood vessels or muscle fibers, along the glomerular basement membrane, and at the dermal–epidermal junction; and (6) chronic inflammatory infiltration by lymphocytes and plasma cells in various tissues including muscle, lung, salivary glands, liver, heart, synovium, and intestine. Autopsy information is limited, but it appears that the chief underlying pathologic lesion in patients with MCTD who proceed to progressive fatal disease is a proliferative intimal and/or medial vascular lesion which results in narrowing of the lumen of large vessels (e.g., aorta, coronary, pulmonary, and renal) and small arterioles of many organs.

TREATMENT AND PROGNOSIS

Although no controlled studies have been conducted, many features of MCTD appear to be responsive to corticosteroid therapy. Mild disease is often controlled with nonsteroidal antiinflammatory drugs or very low doses of corticosteroids. When severe major organ involvement is present, however, an initial dose of 1 mg/kg of prednisone is often employed. Arthritis, serositis, lymphadenopathy, fever, rash, splenomegaly, hepatomegaly, leukopenia, anemia, and myositis are often considerably improved after a few days to a few weeks, at which time the dose of steroids is gradually tapered. Even sclerodermalike skin changes and pulmonary and esophageal function may improve following corticosteroid therapy. If the disease duration is short, the steroid response is apt to be more rapid and complete. Most patients return to normal or near normal activity. Exacerbation of disease, which may occur as corticosteroids are being withdrawn, usually responds to reinstitution of somewhat higher doses.

In patients whose disease has progressed to widespread involvement, more prolonged high-dose corticosteroid therapy, sometimes in combination with cytotoxic drugs, may be associated with clinical improvement; however, the response may not be so complete and the toxicity of the drugs may lead to serious and sometimes fatal complications. In general, the sclerodermalike features of MCTD are least likely to respond. Sustained remissions for several years on little or no maintenance steroid therapy have now been observed in some MCTD patients.

A recent review of over 300 patients with MCTD showed that only 7 percent had died (mean duration of disease was 7 years with a range of 1–25 years), which suggests a rather good prognosis. Causes of death have included renal disease, pulmonary disease, colonic perforation, myocardial infarction, brain hemorrhage, disseminated infection, and suicide.

Because the serologic clue permits early detection, MCTD affords an excellent opportunity to test the effectiveness of early therapeutic intervention through controlled studies in a disease that appears to be very responsive to corticosteroids. If methods can be found for the early detection of those MCTD patients who are going to develop proliferative vascular lesions, it is possible that rational and perhaps effective therapy may also become available for these more complicated patients.

REFERENCES

Oxenhandler R, Hart M, Corman L, Sharp G, Adelstein E: The pathology of skeletal muscle in mixed connective tissue disease. Arthritis Rheum 20:985, 1977

Sharp GC, Irvin WS, Tan EM, Gould RG, Holman HR: Mixed connective tissue disease—An apparently distinct rheumatic disease syndrome associated with a specific antibody to an extractable nuclear antigen (ENA). Am J Med 52:148, 1972

Systemic Arteritis and Related Disorders

John A. Mills

INTRODUCTION

The term *systemic arteritis* refers to a group of diseases in which the primary pathology is inflammation of arteries in multiple organs. Although arteritis is to a variable degree a part of the pathology of many of the other connective tissue diseases, most of them are otherwise identified and are not usually included as forms of systemic arteritis. To be sure, considerable overlapping of clinical manifestations exists and occasionally the precise diagnosis may be uncertain. For example, the clinical course of some patients with systemic lupus erythematosus or rheumatoid arthritis may be dominated by arterial pathology and clinical consequences indistinguishable from those that affect patients with primary arteritis.

CLASSIFICATION

Since systemic arteritis was first described by Rokitansky there has been a progressive delineation of variants that have distinctive clinical and or pathologic features. However, the subject remains confused by different approaches to the problem of classification. That adopted in the following chapters is an extension of the one first proposed by Zeek and is set forth in Table 1. Recently appreciated prognostic and therapeutic distinctions provide additional support for that classification.

ROLE OF IMMUNOLOGIC MECHANISMS

Although familial clustering has been recorded in a few instances, no large study of the association between arteritis and histocompatibility markers has been reported. The arteritis that occurs in animals in the course of serum sickness and the development of arteritis in man in association with drug reactions or circulating hepatitis B antigen–antibody complexes suggest that similiar immunologic mechanisms may be responsible for other forms of arteritis. Systemic arteritis occurs naturally in several kinds of animals in association with viral infection. Examples include equine arteritis, border disease in sheep, and Aleutian disease in mink. Some of these also appear to involve immune complex–mediated vascular damage. However, in only a few instances of human vasculitis have immune complexes or complement con-

Table 1
Major Forms of Systemic Arteritis

Syndrome	Course	Major Manifestations
Periarteritis nodosa	Variable	Infarcts (nervous system, heart, GI tract, kidney)
Cutaneous PAN	Chronic	Subcutaneous nodules, myalgia
Kawasaki disease	Acute	Rash, coronary arteritis (children)
Hypersensitivity angiitis	Acute	Purpura, arthritis, nephritis
Henoch-Schonlein purpura	Acute	Purpura, arthritis, nephritis
Mixed cryoglobulinemia	Chronic	Purpura, arthralgia, nephritis
Allergic granulomatosis	Crescendo	Asthma, pulmonary infiltrates, eosinophilia
Wegener's granulomatosis	Crescendo	Sinusitis, pneumonitis, nephritis
Giant cell arteritis	Acute protracted	Head pain, polymyalgia, loss of vision, high ESR
Takayasu's arteritis	Acute	Young women, aortic arch syndrome

sumption been demonstrated consistently. Thus there is still no direct proof of the role of immunologic mechanisms in most forms of human arteritis.

PERIARTERITIS NODOSA

This relatively rare form of systemic arteritis was first fully described by Kussmaul and Maier as a disease involving muscular arteries. The subsequent recognition of cases in which larger or smaller vessels were involved led to the use of the term *polyarteritis nodosa*. Because it is now appreciated that a number of different forms of arteritis came to be included under that name, the use of the original term, *periarteritis nodosa (PAN)*, for this particular entity is preferred.

PAN mainly affects middle-aged males. Although typical cases have been described in children and females, many of the cases reported in those two patient groups have features that place them in other categories.

CLINICAL MANIFESTATIONS

Most patients consider themselves in good health prior to the first symptoms; in contrast to some other forms of arteritis, a relationship to drug ingestion is rarely evident. The onset is usually abrupt, although the early manifestations may be minor or nonspecific and may persist alone for weeks. They include fever, myalgia, arthralgia, and weight loss. Sooner or later the patient comes to medical attention often because of the advent of peripheral neuropathy, particularly mononeuritis, or an episode of parenchymal organ infarction involving the central nervous system, myocardium, bowel, or kidney. Any combination of these events together or in close sequence should suggest the diagnosis of PAN.

Other patients, after having suddenly developed one of these major manifestations as a seemingly isolated event, do not recover but remain nonspecifically ill with intermittent fever, weight loss, and musculoskeletal pain. Hypertension and/or congestive heart failure may then supervene, neurologic complications may worsen, or a major intracranial, perinephric, or intraabdominal hemorrhage may occur. PAN should be suspected when hyper-

tension develops abruptly during the course of any undiagnosed illness. In contrast to several other forms of vasculitis, petechial or purpuric skin lesions are infrequent; however, ischaemic lesions of the fingers or toes can occur. Tender or nodular swellings along arteries are occasionally palpable on the extremities or trunk and may be found in about 15 percent of cases in the epididymis. In classic PAN pulmonary artery involvement rarely occurs. When it does, it usually leads to pulmonary artery hypertension or occasionally pulmonary infarction or hemorrhage.

PAN has been reported in both adults and children following an acute otitis media. Mononeuritis multiplex and acute episcleritis were the major clinical features in those cases; six of the seven patients had rheumatoid factor in the serum. Two other diseases occasionally associated with PAN-like pathology are regional enteritis and ulcerative colitis. Successful treatment of the bowel disease has resulted in resolution of the arteritis. Retroperitoneal fibrosis is a major manifestation of some cases of PAN. These cases appear to run a more indolent course, characterized chiefly by the renal and gastrointestinal consequences of the retroperitoneal process, which on biopsy shows a widespread necrotizing arteritis of muscular arteries.

DIAGNOSIS

Once the diagnosis of PAN is suspected it can be confirmed only by demonstrating the characteristic arterial pathology by biopsy or arteriography. When practical, biopsies of clinically involved tissues should be attempted. Lesions may be found in the arteries in the deep (fatty) dermis or muscle, or in vessels that accompany nerves such as the sural. Involvement of the temporal arteries has been described and, when there is local tenderness, they may provide a convenient location for biopsy. Blind biopsies at any site carry a 50 percent false-negative rate and should not be relied upon to exclude the diagnosis.

Because the arterial pathology is focal, any biopsy material should be completely sectioned if lesions are not seen initially. Usually lesions are found in all stages of development. The most recent show infiltration of all layers of the arterial wall with leukocytes, the majority of which are neutrophils. A variable number of eosinophils may be present. Fibrinoid necrosis of the vessel wall is an important characteristic to recognize, particularly in the case of smaller vessels where periarterial inflammation as a consequence of other kinds of reaction may resemble an arteritis.

Later lesions show various combinations of thrombosis and destruction of the arterial wall leading to the characteristic aneurysms. In the case of healed arterial lesions, the inflammatory cells are gradually replaced by a mononuclear infiltrate, fibroblast proliferation in the wall, and eventually recanalization of the lumen. In classic PAN the inflammatory reaction is confined to the vessel wall itself unless there has been associated hemorrhage. Inflammation and connective tissue proliferation that form an extensive perivascular reaction are features that are characteristic of other kinds of vasculitis.

The difficulty of obtaining tissue confirmation of a suspected diagnosis has led increasingly to the use of arteriography as a diagnostic method. Because not all vascular beds are affected, arteriographic studies should be performed of organs or tissues where pathology is suspected. Renal, mesenteric, or carotid studies are likely to be of most help. To be diagnostic, arteriograms must show dilatation of arterial segments as well as areas of irregular narrowing. Typically, the aneurysms are multiple and tend to occur at arterial branch points.

Other laboratory studies do not provide reliable diagnostic clues. The erythrocyte sedimentation rate (ESR) is usually but not always elevated. Leukocytosis, often to leukemoid levels, is common, particularly when mesenteric arteritis is present. During acute phases thrombocytosis is often evident. Eosinphilia, although long regarded as a hallmark of PAN, occurs in less than 15 percent of cases.

The urinalysis may be normal or contain only a small amount of protein. Hematuria is usual but is often intermittent, reflecting renal cortical infarction. Glomerulitis is not a feature of classic PAN, although it does occur occasionally in patients whose disease seems otherwise quite typical. Such cases are often those associated with hepatitis B antigenemia.

Immunologic tests such as those for rheumatoid factor or antinuclear antibodies are positive no more frequently than in the general population. A small amount of circulating immune complex may be demonstrated by sensitive methods in about one-half of cases, but serum levels of complement components are almost always normal or elevated. The relationship of circulating immune complexes to the pathogenesis of the disease remains moot. During acute phases of the disease hypoalbuminemia and hyperglobulinemia are present in most patients.

An as yet unknown fraction of patients with classic PAN have hepatitis B surface antigen in their serum. The incidence has varied from 5 to 60 percent in recently reported series. Tests for circulating immune complexes containing the antigen may not be positive in these patients either, although the antigen has been demonstrated in vascular lesions. Most patients do not have acute liver disease. This association of PAN with hepatitis B antigenemia contrasts with the situation encountered in the syndrome of mixed cryoglobulinemia with skin purpura and nephritis (described in the chapter on Other Forms of Arteritis), in which immune complexes containing hepatitis B surface antigen are regularly present.

TREATMENT

Corticosteroid is usually given to control fever and weight loss. Although most patients experience some benefit, there is no evidence that the course of the disease is altered. Such symptomatic benefit can be obtained with doses of prednisone in the range of 20–30 mg/day. Higher doses accomplish no more. Cytotoxic agents, including azathioprine and cyclophosphamide, are widely used in addition to corticosteroid. Although there are isolated reports of both successes and failures with these drugs, no substantial experience has been documented.

An often neglected but important aspect of treatment is the aggressive control of hypertension, which in itself is largely responsible for cardiac and renal failure in some patients. It can also be a factor in the pathogenesis of arterial rupture.

COURSE AND PROGNOSIS

The course of PAN is extremely variable. Patients may suffer fatal myocardial or cerebral infarction at onset. Others survive a number of attacks and live for years. More commonly, the course is one of repeated symptomatic or subclinical vascular episodes with a background of fever and muscle atrophy leading in less than 1 year to hypertensive renal failure, congestive heart failure, or fatal neurologic impairment. Other patients die of internal hemorrhage or an acute abdominal catastrophe.

CUTANEOUS PAN

Another rare form of PAN, often referred to as *cutaneous PAN,* chiefly affects young adults. The disease begins abruptly with the appearance of painful subcutaneous nodules on the extremeties and trunk that on biopsy show an acute necrotizing arteritis of the medium-sized vessels in the deeper layers of the dermis. In males the epididymis is sometimes involved. Fever and leukocytosis may accompany the attacks, which last several weeks and can recur for years. Severe myalgia and joint pain is common in the course of exacerbations of the disease, but objective signs of either myositis or arthritis are rarely encountered. The only other serious manifestation is mononeuritis, resulting in extensive extremity weakness. Neurologic function usually returns with time. Some cases are associated with inflammatory bowel disease and the vasculitis may respond to therapy for the enteritis.

Both salicylate and the nonsteroidal antiinflammatory agents are useful in therapy. Although many of the signs and symptoms are helped, the underlying disease tends to runs its course. Corticosteroids are often no more effective than the aforementioned drugs.

SYNDROMES RESEMBLING PAN

Two additional forms of arteritis of muscular arteries that resemble PAN occur in children: the mucocutaneous lymph node syndrome, or Kawasaki disease, and another extremely rare form that leads to multiple fusiform aneurysms of large vessels.

Kawasaki disease is rare in North America; less than 50 cases have been described. It appears to be epidemic in Japan, where the number of documented cases in the past 10 years exceeds 7000. Nearly all patients are less than 5 years of age; two-thirds are less than 2 years old. Males are somewhat more commonly affected. The disease usually begins abruptly with fever, cervical lymphadenopathy, and macular erythema involving the palms and soles, which desquamate in the convalescent stages. Oropharyngitis with the appearance of a strawberry tongue is a very characteristic finding. Aseptic meningitis occurs in about 10 percent of cases. During the acute phase, tachycardia and electrocardiographic changes indicative of coronary artery disease appear in a majority of patients. Only 2 percent of cases die of arrythmias or congestive failure caused by coronary arteritis, although coronary arteriography has demonstrated characteristic pathology in almost two-thirds of cases studied. The disease lasts 2–3 weeks and does not recur. No effective therapy is known.

Following surgical repair of coarctation of the aorta, particularly in males, an arteritis that closely resembles PAN may develop in the vascular tree below the site of obstruction. Largely on the basis of this observation, some authorities have regarded hypertension as an important element in the pathogenesis of primary PAN.

HYPERSENSITIVITY ANGIITIS

Long considered a variant of periarteritis nodosa, until Zeek pointed out its distinctive clinical and pathologic features, hypersensitivity angiitis is now recognized as a separate and easily identified entity. There are several syndromes that are clinically similar and probably closely related; these include the vasculitis associated with mixed cryoglobulinemia, a syndrome of cutaneous vasculitis and arthritis with hypocomplementemia, and Henoch-Schonlein purpura. The latter is in most respects indistinguishable from hypersensitivity angiitis and accounts for about one-half of all cases. Hypersensitivity angiitis may occur at any age. It effects males slightly more commonly than females. A history of drug administration immediately preceding the onset of symptoms is obtained in about one-half of adult cases. Penicillin, sulfonamide-related drugs, allopurinol, and the thioureas are most commonly implicated. It is often difficult to be sure that the symptoms for which a drug or antibiotic was administered were not in fact the presenting manifestations of the vasculitis. In children with Henoch-Schonlein purpura an upper respiratory infection or streptococcal pharyngitis appears to precede the onset of the vasculitis more often than would be predicted by chance.

CLINICAL MANIFESTATIONS

The first symptoms are usually the sudden onset of malaise and fever followed within 24–48 hours by purpura and arthralgias and frequently by abdominal pain. High fever may occur in the first few days and precipitate convulsions in small children. The purpura begins first about the ankles and spreads proximally to involve the lower thighs and sometimes the arms, neck, and trunk. It is rarely seen on the face or palmar or plantar surfaces. In children particularly, the lesions are sometimes urticarial at first and later become purpuric. The purpura is distinguishable from that of thrombocytopenia or hyperglobulinemia by the fact that most of the lesions are slightly palpable. Arthralgia is an almost constant symptom and about one-half of patients have true arthritis effecting the knees, ankles, wrists, or shoulders. Abdominal pain is particularly common in children but occurs in about one-third of adults as well. Some patients develop signs of bowel infarction, and in children intussusception is a frequent complication. More often, the abdominal pain is related to peritonitis from multiple serosal petechiae without infarction. Fleeting pulmonary infiltrates develop occasionally but produce few symptoms.

In contrast to periarteritis nodosa, the cardiovascular and central nervous systems are rarely affected. A distal sensory neuropathy develops occasionally. Evidence of a glomerulonephritis is found in a majority of patients in all age groups, but related symptoms such as flank pain or gross hematuria are uncommon. In children the process is mild and clears completely without loss of renal function. In adults, however, progressive glomerulonephritis occurs in 20 percent of cases and is the most common cause of death from the disease. Hypertension does not develop until renal failure is severe.

DIAGNOSIS

The diagnosis can be made on clinical grounds. Biopsy of the skin lesion shows a necrotizing arteritis of small arterioles in the superficial dermis. Most of the inflammatory cells are neutrophils. Karyorrexis is usually prominent, a feature which has led to the term *leukoclastic angiitis*. It is important to recognize that there are several forms of purely cutaneous vasculitis that cause palpable purpura in the same distribution but are not associated with other systemic features. The diagnosis of hypersensitivity angiitis or Henoch-Schonlein purpura therefore requires, in addition to purpura, clinical evidence of other vascular involvement. Because hypersensitivity angiitis affects the small arterioles, manifestations related to organ infarction or to gross hemorrhage are not observed, except in the gastrointestinal tract, where extensive purpura may lead to gangrene.

Renal biopsy reveals a focal necrotizing glomerulonephritis. Mesangial proliferation or crescent formation portend a progressive glomerulonephritis with a poorer prognosis.

Leukocytosis, sometimes marked, moderate anemia, often with microangiopathic red cell morphology, and an active urine sediment are the major laboratory features of this disease. Serum complement component measurements are nearly always normal. A syndrome that resembles Henoch-Schonlein purpura has been described in a number of patients who have a congenital absence of the second component of complement. In the case of Henoch-Schonlein purpura, immunofluorescent staining of skin or kidney biopsies often reveals IgA in vascular lesions. Adult cases more often show the presence of IgG, but many cases show only fibrinogen. It is claimed that immunoglobulin deposition is a regular feature but is seen only in the earliest lesions, tending to disappear as fibrinoid necrosis ensues.

The differential diagnosis of hypersensitivity angiitis includes small vessel vasculities of many different kinds, specifically those caused by bacteremia especially chronic meningococcemia, subacute bacterial endocarditis, and rickettsial infection. Thrombotic thrombocytopenic purpura, hemolytic uremic syndrome, and a number of clinical conditions caused by circulating immune complexes also must be considered. Among the last named is the syndrome of mixed cryoglobulinemia. Other forms of cryoglobulinemia, macroglobulinemia of Waldenstrom, and hyperglobulinemic purpura may give rise to similar skin eruptions and occasionally to systemic signs related either to coincident connective tissue disease or plasma hyperviscosity.

COURSE AND PROGNOSIS

The course of the disease is one of several relapses of the entire complex. These recur at 5–10 day intervals with eventual complete recovery in 4–6 weeks. As noted previously, the prognosis is less favorable in adults who develop a chronic glomerulonephritis. Although some children have prolonged albuminuria and microscopic hematuria, less than 2 percent suffer progressive nephritis. Complications of mesenteric arteritis are responsible for a small number of deaths.

TREATMENT

In view of the generally good prognosis, the value of any therapy is difficult to assess. Most drugs are best avoided. Treatment with low-dose corticosteroid usually results in rapid symptomatic improvement, which may be important in children who are febrile and anorexic. There is no evidence that corticosteroid even in massive dosage alters the incidence or severity of the nephritis. The use of cytoxic or immunosuppressive drugs, reported in a small number of cases, has not been uniformly beneficial. A recurrence of hypersensitivity angiitis in the donor kidney following renal transplantation has been described.

Patients with hypersensitivity angiitis should be treated supportively. Occasionally losses of intersitial fluid may be severe and require prompt replacement with albumin or plasma. Symptoms of mesenteric arteritis present a difficult management problem. When there is doubt as to the extent of bowel involvement and ileus or signs of impending shock are appreciated, laparotomy is nearly always indicated.

WEGENER'S GRANULOMATOSIS

Although Wegener's granulomatosis was described as a distinct form of arteritis in 1936, it was not widely recognized as such until more recently. It is a disease of young and middle-aged adults with a male predominance. Cases in children are exceedingly rare.

CLINICAL MANIFESTATIONS

The onset and course may be very abrupt, leading to death in only a few weeks. Other cases may present with indolent granulomatous inflammation of the respiratory tract that shows little change over months. Chronic sinusitis or an inflammatory mass in the nasopharynx is often the first manifestation. The resulting purulent nasal discharge or recurrent epistaxis may antedate other features by years. The process often destroys surrounding bone or cartilage, leading to cranial nerve palsy, sinus tracts to the face, or characteristic collapse of the nasal or tracheal cartilages. When the orbits are involved, proptosis and ocular motor disturbances result. There may be retroorbital cellulitis and scleritis. Ulcerative keratitis is occasionally seen in the absence of other eye manifestations.

Patients present with pulmonary infiltrates that are often multifocal and can resolve and recur or break down to produce ragged thick wall cavities. Mediastinal lymph nodes are not enlarged, which may be a useful point in differentiating the process from tumor or other kinds of inflammation.

A number of other manifestations tend to occur early in the course of the disease, these include polyarthritis (usually of large joints such as the knees, ankles, and elbows), papulonecrotic skin lesions, and peripheral neuropathy. The synovial fluid is moderately inflammatory with a neutrophil predominence. The skin lesions resemble those seen in dissemenated neisserial infections but show a more proliferative arteritis on biopsy. The neuropathy is typically a mononeuritis multiplex; less commonly it is of a symmetric glove or stocking sensory type. Most patients are at least mildly febrile but may not appear otherwise seriously ill.

Signs of nephritis usually appear weeks or months after the onset of the abovementioned manifestations. In about 20 percent of cases nephritis is present from the outset, and these cases tend to run a more rapid course. In a few recorded cases glomerulonephritis has been the only prominent lesion. Vasculitis in other organ systems such as the central nervous system, gastrointestinal, or heart is uncommon in Wegener's, a feature which helps to distinguish this disease from classic periarteritis nodosa.

DIAGNOSIS

The diagnosis depends on the demonstration by biopsy of a proliferative necrotizing arteritis involving medium and small arteries associated with a proliferative inflammatory process in the surrounding tissue. Organized epithelioid cell granulomas containing foreign body giant cells are sometimes present. Because of their tendency to necrosis, repeated biopsies of lesions in the respiratory tract may be necessary before viable tissue suitable for histologic examination is obtained. Inflamed arteries are sometimes hard to locate in the midst of exuberant inflammatory lesions. The polymorphonuclear infiltrate consists of both neutrophils and eosinophils; the latter are likely to be numerous in biopsies of the respiratory tract. The vessels themselves are infiltrated with polymorphonuclear cells and lymphocytes.

Kidney biopsies often show only a focal process within the glomerular tuft, but in other cases the process is markedly proliferative with large epithelial crescents as well as granulomatous interstitial inflammation. This kind of pathology, especially when accompanied by an arteritis, is almost diagnostic of Wegener's granulomatosis. Although arteritis in the cerebral, cardiac, and mesenteric vessels may be found at autopsy, symptoms or signs do not usually result.

There are few diagnostically helpful laboratory investigations. Anemia and an elevated ESR are the rule. Tests for rheumatoid factor are positive in 40 percent of cases. Antinuclear antibody is not present and the levels of serum complement components are usually normal or elevated.

X-rays of the paranasal sinuses may show extensive opacification but are of specific diagnostic value only when bony erosion is seen.

When nephritis is not present the differential diagnosis of Wegener's granulomatosis includes many forms of granulomatous inflammation of the respiratory tract; among them are mycobacterial and fungal infections, aspiration pneumonia, septic pulmonary emboli, and other connective tissue diseases that can cause nodular lung lesions, particularly rheumatoid arthritis. Goodpasture's syndrome presents a special problem in differential diagnosis because pulmonary infiltrates, hemoptysis, and nephritis are cardinal features of that disorder. A kidney biopsy with immunofluorescent staining of the tissue may be required to resolve the problem. Linear staining of the glomerular basement membrane with antibody to IgG is indicative of Goodpasture's syndrome. The staining pattern in Wegener's granulomatosis is either of the "lumpy-bumpy" type or absent.

Both primary and secondary lung tumors must be ruled out. The differential diagnosis of the pulmonary infiltrates may be aided when tomography reveals cavitation that is not otherwise suspected. The biopsy demonstration of granulomatous pathology associated with an acute arteritis is prima facie evidence for the diagnosis of Wegener's granulomatosis. However, tissue necrosis may make the primacy of the arteritis difficult to ascertain. In some cases arterial lesions may not be identified even though characteristic granulomata are present. In contrast to periarteritis nodosa arteriographic studies are not usually helpful. Vascular occlusion may be demonstrated but extensive vessel irregularity and aneurysms are rarely seen. Although the disease called "lethal midline granuloma" was formerly considered by some to be an indolent varient of Wegener's granulomatosis, it now seems clear that it is more in the nature of a lymphoproliferative disorder. Nevertheless, in rare cases of Wegener's when the inflammatory process is of a chronic destructive nature and remains confined to the sinus or nasopharynx, the differential diagnosis may be quite difficult.

TREATMENT

The therapy of Wegener's granulomatosis has been revolutionized by the discovery that the disease is essentially cured by several of the cytotoxic drugs. At the present time cyclophosphamide is most widely used, primarily bcause it has a relatively rapid effect. In view of the sudden onset and swift progression of the nephritis in some patients, the speed of the therapeutic response is an important consideration. Other drugs that have proved effective are azathioprine and nitrogen mustard. Cyclophosphamide and azathioprine are used in doses of 2–3 mg/kg body weight. The induction of leukopenia is not necessary in order to obtain a satisfactory response, but it is the usual practice to give sufficient drug to keep the white blood cell count in the low-normal range. With the use of cyclophosphamide improvement can be anticipated in about 3 weeks.

A feeling of improved health, resolution of fever, and stabilization of renal function are the first signs of a response. This is followed by diminution or clearing of the lung infiltrates. Renal function often improves substantially over the ensuing weeks. There is no consensus as to how long therapy should be continued; however, at least 6 months after a maximum improvement has been obtained is recommended. Occasional patients may relapse after as long as 1 year of therapy and some appear to require long-term treatment at a reduced dose of the drug. As a group, patients with Wegener's granulomatosis seem to tolerate the cytotoxic drugs well. In the author's experience bacterial or fungus infections have not been a major problem nor have malignant tumors been reported with an unusual frequency in treated patients followed to date.

COURSE AND PROGNOSIS

The course of untreated Wegener's granulomatosis is usually rather indolent until nephritis supervenes. The pulmonary lesions may dominate the clinical picture and cause death either from the extent of the pathology or the accompanying complications. As noted previously, severe destruction of normal anatomy can result from lesions in the upper or lower respiratory tract, leading to death from secondary infection. The nephritis may terminate in uremia within several weeks of its discovery.

The long-term prognosis for patients with treated

Wegener's granulomatosis remains unknown. During the acute phase of the disease much depends on the severity of the pulmonary involvement and the risk of superinfection or lung hemorrhage. Peritoneal or hemodialysis has been used to tide patients over a period of renal failure. In some patients otherwise cured of the disease chronic hemodialysis is required and renal transplantation has been successful.

GIANT CELL ARTERITIS

Giant cell arteritis (GCA) is the preferred term for this syndrome, previously called *temporal* or *cranial arteritis*. It is now appreciated that almost any elastic artery can be affected. The distinguishing histologic feature of this form of arteritis is the presence of foreign body–type giant cells in relation to fragmented elastic laminae in the media of involved vessels.

CLINICAL MANIFESTATIONS

The disease is almost entirely confined to those over age 50. Males and females are equally affected. This disease frequently starts so abruptly that the patient can name the day when he or she began feeling achy and often mildly feverish, not unlike the onset of influenza. Pain and stiffness, predominently in the muscles of the shoulder and pelvic girdles, are often worse at night, interfere with sleep, and make arising in the morning very uncomfortable. Some muscular or periarticular tenderness may be present. Weakness is not a feature but myalgia may impair full volition during testing. This syndrome, called polymyalgia rheumatica, is the most common presentation of giant cell arteritis. It is clear, at least in retrospect, that not all patients with polymyalgia rheumatica have GCA. However, because it is often difficult to prove or exclude the presence of GCA, precise diagnosis may be impossible at the time of presentation.

Other patients develop only headache as the first major symptom. This is often associated with localized scalp tenderness so that combing or brushing the hair is painful. Face or tongue pain and particularly jaw claudication are important symptoms. Visual disturbances of any kind are serious and usually portend sudden blindness. The abrupt onset of any pain involving the head or face of an elderly person should alert one to the possibility of GCA. Other less common presentations are fever of unknown origin, unexplained weight loss and malaise, cerebral thrombosis, coronary occlusion, and dissecting aneurysm. The aorta and any of its major branches may be involved. Usually there is some cranial artery involvement when there is clinical evidence of an arteritis at other sites.

The most important finding on physical examination is localized tenderness and thickening of the scalp vessels. Any artery may be affected but the temporal arteries are most commonly involved. The carotid arteries may be tender and local bruits should be sought. Disease in the aorta or its major branches may lead to differences in blood pressure in the extremities. The tongue is occasionally painful or shows localized blanching.

DIAGNOSIS

Most patients with either polymyalgia rheumatica or GCA have an extremely high ESR, frequently in excess of 100 mm/hr. Although one should be reluctant to make the diagnosis in the absence of an elevated ESR, occasional patients show low or even normal values. Other evidence of systemic inflammation is found in an elevated serum globulin level and hypoalbuminemia. A mildly hypochromic anemia is the rule. Serum iron levels and iron-binding capacity are low despite normal or high marrow iron stores. Anorexia is often severe and an elevated serum alkaline phosphatase is found occasionally. Detailed studies of liver pathology are lacking.

The diagnosis of GCA can be made with some assurance when cranial symptoms and scalp vessel thickening are present. When neither feature is detected and the patient has the symptoms of polymyalgia rheumatica proof of an associated GCA is often sought by blind temporal artery biopsy. Because these arteries are not regularly involved, a negative biopsy is inconclusive. Although temporal artery angiography has been proposed as a better screening procedure than blind biopsy, in fact the diagnostic sensitivity is not substantially greater and the specificity is considerably less.

TREATMENT

Because the threat of blindness may be averted only by corticosteroid therapy, which is a form of treatment associated with a high morbidity in this age group, a correct diagnosis is essential. Patients with a compatible history and cranial or eye symptoms should be treated immediately as recommended for GCA. If the only symptoms are those of musculoskeletal aching suggestive of polymyalgia rheumatica, a low-dose prednisone test may be given. A positive test consists of marked improvement of all musculoskeletal symptoms on the morning after taking 7.5–10 mg prednisone one evening at bedtime. A positive test is highly suggestive of polymyalgia rheumatica.

There is no reliable way of excluding the presence of GCA. Therefore, it is probably wise to treat all cases of polymyalgia rheumatica with steroid and maintain it at the lowest dose that controls symptoms and the ESR. This usually requires less than 20 mg/day of prednisone or its equivalent, although higher doses are required initially.

A temporal artery biopsy is necessary only when the diagnosis of GCA is not considered to be strong because there are atypical symptoms and an elevated ESR without cranial symptoms. The patients with only malaise, low-grade fever, and an elevated ESR present an even greater diagnostic problem and its resolution may involve the process of excluding other diagnoses such as infection or occult cancer. A positive biopsy would mandate therapy. If clinically the diagnosis of GCA is considered unlikely, a negative biopsy offers support for the decision not to treat with corticosteroid, but instead to use a nonsteroidal antiinflammatory agent, to which symptoms often respond.

There is relatively little information regarding the long-term prognosis of patients with GCA. In a majority of patients it is possible, after 6–24 months of treatment, to omit steroid therapy gradually without recurrence of disease. In a few patients symptoms return even months or years after therapy has been stopped. In another small group it has not been possible to discontinue treatment even after several years because the ESR immediately rises. The attempt to reduce side effects of corticosteroid therapy by every other day administration has not provided effective control of symptoms in this disease.

OTHER FORMS OF ARTERITIS

ALLERGIC GRANULOMATOSIS OF CHURG AND STRAUSS

In 1951 Churg and Strauss identified syndrome among patients with systemic arteritis; originally named *allergic granulomatosis*, but now often referred to as the *Churg-Strauss syndrome*. Retrospectively, it is possible to identify other patients in the literature with a similiar illness thought to be periarteritis nodosa.

The Churg-Strauss syndrome, in contrast to that of periarteritis nodosa, has a rather stereotyped clinical presentation. Young or middle-aged adults of both sexes give a history of asthma, which may have begun years prior to other features. Allergic rhinitis is common and a majority of patients have marked blood eosinophilia. The vasculitic phase, which begins abruptly, includes severe asthma, fever, polyserositis, skin purpura, and subcutaneous nodules. Arthralgias, abdominal pain, and pulmonary infiltrates are other common features. Asthma is not a major manifestation in all patients. Some present with fever, pulmonary infiltrates, and eosinophilia. In other patients, although respiratory symptoms are mild, signs of mesenteric vasculitis dominate the clinical picture. Peripheral neuropathy in the form of mononeuritis multiplex occurs in about one-half of patients. In contrast to periarteritis nodosa, both central nervous system complications and serious kidney involvement are rare, although a number of the original cases had some evidence of renal disease.

The diagnosis in most cases is easily made on clinical grounds. When skin lesions are present the biopsy reveals a typical arteritis characterized by a predominently eosinophilic infiltrate. Extensive perivascular inflammation is often present. Muscle biopsies may be diagnostic, but there is a high false-negative rate. In other cases the diagnosis may be proven only at laparotomy, when bowel infarction occurs, or when a lung biopsy is undertaken.

Allergic granulomatosis usually responds favorably to corticosteroid therapy. Substantial doses may be required initially. Once controlled, maintenance doses of 10–15 mg prednisone/day or its equivalent are usually sufficient. The drug can often be tapered off after a

number of months but recurrence of the disease at a later date is common. No substantial experience with other drugs has been reported.

If untreated, about one-third of cases prove fatal within 2 years after the systemic phase of the disease supervenes. Death is usually related to myocardial infarction or respiratory causes such as status asthmaticus or pneumonitis. Complete remissions occur in one-half of the survivors. Subsequent episodes of arteritis or persistent asthma may affect others.

MIXED CRYOGLOBULINEMIA

The most common presentation of this syndrome, which occurs predominently in females, is recurrent purpura on the legs and buttocks, often associated with arthralgia that is also episodic in nature. About 50 percent of patients have Raynaud's phenomenon. Other manifestations include Sjögren's syndrome, peripheral neuropathy, and hepatosplenomegaly. Membranoproliferative glomerulonephritis eventually develops in about 20 percent of cases and is the major cause of death. Though it superficially resembles hypersensitivity angiitis, mixed cryoglobulinemia is much less acute. Many patients have recurrent purpura for years before some other feature brings them to medical attention.

Histologic examination of the skin reveals an acute inflammatory infiltrate in the superficial dermis and in the walls of the smaller arterioles and venules. Although fibrinoid necrosis is not usually evident in skin vessels, it can be seen in other locations in occasional patients who develop nephritis, peripheral neuropathy, or mesenteric arteritis.

The hallmark of the disease is the presence of serum cryoprotein, although it is usually not found in large amounts. It consists of a polyclonal and occasionally monoclonal IgM with rheumatoid factor activity complexed to polyclonal IgG. Rarely, the rheumatoid factor activity is an IgA. Rheumatoid factor is also demonstrable in the serum.

Recently it has been found that many of these patients have hepatitis B surface antigen or antibody in both serum and isolated immune complex.

No effective drug therapy is known. Plasmapheresis has been used successfully to control exacerbations of the disease.

CUTANEOUS VASCULITIS WITH ARTHRITIS

An arteriolitis caused by immune complex deposition probably forms the basis of this syndrome. It is characterized by recurrent urticaria, which can involve any part of the body including the face. In some cases lesions may become purpuric. Attacks of arthritis involving both large and small joints accompanied by fever are prominent. Many patients also have episodes of acute abdominal pain, probably reflecting mesenteric vasculitis. Laboratory evidence of a mild membranoproliferative glomerulonephritis is found in this disease, although it rarely becomes clinically significant.

The skin lesions on biopsy reveal a widespread dermal infiltrate of acute inflammatory cells with involvement of smaller arterioles. Immunofluorescent staining shows IgM and often IgA and complement (particularly C3) in the affected vessels. Serum complement levels are reduced in all patients during acute attacks. Hepatitis B antigen has not been found in the serum or vascular lesions in patients with this syndrome.

IMMUNOBLASTIC LYMPHADENOPATHY

Immunoblastic lymphadenopathy is a lymphomalike entity characterized by generalized lymphadenopathy, hepatosplenomegaly, and, frequently, hemolytic anemia. The lymph node histology is characterized by the presence of lymphoblasts and plasma cells, some of which may also be seen in peripheral blood. Lymph node architecture is effaced and marked vascular proliferation is evident within the parenchyma. Most patients have increased levels of polyclonal IgG and IgM. Pulmonary infiltrates occur in some patients and necrotizing arteritis has been seen in skin and muscle biopsies. Because hypocomplementemia has been present in some of these patients, an immune complex pathogenesis has been postulated.

INTRACRANIAL ARTERITIS

A number of reports suggest that there may be a distinct form of granulomatous arteritis largely restricted to the central nervous system. Most cases have run a progressive course over a few months with both focal and more diffuse meningoencephalitic symptoms and signs. A few have had cord manifestations as well. Cerebrospinal fluid protein is nearly always increased and most cases have a lymphocytic pleocytosis.

At autopsy examination cerebral vasculitis is seen. It involves both arteries and venules with a mononuclear infiltrate and sparse but prominent giant cells. Although clinical evidence of pathology has been confined almost entirely to the central nervous system, some involvement of other organ systems has been found post mortem.

MISCELLANEOUS FORMS OF ARTERITIS

A number of rare clinical syndromes exist in which the basic pathologic process is an arteritis. These include Takayasu's aortitis, Cogan's syndrome, and several forms of cutaneous arteritis in which there is apparently no systemic component. The group of cutaneous arteritis syndromes is heterogeneous. Some are associated with other pathology and may reflect an allergic state; these include erythema elevatum diutinum, cutaneous arteriolitis of Ruiter, livedoid vasculitis, nodular vasculitis, and urticaria arteritica. Although they will not be discussed in detail here, the fact that purely cutaneous forms of arteritis exist warrants caution in determining the significance of positive skin biopsies. Systemic arteritis should not be diagnosed unless there is some proof of systemic involvement.

Takayasu's Arteritis

Takayasu's arteritis affects primarily the aorta and its major branches and is predominently a disease of young women. It usually begins with a period of diverse manifestations consisting of low-grade fever, arthralgia or myalgia, anemia, and an elevated ESR. Neck and shoulder pain may be prominent, sometimes with tenderness over the carotid or subclavian vessels. Days to weeks later, manifestations of an aortic arch syndrome are noted. Coldness, cyanosis, or intermittent claudication of an extremity are common symptoms. Syncope, facial numbness, or episodes of dysarthia or loss of vision may indicate carotid disease. Bruits over major vessels and a difference in blood pressure between two extremities should be sought. An important sign in advanced cases is the presence of arteriovenous aneurysms in the retina. The cause of these aneurysms is not understood. They were first described in several of the original cases by Takayasu, an ophthalmologist. A majority of patients complain of dyspnea. The pathogenesis of this is not clear, although 20 percent have pulmonary arteritis or congestive failure related to coronary artery involvement. Although the aortitis is usually most severe in the area of the arch, any part may be affected. Renal artery stenosis leading to hypertension is common, but for some reason the celiac axis is usually spared.

An elevated ESR is present in most patients. There are no specific abnormalities in the laboratory examination. Rheumatoid factors, antinuclear antibody, and cryoglobulin are absent and the levels of serum complement components are normal.

The diagnosis, once entertained, can be confirmed by aortography with particular attention to clinically affected branches. The findings of irregularity of the intimal surface and narrowing of the ostea or lumens of major vessels in a young woman is virtually diagnostic. Affected vessels often show areas of poststenotic dilatation as well.

Treatment with corticosteroids is recommended but long-term proof of benefit is unavailable. Clinical evidence of a response is manifest by the disappearance of fever, fall of ESR, and improved well-being of the patient. Unfortunately, contined narrowing or occlusion of vessels is not uncommon. It has been suggested that this may be related to cicatrization of the inflammatory lesions in the course of healing. The disease usually runs a course of exacerbations and remissions. Treatment with immunosuppressive drugs has not been reported. Although pregnancy is not associated with worsening of the disease, postpartum exacerbations may occur.

Cogan's Syndrome

Cogan's syndrome is characterized by keratitis and nerve deafness. These manifestations may develop in close proximity or as part of a systemic illness in which hypertension, cardiovascular complications, peripheral neuropathy, and other signs of a systemic illness are found. In some cases in which autopsies have been performed or muscle biopsies obtained a widespread arteritis resembling periarteritis nodosa has been found and, in a few instances, an aortitis resembling the Takayasu type. It is not clear that all patients with the clinical complex of keratitis and nerve deafness have an underlying arteritis. A number of patients have survived for years without further complications. The deafness once established is permanent. Nothing is known about the etiology of the syndrome.

Kohlmeier-Degos Disease

Another form of arteriopathy often classified as an arteritic syndrome is atrophic papulosis, also called Kohlmeier-Degos disease. The essential pathology is a sclerosing endarteropathy rather than an inflammatory or destructive process. Kohlmeier-Degos disease is characterized by the appearance on the trunk and extremities of mildly erythematous papules that evolve into unmistakable sharply circumscribed, slightly depressed, 0.5–1-cm alabaster-white scars with a pigmented border. The patients also suffer episodes of abdominal pain related to similar lesions in the mesenteric circulation, and progressive cerebral dysfunction. Unless the cutaneous lesions are recognized the disease is often misdiagnosed as periarteritis nodosa. A favorable therapeutic response to drugs that inhibit platelet adhesion has been reported.

Erythema Elevatum Diutinum

Erythema elevatum diutinum produces crops of purplish papules and nodules distributed on the extensor surfaces of the limbs, particularly in relation to joints and on the buttocks. Malaise and low-grade fever are common. Most patients also have polyarthritis that affects both large and small joints but has not been characterized in other respects. An acute arteriolitis and dermatitis is seen in biopsies of the nodules. Neutrophilic polymorphonuclear leukocytes predominate but some eosinophils are usually also present. Involvement of other organ systems does not occur. The disease runs an indolent course but often responds dramatically to Dapsone, an orally active sulfone.

REFERENCES

Christian CL, Sergent JS: Vasculitis syndromes: Clinical and experimental models. Am J Med 61:385, 1976

Chumbley LC, Harrison EG, DeRemee RA: Allergic granulomatosis and angiitis (Churg-Strauss syndrome). Mayo Clin Proc 52:477, 1977

Cream JJ: Clinical and immunological aspects of cutaneous vasculitis. Q J Med 45:255, 1976

Diaz-Perez JL, Winklemann RK: Cutaneous periarteritis nodosa. Arch Dermatol 110:407, 1974

Fauci AS, Wolff SM: Wegener's granulomatosis: Studies in eighteen patients and a review of the literature. Medicine (Baltimore) 52:535, 1973

Hamilton CR Jr, Shelley WM, Tumulty PA: Giant cell arteritis including temporal arteritis and polymyalgia rheumatica. Medicine (Baltimore) 50:1, 1970

Katz SI, Gallin JI, Hertz KC, Fauci AS, Lawley TJ: Erythema elevation diutinum. Skin and systemic manifestations, immunologic studies and successful treatment with Dapsone. Medicine (Baltimore) 56:443, 1977

Kolodny EH, Rabeiz JS, Caviness VS, Richardson EP: Granulomatous angiitis of the central nervous system. Arch Neurol 19:510, 1968

Levo Y, Gorevic PD, Kassab HJ, Zucker-Franklin D, Franklin EC: Association between hepatitis B virus and essential mixed cryoglobulinemia. N Engl J Med 296:1501, 1977

Lupi-Herrera E, Sanchez-Torres G, Marcushamer J, Mispireta J, Horwitz S, Vela JE: Takayasu's arteritis. Clinical study of 107 cases. Am Heart J 93:94, 1977

McDuffie FC, Sams WM, Maldonaldo JE, Andreini PH, Conn D, Samayoa E: Hypocomplementemia with cutaneous vasculitis and arthritis. Possible immune complex syndrome. Mayo Clin Proc 48:340, 1973

Meadow SR, Glasgow EF, White RHR, Moncrieff SR, Cameron JS, Ogg CS: Schonlein-Henoch nephritis. Q J Med 41:241, 1972

Meltzer M, Franklin EC, Elias K, McCluskey RT, Cooper N: Cryoglobulinemia—A clinical and laboratory study. Am J Med 40:837, 1966

Mowrey FH, Lundberg EA: The clinical manifestations of essential polyangiitis (periarteritis nodosa) with emphasis on the hepatic manifestations. Ann Intern Med 40:1145, 1954

Reza MG, Dornfield L, Goldberg LS, Bluestone R, Pearson CM: Wegener's granulomatosis. Long-term follow-up of patients treated with cyclophosphamide. Arthritis Rheum 18:501, 1975

Sergent JS, Lockshin MD, Christian CL, Gocke DJ: Vasculitis with hepatitis B antigenemia: Long term observation on nine patients. Medicine (Baltimore) 55:1, 1976

Strole WE Jr., Clark WE, Isselbacher KJ: Progressive arterial occlusive disease (Kohlmeier-Degos), N Engl J Med 276:195, 1967

Tanaka N, Sekimoto K, Naoe S: Kawasaki disease. Arch Pathol Lab Med 100:81, 1976

Winklemann RK, Schroeter AL, Kierland RR, Ryan TM: Clinical studies of livedoid vasculitis. Mayo Clin Proc 49:476, 1974

Zeek PM: Periarteritis nodosa: A critical review. Am J Clin Pathol 22:777, 1952

Sjögren's Syndrome

Norman Talal

ETIOLOGY AND MANIFESTATIONS

Sjögren's syndrome (SS) is an autoimmune disease characterized by oral and ocular dryness resulting from the partial to complete destruction of salivary and lacrimal glands by lymphocytic and plasma cell infiltrates. Rheumatoid arthritis (RA) or another connective tissue disease may be present. SS is defined as the triad of dry eyes (keratoconjunctivitis sicca), dry mouth (xerostomia), and a rheumatic disease, though any two of these criteria are sufficient to establish the diagnosis. Approximately one-half of all patients with SS have rheumatoid arthritis; these individuals are also more likely to have other extraarticular manifestations of RA, such as Felty's syndrome, pulmonary lymphoid infiltrates, and vasculitis. SS occurs in 25 percent of patients with RA, but it is also seen with other rheumatic diseases, such as sytemic lupus erythematosus, scleroderma, and polymyositis, or in the absence of any associated disease (the "sicca syndrome").

EPIDEMIOLOGY

SS shows a marked (9:1) preference for females, possibly due to hormonal factors. Onset is usually in the fifth or sixth decade, although the disease has been noted in children and at all ages. In its age and sex preference, SS is similar to organ-specific autoimmune disorders affecting the thyroid gland and the liver.

The exact prevalence of SS is unknown, but it is probably the commonest connective tissue disease after RA, which affects about 1 percent of the population. From the above data, one can reasonably predict a prevalence of 0.5 percent. Autopsy studies support this contention.

ETIOLOGY

Autoimmune disorders have a multifactorial etiology combining elements of (1) *genetic* control, possibly related to the activity of specific immune response genes, (2) *immunologic* control, which may be exerted by regulatory T-dependent lymphocytes (suppressor and helper T cells), (3) possible *viral* influences, although this is yet to be clearly established, and (4) *sex hormone* modulation of immune regulation.

SS is one of several organ-specific autoimmune diseases associated with the histocompatibility antigens HLA-B8 and/or HLA-DW3. (The other diseases include coeliac disease, dermatitis herpetiformis, myasthenia gravis, Grave's disease, chronic active hepatitis, idiopathic Addison's disease, and insulin-dependent diabetes mellitus.) These antigens may be genetically linked to immune response genes that predispose an individual to the development of autoimmune disease. According to this theory, such an individual might be more likely to react immunologically against viral or viral-altered host antigens. Antigenic alteration of salivary gland antigens, for example, could lead to sensitization, lymphocytic infiltration, and production of antitissue antibodies.

The presence of multiple serum autoantibodies is a characteristic feature of SS. Some of these reactions are organ specific, such as the antibody directed against salivary duct epithelium. Others, such as antinuclear antibody and rheumatoid factor, are not specific for salivary gland antigens. Serum antibodies reacting with certain recently described and partially characterized nuclear antigens (called Ha, SS-B, and SS-A) are present in high frequency in SS.

A deficiency of suppressor T cells may predispose to autoimmunity. Suppressor function declines prematurely in NZB and NZB/NZW F_1 mice, strains that spontaneously develop an autoimmune syndrome in which lymphocytic infiltrates of the salivary glands are a feature. Autoimmunity and survival in these genetically susceptible mice are greatly influenced by sex hormones. Androgens suppress disease and prolong survival; estrogens have the opposite effect.

PATHOLOGY

The classic lesion of SS is a lymphocytic and plasma cell infiltrate that can involve salivary, lacrimal, and other exocrine glands in the respiratory tract, gastrointestinal tract, and vagina. Both major (parotid, submaxillary) and minor (gingival, palatine) salivary glands are involved. The term *benign lymphoepithelial lesion* has been applied to describe the characteristic histologic appearance in the salivary glands. These lesions may be present without xerostomia and other features of SS.

Both B and T lymphocytes are present in the tissue lesions, and large amounts of immunoglobulin (particularly IgG and IgM) are synthesized by these infiltrating cells. In patients with coexisting SS and Waldenstrom's macroglobulinemia, the monoclonal IgM may also be synthesized locally in the salivary glands. Rheumatoid factor is produced in the glands, and germinal centers may develop. In these respects, the infiltrated glands in SS resemble the inflamed synovial tissue in rheumatoid arthritis.

The earliest infiltrates may be scattered around small intralobular ducts. The histologic picture is varied and includes acinar atrophy, generally in proportion to the extent of lymphoid infiltration, and proliferative or metaplastic changes in the duct lining cells. The proliferation may progress to form the characteristic epimyoepithelial islets that are seen in about 40 percent of parotid biopsy specimens. In some patients, adipose replacement may be more prominent than lymphoid infiltration. Typically, the lobular architecture is preserved; some lobules may be spared while others are virtually destroyed.

When mucosal glands in the trachea and bronchi are involved, benign appearing lymphoid infiltrates are again a prominent feature. More extensive lymphoid infiltrates may involve the lung, kidney, or skeletal muscle, resulting in functional abnormalities of these organs.

In some patients the lymphoid infiltrates in salivary glands, lymph nodes, or parenchymal organs are more pleomorphic, more primitive, or more invasive, and they raise the possibility of malignancy. Lymph node architecture can be destroyed and lymphoma may be diagnosed if such abnormal cells predominate. It may be impossible to decide between a benign or malignant process, in which case the term *pseudolymphoma* has been employed.

SYMPTOMS AND CLINICAL FEATURES

The manifestations and presentations of SS are protean (Tables 1 and 2). The typical presentation of SS is a middle-aged female with either (1) the insidious development of sicca symptoms complicating chronic RA, or (2) the more rapid onset of distressing oral and ocular sicca symptoms, often with episodic parotid swelling. However, the disease may present in a variety of other ways (Table 2). Lymphoid infiltration of exocrine glands resulting in secretory impairment is the hallmark of SS. This occurs not only in the parotid, submandibular, and lacrimal glands, but also in the labial salivary glands and in the mucus-producing glands throughout the gastrointestinal and respiratory tracts.

Ocular symptoms typical for keratoconjunctivitis

sicca include a foreign body sensation (usually described as "sandy" or "gritty"), burning, smarting, dryness, excess secretion, and inability to tear. Gross conjunctivitis is present only in severe cases, unless complicating bacterial infection is superimposed. The eye generally appears normal. Corneal debris may be present, particularly upon awakening in the morning. Evidence of decreased tearing by Schirmer's test (amount of filter paper moistened by tears when paper is placed in lower conjunctival sac), plus characteristic corneal and scleral staining with rose bengal are strongly suggestive findings. Biomicroscopy is necessary to detect mild involvement and to demonstrate punctate or filamentary keratitis definitively. Evidence of decreased lacrimation with mild ocular staining is not diagnostic but should be reevaluated in a few months' time.

The severity of oral dryness may be indicated by constant rinsing or by carrying fluids or keeping fluids at the bedside. Deficient saliva leads to difficulty in eating and swallowing dry foods such as crackers. Voice fatigue, hoarseness, denture difficulties, oral candidiasis, and rampant caries are frequent consequences of xerostomia.

A history of recurrent or chronic unilateral or bilateral salivary gland swelling is helpful. Suppurative (usually staphylococcal) parotitis can be superimposed and should always be ruled out. Objective findings include parotid or submandibular enlargement and the absence of salivary pooling in the floor of the mouth. Fissuring, erythema, and papillary atrophy of the tongue occur, sometimes resembling avitaminosis. Stimulated parotid flow rate is subnormal (in contrast to many emotional or drug-induced xerostomias).

The involvement of minor salivary glands in the lower lip makes it possible to perform lower lip biopsies and obtain histologic confirmation of the diagnosis in a large number of patients. This procedure is performed with the patient seated in a dental chair under local anesthesia. The specimen is best obtained with a scalpel. Patients will generally experience discomfort for 24–48 hours; approximately 1 percent may complain of more persistent localized numbness. Lymphocytic infiltration can be measured using the focus scoring method, in which the number of foci (defined as 50 or more round cells per 4 mm² of section) is determined on the biopsy specimen. A focus score greater than 1 is a better criterion for the oral component of the syndrome than the subjective evaluation of xerostomia. Although the diagnosis can be made on clinical criteria alone in many instances, the complete evaluation of a patient should include a lip biopsy.

Nasal dryness or bleeding, nonproductive cough, and vaginal dryness mimicking estrogen deficiency are other common and characteristic components of mucous gland impairment in the sicca syndrome.

The arthritis of SS resembles classic RA in its clinical, pathologic, and roentgenographic features. Keratoconjunctivitis sicca develops in about 10–15 percent of patients with RA. Arthralgias and morning stiffness not progressing to joint deformity may occur in patients with

Table 1
Clinical Components of Sjögren's Syndrome
(Exclusive of an Associated Connective Tissue Disease)

Exocrine gland dysfunction
  Keratoconjunctivitis sicca
  Xerostomia
  Enlarged salivary or lacrimal glands
  Dry mucous membranes in nose, pharynx, larynx, bronchi,
    vulva, vagina

Extraglandular features
  Raynaud's phenomenon
  Hepatomegaly
  Spenomegaly
  Pleuritis, pulmonary infiltration
  Vasculitis
  Neuropathy
  Myopathy
  Lymphadenopathy
  Purpura
  Renal tubular dysfunction

Principal laboratory abnormalities
  Rapid erythrocyte sedimentation rate
  Rheumatoid factor
  Antinuclear antibodies
  Hypergammaglobulinemia
  Anemia of chronic disease
  Leukopenia
  Eosinophilia

the sicca syndrome. Fluctuations in the course of the arthritis are not necessarily accompanied by parallel alterations in the sicca symptoms. Splenomegaly and leukopenia suggestive of Felty's syndrome, and vasculitis with leg ulcers and peripheral neuropathy, may appear even in the absence of RA. Raynaud's phenomenon occurs in 20 percent of patients.

Severe proximal muscle weakness and sometimes tenderness may be early symptoms, leading to a diagnosis of polymyositis. Weakness may also be associated with electrolyte imbalance, nephrocalcinosis, and the clinical findings of renal tubular acidosis. Peripheral or cranial neuropathy may cause symptoms of dysesthesia or paresthesia. Facial pain and numbness can accompany trigeminal neuropathy and contribute to the oral discomfort caused by the dryness.

A spectrum of benign to malignant lymphoproliferation occurs, including hyperplastic lymphadenopathy,

Table 2
Clinical Presentation of Sjögren's Syndrome

Sicca complex: dry eyes and dry mouth	Proximal myopathy
Rheumatoid arthritis or other connective tissue disease	Neuropathy, including trigeminal
Parotid tumor	Chronic hepatobiliary disease
Nonthrombocytopenic purpura	Pleural or parenchymal pulmonary disease
Renal tubular acidosis or other tubular disorder	Lymphoma, local or generalized
	Dysglobulinemia

pseudolymphoma, reticulum cell sarcoma, and macroglobulinemia. Visceral organs, especially the lung, liver, and kidney, develop lymphoid infiltrates.

LABORATORY FEATURES

A mild normocytic, normochromic anemia occurs in about 25 percent of patients, leukopenia in 30 percent, eosinophilia (above 6 percent eosinophils) in 25 percent, and an elevated erythrocyte sedimentation rate (greater than 30 mm/hr by the Westergren method) in over 90 percent.

Half of the patients have hypergammaglobulinemia—a diffuse elevation of all immunoglobulin classes. It is most marked in patients who lack RA but have polymyopathy, purpura, or renal tubular acidosis. Monoclonal IgM may be seen. Cryoglobulinemia (often of the mixed IgM–IgG type) may be present, particularly in patients with glomerulonephritis or pseudolymphoma. Hyperviscosity associated with IgG rheumatoid factor and intermediate complexes has been reported. Some patients with reticulum cell sarcoma have hypogammaglobulinemia. A mild hypoalbuminemia is common.

Rheumatoid factor is detected in over 90 percent of sera when pooled human F II gamma globulin is used as antigen, and in 75 percent when rabbit gamma globulin is employed. Thus, many patients who lack RA have rheumatoid factor. Rheumatoid factor may disappear or diminish markedly in titer when reticulum cell sarcoma develops.

The LE cell phenomenon occurs in 20 percent of patients who also have RA. It is otherwise rare unless systemic lupus erythematosus is also present.

Antinuclear factors that give a homogeneous or speckled pattern of immunofluorescence are seen in about 70 percent of patients. Antibodies to native DNA are occasionally present in low titer. An antibody specific for salivary duct epithelium has been observed by indirect immunofluorescence in 50 percent of patients. Thyroglobulin antibodies, detected by hemagglutination, are present in about 35 percent.

Precipitating antibodies to tissue antigens extracted from a human lymphocyte culture line or from calf thymus are present in a majority of patients. Individuals with only the sicca complex have antibodies reactive with nuclear proteins Ha, SS-A, or SS-B. Patients with associated RA have a different antibody (called RAP.) The latter also occurs in 65 percent of patients with RA not accompanied by clinical SS.

Peripheral blood T lymphocytes are decreased in about one-third of patients and increase toward normal following in vitro incubation with thymosin. Immunoglobulin-positive lymphocytes in peripheral blood may be increased slightly. The majority of patients have an impaired lymphocyte response to phytohemagglutinin, particularly when stimulated with a suboptimal concentration of the mitogen. A diminished capacity to develop delayed hypersensitivity to dinitrochlorobenzene may also be present.

β_2-microglobulin is a component of lymphocyte membranes that have a role in immunologic regulation. An increase in salivary β_2-microglobulin concentration correlates with the degree of lymphocytic infiltration found on labial biopsy. Serum β_2-microglobulin levels can be increased, particularly in patients with associated renal or lymphoproliferative complications.

DIAGNOSIS AND TREATMENT

SS can be considered both as an entity unto itself and as a constellation of findings that can occur in any one of the other connective tissue diseases. It is usually benign and is treated with conservative management.

DIAGNOSIS

SS should be suspected in any patient with RA and the diagnosis can be made when any two of the three major clinical features (keratoconjunctivitis sicca, xerostomia, RA or another connective tissue disease) are present. Many patients will present with symptoms of oral and ocular dryness but without an underlying connective tissue disease. Such patients would appear to have sicca syndrome as a primary disease entity. If arthritis does not develop within the first 12 months of the sicca complex, the chances are small (10 percent) that it will appear later.

The patient's history is extremely useful, since the dryness of eyes and mouth produces characteristic symptoms. Subjects complain of a "sandy" or "gritty" feeling in the eyes and experience great discomfort trying to swallow dry foods. Many patients, upon casual questioning, will state that their mouths feel dry or that they awaken at night because of oral dryness. Hoarseness, rampant dental caries, and tracheobronchitis may be presenting problems.

The diagnosis of SS can be made objectively on the basis of oral and ocular findings. Decreased lacrimation is suspected on the basis of an abnormal Schirmer test. Severe desiccation may lead to filamentary keratitis or corneal ulceration. The stimulated parotid salivary flow rate is markedly decreased. Histologic confirmation of SS can be obtained by biopsy of the minor salivary glands of the lower lip, which, like the major salivary and lacrimal glands, are infiltrated by lymphocytes and plasma cells.

The varied clinical presentation and multisystemic nature of the syndrome may make diagnosis difficult (see Table 2 in the preceding chapter). A unilateral or asymmetric glandular enlargement may suggest a possible tumor. Twenty to 30 percent of patients with hyperglobulinemic purpura have other features of SS. The initial symptoms may suggest a severe degenerative or inflammatory muscle disease. Peripheral neuropathy may be a prominent feature, and trigeminal involvement can cause facial discomfort. Pulmonary lymphoid infiltration may result in respiratory insufficiency. Renal infiltrates may cause overt or latent renal tubular acidosis and can lead to renal insufficiency. Liver involvement may present as chronic hepatitis or biliary cirrhosis. The diagnosis of SS can be obscure in such patients if the clinical picture is dominated by a potentially more life-threatening problem.

The suspicion of a neoplasm may be raised by these tissue lymphoid infiltrates or by significant lymph node enlargement. Biopsy of the involved tissue or lymph node may be difficult to interpret. The term *pseudolymphoma* describes a situation in which the clinical suspicion of a malignancy is not confirmed by histologic examination.

PROGNOSIS AND COMPLICATIONS

Most often, SS is a benign disease that does not affect longevity. The prognosis may be the same as for any accompanying disease (e.g., RA). In some patients, lymphoproliferation is not confined to glandular tissue but becomes more generalized, involving sites such as lymph nodes, lung, kidney, spleen, bone marrow, muscle, or liver. The disease may then simulate frankly malignant lymphoproliferative disorders, such as Waldenstrom's macroglobulinemia, reticulum cell sarcoma, or other lymphomas. The subsequent clinical course is frequently that of the lymphoma, ending in death.

TREATMENT

SS generally remains a benign disease, with lymphoproliferation confined to salivary and lacrimal tissue. Consequently, conservative management is the best guide to therapy.

The sicca syndrome is treated with fluid replacement supplied as often as necessary. There are several readily available ophthalmic preparations (Tearisol; Liquifilm; 0.5 percent methylcellulose) that will adequately replace the deficient tears. In severe situations, patients will instill these as often as every 30 minutes. If corneal ulceration is present, eye patching and boric acid ointment may be necessary.

It is more difficult to compensate for the salivary insufficiency. The frequent ingestion of fluids, particularly with meals, is often the best solution. Patients should see their dentists every 4 months and pay scrupulous attention to proper oral hygiene. The careful use of a water pick after eating may reduce the incidence of caries.

Proper humidification of the home environment is helpful in reducing respiratory infections and other complications of the sicca syndrome. Patients should be encouraged to live with their disability. They require sympathetic understanding from those who have never personally experienced the discomfort of the sicca symptoms.

The management of RA or other associated disorders is in no way altered by the presence of SS. There are no controlled studies evaluating the efficacy of corticosteroids or immunosuppressive drugs in the treatment of the sicca complex. In view of the benign nature of this problem, such therapy does not seem justified at this time.

On the other hand, corticosteroids or immunosuppressive drugs seem indicated in the treatment of pseudolymphoma, particularly when there is renal or pulmonary involvement. Cyclophosphamide at a dosage of 75–100 mg/day has diminished extraglandular lymphoid infiltrates and restored salivary gland function in selected patients treated at the National Institutes of Health.

Frank malignant lymphoma should be treated with intensive chemotherapy, surgery, and/or radiotherapy as indicated by the location and extent of disease. These are highly malignant and often fatal lesions which require rapid and skilled intervention.

REFERENCES

Block KJ, Buchanan WW, Wohl MJ, Bunim JJ: Sjögren's syndrome. A clinical, pathological and serological study of sixty-two cases. Medicine (Baltimore) 44:187, 1965

Mason AMS, Gumpel JM, Golding PL: Sjögren's syndrome. A clinical review. Semin Arthritis Rheum 2:301, 1973

Shearn MA: Sjögren's syndrome, in Smith LH (ed): Major Problems in Internal Medicine, Vol. 2. Philadelphia, Saunders, 1971

Talal N: Sjögren's syndrome and connective tissue disease with other immunologic disorders, in Hollander JL (ed): Arthritis and Allied Conditions. Philadelphia, Lea & Febinger, 1972

Talal N, Sokoloff L, Barth WF: Extrasalivary lymphoid abnormalities in Sjögren's syndrome (reticulum cell sarcoma, "pseudolymphoma," macroglobulinemia). Am J Med 43:50 1967

Whaley K, Williamson J, Chisolm DM, Webb J, Mason DK, Buchanan WW: Sjögren's syndrome. I. Sicca components. Q J Med 42:279, 1973

Amyloidosis

Alan S. Cohen

CLASSIFICATION

Amyloidosis has been defined as the extracellular deposition of the fibrous protein amyloid in one or more sites of the body. This protein has unique ultrastructural, x-ray diffraction, and biochemical characteristics. The substance may be local and isolated with no clinical consequences, may grossly involve virtually any organ system of the body and lead to severe pathophysiologic changes, or may fall between these two extremes. The natural history is poorly understood and the clinical diagnosis is often not made until the disease is far advanced.

The following classification is the most useful clinically:

1. primary amyloidosis—no evidence of preexisting or coexisting disease
2. amyloid associated with multiple myeloma
3. secondary amyloidosis—associated with chronic infectious (e.g., osteosteomyelitis, tuberculosis, lep-

rosy) or chronic inflammatory (e.g., rheumatoid arthritis, ankylosing spondylitis, etc.) disease

4. heredofamilial anyloidosis—associated with familial Mediterranean fever and a variety of neuropathic, renal, cardiovascular, and other syndromes
5. local anyloidosis—local, often tumorlike deposits in isolated organs without evidence of systemic involvement
6. amyloidosis associated with aging

With the recent studies delineating the chemical composition of the protein in the various types of amyloidosis, a more exact immunochemical classification is available in part: (1) amyloid associated with tissue deposition of protein AA (secondary amyloidosis; the amyloid of familial Mediterranean fever); and (2) amyloid associated with tissue deposition of protein AL (primary amyloid; amyloid associated with multiple myeloma; possibly some local amyloid). Other chemical types (e.g., that associated with medullary carcinoma of the thyroid, and that associated with old age) may also exist.

PRIMARY AMYLOIDOSIS

Although the term *primary amyloidosis* delineates disease in which no prediposing cause is found, it should not be misconstrued as a peculiar clinical type of amyloid easily distinguishable from other forms. The classic distinctions between primary and secondary amyloidosis based solely upon organ distribution are not completely valid. Histochemical stains cannot distinguish primary from secondary amyloid, and at the electron microscopic level all types of amyloid have an identical fibrillar nature. Only recently has it been shown that the biochemical composition of the amyloid fibril is unique and consists of κ or λ fragments of or of whole immunoglobulin light chains in primary and in myeloma-associated amyloid.

Certain clinical features should alert the clinician to the diagnosis of primary amyloidosis: *unexplained* proteinuria, peripheral neuropathy, progressive numbness and tingling in the feet, enlarged tongue, increased heart size, malabsorption, hepatomegaly, or orthostatic hypotension. Laboratory abnormalities are nonspecific and may or may not include proteinuria, elevated erythrocyte sedimentation rate, or Bence Jones protein or M component in serum or urine. Not infrequently, symptoms have existed for several years before the correct diagnosis has been made and a biopsy of an involved organ is necessary to confirm the diagnosis. All patients who are said to have primary amyloidosis should be thoroughly investigated for evidence of other disease to rule out unsuspected inflammatory disorders and malignant tumors.

AMYLOIDOSIS AND MYELOMA

Multiple myeloma is one of the malignant conditions in which there is an increased prevalence of amyloid disease; 6–15 percent of such patients have amyloidosis, the features of which are often indistinguishable from the primary type. Whereas the overlap of organ involvement in the various types holds true in nearly all cases, involvement of the synovial membrane with amyloid is found almost exclusively in patients with multiple myeloma. Of interest to the rheumatologist is the fact that this joint disease may mimic the features of rheumatoid arthritis.

SECONDARY AMYLOIDOSIS

The frequency of amyloidosis in the general population is not known. Most available data are based on postmortem studies, which are unreliable in that they are performed on a selected group of patients and special stains for amyloidosis are not done routinely. The prevalence of amyloid at autopsy in many general hospitals around the world is about 0.5 percent. In Japan it is low (0.1 percent) and in countries such as Portugal and Israel, where there are known genetic amyloid syndromes, the overall frequency is much greater. However, studies in patients with chronic infectious disease who have an increased risk of developing amyloidosis (e.g. patients with chronic tuberculosis and leprosy) have shown a very high prevalence on postmortem examination (up to 50 percent in some series).

Patients with a number of chronic inflammatory conditions cared for by the rheumatologist may develop amyloidosis. These rheumatic conditions include rheumatoid arthritis, ankylosing spondylitis, juvenile rheumatoid arthritis, Reiter's syndrome, the arthritis associated with psoriasis, and other miscellaneous disorders. Currently, tuberculosis, leprosy, paraplegia, and rheumatoid arthritis have the greatest incidence. The development of secondary amyloidosis in a patient with one of the above-mentioned diseases is often heralded by proteinuria, hepatomegaly, or splenomegaly. The interval between the rheumatic disease and the appearance of amyloid is unpredictable. Secondary amyloid deposits appear to be composed of a new protein moiety, termed *protein AA*, which has a unique amino acid sequence and is distinct from immunoglobulin light chains.

LOCALIZED AMYLOIDOSIS

In addition to systemic deposition, amyloid may be present in small, focal amounts, sometimes in a tumorlike form, in virtually any area of the body. The more common locations are the lung, skin, larynx, eye, and bladder. In nearly all of these cases there has been no evidence for systemic disease. Blood vessel involvement is common in primary and secondary amyloidosis. If present in the local form, further investigation for more widespread disease is indicated.

HEREDITARY AMYLOIDOSIS

Hereditary amyloid syndromes have been described in a number of geographic locations; each family and type described is associated with characteristic organ involvement and clinical manifestations. Generally, the mode of transmission is an autosomal dominant, with the exception of familial Mediterranean fever (a condition seen frequently in the Near East and affecting Sephardic Jews, Armenians, Turks, and Arabs), in which autosomal recessive transmission has been described. The hereditary amyloids represent a new and unfolding chapter in our knowledge of amyloid disease. A gross classification by organ involvement is perhaps the most useful at present. Multiple kinships with hereditary amyloid of the peripheral nervous system are especially prevalent. Such hereditary syndromes have been appearing in the literature at a rate of perhaps one new syndrome or kinship per year and clinically are puzzles that perhaps should alert us in the future pathogenetic mechanisms.

AMYLOIDOSIS AND AGING

For reasons not completely understood, amyloidosis occurs more frequently with increasing age. In one study, virtually all consecutive autopsies of individuals of over 65 years of age demonstrated small deposits of amyloid. Although usually clinically inapparent, small deposits can often be found in the heart, brain, pancreas, and spleen of elderly patients. Occasionally by virtue of its specific location, e.g., the conducting system of the heart, severe symptomatology may result. Although the pathogenesis of amyloid in the process of aging is not clear, the staining properties and ultrastructure of the amyloid found in the elderly is identical to that found in other types.

PATHOBIOLOGY

HISTOPATHOLOGY AND STRUCTURE

Amyloid is an amorphous, eosinophilic, glassy, hyalin extracellular substance ubiquitous in distribution. The involved organs may have a rubbery firm consistency and a waxy, pink, or gray appearance. Organ enlargement (especially liver, kidney, spleen, and heart) may be prominent when the deposits are large. In patients with longstanding renal involvement, however, the kidneys may become small and pale. The heart, in addition to being enlarged due to interstitial myocardial involvement, may have nodular elevations on its pericardial and endocardial surfaces as well as lesions on the valves. Nerves are often normal even when involved, but at times are described as thickened and nodular.

Microscopically, amyloid is pink with the hematoxylin and eosin stain and shows crystal violet or methyl violet ''metachromasia.'' The Congo red stain imparts a unique green birefringence when sections are viewed in the polarizing microscope. This is the single most useful procedure for establishing the presence of amyloid. Under the light microscope, amyloid is almost invariably extracellular in the connective tissue. The deposits may be focal in almost any area of the body but most often perivascular amyloid is present. The heart may show focal or diffuse interstitial deposits in the myocardium, endocardium, or pericardium. In the kidney, the glomerulus is primarily affected, although interstitial, peritubular, and vascular amyloid may be prominent. In early lesions, small nodular or diffuse deposits near the basement membrane appear and, as the disease progresses, the glomerulus may be massively laden with apparent occlusion of the capillary bed.

In the gastrointestinal tract, there may be perivascular deposits only, or irregular or diffuse deposits may be found in the submucosa, in the muscularis mucosa, or the subserosa. The amyloid may appear at any level or portion of the gastrointestinal tract, including the gallbladder and pancreas. Hepatic deposits again may be perivascular only, or, more commonly, diffuse amyloid may be found between the Kuppfer and parenchymal cells. In the nervous system, amyloid has been described along peripheral nerves and in autonomic ganglia, senile plaques, and vessels of the central nervous system. It may be found in any portion of the orbit including the vitreous humor and cornea.

The bronchopulmonary tract may be involved focally or extensively. The unique aspect of pulmonary or pleural involvement is that while amyloid in virtually all areas of the body remains without any evidence of resorption or foreign body reaction, pulmonary amyloid deposits may be accompanied by large numbers of macrophages about and within the lesions. These deposits may also contain islets of cartilage and of ossification. Thus, there is virtually no area of the body that is spared. This ubiquitous distribution elicits a wide variety of clinical symptoms and signs.

All types of human amyloid—primary, secondary, heredofamilial—no matter how classified, consist of fine, nonbranching rigid fibrils that in tissue sections measure approximately 100 Å in diameter. Intracellular fibrils of dimensions comparable to those outside the cell are occasionally observed. Their precise nature has not yet been established. The amyloid fibrils are usually seen in earliest and closest relationship to the mesangial cell in the kidney and Kuppfer cell in the liver.

The amyloid fibrils, when isolated, have a delicate, thin, nonbranching fibrous character. The individual fibril (or filament) has a diameter of about 70 Å and tends to aggregate laterally. Each fibril (filament) has subunit protofibrils 30–35 Å in diameter. The x-ray diffraction picture of the isolated amyloid fibrils is that of a cross beta pattern, the pleated sheet of Pauling and Corey indicating that the polypeptide chain runs transversely to the fiber axis of the specimen.

A second component, the P-component (plasma component or pentagonal unit), with a different ultrastructure, x-ray diffraction pattern, and chemical characteristics, has also been isolated from amyloid and shown to be identical with a circulating alpha globulin present in only very minute amounts. It is not responsible for the characteristic tinctorial properties or ultrastructure of amyloid.

BIOCHEMISTRY OF AMYLOID
FIBRILS

The bulk of amyloid deposits consist of fibrils. The homology of the amyloid fibril of primary and myeloma amyloid to the NH_2-terminal region of the variable fragment of an immunoglobulin light chain and, subsequently, in a limited number of cases, to a homogeneous light polypeptide chain has been demonstrated. These light chain–related proteins range in size from about 5000

Table 1
Helsinki Nomenclature of Amyloid Tissue Isolates

Current Usage	New Nomenclature
Amyloid fibril protein related to immunoglobulin light chains	AL (or A_κ or A_λ) subtype when known, i.e., $A_\kappa I$
Amyloid of unknown origin; nonimmunoglobulin amyloid; amyloid AA protein	AA
Pentagonal unit of amyloid; plasma component of amyloid; P component	AP

Serum isolates: To designate the serum-related component, simply add S as a prefix, i.e., the serum-related AA would now be SAA (instead of amyloid serum component, ASC, etc.). It is recognized that the serum-related component of AL may simply be designated as κ or λ light chains or Bence Jones proteins.

to 25,000 daltons and are now termed *amyloid light chain* (AL) or A_κ or A_λ (Table 1).

It was further demonstrated that amyloidlike fibrils could be formed from Bence Jones proteins isolated from the urines of nonamyloidotic patients. Thus, amino acid sequence analysis indicates that most primary amyloid proteins contain the N-terminal amino acid residue identical to the variable regions of the light chain (Asp–Ile–Gln–Ser–Pro–Ser–Ser–Leu– . . .).

Another protein that is unrelated to any known immunoglobulin has been described in the secondary amyloid deposits. This new protein, amyloid A (AA), can be isolated from patients with secondary amyloidosis, the amyloidosis associated with familial Mediterranean fever, and the amyloid isolated from experimental animals following casein injections. It is a unique protein with a molecular weight of about 8500 daltons made up of 76 amino acid residues arranged in a single chain; the amino acid sequence begins Arg–Ser–Phe. . . . Heterogeneity among the different species has been described, with several additional residues preceding the first residue, suggesting that this may represent the result of proteolysis of a larger precursor.

Antisera to alkali-degraded amyloid fibrils of the protein AA type have detected an antigenically related serum component, SAA. Molecular weights of 80,000–100,000 daltons have been reported, although some techniques have suggested a molecular weight of 180,000. Smaller subunits of 12,000–12,500 or 14,000–15,000 daltons have been isolated. Amino acid analysis, peptide maps, and sequence studies suggest that protein AA is an amino-terminal fragment of SAA and is derived from it by proteolysis. It has been shown that SAA appears to behave as an acute-phase reactant; it is elevated in infection, in inflammation, and with aging. SAA is elevated in amyloid-resistant animals, suggesting that amyloid resistance is related to the processing and catabolism of SAA.

It has been suggested that an SAA-like material is produced by fibroblasts and is a normal constituent of developing extracellular connective tissue. The potential function of SAA has been studied and it appears to suppress antibody response, suggesting that it might act as a regulator of such responses.

P COMPONENT OF AMYLOID

In addition to the characteristic fibrils described above, a minor second component, the P component, has been noted in most amyloid deposits. P component has been recognized by electron microscopy as a pentagonal structured unit with about a 90-Å outside diameter and a 40-Å inside diameter. It consists of five globular subunits of 25–30 Å that may aggregate laterally to form short rods. On immunoelectrophoresis it migrates as an alpha globulin, and it possesses antigenic identity with a constituent of normal human plasma. The amino acid sequence has been described and is distinct from that of the amyloid fibrils. It contains large amounts of aspartic acid, glutamic acid, glycine, and leucine and has an N-terminal histidine. The molecular weight (probably that of a doublet) is about 220,000 daltons and it has subunits of 20,000–25,000. Its pentagonal ultrastructure is similar to C-reactive protein but the latter is one-half the molecular weight of P component and has other well-defined differences despite a similar amino acid sequence.

IMMUNOBIOLOGY OF AMYLOID

The etiology and pathogenesis of amyloidosis is unknown. The advances regarding the characterization of its chemical structure may provide insight into potential mechanisms. Ultrastructural studies of amyloid-laden tissues in the animal model have led to the concept that cytoplasmic invaginations, containing tufts of amyloid fibers at a cell–amyloid interface, are the sites of amyloid formation. Electron microscopic autoradiographic studies have revealed high concentrations of fibrils adjacent to reticuloendothelial cells, suggesting that they may synthesize as well as degrade the fibrils. It has been reported that there are unusual inclusions within the reticuloendothelial cells intimately associated with fresh amyloid deposits. These inclusions are located in the areas rich in the primary lysosome type of dense bodies, and the cytoplasmic invaginations contain well-oriented fibrils. The inclusions may be transitional forms from the usual dense bodies and are believed to afford direct evidence for the involvement of lysosomes in amyloid fibril formation.

Excess antigenic stimulus has been shown to induce amyloid in animals. However, the basic conditions for the experimental induction have not been clearly defined. Marked depression of T cells with maintenance of normal or hyperactive B cell function has been described. These findings suggest that distrubances in immunoregulatory mechanisms may be an important step in the pathogenesis of amyloid disease.

Abundant additional studies have been carried out on aspects of cellular and humoral immunity in amyloidosis by a host of investigators. Most recently, the newly defined M cell has been implicated because its function is abolished in the spleens of amyloidotic CBA/J mice but elevated in the spleens of amyloid-resistant A/J mice. In brief, there are alterations in cellular immune function in humans and in the mouse casein model of amyloid. The latter species has been shown to demonstrate T cell impairment, B cell proliferation, and M cell dysfunction. Immune surveillance is probably a factor, although T cell dysfunction may not be.

CLINICAL ASPECTS

DIAGNOSIS

Although the specific diagnosis of amyloidosis depends upon the appropriate staining of a tissue specimen, one must first clinically suspect the presence of the disease. When a patient who has a disorder predisposing to amyloid (e.g., rheumatoid arthritis, tuberculosis, paraplegia, multiple myeloma, bronchiectasis, leprosy) develops hepatomegaly, splenomegaly, malabsorption, cardiac disease, or, most important, proteinuria, amyloid should be suspected. In addition, in any heredofamilial syndromes, especially those that have a dominant autosomal mode of trasmission and are characterized by peripheral neuropathy (particularly that starting in the lower limb), nephropathy, or cardiopathy, amyloid should be considered in the differential diagnosis. Finally, primary systemic amyloid should be suspected in any individual with a diffuse noninflammatory infiltrative disease involving either mesenchymal tissues (blood vessels, heart, gastrointestinal tract) or parenchymal tissues (kidney, liver, spleen, adrenal).

It is good practice to perform a rectal biopsy when the diagnosis of amyloidosis is suspected. If there is a specific reason for not carrying out this procedure, or if the patient refuses, gingival biopsy is recommended. Recent data indicate that skin biopsy is also useful in both involved and uninvolved skin in all types of amyloid. In patients who show negative results for both these procedures but have renal disease, hepatic disease, or other involvement, biopsy of the appropriate site is undertaken with the standard precautions against bleeding. All tissues obtained must be stained with Congo red and be examined in the polarizing microscope for green birefringence.

GENERAL CLINICAL MANIFESTATIONS

The clinical manifestations of amyloidosis are varied and depend entirely on the area of the body that is involved.

The Renal Involvement

The renal involvement may consist of mild proteinuria or frank nephrosis, or in some cases the urinary sediment may show only a few red blood cells. The renal lesion is usually not reversible and in time leads to progressive azotemia and death. The prognosis does not appear to be related to the degree of proteinuria; when azotemia finally develops, if it is due to the amyloid process and not a reversible superimposed condition, the prognosis is grave. In one group of patients with secondary amyloidosis, however, it was found that patients with small residual renal function could live in a comfortable state for long periods, but once the creatinine was over 3 mgm/dl or the creatinine clearance was under 20 mg/ml the prognosis was poor. In another series, the mean survival of patients with renal amyloid from the time of biopsy was 29 months, but in 5 cases the authors believed evidence of regression of the renal amyloid existed. Hypertension is rare except in longstanding amyloidosis. Serial x-rays of the kidneys may or may not show diminution in size. A picture of renal tubular acidosis or of renal vein thrombosis may be seen. Localized accumulation of amyloid may be noted in the ureter, bladder, or other genitourinary tract tissue.

Hepatic Involvement

While hepatic involvement is common, liver function abnormalities are minimal and occur late in the disease. Hepatomegaly, however, is common. The two tests most useful in indicating hepatic amyloid are the bromsulphthalein extraction and the level of the serum alkaline phosphatase activity. Liver scans produce variable and nonspecific results. Signs of portal hypertension occur but are uncommon. In the author's series, in which liver tissue was available for examination from 54 patients, all 54 (whether the disorder was primary or secondary) had some amyloid present either in the parenchyma or blood vessels. Splenic involvement results in splenomegaly, which may be massive. It usually does not cause symptoms unless traumatic rupture occurs. Amyloidosis of the spleen is not characteristically associated with leukopenia and anemia.

Cardiac Involvement

Cardiac manifestations consist primarily of congestive failure and cardiomegaly (either with or without murmurs) and a variety of arrhythmias. Although the cardiac manifestations reflect predominently diffuse myocardial amyloid, the endocardium, the valves, and the pericardium may be involved. Pericarditis with effusion is very rare, although the differential diagnosis of constrictive pericarditis versus restrictive myocardopathy frequently arises. The clinical features and the demonstration of left ventricular diastolic pressure greater than the right are said to be most useful in distinguishing restrictive myocardopathy from constrictive pericarditis. The techniques of left heart catheterization and quantitative left ventriculography however, have not always been able to distinguish the two. Echocardiography has demonstrated symmetric thickening of the left ventricular wall, hypokinesia and decreased systolic thickening of the interventricular septum and left ventricular posterior wall, and small to normal size of the left ventricular cavities. Hearts that are heavily infiltrated with amyloid may or may not exhibit an enlarged silhouette. Fluoroscopy usually shows decreased mobility of the ventricular wall; angiographic studies usually show a thickened ventricular wall, decreased ventricular mobility, and absence of rapid ventricular filling in early diastole. Cardiac amyloid can present as intractable heart failure.

Electrocardiographic abnormalities include a low voltage in the QRS complex and abnormalities in atrioventricular and intraventricular conduction, often resulting in varying degrees of heart block. The electrocardiographic abnormalities are frequent and often are present in the absence of a previous infarct. Due to the propensity of patients with cardiac amyloidosis to develop conduction defects and arrhythmias, they appear to be especially sensitive to digitalis, and this drug should be used in small doses with caution.

Skin Lesions

Involvement of the skin is one of the most characteristic manifestations of the so-called "primary" amyloidoses. The lesions may consist of slightly raised, waxy, often translucent papules or plaques, usually clustered in the folds of the axillae, anal, or inguinal regions, the face and neck, or mucosal areas such as the ear or tongue. In addition, there may be purpuric areas, nodules or tumefactions, alopecia, a yellowish waxy discoloration, glossitis, and xerostomia. The lesions are seldom pruritic. Involvement of the skin or mucosa may be inapparent, even on close inspection, yet may be disclosed at biopsy. Gentle rubbing of the skin with one's finger may induce bleeding into the skin, leading to purpura. Skin involvement can occur in secondary amyloidosis, and in the author's study was shown to occur in 42 percent of patients (and in 55 percent of a group of patients with primary disease), while all 8 patients with hereditary amyloid neuropathy who were studied had positive skin biopsies for amyloid.

Gastrointestinal Symptoms

Gastrointestinal symptoms in amyloidosis are common. They may result from direct involvement of the gastrointestinal tract at any level or from infiltration of the autonomic nervous system with amyloid. The symptoms include those of obstruction, ulceration, malabsorption, hemorrhage, protein loss, and diarrhea. Infiltration of the tongue occasionally leads to macroglossia, which may become severely incapacitating; alternatively, the tongue, while not enlarged, may become stiffened and firm to palpation. While infiltration of the tongue is especially characteristic of primary amyloidosis or amyloidosis accompanying multiple myeloma, it is occasionally seen in the secondary form of the disease.

Gastrointestinal bleeding may occur from any of a number of sites, notably the esophagus, stomach, or large intestine, and may be extremely severe and even fatal. Amyloid infiltration of the esophagus may lead to motility abnormalities and small bowel lesions may lead to clinical and x-ray changes of obstruction. A malabsorption syndrome is sometimes seen. Amyloidosis may develop in association with other entities involving the gastrointestinal tract, especially tuberculosis, granulomatous enteritis, lymphoma, and Whipple's disease. Differentiation of these conditions from diffuse amyloidosis of the small bowel may be difficult. Similarly, amyloidosis of the stomach may closely mimic gastric carcinoma, with obstruction, achlorhydria, and the radiologic appearance of tumor masses. The patient may exhibit cycles of constipation and diarrhea.

Neurologic Manifestations

Neurologic manifestations are not uncommon. They may include peripheral neuropathy, postural hypotension, inability to sweat, the Adie pupil, hoarseness, and sphincter involvement. These manifestations are especially prominent in the heredofamilial amyloidoses. Cranial nerves are generally spared except for those involving the pupillary reflexes. The protein concentration of the cerebro spinal fluid may be increased. Infiltrates of the cornea or vitreous body may be present in hereditary amyloid syndromes. Certain of these syndromes are characterized by a bilateral scalloping appearance of the pupil. Amyloid may infiltrate the thyroid or other endocrine glands but rarely causes endocrine dysfunction. Local amyloid deposits almost invariably accompany medullary carcinoma of the thyroid. Amyloid infiltration of the muscle may lead to a pseudomyopathy.

Musculoskeletal Manifestations

Amyloid can directly involve articular structures; it may be present in the synovial membrane and synovial fluid or in the articular cartilage. Amyloid arthritis can mimic a number of rheumatic diseases due to the fact that it can present as a symmetric small joint arthritis associated with nodules, morning stiffness, and fatigue. It is clear that the diagnosis of rheumatoid arthritis could be made in error. The condition, although very rare, is important to differentiate from rheumatoid arthritis because it involves a markedly different prognosis. If amorphous material is seen in a diagnostic arthrocentesis, a Congo red stain should be performed and the material should be viewed in the polarized microscope. Amyloid should be suspected in patients with multiple myeloma who have articular manifestations, for most patients with amyloid arthropathy do eventually seem to have multiple myeloma. The synovial fluid usually has a low white cell count and good to fair mucin; most cells are mononuclear and crystals are absent.

The joints most frequently involved have been shoulders, wrists, knees, and fingers. A rather short period of morning stiffness has been associated with the early lesions, The joints are often swollen, firm, and occasionally tender, but redness and severe tenderness are not noted, Shoulders may be prominently involved, giving the appearance of a padded shoulder. Subcutaneous nodules are very common and are present in almost 70 percent of the patients; rheumatoid factor is infrequently present. X-rays show soft tissue swelling. Erosions about the joints have been noted only once among the 20 patients the author studied. Generalized osteoporosis with or without osteolytic lesions, however, is very common and was seen in 80 percent of the patients.

Respiratory Symptoms

The nasal sinuses, larynx, and trachea may be involved by accumulations of amyloid that block the ducts (in the case of the sinuses) or the air passages. Amyloidosis of the lung may include diffuse involvement of the bronchi or alveolar septa. The lower respiratory tract is frequently involved in primary and dysproteinemia-associated amyloidosis. Pulmonary symptoms attributable to the amyloid are present in about 30 percent of the patients and in some are the the most serious disease manifestations. In secondary amyloidosis, pulmonary disease is a frequent histopathologic complication, but very seldom gives rise to clinically significant symptoms. Amyloid may also be localized in the bronchi or alveolar tissue so as to resemble a neoplasm. In these cases, local excision of involved areas should be attempted, when possible, and may be followed by prolonged remissions.

Hematologic Changes

Hematologic changes may include fibrinogenopenia, increased fibrinolysis and selective deficiency of clotting factors.

PROGNOSIS

The course of amyloidosis is difficult to document since it is rarely possible to date the time of origin of the disease, When amyloidosis develops in patients with rheumatoid arthritis, it seldom becomes evident when the arthritis is less than 2 years in duration. In one series, the mean duration of arthritis before amyloidosis was detected was 16 years.

When amyloidosis develops in patients with multiple myeloma, manifestations leading to initial hospitalization are more apt to be related to the amyloid than to the myeloma, In these cases prognosis is very poor and life expectancy is usually less than 6 months,

Instances have been reported of amyloidosis accompanying treatable sepsis, such as osteomyelitis, in which at least partial remission has occurred following treatment of the primary disease. Once established, generalized amyloidosis, while usually progressive and leading to death in several years, may have a better prognosis than once was suspected. The chief cause of death is renal failure. The second most common cause has been sudden death, presumably due to arrhythmias. Occasionally, gastrointestinal hemorrhage, sepsis, respiratory failure, intractable heart failure, etc., may cause death.

TREATMENT

There is no specific therapy for any variety of amyloidosis. Rational therapy should be directed at (1) decreasing chronic antigenic stimuli producing amyloid, (2) inhibiting the synthesis of amyloid fibril, (3) inhibiting its extracellular deposition, and (4) promoting lysis or mobilization of existing deposits.

Eradication of the predisposing disease apparently slows the progression of secondary amyloidosis. However, many such reports are not substantiated by biopsy proof of resorption. Conclusions have been drawn on clinical guidelines or on the basis of the Congo red test, although a few patients have shown biopsy-proven improvement. Despite these occasional reports, amyloidosis is often a progressive disease; however, while the average survival in most large series is 1–4 years, a number of individuals with amyloid have been followed for 5–10 years and more.

A variety of agents have been used to treat amyloidosis. Among the most prominent have been whole liver extract, corticosteroids, and ascorbic acid. Proof of their efficacy is not available. The finding that a portion of the immunoglobulin light chain is incorporated in the amyloid of patients with primary amyloidosis and its presumed synthesis from plasma cells have led to the use of alkylating agents. These agents, however, cause bone marrow depression, and there are reports of acute leukemia developing in patients receiving melphalan. Moreover, there is experimental evidence that immunosuppressive agents may enhance the deposition of amyloid. Hence, the conservative and supportive measures provide the mainstay of management. Rigid adherence to supportive and symotomatic therapy with these patients has led to a more optimistic outlook regarding the quality of life attained.

Two patients with severe renal amyloidosis and azotemia were subjected to bilateral nephrectomy and renal transplantation followed by immune therapy. One patient died of infection 5 months after surgery. The donor kidney showed no evidence of amyloidosis. The second patient is in clinical remission 7 years after receiving a transplanted kidney. Notwithstanding the hazards of operating upon patients with systemic amyloidosis who may have cardiac involvement, a group of patients carefully selected could potentially benefit from transplantation surgery.

Colchicine has been shown to be effective in preventing acute attacks in patients with familial Mediterranean fever. Recently, two groups of investigators have independently reported the inhibition of amyloid deposition in the mouse model by colchicine. It is therefore conceivable that colchicine is effective in blocking amyloid deposition. However, the exact mechanism of its action is not known, and no controlled human clinical study has been reported.

HEREDOFAMILIAL AMYLOIDOSIS

There is no generally accepted nosology for the increasing reports of heredofamilial amyloid syndromes. Some reports emphasize the site of predominant organ involvement (neuropathic versus nephropathic versus cardopathic amyloid), while others stress the genetic aspects. To date, virtually all analyses of pedigrees have shown that, with one major exception, the mode of inheritance is autosomal dominant. The exception, amyloidosis of familial Mediterranean fever, is inherited as an autosomal recessive disorder. Since there are no specific biochemical, hematologic, or immunologic tests that allow the differentiation of one type of amyloid from another, one must rely upon the specific and recognizable

Table 1
Heredofamilial Amyloidoses

Neuropathy
  Lower limb (Portuguese, Japanese, Swedish, other)
  Upper limb (Swiss–Indiana, German–Maryland)

Nephropathy
  Familial Mediterranean fever
  Fever and abdominal pain (Swedish; Sicilian)
  Urticaria, deafness, and renal disease
  Renal disease and hypertension

Cardiopathy
  Progressive heart failure (Danish)
  Persistent atrial standstill (Mexican–American)

Miscellaneous
  Medullary carcinoma of the thyroid
  Lattice corneal dystrophy and cranial neuropathy (Finland)
  Cerebral hemorrhage (Iceland)

clinical patterns for classification. The classification utilized here is tentative and based largely on the major site of organ involvement, in addition to genetic data and ethnic background where available (Table 1).

The heredofamilial amyloidoses include a group primarily involving the nervous system. Among these a lower limb neuropathy, first described in Portugal, has a poor prognosis and is characterized by progressively severe neuropathy, including marked autonomic nervous system involvement. This variety has been described in Japan and in a family of Greek origin in the United States and probably several others. In some of these kinships, bilateral "scalloped" pupils seems to be virtually pathognomonic of the disease. The second type of neuropathy has been found in families of Swiss origin in Indiana and of German origin in Maryland. It is a milder disease, and is often associated with a carpal tunnel syndrome and vitreous opacities. A more severe variety of generalized neuropathy and renal amyloid has been described in Iowa in a family of English–Irish–Scottish ancestry.

Several types of severe familial renal disease in association with amyloid have been described. Possibly the most remarkable is a familial Mediterranean fever. This disorder subdivided into two phenotypes: phenotype I,

with irregularly occurring fever and abdominal, chest, or joint pain, preceding or accompanying renal amyloid; and phenotype II, in which amyloidosis is the first or only manifestation of the disease. This disease is most commonly seen in Sephardic Jews, Armenians, Turks, and Arabs. Sporadically, other hereditary renal amyloids have been described, including the curious association of urticaria, deafness, and renal amyloid.

Severe familial amyloid heart disease has been described in a Danish family, and familial persistent atrial standstill in a family of Mexican-American origin. Miscellaneous hereditary amyloid syndromes include those of hereditary multiple endocrine neoplasias type 2 (including medullary carcinoma of the thyroid with amyloid), and familial lattice corneal dystrophy associated with cranial neuropathy and renal disease in Finland. Finally, a syndrome of hereditary cerebral hemorrhage due to amyloid has been reported from Iceland.

REFERENCES

Brandt K, Cathcart ES, Cohen AS: A prospective study of amyloidosis: Clinical analysis of the course and prognosis of 42 patients. Am J Med 44:955, 1968
Cohen AS: Amyloidosis. N Engl J Med 277:522, 1967
Cohen AS: Inherited systemic amyloidosis, in Stanbury JB, Wyngaarden JB, Frederickson DS (eds): Metabolic Basis of Inherited Disease (ed. 3). New York, McGraw-Hill, 1972
Cohen AS: Diagnosis of amyloidosis, in Cohen AS (ed): Laboratory Diagnostic Procedures in the Rheumatic Diseases. Boston, Little, Brown, 1975, p 395
Cohen AS: Studies of amyloidosis. Arthritis Rheum 20:576, 1977
Cohen AS, Canoso JJ: Rheumatologic aspects of amyloid disease. Clin Rheum Dis 1:149, 1965
Cohen AS, Cathcart ES, Skinner M: Amyloidosis. Current trends in its investigation. Arithritis Rheum 21:153, 1978
Dahlin DC: Classification and general aspects of amyloidosis. Med Clin North Am 34: 1107, 1950
Franklin EC: Amyloidosis. Bulletin on the Rheumatic Diseases 26:832, 1975–1976
Glenner GG, Terry W, Harada M, Isersky C, Page D: Amyloid fibril proteins: Proof of homology with immunoglobulin light chains. Science 172:1150, 1971
Kyle RA, Bayrd ED: Amyloidosis: Review of 236 cases. Medicine (Baltimore) 54:271, 1975
Skinner M, Cohen AS, Shirahama T, Cathcart ES: P-component (pentagonal unit) of amyloid: Isolation, characterization and sequence analysis. J Lab Clin Med 84:604, 1974

Sarcoidosis

John D. Stobo

ETIOLOGY AND PATHOLOGY

Any attempt to define sarcoidosis simply ignores the lack of a demonstrable etiology and the variability of clinical symptoms and course. Perhaps the most complete definition is represented by the description presented by the

Subcommittee on Classification and Definition at the 7th International Congress of Sarcoidosis and Other Granulomatous Disease, which may be paraphrased as follows: Sarcoidosis is a multisystem granulomatous disorder of unknown etiology which most commonly affects young adults. Its presenting manifestations most frequently involve biltaral hilar adenopathy, pulmonary infiltration, and skin or eye lesions. The diagnosis is usually established when clinical and radiographic findings are supported by histologic evidence of widespread noncaseating granuloma. Immunologic features include depressed delayed-type hypersensitivity and raised immunoglobulins. The course and prognosis may correlate with the mode of onset: an acute onset with erythema nodosum heralds a self-limiting course and spontaneous resolution. An insidious onset may be followed by relentless, progressive fibrosis. Corticosteriods relieve symptoms and suppress inflammation and granuloma formation.

ETIOLOGY

The etiology of sarcoid is unknown. Several features, such as the systemic nature of the clinical symptoms, the disseminated granuloma formation, the morphologic similarity of sarcoid granulomas to those formed in response to known infectious agents, the familial and geographic clustering of sarcoid, and the consistent involvement of the pulmonary tree, all suggest an infectious, transmissible etiology; however, direct proof of this is lacking. The frequency with which typical and atypical mycobacteria can be recovered from sarcoid lesions is no higher than the frequency with which these organisms are detected in patients with other, nongranulomatous diseases. No virus has been consistently isolated from sarcoid granulomas. Elevations of antibody titers to viruses such as Epstein-Barr, herpes simplex, rubella, measles, and parainfluenza do not correlate with the stage or activity of disease. Most likely, these increased levels are simply a manifestation of the generalized increases in immunoglobulin and preexisting antibodies known to occur in sarcoidosis.

Experiments performed in animal models, however, indirectly suggest the existence of a transmissible agent in sarcoidosis. Injections of homogenates from sarcoid lymph nodes and spleen into the footpads of mice result, 6–24 months later, in disseminated (footpads, lung, lymph nodes) noncaseating granuloma formation in 60 percent of animals. In contrast, only 1 percent of mice receiving homogenates from normal lymph nodes or spleens showed similar granuloma formation. Successful passage of the granuloma from the infected to normal mice can also be demonstrated. Autoclaved or irradiated sarcoid homogenates do not induce granuloma formation, whereas homogenates passed through fine filters do. In short, a heat- and irradiation-sensitive, small-sized material present in the lymphoid organs from patients with sarcoidosis is capable of inducing noncaseating granulomas in at least one strain of mice. While these experiments require confirmation by others, they do suggest a role for an as yet undefined, transmissible agent in sarcoidosis.

In an attempt to define the etiology of sarcoid further, there has been much interest in immune function of patients with this disorder. In general, there is a dichotomy of immune reactivity. There is augmented humoral or B cell reactivity, manifested by polyclonal elevations of all immunoglobulin classes and the presence of auto-antibodies such as rheumatoid factor, antinuclear antibodies, anticytoplasmic thyroid antibodies, and other preexisting antibodies. The hypergammaglobulinemia persists through both the active and chronic phases of the diseases.

In contrast, cell-mediated or T cell function is depressed. This is most profound during active, progressive disease and is characterized in approximately 75 percent of patients by (1) cutaneous anergy, i.e., low or absent delayed hypersensitivity skin test reactions to any of a panel of antigens such as mumps, trichophyton, streptodornase–streptokinase, *Candida,* and purified protein derivative (PPD), and (2) defective in vitro proliferation of T cells to mitogens and specific antigens. During the chronic stages of sarcoid, true anergy is present in a much smaller proportion (less than 20 percent) of patients.

Two points concerning delayed hypersensitivity skin testing in patients with sarcoidosis should be emphasized. First, a small proportion, approximately 25 percent of patients with active disease, are still capable of demonstrating positive delayed hypersensitivity skin test reactivity. Absence of true anergy does not rule out the diagnosis of sarcoid. Second, although the data are conflicting, it appears that even anergic patients can manifest a positive skin test to PPD if infection with *Mycobacterium tuberculosis* develops. In other words, the development of a positive PPD in sarcoid should not necessarily be taken as evidence of recovery from the basic disease. Instead, it may indicate sensitization to *M. tuberculosis.*

Initially, it was thought that the defective T cell reactivity preceded the onset of sarcoid and thus rendered an individual susceptible to infection with the "sarcoid agent." However, in a large series of sarcoidosis patients previously immunized with bacillus Calmette-Guerin (BCG), it was shown that the inability to respond to PPD occurred only at the onset or shortly after the development of clinically apparent sarcoid. (It is of interest that this study also demonstrated that while BCG vaccination was effective in preventing tuberculosis, it did not alter the subsequent attack rate for sarcoidosis.) It appears then that T cell hyporeactivity does not cause but rather results from the development of sarcoidosis. It is equally clear that the deficiency of T cell function noted in sarcoidosis is a relatively incomplete one and is not as severe as that noted in other disorders such as Hodgkin's disease. In general, viral, fungal (with the exception of *Aspergillus*), and mycobacterial infections are not increased in sarcoidosis. Whereas patients with Hodgkin's disease manifest a prolonged rejection of allogeneic skin grafts, patients with sarcoidosis reject skin grafts normally. Thus, while a negative skin test to PPD has been indicated as the hallmark of sarcoid, true anergy occurs only during active disease. Moreover, deficient reactivity to delayed hypersensitivity skin tests is not accompanied by other stigmata usually associated with defects in cell-mediated immunity.

The mechanisms responsible for the immunologic abnormalities in sarcoidosis are not completely understood but must be considered within the framework of the complex interactions required for full immunologic reactivity. It is known that normal cell-mediated and humoral immune reactivity reflects a complex series of feedback signals occurring between different cell types. For example, while B lymphocytes serve as the precursors for antibody-secreting plasma cells, the amount and type of antibody produced is regulated by T lymphocytes and macrophages. Similarly, the reactivity of effector T cells is modulated by other T cells, macrophages, and B cells. Within this framework, it has been hypothesized that the immune dysfunction in sarcoidosis reflects a breakdown in interactions that normally serve to regulate immune reactivity. Two findings support this hypothesis. First, abnormal in vivo and in vitro T and B cell functions can be demonstrated in the presence of a normal frequency of T and B cells. Second, soluble materials capable of inhibiting T cell reactivity and augmenting immunoglobulin production can be demonstrated to be present in serum or to be released from the lymphocytes of some patients with sarcoidosis. However, this has not been a consistent finding in all patients.

The culmination of delayed hypersensitivity reactions involves the recruitment of lymphocytes and monocytes into the skin test area by "lymphokines" released from antigen-activated T cells. That anergy in some patients with sarcoidosis may reflect a resistance of these potentially recruitable cells to T cell products is supported by the following findings: Systemic or local administration of corticosteroids normally blunts delayed hypersensitivity skin tests; however, similar steroid administration to some anergic sarcoidosis patients paradoxically results in augmented delayed hypersensitivity. Moreover, steroids augment the skin reactivity of patients with sarcoidosis to soluble materials (lymphokines?) liberated during activation of normal cells. The simplest interpretation of these observations is that in sarcoidosis steroids render previously resistant cells susceptible to the action of recruiting factors liberated from T cells.

In summary, the defects resulting in the abnormal T and B cell reactivity noted in sarcoidosis are most likely hetergeneous and vary from patient to patient. Similar defects—i.e., hypergammaglobulinemia and depressed cell-mediated immunity—occur in patients with a variety of other disorders. Again, this observation emphasizes the fact that the abnormal immune reactivity does not cause the disorder but rather is a nonspecific response that can be caused by a variety of stimuli.

The clinical symptoms associated with one form of sarcoidosis are mediated by immune mechanisms. In approximately 90 percent of patients who present with erythema nodosum, bilateral hilar adenopathy, and mi-gratory polyarthralgias, circulating immune complexes can be detected. Moreover, while CH_{50} (Total Hemolytic Complement) and individual complement components are normal or elevated, subtle evidence of complement activation can be detected (elevations in activated products of C_3). The nature of the antigen in the circulating immune complex is unknown. Renal disease is not present and circulating immune complexes are not detectable in other forms of active or chronic sarcoid.

Attempts have been made to determine whether the development of sarcoidosis requires a genetic predisposition. As indicated, familial clusters of sarcoid have been identified. While the incidence of sarcoid among female family members is much higher than that in the general population, and sarcoid is more common in siblings if the mother rather than the father is affected, the expression of the disease is under multigenetic control. Moreover, no significant association between sarcoidosis and either serologically defined or lymphocyte-defined transplantation antigens has been demonstrated. The one exception is a higher frequency of HLA-B8 in patients with erythema nodosum and polyarthralgias.

PATHOLOGY

The histologic finding characteristic of but not diagnostic for sarcoidosis is noncaseating granuloma. The center of the granuloma contains an amorphorous eosinophilic material that is to be distinguished from true caseation present in other granuloma such as those associated with tuberculosis. There are four major cell types present in the granuloma: epithelioid cells, giant cells, lymphocytes, and plasma cells. The epithelioid and giant cells derive from phagocytic macrophages, the latter by fusion of several macrophages. The presence of a prominent Golgi apparatus, endoplasmic reticulum, and vesicles in the cytoplasm of the epithelioid cells indicates that they are secretory rather than phagocytic. Macrophages can secrete a variety of biologically active materials capable of degrading connective tissue and influencing the proliferation of other cell types such as fibroblasts. It is perhaps the net effect of these materials that dictates the extent to which fibrous tissue is deposited in the granuloma.

Among the lymphocytes present, both T and B cells have been described. This might suggest that the granuloma is initiated during an immune response to some foreign agent. However, as previously indicated, no definable agent can be consistently found in sarcoid granuloma. Moreover, it is known that granuloma formation does not require intact cell-mediated or humoral immunity. Granulomas can be demonstrated in individuals with congenital or acquired agammaglobulinemia and can be induced in congenitally athymic mice. From studies of factors involved during granuloma formation in experimental schistosomiasis, it appears that lymphocytes, presumably T cells, can modulate and suppress the size of the granulomas formed. It is likely, therefore, that the presence of lymphocytes in the sarcoid granuloma does not reflect an immunologic assault on an invading foreign antigen; rather, it may represent a process whereby the lymphocytes are crucially involved in regulating the metabolic processes of the epithelioid and giant cells. The nature of these events and their role in determining the life history of the granuloma are not completely understood.

Although granulomas can be detected in almost any organ, a series of postmortem studies on patients with sarcoidosis, 50 percent of whom died from unrelated causes, demonstrated the following distribution: lung, 86 percent; lymph nodes, 86 percent, liver, 65 percent; spleen, 63 percent; heart, 20 percent; kidney, 19 percent; pancreas, 6 percent; and bone marrow, 17 percent. Not only does this finding emphasize the disseminated nature of sarcoid, it also indicates that histologic involvement of any organ may be clinically silent. Only one case of involvement of the adrenal glands has been reported. This contrasts with the higher frequency of adrenal involvement noted in at least two other granulomatous diseases—tuberculosis and histoplasmosis.

The sarcoid granulomas are of relatively low activity; they may remain for years without increasing in either size or number. However, they may cause clinically apparent dysfunction in one or two ways. First, they may directly compress and damage normal tissue parenchyma. This is the mechanism responsible for tissue injury occuring during the acute phases of sarcoidosis. Second, during resolution, they can lead to the deposition of fibrous tissue. This process results in the debilitating decrease in diffusion capacity and restrictive changes seen in chronic pulmonary sarcoid. From clinical studies, it is also apparent that in some cases the granulomas simply resolve without any residua. The precise factors that determine and the clinical signs that can be used to predict the fate of the granulomas are not known.

CLINICAL MANIFESTATIONS

Sarcoidosis affects males and females equally, has a higher frequency among blacks than whites, and is usually first manifest between the ages of 20 and 40 years. Patients first present in one of four ways: (1) with symptomatic thoracic involvement manifested by dyspnea, cough, chest pain, or hemoptysis; (2) with extrathoracic involvement of the skin, eyes, or central nervous system (CNS); (3) with constitutional symptoms of fever, malaise, and weight loss; or (4) with asymptomatic hilar adenopathy detected on a routine x-ray. Although it has been claimed that the manner in which sarcoidosis first appears is dependent on the ethnic and geographic origin of the patient, it is probably more a reflection of physician's awareness of the clinical manifestations of sarcoid and the extent to which routine chest films are performed. In a large study performed in Los Angeles, the first manifestations of sarcoid were asymptomatic hilar adenopathy in 20 percent, respiratory symptoms in 49 percent, and symptoms referrable to extrathoracic involvement in 31 percent of patients.

PULMONARY INVOLVEMENT
Radiographic Staging

Irrespective of the initial signs or symptoms, over 90 percent of patients with sarcoidosis have an abnormal chest film. For convenience, the radiographic picture of sarcoid has been divided into four stages: *Stage 0* shows a normal chest film. *Stage I* exhibits mediastinal adenopathy. Usually, this indicates bilaterial hilar node enlargement. In 5 percent of cases, however, hilar adenopathy may be unilateral (involvement on the right is more frequent than on the left), and less than 1 percent of cases present with isolated right paratracheal lymph node enlargement. *Stage II* shows hilar adenopathy and pulmonary parenchymal infiltrates. These infiltrates may appear as discrete fluffy nodules, confluent opacities, or linear interstitial fibrosis. *Stage III* demonstrates pulmonary parenchymal involvement without hilar or mediastinal lymph node involvement. Although some patients may demonstrate a radiographic progression from stage I to stage III, this is not necessarily the case. The presence of hilar adenopathy does not necessarily indicate that pulmonary parenchymal involvement will ensue. However, a reverse pattern of involvement does not occur. Patients who present with pulmonary parenchymal disease do not subsequently develop concomitant hilar adenopathy. If this does occur, a diagnosis other than sarcoidosis, such as malignancy, should be considered.

The most prominent and crippling symptoms associated with sarcoidosis are usually due to involvement of the pulmonary tree. Histologically, granulomas can be detected around bronchioles, around blood vessels (obliterative vasculitis is rare), or in the interstitium, where they may be accompanied by fibrosis and thickening of the intraalveolar septa. Dyspnea is one of the most prominent symptoms associated with pulmonary sarcoid and is present in one-quarter to one-third of patients at some time during their course. In general, this is usually a sign of advanced parenchymal involvement. However, 5–10 percent of patients radiographically classified as having stage I disease may experience dyspnea. Thus, the radiographic appearance of sarcoidosis, especially in stage I, does not necessarily reflect the extent of pulmonary involvement as measured either by pulmonary function tests or as manifested by clinical symptoms. In stages II and III, dyspnea and abnormal pulmonary function tests are more common. Based on these observations, three general points emerge: (1) The radiographic appearance of sarcoidosis is helpful in supporting the diagnosis and in predicting the course of sarcoid; however, it does not necessarily indicate the pathophysiologic extent of pulmonary involvement. (2) Pulmonary function tests may be a more sensitive indicator of pulmonary parenchymal involvement. They are not useful, however, as prognostigators for the development of pulmonary fibrosis. (3) Clinically manifest dyspnea may be a late manifestation of advanced pulmonary parenchymal involvement.

The usefulness of radiographic staging of pulmonary involvement in predicting the clinical course of sarcoid is supported by the following observations: Approximately 75 percent of patients who present with only bilaterial hilar adenopathy demonstrate spontaneous radiographic and clinical remission within 2 years. Indeed, the complex of bilateral hilar adenopathy and erythema nodosum with or without uveitis (Lofgren's syndrome) indicates a very favorable prognosis, with approximately 90 percent of these patients demonstrating spontaneous disappearance of symptoms. If the radiographic appearance of stage I disease has not improved within 2 years, spontaneous remission is unlikely. The remaining 25 percent of patients with stage I disease will demonstrate progression to pulmonary parenchymal involvement and fibrosis.

In contrast, only 30–50 percent of patients who present with stage II disease will demonstrate radiographic resolution (usually within 2 years), whereas 40–60 percent will demonstrate radiographic progression to stage III and 10 percent will manifest an unchanged pattern. Improvement and not resolution occurs in less than 20 percent in patients with stage III. Unfortunately, there are no definitive criteria for indicating which stage II cases will progress and which will improve. The presence of chronic, extrapulmonary manifestations (infiltrative skin lesions, CNS, and bone sarcoidosis), however, indicates chronic and perhaps progressive disease.

Pulmonary Function Tests

Pulmonary function tests are helpful in indicating the actual extent of pulmonary parenchymal involvement but are not useful prognosticators of the eventual course. Abnormal tests may include a decreased steady-state diffusion capacity, a low vital capacity, and a decrease in maximal midexpiratory flow rates (MMEF). The defect in gas exchange usually is the earliest abnormality. While it has been assumed that this defect represents replacement of interstitial granuloma with fibrosis and subsequent thickening of the intraalveolar septa, this may not be the case. The decreased MMEF most likely represents compression of bronchi by endobronchial granuloma and cellular infiltrates. Clinically, this may be manifested by wheezing.

Other pulmonary findings frequently associated with sarcoid include the following: (1) Vague, substernal chest pain is often present. Pleuritic chest pain and pleural effusions are uncommon, and their presence should suggest another diagnosis such as malignancy or tuberculosis. (2) Bronchiectasis may be found, usually resulting from compression of airways. (3) Cough is a common symptom. (4) Hemoptysis is usually seen in association with bronchiectasis. However, there is an increased frequency of *Aspergillus* "fungus balls" in chronic pulmonary sarcoid. This may present as massive hemoptysis and is a significant cause of death. (5) The upper respira-

tory tract may be involved. Granulomas can effect the nasal turbinates and larynx, usually in association with chronic sarcoidosis of the skin about the face (lupus pernio).

EXTRATHORACIC MANIFESTATIONS

Clinically apparent extrathoracic manifestations of sarcoid include involvement of the lymph nodes (31 percent), joints (25 percent), skin (27 percent), eyes (11 percent), parotid glands (6 percent), CNS (2 percent), bones (4 percent), and heart (variable frequency).

Skin Lesions

Cutaneous manifestations of sarcoid may vary from the transient, relative benign maculopapular eruptions and erythema nodosum to chronic, persistent volaceous—disfiguring lesions about the nose, cheeks, and ears. The latter condition has been termed *lupus pernio* and is associated with a high incidence of granulomatous lesions in the mucosa of the upper respiratory tract and larynx.

Eye Involvement

Ocular sarcoid varies in severity. Anterior uveitis is usually transient. In contrast, chronic iridocyclitis, chrorioretinitis, papilledema, cataract formation and glaucoma may occur. Keratoconjunctivitis sicca with lacrimal and parotid gland enlargement, mimicking Sjögren's syndrome, has been described.

Joint Disease

Symptoms referable to the joints occur in approximately one-fourth of patients with sarcoidosis. Basically, there are two patterns of involvement. The first occurs shortly preceding or just after the development of signs or symptoms indicating sarcoid involvement of other organ systems. Most commonly, this arthropathy is manifested by symmetric polyarthralgias or polyarthritis of the ankles, knees, elbows, wrists, and small joints of the hand in association with fever, uveitis, and erythema nodosum. It is unusual in this early form to have monoarticular arthritis. While symptoms may affect one group of joints (the ankles, for example) and subsequently another (e.g., the wrists) the arthritis usually results in some residual signs or symptoms present in the joints initially affected. Thus, this arthropathy is not a true migratory polyarthritis and is helpful in distinguishing this early pattern of sarcoid joint disease from the joint involvement seen in association with rheumatic fever. Physical findings at this stage usually include periarticular swelling, redness, and tenderness without frank evidence of effusion. Tenosynovitis has been reported. The signs and symptoms, while severe, usually remit within days to weeks (4–6 weeks) after the onset, without any residua or deformity. Radiographic examination of the joints usually reveals only soft tissue swelling with no bony abnormalities. Synovial biopsy demonstrates noncaseating granuloma in the majority of cases (Fig. 1), and in over 90 percent of the patients the chest x-ray shows hilar adenopathy compatible with sarcoidosis.

The second pattern of the joint involvement seen

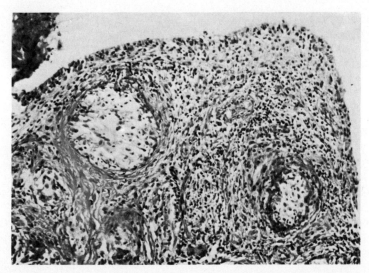

Fig. 1. Granuloma in synovial biopsy of a patient with sarcoid arthropathy. (Reproduced from the Clinical Slide Collection on the Rheumatic Diseases produced by the Arthritis Foundation, New York, copyright 1972.)

with sarcoidosis occurs months to years after the onset of sarcoidosis and is a recurring, episodic polyarthritis that may lead to chronic deformity. Symmetric involvement of the ankles, knees, wrists, and small joints of the hands is the rule, but recurrent monarticular arthritis has been reported. Cutaneous involvement (other than erythema nodosum) is common as is evidence of pulmonary parenchymal sarcoidosis. X-rays of the involved joints usually demonstrate abnormalities, which vary from osteoporosis to narrowing of the joint spaces and frank joint destruction. While there has been a paucity of data delineating the characteristics of the synovial fluid in this form of sarcoid arthropathy, the few published reports indicate an elevated total protein, with white blood cell counts in the range of 15,000–20,000/mm³ and a predominance of lymphocytes.

When seen in association with evidence to support the presence of sarcoidosis in other organ systems, the diagnosis of sarcoid arthropathy is usually not a difficult one. The presence of noncaseating granuloma in a synovial biopsy helps to confirm the diagnosis. Even in the chronic form there are relatively short periods (approximately 4 weeks) of acute exacerbations which help to distinguish sarcoid arthropathy from the more prolonged exacerbations seen in rheumatoid arthritis (early morning stiffness can be a symptom associated with sarcoid arthropathy). It is to be emphasized that approximately one-third of patients with sarcoidosis will have a positive test for rheumatoid factor. This is a manifestation of the aberrant immune reactivity which accompanies sarcoidosis and does not indicate concomitant rheumatoid arthritis.

Occasionally, sarcoid arthropathy may mimic classic podagra. A subsequent migratory pattern of acute arthritis can mimic "migratory gout." The distinction between sarcoid arthropathy and gout is further complicated by two other findings: (1) hyperuricemia is noted in patients with sarcoidosis; and (2) sarcoid arthropathy can have a dramatic response to colchicine. Again, the presence of noncaseating granulomas in other tissues or synovial biopsy and the absence of crystals in the synovial fluid should enable a distinction between two entities.

Psoriasis has also been reported in association with sarcoidosis. However, psoriatic arthritis commonly involves distal interphalangeal joints and the axial skeleton, whereas this pattern of involvement is rare in sarcoidosis.

Therapy for sarcoid arthropathy varies. Aspirin, colchicine, and a short course of steroids have been used to ameliorate symptoms during the self-limited form present early in the course of sarcoidosis. Steriods may be required to treat the more chronic form, although colchicine has also been used during acute exacerbations.

Central Nervous System Manifestations

Sarcoid of the CNS can occur early in the course of the disease and occasionally may be the presenting manifestation. The most common lesions involve the meninges (basilar meningitis), hypothalamus, pituitary, and cranial nerves (cranial nerves VII, II, X, and XII are most frequently affected). Examination of the spinal fluid demonstrates pleocytosis and an elevated protein in 75 percent of the patients, while 10 percent may demonstrate a decreased spinal fluid glucose in the absence of any evidence of concomitant infection. Diffuse encephalopathy, seizures, hydrocephalus (communicating and noncommunicating), and progressive mutifocal leukoencephalopathy may rarely be manifestations of CNS sarcoid. Peripheral neuropathies occur later in the course and may present as mononeuritis, polyneuropathy, or Landry-Guillain–Barré syndrome.

Muscle Involvement

The most common form of myopathic sarcoidosis is an asymptomatic condition in which granulomas can be demonstrated in skeletal muscle in the absence of clinical weakness or elevated muscle enzymes. Both a chronic and an acute myopathy accompanied by weakness, elevated muscle enzymes and abnormal electromyogram can occur.

Cardiac Involvement

Cardiac involvement may be manifested by cor pulmonale, occurring secondary to pulmonary parenchymal sarcoid, or by arrthymias reflecting direct granulomatous involvement of the conducting system. Pericarditis is rare.

Bone Lesions

Three types of bone lesions (usually involving the hands and feet) have been reported in sarcoid: (1) round, lytic lesions occurring in phalanges, metacarpals, and nasal bones; (2) "tunneling" of the cortex and shaft of the phalanx; and (3) destructive lesions with multiple fractures, sequestrum formation, and secondary joint involvement. Eighty-six percent of patients with sarcoid of the bone have radiographic evidence of pulmonary sarcoid.

Other Symptoms

Generalized lymphadenopathy, splenomegaly, and hepatomegaly are not uncommon. However, leukopenia, portal hypertension, and hepatic failure rarely develop (50 percent of patients may have an elevation of hepatic alkaline phosphatase with a normal serum bilirubin suggesting the presence of hepatic granuloma). Hypercalcemia and hypercalcinuria also occur: they reflect increased sensitivity to vitamin D and increased absorption of calcium rather than bone or renal disease.

DIAGNOSIS AND TREATMENT

DIAGNOSIS

The diagnostic criteria for sarcoidosis include (1) a compatible clinical picture, (2) histopathologic evidence of noncaseating granuloma, (3) the presence of supporting data such as positive reactivity to Kveim antigen (see below), elevated serum antiotensin-coverting enzyme (see below), anergy, and hypergammaglobulinemia, and (4) an absence of clinical, histopathologic, bacteriologic, or laboratory evidence to suggest an alternative diagnosis.

The diagnosis of sarcoidosis is usually a process of exclusion as this disease can be mimicked by several others, such as lymphoma, tuberculosis, fungal infection, and vasculitis; therefore, it is important to look for clinical signs or symptoms that may be discordant with sarcoidosis. For example, bilateral hilar adenopathy presenting at age 60 should suggest a diagnosis other than sarcoid since this would be very late for the onset of signs or symptoms in sarcoid. Similarly, while unilateral hilar adenopathy or right paratracheal adenopathy and pleural effusions do occur in sarcoid, they constitute the exception rather than the rule. Constitutional symptoms can be associated with sarcoidosis; however, fever and marked weight loss should suggest an infectious or malignant process rather than sarcoidosis.

The major histologic feature of sarcoidosis, noncaseating granuloma, can also be seen in a variety of other disorders characterized by an infectious, neoplastic, chemical, or immunologic etiology. The value of tissue biopsy in sarcoidosis is not only to support the diagnosis but also to rule out the presence of other, potentially treatable disorders. All biopsies should be subject to meticulous pathologic and bacteriologic examination. Sites chosen for biopsy should depend on the extent of the disease as well as the procedures and expertise available. In a patient with myopathy, skin lesions, lacrimal gland or parotid gland involvement, or palpable peripheral adenopathy, biopsy of these tissue will yield noncaseating granulomas 80–90 percent of the time. Most importantly, such biopsies are low-risk procedures and can be performed with a minimum of morbidity and inconvenience to the patient. Liver biopsy demonstrates noncaseating granulomas in 60–90 percent of patients with sarcoid even in the absence of clinical or biochemical evidence of hepatic involvement.

In patients who manifest only intrathoracic sarcoid, blind biopsy of the scalene fat pad, mediastinoscopy with biopsy of mediastinal nodes, and transbronchial biopsy yield noncaseating granulomas in 60–80 percent. However, these procedures do carry some morbidity, which varies with the experience of the individual performing them. Open-lung biopsy demonstrates noncaseating granulomas in all patients with sarcoid. However, this yield has to be weighed against the higher morbidity associated with the procedure.

Hypergammaglobulinemia and cutaneous anergy are relatively nonspecific findings and can also occur in patients with disseminated fungal and mycobacterial infections. In over 60 percent of patients with stage I or II sarcoidosis, cutaneous injection of a suspension obtained from the spleens or lymph nodes of patients with sarcoidosis (Kveim test) results, 4–6 weeks later, in the presence of a nodule that microscopically contains noncaseating granuloma. Utilizing appropriately prepared "Kveim" antigen, this test is positive in only 3–4 percent of patients with other granulomatous disorders. However, supplies of properly prepared and standardized Kveim antigen are not sufficient to enable its routine diagnostic use.

A recent technique that has tremendous potential usefulness in confirming the diagnosis of sarcoidosis is measurement of angiotensin-converting enzyme (ACE). Recently, it has been demonstrated that circulating levels of this enzyme, which converts angiotensin I to angiotensin II, are elevated in approximately 80 percent of patients with active pulmonary sarcoidosis. This appears to reflect increased synthesis of ACE by epithelioid cells present in granuloma. Studies thus far indicate that consistent, significant elevations of ACE may be expected in only two other disorders, Gaucher's disease and leprosy. ACE measurements may become a useful adjunct to support the diagnosis of sarcoidosis.

The most important consideration in establishing a diagnosis of sarcoidosis is to rule out other diseases. The presence of a compatible clinical syndrome accompanied by biopsy evidence of noncaseating granulomas must be accompanied by a lack of bacteriologic and histologic evidence to suggest an infectious or malignant etiology. Even in this situation, only close, repeated follow-up will indicate whether sarcoidosis is the correct diagnosis.

Two clinical presentations of sarcoidosis deserve special mention. The first is early sarcoidosis in patients who present with bilateral hilar adenopathy, with or without uveitis and erythema nodosum, who are otherwise asymptomatic. It has been suggested that this presentation only rarely occurs in situations other than sarcoidosis and such patients could be spared the inconvenience, cost, and morbidity of tissue biopsy. However, some of the series used to document this concept did not include patients with tuberculosis and fungal infection (especially coccidioidomycosis), both of which can present with hilar adenopathy and erythema nodosum. A decision as to whether the potential risks of biopsy are justified in this situation should be based on an individual assessment of the history, clinical presentation, and facilities available for obtaining biopsy materials.

The second presentation occurs in what has been termed "burnt out sarcoidosis" and is manifest by only severe interstitial pulmonary fibrosis and respiratory distress. Delayed hypersensitivity reactions may be normal, ACE levels are not increased, and reactivity to Kveim antigen may not be present at this stage. Biopsy of pulmonary parenchyma may fail to show granuloma and simply demonstrate fibrosis. Thus, it is difficult to establish the diagnosis of sarcoidosis. In the absence of any evidence to suggest other etiologies, one may be forced to treat symptomatically or with a trial course of corticosteriods (see below).

TREATMENT

Less than 10 percent of patients with sarcoidosis succumb to the disease and its complications. The major causes of death include (1) pulmonary insufficiency, (2) aspergillosis with massive hemoptysis, and (3) myocardial sarcoid. While one- to two-thirds of all patients with sarcoidosis receive corticosteroids at some time during the illness, guidelines for their use and proof of their efficacy are not substantial. The following are general guidelines that are to be modified for the individual case.

Extrapulmonary Sarcoid

A trial of systemic corticosteriods (40–60 mg prednisone/day or its equivalent) should be tried in any individual with severe, extrapulmonary sarcoid. This category includes cases of severe eye disease, infiltrative lesions of the skin and mucous membranes, CNS, musculoskeletal, and myocardial sarcoid, symptomatic hepatic involvement, and hypercalcemia. Steriods are effective in reducing serum calcium levels and in preventing blindness. The results in stemming or reversing CNS, cardiac, and bone lesions are disappointing. Topical corticosteriod therapy or chloroquine has been effective in patients with skin and mucous membrane lesions. Arthralgias, fever, and uveitis usually remit spontaneously and should be treated symptomatically with salicylates.

Pulmonary Sarcoid

Stage I. Since three-quarters of these patients usually demonstrate spontaneous remission within 2 years, initial treatment is not required. If the patient is symptomatic (experiences dyspnea) or if significant pulmonary function abnormalities are present, then the patient should be followed closely for 6 months. If there is clinical, radiographic, or pulmonary function evidence of persistence or progression then corticosteroids should be used.

Stage II. Approximately one-third of these patients will have a spontaneous recovery. If there are no symptoms or abnormal pulmonary function tests, close follow-up is recommended. If dyspnea or abnormal pulmonary function tests are present, corticosteriod treatment should be instituted. Drug-induced improvement can be expected in approximately 50 percent of cases.

Stage III. The incidence of spontaneous resolution at this stage is 0–10 percent. Steriod therapy should be tried early.

Three points concerning steriod treatment for pulmonary sarcoid are to be emphasized: (1) Large doses are not required. A practical regimen is to start with 40 mg of prednisone/day for 4–6 weeks, followed by 15–20 mg/day for 5–6 months, and then gradually taper the dose at the rate of 2.5 mg every other week. (2) During reduction in steriods, relapses are common and require resumption of the higher doses. It can be expected that a substantial percentage of patients will require treatment for longer than 2 years. (3) Corticosteriods are effective in reducing granuloma size. Their ability to prevent fibrosis is not documented. Fluffy or dense radiographic opacities present in pulmonary sarcoid are caused by the granuloma and not by fibrosis. The apparent diminution in the radiographic appearance of pulmonary parenchymal sarcoid may simply reflect the resolution of granuloma with development of fibrosis. Thus, the chest film is not a reliable indicator of the efficacy of steriods. The patient's symptoms (dyspnea) and pulmonary function tests (vital capacity, expiratory flow, and diffusion parameters) are the best reflections of the pathologic process. Side effects from the relatively low doses required to treat pulmonary sarcoid are few.

The usefulness of immunosuppressive therapy is not well studied. Prophylactic use of antituberculous therapy should be individualized for each patient. Overall, the documented efficacy of corticosteriods in preventing the long-term disability associated with pulmonary sarcoid is not very encouraging.

REFERENCES

Epstein WL: Granuloma formation in man. Pathobiol Ann 7:1, 1977

James DG, Carstairs LS, Trowell J, Sharma OP: Treatment of sarcoidosis. Lancet 2:526, 1967

Kaplan H: Sarcoid arthritis, a review. Arch Intern Med 112:162, 1963

Liberman J: Elevation of serum angiotensin-converting-enzyme (ACE) level in sarcoidosis. Am J Med 59:365, 1975

Longcope WT, Freiman DG: A study of sarcoidosis based on a combined investigation of 160 cases including 30 autopsies from Johns Hopkins and Massachusetts General Hospital. Medicine (Baltimore) 31:1, 1952

Mitchell DN, Scadding JG: Sarcoidosis: State of the art. Am Rev Resp Dis 110:774, 1974

Siltzbach LE (ed): Seventh International Conference on Sarcoidosis and Other Granulomatous Disorders, vol 278. New York, New York Academy Sciences, 1976

Spann RW, Rosenow EC, DeRenee RA, Miller WE: Unilateral hilar or paratracheal adenopathy in Sarcoidosis. A study of 38 cases. Thorax 26:296, 1971

Sutherland I, Mitchell DN, Hart P: Incidence of intrathoracic sarcoidosis among young adults participating in trial of tuberculosis vaccines. Br Med J 2:497, 1965

Winterbauer RH, Belic N, Moores KD: A clinical interpretation of bilateral hilar adenopathy. Ann Intern Med 78:65, 1973

Arthritis Associated with Metabolic or Endocrine Disease

Duncan A. Gordon

ARTHRITIS ASSOCIATED WITH HEMOCHROMATOSIS

Hemochromatosis is a disorder of iron metabolism in which deposition of hemosiderin leads to tissue damage and organ dysfunction. The condition rarely appears before age 40 and affects men more frequently than women, who are protected by menstruation. Idiopathic hemochromatosis appears to be hereditary. Although a specific biochemical marker has yet to be discovered, the genes responsible for it may be linked to histocompatibility antigens such as HLA-A3 and HLA-B14. Thus, when hemochromatosis is diagnosed in any individual, other family members should be studied. Increased dietary iron, chronic anemia, cirrhosis, and blood transfusions may also cause iron overload. Without tissue damage this disorder is known as *hemosiderosis,* with tissue damage it is termed *secondary hemochromatosis.* Although the classic features of idiopathic hemochromatosis are skin pigmentation, diabetes mellitus, hepatomegaly, and cardiac disease, arthropathy is also a common and disabling complication.

The arthropathy is characterized by chronic arthritis of the peripheral joints and spine. Half the cases show chondrocalcinosis, and these patients may have pseudogout. Although arthritis develops in more than half the patients showing classic features of hemochromatosis, it should be emphasized that arthritis may be the only early presenting feature of hemochromatosis, and the only clinical feature of it.

Clinically, the main feature is a chronic progressive arthritis affecting predominantly the second and third metacarpophalangeal and proximal interphalangeal joints superficially resembling rheumatoid arthritis (Fig. 1). The dominant hand may be more severely affected. Radiologically, ulnar styloid erosion may suggest rheumatoid disease, but the irregular joint narrowing and sclerotic cyst formation are more indicative of a degenerative process. Although the distal interphalangeal joints may be affected, the carpometacarpal joint changes of generalized osteoarthritis are not a feature. Hip joint involvement has been striking in most series. The radiologic changes are indistinguishable from those in osteoarthritis except that in hemochromatosis there is less osteophytosis.

The diagnosis may be suspected by a raised serum iron level and increased saturation of the plasma iron-binding protein transferrin. These indices many not always be raised and serum ferritin concentrations are not raised in the early stages of primary hemochromatosis. Needle biopsy of the liver may provide the most definitive evidence of iron overload in hemochromatosis. In idiopathic hemochromatosis, iron deposits affect parenchymal hepatic cells, whereas reticuloendothelial cells are most affected in secondary forms. Synovial biopsy in hemochromatosis shows iron deposition in the type B synthetic lining cells of synovium, whereas in rheumatoid arthritis, traumatic hemarthrosis, hemophilia, and villonodular synovitis deposits form in the deeper layers or in the phagocytic type A lining cells. Hemosiderin deposits may also be found in the chondrocytes. Further evidence of iron may be found in biopsies of skin and intestinal mucosa, or in bone marrow, buffy coat, or urine sediment. The amount of iron excreted in the urine after administration of the iron-chelating agent deferoxamine correlates with the presence of parenchymal hepatic iron and a diagnosis of idiopathic hemochromatosis.

Chondrocalcinosis is characteristic of the arthropathy. The hyaline cartilage of the shoulder, wrists, hips, and knees, and the fibrocartilage of the triangular ligament of the wrists and symphysis pubis may be affected.

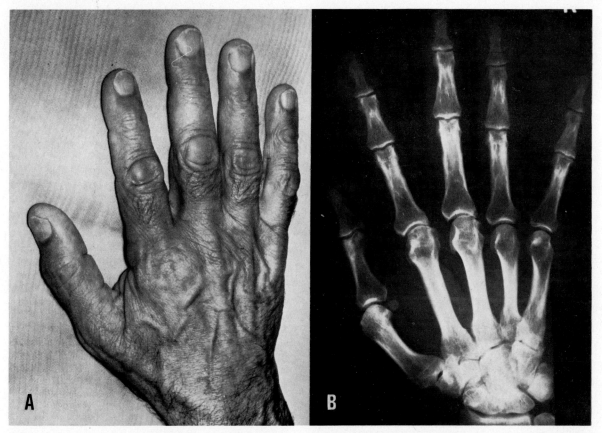

Fig. 1. Arthropathy of hemochromatosis. **A.** Hand shows metacarpophalangeal and proximal interphalangeal joint swelling. **B.** Roentgenogram of same hand shows degenerative changes of second and third metacarpal heads. (From Gordon DA, Clarke PV, Ogryzlo MA: The chondrocalcific arthropathy of iron overload. Arch Intern Med 134:21–28, 1974. Copyright 1974, American Medical Association.)

Superimposed attacks of calcium pyrophosphate dihydrate crystal synovitis occur in these cases.

The pathogenesis of the arthritis is unknown since degenerative joint changes do not necessarily develop in relation to synovial iron. The relationship of chondrocalcinosis to iron overload is also intriguing. The low frequency of chrondrocalcinosis in patients with hemophilia and rheumatoid arthritis weighs against synovial hemosiderin as a cause of chondrocalcinosis. It is speculated that ionic iron might inhibit pyrophosphatase activity and lead to a local concentration of calcium pyrophosphate in the joint. The deposition of calcium in cartilage appears to predispose to inflammatory and degenerative joint disease.

Venesection is the most effective means for removal of excess body iron in hemochromatosis. Deferoxamine administration has not proven to be practical. Venesection may not prevent the progression of arthritis in hemochromatosis, and arthritis may worsen after this therapy. Symptoms may be controlled by nonsteroidal antiinflammatory agents such as indomethacin. Sometimes joint surgery may be required for severe hip disease.

ARTHRITIS ASSOCIATED WITH WILSON'S DISEASE

Wilson's disease (hepatolenticular degeneration) is a rare metabolic disorder in which deposition of copper leads to dysfunction of the liver, brain, and kidneys. It is inherited as an autosomal recessive trait, and patients aged 6 to 40 are affected. Kayser-Fleischer corneal rings, cirrhosis, brain degeneration, psychic disturbances, renal tubular dysfunction, and hemolytic anemia are the classic features, but an arthropathy may also develop in many affected adults.

The arthropathy is characterized by an osteoarthritis of the wrists, metacarpophalangeal joints, knees, or spine. Ossified bodies of the wrists may be associated with subchondral cysts. Chondromalacia patellae, osteochondritis dissecans, or chondrocalcinosis of the knee may be associatedwith mild knee effusions. A few patients show polyarthralgias, possibly from penicillamine therapy. Synovial biopsies show hyperplasia of synovial lining cells with mild inflammation. Neither calcium pyrophosphate nor copper are seen. Unlike hemochromatosis, involvement of the hip and metacarpophalangeal joints are uncommon. Asymptomatic osteopenia is common and pathologic fractures and osteomalacia may occur.

Although Kayser-Fleischer corneal rings are pathognomonic of Wilson's disease, the diagnosis is established by laboratory investigations. Low serum copper and decreased serum ceruloplasmin levels occur in most cases, and in symptomatic patients urinary copper excretion is increased. Microchemical evidence of copper deposition may be obtained from needle biopsy of the liver, but histochemical methods are unreliable. In doubtful cases, specialized studies with radioactive copper may be necessary.

Although the arthropathy is generally milder than that seen in hemochromatosis, its cause may be similar and it may involve deposition of calcium pyrophosphate dihydrate and the development of chronic arthritis.

Copper chelation with penicillamine is the treatment of choice for Wilson's disease. Whether penicillamine can control the arthropathy is uncertain, but arthritis may worsen after the initiation of penicillamine therapy. Otherwise, symptomatic measures suffice to control arthritic symptoms.

ARTHRITIS ASSOCIATED WITH GAUCHER'S DISEASE

Gaucher's disease is a lysosomal glycolipid storage disease in which glucocerebroside accummulates in the reticuloendothelial cells of the spleen, liver, and bone marrow. It is an autosomal recessive disorder caused by subnormal activity of the hydrolytic enzyme glucocerebrosidase. Its clinical subdivisions are as follows: Type 1 is the chronic nonneuronopathic form that develops in adults and involves organomegaly, hypersplenism, conjunctival pengueculae, skin pigmentation, and osteoarticular disease. It has the best prognosis. Type 2, infantile, and type 3, juvenile, both affect the central nervous system. Skeletal involvement is characteristic of type 1 and to a lesser extent type 3 but not type 2 disease.

Rheumatic complaints appear early in the course of Gaucher's disease. Pain in the hip, knee, or shoulder is caused by disease of adjacent bone. Monarticular hip or knee degeneration is typical, and unexplained migratory polyarthritis sometimes occurs. Bony pain tends to lessen with age. Other skeletal features include pathologic long bone fractures, vertebral compression, and aseptic necrosis of the femoral or humeral heads or proximal tibia. The aseptic necrosis can develop slowly, or rapidly with bone crisis. These crises usually affect only one bone area at a time and mimic the clinical picture of acute osteomyelitis. Surgical drainage in these cases commonly leads to infection and chronic osteomyelitis. Because of this increased susceptibility to infection, conservative management of bony lesions is recommended.

Asymptomatic radiologic areas of rarefaction, patchy sclerosis, and cortical thickening are common. Expansion of the distal femur or, less frequently, of the tibia or humerus, produces an Erlenmeyer flask-like contour. Monoclonal gammopathy and multiple myeloma have been reported in cases of adult Gaucher's disease.

Although the total serum acid phosphatase is usually mildly raised in Gaucher's disease, the diagnosis should be confirmed by examination of bone marrow aspirate for the Gaucher cell, a large lipid storage histiocyte. Because there is a risk of secondary infection, bone biopsy is not recommended. Needle biopsy of the liver for assay of glucocerebroside may be performed, but washed leukocytes and extracts of cultured skin fibroblasts are easily obtained for glucocerebrosidase testing. These assays may also be used to detect heterozygous carriers.

Therapy of Gaucher's disease may require periodic control of pain and infection. Hematologic support may require splenectomy. Despite infection, replacement arthroplasty has been successful. Lysosomal enzyme replacement has been tried and has shown promise as a specific therapy, but technical problems must be overcome before it can become a practical therapy.

ARTHRITIS ASSOCIATED WITH ALCAPTONURIA—OCHRONOSIS

Alcaptonuria is caused by one of the classic inborn errors of metabolism. It is a rare autosomal recessive disorder caused by a complete deficiency of the enzyme homogentisic acid oxidase. As a consequence, homogentisic acid, which turns dark on oxidation, is excreted in the urine, and polymers of homogentisic acid (ochronotic pigment) accumulate in connective tissues such as cartilage, sclera, and skin. Because ochronotic pigment is preferentially deposited in cartilage, a degenerative arthropathy is an inevitable complication. Other features of ochronosis include bluish discoloration and calcification of the ear pinnae, triangular pigmentation of the sclera, and pigmentation over the nose, axillae, and groin. Prostatic calculi are common in men and cardiac murmurs may develop from valvular pigment deposits.

The features of the arthropathy include arthritis of the spine (ochronotic spondylosis) and arthritis of the larger peripheral joints, with chondrocalcinosis, formation of osteochondral bodies, and synovial effusions (ochronotic peripheral arthropathy). Symptoms develop by the fourth decade. Initially, the lumbar spine is affected and later the knees, shoulders, and hips deteriorate. In contrast to the picture in primary osteoarthritis, the small peripheral joints are spared. In adults, the first sign of spondylitis may be an acute disc syndrome. Eventually, it resembles ankylosing spondylitis with progressive lumbar rigidity and loss of stature. Knee effusions, crepitus, and flexion contractures are common, and osteochondral bodies are often palpable around the joint. Shoulder and hip restriction develop later.

Radiologically, one of the earliest features is multiple

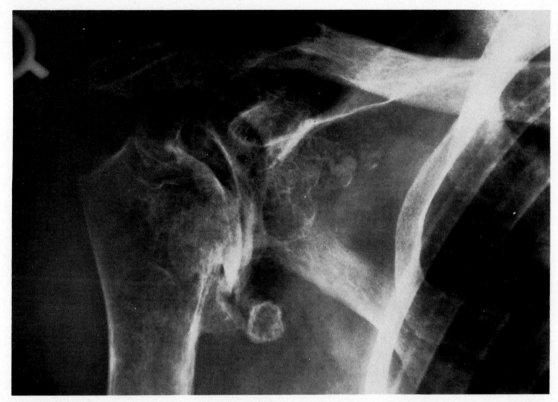

Fig. 1. Arthropathy of ochronosis. Roentgenogram of shoulder joint shows marked degenerative changes and osteochondral bodies. (From Hunter T, Gordon DA, Ogryzlo MA: The ground pepper sign of synovial fluid. J Rheumatol 1:45–53, 1974. Copyright 1974, American Medical Association.)

vacuum discs of the spine. Eventually, the entire spine shows chondrocalcinosis of the discs with narrowing, collapse, and fusion. Chondrocalcinosis may also affect the symphysis pubis, costal cartilage, and ear helix. In contrast to the situation in ankylosing spondylitis, the sacroiliac and apophyseal joints are not affected. The radiographic appearance of the peripheral joints resembles that in primary osteoarthritis, except there is more severe degeneration of the shoulders and hips and osteochondral joint bodies are seen (Fig. 1).

The diagnosis of alcaptonuria is suspected when the patient gives a history of passing dark urine, or when fresh urine turns black on standing, or on alkalinization. Some individuals may not have this typical history, and the diagnosis is made only after the onset of arthritis or the detection of a false-positive test for diabetes mellitus. Although a specific enzymatic method permits quantitation of homogentisic acid in urine and blood, no method allows identification of disease carriers.

Synovial fluid is usually clear, yellow, and viscous and does not darken with alkali. At times the fluid may be speckled with many particles of debris resembling ground pepper. Leukocyte counts of a few hundred cells are predominantly mononuclear. Occasionally, the cytoplasm of mononuclear and polymorphonuclear cells contains dark inclusions of phagocytosed ochronotic pigment. Centrifugation and microscopic examination of

synovial fluid sediment may show fragments of pigmented cartilage. Effusions may contain calcium pyrophosphate dihydrate crystals and show no inflammation. Pathologically, pigmentation of the articular cartilage affects the deeper layers and leads to fibrillation and erosion of cartilage. Tiny shards of pigmented cartilage then penetrate the bone, synovium, and joint cavity. It seems likely that these pigmented cartilage fragments form a nidus for the formation of osteochondral bodies.

Replacement of the missing enzyme is a conceivable therapy for alcaptonuria, but is not yet practical. Although it is possible that large amounts of ascorbic acid might prevent deposition of ochronotic pigment, long-term effects of this therapy are unknown. Current therapy consists of supportive medical and orthopedic measures.

ARTHRITIS ASSOCIATED WITH HYPERLIPOPROTEINEMIA (TYPE II AND TYPE IV)

Type IIa and type IV hyperlipoproteinemia are genetic disorders that are best known for their association with premature arteriosclerosis, but they may also be associated with prominent rheumatic features.

TYPE II

One form of type IIa, or familial hypercholesterolemia, is autosomal dominant, with raised plasma cholesterol in the low-density lipoproteins. Patients with the monogenic form, most of whom are homozygotes, account for only a small proportion of the cases of hyperlipidemia found in the general population. Although xanthomatosis and xanthelasma are common clinical features, they may not appear until age 30, at which time they may present as the sole manifestation. Xanthomas over elbows, dorsal wrists, infrapatellar, and Achilles tendons may easily be overlooked. Episodes of tendinitis or tenosynovitis may recur for a few days several times a year for many years without producing joint deformity or radiographic abnormalities. Although the serum uric acid is normal, these attacks are commonly mistaken for gout. Thus, evaluation of unexplained tendinitis should include the determination of serum cholesterol.

The severe homozygous form of hypercholesterolemia, which mainly affects children, may be associated with a migratory polyarthritis resembling rheumatic fever. Periarticular joint swelling and normal synovial fluid seem unrelated to xanthomas. Although fever and leukocytosis are infrequent, the erythrocyte sedimentation rate is elevated, even without joint symptoms. The diagnosis may also be confounded by xanthomatous infiltration of the aortic valve, which is clinically indistinguishable from rheumatic or calcific aortic stenosis.

Hypercholesterolemia resulting from secondary causes is much more common than the familial variety. These causes include hypothyroidism, nephrotic syndrome, and excessive dietary cholesterol. Hyperuricemia, diabetes mellitus, and obesity do not appear to be directly associated with this form of familial hypercholesterolemia.

TYPE IV

Type IV, or familial endogenous hypertriglyceridemia, is inherited as an autosomal dominant trait and demonstrates raised levels of triglycerides in the very low density lipoproteins. Because there are no unique clinical or biochemical features of endogenous hypertriglyceridemia, the diagnosis can be made with certainty only in patients with affected relatives. Hypertriglyceridemia may also be associated with obesity, hyperuricemia, and insulin-independent diabetes mellitus. It may also be caused by ethanol excess, estrogen therapy, and the nephrotic syndrome.

Polyarthritis may be an uncommon feature of type IV hyperlipoproteinemia. Symptoms affect women, predominantly in middle life. Arthritis affects one or two joints at a time and is associated with considerable tenderness without other signs of inflammation. Metacarpophalangeal or proximal interphalangeal joints may be asymmetrically involved. Synovial effusions may show a mild mononuclear inflammatory reaction without the presence of lipid or crystals. These patients are usually not hyperuricemic. Although the latex fixation test for rheumatoid factors may be mildly positive, serum extraction with cold diethyl ether converts these tests to negative. Radiographic examination shows juxtaarticular rarefaction and cystic lesions affecting the proximal tibia, humeral head, and proximal phalanges. Constitutional symptoms are absent and the arthropathy has not been disabling. Although the pathogenesis is unknown, normalization of serum lipid levels may lead to a decrease in the severity of the arthritis.

ARTHRITIS IN ASSOCIATION WITH MULTICENTRIC RETICULOHISTIOCYTOSIS

Multicentric reticulohistiocytosis is a rare dermatoarthritis of unknown cause. It predominantly affects middle-aged women. The onset is insidious and is characterized by a polyarthritis, skin nodules, and in many cases xanthelasma. Small tumors around the nailfolds are characteristic, and nodulation of the skin of the face, hands, or mucous membranes may ulcerate.

A symmetric polyarthritis resembles rheumatoid disease when proximal interphalangeal joints are affected, and psoriatic arthritis when involvement of distal interphalangeal joints predominates. Tenosynovial involvement may also occur. Radiographs show punched out bony lesions resembling gouty tophi early on, followed by severe joint destruction. Spinal involvement may occur. No specific laboratory abnormality has yet been demonstrated, and the diagnosis is established by examination of biopsies of affected tissues. These samples show histiocytic giant cells of the foreign body type containing periodic acid-Schiff staining material, probably a glycolipid. The pathogenesis is unknown. Although corticosteroids may improve the skin lesions, the arthritis is not affected. Spontaneous remission of skin and arthritis, however, are not uncommon.

ARTHRITIS ASSOCIATED WITH ACROMEGALY, HYPERPARATHYROIDISM, AND HYPOPARATHYROIDISM

ACROMEGALY

Overgrowth resulting from pituitary hypersecretion is the chief manifestation of acromegaly, and arthropathy may be a prominent and disabling feature. While full-blown acromegaly may be obvious, the early diagnosis may be difficult; it may begin with the insidious onset of mild Raynaud's phenomenon, carpal tunnel syndrome, arthralgias, or low back pain.

Clinically, peripheral joint manifestations include pain in the hands, knees, shoulders, and hips associated with marked crepitus and hypermobility. Joint restriction is unusual except in late stages. Painless swelling of metacarpophalangeal, proximal interphalangeal, and carpometacarpal joints may occur. Generally, swelling is periarticular and rarely associated with effusions. Back pain is usually lumbosacral. Dorsal kyphosis is common and spinal mobility is well maintained or increased.

The striking radiologic feature is widened joint spaces of hands and knees due to cartilage hypertrophy. Finger tufting, remodeled phalanges, and new bone formation may be associated with capsular calcification. The knee joint may show chondrocalcinosis and osteophytosis, but rarely attacks of pseudogout. Although the spine may show extensive anterior osteophytosis, disc spaces remain preserved.

While the presence of carpal tunnel syndrome suggests ongoing pituitary overactivity, the severity, duration, and specific therapy of acromegaly do not correlate with the arthropathy. Symptomatic medical measures and joint surgery may be required.

HYPERPARATHYROIDISM

Gastrointestinal, renal, and bone symptoms, along with hypercalcemia, are the classic features of hyperparathyroidism. Several rheumatic syndromes may also be associated with this disorder or may appear after parathyroidectomy.

While primary hyperparathyroidism is an uncommon cause of chondrocalcinosis, patients with hyperparathyroidism frequently develop it. Sites include the hyaline cartilage of peripheral joints, the fibrocartilage of the symphysis pubis, the triangular ligament of the wrist, and the interverterbral discs. Calcific periarthritis may also occur in patients with chondrocalcinosis. The patients with calcium pyrophosphate dihydrate deposition disease are prone to develop pseudogout. Because hyperuricemia and gouty attacks may also occur with primary hyperparathyroidism, examination of synovial fluid by compensated polarizing microscopy is necessary to distinguish calcium pyrophsphate dihydrate from sodium monourate crystals. Sometimes both are present. Attacks of pseudogout or gout may occur shortly after parathyroidectomy, and chondrocalcinosis may then worsen. Arthralgia and morning stiffness may be associated with subperiosteal erosions of fingers and wrists resembling rheumatoid changes. Erosions may also affect the lower outer clavicle, distal ulna, and upper tibia. Less commonly, episodes of traumatic synovitis develop from subchondral collapse of juxtaarticular bone and lead to chronic arthritis.

HYPOTHYROIDISM

Thyroid deficiency may be associated with a variety of musculoskeletal manifestations or may itself complicate connective tissue disorders associated with chronic thyroiditis.

Arthralgias and myalgias of shoulders and hips with pseudomyotonic cramps may be presenting features of myxedema. A proximal myopathy with raised creatine phosphokinase levels may be confused with polymyosi-tis. Carpal tunnel syndrome with tenosynovitis of the flexor tendon sheaths of the hands is common. Polyarthritis of the wrists, fingers, knees, ankles, and feet may be associated with ligamentous laxity, and knee effusions may be overlooked because of a sluggish fluid bulge sign. Synovial fluid shows a noninflammatory exudate, similar to the pleural and pericardial effusions, and ascites of hypothyroidism. Chondrocalcinosis may occur, but without pseudogout. Hyperuricemia with tophaceous gout appears to be commoner than acute gout, and aseptic necrosis of the femoral head may sometimes occur. Thyroid replacement improves all these syndromes, with the exception of chondrocalcinosis, in which attacks of pseudogout may develop with thyroid medication.

CARCINOID ARTHROPATHY

Carcinoid tumors release serotonin and other chemicals, producing a symptom complex of skin flushing, telangiectasia, diarrhea, cardiac valvular lesions, and bronchial constriction known as the carcinoid syndrome. Scleroderma of the legs or polyarthralgias may also be prominent features of the syndrome.

Clinically, polyarthralgias of the fingers are worse with movement, and wrists, shoulders, and knees may be painful. Radiographs show juxtaarticular rarefaction and cystic lesions of the metacarpophalangeal and proximal interphalangeal joints. Blockade of tryptophan hydroxylase with para-chlorophenylalamine may improve the polyarthralgias. Carcinoid scleroderma of the legs may follow pitting dependant edema. Other features of scleroderma, such as acrosclerosis, Raynaud's phenomenon, systemic sclerosis, and antinuclear antibody, are lacking. Thus, the carcinoid syndrome may be included in a list of scleroderma variants such as morphea, eosinophilic fasciitis, vinyl chloride toxicity, porphyria cutanea tarda, and Werner's syndrome.

REFERENCES

Bluestone R, Bywaters EGL, Hartog M, Holt PJL, Hide S: Acromegaly arthropathy. Ann Rheum Dis 30: 243, 1971

Buckingham RB, Bole GG, Bassett DR: Polyarthritis associated with type IV hyperlipoproteinemia. Arch Intern Med 135:286, 1975

Bywaters EGL, Dixon A StJ, Scott JT: Joint lesions of hyperparathyroidism. Ann Rheum Dis 22:171, 1963

Dorwart BB, Schumacher HR: Joint effusions, chondrocalcinosis and other rheumatic manifestations in hypothyroidism. Am J Med 59:780, 1975

Fries JF, Lindgren JA, Bull JM: Scleroderma-like lesions and the carcinoid syndrome. Arch Intern Med 131:550, 1973

Glueck CJ, Levy RI, Fredrickson DS: Acute tendinitis and arthritis of familial type II hyperlipoproteinemia. JAMA 206:2895, 1968

Gordon DA, Clarke PV, Ogryzlo MA: The chondrocalcific arthropathy of iron overload. Arch Intern Med 134:21, 1974

Hunter T, Gordon DA, Ogryzlo MA: The ground pepper sign of synovial fluid: A diagnostic feature of ochronosis. J Rheumatol 1:45, 1974

Kaklamanis P, Spengos M: Osteoarticular changes and synovial biopsy findings in Wilson's disease. Ann Rheum Dis 32:422, 1973

Krey PR, Comerford FR, Cohen AS: Multicentric reticulohis-

tiocytosis: Fine structural analysis of the synovium and synovial fluid cells. Arthritis Rheum 17:615, 1974

Noyes FR, Smith WS: Bone crises and chronic osteomyelitis in Gaucher's disease. Clin Orthop 79:132, 1971

Plonk JW, Feldman JM: Carcinoid arthropathy. Arch Intern Med 134:651, 1974

Stanbury JB, Wyngaarden JB, Fredrickson DS: The Metabolic Basis of Inherited Disease (4th ed). New York, McGraw-Hill, 1978

Arthritis Associated with Hematologic Disease

H. Ralph Schumacher

HEMOPHILIA

The sex-linked recessive inheritance of decreased factor VIII causes deficient clotting in males and, depending on severity, infrequent or severely disabling bleeding. A destructive arthropathy can result from repeated hemarthroses. There are apparently some spontaneous mutations as a family history of hemophilia is not always present.

CLINICAL PICTURE

Pain, stiffness, limitation of motion, and increased warmth usually signal the onset of joint bleeding in the hemophiliac. Swelling need not be detectable, especially with early symptoms. Any joint may be involved, but knees, elbows, ankles, shoulders, and wrists are most common. In established hemarthrosis, these joints can be tensely distended. Blood is resorbed after bouts, but chronic synovial proliferation and contractures can occur with repeated hemarthroses. Involvement may be asymmetric.

RADIOLOGIC FINDINGS

Effusion and synovial thickening are followed by progressive narrowing of the joint space with loss of articular cartilage. The hyperemia appears to stimulate new bone formation and bony overgrowth. Initially this produces increased size, but with premature fusion of ossification centers, mature bone length may actually be less. Prominent trabeculae, juxtaarticular cysts, and erosions develop. Osteopenia may develop from immobilization. There is often widening of the intercondylar notch at the knee.

LABORATORY STUDIES

In addition to prolonged bleeding times, the partial thromboplastin time is prolonged. The whole-blood clotting time may be normal in patients with as little as 5 percent of normal levels of factor VIII. Patients with less than 1 percent of normal factor VIII activity are severely affected and have almost constant bruises, hematomas, and hemarthroses; 2–7 percent activity represents moderate disease; and people with more than 8 percent of normal factor VIII activity tend to have bleeding only with surgery, dental extractions, and major trauma. Syn-

ovial biopsies show iron in phagocytic cells in the deep synovium and lining layer. Macrophages are increased in number and there is often fibrosis and increased vascularity. Cartilage is also pigmented with iron identifiable in chondrocytes.

DIFFERENTIAL DIAGNOSIS

Other known causes of hemarthrosis are defects in other clotting factors such as occur with thrombocytopenia, anticoagulant therapy, factor IX deficiency (Christmas disease or hemophilia B), trauma with or without fracture, articular tumor, pigmented villonodular synovitis, scurvy, aneurysms, arteriovenous malformations or hemangiomas, Charcot's joint, or other destructive or inflammatory arthropathies.

THERAPY

Prompt administration of plasma or factor VIII is effective in shortening the disability time with any bout of hemarthrosis and in decreasing later deformity. Concentrates of factor IX are also available to treat Christmas disease. Infusions carry some risk of acquisition of hepatitis virus. Infusions may often be given at home to allow as near normal activities as possible and to permit prompt treatment. Aspiration of the joint for acute hemarthrosis seems to shorten acute symptoms slightly but not to alter the end result. It may be used in severely distended joints. Immobilization is occasionally advised while the joint is very painful but is often not needed and can lead to muscle wasting. Isometric and range of motion exercises should be started as soon as pain decreases after an acute hemarthrosis. Intraarticular or oral steroids have been advised for acute bleeding but were not found to be effective in all studies.

Synovectomy under coverage of therapy with factor VIII antihemophiliac globulin has been effective in preventing recurrent bleeding in patients with chronic disease. Late contractures may require exercises, serial splinting, or surgery. Although expensive, chronic prophylactic factor VIII can be used to prevent hemarthrosis.

PATHOGENESIS

Abnormal bleeding appears to be caused by the combination of even minor trauma and the clotting factor deficiency. Activation of plasminogen in the joint leads to formation of the proteolytic enzyme plasmin. Collagenase and neutral protease are also produced by the proliferated synovium. Pannus can form and subchondral hemorrhage may contribute to the cartilage changes. Hemorrhage into muscles and fascia, elevated intraarticular pressure, and immobility may also contribute to contracture, cyst formation, and cartilage degeneration.

REFERENCES

Arnold WD, Hilgartner MW: Hemophilic arthropathy. Current concept of pathogenesis and management. J Bone Joint Surg 59A:287, 1977

Kisker CT, Perlman AW, Benton C: Arthritis in hemophilia. Semin Arthritis Rheum 1:220, 1971

Rodnan GP: Arthritis associated with hematologic disorders. Bull Rheum Dis 16:392, 1965

Storti E, Ascari E: Surgical and chemical synovectomy. Ann NY Acad Sci 240:316, 1975

SICKLE CELL DISEASE AND TRAIT

Sickle cell disease, either in the homozygous form or in combination with hemoglobin C or thalassemia, has been associated with a variety of musculoskeletal problems. Associations include bone infarction with aseptic necrosis, acute painful joint effusions, hyperuricemia and gout, osteomyelitis (often due to salmonellae or pneumococci), the hand–foot syndrome in children under age 2, and possibly acute infarctions in soft tissues, including muscle. About 50 percent of patients with sickle cell disease have arthralgias or arthritis at some time.

CLINICAL PICTURE

Infarctions in bone can be the cause of acute pain in single or multiple bony sites. These are usually but not invariably associated with fever and other signs of acute crisis. Aseptic necrosis, which can result when infarctions are near joints, is most prominent in the femoral head where gradually progressive hip pain on weightbearing is the result. Sickle hemoglobin-hemoglobin C (SC) disease may, even more frequently than homozygous sickle cell (SS) disease, result in aseptic necrosis. Infarctions in the phalanges of young children produce diffusely swollen painful hands and feet (the hand–foot syndrome).

Arthralagias or warm, tender, painful joint effusions occur with typical painful crises or occasionally as isolated occurrences. Knees are most frequently involved but elbows or other joints may also have these effusions, which subside spontaneously over 2–14 days. Periarticular bones are often tender. Some chronic synovitis has been seen with sickle cell disease but whether this is coincidental or not will require further study.

RADIOLOGIC FINDINGS

Radiographs may show coarse trabeculae, osteopenia, vertebral indentations, and "hair-on-end" trabec-

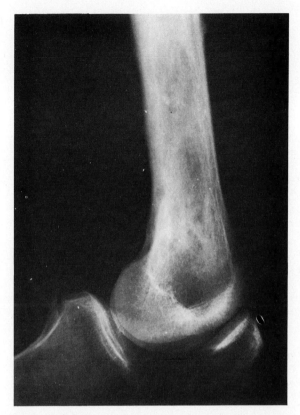

Fig. 1. Radiograph showing mottling of the distal femur due to marrow infarcts in a patient with sickle cell disease. There are also minor periosteal elevations anteriorly and posteriorly at the top of the figure. These are the result of previous cortical infarctions.

ulae in the skull due to expansion of the marrow. Periosteal elevation results from cortical infarcts and aseptic necrosis or medullary dense areas from marrow infarctions (Fig. 1). Focal decreased marrow uptake in otherwise hyperplastic marrow can be detected with technetium-99^m sulfur colloid scans antedating visible x-ray changes in aseptic necrosis or adjacent to joints with effusions. In some cases, detectable changes never appear on routine x-rays despite scan evidence of infarction.

LABORATORY STUDIES

Peripheral blood leukocyte counts are generally elevated during crises. Sedimentation rates are less useful in sickle cell patients than in otherwise normal people as they may be abnormally low even in the presence of inflammation. Serum uric acid levels are often elevated, with both overproduction and impaired excretion of uric acid contributing to the hyperuricemia. Synovial effusions in sickle cell disease usually contain less than 1000 leukocytes/mm^3, although rare leukocyte counts up to 126,000 have been reported in patients who had no evident complicating infection or crystal-induced inflammation. Sickled cells can be seen in effusions but are also seen in joint effusions due to other diseases in patients with sickle cell disease or trait. Synovial biopsies generally show little inflammation but there is focal microvascular thrombosis.

DIFFERENTIAL DIAGNOSIS

Despite the frequent hyperuricemia, gouty arthritis is not especially common in sickle cell disease; however, it should be considered. Septic arthritis must be a frequent concern in the acute warm tender effusions in patients with fever and is an important reason to perform arthrocenteses in sickle cell patients. The periosteal elevation from cortical infarctions might suggest hypertrophic pulmonary osteoarthropathy. Sickle cell patients, however, do not have the typical clubbing. Extensive medullary changes from marrow infarcts may be difficult to distinguish from osteomyelitis.

THERAPY

Acute arthralgias and joint effusion require no specific treatment, for they resolve with the hydration, analgesia, and occasional oxygen used for crises in general. Early aseptic necrosis of weight-bearing joints can be treated with limitation of weight bearing. Joints destroyed by aseptic necrosis have been successfully treated with total hip and knee replacements. Preoperative transfusion to a good level of hemoglobin, hydration, avoidance of hypoxia during surgery, and omission of use of a tourniquet during surgery are suggested precautions.

PATHOGENESIS

Sickling of red cells in the microcirculation is the likely mechanism for the thromboses and infarctions demonstrable in synovium and bone. This microvascular injury is suggested as a factor in the noninflammatory joint effusions. Immune complexes have been detected in sickle cell patients but to date they have not been incriminated in any of the musculoskeletal changes. The occasional unexplained inflammatory and/or chronic arthritis might be related to immunologic mechanisms or to crystals such as apatite that are difficult to detect.

SICKLE CELL TRAIT

Although aseptic necrosis of bone has been reported in sickle cell trait, it is not clear that the association of aseptic necrosis or arthritis with trait (AS or AC) hemoglobins is more than would occur by chance. There is no evidence that the presence of AS or AC hemoglobin interferes with the performance of vigorous physical occupations. Situations causing low oxygen tension may cause attacks of pain at various sites.

REFERENCES

Alavi A, Schumacher HR, Dorwart B, Kuhl DE: Bone marrow scan evaluation of arthropathy in sickle cell disorders. Arch Int Med 136:436, 1976

Dorwart BB, Goldberg MA, Alavi A, Schumacher HR: Absence of increased frequency of bone and joint disease with Hemoglobin AS and AC. Ann Intern Med 86:55, 1977

Schumacher HR: Rheumatological manifestations of sickle cell disease and other hereditary hemoglobinopathies. Clin Rheum Dis 1:37, 1975

Walker BR, Alexander F: Uric acid excretion in sickle cell anemia. JAMA 215:255, 1971

OTHER HEMOGLOBINOPATHIES

Unexplained degenerative changes and "synovitis" have been mentioned in a few patients with β-thalassemia major and thalassemia minor. A single patient with thalassemia minor has been reported with multiple areas of aseptic necrosis. A degenerative arthropathy with iron deposition in synovium similar to that seen in hemochromatosis has been found in one patient with thalassemia and repeated transfusions.

Homozygous hemoglobin C or hemoglobin C trait has not been associated with musculoskeletal problems.

Patients with sickle cell–thalassemia or hemoglobin C have been described with acute and chronic arthritis, infarctions and aseptic necrosis, hand–foot syndrome, and septic complications as described in the preceding chapter.

REFERENCES

Gratwick GM, Bullough PG, Bohne WHO, Markenson AL, Peterson CM: Thalassemic arthropathy. Ann Intern Med 88:494, 1978

Schumacher HR: Rheumatological manifestations of sickle cell disease and other hereditary hemoglobinopathies. Clin Rheum Dis 1:37, 1975

LEUKEMIA

Musculoskeletal manifestations can be early signs, and in fact the mode of presentation, of acute or chronic leukemia. Reports of arthritis are more frequent in children and in acute leukemia than in adults and chronic leukemia.

CLINICAL PICTURE

In acute leukemia, arm and leg pain have been reported to occur in 15 percent or more of patients. Some patients actually have painful, swollen joints. Arthritis is usually polyarticular and sometimes has an additive or migratory pattern. Knees and ankles are most often involved but most joints, including fingers, can be. Joints are symmetrically affected in about 50 percent of cases. Bone pain in the extremities or back may also be present, and bone involvement adjacent to joints can be confused with arthritis. Pain is often severe and out of proportion to the amount of objective arthritis. There may be fever. Leukemic skin infiltrates can superficially mimic rheumatoid nodules or vasculitis. Similar infiltrates in finger tips can resemble clubbing.

In chronic lymphocytic or myelocytic leukemia, joint involvement can be similar to that in acute leukemias. Joints can become involved in early or established disease. Bone tenderness, especially over the sternum, may suggest chronic myelocytic leukemia. Arthritis in both acute and chronic leukemia seems to be related to disease activity but can antedate diagnosed leukemia by more than 1 year.

RADIOLOGIC FINDINGS

X-rays of involved joints are normal in at least 50 percent of cases but can show juxtaarticular demineralization, transverse metaphyseal lucent bands and effusion, or, less often, sclerosis, osteolytic defects, or periosteal elevation. Destructive bone lesions in chronic granulocytic leukemia may be due to infiltration of blast forms and herald the progression into blastic transformation.

LABORATORY STUDIES

Smears of peripheral blood and even bone marrow examinations may not be diagnostic of leukemia in early disease. Occasional low-titer positive tests for rheumatoid factor or antinuclear antibodies are found and hyperuricemia is common. Sedimentation rates are frequently elevated in leukemia with or without arthritis. Hypercalcemia can occur.

Synovial effusions were mildly inflammatory, with a mean leukocyte count of 5500 cells/mm³ and a predominance of polymorphonuclear leukocytes in one series that included both lymphocytic and myelocytic leukemias. A synovial fluid leukocyte count of 90,000 with 99 percent polymorphonuclear leukocytes has been reported in a patient with acute lymphocytic leukemia in whom no crystals were present and cultures were negative. Blast forms seem to be found in synovial fluid very rarely. Synovial biopsies in several studies have shown blastic cells infiltrating synovium, but these are not invariably found. Similar leukemic infiltrates may also involve adjacent bone and periosteum.

DIFFERENTIAL DIAGNOSIS

Acute rheumatic fever is mimicked by the migratory or additive onset of arthritis. Fever and polyarthritis as seen in leukemia may also mimic Still's disease. Systemic lupus erythematosus may be suggested by the arthritis and pancytopenia occasionally seen in leukemia. Infectious arthritis can complicate leukemia, usually in patients already treated with steroids and chemotherapy. Hemorrhage into joints can result from the thrombocytopenia of leukemia. Secondary gout can occur occasionally with chronic myelocytic leukemia and possibly with other leukemias, but it is more common in myeloid metaplasia and polycythemia. Methotrexate has been felt to cause bone pain that resolves with discontinuation of the drug.

THERAPY

Aspirin or indomethacin may give temporary symptomatic relief, but the response of leukemia to chemotherapy almost always is accompanied by resolution of the arthritis. Allopurinol and forcing of fluids should be used with chemotherapy to decrease secondary gout and the risk of uric acid nephrolithiasis.

PATHOGENESIS

Some articular problems in leukemia are clearly associated with local infiltration of malignant cells. Whether other mechanisms such as immune complexes are involved is not known.

Leukemia is not generally felt to be seen with any increased incidence in rheumatoid arthritis, although one series included 7 cases of rheumatoid arthritis and chronic lymphocytic leukemia. Rheumatoid patients treated with azathioprine and cyclophosphamide may well be at an increased risk of developing chronic my-

elogenous leukemia. Patients with ankylosing spondylitis treated with irradiation to the spine have developed chronic myelogenous leukemia.

REFERENCES

Spilberg I, Meyer GJ: The arthritis of leukemia. Arthritis Rheum 15:630, 1972

LYMPHOMA

Bone involvement is common in malignant lymphomas and has been seen at autopsy in up to 50 percent of patients with Hodgkin's disease. Less often, there is invasion of synovial membrane, causing actual arthropathy.

CLINICAL PICTURE

Patients with lymphomas may develop bone pain in late disease or rarely present with bone involvement as an initial or sole manifestation. Joint pain and swelling has been reported to be episodic and unexplained for several years preceding the diagnosis of lymphoma or reticulum cell sarcoma in adjacent bones. Articular manifestations have been mon- or polyarticular and have been sufficiently variable to mimic rheumatoid arthritis, rheumatic fever, and a variety of other systemic diseases with rheumatic manifestations. Relapsing polychondritis has been reported in association with Hodgkin's disease.

RADIOLOGIC FINDINGS

Radiolucent areas at sites of bone pain and adjacent to joint effusions are typical. These may not be detectable on initial films, so that laminograms and sequential x-rays may be needed. Proximal bones tend to be more commonly involved than distal ones. Diffuse osteopenia with compression fractures can result from lymphomatous as well as myeloma bone involvement.

LABORATORY STUDIES

Anemia, hyperuricemia, and mildly elevated sedimentation rates can be seen. Synovial effusions have rarely been studied, but an effusion in one patient with an unspecified lymphoproliferative disease had malignant-appearing cells.

Lymphomatous invasion can be shown in bone and occasionally in synovial membrane. Synovium adjacent to tumors in bone often shows chronic inflammation with both lymphocytes and plasma cells, as well as lining cell proliferation and some fibrin deposition that might superficially be confused with rheumatoid arthritis.

DIFFERENTIAL DIAGNOSIS

The marked lymphadenopathy occasionally seen in rheumatoid arthritis can be confused with lymphoma. Lymph node biopsies in rheumatoid arthritis may be difficult to distinguish from those in chronic follicular lymphoma. Mediastinal Hodgkin's disease has produced hypertrophic osteoarthropathy with joint effusions. Secondary gout can occur in lymphomas and lymphoma may complicate Sjögrens syndrome. Although lymphomas, systemic lupus erythematosus, and other rheumatic diseases have been found to coexist, there is no firm evidence of any increased association. Unusual cerebral and occasionally other lymphomas have been described after immunosupressive therapy in systemic lupus erythematosus.

THERAPY

Radiation to sites of bone and synovial lesions as well as chemotherapy can alleviate pain and cause regression of radiologic changes. Irradiation of small areas of involved bone has been said to decrease pain in other involved areas as well.

REFERENCES

Emkey RD, Ragsdale BD, Ropes MW, Miller W: A case of lymphoproliferative disease presenting as juvenile rheumatoid arthritis. Diagnosis by synovial fluid examination. Am J Med 54:825, 1973

Green JA, Dawson AA, Walker W: Systemic lupus erythematosus and lymphoma. Lancet 2:753, 1978

Reimer RR, Chabner BA, Young RC, Reddick R, Johnson RE: Lymphoma presenting in bone. Ann Int Med 87:50, 1977.

Tumors of Joints and Other Synovial Structures

Juan J. Canoso

SYNOVIAL TUMORAL CONDITIONS

These conditions arise from metaplasia and proliferation of mesenchymal components of the synovial membrane. Joint swelling occurs as a result of synovial growth and effusion. In pigmented villonodular synovitis, the proliferating tissue tends to invade bone, while synovial osteochondromatosis may lead to mechanical derangement of the joint.

PIGMENTED VILLONODULAR SYNOVITIS (PVNS)

This proliferative disorder of the synovial tissue may be diffuse and predominantly villous (DPVNS) or manifest as a single nodule or matted mass of villous projections (PNS). In DPVNS the synovium is reddish brown or chocolate brown and the surface is covered by beard-like villosities and nodules of varying sizes. The nodules of PNS may be sessile or stalked and may be brown to yellow, as are sometimes the largest nodules in DPVNS.

Similar cellular components are seen in the diffuse and nodular forms of the disease, although their relative proportions differ (Fig. 1). These components include (1) masses and sheaths of synovial-like cells that are often polyhedral and have a tendency to dissociate from each other, (2) hemosiderin in synovial cells, both in the lining and in the cellular aggregates, (3) foam cells, (4) multinucleated giant cells with central or peripheral nuclei, (5) fibrosis (which may indicate a tendency to spontaneous regression of the lesion) seen randomly in areas of DPVNS and as the major component of the nodule in

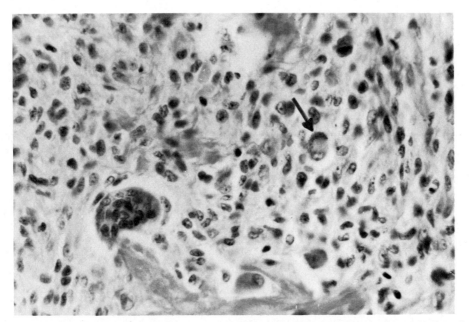

Fig. 1.   Pigmented villonodular synovitis. Synovial-like cells, macrophages containing hemosiderin, collagenous tissue, and a multinucleated giant cell are seen. In other parts of this specimen foam cells are prominent. H&E. ×200.

some cases of PNS, and (6) usually inconspicuous lymphoid and plasma cell infiltrates. Electron microscopic studies have shown a variable proportion of A, intermediate, and B type synoviocytes in the cellular infiltrates.

The etiology and pathogenesis of PVNS are entirely unknown. Its tendency to recur after resection and to invade bone locally led in the past to the consideration of a neoplastic etiology. Metastases, however, have never been demonstrated. Cultures of the lesion are negative. No lipid abnormalities are found to suggest a xanthomatous origin. Repeated intraarticular bleeding, perhaps due to sclerosing hemangiomas, has often been considered a possible pathogenetic mechanism for the lesion. In support of this view are the hemorrhagic characteristics of the synovial fluid, the hemosiderin deposits present in the lesion, and the knowledge that repeated intraarticular bleeding leads to chronic inflammation. However, the pathologic changes in hemophilic arthropathy differ from PVNS in that synovial cell aggregates are not present and foam cells and multinucleated giant cells are not conspicuous.

In one case of DPVNS, filamentous strands similar to myxovirus nucleoprotein were found within endothelial cells; however, they were considered products of autophagic activity and increased transport rather than viral particles. Another intriguing observation is the finding of predominantly type B and intermediate synovial cells in a lesion of PNS in a patient with rheumatoid arthritis suggestive of a B cell hyperplastic stimulus. In a case of DPVNS, there was of a lack of stimulation of peripheral lymphocytes by phytohemagglutinin and autologous synovial fluid, whereas there was significant stimulation when allogeneic rheumatoid arthritis synovial fluid was used.

Diffuse and nodular lesions of PVNS have a tendency to involve bone, probably at the site of entrance of nutrient vessels. Thus, large cystic bony erosions can be seen, usually at both sides of the joint. These cystic lesions are more common in joints enclosed by a tough capsule, such as the hip joint. In more compliant structures, such as the knee, erosions are rare, whereas capsular and ligamentous instability and Baker's cysts can occur.

Clinically, DPVNS occurs most often in females. Usually only one joint is involved, particularly the knee. The history is one of recurrent pain and swelling which may have led to repeated aspirations of brown or serosanguinous fluid. Radiographic studies seldom reveal cystic erosions in the knee; however, they are frequent in the hip, and involve the non-weight-bearing area of the acetabulum and head and neck of the femur. Arthrography delineates the pattern of intraarticular growth and helps to exclude other conditions that can lead to recurrent effusions. Arthroscopy can be extremely helpful for direct observation and biopsy leading to a histologic diagnosis. Angiography can be misleading, however, as the vascular pattern resembles the changes seen in malignant tumors.

DPVNS can also occur in bursae, particularly around the knee (i.e., the popliteal and the anserine bursae), and in the tendon sheaths of the wrist and ankle.

The nodular form of PVNS is uncommon in large joints but is quite prevalent in the distal portion of the limbs, particularly in the hands and feet. In the hand, PNS is the second most common benign tumoral condition, following ganglia, and usually presents as a slowly growing nodule in a finger.

Treatment of DPVNS is difficult and frustrating as synovectomy often fails to remove all the diseased synovium. In the knee, recurrences have been reported up to 40 percent of cases. Recurrent disease can be treated by further surgery, radiotherapy, and injection of radiocolloids. In some cases in which effusions are mild, the lesion is best left alone in the hope that the process will eventually burn out. In the hip, total hip replacement has been followed by apparent cures. When the nodular form of PNS occurs in the knee, surgical resection is generally successful. In the distal part of the limb, local recurrences have occurred in 27–60 percent of cases, particularly when bone invasion was present. A more radical type of excision is indicated in those cases.

SYNOVIAL OSTEOCHONDROMATOSIS

Proliferative changes in the synovial membrane of joints may result in the formation of multiple intrasynovial chondral or osteochondral nodules, a syndrome termed synovial osteochondromatosis. Although sometimes considered to be a form of neoplasia, the simultaneous formation of multiple, distinct lesions supports a reactive process for most cases. Proliferation of cartilage and local calcification as well as ossification are observed intrasynovially. In some patients, free osteochondral bodies appear in the joint space, apparently by detachment from their synovial site of origin. Reabsorption of either intrasynovial deposits or free bodies may occur at any time.

Many cases of this disease probably are undetected during the cycle of intrasynovial proliferation and resorption because symptoms are absent or minimal. The onset is insidious and progression slow. Involvement is characteristically monarticular, mainly in the knee but occasionally in the elbow, ankle, shoulder, and hip. Bursae and tendon sheaths may be affected by the same process. Adult males are usually affected by this uncommon disease. When symptomatic, a longstanding history of solitary joint pain with swelling and decreased range of motion is noted.

On the roentgenogram, multiple small paraarticular, amorphous calcifications are seen with good preservation of the articular surface; these features help distinguish this entity from degenerative joint disease, osteochondritis dissecans, neuropathic joint, tuberculous arthritis, and osteochondral fracture. All of these disorders tend to involve the articulating surfaces and generally produce larger, denser loose bodies. Dye contrast arthrography may be particularly useful when routine films fail to show calcification. In this instance, multiple small, sharply defined defects are observed in the synovium.

Although spontaneous regression has occurred and good results have been reported with simple removal of loose bodies, the treatment of choice is synovectomy. As extensive a procedure as possible is recommended to remove as much as possible of the involved synovium. Recurrences are infrequent, but occasionally local invasion of juxtaarticular bone or soft tissue develops.

BENIGN NEOPLASMS AND MALIGNANT NEOPLASMS

Tumors of joints are quite uncommon. They are usually first encountered by, or referred to, orthopedic surgeons due to symptoms suggestive of internal derangement of a joint or for evaluation of an articular or paraarticular mass. Metastatic involvement of joints is rare and usually occurs in patients with overly disseminated carcinoma.

A simple classification of joint tumors is given in Table 1.

BENIGN NEOPLASMS
Hemangiomas

These vascular tumors predominate in the younger age group and are often associated with cutaneous angiomas. Some are strictly intraarticular, while others involve the capsule and surrounding soft tissues. Synovial hemangiomas may be diffuse or only a single sessile or pedunculated lesion may be found.

The knee is the joint most often involved. Episodic swelling associated with acute pain and repeated aspirations of bloody fluid in the absence of trauma are suggestive of the diagnosis. Radiographic studies may be normal

Table 1
Tumors of Joints and Other Synovial Structures

I. Tumoral conditions
    A. Pigmented villonodular synovitis (articular, bursal, tenosynovial, fascial, ligamentous)
    B. Synovial osteochondromatosis (articular, bursal, tenosynovial)

II. Benign neoplasms
    A. Hemangioma (articular, tenosynovial)
    B. Lipoma
        Arborescens (articular, bursal, tenosynovial)
        Capsular (articular)
    C. Fibroma (articular)

III. Malignant neoplasms
    A. Primary: synovial sarcoma (rarely articular)
    B. Other synovial malignancies
        1. Synovial chondrosarcoma (articular)
        2. Synovial clear cell sarcoma (fascia, tendons)
        3. Synovial epithelioid sarcoma (fascia, tendons, aponeurosis)
    C. Metastatic joint tumors

or may reveal soft tissue shadows in which the presence of phleboliths is virtually diagnostic. Late changes indicative of longstanding, recurrent intraarticular bleeding include enlarged epiphyses, joint narrowing, and enlargement of the intercondylar notch, resembling the findings in hemophilic arthropathy.

Arteriography is useful for determining the extraarticular extent of the lesion, while arthrography allows delineation of its intraarticular contour, thus facilitating the treatment (i.e., surgical excision).

Lipomas

Articular lipomas are exceedingly rare. Chronic irritation of the subsynovial fat, however, can lead to hyperplastic and inflammatory changes in the fat pad (Hoffa's disease). Another condition occasionally seen is the "lipoma arborescens," which is characterized by fatty villous projections of the synovial membrane. It may occur in joints, bursae, and tendon sheaths. Fibromas are also quite rare.

MALIGNANT NEOPLASMS
Synovial Sarcoma

This is a relatively rare example (occurring in about 10 percent of cases) of soft tissue sarcomas. Its synovial origin has been assumed based on its appearance upon light microscopy. However, the rare articular location of the tumor plus certain ultramicroscopic findings not present in synovium raise some questions about its histogenesis.

Histologically, synovial sarcoma is a biphasic sarcoma comprised of an epithelial-like component resembling synovial cells, lining clefts and cysts with a mucinous content, and a spindle cell stroma with the appearance of fibrosarcoma (Fig. 1). The relative proportions of these two components vary within a tumor and among different tumors. Electron microscopic studies have shown that the epithelial-like cells have maculae adherentes and desmosomes in their attachments with neighboring cells, and a basal lamina separates the epithelial-like cells and the spindle cell stroma. None of these structures are present in normal synovium, although some can appear in reactive situations.

Clinically, synovial sarcoma can appear at any age, although it predominates in young adults. Males are slightly more frequently affected than females. Patients present with a growing mass in a lower or upper extremity, pain and diffuse swelling when the lesion is deep seated, or clinical evidence of neck, chest, retroperitoneal, or abdominal wall tumor.

Diagnosis and treatment of synovial sarcoma follows the guidelines applicable to soft tissue sarcomas in general. When such a lesion is suspected, an open-wedge biopsy is the best method for diagnosis. If positive, wide resection is undertaken. The extent is dictated by the anatomic position of the tumor. Radical lymph node dissection is usually included. Preoperative radiotherapy, as well as perfusion chemotherapy, may allow preservation of a functional limb. Postoperative chemotherapy

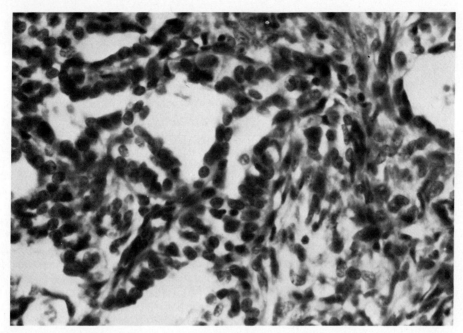

Fig. 1. Synovial sarcoma. Cavities lined by epithelial-like cells contain trace of mucinous material. The stroma has the appearance of fibrosarcoma. H&E. ×200.

and chemoimmunotherapy may be of value. Local recurrences and metastatic disease are treated by irradiation and chemotherapy (Adriamycin has been the agent most often used) as well as by resection of isolated metastases.

The prognosis of synovial sarcoma appears to relate to host and tumor factors. Sarcomas in the very young or very old, tumors located in "exposed" areas, and small tumors (less than 5 cm in diameter) carry a more favorable prognosis. Recent experience has indicated a 5-year survival rate of 28–50 percent and a 10-year survival rate of up to 30 percent.

Other Malignant Neoplasms Related to Synovial Structures

Synovial chondrosarcoma.   This lesion has most infrequently arisen from what appears to have been a bona fide preceding synovial chondromatosis.

Clear cell sarcoma.   This sarcoma occurs predominantly in tendinous or aponeurotic structures of the foot. Monomorphous nests or sheaths of pale, polyhedral cells usually containing glycogen characterize this highly malignant tumor.

Epithelioid sarcoma.   This is a polymorphic tumor which at times has been confused with inflammatory granulomas or metastatic carcinoma. It occurs preferentially in the distal portions of the upper extremity in relation to tendinous and aponeurotic structures. It has a high degree of malignancy.

Metastatic Joint Tumors

Metastatic involvement of joints is unusual, considering the enormous vascular supply of synovial tissue and its proximity to bone, which is a prime site for metastases. Most reported cases have involved the knee. In general, metastatic disease has been obvious at the time the pain or effusion developed. Radiographic studies are helpful in that lytic lesions of the patella, femoral condyle, or proximal tibia are often found. Synovial fluid aspiration has allowed identification of malignant cells in some cases, and needle synovial biopsy may reveal the structural features of the tumor.

REFERENCES

Ackerman LV, Spjut HJ, Abell MR (eds): Bones and Joints. Baltimore, Williams & Wilkins, 1976

Cohen AS, Canoso JJ: Tumors of synovium and related structures; Rheumatologic syndromes associated with nonhematologic malignances, in McCarty DJ Jr: Arthritis. Philadelphia, Lea & Febiger (in press)

Goldenberg DL, Kelley W, Gibbons RB: Metastatic adenocarcinoma of synovium presenting as an acute arthritis. Diagnosis by closed synovial biopsy. Arthritis Rheum 18:107, 1975

Granowitz SP, D'Antonio J, Mankin HL: The pathogenesis and long-term end results of pigmented villonodular synovitis. Clin Orthop 114:335, 1976

Hajdu SI, Shiu MH, Fortner JG: Tendosynovial sarcoma. A clinico-pathological study of 136 cases. Cancer 39:1201, 1977

Jaffe HL: Tumours and Tumorous Conditions of the Bones and Joints. Philadelphia, Lea & Febiger, 1958

Milgram JW: Synovial osteochondromatosis. A histological study of thirty cases. J Bone Joint Surg 59A:792, 1977

Hypertrophic Pulmonary Osteoarthropathy

H. Ralph Schumacher

CLINICAL AND LABORATORY FINDINGS

Hypertrophic osteoarthropathy (HOA) occurs in about 4 percent of primary pulmonary neoplasms but it is also occasionally associated with other diseases in the lung and a variety of other sites. Presently about 90 percent of cases are due to bronchogenic carcinoma. The condition is characterized by clubbing of the fingers and toes, tender periosteal reaction with new bone formation, and frequent joint effusions. HOA is often a clue to important underlying diseases, such as bronchogenic carcinoma, and must be differentiated from a similar idiopathic hereditary condition, pachydermoperiostitis. Clubbing alone also should be distinguished from the full-blown syndrome of HOA, as the former may be seen with pulmonary fibrosis, uncomplicated tuberculosis, biliary cirrhosis, sarcoidosis, local trauma, inflammatory bowel disease, and vascular anomalies without later HOA.

Clubbing of the fingers was recognized by Hippocrates but the first description of HOA is attributed to Bamberger in Germany and Marie in France in 1889–1890. Despite widespread interest in HOA the mechanisms involved in pathogenesis are not known.

CLINICAL AND RADIOLOGIC
PICTURE

Clubbing of the fingers is characterized by softening and increased thickness of the nail bed. Loss of the normal angle between the nail and nail bed is almost always present. However, since clubbing may be subtle and a subjective bedside diagnosis, it is important not to exclude the possibility of HOA in patients felt not to have clubbing. Do not expect to see radiographic bone or periosteal changes at the clubbed digits in the absence of very advanced HOA. Clubbing is usually neither painful nor tender except when it develops extremely rapidly. Usually it occurs gradually and tends to antedate the other manifestations of HOA.

Joint pain and effusions also appear gradually and initially involve knees, ankles, wrists, and elbows. Joints may be warm, tender, or painful on motion, but there is also periarticular tenderness. Some patients have morning stiffness lasting up to 1 hour, making rheumatoid arthritis important in differential diagnosis. In chronic HOA, effusions can be large and very painful and there can be swelling around the small bones and joints of the hands and feet as well as more proximal sites such as the clavicles. Tenderness adjacent to joints can progress to identifiable swelling and induration. Gynecomastia has been reported in about 5 percent of cases of HOA.

X-rays almost always show periosteal elevation with a thin line of new periosteal bone at the distal ends of the long bones although this is occasionally not detectable at the onset of arthropathy (Fig. 1). Bone scans with ^{99m}Tc-diphosphonate may suggest periosteal involvement before x-ray changes are identifiable. Periosteal elevation in the hands and feet occurs in severe cases. Articular manifestations are chronic and are not migratory; they often persist for months without chest symptoms. Chest x-rays may be normal or nondiagnostic in early HOA due to a bronchogenic carcinoma detectable only by bronchoscopy or surgery.

A variety of diseases are less common causes of HOA; these include Hodgkin's disease in the mediastinum, metastatic tumors (predominantly sarcoma), pleural mesotheliomas (HOA is seen in 50 percent of patients with this uncommon tumor), cyanotic congenital heart disease, cystic fibrosis with pulmonary involvement, upper gastrointestinal neoplasm, endocarditis, infected vascular grafts (HOA is localized distally to the graft), bronchiectasis, lung abscess, and rarely with other hepatic and abdominal lesions.

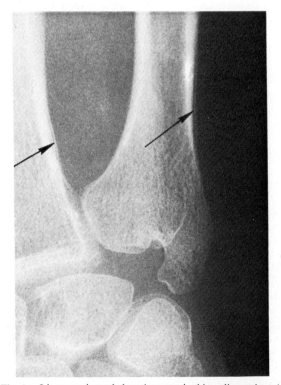

Fig. 1. Linear periosteal elevation seen in this radiograph at the arrows along the distal ulna and radium is typical of the moderate periosteal change in early hypertrophic pulmonary osteoarthropathy.

LABORATORY STUDIES

Sedimentation rates are almost always elevated in HOA due to bronchogenic carcinomas; they varied from 26 to 130 mm Westergren in one series. There are no specific laboratory abnormalities. Rheumatoid factor and antinuclear antibody are negative or only coincidentally positive.

Synovial effusions can be voluminous but tend to be clear, yellow, and normally viscous. The leukocyte count is usually less than 1000 cells/mm^3 and there are predominantly mononuclear cells. Some effusions clot spontaneously. Synovial biopsies early in HOA show mild lining cell proliferation, some congested and other occluded vessels, and only small numbers of lymphocytes. Lymphocytic infiltration can increase with chronic arthropathy.

DIFFERENTIAL DIAGNOSIS

Clubbing of the fingers can be confused with thyroid acropachy, which produces digital swelling and periosteal elevation along the phalanges but not at the distal long bones. Acromegaly must be distinguished because it may be mimicked by the diffuse thickening of extremities and occasional facial furrowing in HOA. Leukemic infiltrates in distal phalanges are rare but can produce a clubbed appearance.

The joint effusions of HOA must be distinguished from those of rheumatoid arthritis or other inflammatory rheumatic diseases. HOA especially mimics rheumatoid arthritis due to its symmetric warm, tender swelling of multiple joints, occasional morning stiffness, elevated sedimentation rates, and, as noted below, improvement with aspirin. Joint effusions in HOA however, have low leucocyte counts in contrast to rheumatoid arthritis. The low leucocyte counts may cause confusion with osteoarthritis and other noninflammatory arthropathies if the full clinical picture is not considered.

Other causes of multiple areas of periosteal new bone formation to be differentiated from the periosteal reaction of HOA include local trauma or inflammation, vasculitis, syphilis, hypervitaminosis A, Caffey's disease, leukemia or lymphoma, dysproteinemias, renal osteodystrophy, enterocolitis, and hyperphosphatemia. Periostitis occurs in psoriasis and Reiter's syndrome.

Pachydermoperiostitis is a familial condition with clubbing, periosteal elevation, and occasionally joint effusions clinically appearing identical to that of HOA. Patients with pachydermoperiostitis, as suggested by the name, also have varying degrees of thickening and furrowing of the skin that is more prominent on the forehead, scalp, and neck. Onset is usually gradual in adolescence but patients may not be aware of the findings until detected in later age on a medical examination. This syndrome is important to consider as it is not associated with underlying tumor. Mild joint stiffness is often the only symptom. Pachydermoperiostitis appears to be more common or at least more severe in men. Skin changes may not be evident in all cases with a familial syndrome resembling HOA. Excessive sweating may be seen with pachydermoperiostitis and also in some patients with hypertrophic pulmonary osteoarthropathy.

THERAPY AND PATHOGENESIS

Symptomatic relief of the painful arthropathy and periostitis can be dramatic with aspirin, indomethacin, or adrenocorticosteroids. Resection of lung tumors results in dramatic relief of joint and extremity pain in the first 24 hours. Swelling of joints and clubbing also rapidly decrease with successful tumor removal or improvement with radiation therapy. Periosteal changes on radiographs have been reported to decrease but only rarely disappear completely after removal to decrease but only rarely disappear completely after removal of tumors or vagotomy. Vagotomy, thoracotomy, or even laparotomy have been claimed to relieve symptoms promptly in some cases of HOA, but benefits from these procedures are not invariable. Periosteal changes may advance despite symptomatic improvement after vagotomy. Atropine, lumbar sympathectomy, or sympathetic blockade does not help in HOA. HOA may or may not exacerbate with tumor recurrence after surgery.

The relief of pain and decreased peripheral blood flow after vagotomy in patients with lung tumors have suggested that neurogenic factors may be involved in pathogenesis. Humoral mechanisms have also long been considered. The occurrence of HOA in patients with intrathoracic shunting of blood flow might be due to failure of removal of some humoral factor by the lungs. Cross-circulation studies in dogs with HOA were carried out for only 30 minutes and did not produce HOA in the recipient dog.

Electron-dense deposits have been seen in vessel walls in some synovial biopsies examined by electron microscopy in patients with bronchogenic carcinoma. Limited study with immunofluorescent techniques has not identified immunoglobulins in HOA synovium. It is still intriguing to speculate that these deposits might represent tumor antigen–antibody complexes (as have been seen in kidneys in patients with tumors and nephrotic syndrome) or some other tumor-related material.

Estrogen and growth hormone were considered in the past as possible humoral factors in HOA but they do not seem adequate explanations. There is an intriguing increased frequency or HOA with tumors in the periphery of the lung and pleura and with histologic types other than oat cell carcinoma. The development of HOA only distal to infected and possibly infected aortic grafts may favor a circulating factor.

Note that different mechanisms may be involved in clubbing and HOA as each can at least occasionally occur without the other. Digital capillary blood flow as measured by ^{85}Kr has been said to be increased in clubbing but studies using microspheres injected into the brachial artery of one patient with HOA suggested decreased blood flow to the area with periosteal change.

REFERENCES

Gall EA, Bennett GA, Bauer W: Generalized hypertrophic osteoarthropathy. A pathologic study of seven cases. Am J Pathol 27:349, 1951

Ginsburg J: Hypertrophic pulmonary osteoarthropathy. Postgrad Med J 39:639, 1963

Hammarsten JF, O'Leary J: The features and significance of hypertrophic osteoarthropathy. Arch Intern Med 99:431, 1957

Holling HE, Brody RS: Pulmonary hypertrophic osteoarthropathy. JAMA 178:977, 1961

King JO: Localized clubbing and hypertrophic osteoarthropathy due to infection in an aortic prosthesis. Br Med J 4:404, 1972

Lauter SA, Vosey FB, Höttner I, Osterland CK: Pachydermoperiostosis: Studies on the synovium. J Rheumatol 5:85–94, 1978

McLaughlin GE, McCarty DJ, Downing DF: Hypertrophic osteoarthropathy associated with cyanotic congenital heart disease. Ann Intern Med 67:579, 1967

Mendlowicz M: Clubbing and hypertrophic osteoarthropathy. Medicine (Baltimore) 21:269, 1942

Schumacher HR: Articular manifestations of hypertrophic pulmonary osteoarthropathy in bronchogenic carcinoma. A clinical and pathologic study. Arthritis Rheum 19:629, 1976

Vogel A, Goldfischer S: Pachydermoperiostosis. Am J Med 33:166, 1962

Crystal-induced Arthritis: Gout

HYPERURICEMIA

Gerald P. Rodnan

"Among all the Diseases that infect our Human Bodies, there is not one known hitherto, that more deservedly is called Opprobrium Medicorum, the Reproach of Physicians, than the Gout."
John Marten, *The Attila of the Gout*, 1713

Gout, a disease of long and distinguished lineage, is characterized by recurrent paroxysms of violent acute arthritis associated with the presence of microcrystals of monosodium urate monohydrate in the synovial fluid, and, in many cases, by the development of gross deposits of sodium urate (tophi) in joints, paraarticular tissues (including certain subcutaneous areas), and the kidneys. Approximately 15–20 percent of the patients have urinary calculi (uric acid). The term *gout* is derived from the Latin *gutta*, "a drop," and reflects the ancient belief that the disease was caused by a malevolent humour dropping into the weakened joints. Gouty arthritis represents a complication of prolonged hyperuricemia. In man who, unlike most other mammals, lacks the enzyme uricase, uric acid constitutes the major end product of the catabolism of purine. Uric acid is only sparingly miscible in body fluids, its solubility in plasma (and synovial fluid) being approximately 8.0 mg-dl. The often higher concentrations of serum urate found in gout and other hyperuricemic states are the result of supersaturation. The deposition of sodium urate (the chief compound of uric acid existing at body pH) takes place not only in gouty humans, but also occurs in those species of animals in which uric acid represents the major end product in the catabolism of amino acids as well as purine nitrogen. Thus, man finds himself in the company of uricotelic phyla—Insecta,

Aves, and Reptilia—the members of which are also subject to the development of tophaceous disease.

Gouty arthritis can be treated so effectively nowadays (see below) that it may be difficult to appreciate the dread once inspired by this disease. The "classic" case of far advanced disease has become increasingly uncommon and it is unusual now to see examples of the massive tophaceous deposits of the sort which gouty English clubmen boasted could be used to chalk their game scores. Every so often, however, one encounters patients in whom failure in diagnosis and/or lack of proper treatment have permitted the full expression of the disease, and one understands why in ages past the gout was known as the *opprobrium medicorum* (Fig. 1).

NORMOURICEMIA

The normal values for serum urate concentration in the adult are 5.1 ± 1.0 mg/dl in men and 4.0 ± 1.0 mg/dl in women (enzymatic uricase spectrophotometric method). The concentration is lower in children (3.5–4.0 mg/dl). In boys it rises to the adult level during puberty. There is little or no change in the concentration of serum urate in girls. As noted above, the value in mature women is normally slightly lower than that in men; this difference is attributable, at least in part, to the promotion of renal uric acid excretion by estrogenic hormones. Following cessation of the menses the serum urate level tends to rise and approaches that found in the male.

EPIDEMIOLOGY

In the population at large, serum urate levels fall on a bell-shaped distribution curve, with skewing toward the higher values. Serum urate concentration constitutes a continuous variable, similar to blood pressure, and represents the result of a complex multifactorial inheritance modified and influenced by numerous other factors, including diet, body weight, and hemoglobin level, as well as social class and drive. The interplay of genetic and

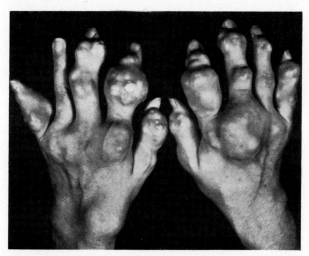

Fig. 1. Striking tophaceous deposits in the hands of a 38-year-old chef with inadequately treated gouty arthritis of many years duration. Such "textbook cases" have become rare, fortunately, but serve to explain the dread inspired by the gout in ages past.

environmental factors in the determination of hyperuricemia is illustrated by the observation of a significantly higher mean serum urate level in Filipinos in the United States compared to racially identical individuals living in the Philippines. The basis for this difference appears to lie in a limited ability to excrete uric acid which cannot compensate for the increased purine content in the usual U.S. diet.

In large-scale investigations of the serum urate concentrations in adult populations approximately 5 percent of those surveyed have been found to have hyperuricemia (most often of mild degree) at some time or another during the study period. Only a small minority of these individuals, however, have developed or are likely to develop gouty arthritis. It has been demonstrated that there is a direct relationship between the level of serum urate and both the likelihood of subsequent development of gouty arthritis and age at time of the initial attack. In many instances the absence of gout in hyperuricemic populations can be explained by a lack of sufficient severity and persistence in the hyperuricemia (various drugs and dietary factors may account for transient hyperuricemia). In other cases, however, the lifelong protection from deposition of urate in the tissues and freedom from gout in individuals with severe and prolonged hyperuricemia remains unexplained.

SERUM URATE LEVELS

All patients with gout, unless treated, have an increased quantity of dissolved urate in their extracellular fluid. Characteristically, and almost if not quite invariably, this is manifested by an elevated serum urate level—first detected by A. B. Garrod in 1848. The mean average level in untreated patients is 9–10 mg/dl. Individuals with chronic joint disease and those in whom the gout is secondary to a blood dyscrasia (see below) have signifi-

cantly higher concentrations of serum urate than the remainder.

REFERENCES

Hall AP, Barry PE, Dawber TR, McNamara PM: Epidemiology of gout and hyperuricemia. A long-term population study. Am J Med 42:27, 1967

Klinenberg JR (ed): Proceedings of the Second Conference on Gout and Purine Metabolism. Arthritis Rheum 18[Suppl]:659, 1975

Wyngaarden JB, Kelley WN: Gout and Hyperuricemia. New York, Grune & Stratton, 1976

METABOLIC ABNORMALITIES

Gerald P. Rodnan

URIC ACID METABOLISM IN NORMAL MAN

Uric acid is derived chiefly from the catabolism of purine formed in the de novo biosynthesis of nucleic acids (Figs. 1 and 2) and, to a lesser extent, from the breakdown of preformed purines taken in the diet. At the pH of body fluids, uric acid is present almost entirely in the ionized form as a monovalent urate ion. Since sodium is the principal extracellular cation, the solubility properties of uric acid in the body fluids will be predominantly those of monosodium urate. As estimated by the isotope-dilution method, the miscible pool of uric acid in a normal man averages about 1.20 g, with a range of 0.87–1.60 g.

In healthy individuals on a purine-free diet approximately 60 percent of this amount, or an average of 700 mg, is replaced daily by freshly elaborated uric acid (10 mg/kg body weight) resulting from the catabolism of adenine and guanine. This endogenous production of uric

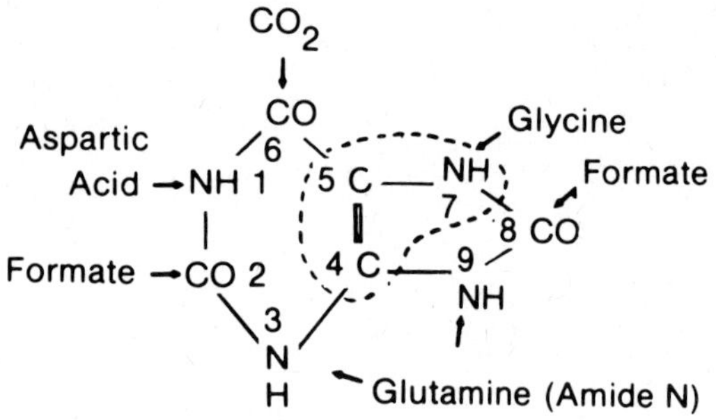

CO_2
↓
CO
Aspartic   ⁶
Acid → NH 1   5 C ——— NH   Glycine
| ‖   7   Formate
Formate → CO 2   4 C   8 CO
‖   9
3
N   NH
H   Glutamine (Amide N)

Fig. 1. Structure of uric acid, indicating the source of each carbon and nitrogen atom in the biosynthesis of purine.

acid is augmented by purine contained in foodstuffs (exogenous purine). Since the serum urate level in normal man is nearly twice that calculated to be present were the total body pool of uric acid uniformly distributed in body water, it is apparent that there are some intracellular compartments that contain relatively little uric acid. The concentration of urate in erythrocytes, for example, is about one-half that in plasma.

Approximately two-thirds of the uric acid formed each day is eliminated by the kidney. Following glomerular filtration, all or nearly all of the urate is reabsorbed in the proximal tubule. Urate is then excreted by a process of active tubular secretion, following which there may be some further postsecretory reabsorption. The quantity of uric acid found in the urine depends in part on the amount of ingested purine. In normal man taking a purine-restricted diet, urinary uric acid amounts to 420 ± 70–80 mg/24 hours; individuals whose food includes meat and

other purine-rich comestibles may excrete as much as 1000 mg/24 hours. Most of the remaining uric acid elaborated each day is excreted via the gastrointestinal tract. Normally little or no uric acid is found in the feces, however, since it is promptly degraded by the intestinal bacteria.

The pathways of both biosynthesis and reutilization of purine are controlled by feedback inhibition, a mechanism whereby the end product (in this case guanylic acid and adenylic acid) regulates its own rate of production by inhibiting the catalytic activity of the first enzyme, which is unique to the metabolic pathway in question. In this case the enzyme is amidophosphoribosyltransferase, which catalyzes the reaction between α-5-phospho-D-ribosyl-1-pyrophosphate (PP-ribose-P) and L-glutamine, the rate-limiting step in purine biosynthesis (Fig. 2). The basis for this inhibition has now been elucidated. Under the influence of purine nucleotides, two of the catalytically active, monomeric molecules of amidophosphoribosyltransferase join to form an inactive dimer. The latter in turn dissociates into active monomers upon the addition of PP-ribose-P.

ORIGINS OF HYPERURICEMIA

Although hyperuricemia which persists on a purine-free diet may thus theoretically be produced by a number of different mechanisms, in the great majority of cases it is the result of either an increase in the de novo (endogenous) biosynthesis of purines or faulty elimination of uric acid by the kidney, or a combination of these mechanisms (Table 1). Alterations in purine intake and the extrarenal disposal of uric acid generally have relatively little influence on the serum urate level, although in some

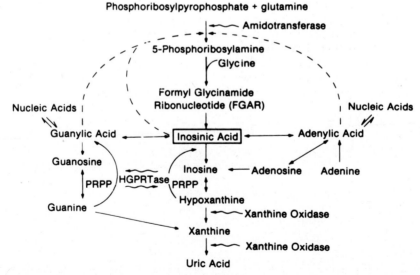

Fig. 2. Purine biosynthesis. The conjugation of α-5-phospho-D-ribosyl-1-pyrophosphate (PRPP) and L-glutamine, the first irreversible step in the de novo synthesis of purines, is catalyzed by the enzyme PRPP-glutamine amidotransferase and is regulated through feedback inhibition by purines and ribonucleotides, including guanylic acid, inosinic acid, and adenylic acid. Note the importance of the enzyme hypoxanthine–guanine phosphoribosyltransferase (HGPRTase) in the reutilization (salvage) of hypoxanthine and the feedback control mechanism.

Table 1
Origins of Hyperuricemia

I. Primary hyperuricemia
  A. Increased production of purine
    1. Idiopathic
    2. Specific enzyme defects (see Fig. 2)
      a. Enzymatic abnormalities leading to an increase in the availability of α-5-phospho-D-ribosyl-1-pyrophosphate (PP-ribose-P)
        i. Increase in the rate of synthesis of PP-ribose-P
          (a) PP-ribose-P synthetase, increased activity
          (b) Glucose-6-phosphatase deficiency [glycogen storage disease (GSD), type 1]
          (c) Glutathione reductase, increased activity (?)
        ii. Decrease in the rate of utilization of PP-ribose-P
          (a) Hypoxanthine-guanine phosphoribosyl-transferase (HGPRTase) deficiency complete deficiency (Lesch-Nyham syndrome) partial deficiency
      b. Enzymatic abnormalities leading to an increased concentration of L-glutamine
        i. Renal glutaminase I deficiency (?)
        ii. Glutamate dehydrogenase deficiency (?)
      c. Enzymatic abnormalities leading to a decrease in the intracellular pool of purine ribonucleotides
        i. Decrease in the production of purine nucleotides
          (a) HGPRTase deficiency
          (b) Xanthine oxidase, increased activity (? secondary alteration)
          (c) Adenosine kinase deficiency
        ii. Increase in the catabolism of purine nucleotides (no definite examples to date)
      d. Glutamine PP-ribose-P amidotransferase feedback resistance
  B. Decreased renal clearance of uric acid (idiopathic)

II. Secondary hyperuricemia
  A. Increased catabolism (turnover) of purine
    1. Myeloproliferative disorders
      a. Polycythemia, 1° or 2°
      b. Myeloid metaplasia
      c. Chronic myelocytic leukemia
    2. Lymphoproliferative disorders
      a. Chronic lymphatic leukemia
      b. Multiple myeloma
    3. Disseminated carcinoma and sarcoma
    4. Sickle cell anemia and other forms of chronic hemolytic anemia
    5. Psoriasis (uncommon)
    6. ? Paget's disease of bone
    7. Cytotoxic drugs
  B. Decreased renal clearance of uric acid
    1. Intrinsic disease of the kidney
      a. Chronic renal insufficiency of diverse cause
      b. Saturnine gout (lead nephropathy)
      c. Sickle cell anemia
      d. ? Hyperparathyroidism
    2. Functional impairment in tubular transport of uric acid
      a. Drug-induced; thiazide diuretics; furoseamide; ethacrynic acid; ethambutol; pyrazinamide; low doses of aspirin and probenecid
      b. Hyper-lactic-acidemia; lactic acidosis; ethanolism; preexlampsia; GSD, type I; chronic
      c. Hyperketoacidemia (acetoacetic and β-hydroxybutyric acids); diabetic ketoacidosis; starvation; GSD, type I
      d. Congenital vasopressin-resistant diabetes insipidus
      e. Bartter's syndrome (hyperaldosteronism and hypokalemic alkalosis)
      f. ? Hypoparathyroidism
      g. ? Hypothyroidism
      h. Down's syndrome

---

instances severe reduction in the dietary intake of purine may lead to correction of hyperuricemia (see below).

Glycine is one of the major precursors of the purine molecule (Fig. 1) and determination of the rate of incorporation of a labeled tracer dose of glycine into urinary uric acid provides a measure of de novo synthesis of purine. By use of this technique the hyperuricemia in approximately 75 percent of individuals with primary familial gout has been found to involve a defect in the regulation of purine metabolism which leads to the chronic overproduction of uric acid from simple nonpurine precursors. There is an increased proportion of intermediate nucleotides which appear to be shunted directly into metabolic pathways leading to uric acid formation without prior incorporation into nucleic acids. In only 10–25 percent of cases, however, is this overproduction reflected in an abnormally large excretion of urinary uric acid (>600 mg/24hours). In the others the overproduction of purine is combined with a disturbance in the renal disposal (tubular secretion) of uric acid; an inappropriately low rate of tubular secretion of urate in this group becomes increasingly apparent as the concentration of plasma urate rises.

An inability to compensate for urate load by increasing tubular secretion may be the abnormality responsible for hyperuricemia in those patients with primary gout who fail to present evidence of uric acid overproduction. In a recent study of this question the renal clearance of uric acid in a group of 46 gouty subjects with (otherwise) nearly normal kidney function (mean creatinine clearance 97 ± 26 ml/min) was found to be significantly lower (3.6 ml/min) than that of an equal number of controls (5.8 ml/min). The molecular mechanisms underlying this alteration in active urate transport have not been established.

PRIMARY VERSUS SECONDARY
GOUT

The term *primary gout* (or *primary familial gout*) is applied to those cases in which the underlying hyperuricemia is due to an inborn, genetically determined metabolic error leading to a pathologic increase in the de novo biosynthesis and/or retention of uric acid (*primary hyperuricemia*). In these cases, which constitute the great majority of patients with gout, there is a tendency toward familial aggregation of the disease and an increased prevalence of hyperuricemia (about 25 percent) in close relatives. The term *secondary gout* designates those cases in which the hyperuricemia responsible for development of the disease is the result of some other, acquired disorder or condition (*secondary hyperuricemia*) in which there is overproduction of uric acid consequent to an accelerated turnover of nucleic acid—e.g., polycythemia, myeloid metaplasia, sickle cell anemia and other hemoglobinopathies, and various other myeloproliferative diseases—and/or impairment in the disposal of uric acid by the kidney—e.g., various disorders in which there is an overall decrease in renal function or a specific defect in the tubular secretion of urate, or conditions leading to the generation of substances (e.g., certain small organic acids) that compete with urate for tubular secretory sites (Table 1).

Although the hyperuricemia found in individuals with primary gout is believed to be most often polygenic in origin, a number of specific single gene defects have

Table 2
Disorders Associated with Hypouricemia

Increased urinary excretion of uric acid
Healthy individuals with isolated defect in tubular reabsorption of uric acid (Dalmation dog mutation)
Diminished reabsorption of urate: Fanconi syndrome, Fanconi syndrome associated with Wilson's disease, carcinoma of the lung, acute myelogenous leukemia, light chain disease, out-dated tetracycline, ? alcoholism
Malignant neoplasm: carcinoma, Hodgkin's disease, sarcoma
? Excessive tubular secretion of uric acid: Hodgkin's disease, hyperparathyroidism
Hypervolemia 2° to inappropriate antidiuretic hormone secretion
Drugs: aspirin, probenecid and other uricosuric agents, allopurinol, glyceryl guaiacholate
Radiographic contrast agents: iopanoic acid (Telopaque), iodipamide meglumine (Cholografin), diatrizoate sodium (Hypaque)
Severe liver disease, ? hyperbilirubinemia

Decreased production of uric acid
Heritable deficiencies in enzymes involved in purine biosynthesis: PP-ribose-P synthetase deficiency, adenosine deaminase deficiency, purine nucleoside phosphorylase deficiency, xanthine oxidase deficiency (xanthinuria)
Acquired deficiency in xanthine oxidase activity (metastatic adenocarcinoma of lung)
Acute intermittent porphyria
? Pernicious anemia

now been identified which account for the accelerated rate of purine biosynthesis underlying the hyperuricemia in a small proportion of cases (Table 1). An example is the enzyme defect responsible for the Lesch-Nyhan syndrome (M. Lesch and W. L. Nyhan, 1954), a rare sex-linked disorder of young boys characterized by choreoathetosis, spasticity, mental retardation, and compulsive self-mutilation, which has been traced to a virtually complete absence of activity of the enzyme hypoxanthine–guanine phosphoribosyltransferase (HGPRTase). This enzyme is responsible for the conversion of hypoxanthine and guanine into nucleotides that normally serve to control the rate of de novo purine biosynthesis (Fig. 2). In the child who lacks this enzyme there is strikingly excessive generation of uric acid, which eventually gives rise to severe tophaceous gout. A heritable *partial* insufficiency of HGPRTase has been shown to be responsible for 1–2 percent of primary familial gout. In the great majority of cases, however, the etiology of the hyperuricemia in primary gout is as yet unexplained.

There are several varieties of secondary hyperuricemia and gout in which the role of renal underexcretion is now clearly established. In type 1 glycogen storage disease (glucose-6-phosphatase deficiency) there is evidence of both an abnormally increased synthesis of uric acid and a diminished renal clearance of uric acid, the latter ascribable to a chronic elevation of plasma lactate and ketoacids (acetoacetic and β-hydroxybutyric acids) which inhibit the tubular secretion of uric acid. Gouty arthritis and gouty nephropathy (see below) often develop into major clinical problems in these patients when they reach adulthood. A renal mechanism is also responsible, at least in part, for the hyperuricemia in sickle cell disease and saturnine gout and that which develops in patients who are being treated with certain drugs, most notably thiazides (Table 1).

The gout that occurs in the wake of various myeloproliferative disorders is similar to primary gout in its clinical characteristics, although the average age of onset and relative frequency with which women are affected are both greater in the secondary form of the disease. In further contrast, a history of familial involvement is unusual in secondary gout and there is a tendency toward higher serum urate levels and greater urinary uric acid excretion. Accordingly, there is a much higher incidence of tophus and uric acid stone formation. Despite the similarities in the clinical and pathologic features of primary and secondary gout, there is a basic difference in the origin of the hyperuricemia in the two conditions. When patients with secondary gout due to polycythemia or myeloid metaplasia are given labeled purine precursors, the amount of isotope that accumulates in urinary uric acid is much greater than that observed in normal subjects. The rate at which this incorporation occurs is slower than the rapid enrichment of urinary uric acid often found in primary gout, which has been attributed to de novo synthesis of uric acid without prior incorporation of the isotope into nucleic acids. In secondary gout the findings are consistent with the belief that the hyperuricemia is the result of hyperactive turnover of nucleoprotein.

HYPOURICEMIA

Either a decreased production of uric acid (resulting most often from a heritable deficiency in various enzymes involved in the biosynthesis of purine) or a pathologic urinary loss of uric acid (resulting in most cases from defective tubular reabsorption of urate) may give rise to hypouricemia (Table 2). In the great majority of instances, however, hypouricemia is the result of the use of various uricosuric drugs and is of little or no clinical consequence.

REFERENCES

Dwosh IC, Roncari DAK, Marliss E, Fox IH: Hypouricemia in disease: A study of different mechanisms. J Lab Clin Med 90:153, 1977

Klinenberg JR (ed): Proceedings of the Second Conference on Gout and Purine Metabolism. Arthritis Rheum 18[Suppl]:659, 1975

Rieselbach RE, Steele TH: Influence of the kidney upon urate homeostasis in health and disease. Am J Med 56:665, 1974

Sorensen LB, Levinson DJ: Origin and extrarenal elimination of uric acid in man. Nephron 14:7, 1975

Wyngaarden JB, Kelley WN: Gout and Hyperuricemia. New York, Grune & Stratton, 1976

CLINICAL FEATURES AND PATHOGENESIS

Gerald P. Rodnan

In the majority of cases of gout, recurring bouts of acute joint inflammation constitute the first manifestation of the disease; in approximately one-fifth of the patients, arthritis is preceded by evidence of nephrolithiasis (see below). Gouty arthritis is a disorder chiefly of middle-aged and older men (who constitute 85–90 percent of patients) and of postmenopausal women; there is often a family history of the disease. It is the most common form of inflammatory joint disease in men past 40 years of age. Although the disease may commence as early as the second decade of life in the rare individuals with a heritable deficiency in HGPRTase or some other enzymatic disturbance leading to congenital hyperuricemia, the peak period of onset of gouty arthritis falls in the fourth and fifth decades, and it is not unusual for individuals to first experience gout as septuagenarians.

ACUTE GOUTY ARTHRITIS

The inaugural attacks are typically monarticular (uncommonly oligoarticular) and tend to affect first the lower extremities, particularly the first metatarsophalangeal (MTP) and tarsal joints, the ankles, and the knees. The great toe is the most common site of initial involvement, and inflammation of the first MTP (podagra) occurs in 75 percent or more of all patients.

In the beginning there may be intervals of many months or years between the paroxysms of gouty inflammation, but in time there is a tendency toward increasingly frequent and severe attacks that come to affect more and more parts, including the finger joints, wrists, and elbows; olecranon bursitis develops with notable frequency. Inflammation of the shoulder and hip are uncommon, however, and involvement of the sacroiliac and other intervertebral articulations is rare. At first, the joints appear to return to a quite normal state between attacks, but in time, as the disease tightens its grip, swelling and disability persist for longer and longer periods and eventually become permanent (chronic gouty arthritis). In this later stage of the disease erosion of articular cartilage and subchondral bone caused by the inflammatory reaction to tophaceous matter may lead to severe joint deformity and disability (Figs. 1–3).

In contrast to most other types of arthritis, the onset of joint inflammation in acute gout (which often occurs at night) is very abrupt, and, typically, maximal pain and swelling are reached within 24 hours. The affected joint tends to be markedly swollen and exquisitely painful and tender. There is generally a considerable degree of periarticular swelling and erythema (dusky redness in the case of the great toe). This feature, combined with the low-grade fever and leukocytosis which often accompany the attack, frequently gives rise to the mistaken impression of cellulitis or thrombophlebitis. Thomas Sydenham, himself a victim of the disease, described (1683) the attack as follows:

The victim goes to bed and sleeps in good health. About two o'clock in the morning he is awakened by a severe pain in the great toe; more rarely in the heel, ankle, or instep. This pain is like that of a dislocation, and yet the parts feel as if cold water were poured over them. Then follow chills and shivers, and a little fever. The pain, which was at first moderate, becomes more intense. With its intensity the chills and shivers increase. After a time this comes to its height, accommodating itself to the bones and ligaments of the tarsus and metatarsus. Now it is a violent stretching and tearing of the ligaments—now it is a gnawing pain, and now a pressure and tightening. So exquisite and lively meanwhile is the feeling of the part affected, that it cannot bear the weight of the bedclothes nor the jar of a person walking in the room. The night is passed in torture, sleeplessness, turning of the part affected, and perpetual change of posture.

Mild attacks of the gout usually last for several days if untreated, while more severe seizures may persist for several weeks. Desquamation of the overlying skin may occur with resolution of the inflammation, following which the joint returns to its previous state. Many patients experience numerous minor fits of joint inflammation in addition to the classically florid attacks.

INTERCRITICAL GOUT

During the interval between attacks the patient with early gout is usually entirely asymptomatic and no abnormalities may be found on examination of the joints. Several years may elapse between the first and second episodes of gouty arthritis, but as the years pass these paroxysms tend to become more frequent and more severe, often involving more than one joint at a time and persisting for longer and longer periods.

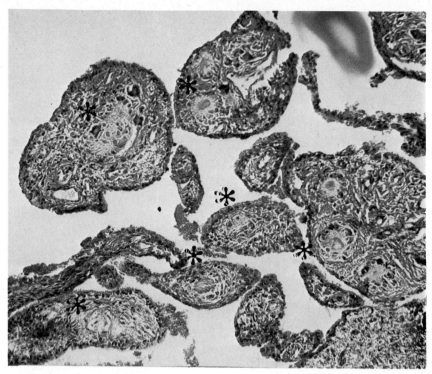

Fig. 1. Photomicrograph of synovium (knee) of a 46-year-old man who had sustained repeated attacks of gouty arthritis for 15 years. Note numerous small tophaceous deposits with surrounding giant cell reaction (asterisks).

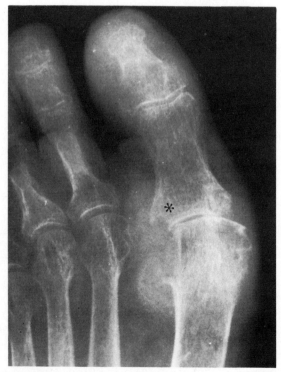

Fig. 2. Roentgenogram of left great toe of a 52-year-old man with chronic tophaceous gout. Note erosion at base of the proximal phalanx (asterisk) with overhanging edge of bone.

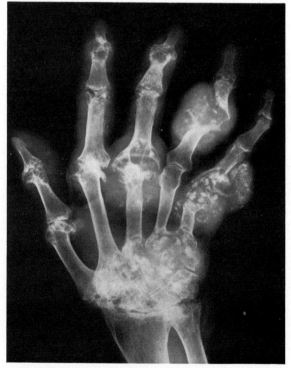

Fig. 3. Roentgenogram demonstrating severe destructive changes in the right hand of a 62-year-old man with chronic tophaceous gout who had been erroneously thought to have rheumatoid arthritis for many years.

CHRONIC TOPHACEOUS GOUT

Prior to the introduction of effective drugs for the control of hyperuricemia, approximately 50–60 percent of gouty patients developed clinically or radiographically detectable deposits of monosodium urate monohydrate in their tissues (Figs. 1–3; also see Fig. 1 in the chapter on Hyperuricemia). The ancients referred to these concretions or "articulation badges" of the gout as tophi (from the Greek, "chalk stone") in the belief that they represented an inspissated earthy humour. In 1797 W. H. Wollaston announced that the principal constituent of tophi was "a neutral compound, consisting of lithic [uric] acid and mineral alkali [sodium]." This epochal discovery provided the first direct evidence linking uric acid to the gout.

Tophi are rarely apparent at the time of the initial attack of gouty arthritis; they are generally first noted some time after onset, on an average of 10 years later. They occur most commonly in the synovium (Fig. 1), subchondral bone (Figs. 2 and 3), olecranon bursa, infrapatellar and Achilles tendons, and subcutaneous tissue on the extensor surface of the forearm and overlying the joints (see Fig. 1 in the chapter on Hyperuricemia). The traditional location, namely, the cartilage of the helix of the ear, is a relatively infrequent site for these deposits.

Histologically, the tophus consists of a nodular core of monosodium urate with a surrounding inflammatory reaction that includes foreign body type giant cells (Fig. 1). It may be difficult to distinguish tophi from rheumatoid nodules clinically. The former tend to be harder and may grow to be large and more irregular in shape; occasionally, the whitish contents of the tophus are apparent. The skin overlying bulky, more superficial tophi may ulcerate, with prolonged drainage of uratic matter. When there is any doubt concerning the tophaceous nature of a given subcutaneous nodule, it should be aspirated and examined for the typical needle-shaped crystals of monosodium urate monohydrate (first described by Leeuwenhoek) or removed in its entirety, fixed in absolute alcohol to prevent dissolution of the deposit, and scrutinized microscopically and chemically.

The presence of tophaceous deposits is associated with a tendency toward more frequent and severe episodes of acute gouty arthritis. Chronic gouty arthritis, with deformity of the joints, develops as a result of the erosion of cartilage and subchondral bone caused by the inflammatory reaction to articular tophaceous matter. Tophaceous deposits may also be responsible for carpal tunnel syndrome and trigger finger deformity as a result of infiltration of the flexor tendons and their sheaths. In exceptional instances tophi have been observed in the nasal cartilage, tongue, vocal cords, aorta, and myocardium. The destruction of joint cartilage in chronic gout may lead to severe secondary osteoarthritis with or without chondrocalcinosis.

Tophus formation is related to the serum concentration of urate, as well as to the local tissue factors. In general, the higher the serum urate level, the earlier the appearance and more extensive the development of tophi. These deposits are relatively uncommon in those individuals with gout whose serum urate concentration (untreated) is less than 8.5 mg/dl (enzymatic method).

GOUTY NEPHROPATHY

Individuals with longstanding gout often have kidney disease which is marked by proteinuria, diminution in concentrating capacity, and ultimately a decrease in creatinine clearance and azotemia. Uncommonly, severe renal insufficiency may develop. However, even in the era prior to the availability of highly effective serum urate–lowering treatment, only a small minority of gouty patients succumbed to renal failure; most died of cardiovascular or cerebrovascular disease after a life span similar to that of nongouty individuals. Histologic examination of the gouty kidney reveals a variety of abnormalities, the most distinctive and consistent of which is the presence of tophaceous masses in the interstitium of the renal medulla. Other pathologic changes, including calculus formation and pyelonephritis, are believed to be secondary to these deposits. In addition, it is common to find nephrosclerosis and other evidence of hypertensive disease. Recent studies indicate that the earliest abnormality is that of tubular damage (the result of intratubular deposition of uric acid) associated with an interstitial inflammatory reaction.

Striking increases in serum urate levels (40–60 mg/dl) may occur in patients with leukemia or lymphoma as a result of the rapid breakdown of cellular nucleic acid following aggressive treatment with corticosteroids, x-irradiation, and alkylating agents. The precipitation of uric acid in the renal tubules of such patients may lead to severe urinary obstruction with prolonged oliguria. This hazard can be prevented or reversed by treatment with allopurinol (see below).

URIC ACID STONE

In the United States uric acid stones represent about 10 percent of all urinary calculi. Such stones occur in approximately 15–20 percent of all patients with gout (and 40 percent of those with secondary gout). Uric acid stones are usually relatively small, smooth, and rounded and range in color from pale yellow through dark red to black. They are characteristically radiolucent, but some, particularly the larger ones, may contain calcium salts and hence may be radiopaque.

At customary urinary pH, uric acid is largely or completely nondissociated. Nonionized uric acid is less soluble than sodium urate and is markedly less soluble the more acid the pH. Normally the urine is most acid at night and in the early morning; the pH rises sharply in the morning and remains at only mildly acid levels for most of the day. In many patients with gout and uric acid nephrolithiasis the urine pH remains persistently low throughout the day, an abnormality which has been related to a deficiency in the production of ammonia buffer by the kidney. Other factors that contribute to uric acid stone formation are hyperuricosuria and contraction of urine volume. Urinary uric acid content varies with dietary purine intake (see preceding).

COMPLICATIONS AND ASSOCIATED DISEASES

Patients with gout have a higher frequency of arterial hypertension and renal malfunction than do nongouty individuals, and they are often found to have nephrosclerosis. The development of hyperuricemia in arterial hypertension appears to be related to an abnormality in uric acid transport by the renal tubules.

Diabetes mellitus, cardiac and cerebral atherosclerosis, and hypertriglyceridemia all occur more frequently among the gouty. The precise mechanism for these associations is not known, although a common connection with obesity has been suggested.

Avascular necrosis of bone, involving particularly the head of the femur, occurs with increased frequency in gouty individuals. In some instances this association may be related to chronic alcoholism (Chandler's disease). The presence of lipoprotein abnormalities (hyperlipoproteinemia types II and IV) in a number of these cases has led to the suggestion that the bone necrosis may be caused by fat emboli.

ROENTGENOGRAPHIC FINDINGS

At the time of the initial attack of gouty arthritis in younger individuals roentgenographic examination of the affected joint (most often the first MTP juncture) is usually normal. In older individuals there frequently are signs of (preexisting) osteoarthritis in this area. Later there is evidence of progressive damage of the articular cartilage and subchondral bone (Figs. 2 and 3). Emphasis has been placed on the presence of sharply defined marginal erosions of the subchondral bone at the periphery of which there may be a thin shell-like overhanging edge of bone (Fig. 2). Such erosions occur most commonly in the first MTP (particularly in the base of the proximal phalanx) but are also found in the finger joints and other articulations affected by the disease.

PATHOGENESIS OF ACUTE GOUTY ARTHRITIS

As noted above, monosodium urate is only sparingly soluble in body fluids and tends to precipitate in the tissues when the concentration in the plasma exceeds 8–9 mg/dl. There is a striking predilection for these deposits to form on the surface and within the substance of the articular cartilage as well as in the synovium and related paraarticular structures, including bursae, tendons, and tendon sheaths. The basis for this affinity, which may be related in some way to a preferential binding of urates to proteoglycans and other components of connective tissue, remains to be determined.

Attacks of joint inflammation (acute gouty arthritis) occur when microcrystals of monosodium urate monohydrate form within the joint cavity or, as is probably more common, are discharged into this cavity from preexisting intraarticular (cartilaginous) urate deposits ("crystal shedding"). Such crystals are invariably present (usually in abundance) in the synovial fluid of acutely inflamed joints, either contained within the cytoplasm of neutrophilic leukocytes or floating free. The volume of synovia in the swollen joint tends to be large (often 50 ml or more in the case of the knee) and characteristically there is a very high white cell count (often 15,000/mm^3 or greater) with a striking predominance of polymorphonuclear leukocytes. The crystals of monosodium urate monohydrate, which are rodlike or acerose (needle-shaped), average about 10 μm in length; they are best seen by means of polarized light and are negatively birefringent (Fig. 4). Experimental intrasynovial injection of these crystals produces inflammation closely similar to natural gout.

It has been shown that microcrystals of monosodium urate monohydrate (as well as other substances involved in the production of crystal-induced synovitis) are coated with plasma proteins, including immunoglobulins. The pesence of IgG on these crystals is believed to enhance their phagocytosis by neutrophilic leukocytes which carry Fc receptor sites on their surface. Once the microcrystals have been incorporated into phagolysosomes within the neutrophil the surface proteins are removed, restoring the microcrystals' membrane-disrupting capacity.

The phagocytosis of these microcrystals by polymorphonuclear leukocytes (and probably by phagocytic synovial lining cells as well) leads to the formation of a chemotactic factor that recruits additional leukocytes. Ingestion of urate crystals is followed by the rapid degranulation and disintegration of these cells, with release of both cytoplasmic and lysosomal enzymes that are responsible for dissolution of articular cartilage as well as injury to the soft tissue. (Note that urate crystals are *not* chemotactic per se but will increase random motility of leukocytes; phagocytosis is necessary for the production of chemotactic factor, which has been found to be a heat-labile glycoprotein with a molecular weight of 8400 daltons.)

The immediate mechanism of the initial crystallization is not fully known. In some instances gouty attacks take place after local trauma, which may rupture tophaceous deposits in the synovium and articular cartilage. More often, joint inflammation develops in the wake of rapid fluctuations in serum urate levels (see below). A sudden increase in serum urate concentration may lead to crystal precipitation in the already supersaturated synovial fluid, while a drop in serum urate concentration may give rise to the irregular dissolution of the surface of intraarticular tophi and the release of undissolved crystals. Gouty patients are also prone to develop acute arthritis following surgical procedures (postoperative gout), usually within a period of 72 hours.

EATING, DRINKING, AND THE GOUT

The connection of gout with gluttony and the belief that attacks of articular inflammation followed upon sacrifice at the altar of Bacchus and Venus—that is to say, intemperance and venery—date to ancient times and serve as the basis for the extensive use of the gouty foot

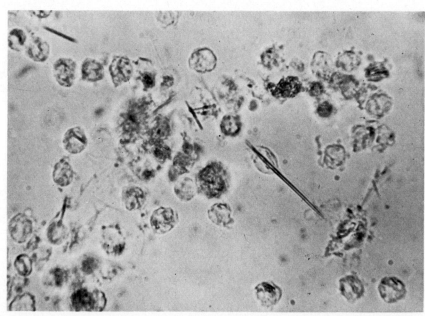

Fig. 4. Photomicrograph of fresh preparation of synovial fluid obtained from the inflamed knee of a 45-year-old man with acute gouty arthritis. Note numerous small and large needle-shaped crystals of monosodium urate monohydrate which have been engulfed by neutrophilic leukocytes.

as a symbol of overindulgence and ill-gotten gain in satirical works throughout the centuries. The association of primary gout with overeating and alcoholism is well documented. Approximately one-half of gouty individuals weigh 15 percent or more in excess of ideal weight, and 75 percent or more exhibit hypertriglyceridemia which appears to be correlated with the presence of obesity. It has been aptly noted that "the associates of a high [serum] uric acid are the associates of plenty."

The observation that uric acid synthesis (as measured by the incorporation of glycine into urinary uric acid) is accelerated when the diet is fortified with protein and reports of the occasional correction of hyperuricemia in obese individuals by severe weight reduction suggest that chronically excessive food intake may be of importance, at least in some cases, in the elevation in serum urate level. It is possible that the heightened synthesis of purine associated with obesity results from an increased availability of PP-ribose-P derived from ribose-5'-phosphate produced by stimulation of the pentose phosphate pathway during lipogenesis. This pathway is involved in the regeneration of reduced nicotinamide adenine dinucleotide (NADPH), which is consumed in the synthesis of fatty acids. In general, however, adherence to a strict low-purine diet is followed by only a modest reduction in the concentration of serum urate, usually amounting to no more than 2 mg/dl.

The effects of heavy drinking, on the other hand, can be much more striking. The metabolism of ethanol gives rise to an increase in the concentration of blood lactate, which is formed from pyruvate in a reaction linked to the oxidation of ethanol to acetaldehyde and the generation of NADPH. Like a number of other small organic acids, lactic acid blocks the renal excretion of uric acid (presumably through inhibition of tubular secretion), and if the blood lactate level rises and remains above 20–25 mg/dl for a sufficient period of time there will be a sharp reduction in uric acid output by the kidney. In a like manner, the hyperuricemia attendant upon fasting is traceable to an increase in the plasma level of acetoacetic and β-hydroxybutyric acids. When gouty patients take whiskey while fasting—a combination of circumstances not uncommon in real life—there is a substantial rise in serum urate levels, with evidence that the effects of these factors on uric acid excretion are additive or potentiating. The consumption of moonshine whiskey presents the additional hazard of lead poisoning (the lead derived from automobile radiators used in the distillation of this brew) and subsequent saturnine gout.

When a large purine- and protein-rich meal is accompanied by the imbibition of copious amounts of ethanol, the lactic acid produced in the course of the metabolism of the ethanol temporarily blocks the disposal of uric acid by the kidneys and leads to a greater rise in serum urate concentration than that produced by the same meal taken without spirituous fluids. The rapid fluctuations in serum urate concentration induced by fasting, by the consumption of large amounts of spirits or ethanolic beverages, or, especially, by the combination of heavy drinking and a protein- and purine-rich meal, are often followed by flares in gouty arthritis (aldermanic gout). Similar swings in the level of serum urate precede the crises of gouty arthritis which often occur early in the course of treatment with uricosuric drugs or allopurinol (see below) or after the administration of various other drugs that affect the renal handling of uric acid, e.g., thiazides, furoseamide, and ethacrynic acid.

COURSE

The severity and the rate of progression of untreated gouty arthritis are extremely variable. Some individuals experience no more than a few attacks in a lifetime. More often, however, these paroxysms tend to recur with increasing frequency and intensity and are associated with the gradual development of slowly progressive disability as a result of loss of articular cartilage and erosion of the subchondral bone and related paraarticular structures. In extreme cases highly destructive joint disease and massive tophaceous deposits arise within a period of a few years, associated at times with severe renal insufficiency.

REFERENCES

Bluestone R, Waisman J, Klinenberg JR: The gouty kidney. Semin Arthritis Rheum 7:97, 1977

Kozin F, McCarty DJ: Protein absorption to monosodium urate, calcium pyrophosphate dihydrate, and silica crystals. Relationship to the pathogenesis of crystal-induced inflammation. Arthritis Rheum 19:433, 1975

Maclachlan MJ, Rodnan GP: Effects of food, fast and alcohol on serum uric acid and acute attacks of gout. Am J Med 42:38, 1967

McCarty DJ, Kozin F: An overview of cellular and molecular mechanisms in crystal-induced inflammation. Arthritis Rheum 18[Suppl]:757, 1975

Resnick D: The radiographic manifestations of gouty arthritis. Crit Rev Diag Imag 9:265, 1977

Spilberg I, Gallacher A, Mehta JM, Mandell B: Urate crystal-induced chemotactic factor. Isolation and partial characterization. J Clin Invest 58:815, 1976

Wyngaarden JB, Kelley WN: Gout and Hyperuricemia. New York, Grune & Stratton, 1976

DIAGNOSIS AND CLASSIFICATION

Stanley L. Wallace

Acute gout is not usually difficult to diagnose. Monarticular arthritis (particularly involving the first metatarsophalangeal joint) of rapid onset in an otherwise healthy adult male is the classic clinical picture. This syndrome is usually associated with hyperuricemia and most commonly clears dramatically after the administration of a full therapeutic dose of colchicine.

CRYSTALS

In 1961, the diagnostic significance of negatively birefringent monosodium urate monohydrate crystals (as seen with the use of polarized light) within synovial fluid leukocytes during the acute attack of gout was rediscovered. In 1977, the Gout Criteria Subcommittee of the American Rheumatism Association evaluated this and other clinical, radiologic, and laboratory criteria in the classification of acute primary gout, comparing 178 patients with gout with a total of 528 patients with pseudogout, rheumatoid arthritis, or septic arthritis. It was con-

firmed that the best single criterion for gout was the demonstration of the characteristic crystal. A search for the crystal was made in only 90 of the 178 patients with gout. Typical crystals were found in 76 (84.4 percent) of the 90. Urate crystals were not seen in the joint fluid in any patient with the control disorders in the study. This criterion, when present, is therefore absolutely specific for acute gout.

TOPHI

The presence of tophi, proved on aspiration to contain sodium urate crystals either chemically or by polarized light microscopy, was also useful in categorizing patients. The proven tophus was found in 52 (30.2 percent) of 172 patients with gout; tophi were not seen in rheumatoid arthritis or in pseudogout, but 4 of 112 patients with septic arthritis were also shown to be tophaceous. As a criterion for classification, proven tophi were much less sensitive but were nearly as specific as synovial fluid urate crystals. Fewer than 1 percent (4 of 521) of the control patients with the other articular disorders had proven tophi.

PROPOSED CRITERIA

There were 102 patients with primary gout in the study (57.3 percent of the total) in whom joint fluid urate crystals were either not searched for or not found when sought; 71 (39.9 percent of the total) had neither crystals demonstrated in synovial fluid nor proven tophi. Classification of gout in the patients without synovial fluid crystals or proven tophi was accomplished with the use of a set of clinical, radiologic, and laboratory criteria (Table 1).

Five or more of the criteria in Table 1 were found in 95.5 percent of patients with primary gout, 7.7 percent of the patients with rheumatoid arthritis and 6.7 percent of the patients with septic arthritis. However, 27.3 percent of patients with pseudogout also demonstrated five or more criteria, an unacceptable lack of specificity. Six or more criteria were present in 87.6 percent of patients with gout, 2.0 percent of rheumatoid arthritics, 2.5 percent of patients with septic joint disease, and 10.9 percent of those with pseudogout. Requiring seven or more criteria reduced sensitivity in acute gout; only 74.1 percent of patients satisfied this number. The specificity, however,

Table 1
Proposed Criteria for the Acute Arthritis of Primary Gout

More than one attack of acute arthritis
Maximum inflammation developed within 1 day
Monarticular attack of arthritis
Redness observed over joints
First metatarsophalangeal joint painful or swollen
Unilateral attack in first metatarsophalangeal joint
Unilateral tarsal joint attack
Suspected tophus (not proven)
Hyperuricemia
Asymmetric swelling within a joint on x-ray
Subcortical cyst without erosions on x-ray
Joint fluid culture negative for organisms during attack

Gout { 15% ⊖ crystals in fluid
8% nl uric acid levels

was improved enormously: only 0.3 percent of patients with rheumatoid arthritis, 0.8 percent of those with septic arthritis, and 2.7 percent of pseudogout patients met seven criteria. The most useful combination of sensitivity and specificity seemed to be 6 of the total of 12 criteria in Table 1.

Hyperuricemia was shown to be present at some time in the course of the disease in only 92.2 percent of the gout patients in the study. In addition, 18.4 percent of the patients with septic arthritis, 17.5 percent of those with pseudogout, and 10.2 percent of the rheumatoid arthritics had elevated urate levels. Hyperuricemia therefore was an unreliable criterion considered alone.

There are other clinical phenomena that occur frequently enough in acute gout to have value as criteria. The duration of an untreated or inadequately treated attack, at least early in the course of gout, is fairly short, averaging 2 weeks, with a range of 2 days to 6 weeks. The patient with early gout is usually completely free of all joint pain, discomfort, and stiffness between attacks. The acute episode may be precipitated by certain triggers, such as major medical illness, general surgery, and physical or psychic trauma; however, an equal proportion of patients with pseudogout have acute episodes initiated by these same triggers.

First metatarsophalangeal joint involvement occurs in 75 percent of patients at some time during the course of recurrent episodes of acute gout. Other commonly attacked joints include the knee, ankle, and tarsus, in that order of frequency.

An objective dramatic, rapid response to colchicine occurs in about 75 percent of patients with acute gout; it occurs less consistently in pseudogout, the other calcium salt inflammatory processes, and sarcoid arthritis, and rarely, if ever, in other kinds of joint disease. Finally, a positive family history of gout, when present, is useful. The typical crystal remains the best criterion.

REFERENCES

McCarty DJ Jr, Hollander JL: Identification of urate crystals in gouty synovial fluid. Ann Intern Med 54:452, 1961

Wallace SL, Robinson H, Masi AT, et al: Preliminary criteria for the classification of the acute arthritis of primary gout. Arthritis Rheum 20:895, 1977

TREATMENT

Stanley L. Wallace

Gout is the most treatable form of arthritis. When recognized early, the acute attack can be eradicated rapidly and completely. Gouty recurrences can be prevented and tophaceous deposition dissolved. The treatment of gout is classically divided into three parts: (1) antiinflammatory therapy of the acute episode; (2) prevention of subsequent attacks; and (3) prevention or dissolution of tophaceous deposition by reducing the serum urate level to normal.

Table 1
Drugs Useful in the Treatment of Acute Gout

Colchicine (orally or intravenously)
Phenylbutazone or oxyphenbutazone
Indomethacin
Other nonsteroidal antiinflammatory agents, including ibuprofen, fenoprofen, and naproxen
Adrenocorticotropic hormone
Adrenocortical steroids (orally or intraarticularly)

TREATMENT OF ACUTE GOUT

Colchicine is the only one of the drugs that can be used in the therapy of acute gouty arthritis that has both diagnostic and therapeutic value (Table 1). A dramatic, objective response to colchicine administration is most compatible with the diagnosis of acute gout, although occasionally patients with calcium salt crystal–induced arthritis and sarcoid arthritis show similar benefit.

The earlier that any agent is given in the course of an acute attack of gout, the more effective it will be. Colchicine is usually administered in multiple small oral doses in order to minimize ultimate gastrointestinal toxicity. Initially, 0.5 mg or 0.6 mg is given hourly until therapeutic benefit or toxic side effects occur; if neither of these occurs first, it is given until the completion of an arbitrarily chosen maximal dose. This maximal dose ranges from 5 to 10 mg, according to body weight, given over a period of 8–16 hours. About 75 percent of patients respond to full doses of colchicine. Gastrointestinal toxicity (hyperperistalsis, diarrhea, cramping abdominal pain, nausea, and/or vomiting) most commonly appears within 12 hours of starting oral colchicine therapy; benefit is typically delayed until 12–48 hours after treatment is begun.

Colchicine is as effective intravenously as it is by mouth. The major advantage of the intravenous route is that it avoids the gastrointestinal side effects associated with oral use. Benefit generally comes more rapidly, usually in 6–24 hours after a single dose of 3 mg. The major risk associated with intravenous colchicine therapy is that of extravasation and local tissue damage. Colchicine solutions are very irritating and should be administered slowly. Since intravenous administration of colchicine is rarely, if ever, associated with gastrointestinal side effects, the dose need not be fractionated. The single bolus of 3 mg is as effective as multiple smaller ones. Colchicine is excreted very slowly; frequently repeated intravenous doses raise the possibility of profound systemic toxicity and should be avoided.

Phenylbutazone and its analog, oxyphenbutazone, are very effective drugs in the treatment of acute gout; they are more effective than colchicine. They have no diagnostic value, but once the diagnosis is made, and especially if intravenous preparations of colchicine are not available, phenylbutazone or its analog is the drug of choice in treating acute gout in suitable patients. The optimal dose of either drug is about 600 mg/day, usually as 200 mg three times daily with meals. These drugs act in the liver as enzyme inducers, accelerating their own me-

Table 2
Drugs that Can Effect a Reduction in Serum Urate Levels

Uricosuric agents
   Probenecid
   Sulfinpyrazone
   Acetylsalicylic acid (in doses greater than 3 g/day)
   Benzbromarone
   X-ray contrast agents, including iopanoic acid, sodium
      ipodate, iodipamide, and sodium diatrizoate

Xanthine oxidase inhibitors
   Allopurinol
   Oxipurinol

tabolism, so that large loading doses or total daily doses greater than 600 mg are of no advantage. Three to five days of therapy are generally necessary to overcome the attack of gout and to minimize the likelihood of a recurrence.

Phenylbutazone and oxyphenbutazone are capable of producing infrequent but serious toxic effects. In treatment lasting only 3–5 days, the most likely problems are worsening an already present peptic ulcer or increasing fluid accumulation in a patient in congestive heart failure. The presence of peptic ulceration or of severe congestive failure are absolute contraindications to therapy with these agents. Marrow depression, skin rashes, and hepatocellular damage are rare during brief therapy.

A number of acidic drugs compete with phenylbutazone and oxyphenbutazone for the same albumin-binding sites; these include warfarin, other coumarin anticoagulants, the sulfonamides, and tolbutamide, among other agents. Phenylbutazone or its analog can displace these other drugs from albumin and potentiate their effects. Phenylbutazone and oxyphenbutazone are also hepatic microsomal enzyme inducers and may increase the liver metabolism of (or have their own metabolism increased by) a wide variety of other drugs, including the barbiturates, certain sedatives, tranquillizers, anticonvulsants, and antidiabetic agents. These problems in drug interference must be considered when administering phenylbutazone and oxyphenbutazone.

Indomethacin in large doses (150–200 mg/day or more for 5 or 6 days) is effective in the treatment of acute gout. However, such large doses may produce an inordinate frequency of gastrointestinal or central nervous system side effects. Experience with the other nonsteroid antiinflammatory agents is still limited. One would expect them to be moderately effective in the treatment of acute gout, with a relatively low frequency of toxicity.

PREVENTION OF GOUTY RECURRENCES

Colchicine alone in small daily doses (0.6 or 1.2 mg) will reduce the frequency of subsequent attacks in nearly all patients and will completely abolish recurrences in many. Maintainance of the miscible pool of urate at a normal level in the patient with gout will ultimately lead to the disappearance of new episodes. Both xanthine oxidase inhibitors and uricosuric drugs are capable of accomplishing this result. However, an increased fre-

quency of gouty attacks is likely to occur early in such therapy; small doses of colchicine must be given in conjunction with the drug reducing the serum urate level, at least until the miscible pool of urate has been normal for a protracted period and all precipitated urate is dissolved.

TREATMENT OF TOPHACEOUS GOUT

The dissolution of tophi depends upon reducing the serum urate level to well within the normal range. Both uricosuric drugs and xanthine oxidase inhibitors are capable of accomplishing this result in most patients with gout (Table 2). The uricosuric agents, however, have the disadvantage that they must be delivered to the renal tubule to be effective, and therefore do not work in some gouty patients with severe renal insufficiency. In addition, they increase the urinary urate load and increase the risk of gravel or stone in the uncooperative patient who is unwilling or unable to drink adequate quantities of fluids.

Allopurinol is an analog of hypoxanthine and a potent inhibitor of xanthine oxidase, which catalyzes the conversion of hypoxanthine to xanthine, and xanthine to uric acid; allopurinol therby lowers both serum and urinary levels of urate, increasing urinary xanthine and hypoxanthine at the same time. In addition, allopurinol and its metabolite, oxipurinol, inhibit early steps in de novo purine synthesis. Allopurinol doses range from 200–800 mg/day and must be carefully individualized. Most patients require 300 or 400 mg/day. Colchicine in small doses should be given along with allopurinol (see above).

Toxicity with allopurinol is frequent and includes diarrhea, upper gastrointestinal irritation, hepatocellular chemical changes, and rash. The last may be a harbinger of an allopurinol-induced disseminated vasculitis and is an indication for total cessation of therapy. Because the ultimate risk of allopurinol is not yet clear, caution in its use is necessary. At present, it is particularly indicated in those tophaceous patients with stones or with marked overproduction of urate, in those with severe enough renal malfunction to make them unresponsive to uricosuric drugs, and in those unable to tolerate the uricosuric drugs. Allopurinol is also especially useful in the prevention of acute uric acid nephropathy following cytolytic therapy in neoplasms.

Probenecid has been in use as a uricosuric agent for many years. Effective doses vary greatly from patient to patient and must be determined by trial and error. The most commonly used dose is 1.5 g/day; a significant minority of patients need 2.5 g/day or more. Toxicity is infrequent with probenecid; gastrointestinal irritation is possible, but the risk of gravel or stone is of greater importance. Urate stone can usually be prevented by forcing fluids. Colchicine must be given along with probenecid until the risk of acute gouty recurrences is gone. Sulfinpyrazone and benzbromarone are other effective uricosuric drugs.

PREVENTION OF TOPHACEOUS DEPOSITION

Approximately 40 percent of patients with acute recurrent gout ultimately become tophaceous. There is a significant question as to whether every patient with acute recurrent gout must be treated with a urate-lowering agent to prevent deposition. Those at greatest risk of stone formation or urate deposition certainly should be so treated; this category includes those who are major overproducers of urate, those who excrete large amounts in the urine, and those who already show renal function abnormalities. The remaining patients should be watched very carefully, and xanthine oxidase inhibitor or uricosuric therapy should be started only if urate is found to be depositing.

REFERENCES

Brodie BB: Displacement of one drug by another from carrier or receptor. Proc R Soc Med 58:946, 1965

Gutman AB: Uricosuric drugs, with special reference to probenecid and sulfinpyrazone. Adv Pharmacol 4:91, 1966

Rundles RW, Wyngaarden JB, Hitchings GH, et al: Effects of a xanthine oxidase inhibitor on thiopurine metabolism, hyperuricemia and gout. Trans Assoc Am Physicians 76:126, 1963

Wallace SL: Colchicine. Semin Arthritis Rheum 3:369, 1974

Crystal-induced Arthritis: Pseudogout and Hydroxyapatite

Daniel J. McCarty

PSEUDOGOUT

Calcium pyrophosphate dihydrate (CPPD) crystal deposition disease was originally described as *pseudogout* because it is associated with acute goutlike episodes of arthritis. Subsequent observations show that it can also resemble rheumatoid arthritis, osteoarthritis, traumatic arthritis, neuropathic joints, and, rarely, ankylosing spondylitis, rheumatic fever, or psychogenic rheumatism.

Anatomic and radiologic studies of the prevalence of knee cartilage calcification suggest that CPPD deposits occur in 5 percent of the adult population at the time of death. One study showed three different types of crystals and four distinct radiologic patterns in excised fibrocartilaginous menisci. The deposits in at least 7 percent of the cadavers would almost certainly have been seen on high-quality radiographs. Vascular calcifications, composed of apatite and usually involving the outer third of all four menisci, were common and most would probably have been visible on x-ray examination.

One study using high-resolution film showed that 27.6 percent of ambulatory elderly Jewish volunteers had calcific deposits, suggesting that age per se is an important factor in disease expression. These elderly subjects had only increased wrist complaints as compared to controls in the same population. On the other hand, our clinical experience suggests a greater frequency of symptomatic disease; over a 19-year period we have seen approximately one patient with symptomatic arthritis associated with CPPD for every two patients with clinical gout, and a similar ratio was seen at the Mayo Clinic.

PATHOGENESIS

The initial site of CPPD crystal deposition is probably articular cartilage, although precipitation in synovial tissue or synovial fluid cannot be excluded. CPPD crystals are found in these sites. The smallest deposits appear around the chondrocyte lacunae in the midzone of hyaline cartilage. Crystals also occur in fibrocartilage, ligaments, and tendons. The only exception to an articular or

periarticular localization is a single case showing monoclinic CPPD in the dura mater in a patient with gout, pseudogout, and hyperparathyroidism.

CPPD crystals are found in a granular matrix staining more densely than surrounding cartilage with alcian blue, colloidal iron, and PAS and appearing to be largely mucopolysaccharide. The primary change may occur in the ground substance—the "soil" that permits nucleation and growth of the crystals. This is also true in gout, where hyperuricemia is a necessary but not sufficient cause of monosodium urate crystal formation.

A gradient of inorganic pyrophosphate (PPi) exists between joint fluid and plasma in most patients with CPPD deposition or with osteoarthritis, and in some patients with other joint diseases. Levels of PPi in joint fluid correlate with the degree of osteoarthritis as judged radiographically, irrespective of the clinical diagnosis. The joint fluid PPi levels were lower during an acute attack and rose as the attack subsided, probably due to increased blood flow during the acute inflammatory phase, so that synovial fluid levels were more closely equilibrated to those of plasma.

Articular chondrocytes are the most likely source of synovial fluid PPi. Immature, but not adult, rabbit articular cartilage slices, incubated in vitro, liberate PPi into the surrounding medium. Human osteoarthritic, but not normal, adult cartilage liberates PPi similarly. Derivation of joint fluid inorganic pyrophosphate from other tissues such as bone remains an open question. The sites of CPPD crystal deposition are perilacunar, in large tophuslike masses, along clefts in degenerated cartilage, scattered in normal appearing cartilage matrix, and in the synovium.

As mentioned already, CPPD crystals lay in a "mold" of ground substance. Assuming a thermodynamic equilibrium with Ca^{2+} and $(P_2O_7)^{-4}$, the ions from which they were formed, events that either lower ionized calcium or bind $(P_2O_7)^{-4}$ by chelation may dissolve the CPPD crystals slightly, allowing some to escape into the adjacent joint fluid. Decreased Ca^{2+} lowers CPPD crystal

Table 1
Mechanisms of "Autoinjection" of CPPD Crystals from
Cartilage to Joint Fluid

Trigger	Mechanism	Clinical Circumstance
Fall in (Ca^{++}) level	CPPD dissolution, crystal shedding	Postoperative or acute medical illness
Mechanical disruption of cartilage architecture	Microfractures of subchondral bone	Trauma, neuropathic joint
Increased activity of enzymes degrading cartilage matrix	Removal of matrix by "enzymatic strip mining"	Pseudogout superimposed on another type of arthritis
Hypothyroidism with treatment	Loosened cartilaginous "mold" with crystal shedding	Joint symptoms after thyroid hormone replacement

solubility in vitro, and acute CPPD crystal-induced inflammation has been induced by lavage of joints with crystal solubilizers like EDTA- or Mg^{2+}-containing buffers. Acute arthritis associated with suddenly lowered calcium blood concentrations has also been reported. All support the concept of "crystal shedding."

Other mechanisms have been postulated to explain the "autoinjection" of CPPD crystals thought to precede an acute attack of pseudogout (Table 1). Mechanical disruption of cartilage architecture accompanying the collapse of the supporting subchondral bone has been implicated as etiologic in an acute attack occurring for the first time in a joint developing acute neuropathic changes.

"Enzymatic strip mining" has been proposed to explain the finding of CPPD crystals in joints showing osteoarthritis, acute gout, or acute pyogenic arthritis. Several cases of concomitant pseudogout and septic arthritis have been described, and simultaneous urate gout and pseudogout is not unusual. A common early histopathologic change in osteoarthritis is loss of the normal staining properties of superficial articular cartilage, interpreted as loss of matrix. Thus the finding of CPPD crystals in joint fluid must be interpreted in the light of the clinical picture as they might be a result, as well as a cause, of joint inflammation. The recent observations on the association of silent CPPD deposition and hypothyroidism, with the onset of acute pseudogout only after thyroid hormone replacement, suggests that a metabolically induced change in the cartilaginous ground substance may also free crystals.

Thus crystal shedding is possible when the crystals dissolve slightly, loosening them from their mold, or when the components of the mold itself are removed.

Once released into the synovial tissue space, the CPPD crystals are coated with protein, mostly IgG, which is oriented on the crystal surface with the Fc groups exposed. This promotes phagocytosis by polymorphonuclear leukocytes and monocytes, cells with Fc receptors. A low molecular weight chemotactic factor, identical to that released by polymorphonuclear leukocytes after phagocytosis of many different particles, including urate crystals, is released after CPPD phagocytosis. Lysosomal discharge then accounts for the acute inflammation of pseudogout, as this will not occur in the absence of polymorphonuclear leukocytes.

DIAGNOSIS AND CLINICAL PICTURE

Crystal-induced inflammation is related to "dose," and CPPD crystal deposits are usually polyarticular, symmetric, and related to concurrent or subsequent cartilage degeneration. Various combinations of inflammatory and degenerative arthropathies are seen (Fig. 1). The following five clinical patterns are seen.

Type A: Pseudogout

This pattern is marked by inflammatory episodes lasing approximately 1 day to 4 weeks. Such episodes are self-limited and usually involve only one or few peripheral joints. These attacks may be as severe as those of urate gout, but the average attack takes longer to reach peak intensity and is usually less painful and disabling. Inflammation may begin in a single joint, spreading to involve neighboring "daughter" joints—the "cluster" attack. These attacks occur in true urate gout as well. Mild attacks occur in both crystal deposition dieases and many often outnumber full-blown attacks.

Provocation of attacks by surgery or by acute medical illness is common in both gout and pseudogout. The percentage of patients with either disease who had at least one episode after surgery was nearly identical—8.3 percent of 168 gouty patients versus 9.4 percent of 106 patients with pseudogout. Severe medical illness, such as pneumonia or acute vascular occlusions, provoked attacks in 20.3 percent of 167 gouty patients versus 24 percent of 104 patients with pseudogout. Trauma may provoke acute arthritis in either gout or pseudogout. As mentioned above, both types of crystals are often found in the same subject; joint aspiration and specific crystal identification are absolutely necessary for precise differential diagnosis.

The knee joint is to pseudogout what the bunion joint is to gout. First metatarsophalangeal joint involvement—"pseudopodagra"—occurs rarely. Although not nearly as predictably effective as in urate gout, colchicine may provide dramatic relief in pseudogout. The release of chemotactic factor by polymorphonuclear leukocytes after phagocytosis of either urate or CPPD crystals is inhibited by colchicine in concentrations easily obtained in serum by the usual doses. Inhibition of urate crystal-induced release is more predictable than that induced by CPPD crystals, providing an in vitro parallel to the clinical experience in patients.

Approximately 20 percent of patients with CPPD deposits have hyperuricemia and about 5 percent have monosodium urate crystal deposits. About 25 percent of patients show this goutlike type A pattern. Men predominate. As in gout, the patient is completely asymptomatic between attacks. Radiographic evidence of CPPD crystal deposits is found in most patients showing this pattern.

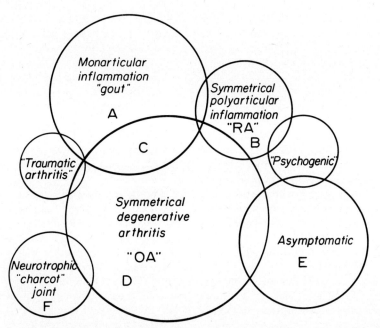

Fig. 1. Diagnoses most commonly affixed to patients with articular CPPD crystal deposits. The letters represent the types of clinical patterns referred to in text: OA, osteoarthritis; RA, rheumatoid arthritis. Although true association of CPPD deposition with arthritis of other etiology does occur, in most cases the CPPD-induced inflammation and/or associated cartilaginous and bony degeneration have resulted in a pattern of disease that misleads the clinician. (Reproduced by permission of the publisher from *Bulletin on the Rheumatic Diseases* 25:804, 1974–75.)

Type B: Pseudorheumatoid Arthritis

Approximately 5 percent of patients have multiple joint involvement with subacute attacks lasting for weeks or even months. Nonspecific symptoms of inflammation, such as morning stiffness and fatigue, are found. Signs such as synovial thickening, localized pitting edema, limitation of joint motion due to inflammation and/or to flexion contractures, and elevated acute phase reactants are usually found. Such patients are often thought to have rheumatoid arthritis. About 10 percent of patients with CPPD-related arthritis have positive tests for rheumatoid factors, usually in low titer. Urate gout may present with polyarticular involvement or rheumatoid factors (in 10 percent of cases), and may mimic rheumatoid arthritis.

CPPD deposits have been described both histologically and radiographically in patients with presumably bona fide rheumatoid arthritis. By chance, about 1 percent of patients with CPPD joint deposits would be expected to have rheumatoid arthritis. The author has seen 3 cases of true rheumatoid arthritis among 300 patients with CPPD crystal deposition. Over 600 cases of crystal-proved urate gout were studied during the same time, and only 1 instance of the coincidence of the two diseases was found. This case showed rheumatoid nodules and factor, hyperuricemia, and an ear tophus, but the articular disease was entirely due to the rheumatoid arthritis. This apparent negative association of urate gout and rheumatoid arthritis does not hold for CPPD deposits and rheumatoid arthritis.

The type B pattern differs from rheumatoid arthritis in several respects: the joints are inflamed "out of phase"

with one another, as in gout, rather than "in phase," as in rheumatoid arthritis. There is osteophyte formation and CPPD crystals are found in joint fluid leukocytes.

Types C + D: Pseudoosteoarthritis

Approximately one-half of these patients have progressive joint degeneration. Women predominate. The knees are most commonly affected, followed by the wrists, metacarpophalangeal joints, hips, shoulders, elbows, and ankles. Involvement is generally bilateral, although the degenerative process may be much further advanced on one side, especially in joints subjected to trauma. Flexion contractures are very common, especially of the knees, wrists, and elbows. CPPD crystal deposition should be suspected in patients with bilateral varus deformities and/or flexion contractures of the knees, especially when associated with osteophytes and flexion contractures of other joints not usually affected in primary generalized osteoarthritis.

About one-half of these patients have a history of episodic, superimposed acute attacks and have been classified as type C. Those without a clinically apparent inflammatory component have been classified as type D.

Characteristic calcific deposits may or may not be visible on x-ray examination. CPPD crystals are often found in radiographically negative joints, especially those with extensive degenerative change. Serial studies have shown examples of joints with obvious CPPD deposits at an early phase of the disease that are difficult to discern when severe degeneration has supervened. "Fine-detail" radiographs are helpful in detection of small or faint deposits.

"Squaring" of bone ends, subchondral cystic changes, and hooklike osteophytes, especially in the metacarpophalangeal joints—degeneration in sporadic CPPD crystal deposition disease is similar to that associated with hemochromatosis.

The pattern of joint degeneration in types C + D (i.e., wrists, metacarpophalangeal, elbow, and shoulder) is clearly different from that seen in primary osteoarthritis, which affects chiefly proximal and distal interphalangeal joints and the first carpometacarpals. The knees and hips are commonly affected by both conditions. Heberden's and Bouchard's nodes as well as other findings of primary osteoarthritis often coexist with the pattern of joint involvement peculiar to CPPD crystal deposition—probably a chance association of two very common conditions.

Type E: Asymptomatic CPPD Crystal Deposition

This type may be the most common of all. Most joints with CPPD deposits plainly visible on x-rays are not symptomatic, even in patients with acute or chronic symptoms in other joints.

Type F: Pseudoneurotrophic Joints

Recently, 4 cases of "neurotrophic" arthritis of the knees associated with polyarticular CPPD deposition have been reported. Three of these cases had mild tabes dorsalis and tertiary syphilis, but a fourth case also had late latent syphilis but no neurologic abnormality. Other reports of destructive, neurotrophiclike arthropathy in patients with CPPD deposits and normal neurologic examination underscore this association. All reported series of tabes dorsalis state that Charcot's knees develop in only 5–10 percent of cases. It is postulated that neurotrophic joints actually develop in that 5 percent of the tabetic population that happens to have underlying CPPD crystal deposition. The fact that CPPD alone can be associated with a very destructive arthropathy, without any neurologic deficit, reinforces this hypothesis.

Other Patterns

Stiffening and straightening of the spine have been described, especially in familial cases, and these cases may be confused with ankylosing spondylitis. True bony ankylosis has been described, and the author has seen several examples in very elderly patients.

It is clear from the long-term observations of the natural history of CPPD joint deposition that a patient may show one pattern of arthritis early in the course of the disease and a different pattern later. Many type A or E patients might later show patterns C, D, or F, for example.

RADIOLOGIC FINDINGS

The appearance of CPPD crystal deposits in joint cartilage is usually characteristic (Fig. 2). Punctuate radiodensities are seen first, and later, linear radiodensities

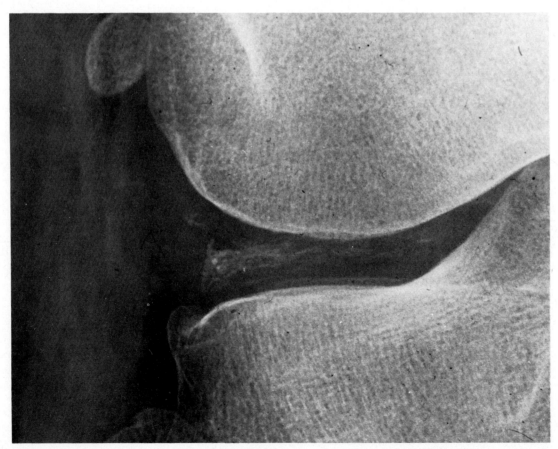

Fig. 2. Characteristic linear radiopacities due to CPPD crystals are seen in the fibrocartilaginous lateral meniscus and in the hyaline articular cartilage as a radiodense line in hyaline articular cartilage paralleling the density of the underlying tibial cortex.

are visualized. Views of both knees and the pelvis in the anteroposterior projections and single anteroposterior views of both hands will suffice to identify nearly all patients with radiographic CPPD deposits. Additional views will not uncover any patient if the above views are negative for CPPD.

The degenerative changes that frequently coexist with CPPD crystal deposits are sufficiently characteristic to suggest the underlying presence of CPPD. Thus "osteoarthritis" of metacarpophalangeal, wrist, elbow, or shoulder joints, or isolated patellofemoral osteoarthritis (patella "wrapped around" the femur) are suggestive. Joint aspiration and specific crystal identification by polarized light may then confirm the diagnosis.

CLASSIFICATION

A classification of CPPD crystal deposition disease is given in Table 2. None of the hereditary cases have had associated metabolic conditions, such as hyperparathyroidism. Nearly half of the offspring of a heterozygote get the disease, so penetrance is nearly complete.

The "sporadic" or "idiopathic" cases are generally cases in which there has been no systematic search for the condition among blood relatives and in which none of the putative metabolic disease associations has been found. It is probable that a thorough study of "sporadic" cases would result in their reclassification as being either hereditary or associated with metabolic disease.

All of the metabolic disease associations are unproved statistically, because appropriate controlled comparisons either have not been done or have run into a problem of small numbers, invalidating appropriate statistical comparisons. As the prevalence of CPPD appears to rise sharply with age, the question of aging per se as an associated condition arises. The metabolic conditions listed in Table 2 may directly affect CPPD crystal deposition or they might bring about a premature phenotypic expression of an underlying heterozygous state.

TREATMENT

Treatment of the acute attack generally poses no great difficulty. Thorough aspiration of a large joint is often sufficient treatment. Instillation of corticosteroid

Table 2
Classification of CPPD Crystal Deposition Disease

Hereditary (relatively rare)
  Czechoslovakian
  Chilean
  Dutch
  Other

Sporadic (idiopathic) (most common)

Associated with metabolic disease (common)
  Hyperparathyroidism
  Hemochromatosis
  Hypothyroidism
  Gout
  Aging
  Ochronosis
  Wilson's disease
  Hypophosphatasia
  Hypomagnesemia

crystals after aspiration may be indicated in very severe attacks. Usual doses of nonsteroidal antiinflammatory drugs will control attacks in small joints or inflammation occurring in multiple joints.

REFERENCES

McCarty DJ: Pathogenesis and treatment of crystal induced inflammation, in McCarty DJ (ed): Arthritis and Allied Conditions (ed 9). Philadelphia, Lea & Febiger, 1979

McCarty DJ: Calcium pyrophosphate crystal deposition disease, in McCarty DJ (ed): Arthritis and Allied Conditions (ed 9). Philadelphia, Lea & Febiger, 1979

McCarty DJ: Proceeding of a Conference on Pseudogout and Pyrophosphate Metabolism. McCarty DJ (ed): Arthritis Rheum 19:275, 1975

HYDROXYAPATITE DEPOSITION DISEASE

Perhaps the commonest, yet least understood, crystal deposition disease is that associated with hydroxyapatite crystals. Calcific tendonitis or bursitis is a clinical entity familiar to most physicians. Sometimes familial and often affecting multiple periarticular sites, this condition is associated with the sudden onset of pain and the signs of acute inflammation.

LABORATORY AND RADIOLOGIC FINDINGS

Microscopically, small round bodies ranging in size from 0.5 to 100 μm are seen. Many of these bodies, which have characteristic eccentric or concentric laminations, are phagocytosed by polymorphonuclear leukocytes. The acute attack is presumed to occur when preformed crystal deposits in dense connective tissue rupture into vascular tissue spaces, such as tendon sheaths or bursa. By electron microscopy, the round bodies are seen to consist of clumps of needle-shaped crystals in an organic matrix.

The calcific deposits are easily seen by x-ray if care is taken to rotate the extremity so that their radiodensity does not overlap with that of contiguous bony structures (Fig. 1); as crystals comprise only 5–10 percent of the round bodies, radiodensity is sometimes modest.

OTHER SYNDROMES

Recently, additional articular apatite crystal deposition disease syndromes have been described. Here the aggregates of crystals are much smaller, identification being made only by transmission or scanning electron microscopy. Such crystals have been identified both free in joint fluid and in joint fluid leukocytes in cases of osteoarthritis.

It is likely that there are a number of clinical conditions wherein apatite crystals play a role. These include calcific tendonitis, calcinosis ("kalkgicht") associated with scleroderma or dermatomyositis (where calcific material may rupture through the skin or into joints), periarthritis in uremic patients (Caner-Decker syndrome), synovial calcification associated with hypercalcemic states, and, lastly, as mentioned above, the inflammatory component of osteoarthritis. Much more data are needed to establish the last condition as a clinically important phenomenon.

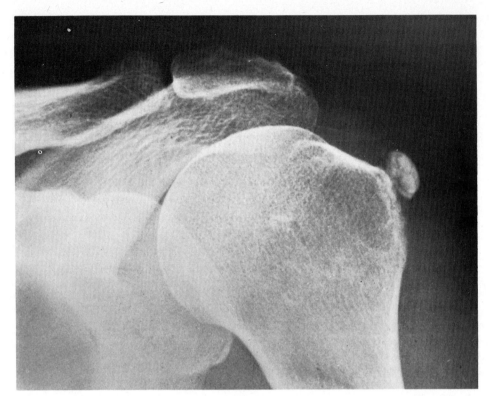

Fig. 1.   Typical hydroxyapatite calcification in the rotator cuff of the shoulder.

TREATMENT

Treatment of the periarticular calcific syndromes is ordinarily successful with phenylbutazone 100 mg, or indomethacin 50 mg four times daily, with or without concomitant injection of a corticosteroid ester suspension mixed with a local anesthetic directly into the inflamed area. Recalcitrant or chronic lesions may require surgical removal of the calcific deposits.

REFERENCES

Schumacher HR, Somlyo AP, Tse RL, et al: Ann Intern Med 87:411, 1977

Osteoarthritis

Alfred Jay Bollet

PATHOGENESIS

Osteoarthritis is the most common form of symptomatic joint disease. The terms *degenerative joint disease* and *osteoarthrosis,* the latter most frequently used in Britain, are synonymous with *osteoarthritis;* although inflammation plays a negligible role in pathogenesis, *osteoarthritis* is the term generally used in this country.

Every form of animal life that has left skeletal remains for examination has shown the characteristic alterations of osteoarthritis, including all known early hominids. The disease is thus one of the oldest known to exist on this planet. Osteoarthritis increases in prevalence with increasing age; it is an ancient disease primarily affecting the elderly, but its relationship to aging as a biologic phenomenon is unclear. Recent developments in the understanding of the pathogenesis of osteoarthritis have focused attention on primary physical stresses causing alterations in metabolic phenomena in articular cartilage, making it more susceptible to wear. Alterations in cartilage and bone structure result. This new understanding offers hope of increased means of influencing the development and progression of this common cause of serious disability.

Loss of substance of the articular cartilage is the initial grossly apparent lesion in osteoarthritis. Irregularities appear in the surface of the cartilage and progress to roughness, cracks, and fissures which extend into the cartilage; subsequently fraying and loss of the cartilage substance occur. Erosion of the cartilage may occur in small well-defined loci or in large irregular patches. This destruction of the cartilage is the basic lesion in osteoarthritis but it does not cause symptoms directly since there are no nerve endings in cartilage. Pathologic changes also occur in the underlying subchondral bone, which becomes subject to altered mechanical stresses since the thinned, abnormal articular cartilage no longer performs its functions properly. In addition, proliferation of cartilage and bone occurs at the margins of the articular cartilage, producing outgrowths known as osteophytes; these lesions are often called "spurs" because of their appearance on radiographs.

COMPOSITION AND FUNCTION OF ARTICULAR CARTILAGE

Studies of the mechanism of cartilage erosion in osteoarthritis have concentrated on the structure and composition of the articular cartilage and the function of various locomotor structures during joint movement.

Cartilage is a highly differentiated form of connective tissue in which the cells, chondrocytes, have produced a gelatinous extracellular matrix rich in characteristic protein–polysaccharides and collagen fibers. The collagen fibers form a supporting framework in which the matrix and the sparsely distributed cells are embedded. The collagen fibers form arcades; in the deeper portions of the cartilage the fibers lie perpendicular to the joint surface, running from the underlying bone toward the surface, but superficially they form arches and become parallel to the joint surface and more closely packed.

The gelatinous matrix between the collagen fibers is rich in the complex protein–polysaccharides or proteoglycans of connective tissue. The specific proteoglycans of cartilage are protein–chondroitin-4-sulfate, protein–chondroitin-6-sulfate, and protein–keratan sulfate. These polysaccharide (glycosaminoglycan) chains are now thought to be linked to the same protein core, the linkage region consisting of a short chain of an oligosaccharide containing two galactoses and one xylose; the latter is covalently linked to an amino acid (usually serine or threonine) residue in the core protein. These protein units, with their radiating chains of polysaccharide, are aggregated together by a distinct protein moiety, called *link protein*, and the large masses of protein–polysaccharide thus created are formed into huge complex molecules by a long chain of another polysaccharide, hyaluronic acid.

There is also a small amount of glycoprotein present in the matrix; this protein shows immunologic species specificity and may serve to contribute to the aggregation of these complex protein–polysaccharides. The protein in the proteoglycan units is not species specific.

These proteoglycans and proteins are synthesized by the chondrocytes, which are embedded in lacunae in the cartilage matrix. Embryonic cartilage and epiphyseal cartilage have blood vessels, but in later childhood and adulthood the articular cartilage is avascular. Since the cells in mature cartilage are distant from any blood supply, they exist in an environment that is almost totally devoid of oxygen; glycolysis is therefore almost totally anaerobic and large amounts of lactate are produced. Nutrients must reach the chondrocytes and wastes leave them by diffusion across the matrix into the synovial fluid bathing the surface or into the bone marrow beneath the articular cartilage. Waste products, particularly lactate, are most concentrated around the cells and the pH in these loci can be strikingly acidic.

Cartilage is very rich in water, since the proteoglycans are extremely hydrophilic. This very wet gelatinous matrix is important to the function of articular cartilage, both in avoiding friction during joint motion and in absorbing strong compressive forces during muscle contraction or weight bearing. Because of its composition the articular cartilage can behave as a sponge, deforming when compressed as water is squeezed away from the point at which the pressure is applied. The cartilage can return to its original shape, in the fashion of tissues that have elastic fibers, when the pressure is released and the water is attracted back into the matrix. The elasticity of the cartilage spreads the area subject to the loading forces that develop during weight bearing or muscle pull. The fluid squeezed out of the surface of the cartilage at the site where the force is applied keeps opposing cartilage surfaces from touching each other and thus contributes to lubrication, keeping friction extremely low. Other as yet ill-defined lubricants may exist, but the articular cartilage itself functions as a deformable, self-lubricating bearing; these properties permit normal joint function without significant wear.

The primary function of articular cartilage is to prevent friction during joint motion. Measurements of the coefficient of friction of animals joints have shown values far lower than those obtainable with mechanical structures and excellent synthetic lubricants. These functional properties of cartilage are dependent on the presence of the proteoglycans. The elastic deformation of the cartilage that occurs when a load is applied is proportional to the concentration of the proteoglycans in the matrix.

There is considerable variation in the chemical composition and the function of different types of cartilage. Articular cartilage is richer in complex proteoglycans than other forms of cartilage, and there are differences in the concentration of these components and therefore the properties of articular cartilage in different sites. These differences may influence the normal properties of the articular cartilage in different joints and thus the ability of the cartilage in specific sites to withstand mechanical stresses in that joint without degeneration.

Although cartilage is elastic and capable of absorbing impact stress very well, the layer of articular cartilage covering the joint surface is too thin to have much effect. Bone is rigid and absorbs stress relatively poorly, but there is a great deal of it. Measurements have shown that impact stresses applied to an extremity are absorbed primarily by the large amount of trabecular bone rather than by the articular cartilage. In this sense, the bone protects the cartilage rather than vice versa, and alterations in the bone which makes it thicker and even less elastic may cause excessive physical stresses on cartilage, resulting in osteoarthritic breakdown. Conversely, some studies have suggested that osteoporosis, with thinner more elastic bone, is better able to absorb impact stresses and is associated with a lower incidence of osteoarthritis.

Other structures involved in locomotion also protect joints, and the articular cartilage in particular, from injury. This phenomenon was illustrated during a study of neuromuscular physiology performed by suspending subjects above the floor by means of an electromagnet, and dropping them unexpectedly by turning off the power. Measurements were made of the lag time before electromyographic evidence of activation of the gastrocnemius, as well as of the force of the impact. A fall of less than 7 cm resulted in impact before the neuromuscular apparatus could be activated, and a hard, uncomfortable impact occurred with the heel striking the floor. A fall of 15 cm allowed time for the neuromuscular apparatus to be activated to cushion the impact, and a softer, comfortable landing resulted; the heel was prevented from striking the floor. This experiment demonstrates that the neuromuscular apparatus protects joint structures from injurious stress; it resembles the common experience of an unexpected extra step at the bottom of a flight of stairs. The unexpected step is no higher than the others, but the impact stress is much greater.

Analysis of joint stress is primarily analysis of the ability of the rest of the locomotor system to absorb that stress normally. Fatigue, neural dysfunction, muscle atrophy, and bone pathology are important in the consideration of the nature of abnormal physical stresses on joints, as are joint instability, incongruity of articular surfaces, and the physical magnitude of the stresses.

MORPHOLOGIC AND BIOCHEMICAL PATHOLOGY

The earliest morphologic lesions in osteoarthritis consist of irregularities in the cartilage surface. Although articular cartilage appears smooth in gross appearance, ultramicroscopically the surface of articular cartilage has fine irregularities and undulations; osteoarthritis begins as an increased irregularity of the surface, followed by fissures or cracks extending into the cartilage substance. As the process proceeds the irregularities become greater and deeper; the resulting fibrillation then proceeds to loss of substance of the cartilage. Simultaneously with the process of erosion, new growth of cartilage and bone at the articular margins gives rise to ostephytes. In advanced lesions the cartilage may be completely lost, exposing underlying cortical bone, which becomes thickened into an ivorylike density called *eburnation*.

Accompanying the changes in surface texture of the cartilage, there is softening (chondromalacia) and increased friability of the substance of the cartilage. Chemically, in most sites of experimental osteoarthritic lesions in animals a loss of glycosaminoglycan content occurs. The earliest and most marked losses occur in the concentration of the chondroitin sulfates, but loss of keratan sulfate also occurs. In osteoarthritic lesions there is disaggregation of these huge, complicated protein–polysaccharide molecules, but the exact alterations in chemical structure responsible for the loss of these compounds is not yet clear.

Histochemically, the loss of the glycosaminoglycans results in a loss of matrix staining for polysaccharides, most marked in the superficial zones of the cartilage near the articular surface. As loss of staining becomes more marked, it extends into the deeper zones. The polysaccharide stains most intensely around the chondrocytes, where it is being synthesized. Concomitantly with progression of the biochemical changes, the surface of the cartilage becomes irregular and proliferation of the chondrocytes occurs, especially in the superficial zones near the joint surface of the cartilage. As a result the lacunae become larger and contain clusters of several cells.

The collagen present in cartilage differs chemically from that found in skin and bone and is known as *type II collagen*. The concentration of collagen, measured by the hydroxproline content of the cartilage, is not altered in the abnormal osteoarthritic sites and no abnormalities of collagen metabolism have been identified in osteoarthritic lesions. Collagen as well as matrix is lost when the cartilage becomes eroded due to mechanical abrasion or wearing away; the wear occurs at sites in which the matrix glycosaminoglycans were decreased.

The chemical changes are accompanied by alterations in the physical properties of the cartilage and therefore of its functional properties. The compressibility and ability of the cartilage to return to its original shape (elasticity) when force is applied is dependent on the high glycosaminoglycan content; elasticity decreases as glycosaminoglycan content decreases, as does the "weeping" of fluid at the sites of application of load. The ability of the articular cartilage to function as a deformable, weeping bearing that keeps friction low during joint motion is thus progressively lost as these chemical changes become more marked. Mechanical factors are fundamental to the development of osteoarthritis, and the mechanical stresses in the joint change as the abnormal cartilage becomes less able to tolerate them by spreading the load and keeping friction low.

METABOLIC ALTERATIONS IN OSTEOARTHRITIS

The decreased content of proteoglycans in the cartilage matrix is accompanied by an increase in the rate of synthesis of these compounds. At the sites of the lesions there is an increased rate of incorporation of radiosulfate and other labeled components into the cells and into glycosaminoglycans. Increased incorporation of labeled amino acids into proteoglycans also occurs. There is also an increase in the rate of synthesis of ribonucleic acid as part of the increased metabolic activity of the chondrocytes in osteoarthritic lesions. Increased synthesis of deoxyribonucleic acid has also been demonstrated as a concomitant of the increased proliferation of these cartilage cells.

Thus there is an increase in the rate of synthesis of the matrix components in osteoarthritic cartilage lesions. Since there is a decrease in their concentration, a greater increase in the rate of loss of these compounds must be occurring. An understanding of the mechanism of the increased degradation of the proteoglycans seems to be fundamental to understanding the pathogenesis of the cartilage degeneration in osteoarthritis. The increase in

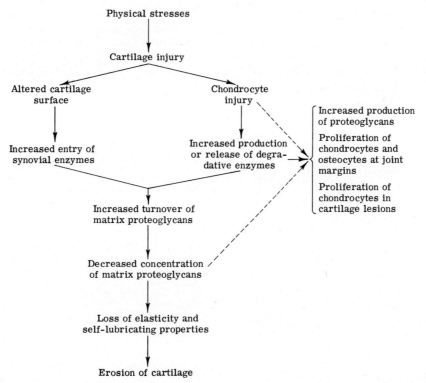

Fig. 1.   Events in the pathogenesis of osteoarthritis. Physical injury starts the process leading to loss of matrix components and erosion of the cartilage substance. Concomitantly a response occurs that can be considered an attempt at healing, including cellular proliferation. Outgrowth of bone and cartilage at the joint margins (osteophyte formation) results.

the rate of synthesis of these compounds is an attempt to replace the matrix components in response to the initial losses which have altered mechanical properties of the cartilage, thereby altering physical stress on the chondrocytes. These metabolic changes and the proliferation of the chondrocytes. These metabolic changes and the proliferation of the chondrocytes are thus attempts at healing (Fig. 1).

Degradation of the proteoglycans can occur by proteolytic breakdown of the protein core or aggregating units, by depolymerization of the polysaccharide chains, or by hydrolysis of the linkage regions whereby polysaccharide chains are attached to the peptides. The exact role of each of these possible mechanisms is not clear, and the list of possibilities may not be complete since the structure of these complex compounds is not yet fully understood. Some clues, however, do exist.

The enzymes that are capable of these degradative reactions are located primarily in lysosomes. Chondrocytes contain abundant lysosomal protease, primarily cathepsin B, which can degrade the protein components of the cartilage proteoglycans. Neutral protease activity has also been described in chondrocytes. β-Glycosaminidase and β-glucuronidase are present in chondrocytes and can degrade the chondroitin sulfate chains, alternately hydrolyzing terminal groups of the polysaccharide chains; this reaction process, however, would be rela-

tively slow and it seems unlikely that it occurs in vivo. Although enzymes that can degrade the chains of keratan sulfate have not been demonstrated in these tissues, this glycosaminoglycan would be lost if the protein core were degraded, permitting the peptide remnants with their attached polysaccharide chains to diffuse out of the cartilage. In addition there are enzymes that can split the sites of attachment of the polysaccharide chains to the polypeptides; this may occur at the xylosylserine linkages, at the links between xylose and galactose, between the two galactose residues, or between the galactose and the start of the disaccharide repeating units. These enzymes have been demonstrated in several tissues, including cartilage, but their pathophysiologic importance has not yet been demonstrated.

In addition, the chondroitin sulfate chains may be interrupted by hyaluronidase, which is an endo-β-glucosaminidase capable of depolymerizing hyaluronic acid or the chondroitin sulfates. Hyaluronidase has not been demonstrated in cartilage cells, but it is present in synovial cells and synovial fluid. The chondroitin sulfates in partially eroded or softened osteoarthritic cartilage have been shown to be qualitatively abnormal, having shortened chains. This decrease in average chain length could result from depolymerization or synthesis of shorter chains. If it is due to depolymerization it means that the chains have been degraded in the regions in which the chondroitin sulfate concentration is decreased; action of an enzyme such as hyaluronidase is implied by these data. Since loss of glycosaminoglycans occurs first near the cartilage surface, which is bathed by synovial fluid, and hyaluronidase is demonstrable in synovial fluid, it is possible that this enzyme reaches the cartilage matrix along with the nutrients that enter from synovial fluid. The entry of substances from the synovial fluid and egress of wastes is augmented by intermittent compression of the cartilage during joint use. High molecular weight substances such as enzymes do not enter the cartilage matrix as freely as do small nutrients.

The earliest changes in osteoarthritic cartilage, confirmed by scanning electron microscopic studies, occur at the synovial surface and include disruption of the surface collagen fibers. The exposed matrix thus is more accessible to the entry of larger molecules. Excessive physical stresses on the cartilage surface apparently initiate the metabolic alterations seen in osteoarthritis. These stresses may achieve this result by disrupting the cartilage surface, thereby allowing increased entry of synovial hyaluronidase, or by directly altering the metabolism of the cartilage cells to activate degradative enzymes. An increase in the breakdown of matrix protein–polysaccharide results. Either or both of these mechanisms may thus start the cycle of events leading to loss of the cartilage substance.

Collagenase has not yet been demonstrated in chondrocytes but does exist in synovial tissue. There is no evidence that collagenase plays a role in the pathogenesis of the cartilage breakdown in osteoarthritis. The collagen loss occurs late and probably is due to mechanical erosion after the framework of collagen fibers has been exposed to increased physical stress by the loss of the normal resiliency provided by its high concentration of proteoglycans.

EPIDEMIOLOGIC OBSERVATIONS

A large number of genetic, occupational, and population studies of the frequency of osteoarthritis have revealed evidence that physical stresses play a role in the genesis of this disease. Although genetic factors play a role in certain instances, especially in the familial frequency of Heberden's nodes (osteoarthritic lesions of the distal interphalangeal joints), it has not been possible to identify genetic determinants in the development of osteoarthritis in other joints. A rare syndrome, primary generalized osteoarthritis, or Kellgren's disease, is familial; in this disease distal and proximal interphalangeal joints, the carpometacarpal joints at the base of the thumb, and, less frequently, other joints can become affected by a process resembling typical osteoarthritis. The etiology of this syndrome is not clear. Familial or congenital postural or bony abnormalities or other locomotor phenomena that increase physical stresses on joints, such as capsular laxity and joint hypermobility, seem to be responsible for the early appearance of some cases of osteoarthritis.

In many instances local mechanical stresses, often of an occupational nature, stand out as important in the pathogenesis of this disease. Coal miners, who work in 4-ft-high mine shafts and work with their knees bent all day, have a very high incidence of osteoarthritic lesions of the knees but the same frequency of cervical spine osteoarthritis as do contemporaries in mine offices. In mines in which the shafts are 18 inches high, however, miners work prone, with the neck markedly hyperextended, shoveling coal over the shoulder; these miners have a high frequency of osteoarthritis in the cervical spine but not in the knees. Football players and other individuals with meniscus injuries develop early and severe osteoarthritis of the knees. Diseases that change the contour of the femoral head or of the acetabulum (e.g., asceptic necrosis of the femoral head, slipped epiphyses, epiphysitis, congenital dislocations of the hip, and Paget's disease of the acetabulum) lead to early and severe osteoarthritis of the hip. Epiphyseal diseases or intraarticular fractures that alter the contour of other joints also lead to the early development of osteoarthritic lesions in those joints.

Similar studies of naturally occurring osteoarthritis in animals suggest that local physical stresses are involved in the pathogenesis of osteoarthritis, although breeding customs in the carefully studied species leave open the possibility that genetic factors are important. Thoroughbred racehorses, for example, have a very high incidence of osteoarthritic lesions in the distal interphalangeal joints of the forelegs in relatively young animals. German shepherd dogs and some other breeds have a high frequency of osteoarthritis of the hips, apparently secondary to congenital dysplasia of these joints. Biochemical studies of natural and experimental osteoarthritis in animals reveal alterations similar to those found in the human disease. Genetic analyses in several species have failed to reveal a definable single-gene mechanism of inheritance.

These epidemiologic and clinical observations indicate that local mechanical factors within joints or portions of joints lead to local cartilage breakdown. Thinning of the cartilage as well as the altered biophysical properties of the cartilage which result from the chemical pathology produce further alterations in the mechanical stresses within the joints; progression of the disease results. These observations thus have important clinical implications regarding prevention and management of osteoarthritis.

It is entirely possible that more than one type of osteoarthritis, in terms of initial pathogenetic mechanism, exists. Loss of cartilage becomes the major pathway in the progress of the disease, but the initial mechanism leading to the loss of cartilage can vary. For example, experimental agents that kill chondrocytes lead to loss of cartilage, but this is not the mechanism of ordinary human osteoarthritis. However, damage to the chondrocytes may be the mechanism responsible for the osteoarthritis that appears in ochronosis (alcaptonuria). Damage to cartilage occurs with repeated hemorrhage into joints, and an osteoarthritic process is part of the pathology in hemophilic arthopathy. In eastern Siberia a nutritional disease, called *Kashin-Beck disease,* leads to osteoarthritis. Although the mechanism is not clear, a toxin from a fungus contaminating grain supplies has been suggested as the cause of defective epiphyseal growth and maturation that leads to secondary joint changes.

The frequency of osteoarthritis increases with increasing age. The relationship of the fundamental pathogenetic mechanism to aging as a biologic phenomenon remains obscure. No alterations in proteoglycan or collagen metabolism with increasing age have been demonstrated. One relevant observation, however, pertains to the increased cross-linking of collagen fibers which appears with time and thus with age. This increased cross-linking results in a decrease in tensile strength of the collagen fibers in articular cartilage with increasing age. The loss of tensile strength presumably makes the cartilage more susceptible to injury from impact stress. This phenomenon and compromised neural and muscular function (and thus decreased ability of the neuromuscular apparatus to protect cartilage from injury) are both components of the normal process of aging and may be important factors contributing to the development of osteoarthritic cartilage lesions in older individuals.

CLINICAL FEATURES

Osteoarthritis most frequently affects older people, increasing in frequency with increasing age. The most frequent age of onset of symptoms is in the fifth decade and later. When special mechanical problems affect specific joints, symptoms may begin in the 20s or even earlier; this occurs, for example, following alterations in the contour of the femoral head by aseptic necrosis in childhood. Occupational stresses are another frequent cause of the early onset of symptoms of osteoarthritis. Lesions of the finger joints often appear in women shortly after menopause, although the relationship to the change in endocrine function is unknown.

Symptomatic osteoarthritis occurs with similar frequency in men and women, although there is a sex difference in the distribution of the disease. Lower spine and hip disease are more common in men, whereas cervical spine and finger lesions are more frequent in women.

The most commonly affected joints in osteoarthritis are the distal interphalangeal joints of the fingers (Heberden's nodes), the proximal interphalangeal joints of the fingers (Bouchard's nodes), the first metatarsophalangeal (bunion) joints of the feet, the spine, the hips, and the knees. Several finger joints (Fig. 2) or numerous joints in the spine may be affected in a single individual but the disease is usually limited to one or two axial joints. There is no increased incidence of osteoarthritis in the hips or knees of patients with Heberden's nodes; local physical factors produce the disease and thus are not necessarily associated with pathogenetic local factors in other sites.

Pain is the cardinal symptom of osteoarthritis. The pain initially occurs on motion or weight bearing and is relieved by rest. As the disease progresses a minimal

motion produces pain and use of the joint becomes very limited, producing serious disability. In severe exacerbations accompanied by muscle spasm, pain may be continuous, unrelieved by rest, and can awaken the patient at night when any movement occurs. Stiffness after periods of rest, especially on arising in the morning, is frequent but not as consistently present as in rheumatoid arthritis and usually is brief unless the process is far advanced. Pain may be local in the region of the affected joint or may radiate along the muscles that move that joint, especially in the case of spinal and hip osteoarthritis.

It is important to try to decipher the mechanism responsible for the pain in each patient. Since there are no nerve endings in cartilage the degenerative process in that tissue does not cause the pain. Much of the pain in osteoarthritis is the result of muscle spasm, especially in the extensor muscles of the spine in spinal osteoarthritis or in adductors and flexors of the hip in osteoarthritis of that joint. In other cases pain seems to result from abnormal stresses on the underlying bone, which is rich in nerve endings and is exposed to increased stresses as a result of the loss of its covering of articular cartilage. Pain in osteoarthritis can also arise from the joint capsule, surrounding ligaments, or soft tissue, again due to abnormal mechanical stresses on these tissues, or from periosteal elevation and inflammation at sites at which osteophytic new growth is developing. At times there is also superimposed low-grade synovitis; this synovial inflammation may be persistent and can contribute significantly to the symptoms. Antiinflammatory measures thus can give significant relief to some patients with osteoarthritis even though the disease is not primarily an inflammatory form of arthritis.

Objectively, signs of inflammation or joint effusion are usually minimal in osteoarthritis, but tenderness is often present, especially focally over joint margins where osteophytes are forming. Crepitus may be palpable during joint motion due to roughened cartilage surfaces. Muscle atrophy, weakness, limitation of motion, and contractures appear as the process progresses. Joint deformities due to altered bony alignment may be present, producing knock-knees or bowlegs.

Since osteoarthritis is a local process it is not associated with systemic manifestations such as those that occur with inflammatory joint disease. Thus there is no associated anorexia, weight loss, fever, leukocytosis, elevated sedimentation rate, or immunologic abnormalities (such as immunoglobulin elevations or complement depletion). Osteoarthritis is very common, however, and may coexist with other diseases that do produce such phenomena.

Early in the development of osteoarthritis of the distal interphalangeal joints there may be a great deal of swelling, redness, warmth, and tenderness at the sites where the bony swellings of the Heberden's nodes later appear. During the period when these inflammatory findings are present there is considerable local pain. These findings may be diagnostically confusing and an inflam-

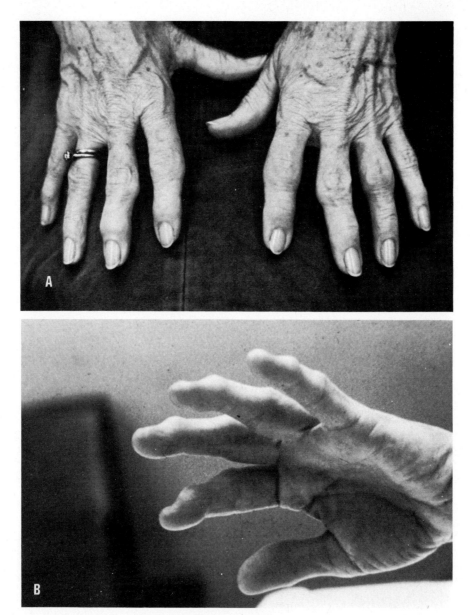

Fig. 2. Hands of a patient with osteoarthritis showing Heberden's nodes at the distal interphalangeal joints and Bouchard's nodes at the proximal interphalangeal joints.

matory form of joint disease or even a neoplasm may be suspected. This local inflammation apparently occurs when the cartilage and bone proliferation (osteophyte formation) begin, before there is any radiologic abnormality. Later, after the osteophyte is fully formed, the inflammatory phenomena are completely absent but the joint is deformed by the bony swelling and often some lateral deviation of the distal phalanx, producing the typical "gnarled" fingers of the aged. X-rays at this point show narrowing of the joint space, osteophytes, and the deformity, but there are few symptoms at this time.

This course of events may be easily observed in the distal interphalangeal joints since they are superficial, but the same sequence of events may occur in other joints where the process is not visible due to overlying muscle and soft tissue, such as the spine or hips. This phenomenon may account for many patients with early osteoarthritis whose symptoms are not accompanied by demonstrable radiologic changes. It must also be kept in mind that x-rays are relatively insensitive indicators of cartilage degeneration, and thus symptoms can appear for any of the reasons mentioned without radiologic abnormality. As a result, some patients with osteoarthritis are told they have no disease or they have psychogenic rheumatism because x-rays are read as negative. On the other hand, many individuals with advance x-ray evidence of osteoarthritis of the spine do not have symptoms, apparently because no nerves are compressed and no muscle spasm is occurring. A mild episode of trauma can upset a precarious balance, however, and persistent symptoms may develop suddenly.

A notable group of patients with osteoarthritis of the distal and proximal interphalangeal joints, mostly women, have a marked inflammatory reaction over the joints at the onset and proceed to develop extensive destruction of cartilage and bone in these joints. Mucous cysts may occur over the joints. Narrowing of joint space occurs early, and destruction of bone of the articular cortex and juxtaarticular erosive lesions also occur. The destruction of the joint surfaces can also lead to subluxation of the digits. This inflammatory, destructive process is often referred to as *erosive osteoarthritis*. Differentiation from rheumatoid arthritis may be difficult on clinical grounds, but the sedimentation rate remains normal or low and rheumatoid factor is absent in these cases.

Advanced osteoarthritis can cause deformities of affected joints due to distorted alignment of joint surfaces. Loss of joint motion is common in advanced disease, mostly due to muscle spasm or contractures, but occasionally due to the bony deformity, joint surface incongruity, or impingement of large osteophytes on other bony surfaces.

Other local complications can have more extensive functional consequences; for example, nerve root or spinal cord compression can produce widespread neurologic disease. Proliferation of cartilage and bone around affected joints of the cervical spine may be particularly marked along the posterior surface of the vertebral bodies and may encroach on the spinal canal. This new bone formation can press into the ventral surface of the spinal cord; segmental anterior horn compression can produce loss of motor function of that segment and long-tract sensory loss or motor abnormalities can occur below. This process is often labeled *cervical spondylosis*.

Osteophytes forming around the nerve root foramina, which result from osteoarthritic changes in the apophyseal joints between the vertebral articulating facets, can cause dysfunction of the nerve roots. Pain, muscle weakness, atrophy, and loss of deep tendon reflexes can occur. Pain radiation may follow specific nerve root distribution and cause objective changes in muscle groups served by those roots. For example, root compression at L_3 will cause sensory change in the anterior surface of the lower thigh and medial surface of the knee and weakness in abduction of the hip and extension of the knee. Compression of the nerve root at L_4 can result in quadriceps weakness and loss of the knee jerk, as well as sensory change along the anteromedial surface of the leg. A lesion at L_5 can cause loss of dorsiflexion of the foot and toes, weakness of extension and abduction of the hip, and sensory changes anterolaterally. When the lesion is at S_1 the ankle jerk can be lost, weakness occurs in flexion of the knee and foot, and there are sensory changes posterolaterally in the calf and foot.

The compression of nerve roots in osteoarthritis correlates with the presence of osteophytes encroaching on the neural foramina, but not necessarily with the degree of impingement on this space seen radiologically. The lack of correlation between symptoms and x-ray findings occurs because the cartilaginous component of the osteophyte is radiolucent and because symptoms can result from kinking or compression of the vascular supply to the nerve root and are not solely due to actual compression of the nerve tissue by the newly formed bone itself.

Examination of the synovial fluid in uncomplicated osteoarthritis usually shows normal viscosity, relatively few cells (which are mostly mononuclear), and low total protein. No pathologic crystals are present, but the spun sediment may show fragments of cartilage worn off the abnormal surfaces. No significant antibodies, lowering of complement, or other immunologic abnormalities are found. The synovial fluid reflects the fact that the basic processes are mechanical and metabolic rather than immunologic or inflammatory.

X-rays may show narrowing of the "joint space," a result of the loss of cartilage substance (the radiologic space between the bones is due to the presence of the radiolucent cartilage).The proliferation of bone and cartilage at the joint margins produces radiologically visible osteophytes. Occasionally subcortical bone cysts occur in osteoarthritis; when numerous they can confuse the radiologic diagnosis since they resemble lesions seen in rheumatoid arthritis or gout. The pathogenesis of these cysts is unclear; according to a popular theory tiny fratures through the cartilage substance and the articular cortex allow synovial fluid to be forced down into narrow spaces under pressure, producing cysts.

Flare-ups of pain and inflammation in osteoarthritic joints can occur because of superimposed pseudogout. Crystals of calcium pyrophosphate can be found in the joint fluid in such instances and occasionally there is radiologically demonstrable calcification in the articular cartilage. These attacks of crystal-induced synovitis resemble attacks of gout and on occasion respond to colchicine. Patients with osteoarthritis have the usual frequency of other diseases, including other forms of arthritis. Urate crystal-induced synovitis, true gout, can thus appear as well.

SECONDARY OSTEOARTHRITIS

Since other forms of joint disease can alter the articular surfaces and change mechanical forces in the joint, osteoarthritic changes can develop secondary to other forms of arthritis. Clinically it is necessary to determine which aspects of the patient's problem result from which type of joint pathology. The radiologic report usually describes "mixed arthritis," which is technically correct, but the symptoms are usually due to the primary form of joint disese and the osteoarthritis is more apparent radiologically than clinically. In some instances the primary process, perhaps rheumatoid arthritis, may be inactive or burnt out and the symptoms may be due to the secondary osteoarthritis which now does not respond to the antirheumatic agents that controlled the rheumatoid arthritis when it was active.

The concept of secondary osteoarthritis also includes instances in which an earlier form of bone pathology has altered physical stresses in the joint, resulting in the development of osteoarthritic lesions. The osteoarthritis is thus secondary to the preexisting joint abnormality. For example, secondary osteoarthritis commonly develops in a hip joint following aseptic necrosis of the femoral head; the collapse and distortion of the femoral head results in incongruity of the joint surfaces and altered physical stresses develop during motion of the hip.

Osteoarthritis may follow other causes of altered mechanical forces in the joints. Specific instances of trauma may cause altered physical stresses of a joint, perhaps as a result of fracture of a joint surface, damage to other intraarticular structures (e.g., the menisci of the knee), or tearing of ligamentous structures, thus producing instablity of the joint and subsequently unusual stresses with joint motion.

Sensory neuropathies, especially if position sense is impaired, result in severe forms of osteoarthritis which can develop rapidly and cause gross disorganization of the joint. The typical "Charcot's joint" which develops in these instances may have a more complex etiology, due to loss of as yet undefined neural influences on joint integrity, but much of the pathogenesis is the consequence of the abnormal physical stresses which result from loss of protective neuromuscular functions. Spinal cord syphilis used to be the most common cause of neuropathic arthritis, but diabetic and other forms of peripheral neuropathy and syringomyelia are the most common causes at the present time. Since the neuropathy affects transmission of pain sensation, this process may be painless; instability of the joint, bony deformity, swelling and large effusions due to traumatic synovitis, and disability are the usual clinical manifestations.

TREATMENT

Therapy of osteoarthritis initially consists of attempts to prevent the cartilage injury or to delay progression of wear of the joint structures in established cases. Relief of pain and preservation of joint motion are the main objectives of treatment. There are no agents currently available that can influence the progression of the basic process of cartilage erosion, although progress in our understanding of the biochemical mechanisms offers hope of the development of agents to delay loss of cartilage matrix components or to hasten their replacement.

Prevention of osteoarthritis currently consists of efforts to prevent or minimize the mechanical factors important in initiating or causing progression of the cartilage breakdown. Thus postural abnormalities, instability of joints, meniscus tears, etc., should be corrected as soon as possible. Avoidance of excessive fatigue during exercise is also important since protection of joint structures from injury requires normal function of the neuromuscular apparatus. Prevention of progression of the disease can sometimes be accomplished through measures aimed at the same mechanical factors that are important in pathogenesis, such as joint instability. Weight is a major form of stress on most osteoarthritic joints; if a patient is obese, measures to reduce weight, if successful, can give significant symptomatic improvement and presumably delay progression of the basic process. Use of mechanical assistive devices, such as a cane or crutches, can also derease the load and thus the physical stresses on abnormal joint surfaces.

An analgesic dosage of aspirin constitutes the initial basis of drug treatment in most instances. Other nonsteroidal antirheumatic drugs are also useful if the patient does not tolerate aspirin well. Indomethacin, phenylbutazone, Tylenol, and newer agents such as ibuprofen, naproxen, and flufenamic acid have been found to be useful adjuncts in the therapy of osteoarthritis. Since much of the pain experienced by patients with osteoarthritis is due to muscle spasm, measures directed at this problem, such as heat, massage, and traction, may give greater relief than analgesics. Agents directed specifically at relief of pain, such as propoxyphene hydrochloride (Darvon) can also be useful, but addictive narcotics such as codeine should be avoided. Since the disease requires prolonged, indefinite therapy, narcotic agents can cause major problems and the avoidance of toxicity of any agents used must be given careful consideration.

Rest is helpful during exacerbations of pain. Exacerbations of pain resulting from traumatic synovitis may respond to local heat and antiinflammatory doses of aspirin or other antirheumatic agents. Some patients experience considerable temporary improvement from intraarticular injections of steroidal antiinflammatory agents. However, intraarticular steroids should be used sparingly in osteoarthritis and rarely should be given more than once or twice in a single joint without several months between injections as these steroids can suppress synthesis of proteoglycans by the chondrocytes; decreased synthesis of the proteoglycans could hasten the loss of these vital matrix components, accelerating the pathogenetic process. Severe disorganizing osteoarthritis, called *Charcot-like arthropathy* has been reported following frequent intraarticular steroid injections.

Prevention of secondary muscle atrophy and contractures can minimize the disability that occurs in osteoarthritis. Passive and active exercises directed at these objectives is therefore of special importance in osteoarthritis of the hips and knees since flexion contractures of these joints are particularly disabling. Quadriceps weakness and atrophy should be prevented or corrected as soon as possible by specifically designed exercises.

Surgical procedures can be of great benefit to patients with osteoarthritis. At times minor operations, such as removal of joint mice or a torn meniscus causing locking or pain, can be of value. Major orthopedic procedures are necessary to relieve pain and restore function when the destructive lesions have progressed to the point of severe unremitting pain, especially pain at night, and marked disability. The decision concerning the appropriate time of surgery can usually be left to the patient; when the pain and disability are severe enough the patient requests it. At this stage there is usually very marked deformation of the femoral head or the knee joint—the two most frequent sites of arthroplasty using prosthetic devices.

Older operative procedures, such as muscle-splitting operations around the hip, gave a great deal of relief to some patients with minimal surgery. Joint fusion can also be valuable in selected instances. These procedures are still useful when the condition of the patient precludes more extensive surgery, but results with prosthetic replacement of the hip joint are so successful that other procedures have largely been discontinued. Success rates of 90–95 percent are being achieved in most centers; the rare occurrence of late postoperative infection is the main reason for poor results. Attempts to achieve similar results with prosthetic replacement of other joints are in earlier phases of development but promising results are being achieved.

Osteoarthritic chondromalacia of the patella can cause a great deal of pain and a simple procedure such as a patellectomy can give relief in such instances. Osteoarthritis of the spine, especially of the cervical spine, may benefit from fusion if traction and analgesics fail. Patients with cervical spondylosis with neuropathy usually improve following surgical removal of the bony overgrowth compressing the spinal cord.

REFERENCES

Bennett GA, Waine H, Bauer W: Changes in the Knee Joint at Various Ages. New York, Commonwealth Fund, 1942

Bollet AJ: An essay on the biology of osteoarthritis. Arthritis Rheum 12:152, 1969

Mankin H: The reaction of articular cartilage to injury and osteoarthritis. N Engl J Med 291:1285, 1335, 1974

Radin EL: Mechanical aspects of osteoarthrosis. Bull Rheum Dis 26:862, 1976

Sokoloff L: The Biology of Degenerative Joint Disease. Chicago, University of Chicago Press, 1969

Wright V (ed): Osteoarthrosis. Clinics in Rheumatic Diseases, vol 2. Philadelphia, Saunders, 1976

Neuropathic Joint Disease

J. Donald Smiley

PATHOGENESIS AND PATHOLOGY

ETIOLOGY AND PATHOGENESIS

The diabetic patient with peripheral neuropathy can stand without discomfort in one position for so long that he causes a pressure necrosis of the skin of the foot leading to deep ulceration and indolent infection. The same defect in deep pain or position sense can affect joints by producing cartilaginous damage. Chondrocytes in the deeper cartilage layers then proliferate in an attempt to repair the cartilage injury, and degenerative joint changes that resemble osteoarthritis develop. A small fraction of patients with diabetes—about 1 of 600—go on to develop a rapidly destructive arthritis of the involved joint. Diabetic neuropathic arthropathy is clinically similar to that described by Jean Martin Charcot in patients with neurosyphilis in 1868, except for differences in joint distribution.

Since most diabetic or syphilitic patients with severe neuropathy do *not* develop the destructive arthritis, other contributing factors must be necessary. Recently, McCarty and his co-workers have observed that chondrocalcinosis caused by the deposition of calcium pyrophosphate dihydrate (CPPD) crystals in cartilage is an almost universal accompaniment of neuropathic arthropathy. Chondrocalcinosis is many times more frequent in diabetic patients than in nondiabetic controls and is usually associated with roentgenologic and histologic changes of osteoarthritis. It is reasonable to suggest, therefore, that the neuropathy of diabetes predisposes the joints of the

foot to cartilage injury, that the injured, now dividing chondrocytes release inorganic pyrophosphate, and that this leads to CPPD deposition. The CPPD further alters the physical properties of cartilage and degenerative changes result. The remarkable similarity of the early histopathology in cartilage and synovial tissue of neuropathic arthropathy to that found in osteoarthritis emphasizes cartilage degeneration as a common initiating event in both conditions.

Thus, it is suggested that Charcot's joints occur in those occasional patients whose CPPD deposition exceeds a critical level. Since pain recognition is impaired, the patient continues to use the affected joint and cartilage surface is lost, shedding CPPD crystals into the joint space and thus generating inflammation and synovitis. With absent cartilage the noncushioned bone then develops microfractures, joint surface destruction, and fragmentation. Intraarticular hemorrhages follow and the *destructive phase* of Charcot's joint is seen. The degree and location of sensory loss, the relative intensity of physical use of the desensitized joint, the level of cartilage injury and repair, and probably other variables in cartilage metabolism all influence the development of neuropathic arthropathy. Very rare patients without demonstrable neuropathology have been described in whom destructive arthritis indistinguishable from Charcot's joints has developed. Perhaps other genetic or metabolic disorders that predispose cartilage to CPPD deposition could explain the joint pathology found in these otherwise normal patients.

Table 1
Causes of Neuropathic Arthropathy

Syphilitic tabes dorsalis	Familial dysautonomia* (Riley-
Diabetic polyneuropathy	Day)
Syringomyelia	Other hereditary neuropathies*
Spina bifida with	including Djerine Sottas
meningomyelocele*	disease
Alcholic neuropathy	Thalidomide-induced injury*
Trauma to or surgery of the	Pernicious anemia
spinal cord	Hemiplegia
Tumors of the spinal cord	Arachnoiditis after tuberculosis
Leprosy	or spinal anesthesia
Peroneal muscle atrophy*	Amyloidosis
(Charcot-Marie-Tooth)	Acromegaly
	Intraarticular steroid therapy

*More common in children.

Charcot's joints may develop in patients with almost any cause of significant sensory loss except those associated with increased spastic muscle tone. Table 1 is a list of the more common causes in the order of their relative frequency in the United States. The rapid decline in the incidence of syphilis will eventually make diabetes the leading cause of neuropathic arthropathy.

PATHOLOGY

The underlying disease processes responsible for neuropathic arthritis are often present a number of years prior to the onset of the joint disease. For example, diabetes and syphilis usually require 15–20 years before sufficient neuropathy develops to cause Charcot's joints to appear. The location of the greatest sensory loss determines the site of the joint destruction. In patients with syphilitic tabes dorsalis, the knee is the most frequent joint involved, but 40 percent of patients show multiple joint involvement reflecting the widespread nature of the sensory loss. Ankle, foot, and hip involvement are common, and 6 percent of patients develop axial spine arthropathy.

Diabetic patients tend to develop Charcot's joints primarily in the forefoot in the metatarsophalangeal and tarsometatarsal joints; only 12 percent of patients show ankle involvement. Only an occasional diabetic patient develops a Charcot's joint in the knee, hip, or spine. Syringomyelia, which creates sensory loss primarily in the upper extremities, selects the shoulder joint most frequently, followed by the elbow and the wrist—altogether accounting for 80 percent of affected joints. The cervical spine is the next most frequent location and multiple joint involvement is also common in syringomyelia. In leprosy, the joints involved most frequently are the small joints of the hands and feet, including the tarsus and wrist joints—again emphasizing the selective nature of the neuropathy in various conditions.

Syringomyelia and leprosy have a high frequency (25–29 percent of patients) of Charcot's joint development. Between 4 and 10 percent of patients with syphilitic tabes dorsalis develop Charcot's joints. In diabetes, a wide range (0.11–6.8 percent) of estimates of the frequency of neuropathic arthropathy have been reported. Because many of the joints involved in the diabetic foot coexist with adjacent infected ulcers, a number of series have excluded these patients, thereby underestimating the true incidence of Charcot's joints in diabetic subjects. Neuropathic arthropathy probably occurs in about 0.2 percent of adult diabetic patients. Congenital abnormalities of the spine associated with spina bifida and meningomyelocele are the most frequent causes of Charcot's joints in children. These defects, even when surgically repaired, often produce damage to nerves serving the lower extremities and predispose these children to neuropathic arthropathy.

The histopathology of the different types of neuropathic arthropathy is similar. Early the features resemble those of osteoarthritis. The *destructive phase,* however, rapidly creates such fragmentation of the joint surface and surrounding bone tissue that particles of calcium are implanted in the synovium even at some distance from the major joint surface. An "autoarthrogram" is occasionally generated in the suprapatellar space or in bursae surrounding the joint.

The synovium proliferates and becomes invasive, with large numbers of capillaries in the deeper layers. The macrophages lining the synovial membrane pick up fragments of cartilage and bone, and in some areas these cartilage fragments calcify or even ossify. During the *hypertrophic phase,* osteophytes develop and can be fractured to generate large loose bodies which may be numerous. This phase represents an effort to repair the instability generated during the destructive phase. Once the patient has passed through the hypertrophic phase, the joint gradually becomes more stable and rarely reverts to the destructive phase of the disease. At this point, essentially all cartilage surface has been lost and further generation of CPPD is decreased.

CLINICAL ASPECTS AND TREATMENT

CLINICAL ASPECTS

An unexpected dislocation of a weight-bearing joint should strongly suggest the diagnosis of neuropathic arthropathy. After a thorough neurologic examination which demonstrates the loss of sensation, the diagnosis of Charcot's joints involves evaluation of laboratory parameters related to the causes of the disease. Laboratory studies should include serum tests for syphilis, spinal tap with spinal fluid Wasserman, blood sugar determination, glucose tolerance curves, serum B_{12} determinations, skull x-rays, myelograms if syringomyelia is suspected, nerve conduction studies in the peroneal nerve area for Charcot-Marie-Tooth disease, and nerve biopsies if Djerine-Sottas disease is suspected.

Since the fluid from the neuropathic joint is often present in large amounts and reaccumulates rapidly after arthrocentesis, this procedure may be useful in suggesting the diagnosis. Initially it resembles the fluid obtained from an osteoarthritic joint with high viscosity and little tendency to clot. This joint fluid usually has a low white blood cell count ranging from a few hundred to 2000 cells/mm³, although rare effusions have been described that resemble sterile pus. Fragments of cartilage and collagen fibers are often present and CPPD crystals can usually be demonstrated by careful examination under polarized light. As time progresses, there is a greater tendency to bleed into the damaged joint, producing an inflammatory reaction similar to that seen in hemophilia. The blood flow to the joint, and indeed the entire extremity, may be significantly increased and tense swelling and erythema may appear. The pain is much less than would be expected from the amount of the swelling and inflammation present. In some patients, the joint hemorrhage and bony destruction occur in the complete absence of pain.

Involvement of the spine is particularly likely to occur without symptoms until spinal cord compression supervenes. Excessive doses and/or too frequent use of intraarticular steroids may produce joint changes closely resembling Charcot's joints. The pain relief produced by steroids followed by overexercise of injured joints may mimic a neuropathic process.

Because the large synovial effusion that occurs in a neuropathic joint may dissect into the adjacent soft tissues, causing inflammation, this condition may also resemble acute thrombophlebitis in an occasional patient.

Conditions that mimic neuropathic arthropathy include coagulation disorders which cause bleeding into the joint space, infections with tuberculosis or staphylococci, and neoplasms such as osteogenic sarcoma or chondrosarcoma, which may cause extensive bone destruction and also produce hemorrhage into the joint space. Less commonly, gout, pseudogout, rheumatoid arthritis, or psoriatic arthritis may be so severe that they cause rapid joint destruction in a weight-bearing joint.

TREATMENT

Treatment of the patient with a Charcot's joint should be primarily directed at stabilization of the joint involved and thorough instruction of the patient to avoid joint trauma. Sometimes this is very difficult because the patient has relatively little pain in the area of the joint involvement. Reduction in the amount of walking, use of protective shoes, special boots or splints, or even a hip spica to stabilize disintegrating joints allows healing of the numerous microfractures that are present. Control of the underlying disease in syringomyelia by surgical decompression of the syrinx may allow improvement in the arthropathy. Careful management of the diabetes may also be beneficial in some patients. Treatment of syphilis with high doses of penicillin does not reverse the progression of destructive Charcot's joint changes. Careful treatment of skin ulceration with eradication of local infection is necessary to care for the diabetic foot that develops a neuropathic joint.

In patients who have gross anatomic dislocations of joints, transplantation of peripheral nerves or decompression of the spinal cord may be necessary. In occasional patients, the judicious removal of large loose bodies may allow the involved joints to become more stable. Rarely, more extensive surgery may be necessary. Arthrodesis using Charnley's compression clamps or prolonged immobilization in a cast can be beneficial. The use of glenohumeral joint replacement in the shoulder of syringomyelia patients has been evaluated and may be helpful. Weight-bearing prostheses in the lower extremity for hip, knee, or ankle joint replacement are of doubtful usefulness because of the tendency of these patients to traumatize and fragment bone adjacent to the artificial joint because of the loss of deep pain sensation.

REFERENCES

Bruckner FE, Howell A: Neuropathic joints. Semin Arthritis Rheum 2:47, 1972

Clouse ME, Gramm HF, Legg M, Flood: Diabetic osteoarthropathy. Clinical and roentgenographic observations in ninety cases. Am J Roentgenol Radium Ther Nucl Med 121:22, 1974

Jacobelli S, McCarty DJ, Silcox DC, Mall JC: Calcium pyrophosphate crystal deposition in neuropathic joints. Four cases of polyarticular involvement. Ann Intern Med 79:340, 1973

Sinha S, Munichoodappa CS, Kozak GP: Neuro-arthropathy (Charcot joints) in diabetes mellitus (clinical study of 101 cases). Medicine (Baltimore) 51:191, 1972

Heritable Disorders of Connective Tissue

The heritable disorders of connective tissue are a group of disorders in which pathology is the result of abnormal metabolism of molecules of the extracellular matrix, collagen, elastin, proteoglycans, and glycoproteins. Those disorders, in which biochemical abnormalities have been identified, are primarily defects in proteoglycan and collagen metabolism, the former among the mucopolysaccharidoses, the latter among the Ehlers-Danlos syndromes.

REFERENCES

Bornstein P, Byers PH: Disorders of collagen metabolism, in Bondy P, Rosenberg, L (eds): Duncan's Diseases of Metabolism (ed 8). Philadelphia, Saunders, (in press).

McKusick VA: Heritable Disorders of Connective Tissue. St. Louis, Mosby, 1972

Uitto J, Lichtenstein JR: Defects in the biochemistry of collagen in diseases of connective tissue. J Invest Dermatol 66:59, 1976

EHLERS-DANLOS SYNDROMES

Peter H. Byers
and Karen A. Holbrook

The Ehlers-Danlos syndromes (EDS) are a group of disorders characterized by skin fragility and hyperextensibility, joint hypermobility, and marked increase in bruising. There are at least seven varieties that can be distinguished clinically; biochemical, genetic, and morphologic studies have demonstrated further discrimination within the broad clinical categories.

TYPE I: GRAVIS

Type I EDS is the severe, classic form of EDS and is characterized by thin, soft skin that has a velvety texture, marked large and small joint hypermobility, hyperextensible and fragile skin that results in gaping wounds when cut, and marked increase in bruisability. Wounds heal with papyraceous scars—the "cigarette paper" scars associated with the syndrome. In areas of repeated trauma, hyperpigmentation is common and "pseudotumor molluscum," accumulations of soft connective tissue, may occur. Although the skin may be the most dramatically affected tissue, many other systems may be affected.

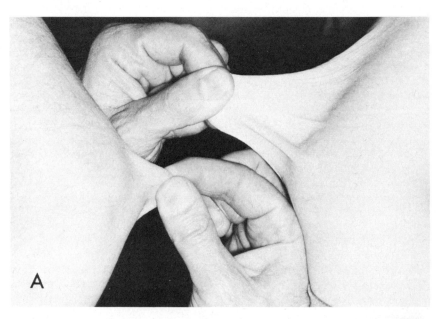

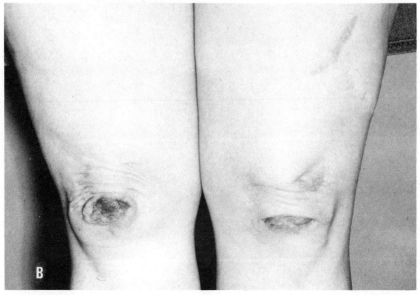

Orthopedic problems such as severe pes planus, kypho-scoliosis, and early onset osteoarthritis may occur. Inguinal hernia is common, as well as cardiac valvular abnormalities. Indeed, mitral valve prolapse may affect the majority of individuals with type I EDS. Prematurity is frequent and is apparently due to abnormalities in fetal membrane structure (Fig. 1).

Histologically, in Type I EDS the dermis usually contains collagen bundles that appear in whorls. At the ultrastructural level collagen fibrils are 15–50 percent larger than normal and may be branched and twisted but still retain a normal banding pattern (Fig. 2, page 346).

Inheritance of the disorder is in an autosomal dominant manner and, unlike some other dominant disorders, there is very little variability within families among those affected. The risk to an affected individual for having a similarly affected child is 50 percent, as it is with all dominantly inherited disorders.

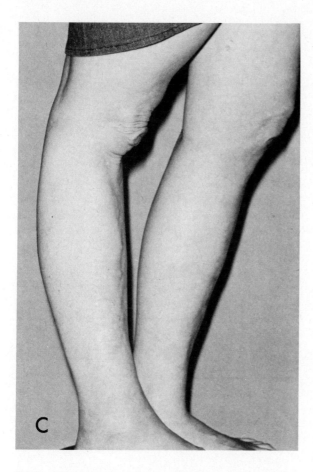

Fig. 1. Woman with type I EDS. **A.** Skin extensibility. Skin over the elbow of a woman with EDS (right) stretches considerably farther than that of a control (left). **B.** Scars are often hyperpigmented and generally have an atrophic or "cigarette paper" quality. **C.** Large joints are frequently hypermobile, as illustrated here by genu recurvatum.

TYPE II: MITIS

Type II EDS shares many of the clinical features of type I but is milder in all respects. Thus, skin fragility, hyperextensibility, joint hypermobility, and bruising, while all present, are much less severe than in type I and scarring is more normal. This, too, is a dominantly inherited disorder but is distinct from type I since families with type II do not contain individuals with the clinical manifestations of type I. Possibly they are allelic disorders, that is, different mutations at the same genetic locus. The histologic and ultrastructural findings are similar to those seen in type I.

TYPE III: BENIGN FAMILIAL HYPEREXTENSIBILITY

Type III EDS is another dominantly inherited disorder in which the major manifestations are those of joint hypermobility, particularly of the large joints. While the skin may be somewhat soft, it is generally not hyperextensible and scarring is usually normal. In contrast to types I and II, there may be moderate variability among family members with this disorder.

The biochemical basis of EDS types I, II and III is unknown, although the similarity of clinical findings to those in other disorders in which collagen metabolism is known to be affected, and the ultrastructural findings that demonstrate abnormal collagen, suggest strongly that the basic defect probably lies in type I collagen. It is possible, however, that molecules such as matrix proteoglycans, which affect the arrangement of collagen in tissues, could be defective.

TYPE IV: ECCHYMOTIC

Type IV EDS (ecchymotic type, Sach-Barabas type, or arterial variety) is characterized by extreme thinness of skin, severe bruising, and a high frequency of rupture of bowel and large arteries. This disorder is genetically heterogeneous and both dominant and recessive inheritance has been noted. The dominantly inherited variety appears to be less severe; longevity is near normal, although death may be due to a catastrophic event such as rupture of the bowel or an artery. The recessive variety is more severe and survival beyond the third decade of life is rare. Skin is extremely thin and the venous pattern may be visible throughout the body; the subcutaneous tissues are normal and the thin skin is due to marked decrease in dermal collagen. The dermis may be fragile, but healing and scar formation are usually normal; joint hypermobility, when present, is limited to the small joints of the hands and fingers, and skin is not hyperextensible. Minor trauma often produces large hematomas (Fig. 3).

Biochemical investigations of one individual with a sporadic variety of type IV EDS indicated that no type III collagen was produced by cells in culture and that none could be found in any of the tissues investigated. It seems likely that this phenotype is due to abnormalities in the production or stability of type III collagen and that the tissues most severely affected are those rich in that collagen.

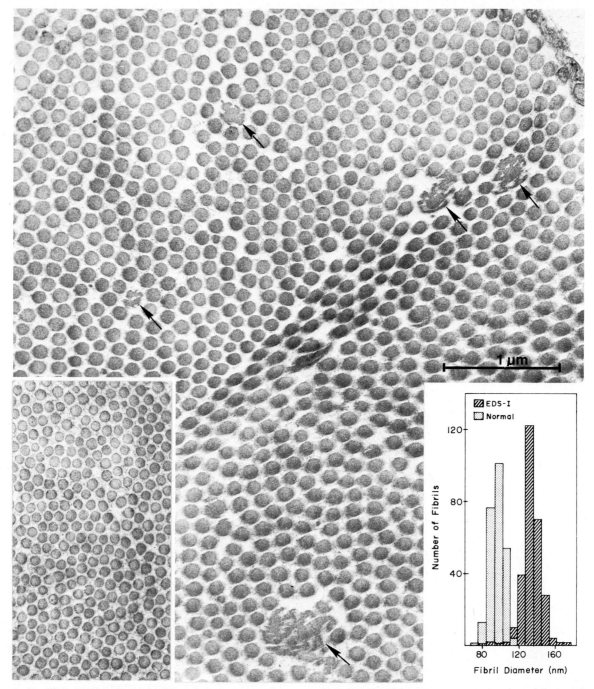

Fig. 2.   Electron micrograph of collagen fibrils in dermis of a 16-year-old male with EDS-I. When compared to normal (lower left), fibril cross-sections are larger and many fibrils are large and irregular in outline (arrows). At lower right is a histogram of fibril diameters. The fibrils in this patient with EDS-I have a mean diameter of 134 nm; normal is 95 nm. [Reproduced by permission from Vogel, Holbrook, Steinman, Gitzelman, Byers: Abnormal collagen fibril structure in type I (gravis) Ehlers-Danlos syndrome. Lab Invest 40:201–206, 1979.]

TYPE V: X-LINKED

Type V EDS is an X-linked variety in which the clinical findings are similar to those in type II. Several families have been described in which the disorder affects only males. In one family in which the additional abnormalities of short stature and cardiac defects have been described, it has been suggested that lysyl oxidase, the enzyme involved in collagen cross-link formation, may

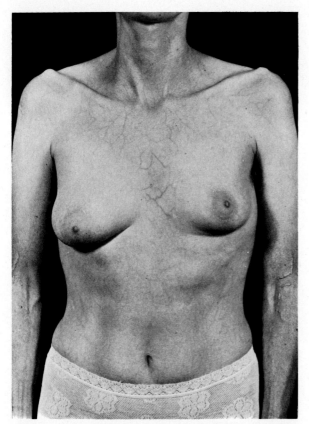

Fig. 3. Woman 26 years old with type IV EDS. She has extremely prominent vasculature, which is visible over her chest, abdomen, and arms. Elastosis perforans serpiginata is visible on her arms. (Courtesy of Dr. B. McGillivray and Dr. P. M. MacLeod.)

TYPE VII: ARTHROCHALASIS MULTIPLEX CONGENITA

Type VII EDS is a rare, recessively inherited disorder characterized by short stature and severe large and small joint hypermobility, commonly with recurrent dislocation; skin is soft and mildly hyperextensible. Deficiency of the enzyme that cleaves the NH_2-terminal extensions from procollagen appears to be the biochemical disorder in this type of EDS. Failure to normally convert procollagen to collagen appears to interfere with normal fibril formation, stability, and function.

It is likely that the EDS will be further subdivided as more biochemical defects are found. At present the common pathologic process appears to be interference with normal collagen fibril stability.

REFERENCES

Beighton P: The Ehlers-Danlos Syndrome. London, William Heinemann, 1970

Di Ferrante N, Leachman RD, Angelini P, Donnelly PV, Francis G, Almazan A: Lysyl oxidase deficiency in Ehlers-Danlos syndrome type V. Connect Tissue Res 3:49, 1975

Lichtenstein JR, Martin GR, Kohn L, Byers PH, McKusick VA: Defect in conversion of procollagen to collagen in a form of Ehlers-Danlos syndrome. Science 182:298, 1973

Pinnell SR, Krane SM, Kenzora JE, Glimcher MJ: A heritable disorder of connective tissue. Hydroxylysine-deficient collagen disease. N Engl J Med 286:1013, 1972

Pope FM Martin GR, Lichtenstein JR, Penttinen RP, Gerson B, Rowe DW, McKusick VA: Patients with Ehlers-Danlos syndrome IV lack type III collagen. Proc Natl Acad Sci USA 72:1314, 1975

OSTEOGENESIS IMPERFECTA

Peter H. Byers

be abnormal. In another disorder, an X-linked variety of cutis laxa, lysyl oxidase is abnormal.

TYPE VI: OCULAR

Type VI EDS is the best biochemically characterized of the human disorders. The clinical findings are similar to those of type I EDS, although scarring may be less prominent. Joint hyperextensibility is marked, scoliosis may be prominent, and there may be keratoconus and ocular globe fragility. One affected individual died in her late forties as the result of aortic rupture. At the ultrastructural level, collagen fibrils are described as normal, although organization of collagen bundles in dermis may be abnormal. This disorder is biochemically and clinically heterogeneous, perhaps because of multiple allelic abnormalities. The mechanical abnormality of skin and other tissues is due to a lack of lysyl hydroxylation, caused by decreased lysyl hydroxylase activity, and leads to altered crosslink formation. This disorder is recessively inherited. A similar clinical disorder has been described in which lysyl hydroxylase is apparently normal. Apparently, the major cross links in collagen contain hydroxylysine rather than lysine.

Osteogenesis imperfecta (OI) is a group of genetically, clinically, and biochemically distinct disorders that have in common decreased bone mineralization and increased bone fragility. They are, however, generalized connective tissue disorders in which blue sclerae, diminished hearing due largely to otosclerosis, dentinogenesis imperfecta, and thin skin are common findings; indeed, the triad of brittle bones, blue sclerae, and deafness is common among affected individuals.

The most common form of OI is the dominantly inherited variety, in which affected individuals have the characteristic group of findings just described. There is considerable variability in expression such that even within a single family some members may have multiple fractures (as many as 100 prior to puberty) and the majority of associated clinical findings, while others may have only blue sclerae. Severely affected individuals may be dwarfed as a result of shortened long bones secondary to multiple fractures. Intelligence is usually normal unless birth is complicated by intracranial bleeding; this results occasionally because of the enlarged cranial vault and multiple wormian bones. The characteristic triangular faces of individuals with the dominant form of OI is the result of small basal bones in the skull and the enlarged calvarium.

The dominant forms may be symptomatic at or prior to birth with multiple in utero fractures often found. Characteristically, fracture frequency is highest in childhood and decreases after puberty. There may be two dominantly inherited varieties of OI: one, the congenita form, is manifest at or prior to birth; in the other, the tarda form, fractures do not occur until later in childhood. On x-ray examination in the severe variety the long bones are characteristically extremely thin and decreased mineralization is generally apparent. Areas of multiple healing fractures may be seen and callus may be exuberant.

One other form of OI present at birth may be recessively inherited. In these infants perinatal death is common. Bones are extremely brittle but are usually broad and wavy in contrast to the thin bones of the dominant variety. Characteristically, there is marked proximal limb shortening, and with survival extremely short stature is seen.

The biochemical basis of OI is not yet certain; in view of the several varieties, multiple abnormalities can be expected. Abnormalities in synthesis or stability of type I collagen have been detected in cultures of dermal fibroblasts from several individuals. Increased amounts of type III collagen relative to type I in skin support such a mechanism. Increased lysyl hydroxylation of bone type I collagen has also been observed. Similar alterations of collagen in bone are seen in vitamin D deficiency, in which bone mineralization is markedly abnormal. It is likely that multiple mechanisms that ultimately affect bone mineralization will be found to explain the genetic and clinical heterogeneity in OI.

REFERENCES

Ibsen KH: Distinct varieties of osteogenesis imperfecta. Clin Orthop 50:279, 1967

Penttinen RP, Lichtenstein JR, Martin GR, McKusick VA: Abnormal collagen metabolism in cultured cells in osteogenesis imperfecta. Proc Natl Acad Sci USA 72:586, 1975

Sykes B, Francis MJ, Smith R: Altered relation of two collagen types in osteogenesis imperfects. N Engl J Med 296:1200, 1977

Trelstad RL, Rubin D, Gross J: Osteogenesis imperfecta congenita. Evidence for a generalized molecular disorder of collagen. Lab Invest 36:501, 1977

THE MARFAN SYNDROME

Peter H. Byers

The characteristic clinical features of the Marfan syndrome include arachnodactyly (long thin fingers), dolichostenomelia (long thin extremities), ectopia lentis, pectus excavatum or carinatum, scoliosis, high-arched palate, soft skin, loose jointedness, and cardiovascular abnormalities. As many as 80 percent of affected individuals have ectopia lentis and more may have cardiovascular disorders. Mitral valve prolapse and incompetence affect more than 90 percent of individuals with a confirmed diagnosis; somewhat fewer have aortic valvular abnormalities. Because of the more severe hemodynamic consequences of aortic valvular insufficiency, these lesions are of greater clinical concern than the mitral valvular ones. Aortic dissection is far more common in the Marfan syndrome patients than in normals; dissection usually begins in the ascending aorta and may progress both proximally and distally. The increased frequency of dissection accounts, in part, for the decreased life expectancy of individuals with this disorder. The generalized abnormality of connective tissue makes repair of valvular abnormalities and of structural large vessel damage difficult.

The Marfan syndrome is inherited in an autosomal dominant manner but there is considerable variation in expression. Thus, while some individuals have the severe findings, other affected members of the same family have only ectopia lentis or mild mitral valvular abnormalities.

Several disorders with similar clinical findings are grouped with the Marfan syndrome and include both the aesthenic (classic) and nonaesthenic varieties, contractural arachnodactyly, and the marfanoid hypermobility syndrome. Individuals with the nonaesthenic habitus nonetheless are at risk for major cardiovascular complications. Those with contractural arachnodactyly have tight joints and usually do not have ectopia lentis or major cardiovascular problems. The marfanoid hypermobility syndrome includes individuals with markedly hypermobile large joints, a marfanoid habitus, who may have valvular heart disease. Other conditions to be differentiated from the Marfan syndrome include homocystinuria (see the next chapter), homozygous sickle cell anemia, and Klinefelter's syndrome; in each, characteristic laboratory tests make the distinction. Ectopia lentis, often used as a major diagnostic criterion in the Marfan syndrome, is a feature of homocystinuria and the Weil-Marchesani syndrome but may appear as an isolated dominantly inherited disorder, in which case the differentiation from the Marfan syndrome may be difficult. It is frequently necessary to examine other family members in order to make the correct diagnosis in the proband.

The basic defect(s) in the Marfan syndrome remain unknown. The clinical similarity to animals treated with agents that inhibit collagen cross-link formation has suggested that abnormalities in collagen metabolism may be fundamental. In some patients an abnormality of proteoglycan metabolism may be important.

REFERENCES

Brown OR, DeMots H, Kloster FE, Roberts A, Menashe VD, Beals RK: Aortic root dilation and mitral valve prolapse in Marfan's syndrome: An echocardiographic study. Circulation 52:651, 1975

Lamberg SI, Dorfman A: Synthesis and degradation of hyaluronic acid in the cultured fibroblasts of Marfan's disease. J Clin Invest 52:2428, 1973

Murdoch JL, Walker BA, Halpern BL, Kuzman JW, McKusick VA: Life expectancy and causes of death in the Marfan syndrome. New Engl J Med 286:804, 1972

HOMOCYSTINURIA

Peter H. Byers

Homocystinuria is a group of recessively inherited disorders of methionine metabolism in which high circulating levels of homocysteine apparently produce multiple abnormalities. The clinical features include a marfanoid habitus with arachnodactyly and dolichostenomelia, ectopia lentis, kyphoscoliosis, and joint contracture, in contrast to the joint laxity of Marfan's syndrome. Mild mental retardation is common, and osteoporosis may be marked. There is an increased incidence of thrombosis in intermediate caliber arteries which can produce stroke, coronary artery occlusion, renal impairment and hypertension, claudication, and gastrointestinal hemorrhage. Although less frequent, venous thrombosis and pulmonary embolism do occur.

Some individuals with cystathionine synthetase deficiency, the most common enzymatic deficiency, respond to dietary B_6 (a cofactor of the enzyme) supplementation by a decrease in circulating homocysteine. In addition, some protection from vascular thrombosis may be afforded by platelet-directed anticoagulants.

The mechanisms by which homocysteine accumulation produces vascular abnormalities and connective tissue alterations are probably different. Homocysteine may directly injure endothelial cells and locally denude vessels, leading to thrombosis. In addition, homocysteine appears to interfere with collagen, and probably elastin, cross-link formation, although the precise manner in which this occurs is not known.

REFERENCES

Harker LA, Ross R, Slichter SJ, Scott CR: Homocystine-induced arteriosclerosis. The role of endothelial cell injury and platelet response in its genesis. J Clin Invest 58:731, 1976
Siegel RC: Collagen cross-linking. Effect of D-penicillamine on cross-linking in vitro. J Biol Chem 252:254, 1977

PSEUDOXANTHOMA ELASTICUM

Peter H. Byers

Pseudoxanthoma elasticum (PXE) is a group of inherited disorders characterized by age-dependent alterations in skin, angioid streaks of the retina, arterial calcification, and hemorrhage. Typically, the disorder is inherited in an autosomal recessive manner, although dominantly inherited forms are known.

Onset of skin changes is usually from the second to fourth decade with the appearance of yellow-colored macular or slightly raised and thickened areas along or near lines of folding. Thus the neck, axillae, and inguinal grooves are characteristic locations. The skin lesions have the texture of orange peel ("peau d'orange"). Angioid streaks, nonvascular markings on the retina that do not follow the usual vascular course, are frequently seen, with onset about the time of that of the skin lesions. Such lesions are occasionally seen in other of the inherited connective tissue disorders.

The major complications in PXE arise as a result of arterial occlusion or rupture, both consequences of early and progressive arterial calcification. Thus angina, stroke, hypertension, and gastrointestinal hemorrhage are frequent occurrences, the latter perhaps most common.

The basic biochemical defects in PXE are not known. Histologically, there is calcification in arterial vessels and in skin. The calcification appears limited to elastic fibers in the skin and in the artery walls. Whether the basic abnormalities involve the protein elastin or other connective tissue elements important for its organization has not been determined. Carriers of the recessive type cannot be detected by histologic examination, even at the electron microscopic level, but affected individuals with the dominant types can be detected occasionally prior to emergence of clinical signs.

REFERENCES

Dorfman A, Matalon R: The mucopolysaccharidoses. Proc Nat Acad Sci US 73:630, 1976

MUCOPOLYSACCHARIDOSES

Peter H. Byers

The mucopolysaccharidoses are a group of disorders in which the intracellular, lysosomal breakdown of polysaccharide chains derived from proteoglycans is defective. Because one or more of the acid hydrolases that normally function in lysosomes is abnormal, orderly degradation does not occur and large amounts of polysaccharide chains accumulate in lysosomes and appear in extracellular spaces and in urine.

Further complexity is introduced when it is recognized that certain of the lysosomal hydrolases may also degrade some glycolipids. Thus, abnormalities in those enzymes may also lead to lipid storage and additional symptomatology. Some attempts to treat these disorders have been made either by infusion of the missing enzyme directly or infusion of enzyme incorporated into liposomes; the results are still too preliminary to assess but the possibility of treatment remains (see the section on Lysosomal Diseases in the fascicle on Specific Articular and Connective Tissue Diseases for the clinical classification of these lysosomal disorders).

REFERENCES

Pope FM: Autosomal dominant pseudoxanthoma elasticum. J Med Genet 11:152–157, 1974

Relapsing Polychondritis

Charles D. Tourtellotte

PATHOGENESIS AND CLINICAL FEATURES

Relapsing polychondritis (RP) is an uncommon disorder characterized by inflammation of tissues that contain proportionately large amounts of sulfated glycosaminoglycans (mucopolysaccharides). Cartilagenous structures such as ear, nose, trachea, and rib, therefore, are prominently affected. The course is generally episodic and progressive. Arthritis, varied forms of ocular inflammation, audiovestibular impairment, cardiovascular lesions, and fever further characterize the disease. Mortality is moderately high due to involvement of the respiratory tract (tracheobronchial collapse) and cardiovascular structures (valvular or vasculitis). RP usually is recognized as an independent entity, but one-third of cases coexist with a broad range of other rheumatic and immunologically mediated disorders. Most patients are between the ages of 20 and 60, although the range extends from newborn infants to the elderly. A racial or sex predominance has not emerged.

PATHOGENESIS

The pathogenesis of RP is not entirely clear, however, it is generally regarded as a form of connective tissue disease in the spectrum of vasculitides with an immunologic mediation. Despite the low antigenicity of cartilage proteoglycans, antibodies and delayed hypersensitivity have been demonstrated in patients with RP. Histopathologically, during active phases there is focal perichondral chronic inflammation leading to matrix depletion of proteoglycans, probably mediated by lysosomal hydrolytic enzymes.

CLINICAL FEATURES

Painful erythematous swelling of one or both ears is the most common clinical presentation of this disorder. The noncartilagenous portion of the ear or the ear lobe is spared. Arthralgia and overt arthritis are common manifestations, but are somewhat variable in pattern and character. RP may resemble rheumatoid arthritis with small joint involvement of the hands. Alternatively, joint inflammation may be migratory, asymmetric in distribution, and intermittently acute. Arthritis, although usually nonerosive in character, may be extensive, mutilating, and otherwise indistinguishable from coexisting rheumatoid disease or ankylosing spondylitis. Polytendonitis has been reported.

Somewhat less commonly, laryngotracheitis and nasal and ocular inflammation occur. There may be laryngeal and tracheal tenderness, hoarseness, cough, and dyspnea secondary to collapse of the cartilagenous tracheal rings and granulation tissue proliferation within the tracheobronchial tree. The nasal chondritis, as in the ear, is often of sudden onset, very painful, and associated with a feeling of fullness in the bridge of the nose and surrounding tissues. The process subsides over several days, but involvement of the cartilaginous portion of the nose ultimately leads to saddle nose deformity. Episcleritis is the most common form of ocular involvement and can be readily seen as vascular proliferation overlying the sclerae. Other forms of ocular involvement that occur are iritis, conjunctivitis, keratitis, keratoconjunctivitis sicca, painful exophthalmos, ophthalmoplegia, and retinitis.

The external auditory meatus may be obstructed by edema and contribute to auditory impairment, but perceptive deafness and vertigo as a result of labyrinthine involvement also occur. Vertigo has not been reported in the absence of hearing loss. Back pain reflecting spinal involvement affects all levels of the spine. Chest pain may indicate affection of costochondral junctions or sternomanubrial or sternoclavicular joints.

Typically, RP is characterized by episodic attacks in which the cartilagenous structures are ivolved by inflammation. The hallmark of the disorder is bilateral auricular chondritis appearing abruptly with marked erythema, swelling, warmth, and pain. The ears become thickened and flabby and they flop with ambulation.

Most RP exists as an independent entity, however, one-fourth of cases are associated with other rheumatic diseases (adult and juvenile rheumatoid arthritis, Sjögren's syndrome, systemic and discoid lupus erythematosus, progressive systemic sclerosis, Reiter's/psoriatic arthritis, Raynaud's syndrome), autoimmune diseases (thyroid disease, ulcerative colitis, glomerulonephritis, dysgammaglobulinemia, pernicious anemia), malignancy, and miscellaneous disorders (sinusitis/mastoiditis, diabetes mellitus, sarcoidosis).

Nearly one-fourth of reported RP patients have had cardiovascular involvement, which contributes to the serious and sometimes fatal nature of the disease. Aortic valvular insufficiency, primarily due to annular dilatation, is most common, but the mitral and tricuspid valves may also be affected. The floppy mitral regurgitant valve or Barlow's syndrome has been observed. Cardiac conduction defects and myocardial abnormalities with cardiomegaly and pericarditis may occur. Large arterial dissecting aneurysms, arteritis, and central nervous system vasculitis further indicate the grave character of RP. Cutaneous vasculitis or nodular erythematous lesions that ulcerate and heal poorly may be troublesome.

DIAGNOSIS AND THERAPY

DIAGNOSIS

The most definitive diagnostic procedure in RP is biopsy of cartilage. Where the diagnosis is clinically obvious, it is probably not essential to obtain a cartilage biopsy. Recent observations suggest that detection of anticartilage antibodies in serum of affected patients may prove to be helpful in diagnosis. The most consistent laboratory abnormality is an elevated erythrocyte sedimentation rate, which generally parallels disease activity. Other laboratory abnormalities are wholly nonspecific and of the sort associated with chronic inflammatory and rheumatic diseases.

Pulmonary function testing may reflect airway obstruction. Electrocardiogram phonocardiography and echocardiography, as well as catheterization studies, may be called upon to document cardiovascular complications.

Audiometric and vestibular function tests (calorimetry and electronystagmography) may be expected to confirm conductive and/or perceptive deafness and labyrinthine dysfunction. Ophthalmologic examination with slit lamp evaluation delineates the range of ocular involvement.

Radiographic studies may demonstrate various complications of RP. Tracheal cartilage collapse can be seen tomographically. Ear cartilage calcification is visualized with the soft tissue technique. Plain films and specialized audiographic studies elucidate cardiovascular sequelae.

It has been proposed that the diagnosis of RP is most reliably made when there is evidence of recurrent inflammation of at least two cartilagenous sites, involvement of an organ of special sense, and a compatible biopsy of cartilage reflecting focal inflammatory involvement.

DIFFERENTIAL DIAGNOSIS

For this relatively uncommon disease, a rather broad range of differential diagnostic possibilities exist. Rheumatoid disease is most commonly considered; however, inflammation of ear, nose, and laryngotracheal cartilage does not occur except where the two disorders may coincidentally coexist. In addition, RP is not associated with rheumatoid nodules and rheumatoid factor is not present in high titer. Rheumatic fever requires evidence of antecedent streptococcal infection, which usually does not pertain in RP. Ankylosing spondylitis may present problems in differentiation with respect to ocular inflammation, aortic valvular insufficiency, peripheral arthritis, and back involvement, but again the ear and airway cartilages are uninvolved. As with rheumatoid disease, however, there may be coexistence or overlap of RP with ankylosing spondylitis.

Chondrodynia costosternalis, a variant of Tietze's syndrome, is usually self-limited and unassociated with further systemic manifestations. Gout and pseudogout are most readily and definitively distinguished by recovery of urate or calcium pyrophosphate dihydrate crystals from joint fluid or tissue deposits. The arthritis and conjunctivitis of Reiter's syndrome may cause confusion, but urethritis and distinctive skin and nail changes of this disorder do not occur in RP. Wegener's granulomatosis and lethal midline granuloma with a presentation of upper airway involvement and otitis media may be difficult to distinguish; in fact, several case reports suggest that these entities may also coexist. Typically, however, in granulomatous vasculitis the external ear is not involved.

Ulcerative granulomas of the upper airway due to syphilis or tuberculosis can best be distinguished by culture, biopsy, and/or other laboratory tests.

Aortitis or aortic aneurysms with dissection secondary to or associated with syphilis, Marfan's syndrome, Ehler-Danlos syndrome, idiopathic cystic medial necrosis, or arteriosclerosis are all far more common than the cardiovascular complications associated with RP, but an association may be entertained when cartilagenous inflammation and special sense organ involvement exist. The posttraumatic cauliflower ear one used to see typically in professional wrestlers is different from the early inflamed and swollen and later floppy ear of RP. The valvulitis of rheumatic fever results in thickened, calcified, and retracted valves, whereas RP typically results in valvular insufficiency due to valvular ring dilatation. Ear cartilage calcification of Addison's disease, hyperparathyroidism, and hypervitaminosis A require distinction. Chondrodermatitis nodularis chronica helicis is a distinctively localized nodular affliction of the ears. Meniere's syndrome will not have the cartilagenous abnormalities listed above. Cellulitis of the ears and/or nose as with recurrent syphilis seldom damages the cartilagenous tissues and an appropriate organism may be found.

Various forms of ocular disease must be distinguished, but usually lack an association with cartilagenous inflammation. Cogan's syndrome, an ocular lesion of interstitial keratitis associated with vestibuloauditory symptoms leading to deafness, is considered to be a localized form of polyarteritis nodosa, but again there is a lack of cartilagenous inflammatory involvement.

THERAPY

Due to the variable severity and episodic nature of RP, careful, prolonged follow-up and individualized therapy is required for optimal management. Corticosteroids are usually utilized to suppress disease activity. Usual initial doses are 30 mg/day of prednisone or its equivalent, subsequently tapered over many weeks to the lowest effective dosage. Clinical manifestations supplemented by laboratory data are the basis of subsequent steroid dosage adjustment. Protracted therapy may be required, but steroids may not be expected to be very efficacious at a late stage of cartilage loss. Indomethacin has been found to be particularly useful by some observers. Supplemental immunosuppressive or cytotoxic agents such as azathioprine or cyclophosphamide have been successfully utilized when corticosteroid sparing is desired or serious complications exist not entirely responsive to corticosteroids. Very limited experience suggests that dapsone may be effective therapy for RP by inhibiting lysosomal enzyme–mediated cartilage damage.

Even though the glotic airway may seem normal, early consideration of tracheostomy has been advised due to frequent subglotic involvement. Intubation and endoscopy can be hazardous, but may be undertaken for aspiration of crusts and secretions. Very limited experience exists with surgical reconstructive repair of airways. Satisfactory replacement of aortic and mitral valves has been undertaken as well as aneurysmal repair.

REFERENCES

Dolan DL, Lemmon GB, Teitelbaum SL: Relapsing polychon-
    dritis, analytical literature review and studies on pathogen-
    esis. Am J Med 41:285, 1966
Herman JH, Dennis MV: Immunopathologic studies in relapsing
    polychondritis. J Clin Invest 52:549, 1973
Hughes RAC, Berry CL, Seifert M, Lessof MH: Relapsing

polychondritis, three cases with a clinico-pathological study
    and literature review. Q J Med 41:363, 1972
McAdam LP, O'Hanlan MA, Bluestone R, Pearson CM: Relaps-
    ing polychondritis: Prospective study of 23 patients and a
    review of the literature. Medicine (Baltimore) 55:193, 1976
Rogers PH, Boden G, Tourtellotte CD: Relapsing polychondritis
    with insulin resistance and antibodies to cartilage. Am J
    Med 55:243, 1973

Paget's Disease

Robert B. Zurier and Gregory R. Mundy

PATHOGENESIS AND CLINICAL FEATURES

Paget's disease (osteitis deformans) is a very common
skeletal disorder of the elderly in which there is excessive
resorption and formation of bone. The early asymptomatic phase is encountered frequently due to widespread
application of routine screening blood and roentgenographic studies. A century after the description of the
disease, effective agents for its control are being
developed.

EPIDEMIOLOGY

Paget's disease affects men and women almost
equally. Patients younger than 40 years of age are rare,
and the prevalence increases steadily with age. Autopsy
and radiologic studies indicate that the disease affects 3–4
percent of people over the age of 40 years and 11 percent
of individuals over the age of 80. The disease appears to
be most common in Anglo-Saxon countries, but since
large-scale epidemiologic studies have not been reported
from areas with alleged low incidences (Asia, Africa,
Middle East), the accuracy of that information is not
clear. Certainly, Paget's disease is not uncommon in
black Americans. Although a family history of Paget's
disease is frequently noted, a genetic basis for the disease
has not been demonstrated.

ETIOLOGY

The etiology of Paget's disease is unknown. Paget
considered it to be a chronic inflammation of bones, but
inflammatory cells are rarely seen in affected bone. A
series of studies has failed to provide evidence for disordered hormone (pituitary, parathyroid, adrenal) secretion
as its cause. Abnormal immune responses are not known
to be associated with the disease. The evidence for an
inborn error of connective tissue metabolism is controversial: abnormal collagen has been found in skin of some
patients and the association of Paget's disease with retinal angioid streaks, pseudoxanthoma elasticum, and vascular calcification suggests the existence of a subtle abnormality in collagen metabolism. Nuclear inclusions that
most closely resemble viral nucleocapsids of the para-
myxovirus type have been observed in osteoclasts from
patients with Paget's disease. Their significance is not
known. Similar structures have been seen in brain tissue
from patients with subacute sclerosing panencephalitis, a
central nervous system disorder that is recognized clini-

cally after a long latent period following measles
infection.

PATHOGENESIS

The histopathology of Paget's disease is characterized by abundant osteoclasts and osteoblasts, an increase
in vascular fibrous tissue in the marrow, and disordered
architecture of both medullary and cortical bone. The
earliest lesions appear to be osteolytic and the initial
abnormality is probably an increase in osteoclastic activity, to which bone cells respond locally with increased
and inappropriate bone formation. The new chaotic
weakened bone consists of a mosaic of irregular pieces of
lamellar bone, interspersed with woven bone. The latter
is a more primitive bone present in the embryo and during
childhood but not normally found in adults. It is associated with rapid bone remodeling and characterized by a
disorganized pattern of collagen fibers. The histopathologic process does not traverse cartilaginous structures
such as joints, but the sutures of the skull may become
obliterated. The accelerated bone turnover affects both
mineral and organic matrix and the increase in both
osteoblastic and osteoclastic activity can be monitored.

CLINICAL FEATURES

Patients with Paget's disease may present with a
wide spectrum of findings. Osseous involvement is often
detected unexpectedly by x-ray or alkaline phosphatase
determination in asymptomatic patients. The vertebrae,
skull, and pelvis are most often affected, but single localized or multiple lesions may occur in any bone. Extensive
bony involvement with Paget's disease is usually associated with deep aching pain which may be aggravated by
walking if the axial skeleton and hips are affected. However, such patients may be pain free, or severe bone pain
may be present in the early osteolytic phase of disease
when there is no radiographic evidence of new bone
formation. Increased warmth of tissue overlying involved
bone is due to increased cutaneous blood flow.

Articular pain is common in patients with Paget's
disease, particularly in joints adjacent to involved bone.
Acute inflammatory episodes often occur at sites of periarticular calcification. Paget noted the association with
gout in his initial report. Recent studies indicate a high
frequency of increased serum uric acid concentrations
and gouty arthritis in patients with extensive Paget's
disease (mostly males). Involvement of the spine may

result in dorsal kyphosis and stooped posture. The clavicles and humerus may enlarge. Bowing of the femur and tibia may be so marked as to limit mobility. Structurally inadequate new bone may result in complete and incomplete fractures of the long bones Incomplete (fissure) fractures usually occur on the convex aspect of the femoral or tibial cortex, and may account in part for bowing of the lower limbs. Complete fractures occur most commonly in the femur.

With progressive disease the skull enlarges and temporal arteries may become engorged and tortuous. Thickening of the petrous portion of the temporal bone may lead to cochlear dysfunction and sensorineural hearing loss. Conductive hearing loss also occurs following ankylosis (otosclerosis) of the ossicles. Rarely, excessive cranium weight and softening of the base of the skull can result in basilar invagination and spinal cord compression. Cardiac failure in elderly patients with Paget's disease may be due in part to increased skeletal blood flow, which results in high cardiac output.

A much feared complication of Paget's disease is the development of osteogenic sarcoma, which probably occurs in only 1 percent of all patients. However, approximately 30 percent of all osteosarcoma is associated with Paget's disease, and such patients are at a 30-fold greater risk of harboring an osteosarcoma. The tumor appears always to originate in pagetic bone.

DIAGNOSIS AND TREATMENT

DIAGNOSIS

In patients with generalized involvement, the x-ray picture is virtually diagnostic. The radiologic appearance includes radiolucent areas adjacent to coarsely striated sclerotic bone (Fig. 1). The classic radiologic feature of early Paget's disease in a long bone is that of an advancing resorption front (osteolytic lesion) that has a V-shaped configuration. Radionuclide bone scans using agents such as technetium-labeled diphosphonates show increased uptake at the site of active lesions and are a good measure of extent of disease.

There is a marked increase in serum of heat-labile (bone isoenzyme) alkaline phosphatase activity, proportional to the extent and activity of disease. Total urine hydroxyproline is also increased in most patients with Paget's disease. Hydroxyproline accounts for 10 percent of the total amino acid composition of bone collagen. It is formed by hydroxylation of proline after its incorporation into the collagen molecule. During the synthesis of collagen, some of the newly synthesized material is not deposited in bone, but is partially degraded to nondialyzable peptides. During bone resorption, collagen is degraded more completely to low molecular weight peptides, two or three amino acids of which (including hydroxyproline) are dialyzable. Both dialyzable and nondialyzable com-

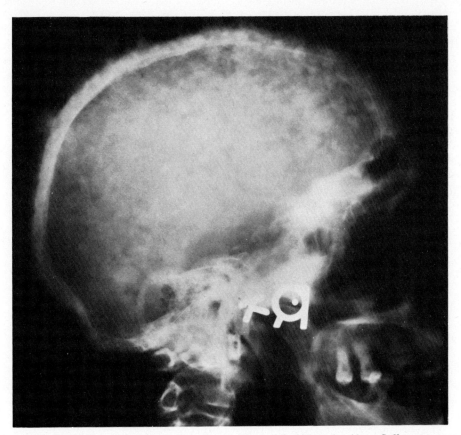

Fig. 1. Skull x-ray from patient with Paget's disease. The vault is thickened and has a fluffy appearance. Mottling is due to areas of osteolysis and osteosclerosis.

ponents are increased in the urine of patients with Paget's disease. Despite the remarkable increase in metabolic activity of bone, most patients with Paget's disease have normal serum concentrations of calcium and phosphate, suggesting that rates of bone formation and resorption are closely coupled, as in normal individuals.

DIFFERENTIAL DIAGNOSIS

In general, the manifestations of advanced Paget's disease should not be confused with other diseases, but diagnostic problems do exist. In the occasional patient who exhibits hypercalcemia, the additional diagnosis of hyperparathyroidism must be considered. Monoostotic Paget's disease may be confused with osteoblastic metastases from carcinoma of the prostate. Assay of the prostatic fraction of acid phosphatase is readily available and can be helpful. Pelvic enlargement and thickening of the pelvic rim ("brim sign") also helps differentiate localized Paget's disease from osteoblastic metastases. Occasionally, bone biopsy may be required to make the diagnosis or, when pain is an especially prominent finding, to search for sarcoma.

Although several bone disorders exist in which both increased bone formation and resorption occur (severe hyperparathyroidism, osteoblastic metastases, Brodie's abscess, hereditary hyperphosphatasia), none produce the striking mosaic pattern of Paget's disease. The disease is slowly progressive, usually over a period of years, and it is difficult to predict the course in an individual patient.

TREATMENT

The major indication for therapy of Paget's disease is pain and the treatment of choice is calcitonin. This hormone, secreted by the parafollicular (C) cells of the thyroid gland, inhibits osteoclastic bone resorption. In Paget's disease calcitonin treatment results in rapid reduction in osteoclastic and osteoblastic activity and decreased bone turnover. Ultimately, the lesions may be replaced by normal bone, but complete histologic healing has not been demonstrated. The clinical benefits of calcitonin are usually greatest during the first 6–12 months; relapses occur with increasing frequency during subsequent years of treatment. Bone pain improves gradually over several months. Serum alkaline phosphatase activity and urinary hydroxyproline excretion may fall after only

2 weeks of therapy and continue to decrease, but usually not to normal levels. Calcitonin must be given parenterally and is expensive. Adverse effects include nausea, anorexia, flushing, hand swelling, and skin rashes. It is not known why the beneficial effects of calcitonin, noted in approximately 75 percent of patients during the first year of therapy, do not persist.

Diphosphonates are compounds structurally related to pyrophosphate, but resistant to degradation by pyrophosphatase. They bind strongly to crystals of hydroxyapatite, block the growth and dissolution of such crystals in vitro, and slow bone turnover rate in experimental animals. The compound used clinically, edathimil, delays mineralization. Although some patients have shown good early response to therapy, subsequent development of osteomalacia has proved troublesome. Treatment with lower doses is being evaluated.

Mithramycin is an antibiotic that inhibits DNA-dependent RNA synthesis. It appears to inhibit bone resorption—perhaps by killing bone cells—and has been used successfully to control hypercalcemia and in a few patients with Paget's disease. The drug has serious potential toxic effects, but continued studies with low doses given to selected patients do seem warranted.

Salicylates and other nonsteroidal antiinflammatory drugs may be sufficient for alleviation of pain, including joint pain. However, hips of some patients with involvement of both femoral head and acetabulum undergo abnormal remodeling; total hip replacement may then be necessary for pain relief. Early ambulation and high fluid intake postoperatively is essential since immobilization favors bone resorption, which is reflected in increased urinary calcium excretion and occasionally in hypercalcemia.

REFERENCES

Franck WA, Bress NM, Singer FR, Krane SM: Rheumatic manifestations of Paget's disease of bone. Am J Med 56:592, 1974

Haddad JG: Paget's disease of bone: Problems and management. Orthop. Clin North Am 3:775, 1972

Nagant de Deuxchaisnes CN, Krane S: Paget's disease of bone: Clinical and metabolic observations. Medicine (Baltimore) 43:233, 1964

Singer FR: Paget's Disease of Bone. New York, Plenum, 1977

Miscellaneous Disorders

Frank R. Schmid

OSTEOCHONDRITIS DISSECANS

In osteoarthritis dissecans, tangential and twisting forces applied to the convex member of opposing joint surfaces in a diarthrodial joint can precipitate a fracture with release of a bony fragment and its articular cartilage into the joint space. The bone fragment can remain as a loose body within the joint or become attached to the synovial membrane. In either location, reabsorption may occur or the fragment may increase in size or change its configuration due to proliferation of its chondroblasts and osteoblasts. The occasional appearance of the disease in several joints and in other members of the same family suggests a genetic tendency, but the inherited structural defect in bone that predisposes to the separation is not known.

The disease is several times as common in males as in females. An overall incidence of 10–15/100,000 persons has been found in one survey, with twice the number occurring between the ages of 10 and 20 years. The process most commonly involves the femoral condyles. Other sites are the capitellum of the elbow and the femoral head at the hip, but almost any diarthrodial joint may be involved.

Symptoms may be absent during the development of the fracture line. When present, pain or decrease in range of motion or locking are related to the loose body in the joint. Sometimes a bland, clear effusion may occur. In one case observed personally, the joint fluid was milky due to the presence of myriads of micalike chips of articular cartilage.

Diagnosis requires the demonstration of a defect in the joint surface in which the fragment sits or from which it has become dislodged. Rarely, however, is it possible to detect the fragment in situ. The defect is usually recognized on conventional roentgengrams, but tomograms permit a clearer definition of the lesion. Arthroscopy also can reveal the defect.

Osteochondritis dissecans may be a complication of the late onset of Legg-Perthes disease at the hip (see the chapter on Juvenile Osteochondroses) if non-union of the fragment produced by the osteonecrosis of this disease has occurred. The superior lateral aspect of the femoral head is most often involved. At this weight-bearing site, the fragment may remain in place or even become impacted, perhaps for years, before being shed into the joint space.

Treatment is directed toward protection of the damaged joint surface from stress or weight-bearing until healing has been accomplished; in those instances of repeated locking or pain, the loose bodies are surgically removed. Analgesics, rest, and heat are helpful during a flare. Some patients may subsequently develop degenerative joint disease.

REFERENCES

Green JP: Osteochondritis dissecans of the knee. J Bone Joint Surg 48B:82, 1966

Linden B: The incidence of osteochondritis dissecans in the condyles of the femur. Acta Orthop Scand 47:664, 1976

TIETZE'S SYNDROME

Costochondritis or Tietze's syndrome is a benign, often self-limited condition of unknown cause and of uncertain pathogenesis involving the costochondral junctions of the anterior ribs or sternum or the manubriosternal joint. The disease most often afflicts middle-aged adults. Its commonest feature is localized pain confined exclusively to the afflicted site. The pain may be spontaneous, but usually it is made worse by pressure. Sometimes swelling of the underlying joint structure can be noted, but the overlying skin and subcutaneous tissue are normal. Other conditions such as infection, tumor, trauma, or systemic rheumatic diseases such as rheumatoid arthritis or ankylosing spondylitis must be excluded.

The diagnosis is made entirely on clinical evidence. Swelling, if present, would make the diagnosis secure but is not an absolute requirement. Usually, the process is unilateral and confined to one or two joints. No laboratory or radiologic findings are associated with this disease, but care must be taken to exclude cardiac, pleural, or lung causes of chest pain. Referred pain to the chest wall from the upper or midthoracic spine presents difficulties. In these cases the pain in the anterior chest wall is of the referred type; that is, it is not made worse by local pressure and sometimes is aggravated by or associated with spinal motion.

Reassurance is the key component of therapy, particularly with regard to concern over intrathoracic disease. Heat, nonsteroidal antiinflammatory drugs such as aspirin, and local infiltration with analgesics such as procaine and corticosteroid drugs are beneficial during disease activity.

REFERENCES

Levey GS, Calabro JJ: Tietze's syndrome: Report of two cases and review of the literature. Arthritis Rheum 5:261, 1962

NODULAR PANNICULITIS

Classification of inflammatory diseases of adipose tissue is difficult because so little is known of initiating events or subsequent pathogenesis. Some disorders, such as nodular, nonsuppurative panniculitis (Weber-Christian disease) and the disseminated fat necrosis associated with pancreatitis (see the next chapter), appear to have their primary origin in this tissue. Others, such as erythema nodosum, are the result of a vasculitis in the deep dermis and subcutis with secondary reactive changes in subcutaneous fat.

Nodular panniculitis is characterized by recurrent bouts of fever accompanied by the appearance of crops of subcutaneous nodules that range in size from 1 cm or less to larger confluent masses. While sometimes painless, they usually are tender and erythematous. They favor the subcutaneous areas of the proximal extremities and trunk. Necrosis may result, leaving behind an area of atrophy. Most forms of the disease are localized to the skin, but in some patients a more systemic form is seen with involvement of mesenteric, pericardial, pleural, and retroperitoneal tissues; in such patients the skin involvement can be extensive. The course of the illness tends to be benign but fatalities have occurred in the systemic type.

Apart from these essential forms of nodular panniculitis, a similar type of involvement infrequently occurs as part of a multisystem disease such as systemic lupus erythematosus, the fat necrosis of which is called *lupus profundus*. Withdrawal from large doses of steroids, such as occurs as in the treatment of rheumatic fever, has also been associated with panniculitis.

The basic mechanism for panniculitis remains obscure. No direct evidence for an initiating event, such as infection or an altered immune response, have been found. In two patients with fatal systemic panniculitis, an absence of α_1 antitrypsin was found, suggesting that this inhibitor may ordinarily act to prevent dissemination of localized forms of panniculitis.

Diagnosis is based upon the clinical presentation, with confirmation by biopsy of the nodule. Acute phase reactants such as the erythrocyte sedimentation rate may be elevated, but no other laboratory findings are specific.

Treatment is supportive. Corticosteroid drugs may be used during the acute phase to control the inflammatory process.

REFERENCES

MacDonald A, Feiwel M: A review of the concept of Weber-Christian panniculitis with a report of five cases. Br J Dermatol 80:355, 1968

Rubenstein HM, Jaffer A, Kudrna JC, Letratanakul Y, Chandrasekhar AJ, Slater D, Schmid FR: α_1 antitrypsin deficiency with severe panniculitis. Report of two cases. Ann Intern Med 86:742, 1977

ARTHRITIS OF PANCREATIC DISEASE

As the pancreas is an organ with both an exocrine and endocrine function, its diseases fall into two categories. Pancreatitis and pancreatic carcinoma may occasionally be associated with a syndrome of subcutaneous nodules, arthritis, and bone lesions. Diabetes mellitus also has an association with a rheumatic syndrome, although less well recognized, which is related to some aspect of a disturbed insulin metabolism.

The syndrome of disseminated fat necrosis stands apart from other instances of panniculitis on both clinical and pathologic grounds. Patients with this disease either have chronic pancreatitis or a pancreatic malignancy. Although a variety of explanations have been postulated to account for systemic fat necrosis, including dissemination of lipase or proteolytic enzymes from the pancreas, none have been proven. The telltale mark of the disease is the appearance of discrete, raised, red subcutaneous lesions that are sometimes painful and are often accompanied by an arthritis. The arthritis most likely results from involvement of subsynovial fat with extension of the process into the joint space. Usually one or only a few joints are involved. The joint fluid may contain necrotic debris or may be relatively clear, showing few cells and, at least in a few instances, fat globules. Medullary fat necrosis may occur more often than subcutaneous lesions but, because of lack of pain in many instances, may be overlooked. The necrosis can cause osteolysis of long bones and phalanges, the latter producing punched-out lesions with an adjacent periosteal reaction.

Diagnosis depends on the demonstration by a biopsy of the characteristic liquefaction necrosis of adipose tissue obtained from a subcutaneous nodule. Such a biopsy finding often calls attention to the true nature of the disease, which otherwise would have been considered to be an instance of erythema nodosum with arthritis. Elevated serum amylase or lipase levels and demonstration of calcification in the pancreas or other evidence of pancreatic disease are usually not recognized until fat necrosis has been proven.

The prognosis depends upon the outcome of the underlying pancreatic disease. Fat necrosis per se has little or no effect on mortality. In patients with pancreatitis, recurrences of fat necrosis have been reported. Most patients with tumor have advanced metastatic disease at the time fat necrosis becomes apparent. Treatment is supportive. Corticosteroid therapy is often used, but its effect upon the disease is unproven.

The diabetic state is associated with several musculoskeletal syndromes: osteoporosis and osteolysis of the forefoot, neuropathic arthritis, ankylosing hyperostosis of the spine, and Dupuytren's contracture. Less often appreciated is the relationship of diabetes, particularly insulin-dependent diabetes, with periarthritis about the shoulder or with contracture of the finger joints. The latter complication appears to be due to tendon or subcutaneous skin involvement and is more often seen in teenage or young adults who may have short stature. The skin of the hands is thickened and waxy in appearance, a finding that bears a resemblance to the changes of scleroderma. Raynaud's phenomenon, vascular calcification, or neuropathy, except for an occasional instance of a carpal tunnel syndrome, are not found. Function may remain adequate, but no specific treatment is known.

REFERENCES

Good AE, Schnitzer B, Kawanishi H, Demetropoulos KC, Rapp R: Acinar pancreatic tumor with metastatic fat necrosis. Report of a case and review of rheumatic manifestations. Am J Dig Dis 21:978, 1976

Grgic A, Rosenbloom AL, Weber FT, Giordano B, Malone JI, Schuster JJ: Joint contracture—common manifestation of childhood diabetes mellitus. J Pediatr 88:584, 1976

Immelman EJ, Bank S, Krige H, et al: Roentgenologic and clinical features of intramedullary fat necrosis in bones in acute and chronic pancreatitis. Am J Med 36:96, 1964

Mullen GT, Caperton EM, Crespin SR, et al: Arthritis and skin lesions resembling erythema nodosum in pancreatic disease. Ann Intern Med 68:75, 1968

Pasten RS, Cohen AS: The rheumatologic manifestations of diabetes mellitus. Med Clin North Am 62:829, 1978

RHEUMATIC DISEASES IN HEMODIALYSIS AND RENAL HOMOTRANSPLANTATION PATIENTS

A wide variety of musculoskeletal abnormalities are recorded in patients who suffer the complications of treatment of chronic renal failure. The metabolic changes associated with uremia are diverse and include alteration in bone mineral resorption and deposition, impairment of host defense mechanisms, vascular calcification, and neuropathy. Treatment by dialysis rectifies some of these aberrations, but imposes other risks such as infection. Treatment by homotransplantation creates additional problems, particularly by stimulation of the host's immune system and by the still crude use of immunosuppressive drugs employed to control this response. Therefore, in patients of this group who present with a rheumatic complaint, an interwoven set of factors determines the nature of the process.

ARTHRITIS WITH HEMODIALYSIS

In hemodialysis patients, two main articular syndromes are recognized: crystal-induced synovitis and pyogenic bone or joint infection.

Synovitis due to several types of crystals is one of the commonest problems encountered. Calcium hydroxyapatite microcrystals can be the responsible agent for acute painful swelling and redness of the connective tissues of patients with soft tissue calcification. Synovial inflammation of nearby tendons, joints, or bursae may develop with effusions. These tiny crystals are not seen in the joint fluid by conventional techniques but can be demonstrated by electron microscopic examination of sediments of the fluid. Clues to the diagnosis are the demonstration of an aseptic inflammatory joint fluid containing mainly polymorphonuclear cells in a patient with nearby periarticular soft tissue calcification as demonstrated by the roentgenogram. The serum calcium–phosphorus ion product usually exceeds 75. Crystals associated with gout (sodium urate) and with pseudogout or articular chondrocalcinosis (calcium pyrophosphate dihydrate) are easily recognized by ordinary light or polarizing microscopy. In chondrocalcinosis, evaluation of the patient for hyperparathyroidism should be made. The presence of hyperuricemia, which is common in all patients of this group, cannot be taken as a diagnostic finding for gout in the absence of appropriate crystal demonstration.

Management includes immobilization and the short-term use of any one of several nonsteroidal antiinflammatory compounds such as phenylbutazone or indomethacin. In gout, colchicine may be used for the acute episode and allopurinol for the long-term control of hyperuricemia. In hydroxyapatite disease, aluminum hydroxide is used to lower serum phosphorus.

Problems with infection pose a serious threat and need to be carefully excluded by a suitable culture of joint fluid in any patient with an effusion. Osteomyelitis also must be considered. Details of diagnostic procedures and management for this complication are recorded elsewhere (see References).

An unusual syndrome of progressive ischemic skin ulcerations of fingers, toes, and extremities has been noted in patients with renal failure. The illness is closely linked to the development of secondary hyperparathyroidism—so much so that subtotal removal of these glands is required for control of the process.

OTHER MUSCULOSKELETAL DISORDERS WITH HEMODIALYSIS

Peripheral neuropathy may sometimes be confused with bone or joint pain. In addition, the neuropathy may expose the less sensitive limb to undue strain, leading to a noninflammatory pain syndrome about the joints, sometimes with effusion. Neuropathic joint changes have not been reported. Sometimes a diffuse painful myopathy may accompany vascular calcification as an additional musculoskeletal complaint in this group of patients.

More prominent in this category of patients are complaints due to renal osteodystrophy. Bone pain with or without fractures ensues. The pathogenesis of this process varies. In some patients, defective mineralization (osteomalacia), probably due to abnormal metabolism or action of vitamin D, is responsible. In others, enhanced osteoclastic activity with increased bone resorptive surfaces develops from parathyroid hyperplasia. Usually some element of each of these processes exists in each patient. Additional factors are immobilization, calcium deficiency, or chronic protein depletion, all features of osteoporosis. Radiographic techniques are helpful in diagnosis. In particular, fine-grain films can reveal early subperiosteal reabsorption and increased intracortical striations due to enhanced endosteal reabsorption. Therapy is directed toward maintenance of the normal blood concentrations of calcium and phosphorus, suppression of hyperactivity of the parathyroid glands, restoration of skeletal defects toward normal, and correction or prevention of soft tissue calcification.

RHEUMATIC DISEASES IN HOMOTRANSPLANTATION

Patients who receive a donor kidney (or, in the future, those who may receive other organ transplants) have usually been exposed to dialysis for varying periods of time before a graft is used. They can be victims, therefore, to the same set of musculoskeletal problems already discussed. In addition, unique problems occur related to the graft itself.

Patients undergoing acute rejection of a renal graft may have an illness resembling serum sickness with severe arthritis. Those with late rejection may have severe myalagia and arthralgia, although frank arthritis is rare. Associated with these clinical features are the presence of serum antibodies such as antiglobulin or rheumatoid factors and antinuclear antibodies. These antibodies are nonspecific and are not indicative of the development of one of the major connective tissue diseases. Treatment with corticosteroid drugs to control the rejection phenomenon usually controls these complaints; rapid reduction of dose can sometimes cause a flare of the joint complaint.

Treatment of graft rejection imposes two risks on the patient. Infection, as discussed above with hemodialysis patients, may be facilitated and septic arthritis may result. Ischemic necrosis of subchondral bone with subsequent collapse of the articular surface usually, but not always, follows long-term and high-dosage corticosteroid administration. Weight-bearing joints, such as the femoral head of the hip, the femoral condyle at the knee, and sometimes the ankle talus, are especially involved. Radiologic features are pathognomonic (see the chapter on Avascular Necrosis of Bone). Treatment is supportive and symptomatic with avoidance of weight bearing, use of analgesics, and, in selected patients who have been well maintained on treatment, the use of artificial joint replacement.

REFERENCES

Irby R, Edwards WM, Gatter R: Articular complication of homotransplantation and chronic renal dialysis. J Rheumatol 2:91, 1975

Massry SG, Bluestone R, Klinenberg JR, Coburn JW: Abnormalities of the musculoskeletal system in hemodialysis patients. Semin Arthritis Rheum 4:321, 1975

MUSCULOSKELETAL SYNDROMES IN INTRAVENOUS HEROIN USERS

Parenteral drug abuse can cause infectious arthritis from bacteria, fungi, or the hepatitis virus, or a sterile arthritis can result from subacute bacterial endocarditis or arthralgia and myalgia during the withdrawal of the addicting drug or from systemic vasculitis. Recently, a unique musculoskeletal complication has been described. Fever, paraspinal myalgias, and arthralgias were noted in addicts who had been using a type of "street" heroin with a brown color. Examination disclosed cervical and lumbosacral muscle tenderness and spasm. Two or more joints, e.g., knees, ankles, shoulders, elbows, or wrists, were painful but not swollen or red. Symptoms were maintained while the drug was being used and all remitted promptly during hospitalization with cessation of the drug. None of the patients had evidence of infection. Autoimmune phenomena were not striking. Whether an altered immune response to a product in the heroin mixture or a toxic reaction to an adulterant was responsible could not be determined.

REFERENCES

Pastan RS, Silverman SL, Goldenberg DL: A musculoskeletal syndrome in intravenous heroin users. Association with brown heroin. Ann Intern Med 87:22, 1977

AVASCULAR NECROSIS OF BONE

Ischemic destruction of bone preferentially occurs in those locations where collateral vessels are insufficient to compensate for loss of the main arterial blood supply. These locations include the femoral (by far the commonest site) and humeral heads, the proximal portion of the carpal navicular and lunate bones, the talus of the foot, and the femoral condyles. As long as the bony structure is preserved, few or no symptoms result, but when fragmentation occurs or the joint surface becomes deformed due to loss of support of the subchondral bone, pain appears at rest and is worsened with motion or weight

Table 1
Conditions Associated with Avascular Necrosis

Fracture (e.g., neck of femur, carpal navicular)
Slipped capital femoral epiphysis
Dislocation
Caisson disease
Sickle cell disease and trait
Sickle cell–hemoglobin C disease
Systemic lupus erythematosus
Progressive systemic sclerosis
Rheumatoid arthritis
Cushing's syndrome
Treatment with corticosteroids
Alcoholism
Pancreatitis
Renal homotransplantation
Gaucher's disease
Fabry's disease
Radiation therapy
Infection

bearing. In the hip, pain may be referred to the knee. Limitation of motion can be profound.

A large number of otherwise unrelated conditions may cause avascular necrosis. They all share in common potential end-artery obstructive disease (Table 1).

Radiologic features are pathognomonic: early, a translucent air crescent immediately beneath the articular surface is seen when the necrosed bone has started to collapse; later increased sclerosis occurs around the subchondral bony infarct; and finally, the subchondral bony plate may become fragmented or compacted. The translucent air crescent can be more effectively demonstrated at the hip by exerting traction on the affected limb. Severe degenerative changes may be the end result. Unfortunately, even the earliest stage visible on the roentgenogram may be seen only weeks or months after the bone has become ischemic. Radioisotopic scanning techniques using a bone-seeking polyphosphonate compound may reveal earlier changes than conventional roentgenograms. These may show a central area free of isotope surrounded by a dense zone of isotope accumulation.

If a joint could be protected from stress or weight bearing during evolution of the process, the ischemic tissue could be revascularized, necrotic bone reabsorbed, and new bone layed down. Such restriction would have to be maintained for months since the process is slow. This feature, combined with the almost inevitable late recognition of the process, almost always results in destruction of the subchondral bone. In these far advanced lesions, joint replacement or other reconstructive procedures may be the only means to restore function and relieve pain.

REFERENCES

Herndon JH, Aufranc OE: Avascular necrosis of the femoral head in the adult: A review of its incidence in a variety of conditions. Clin Orthop 86:43, 1972

Jones JP Jr, Engelman EP: Osseous avascular necrosis associated with systemic abnormalities. Arthritis Rheum 9:728, 1966

Table 1
Juvenile Osteochondroses

Eponym	Site	Clinical Aspects	Pathogenesis
Legg-Calve-Perthes	Proximal femoral capital epiphysis	Mainly boys, ages 3–8	Osteonecrosis
Freiberg's	Head 2nd metatarsal	Children, ages 12–15	Osteonecrosis
Panner's	Capitellum humerus	Teenage	Osteonecrosis
Kienböck's	Carpal lunate	Variable age	Osteonecrosis
Preiser's	Carpal navicular	Variable age	Osteonecrosis
Osgood-Schlatter	Tibial tubercle at insertion of patella tendon	Mainly boys, ages 9–16 often bilateral	Avulsion by stress
Blount's	Medial side proximal tibial epiphysial plate	Variable, infants/adolescents	Abnormality of endochondral ossification
Sever's	Calcaneal apothysis at insertion of Achilles tendon	Children, ages 6–10	Avulsion by stress
Scheuermann's	Thoracic/lumbar vertebrae (multiple)	Ages 8–16	Defect at endochondral ossification
Calve's	Vertebral body (single)		Eosinophilic granuloma
Kohler's	Tarsal navicular		Osteonecrosis/defect of endochondral ossification

JUVENILE OSTEOCHONDROSES

A large variety of syndromes, each involving a particular site and identified with a time-honored eponym, have been grouped under heading of *juvenile osteochondroses,* or sometimes, *osteochondritis* (Table 1). The disease characteristically affects growing bones and in most cases it is attributed to aseptic necrosis of an apophyseal or epiphyseal growth center that results in a disturbance of development of the affected bone. Trauma may be a precipitating factor. Symptoms include pain or diminished function of the affected part. In some cases the process is bilateral. Roentgenographic findings are usually sufficient to confirm the diagnosis, but occasionally a biopsy is required to exclude an infectious lesion. Treatment is geared to limitation of stress or weight bearing until healing has occurred, which usually takes months to a year or so.

REFERENCES

Rodnan GP (ed): Primer on the Rheumatic Diseases (ed 7). JAMA[Suppl] 224, 1973

FAMILIAL MEDITERRANEAN FEVER

Articular manifestations of familial Mediterranean fever (FMF) represent a key feature of one of its two major clinical presentations, that of periodic and brief attacks of fever accompanied by joint pain or pleurisy or peritonitis. The other presentation is the development of amyloidosis (see the section on Amyloidosis). FMF is a hereditary disorder affecting certain ethnic groups that traditionally come from the eastern Mediterranean littoral. Sephardic Jews, Armenians and, to a lesser extent, Anatolian Turks and Arabs of the Levant are afflicted. The disease is transmitted by a single recessive autosomal gene, an observation consistent with the presence of consanguinous marriages in some of the parents of families with this disease.

Attacks of FMF are usually brief, each marked by a sudden and acute onset of fever and pain in the abdomen, chest, or joints, or rarely fever alone. In the interval between attacks, no residua remain. The disease, however, is characterized by the almost inevitable development of renal amyloidosis at a very young age. Attacks occur at irregular intervals without periodicity with a wide variation from months to years between each episode. Peritonitis occurs most frequently, in almost 95 percent of patients, articular pain is next most common, and pleurisy is the least common, in about 40 percent of patients. The intensity of the pain is usually quite severe, although milder attacks do occur. Each episode lasts 1–2 days, except for the joint disease, which may be protracted. A very characteristic erythema that resembles erysipelas may develop on the skin of the lower extremities, usually below the knees.

No pathognomonic test or finding exists, so that the diagnosis is based upon a cluster of findings: the typical short attacks of fever in persons of Mediterranean ancestry; a painful abdomen, chest, or joint; the erythematous skin lesion; and a family history of similar disease. The exclusion of other arthritic processes is important, particularly gout or infection. Laboratory findings are meager. Acute phase reactants such as the sedimentation rate are elevated. Greater confidence in the diagnosis is usually obtained after several attacks have occurred.

The arthritis characteristically involves the larger joints of the lower extremities. The sacroiliac joint may also be involved. Usually only one joint is affected at a time. The height of the attack is reached in 1–2 days, then resolution is achieved in 1 week, sometimes longer. About 5 percent of patients may have a more protracted course with persistent swelling and pain often in the hip or knee. The synovial fluid may be noninflammatory in type with few cells or a grossly inflamed fluid with counts of over 100,000 white cells/mm³, usually polymorphonuclear leukocytes. Glucose may be normal or low but bacteria are not found. The synovial membrane shows a nonspecific synovitis. On roentgenograms, osteoporosis may develop rapidly, and in protractic cases loss of cartilage and juxta-articular erosions may occur. In the hip, a picture of avascular necrosis can be seen. In spite of the intensity or even the duration of each attack, recovery is the rule, except occasionally in the hip, which may show destructive changes. Total hip replacement has been carried out successfully for this complication.

Treatment is supportive. Corticosteroid drugs have been used along with nonsteroidal antiinflammatory compounds. Rest and splints may be useful.

Of special interest is the now well-documented evidence that prophylactic use of colchicine prevents the disabling attacks of fever and pain. Whether it would also influence the development of amyloidosis is still not known but under investigation. Treatment consists of the use of 0.5 mg colchicine twice a day.

REFERENCES

Dinarello CA, Wolff SM, Goldfinger SE, Dale DC, Alling DW: Colchicine therapy for familial Mediterranean fever. N Engl J Med 291:934, 1974
Goldfinger SE: Colchicine for familial Mediterranean fever. N Engl J Med 287:1302, 1972
Sohar E, Pras M, Gafni J: Familial Mediterranean fever and its articular manifestations. Clin Rheum Dis 1:195, 1975
Zemer D, Revach M, Pras M, Modan B, Schor S, Sohar E, Gafni J: A controlled trial of colchicine in preventing attacks of familial Mediterranean fever. N Engl J Med 291:932, 1974

FOREIGN BODY REACTIONS IN JOINTS

Foreign bodies may penetrate the joint capsule or tendon sheath and produce inflammation. Sepsis may occasionally result, as is the case in sporotrichosis, which is introduced by penetration of a rose thorn. In other cases the inflammation can be sterile. If the object is radiopaque it can be readily demonstrated on the roentgenogram; if not, detection may depend upon an accurate history. Unfortunately, the injury made may often be overlooked or full realization of the depth of the injury may not be recognized. Persistence of synovitis in the absence of other known cause or late suspicion of foreign body penetration calls for adequate surgical exploration. If debridement is not extensive enough, the foreign body may be missed, whereas careful and extensive debridement results in a complete cure.

In one series of 8 patients, 3 had a black thorn in the joint, 1 glass, 1 a brick fragment, 1 stone chips, 1 wood fragments, and 1 rubber particles from a nail wound that had penetrated the rubberized sole of the shoe. In warmer climates, the thorn from the palm tree may penetrate the joint. The lesson to be learned is that on suspicion of a penetrating injury into the joint, an adequate synovectomy must be performed in the face of persistent synovitis. The tissue specimen should be carefully examined for evidence of the foreign body. Its detection leads to an exact diagnosis and its removal to eradication of the problem.

REFERENCES

Goodnough CP, Frymoyer JW: Synovitis secondary to nonmetallic bodies. J Trauma 15:960, 1975

Infectious Arthritis

Don L. Goldenberg

GENERAL COMMENTS

PATHOGENESIS

Joints may be infected by any microorganism. Bacterial infections are the most readily diagnosed and the most virulent. Infectious agents probably account for far more cases of arthritis than are currently recognized. For instance, the association of hepatitis antigen and rheumatic disease has only recently been clearly identified. As diagnostic techniques for the detection of viruses and other microorganisms improve, more infectious agents will be found to be associated with specific rheumatic diseases.

The relationship of microorganisms to the etiology of the common rheumatic diseases such as systemic lupus erythematosus and rheumatoid arthritis is speculative and beyond the scope of this chapter. However, other rheumatic diseases are associated with an infectious agent, since the organism can be recovered from the joint or the arthritis is a manifestation of systemic disease related to a specific microbial agent (Table 1). Bacterial arthritis is an example where an infectious agent can be recovered from the joint. In classic suppurative arthritis, the organism enters the joint by direct intraarticular penetration or by hematogenous seeding to the synovium. The organisms then multiply and penetrate into the synovial fluid, resulting in the inflammation and necrosis characteristic of a purulent joint. In the second category, a systemic or localized infection results in subsequent synovitis, but the infectious agent cannot be recovered from the synovial fluid or synovial membrane. There is some evidence that immune mechanisms or hypersensitivity reactions may account for the subsequent synovitis. The specific antigens involved as well as definitive data incriminating immune mechanisms are generally not yet defined.

The mechanics of joint destruction in bacterial arthritis have been partially elucidated, although experi-

Table 1
Varieties of Infectious Arthritis

Type I: Organism is recovered from the synovial fluid or membrane
    Bacteria
    Tuberculosis and other mycobacteria
    Fungus
    Possibly some viruses
	Type II: Joint fluid is sterile, but there is evidence of preceding or coexistent systemic infection
	    Hepatitis
	    Bacterial endocarditis
	    Reiter's syndrome (post-salmonella or -Shigella dysentery)
	    Acute rheumatic fever
	    Whipple's disease
	    Yersinia, salmonella, or meningococcal arthritis
	    Lyme arthritis

mental data for many clinical observations are lacking. Within an hour after bacteria are experimentally injected into rabbits' joints, they are phagocytized by the synovial lining cells and by polymorphonuclear leukocytes which have migrated to the site of infection. Bacteriolysis occurs within these cells, thereby releasing lysosomal enzymes that result in synovial membrane necrosis. Further inflammatory cell influx occurs, resulting in abscess formation. Synovial lining cell regeneration and hyperplasia results in chronic inflammation with the invasion of cartilage and bone by granulation tissue. If left unchecked, marked articular destruction will occur and, ultimately, fibrous or bony ankylosis.

Certain bacteria, such as *Neisseria gonorrhoeae*, seem to have a propensity to spread to joints during bacteremia. Some bacteria are obviously more destructive once they enter the joint. For example, permanent joint destruction rarely follows gonococcal arthritis, yet it is quite common following arthritis due to gram-negative bacilli.

The relationship of bacteria, viruses, and other microbes to "reactive" or "sterile" synovitis is much less clearly understood. As noted above, hepatitis-associated antigen is implicated in the development of an acute arthritis, as well as a chronic necrotizing vasculitis (see the section on Systemic Arteritis and Related Disorders). There is evidence that immune activation plays a role in the development of hepatitis-associated rheumatic disease. The possible association of specific microorganisms with chronic rheumatic diseases, such as Reiter's syndrome, Whipple's disease, and acute rheumatic fever, will not be covered in this section. However, in certain rheumatic diseases a microorganism is clearly involved in pathogenesis and these will be reviewed (Table 1).

CLINICAL CHARACTERISTICS

The classic presentation of septic arthritis is an abrupt onset of a single, swollen, red, hot, and extremely tender joint that is very painful with any active or passive motion. For reasons not well understood, the large weight-bearing joints, especially the knee, are most often affected. The differential diagnosis generally includes gout and pseudogout, but other illnesses may mimic septic arthritis (see the section on Acute Monarticular Arthritis in the fascicle on Differential Approach to Major Rheumatic Syndromes).

Certain bacteria, especially *Neisseria gonorrhoeae*,

may cause polyarthritis as well as signs of bacteremia (i.e., high fever, chills, embolic skin lesions, polyarthralgias, and tenosynovitis). Florid fever, chills, and skin lesions, however, are not prominent features of acute monarticular septic arthritis. Signs and symptoms of infection elsewhere in the body are common and should be sought. Thus, a patient with probable gonococcal arthritis usually has evidence of a genitourinary infection; a patient with staphylococcal arthritis may have a coexistent skin infection; a patient with gram-negative bacilli in the joint often has a urinary tract infection; and a patient with pneumococcal arthritis often also has pneumonia. These extraarticular sites of infection may give a clue as to which organism has infected the joint.

LABORATORY ANALYSIS

A peripheral blood leukocytosis is common, but not always present. An elevated erythrocyte sedimentation rate reflects the inflammatory response but is not specific. Radiographs of the affected joint must always be ob-

Table 2
Diagnostic Procedures Useful in Septic Arthritis

Peripheral blood
    Leukocytosis—often but not always present
    Erythrocyte sedimentation rate—elevated but not specific
    Culture—if positive, very helpful; may be only source of
        microbial identification

Other sites of infection—culture and gram stain all possible
    sources of infection

Synovial fluid analysis
    Culture—definitive if positive
    Leukocytosis—greater than 50,000 cells/mm³ is suggestive
    Synovial fluid glucose—less than 40 mg/dl of blood glucose is
        suggestive
    Gram stain—diagnostic, but positive in less than one-half of
        cases
    Poor mucin clot—almost always, but not specific
    Elevated protein—almost always, but not specific

X-ray of joint—Generally not helpful unless there is coexistent
    osteomyection that has caused erosion(s)

Immunologic data (serum as well as synovial fluid)
    Evidence of immune complex activation may point toward
        "sterile" synovitis (depressed complement, etc.)
    Identification of bacterial antigen may be useful in culture-
        negative cases.

tained to help rule out a site of contiguous osteomyelitis, but generally are unremarkable early except for soft tissue swelling or evidence of an effusion. If the joint infection has been present for 2–3 weeks, bone destruction may have already occurred. Blood cultures and cultures from other possible sites of infection may yield the organism.

The diagnosis can only be definitive if the microorganism is found in the synovial fluid with gram stain of a smear or culture. Therefore, if septic arthritis is suspected, immediate synovial fluid aspiration and analysis must be done. A positive gram stain is present in only about one-half of cases in which the organism is recovered from the synovial fluid. The following synovial fluid characteristics should alert the physician to the likelihood of septic arthritis: a synovial fluid leukocyte count greater than 50,000 cells/mm^3, of which greater than 90 percent are polymorphonuclear cells; and a greater than 40 mg/dl difference between the synovial fluid glucose in comparison to a simultaneous blood glucose (Table 2).

In certain cases of presumed septic arthritis, the organism cannot be recovered from the synovial fluid. Occasionally, this may be due to prior use of antibiotics or to improper culture techniques. Certain organisms, however, especially *Neisseria gonorrhoeae,* are very difficult to grow in vitro, accounting for the frequency of negative culture results. In certain cases, immunologic identification of bacterial antigens may prove useful. Recently, counterimmunoelectrophoresis has been used in the diagnosis of septic arthritis due to *Hemophilus influenzae, Neisseria* species, and *Streptococcus pneumoniae* and may be extended to the identification of other bacterial antigens.

PRINCIPLES OF THERAPY

Successful treatment of septic arthritis requires the administration of effective antibiotics as well as mechanical drainage of purulent joint effusions. If the large puru-

Table 3
Principles of Treatment of Septic Arthritis

1. Be aware of possible septic arthritis.
2. Perform immediate arthrocentesis.
3. If grossly purulent synovial fluid present or gram stain of smear is positive, start antibiotics after all cultures have been obtained.
4. Identify the specific microorganism in the synovial fluid and use the most effective antibiotic on the basis of culture and sensitivity results.
5. Drain the infected fluid.
   a. Initially closed needle aspiration should be adequate.
   b. In hip infection or if the joint is difficult to drain by closed aspiration, open surgical drainage is necessary.
6. Continually assess response to treatment.
   a. Assess antimicrobial activity in synovial fluid.
   b. Follow synovial fluid culture, leukocyte count, and glucose concentration.
7. Rest the affected joint (articular splints).
8. Exercise periarticular muscles to prevent atrophy.

lent effusions are not removed from the joint, the continuous release of proteolytic enzymes and the increased pressure will cause articular cartilage damage despite sterilization of the joint. Moreover, the purulent exudates retard bacterial cell growth, allowing the survival of dormant bacteria that are more resistant to bactericidal activity. The effusions may be removed by closed needle aspiration or open surgical joint drainage. Most joints, such as the knee and wrist, can be drained effectively and most easily by needle aspiration, although daily or even more frequent aspirations may be initially required. Closed aspiration also enables the physician to assess the therapeutic response by following the serial synovial fluid leukocyte count, glucose, culture results, and antimicrobial levels obtained in the synovial fluid. Joints that are more difficult to drain by needle aspiration, such as the hip or joints that have not responded adequately to closed needle aspiration, should undergo open surgical drainage with debridement of necrotic tissue. There is no conclusive evidence that continuous irrigation or other special drainage procedures affect the outcome.

There is evidence that most currently used antibiotics are transported into inflamed joints following bactericidal concentrations. Therefore, antibiotics do not need to be injected intraarticularly. The duration and route of administration, as well as the antibiotic of choice, varies with the microorganism and will be discussed in the ensuing chapters.

REFERENCES

Curtiss PH Jr, Klein L: Destruction of articular cartilage in septic arthritis. J Bone Joint Surg 45A:797, 1963

Parker PH, Schmid FR: Antibacterial activity of synovial fluid during treatment of septic arthritis. Arthritis Rheum 14:96, 1971

Shaffer MF, Bennet GA: The passage of type III rabbit virulent pneumococci from the vascular system into the joints and certain other body cavities. J Exp Med 70:293, 1939

Goldenberg DL, Cohen AS: Acute infectious arthritis. A review of patients with non-gonococcal joint infections, with emphasis on therapy and prognosis. Am J Med 60:369, 1976

GONOCOCCAL ARTHRITIS

CLINICAL SPECTRUM

The most common acute previously undiagnosed arthritis requiring hospitalization is gonococcal arthritis. The incidence of gonococcal infection has increased in the past two decades. An estimated three million patients were treated for gonococcal infection in 1975. Disseminated gonococcal infection (DGI) complicates approximately 1 percent of such infections and may follow local infection of the genitourinary tract, anorectum, oropharynx, eyes, and skin. Extragenital infection may also involve the peritoneal cavity, liver, heart, and meninges. However, DGI typically involves the joints and the skin.

The clinical spectrum of DGI has changed in the past

Table 1
Differential Features of Gonococcal Versus Gram-Positive Coccal Arthritis

Features	Gonococcal Arthritis	Gram-Positive Coccal Arthritis
Prodromal polyarthralgia	Frequent	Rare
Number of joints	Usually polyarticular	Usually monarticular
Tenosynovitis	Frequent	Rare
Skin lesions	Common (20–50%)	Rare
Positive gram stain	Rare (less than 25%)	50%
Positive synovial fluid culture	50%	Nearly always
Diagnostic trial with antibiotics	Helpful	Not an important initial diagnostic criteria
Repeated mechanical drainage	Helpful but not usually necessary	Important

half-century. In the preantibiotic era the great majority of patients were male. Presently, most symptomatic males receive antibiotics shortly after the development of a urethral discharge. Therefore, over 60 percent of cases of DGI now occur in women. Documented bacteremia, skin lesions, and arthralgias occur more in DGI today and recovery of organisms from the joint is more frequent. Although osteomyelitis occurred in 10 percent of DGI cases in the preantibiotic era, gonococcal osteomyelitis is now rare.

The clinical manifestations of gonococcal arthritis can be differentiated from other types of infectious arthritis (Table 1). Skin lesions occur in 10–90 percent of patients with DGI. The characteristic lesions are maculopapular eruptions, often over the dorsum of the hands or feet. However, vesicles, pustules, or bullae may also be present. Although gram stain smears of the lesions may reveal gram-negative diplococci, the cultures of these lesions are rarely positive. Unlike gram-positive coccal arthritis, gonococcal arthritis is often associated with arthralgias, tenosynovitis, and migratory polyarthritis. Monarticular infection occurs in less than one-third of patients. In a recent survey of 31 patients with acute arthritis and proven gonococcal infection, as many as 7 joints and a mean of more than 3 joints per patient were involved.

Most patients have had significant fever, chills and leukocytosis. Unlike most cases of gram-positive septic arthritis, which often occur in elderly, debilitated patients with chronic disease, the typical case of gonococcal arthritis develops in young, healthy individuals.

There is some evidence that DGI is more common in pregnant and menstruating women. Various factors have been proposed to account for this: (1) maximal shedding of organisms occurs during menstruation; (2) the pH of cervical secretions is alkaline and the gonococcus is sensitive to acid surroundings; and (3) the pH-dependent peroxidase-mediated bactericidal system of cervical secretions does not function optimally at alkaline pH.

Two sequential stages in DGI were first described in 1968. A bacteremic stage, identified by positive blood cultures and typical skin lesions, occurred after a mean of 3 days of symptoms. Although polyarthralgias and tenosynovitis were present, large purulent effusions and positive synovial fluid cultures were not obtained. Shaking chills and fever were prominent. A number of patients were also observed whose symptoms had been of longer duration. These patients presented with purulent monarthritis and positive synovial fluid but negative blood cultures. Chills, fever, and skin lesions were not present. It was postulated that this later septic joint stage developed after a relatively asymptomatic bacteremic episode, allowing the gonococcus enough incubation time in the synovial membrane to produce a purulent effusion.

In 1974, 31 patients with gonococcal arthritis were similarly evaluated but sequential clinical stages of DGI were not confirmed. In this study 7 patients with positive blood cultures were compared to 15 patients with positive synovial fluid cultures. None of the patients had both positive blood and synovial fluid cultures. Articular pain was the initial manifestation in all but 1 patient. The interval between the onset of illness and initial evaluation was brief in both groups, 2.3 and 3.4 days, respectively. Two of the 7 with positive blood cultures and 4 of the 15 with positive synovial fluid cultures had symptoms for 24 hours or less prior to hospitalization. The mean temperature and initial peripheral blood leukocytosis was higher in the patients with positive blood cultures (103.4° versus 101.9°F, and 17,500 versus 12,000 cells/mm^3). However, only 1 of 7 patients with positive blood cultures (group I), but 7 of 15 with positive synovial fluid cultures (group II) had migratory polyarthritis. Only 2 patients in group I and group II had monarticular involvement. Purulent effusions were typical in both groups, with an average synovial fluid count of 82,000 leukocytes/mm^3.

There was no relationship found between the synovial leukocyte count and the duration of illness or the number of joints involved. Similarly, no correlation was observed between the synovial fluid leukocyte count and the results of synovial fluid cultures. Two effusions with leukocyte counts greater than 100,000 cells/mm^3 were sterile, whereas gonococci were recovered from three fluids containing fewer than 30,000 cells/mm^3.

Thus, the patients in this series could not be clinically distinguished into a bacteremic and septic joint stage, but rather demonstrated features of both. There was no evidence that patients with a septic joint stage have a prolonged asymptomatic bacteremic stage.

DIAGNOSIS AND MICROBIOLOGY

Any patient suspected of DGI should be evaluated with gram staining of smears and cultures of genitourinary foci, skin, or synovial fluids. Blood, oropharyngeal, and anal cultures should be obtained. Thayer-Martin media containing antibiotics that enable *Neisseria* to grow but suppress the growth of other common contaminants should be used for genitourinary or throat cultures. All other cultures should be directly plated in broth and onto chocolate agar, and the laboratory should be alerted so that the organism will be cultured in 5–10 percent CO_2.

However, even in the best of laboratories, gonococci are recovered from the joints in only about 50 percent of suspected gonococcal arthritis cases. Attempts to improve the culture media, including the use of a high-sucrose media to allow L-forms to grow, have met with limited success. Gram staining of smears is even less reliable.

Antigenic identification may be helpful in the future. Currently, the direct fluorescent antibody test has been useful in confirming the presence of gonococci in clinical materials. However, existing serologic tests are only 80–90 percent effective when compared to cultures. They do not distinguish between current and previous infections and the antigens employed cross-react with other *Neisseria* species. More specific yet sensitive serologic tests will depend on the identification of antigen specificity. Most interest regarding antigenic classification currently centers around the outer membrane proteins and pili of the gonococcus.

TREATMENT

DGI is exquisitely sensitive to antibiotics. There are no reports of penicillin-resistant strains causing DGI. In Seattle, 85 percent of strains isolated from patients with DGI have mean inhibitory concentrations to penicillin one-tenth of that of isolates from persons with uncomplicated gonococcal infection. This indicates that the strains causing DGI are much more sensitive to penicillin than the strains that result in isolated genitourinary infection.

Although traditionally DGI and gonococcal arthritis have been treated with large doses of parenteral antibiotics, recent evidence suggests that DGI may respond to lower doses of parenteral antibiotics or oral antibiotics. In one study, 98 patients with DGI were treated with various antibiotic regimens: 33 received 10 million units of penicillin G intravenously per day, followed by oral ampicillin for at least 10 days; 29 received 3.5 ampicillin orally with probenecid, followed by 2 g/day for at least 7 days; 20 received lower doses of parenteral penicillin; 6 received oral tetracycline; 5 received parenteral cephalosporins; and 5 received other regimens. The response to treatment was equally rapid and complete within each group. At least 90 percent of the patients in each group had subjective improvement and defervescence within 2 days, and all patients followed for at least 2 weeks achieved complete clinical and bacteriologic cure. Skin lesions resolved after a mean of 3 days of treatment, but synovial effusions took slightly longer to resolve.

This study and others document the sensitivity of DGI to antibiotics and lend more credence to the use of antibiotics for diagnostic as well as therapeutic value.

Thus, within 24–48 hours after antibiotics are initiated, fever should abate and marked subjective improvement should occur if the patient does have DGI. The rate of resolution of the arthritis is more closely related to the initial presence or absence of a purulent joint effusion than to the antibiotic regimen used. Those patients with purulent effusions had a longer duration of effusion (mean of 8.5 compared to 2 days) and a longer duration of hospitalization (8.4 compared to 4.1 days). Thus, gonococcal arthritis must be managed like any gram-positive coccal arthritis if purulent joint effusions are present. Frequent needle aspirations may be required to decompress large purulent effusions. Open surgical drainage should rarely be necessary.

REFERENCES

Brandt KD, Cathcart ES, Cohen AS: Gonococcal arthritis. Arthritis Rheum 17:503, 1974

Holmes KK, Counts GW, Beaty HN: Disseminated gonococcal infection. Ann Intern Med 74:979, 1971

Keiser HL, Ruben FL, Wolinsky E, Kushner I: Clinical forms of gonococcal arthritis. N Engl J Med 279:234, 1968

NONGONOCOCCAL BACTERIAL ARTHRITIS

The bacteria recovered from patients with septic arthritis vary with the age of the patient (Table 1). In children less than 2 years old, *Hemophilus influenzae* is the most prevalent bacterium, but in older age groups the spectrum of bacteria isolated in septic arthritis is similar to that in adults. In adults, *Staphylococcus aureus* and streptococci have been most frequently recovered from infected joints, but in the past decade gram-negative bacilli have become an important cause of acute infectious arthritis.

PREDISPOSING FACTORS

In adults, host factors that seem to predispose patients to the joint infection include serious chronic illness, such as malignancy, cirrhosis, or diabetes mellitus, or

Table 1
Bacteria (Nongonococcal) Isolated from Synovial Fluid*

Bacteria	Percentage of Patients with Septic Arthritis (Grouped by Age)		
	< 2 Years	2–10 Years	Adults
Staphylococcus aureus	27	35	62
Streptococcus hemolyticus	12	21	15
Streptococcus pneumoniae	8	14	8
Gram-negative bacilli†	14	12	12
Hemophilus influenza	34	12	2
Other	5	6	1

*A total of 329 cases from our experience (1967–1977) and selected reports (1947–1967).

†*Escherichia coli, Pseudomonas, Klebsiella, Serratia,* and *Salmonella.*

factors that interfere with host defense mechanisms, such as prior immunosuppressive treatment. An important predisposing factor is prior arthritis in the infected joint. Patients with rheumatoid arthritis have an increased incidence of septic arthritis when compared to control populations. Whether a local factor enables bacteria to penetrate the previously damaged joints more readily is not clear. In addition, patients with rheumatoid arthritis have an increased incidence of bacterial infections. This may be related to impairment in chemotaxis because of phagocytosis of rheumatoid factor complexes and other factors. *Staphylococcus aureus* is recovered from the infected joint in the majority of such patients.

The results of treatment in these patients are significantly worse than in patients who develop septic arthritis but who do not have underlying chronic joint disease. Multiple factors probably account for these poor results, including prior articular damage and previous immunosuppressive therapy, which may depress the inflammatory response. However, the most important factor is a delay in diagnosis and therapy. The physician, if not alert to the possibility of superimposed septic arthritis, may attribute the patient's joint inflammation to a local flare-up of rheumatoid arthritis. There are reports of bacterial arthritis complicating many other rheumatic diseases, including systemic lupus erythematosus, gout, pseudogout, osteoarthritis, and Charcot's arthropathy. It is therefore necessary to be aware of the possibility of septic arthritis superimposed on a chronic arthritis and to aspirate the joint in question.

In the past decade, the incidence of gram-negative bacilli bacteremia has increased alarmingly. Gram-negative bacilli cause the most serious infectious diseases requiring hospitalization. Similarly, the incidence of gram-negative bacilli arthritis has increased. Whereas only 7 percent of septic arthritis was caused by gram-negative bacilli during reports from 1947 to 1967, 26 percent of septic arthritis during the past decade has been caused by gram-negative bacilli at our medial center. *Escherichia coli, Pseudomonas,* and *Serratia* are most often involved. The two most important predisposing factors identified are intravenous drug use and impaired host defense response. Intravenous heroin users seem prone to develop septic arthritis due to *Pseudomonas* and *Serratia.* Unusual sites of infection, including the sternoclavicular and sacroiliac joints, are commonly identified in these infections. The reason that intravenous drug users develop these unusual infections is not clear, although contamination from skin, tap water, or the injection paraphernalia used may be the source. The other patients who have developed gram-negative bacilli arthritis almost all had serious underlying diseases or other predisposing host factors.

CLINICAL FEATURES

There are no remarkable clinical features to distinguish the varieties of non-gonococcal bacterial arthritis. A single joint or occasionally two joints are infected and the onset is abrupt. Fever is almost always present, but may be low-grade. Peripheral blood leukocytosis is present in only 60 percent of patients. The synovial fluid characteristics are similar to those described above, a mean of 70–100,000 leukocytes/mm^3 with greater than 90 percent polymorphonuclear cells and a depressed synovial fluid glucose.

TREATMENT

The treatment and results of therapy in nongonococcal bacterial arthritis depend on multiple factors. Appropriate antibiotics, adequate joint drainage, and continuous assessment of the effect of therapy are essential. Rapid initiation of antibiotics is important and often should be started prior to the identification of the microorganism in culture. If the gram stain of the smear is positive, a rational initial antibiotic regimen can be started. However, if the gram stain of the smear is not helpful, antibiotic choice must rest on the likelihood of certain bacteria infecting certain hosts. For example, in intravenous drug users or in immunosuppressed hosts, the antibiotics should be effective against *Staphylococcus aureus* as well as gram-negative bacilli. In children under the age of 2 years, antibiotics effective against *Hemophilus influenzae* should be initiated. Once the culture results and sensitivities of the organism to various antibiotics are identified, the most specific and least dangerous antibiotic should be utilized, and the intravenous route should be used whenever possible. The optimal dose and duration of treatment are not known, although most authors recommend at least 2 or 3 weeks of parenteral antimicrobial therapy.

Even with optimal management, complete recovery occurs in less than 50 percent of patients with gram-negative bacilli arthritis and about 75 percent of patients with staphylococcus aureus arthritis. The serious underlying disease in many of these patients adversely effects the outcome. For example, the young healthy intravenous drug users who develop gram-negative bacilli arthritis generally recover completely when adequately treated, whereas elderly chronically ill patients who develop this joint infection usually develop serious residual joint destruction. The rapidity with which therapy is initiated is the single most important variable in determining the outcome of patients with nongonococcal bacterial arthritis.

REFERENCES

Bayer AS, Chow AW, Louie JS, Nies KM, Guze LB: Gram-negative bacillary septic arthritis: Clinical, radiographic, therapeutic, and prognostic features. Semin Arthritis Rheum 7:123, 1977

Chartier Y, Martin WJ, Kelly PG: Bacterial arthritis: Experiences in the treatment of 77 patients. Ann Intern Med 50:1462, 1959

Goldenberg DL, Brandt KD, Cathcart ES, Cohen AS: Acute arthritis caused by gram-negative bacilli: A clinical characterization. Medicine (Baltimore) 53:197, 1974

Myers AR, Miller LM, Pinals RS: Pyarthrosis complicating rheumatoid arthritis. Lancet 2:714, 1969

ARTHRITIS DUE TO MYCOBACTERIA

TUBERCULOUS ARTHRITIS

Tuberculous arthritis usually develops secondary to reactivation of a hematogenously seeded primary pulmonary infection. About 1 percent of patients with tuberculosis develop skeletal involvement. Patients generally present with chronic, insidious monarthritis. The most frequently affected sites are the spine, knee, and hip. Tenosynovium may be infected and tuberculosis may produce a carpal tunnel syndrome. Systemic features typical of pulmonary tuberculosis such as severe chills, high fever, and night sweats are not common. Active pulmonary tuberculosis is present in less than 20 percent of patients with articular tuberculosis; however, nonpulmonary extraarticular sites such as the lymph nodes, urinary tract, liver, and skin may be infected.

A positive skin test to intermediate-strength purified protein derivative is generally present despite the absence of chest x-ray evidence of active tuberculosis. Articular roentgenograms are often abnormal, probably reflecting the insidious onset of arthritis. Therefore, osteoporosis, metaphyseal erosions, and joint space narrowing may have already developed before the diagnosis is considered. Synovial fluid analysis generally reveals an inflammatory fluid, although the total leukocyte count has ranged from 40 to 136,000 cells/mm^3. Synovial fluid glucose is depressed, the total protein is elevated, and the mucin clot is poor.

Synovial fluid smears demonstrate acid-fast bacilli in 20 percent of cases and synovial fluid cultures are positive in 80 percent. However, synovial membrane biopsy is the procedure of choice since either typical histology or positive culture are present in greater than 90 percent of tuberculous synovia examined.

Combination chemotherapy is generally successful. Isoniazid, streptomycin, ethambutol, and rifampin are currently used in various combinations. Extensive surgery was necessary in the preantibiotic era, but more recently limited procedures such as synovectomy or just immobilization have been advocated.

ATYPICAL MYCOBACTERIAL ARTHRITIS

The atypical mycobacteria are a heterogenous group of organisms that are similar to *Mycobacterium tuberculosis* and *bovis* but represent distinct organisms. Although there are numerous classifications, the most widely used is the Runyon classification, which depends upon biologic laboratory characteristics: group I, photochromogens; group II, scotochromogens; group III, nonchromogens; and group IV, rapid growers. The disease produced by atypical mycobacteria is generally indistinguishable clinically, radiologically, and histologically from tuberculosis. Definitive diagnosis depends on isolation of the organism by culture or identification by special laboratory tests.

The arthritis generally results from hematogenous spread. Most patients have had preexisting joint disease or trauma and were compromised hosts. Chest x-rays are generally unrevealing except for old calcification. Intermediate-strength purified protein derivative reveals less than 8 mm induration at 48 hours, although second-strength skin testing with material prepared from atypical mycobacteria is usually positive. Unlike the arthritis due to *Mycobacterium tuberculosis,* the atypical mycobacteria not uncommonly cause polyarthritis. Synovial fluid and synovial membrane pathologic changes are similar to those described above in tuberculous arthritis. Treatment has consisted of synovectomy and antimicrobial agents based on sensitivities of the organism. Since many organisms are resistant or partially resistant to the major antituberculous drugs, multiple medications must be tested and used in combination to obtain an effective therapeutic response.

REFERENCES

Berney S, Goldstein M, Bisko F: Clinical and diagnostic features of tuberculous arthritis. Am J Med 53:36, 1972

Davidson PT, Horowitz I: Skeletal tuberculosis. Am J Med 48:77, 1970

Goldenberg DL, Cohen AS: Arthritis due to tuberculous and fungal microorganisms. Clin Rheum Dis 4:211, 1978

Wallace R, Cohen AS: Tuberculous arthritis. A report of two cases with review of biopsy and synovial fluid findings. Am J Med 61:277, 1976

FUNGAL ARTHRITIS

Mycoses are unusual causes of systemic infections and fungal arthritis is rare. Therefore, the diagnosis is often not considered and specific treatment is delayed for months or years, resulting in irreversible joint destruction. The mycoses most frequently causing arthritis are coccidioidomycosis, blastomycosis and sporotrichosis.

COCCIDIOIDOMYCOSIS

Coccidioidomycosis, which is endemic in the southwestern United States, is associated with two forms of arthritis. During acute primary coccidioidomycosis, transient joint symptoms may develop. The symptoms usually subside within 1 month without residual joint disease and may represent a hypersensitivity synovitis. Disseminated disease occurs in 0.1–0.2 percent of patients and approximately 20 percent of cases involve bones or joints. Joint involvement secondary to contiguous osteomyelitis is not unusual, although primary granulomatous coccidioidal arthritis is rare. The arthritis may fluctuate in activity for many years and may cause years of minimal morbidity. If untreated, however, permanent destruction will result. The chronically infected joints reveal a thickened gray synovial membrane which may contain serous or purulent fluid.

The diagnosis should be suspected in patients with a chronic, destructive arthritis, especially if the patient has lived in or traveled to endemic areas. Skin tests and especially serologic tests are helpful diagnostically, but a specific diagnosis can be made only by the recovery of the organism from joint fluid culture or from biopsy specimens. The treatment of choice is intravenous amphotericin B. Although some authors advocate synovectomy, the role of surgery in treating focal articular coccidioidal infection is not clear. In patients with far advanced joint damage, surgical fusion or amputation may be necessary. Intraarticular amphotericin has been used with limited success and may prove a useful alternative to intravenous therapy in cases with evidence of local disease. A severe, local reaction to the intraarticular injection may be diminished by combining the amphotericin with a local anesthetic.

BLASTOMYCOSIS

Blastomyces dermatitidis generally causes pulmonary or cutaneous manifestations, but it may cause widespread disease involving bones and joints. Osteomyelitis occurs in 30–50 percent of patients with disseminated blastomycosis and often results in secondary septic arthritis. Primary arthritis without bone disease most often affects the knees and ankles. The arthritis is almost always accompanied by skin lesions and lung involvement. Synovial fluid microscopic examination usually reveals the organisms, as they are numerous. Treatment with parenteral amphotericin B is usually successful.

SPOROTRICHOSIS

Sporotrichum schenckii infections follow direct implantation of the fungus and generally are limited to the skin and regional lymphatics. However, 8 percent of disseminated infections involve musculoskeletal sites. Widespread systemic sporotrichosis usually occurs in compromised hosts, but focal articular sporotrichosis may develop in healthy adults. Outdoor occupations and alcoholism seem to predispose patients to this fungal infection.

Sporotrichosis arthritis most commonly affects the knees, ankles, wrists, and elbows, although any joint or tenosynovium may be involved. The synovitis is usually monarticular or pauciarticular and generally is insidious in onset. The synovial fluid is inflammatory; the leukocyte counts range from 8000 to 23,000/mm³. The diagnosis is best established by culture of both the synovial fluid and tissue. Roentgenograms generally reveal osteoporosis and bony erosions. Amphotericin B, either alone or with surgical debridement, is the therapy of choice.

CANDIDIASIS

Candida arthritis is rare, but with the increased incidence of disseminated candidiasis more cases are being reported. The arthritis develops during the course of hematogenous infection. Most patients with candida arthritis have had significant underlying diseases and factors predisposing to infection. Neonates with candida arthritis have had low birth weights, prematurity, bacterial sepsis, pulmonary disease, and intravenous catheters. Adults have had chronic disease such as carcinoma, rheumatoid arthritis, or systemic lupus erythematosus,

and often have been receiving antibiotics, corticosteroids, or cytotoxic drugs and were maintained on intravenous or urinary catheters. The arthritis most often is monarticular but may be polyarticular. Joint roentgenograms are generally unrevealing. Synovial fluids have been seropurulent or purulent; the leukocytes have ranged between 10,000 and 150,000/mm³. Synovial fluid culture is usually adequate for diagnosis. Organisms may be seen on gram stain. Intravenous amphotericin B has been successful in most patients, although intraarticular amphotericin B or surgery may be necessary adjuncts. Fluorocytosine has also been used successfully.

OTHER ORGANISMS

Histoplasmosis rarely causes bone and joint disease. An acute, migratory polyarthritis as the predominant manifestation of primary histoplasmosis has, however, been described. It was postulated that this represented an allergic type of manifestation similar to that in primary coccidioidomycosis. However, the diagnosis was made solely on the basis of serologic tests for histoplasmosis and synovial fluid was not evaluated.

Arthritis may occur in association with the bone lesions of cryptococcosis. Treatment with either amphotericin B or 5-fluorocytosine as been used. *Actinomyces israelii,* which is actually a bacterium, may also cause bone infections and may secondarily infect joints. Treatment with penicillin is successful. Rare cases of arthritis associated with *Nocardia* and *Cephalosporium* species have been reported.

REFERENCES

Crout JE, Brewer NS, Tompkins RB: Sporotrichosis arthritis. Ann Intern Med 86:294, 1977

Greenman R, Becker J, Campbell G, Remington J: Coccidioidal synovitis of the knee. Arch Intern Med 135:526, 1975

Murray HW, Fialk MA, Roberts RB: Candida arthritis. A manifestation of disseminated candidiasis. Am J Med 60:587, 1976

VIRAL ARTHRITIS

HEPATITIS-ASSOCIATED VIRUS

Until recently, the spectrum of viral arthritis was narrow and poorly defined. However, the association of distinct rheumatic diseases and hepatitis B antigen (HBsAg) has expanded our knowledge. The HBsAg is associated with an acute, transient polyarthritis and two chronic rheumatic diseases—polyarteritis nodosa and mixed cryoglobulinemia (Table 1). These represent the best studied examples of a virus or viral particle associated with arthritis.

The association of arthralgias and arthritis with hepatitis has been recognized for over a century. However, not until specific immunologic markers of hepatitis infection became available was this association clearly identi-

Table 1
Characteristic Features of Rheumatic Disease Associated with Hepatitis Antigen (HBAg)

Feature	Transient Illness	Chronic Multisystemic Illness
Onset	Acute	Insidious
Systemic features	Minimal	Fever, leukocytosis, anemia
Arthritis	Acute, symmetric, additive, or migratory polyarthritis	Chronic polyarthritis, possibly osteoporosis and erosions on x-ray
Rash	Maculopapular, urticarial	Petechiae, nodules
Jaundice	Generally present at or soon after onset of arthritis	Rare
Other organ involvement	Rare	
Renal		Hypertension, azotemia
Nervous system		Mononeuritis, cerebritis
Gastrointestinal		Vasculitis
Heart		Myocarditis, pericarditis
Liver		
Hepatocellular function	Markedly increased enzymes	Normal or moderately increased enzymes
Biopsy findings	Acute viral hepatitis	Chronic persistent or viral hepatitis, no specific diagnosis
HBsAG	Present acutely, then often disappears with presence of antibody	Persistent

fied. The serologic evaluation of hepatitis antigens (HBAg) and antibody (HBAb) has been especially useful in characterizing an acute polyarthritis associated with a hepatitis.

Acute Polyarthritis

Most of the patients have developed an acute migratory or additive polyarthritis as a prodrome of clinical hepatitis. Thus, at initial presentation the patients are not jaundiced and may not yet have developed anorexia, fatigue, or liver tenderness. Although the bilirubin may be normal, the hepatocellular enzymes such as the SGOT are usually elevated.

The arthritis generally involves multiple joints, including the small joints of the hands, and may resemble rheumatoid arthritis. Polyarthralgias and tenosynovitis occur frequently. Differential diagnosis may include acute rheumatic fever and gonococcal arthritis. The results of synovial fluid analysis have been variable. Some authors have described noninflammatory joint fluid, whereas others report purulent fluids. A recent report of 10 such fluids included a leukocyte range of 465 to 90,000 cells/mm³ with a mean of 24,000 cells/mm³. The differential cell count revealed a predominance of neutrophils in 6 and mononuclear cells in 4 fluids. The mean protein concentration was 4.2 g/dl and the mean glucose level was 114 mg/dl. C3 levels were depressed in only 2 of the 10 synovial fluids in this series. Four of 8 synovial fluids were positive for HBsAg and 2 were positive for HBAb only.

The few synovial membranes evaluated have revealed little evidence of inflammation. Moderate vascular inflammation has been present. Immunofluorescent and electron microscopic evidence of HBsAg in the synovium has been demonstrated. The arthritis is generally responsive to salicylates.

A skin rash, maculopapular or urticarial, often accompanies the arthritis. The arthritis and rash are similar to that which occurs in acute serum sickness. Indeed, there is now evidence to conclude that this syndrome is due to circulating immune complexes and that complement activation is triggered by the hepatitis virus. The sera and synovial fluid both have been shown to contain HBAg during the acute arthritis as well as depressed levels of total hemolytic complement and various complement components. Antigen–antibody complexes containing HBAg and HBAb have been identified by immunologic techniques and with electron microscopy in both the sera and synovial fluid. The arthritis and rash generally resolve with the appearance of jaundice, coincident with the disappearance of HBAg in the sera and the appearance of HBAb. Liver histology during this transient polyarthritis is characteristic of acute viral hepatitis.

Chronic Multisystem Disease

In addition to the transient polyarthritis, HBsAg is associated with chronic multisystem disease, including necrotizing arteritis and essential mixed cryoglobulinemia (see the section on Systemic Arteritis and Related Disorders in the fascicle on Specific Articular and Connective Tissue Diseases). Histologic evidence of arteritis and glomerulonephritis are present. The arteritis resembles chronic serum sickness and circulating immune complexes, decreased complement, and HBsAg and HBAb have been identified in the serum. HbsAg, immunoglobulins, and complement on vascular membranes of target organs have been detected. Evidence of HBsAg or HBAb has been found in the serum and/or cryoprecipitates of over 50 percent of patients with essential mixed cryoglobulinemia. The chronic illness is characterized by severe organ system arteritis with resultant hypertension, azotemia, proteinuria, hematuria, abdominal pain, carditis, purpura, and mononeuritis multiplex typical of idiopathic polyarteritis nodosa.

OTHER ASSOCIATIONS

Many of the other proposed associations of a virus with arthritis are speculative. Viruses have not been recovered from synovial fluid or synovial membranes in most of these cases, and the diagnosis rests on clinical grounds plus serologic evidence of a recent rise in antibody levels to the specific virus. Case reports have described an acute, transient mon- or polyarthritis in association with clinical and serologic evidence of adenovirus, coxsackievirus, varicella, and arbovirus. Suppurative arthritis and osteomyelitis associated with smallpox have been verified by the demonstration of the organism in tissue culture.

Rubella is complicated by joint symptoms in 15–30 percent of cases. Migratory polyarthralgias are most common. The arthritis may resemble rheumatoid arthritis and typically consists of acute transient symmetric polyarthritis of the small joints of the hands and the knees. Articular manifestations may even precede the typical rash, but the synovitis generally disappears within a few weeks. Rubella vaccinations may cause similar articular symptoms. The synovial fluid in rubella arthritis is inflammatory in nature. Salicylates are usually sufficient treatment until the arthritis spontaneously resolves. Joint manifestations associated with many other viral diseases, including infectious mononucleosis and mumps, have been described.

REFERENCES

Duffy J, Lidsky MD, Sharp JT, Davis JS, Person DA, Hollinger FB, Min K-W: Polyarthritis, polyarteritis and hepatitis B. Medicine (Baltimore) 55:19, 1976

Onion DK, Crumpacker CS, Gilliland BC: Arthritis of hepatitis associated with Australia antigen. Ann Intern Med 75:29, 1971

"REACTIVE" ARTHRITIS

As mentioned in the introduction to this section, certain rheumatic diseases are associated with systemic infections, but there is no evidence that the microorganism is directly responsible for the subsequent arthritis. The term *reactive arthritis* refers to rheumatic diseases following a systemic infection, but the microorganism responsible for the infection cannot be recovered from the joint (see Table 1 in the chapter on General Comments on Infectious Arthritis). Various reasons are postulated to account for why the joint is "sterile." For example, the microorganism may be very difficult to recover by standard culture techniques, or the organism may exist in an altered form in the joint, thus escaping detection. Alternatively, these organisms may trigger some immune process that causes the synovitis. Examples of an association of a systemic infection and subsequent immune synovitis include both acute rheumatic fever and hepatitis.

Three rheumatic diseases are notable examples of

reactive arthritis. Of special interest is the observation that each of these organisms may infect the joint by hematogenous seeding, but also may be associated with a chronic "sterile" synovitis which may be secondary to immune or hypersensitivity mechanisms. These three organisms, *Salmonella, Yersinia,* and meningococci, thus have the potential, like streptococci, to cause either a classic, suppurative septic joint or to be associated with reactive arthritis.

Salmonella may cause a septic arthritis and be recovered from the joint. Most patients with suppurative salmonella arthritis have had serious underlying illness. More often, salmonella arthritis is a transient, sterile, serous synovitis which follows a diarrheal illness by a week or a few months. The arthritis is typically polyarticular and the synovial fluid is sterile, but the organism can be recovered from the stool or the blood.

Similarly, the arthritis associated with *Yersinia enterocolitica* infections has been described as a sterile synovitis occurring 1–14 days following acute enteritis. The arthritis may be monarticular or polyarticular, involving any joint. The diagnosis usually depends upon recovering the organism from stool cultures and/or serologic evidence (rise in serum agglutination titer). However, the organism has also been recovered from the synovial fluid following *Yersinia enterocolitica* septicemia in a 69-year-old man who developed classic suppurative polyarthritis.

Meningococcal arthritis may also cause classic suppurative arthritis or a sterile, intermittent migratory polyarthritis. Acute meningococcemia may be associated with transient polyarthralgias or inflammatory sterile synovitis, and chronic meningococcemia may be associated with either a transient polyarthritis or a chronic monarthritis.

It is intriguing to speculate why certain infections are associated with the spread of the microorganism into the joint, whereas other infections seem to only indirectly stimulate a joint "reaction." A further understanding of these observations may shed light on the pathophysiology of many of the chronic rheumatic diseases.

REFERENCES

Warren CPW: Arthritis associated with salmonella infections. Ann Rheum Dis 29:483, 1970

Winblad S: Arthritis associated with Yersinia enterocolitica infections. Scan J Int Dis 7:191, 1975

LYME ARTHRITIS

A newly recognized form of inflammatory arthritis, named after the Lyme, Conn., community where it was first described, may also be caused by an infectious agent. Fifty-one residents (mainly children and young adults) of three Connecticut communities developed brief but generally recurrent episodes of mon- or oligarthritis. Subsequently, 32 patients were studied prospectively.

The arthritis usually began suddenly in one or two joints, most often the knee or other large joints. The synovial fluid was inflammatory, with a median leukocyte count of 24,000 cells/mm³. Synovial biopsies revealed hypertrophy, vascular proliferation, and mononuclear cell infiltration. Permanent joint deformities did not occur. Associated findings included headache, stiff neck, backache, myalgias, lymphadenopathy, aseptic meningitis, myocardial conduction abnormalities, serum cryoprecipitates, elevated erythrocyte sedimentation rate, and elevated serum IgM levels.

The clues to diagnosis as well as to possible infectious etiology are (1) a geographic clustering of cases and (2) a skin lesion which heralds the onset of arthritis. The cluster of cases in rural communities and the absence of a common water supply suggested a possible arthropod vector spread. Seventeen of the first 39 patients reported lived on four country roads where 1 in 10 residents developed the illness. Six families had more than one affected member. Cultures of synovial fluid and membrane revealed no growth of any microorganism and no cytopathic effects, and serologic tests were unrevealing.

The best clue to diagnosis was the onset of skin lesions which began about 3–4 weeks prior to the onset of arthritis. The lesion began as a red macule or papule that expanded to form a large ring with central clearing. Multiple lesions were common, but usually smaller than the initial one (median diameter 16 cm). The lesions faded in an average of 3 weeks. These lesions are typical of erythema chronicum migrans, which is believed to be transmitted by the sheep tick, *Ixodes ricinus*. However, no causative agent, including rickettsiae, have been isolated in individual patients.

Some authors have felt that antibiotics may result in prompt disappearance of the skin lesion, but it is not clear that antibiotics have any effect on the development of arthritis or other symptoms. Antiinflammatory agents may help during the attacks of arthritis.

REFERENCES

Steere AC, Malawista SE, Hardin JA, Ruddy S, Askenase PW, Andiman WA: Erythema chronicum migrans and Lyme arthritis. Ann Intern Med 86:685, 1977

IMMUNOLOGY: CONCEPTS AND DIAGNOSTIC PROCEDURES

Immunoglobulins

Edward C. Franklin

GENERAL NATURE

The defense of the host against a variety of infectious and other noxious agents, and perhaps also against the development of malignancy, is a complex process involving both cellular and humoral factors. Prominent among these are antibodies, or as they are now known, immunoglobulins, which are the major humoral constituent of this defense system. Because animals need to produce an almost infinite number of antibodies having specificities against the many antigens that they are exposed to, immunoglobulins represent the most heterogeneous group of proteins known to man.

Structural Heterogeneity

The structural heterogeneity of immunoglobulins exists on three levels. Foremost and most complex are the structural differences related to antibody specificity (*idiotypy*). It is now generally accepted that antibody specificity is a reflection of amino acid sequence differences limited to a part of the immunoglobulin molecule and that all antibodies differ from each other in their amino acid sequence. The second level of heterogeneity is due to the existence of several classes and subclasses of immunoglobulins that are present in all members of the species and presumably have evolved to fulfill certain specific functions. This heterogeneity, known as *isotypy,* is most easily recognized by immunologic techniques that readily recognize the antigenic determinants related to the amino acid sequence differences among the different classes and subclasses. Comparison of the structural and antigenic similarities and differences between classes and subclasses provides an excellent measure of the evolutionary relationships among them. Third, there are the subtle and very limited structural differences that reflect genetic polymorphisms among individuals of a species. This heterogeneity, known as *allotypy,* is analogous to the polymorphisms previously recognized primarily for the red cell antigens, white cells, and many serum proteins, such as the haptoglobins, lipoproteins, and transferrins. At the present time, the biologic significance of allotypy is not fully understood since it has not been shown to play a significant role in regulating the immune response, in affecting the biologic properties of antibodies, and in influencing susceptibility to disease.

Before discussing in detail the structure and function of antibody molecules, two general points deserve emphasis. First, although antibodies are produced primarily in response to foreign antigens, most commonly infectious agents, and play a major role in protecting us against them, we have become aware of an ever-increasing number of instances in which the immune system, either because of genetic or other influences, is diverted to react against constituents of the host. This phenomenon of "autoimmunity" is of significance primarily because some of these antibodies, such as those seen in systemic lupus erythematosus, myasthenia gravis, rheumatoid arthritis, and certain other diseases, play a significant role in the pathogenesis of the lesions associated with these diseases. In addition, detection and sometimes quantitation of antibodies against certain tissue constituents, such as DNA, gamma globulin, thyroglobulin, or mitochondria, is often of value in the diagnosis of a variety of different diseases.

The second point that warrants mention, and will not be discussed in detail subsequently, deals with the recently recognized phenomenon that, in addition to the circulating antibodies that constitute the major immunoglobulin component, similar or closely related proteins occur on the surfaces of lymphoid cells, especially those of the B cell series but perhaps also those of the T cell series, where they appear to function as specific antigen receptors. Consequently, antibodies serve not only as the major effector molecules in the immune response, but are also exceedingly important in antigen processing and in triggering and regulating the immune response. The utilization of the same type of molecule as receptors on cells and effectors in serum is obviously a very simple and economical mechanism that avoids the creation of a dual system requiring a similar degree of specificity.

Clinical Implications

Although changes in immunoglobulin concentration are associated with a variety of diseases, evaluation of immunoglobulin levels and distribution among classes and subclasses is significant and useful only in a limited number of instances. Among these are diseases associated with a failure of immunoglobulin production, such as the various types of a- and hypogammaglobulinemia,

A. Structure

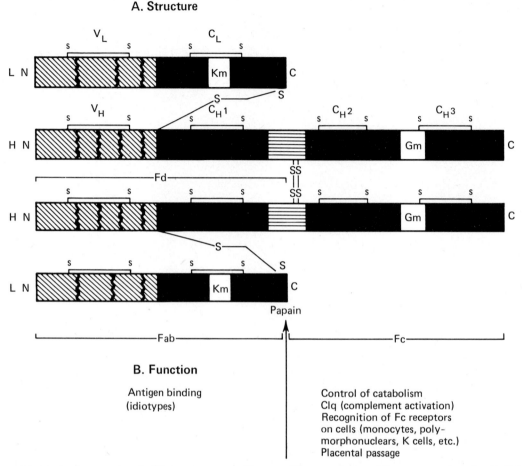

B. Function

Antigen binding
(idiotypes)

Control of catabolism
Clq (complement activation)
Recognition of Fc receptors
on cells (monocytes, poly-
morphonuclears, K cells, etc.)
Placental passage

Fig. 1.   A. Model of an immunoglobulin. ■, Constant region; ⊟, hinge; ◩, variable region; ⟩⟩⟩, hypervariable region; L, light chain; H, heavy chain; Km and Gm, genetic markers; S-S, disulfide bridge; N, amino-terminus; C, carboxy-terminus. **B.** Localization of functional properties of immunoglobulin molecules. (Reproduced by permission of the publisher from Franklin EC, in McCarty DJ (ed): Arthritis and Allied Conditions. Philadelphia, Lea & Febiger, 1978.)

diseases of a neoplastic nature in which monoclonal proteins are produced (such as multiple myeloma and macroglobulinemia), and disorders in which antibodies are produced that are involved in the pathogenesis of the lesions
or that are of diagnostic value (for example, systemic
lupus erythematosus, rheumatoid arthritis, and the other
connective tissue diseases). In the remainder of the illnesses associated with immunoglobulin changes, there is
simply a diffuse increase in immunoglobulins which is of
little specific diagnostic value. These aspects of immunoglobulin alterations will be discussed in detail in the
section on hypergammaglobulinemia in the next fascicle.

STRUCTURE OF ANTIBODY
MOLECULES

Since they appear to have evolved from a common
primitive immunoglobulin molecule, the basic structure
of all classes and subclasses of antibodies is the same; the
types that exist as polymers are composed of two to five
immunoglobulin subunits. Much of the structural information has been derived from studies of homogeneous
monoclonal proteins produced by patients with plasma
cellular and lymphoid neoplasms, which appear to be

identical in structure and often also in function to the
heterogeneous immunoglobulins that occur in normal
serum. The latter are much more difficult to study because they represent mixtures of many different
antibodies.

Domains and Regions of Heavy and Light
Chains

All immunoglobulins consist of four polypeptide
chains generally held together by disulfide bridges (Fig.
1). Two of these are known as the heavy chains because
of their large size, and two are known as light chains. The
light chains, of which there are two major types, known
as kappa and lambda, are common to all types of immunoglobulins; they have molecular weights of approximately 25,000. The heavy chains, whose structure is
characteristic for each class and subclass, have molecular
weights of 55,000–65,000. Both types of polypeptide
chains can be further divided into domains, each consisting of about 110 residues and characterized by an invar-
iant intrachain disulfide bridge. The light chains have two
domains known as the variable (V_L) and constant (C_L)
domains, while the heavy chains have four or five do-

mains depending on the class. In the heavy chains there is a variable domain (V_H) and three or four constant region domains known as C_H1, C_H2, C_H3, and C_H4. The striking degree of homology in the amino acid sequences of the constant region and also the variable region domains points to a common evolutionary origin.

Because each of the domains contains an intrachain disulfide bridge spanning approximately 60 residues, they are tightly folded into globular structures that are separated by the more flexible and open interdomain regions. Studies of the localization of various biologic properties characteristic of immunoglobulins suggest that the domains have evolved to serve different biologic functions. Unique to the heavy chains of most of the classes and subclasses is a region in the middle known as the interdomain or "hinge" region. This stretch has no homology with any other part of the immunoglobulin molecule, varies in size from 15 to 65 residues, contains between 1 and 11 cysteine residues, and is usually very rich in proline residues. The hinge region is the site of the interchain disulfide bridges joining the heavy chains to each other and occasionally also to the light chains. Variations in its size are responsible for some of the differences in the molecular weights of certain of the subclasses of IgG. It is of interest that there are striking homologies in the structure of the hinge regions of different classes and subclasses of immunoglobulins; in several instances there is evidence of gene duplications. These features, coupled with a lack of homology to the remainder of the heavy chain, suggest that the hinge may have evolved independently and may perhaps be under separate genetic control.

The larger size of the ϵ and μ chains of the IgE and IgM classes of immunoglobulins is not due to the presence of an extended hinge but rather to the existence of an extra domain (C_H4). The disulfide bridges linking the heavy chains to the light chains join the carboxy terminal cysteine of light chains to a cysteine residue in the second heavy chain domain, i.e., the C_H1 domain, except in one of the subclasses of IgG, in which the light chain is linked to the amino-terminal cysteine of the hinge.

Structural and functional studies during the past 15 years have led to the concept that the antibody molecule consists of an amino-terminal quarter, which contains the two antigen-binding sites found in every immunoglobulin, and a carboxy-terminal region responsible for the secondary properties characteristic of the different classes and subclasses of antibody molecules. This division was initially based on the finding that several proteolytic enzymes cleaved the molecule at the hinge into two types of fragments, one of which (Fab) contained the antigen-binding sites while the other (Fc) possessed all the other properties of antibodies. This concept has been conclusively proven by structural studies of a large number of homogeneous immunoglobulins.

The first 115 residues of both heavy and light chains differ significantly for diferent myeloma proteins and antibodies. This feature is responsible for the term *variable region,* which has been applied to this part of the

heavy and light polypeptide chains. In contrast, the remaining half of the light chains and the remainder of the heavy chains are identical for every immunoglobulin belonging to a particular class and subclass, with the exception of minor genetic (allotypic) differences. They are therefore known as the *constant regions* of the respective polypeptide chains.

In the variable regions, the structural variability is particularly pronounced in three or four short stretches known as the *hypervariable regions* and much less obvious in the remainder known as the *framework regions.* Abundant structural, functional, and x-ray diffraction data place the antibody-combining sites in the variable regions, and implicate in particular the hypervariable stretches. There are three hypervariable regions in the light chains and four in the heavy chains; although separated in the linear sequence by the larger framework regions, they are in close proximity at the tips of the fully folded molecule as determined by x-ray diffraction studies. Amino acid sequence studies of the hypervariable regions of a limited number of antibodies or myeloma proteins with a given specificity, taken together with common antigenic (idiotypic) determinants, suggest that frequently they may be virtually identical for antibodies having the same specificity.

Since it is difficult to study large numbers of these molecules chemically, antisera have been employed often to define these determinants in the hypervariable regions, which are known as *idiotypic determinants.* Common or shared idiotypes are frequently encountered in murine or rabbit antibodies and myeloma proteins having the same specificity; in man they are most often found in cold agglutinins, rheumatoid factors, and certain red cell antibodies. This phenomenon, which is called *cross idiotypy,* has been very useful in defining the structural basis of antibody specificity. The more highly conserved framework regions which separate the hypervariable regions permit the division of the variable regions of both heavy and light chains into several immunologically and structurally recognizable subclasses. On the basis of currently available information we recognize five variable region subclasses for the λ chains, three for the κ chains, and at least four for the heavy chains. It is of particular interest that the same variable regions are associated with all of the classes and subclasses of immunoglobulins, and that in myeloma patients producing two myeloma proteins the variable regions usually tend to be identical. This feature has given rise to the concept that both the light and heavy chains may be under the control of more than one gene. Although the antigen-binding sites involve both the heavy and light chain variable regions, the heavy chain generally appears to play the predominant role in determining the specificity of the antibody.

Localization of Functions

Although the primary effector function of an antibody is its combination with antigen, this interaction by itself is usually not sufficient to allow it to fulfill its role in the defense of the host. In order for it to be effective, it is necessary for the antibody molecule to reach the proper site and to initiate a number of secondary reactions, such as the activation of the complement cycle and the generation of an inflammatory response, both designed largely to remove antigen–antibody complexes. All of these secondary properties, which are characteristic for each class and subclass of immunoglobulin, have been localized in the constant region of the molecule (see Fig. 1B).

The structural basis of most of the biologic functions characteristic of the different classes and subclasses has been difficult to define precisely since there is a great deal of structural homology among the constant region domains (it can exceed 95 percent identity among the constant regions of the various subclasses of IgG) and because it is generally not possible to recover smaller biologically active peptides. Nevertheless, most of these functions have been localized to different parts of the heavy chains. Studies to date, though far from complete, suggest that C_H2 is responsible for complement fixation and regulating the catabolic properties of antibodies, while the C_H3 domain is important in its interaction with receptors of many cells, including monocytes, polymorphonuclear leukocytes, lymphocytes, and endothelial cells. These interactions with a variety of cells are important in allowing the antibody to reach various sites in the body, in permitting certain classes to traverse the placenta to provide passive immunity to the newborn, and in initiating the inflammatory response involving polymorphonuclear lymphocytes, platelets, and other cells in response to antigen–antibody reactions.

Localization of these biologic functions has been achieved largely by means of fragments of immunoglobulin molecules obtained with proteolytic enzymes such as papain, pepsin, and trypsin, which cleave the molecule at selected sites. The most susceptible site of cleavage is in the middle of the hinge. Digestion at this site yields two types of fragments—Fab, which is able to bind antigen, and the carboxy-terminal Fc fragment, which possesses most of the other properties. Other conditions of digestion expose different cleavage sites that permit the isolation of individual domains such as the C_H3 domain and V_H domains and thus allow clear-cut positioning of many of the important biologic functions.

Although the basic structure of all immunoglobulin subunits can be depicted as H_2L_2, certain classes of immunoglobulins or certain immunoglobulins in given locations contain additional polypeptide chains. Specifically, those immunoglobulins that exist in the form of polymers contain the joining (J) chain, which is a peptide of about 15,000 daltons that has no structural homology with any immunoglobulin. Like the immunoglobulins, it appears to be synthesized by plasma cells and to be incorporated into the polymer in a ratio of 1 mole of J chain per polymer. It has been proposed that in the polymer the J chain links two subunits by a disulfide bridge, perhaps thus initiating the self-association. The other additional component that is found in immunoglobulins in external sections, especially IgA, is the secretory component, a 70,000-dalton peptide synthesized by epithelial cells. The secretory component may play a dual role: it has been shown to protect the immunoglobulin against proteolytic digestion in the external secretions and to serve as a receptor on the surface of cells in certain locations to attract IgA molecules or IgA-producing cells to the sites of external secretion.

Three-Dimensional Structure

A greal deal of information about the three-dimensional structure of the immunoglobulin molecule has been obtained from x-ray diffraction studies. There is now little question that the domains are folded and globular, that the hinge is a region of flexibility which allows the two arms of the Y to change in relation to the Fc fragment, and that the antigen-binding sites are composed of the hypervariable regions that are in close proximity to each other and at the tips of the Y. In three dimensions, the hypervariable regions of the heavy chains and the light chains are in close apposition to each other. There is some question at the moment as to whether each antigen-binding site is specific for only one antigenic determinant or whether it can combine with more than one antigenic determinant.

CLASSIFICATION

On the basis of the structural differences of the constant regions, which are reflected in their antigenic properties and hence readily recognized with antisera, antibodies can be divided into five major classes and a number of subclasses (Table 1). Since both the classes and subclasses are under the control of a series of closely linked genes, the distinction between a class and a subclass is a rather arbitrary one and reflects perhaps little more than the closeness of their relationship on the evolutionary scale. Since each of the classes and many of the subclasses fulfill unique biologic functions, it seems likely that the evolutionary forces that have led to their development are basically related to their fulfilling specific biologic functions. Table 1 lists the five major classes of immunoglobulins, describes some of their physical and chemical properties, indicates that for each class there exists a homogeneous immunoglobulin which is useful in studying its properties, and identifies, for IgG and IgA and perhaps also for IgM and IgD, the existence of a series of subclasses.

The subclass-specific properties listed in Table 1 reside entirely in the constant region of the heavy chain. Since the structural differences between them are also reflected by their antigenic properties, it is relatively easy to identify the classes, and to some extent the subclasses, using antisera that are prepared against myeloma proteins and appropriately absorbed. When this is not possible or proves difficult due to the subtleness of the antigenic differences, they can be characterized chemically on the basis of characteristic differences in their interchain disulfide bridges. This is most easily done by the technique of chemical typing, a procedure designed to label and to identify the cysteine-containing peptides involved in linking the heavy and light chains to each other. It should be emphasized that the heavy chain variable regions are similar for all classes and subclasses of immunoglobulins and, as a consequence, all immunoglobulins share the

Table 1
Classes and Subclasses of Immunoglobulins

Feature	IgG	IgM	IgA	IgD	IgE
Molecular weight	160,000	900,000	170,000	180,000	200,000
Structure	$\gamma_2 L_2$	$(\mu_2 L_2)_5$	$(\alpha_2 L_2)_{1-5}$	$\delta_2 L_2$	$\epsilon_2 L_2$
Valence	2	10(5)*	2†	2	2
Homogeneous component in neoplasms	G myeloma	Macroglobulin	A myeloma	D myeloma	E myeloma
Subclasses	γ1,2,3,4	Several	α1, 2	δ1, 2	?
Special properties	Placental passage Strong immunologic memory Cytophilia Complement fixation	Primary response IgM's ($\mu_2 L_2$) on lymphocytic membrane Complement fixation	Secretory immune system local protection	Lymphocyte membrane	Reagins ? Defense against parasitic infections
J chain	—	+	+	—	—
Secretory component	—	—	+	—	—
Genetic factor	Gm	—	Am	—	—

*There are 10 potential sites, but only 5 are accessible with large antigens.
†There are 2 per 4-chain subunit.

same repertoire of variable regions. In contrast, the κ light chain and λ light chain each has its own unique repertoire of V_L subclasses. Any one immunoglobulin molecule contains only one type of light chain and one type of heavy chain, even in the rare instances in which a plasma cell can be shown to make more than one kind of heavy or light chain.

Subclasses of the light chain constant regions, although recognized especially for λ chains, have not been defined with nearly the same degree of precision as those for the heavy chains and will not be discussed. Since the importance of the subclasses is related primarily to their biologic rather than their structural properties, their functional properties will be emphasized (Table 2).

IgG

IgG, the major class of immunoglobulins, consists of molecules of 160,000 daltons and the structure $\gamma_2 L_2$. There are four subclasses, known as γ1, γ2, γ3, and γ4, which are strikingly similar in structure and function; they differ primarily in the number and location of the interchain disulfide bridges. Since the preparation of monospecific antisera recognizing them is exceedingly difficult, the procedure of chemical typing is particularly useful in their classification and recognition.

The differences in the interchain disulfide bridges are particularly striking for the γ1 subclass, in which the heavy–light disulfide bridge is associated with the hinge instead of the C_H1 domain, and the γ3 subclass, which

Table 2
Distribution and Biologic Functions of Human Immunoglobulins

Property	IgG	IgA	IgM	IgD	IgE
Concentration (mg/ml)	12	3	1	0.03	0.0001
Half-life (days)	23	6	5	3	3
Distribution					
Intravascular (%)	50	50	75	75	50
Extravascular (%)	50	50	25	25	50
Synthetic rate (mg/kg/day)	33	24	6.7	0.4	0.0038
Lymphocyte membrane*			+ (monomer)	+	
Secretions*		++			
Complement activation					
Classic pathway	+	—	+	?	—
Alternative pathway	—	+	—	?	±
Placental transfer	++	—	—	—	—
Sensitization of mast cells and basophils*					++

*Predominant, but perhaps not exclusive.

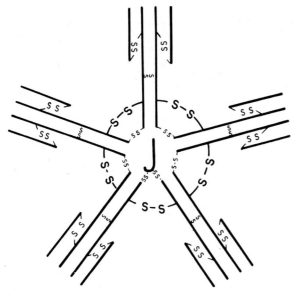

Fig. 2. Model of IgM made up of 5 IgM subunits and 1 molecule of J chain. (Reproduced by permission of the publisher from Frangione et al: Scand J Immunol 5:624–627, 1976.)

has a triplication or perhaps a quadruplication in the hinge region, which accounts for its larger molecular weight.

IgG activates complement by the classical pathway with the IgG1 and IgG3 subclasses most effective; IgG4 does not fix complement effectively in the native state but does so after proteolytic cleavage. This property is thought to be associated primarily with the C_H2 domain, although its precise biochemical basis remains to be defined. All four subclasses of IgG cross the placenta, and IgG is the only immunoglobulin fraction that provides passive immunity to the newborn. While this is of great value for the immunologically inert newborn infant in defending itself against neonatal infections, the transplacental passage of immunoglobulins can also be harmful in those instances in which there are ABO or Rh incompatibilities.

In addition to activating complement, several IgG subclasses interact with varying efficiencies with cell receptors for the Fc fragment on platelets, lymphocytes, polymorphonuclear cells, mononuclear cells, and macrophages, a property which is of great importance in initiating the inflammatory response and, like complement fixation, occurs predominantly in the $\gamma 1$ and $\gamma 3$ subclasses. This property is associated predominantly with the C_H3 domain.

IgG has a slow catabolic rate; the half-time is approximately 20 days, and only IgG3 is degraded more rapidly. The observation that the turnover of IgG is proportional to its concentration has led to the theory that a limited fraction is bound to receptors that protect it from degradation, whereas the remainder, which is free in the circulation, is degraded.

All types of antibody activity have been associated with the IgG fraction. In most species, immunologic memory resides primarily in the IgG fraction, so that the long-term immune response resides primarily in these

molecules. Certain antigens elicit a preferential response of one or another of the subclasses.

IgM

Historically, IgM was the second immunoglobulin class to be discovered, although its concentration is less than that of IgA (Table 1). IgM exists primarily in the form of a pentamer of a 180,000-dalton subunit with a molecular formula μ_2L_2; however, generally a minor fraction also exists in a monomeric form. It is of interest that the IgM monomer, or a molecule closely related to it structurally and functionally, appears to be one of the two major immunoglobulins on the surface of lymphocytes. The major 900,000-dalton pentameric IgM has a molecular formula $(\mu_2L_2)_5J$ (Fig. 2), the J indicating that one molecule of the J chain is disulfide bridged to each pentameric subunit. It seems probable that the J chain is involved in initiating the formation of the polymer.

IgM appears to serve a specific role in the primary immune response in most species since it is often the predominant immunoglobulin produced shortly after antigen stimulation. Although certain antigens, such as the I antigen, immunoglobulins, and certain red cell antigens, stimulate a predominant and persistent IgM response, most classic antigens result in a switch to IgG following the initial burst of IgM. Nevertheless, there is now abundant evidence for the persistence of a long-lasting IgM memory response as well. IgM activates complement via the classic pathway and initiates complement activation through some structure located in the C_H4 domain.

Unlike IgG, which is distributed approximately equally between the intravascular and extravascular space, IgM is located predominantly in the intravascular space. Its turnover is significantly faster than that of IgG and is unrelated to its serum concentration. Although most inflammatory cells do not appear to have receptors for IgM, recent studies suggest that helper T cells interact with IgM. IgM resembles the other immunoglobulins, with the exception of IgG, in not being able to cross the placenta.

As indicated by its pentameric structure, the macroglobulin molecule has 10 potential antigen-binding sites. However, as originally described for rheumatoid factors, the actual valence when reacting with large protein antigens may be 5, since half of the combining sites may be inaccessible. To date, all attempts to clearly define subclasses of IgM have met with failure.

Of great interest is the recent finding that the monomer of a protein similar to IgM appears to be, together with IgD, the major immunoglobulin on the surface of B cells and perhaps also on T cells. The idiotype on the surface-associated immunoglobulin appears to be identical to that found in the serum and the evidence strongly suggests that the immunoglobulin molecules on the lymphocytes act as receptors for both soluble antigens and antigens associated with another cell, such as the macrophage or T cell.

IgA

Next in concentration to the IgG fraction is IgA, which exists in serum predominantly as a monomer but occasionally also in a polymeric form. It appears to serve no unique function in the circulation; in fact, it is rather inefficient in its activation of complement, which it achieves only by the alternative pathway and its interaction with cell receptors. Thus it is not as effective as other immunoglobulins in initiating some of the secondary manifestations of antigen–antibody reactions such as phagocytosis and antigen removal. Its major role appears to be in the so-called secretory immune system, which was recognized functionally in the 1930s but was not clearly related to the IgA fraction until the 1960s.

IgA exists in two forms: IgA1 is a disulfide-bonded $\alpha_2 L_2$ molecule, while the minor subclass IgA2, with the exception of a minor A2m2 allotype, lacks the usual heavy–light disulfide bridge and consists of a noncovalently linked molecule composed of $\alpha_2 L_2$. Although the IgA2 component constitutes less than 5 percent of the IgA present in serum, it seems to make up a significantly larger fraction of the secretory IgA. The secretory IgA is synthesized largely in the plasma cells located in the organs of external secretion, such as the intestinal tract and respiratory tract, and there is good evidence that lymphoid cells originating in these sites will ultimately return to the gut-associated organs to fulfill their role in immunologic defense against infectious agents.

The IgA that is found in the external secretions is unusual because it exists as a polymer that is bound to an additional component known as the secretory component, a 70,000-dalton molecule that is synthesized by the epithelial cells and has no structural homology to IgA (Fig. 3). The secretory component is disulfide bridged to the heavy chain of IgA and appears to protect it against proteolytic digestion in those sites where IgA normally functions. In addition, since the secretory component has been found on the surface of the cells in the gut, it may play a role in attracting IgA producing cells or circulating IgA back to the gastrointestinal tract. The recent observation that several bacterial enzymes readily digest IgA1 but not IgA2 in the hinge region may perhaps explain the relative predominance of IgA2 in the external secretions.

The biologic significance of the IgA system cannot be overestimated if it is remembered that most bacterial and viral infections enter the body via the respiratory, gastrointestinal, and genitourinary tracts. As a consequence, the IgA system provides a first line of defense against a variety of infections, a fact that has proven to be exceedingly important in designing immunization programs (for example, in the case of polio vaccination, in which the oral route was found to be much more effective than the systemic).

IgD

IgD is a minor immunoglobulin fraction in the serum. It appears to have no unusual function in serum, although a few antibodies have recently been shown to be associated with this fraction. However, together with IgM, it appears to be the major immunoglobulin on the surface of lymphoid cells. Recent studies suggest that triggering of IgD and IgM on the surface of the cells by antigen results in a primary response of both T and B cells.

IgD in serum is the same size as IgG, but differs from IgG in that it is unusually susceptible to digestion by a

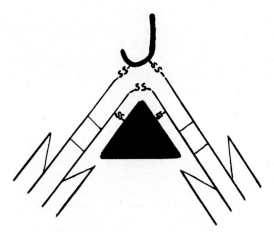

Fig. 3. Model of secretory IgA. ▲, secretory component: J, J chain. (Courtesy of Dr. Blas Frangione.)

variety of proteolytic enzymes. Its half-life is short, and consequently the number of cells engaged in IgD immunoglobulin synthesis is larger than would be expected on the basis of its serum concentration.

IgE

The most recently described immunoglobulin and the one present in the lowest concentration is the IgE fraction, which contains the reaginic antibodies. The heavy chain of IgE resembles the μ chain in that it does not have a true hinge and possesses an extra domain. Because of its unusually fast turnover, its synthetic rate is greater than would be expected.

Reaginic antibodies of the IgE type are responsible for the immediate hypersensitivity response that is initiated by their ability to interact with receptors on mast cells and basophils. This response is followed by the degranulation of these cells, which results in the release of histamine and various vasoactive substances responsible for the clinical manifestation of their allergic states.

Until recently, no clear-cut beneficial role for IgE had been defined. It seems probable, however, that IgE antibodies play a protective role in a variety of parasitic infections, perhaps by increasing vascular permeability and thus permitting other antibodies to arrive at the site of inflammation. In addition, IgE seems to have the ability to interact with eosinophils and macrophages and to initiate phagocytosis of complexes. The unique properties of IgE, like those of other classes of immunoglobulins, are located in the Fc fragment. Fortunately, IgE does not cross the placenta. IgE activates the complement pathway only by the alternative pathway.

GENETIC POLYMORPHISMS

The third level of heterogeneity, and probably the most subtle one, involves the differences among immunoglobulins based on genetic differences among the members of a species. Because they were originally discovered by immunologic techniques, these polymorphisms for immunoglobulins are called *allotypes* and are recognized most readily by serologic techniques. However, the biochemical basis for several of the allotypes of the γ heavy and κ light chains has been clearly delineated. Among human immunoglobulins, allotypic specificities have been recognized for the light chains (Km), $\gamma1$, $\gamma2$, $\gamma3$, and $\gamma4$ chains (Gm), and the $\alpha2$ chains (A2m). Thus far, no clear-cut allotypic differences have been demonstrated for the δ, the ϵ, and the μ chains. Population and genetic studies of myeloma proteins suggest the existence of a series of closely linked heavy chain loci (in the following order: $\gamma1$, $\gamma4$, $\gamma2$, $\gamma3$, α, μ, δ, and ϵ) and two unlinked light chain loci (κ and λ) which may not even be present on the same chromosome. It is quite likely that not all of the loci have been defined and that additional ones will ultimately be recognized corresponding to every class and subclass of immunoglobulins.

The biochemical basis of the allotypic specificities of the Km type has been defined and shown to result from the exchange of leucine for valine at position 191. Amino acid residues specific for some of the Gm factors have also been found in the Fc fragment of IgG but, for unknown reasons, they often differ by more than a single amino acid residue. In the case of many of the G3m allotypes, serologic differences have been recognized in the absence of distinct structural differences, a finding that is difficult to explain.

Although these genetic differences have proven of great interest in serology, rheumatology, and forensic medicine, they have been of little significance clinically as markers of disease susceptibility or immune response, or as causes of transfusion reactions; in clinical practice, these subtle differences can be ignored.

CELLULAR ORIGIN AND SYNTHESIS

There is little doubt that immunoglobulins are synthesized almost exclusively in the rough endoplasmic reticulum of plasma cells and then secreted via the Golgi apparatus. It seems probable that mature plasma cells are derived from circulating lymphocytes that are able to synthesize small amounts of immunoglobulins, which can be incorporated into their surface membranes, but have not developed the mechanisms required for secreting them. The plasma cells are well equipped to fulfill the synthetic function since they have a prominent rough endoplasmic reticulum that is replete with antibody-synthesizing polyribosomes. Up to 20 percent of the protein synthesized by plasma cells appears to consist of immunoglobulins.

Antibody synthesis is triggered by a multitude of factors, such as contact with antigen or mitogens. These stimuli initiate the synthesis of mRNA, followed by protein synthesis. Light and heavy chains are synthesized on separate polysomes and are joined by disulfide bridges prior to secretion. In general, as yet unknown factors exist that ensure approximately balanced synthesis of heavy and light polypeptide chains.

Immunoglobulin synthesis is unique in that a single mature plasma cell can synthesize only one type of immunoglobulin at a time. In a few rare instances, a clone of a plasma cell that may have undergone malignant changes at a time when it was in a stage of transition in its immunoglobulin synthesis is able to synthesize two types of immunoglobulins. While such a degree of specialization is characteristic of molecules under the control of X-linked genes, it has never before been noted for those controlled by autosomal genes. The reasons for this specialization and its significance in the control of antibody synthesis remain unknown. The pathways of assembly for immunoglobulins have been studied in some detail and appear to differ for different types of immunoglobulins.

REFERENCES

Capra JD, Kehoe JM: Hypervariable regions, idiotypes and the antibody combining site. Adv Immunol 20:1, 1975

Davies DR, Padlan EA, Segal DM: Immunoglobulin structure at high resolution. Contemp Top Mol Immunol 4:127, 1975

Frangione B: Structure of human immunoglobulins and their variants, in Benacerraf B (ed): Immunodeficiency and Immunogenetics. London, Medical & Technical, 1975, pp 2–53

Fudenberg HH, Pink JRL, Wang A-C, Douglas SD: Basic Immunogenetics (ed 2). New York, Oxford University Press, 1970

Gally JA: Structure of immunoglobulins, in Sela M (ed): The Antigens. New York, Academic Press, 1973, pp 162–298

Metzger H: Structure and function of γM macroglobulins. Adv Immunol 12:57, 1970

Spiegelberg H: Biological activities of immunoglobulins of different classes and subclasses. Adv Immunol 19:259, 1974

Tomasi TB Jr: The gamma A globulins; First line of defense, in Good RA, Fisher DW (eds): Immunology. Stamford, Conn., Sinauer, 1971, pp 76–83

Cellular Basis of the Immune Response

Leonard Chess

INTRODUCTION

The immune response is generated by a complex array of cellular interactions between an extraordinarily heterogeneous group of cells, predominantly the small lymphocytes and macrophages. These cellular interactions evolved to protect man from foreign invaders whether they are in the form of bacteria, viruses, or other microorganisms or whether they arise endogenously in the host as a consequence of neoplastic transformation. The interaction of these foreign antigens with the cells of the immune system results in the triggering of two distinct effector pathways. On one hand, there is the synthesis of antibody molecules with precise specificity for the triggering antigens. On the other hand, there is the activation of immunospecific lymphocytes that differentiate into specifically cytotoxic cells and synthesize and secrete a variety of soluble molecules (lymphokines). Together the cytotoxic cells and the soluble lymphokines are critically important in cell-mediated immune responses, including delayed hypersensitivity reactions, graft rejection, graft-versus-host phenomenon, tumor rejection, and certain tissue-specific autoimmune lesions.

It is well recognized now that the two major types of immune responses, i.e., antibody production and cell-mediated immune responses, are carried out by two discrete major classes of lymphocytes. For example, the predominant cell types responsible for antibody production reside in a group of lymphocytes that arise in the bone marrow and differentiate independent of the thymus gland; they are called *B lymphocytes*. Cell-mediated immune responses depend, in large measure, on morphologically identical lymphocytes that have differentiated under the influence of the thymus gland; they are called *T lymphocytes*.

More recently, it has become evident that there is microheterogeneity among the major T and B cell classes and that subclasses of T and B cells interact with one another, both in the generation of antibody molecules and in the phenomena associated with cell-mediated immunity. Moreover, the cells of the monocytic–macrophage lineage interact with T and B cells in the induction and effector pathways of immune responses. In order to understand the mechanisms involved in these cellular interactions, it is important first to understand the differentiative history and function of the individual cell populations themselves, and finally to delineate cell–cell interactions that are critically important to an intact immune response.

MACROPHAGES AND THE MONONUCLEAR–PHAGOCYTIC SYSTEM

Macrophages or phagocytes constitute a diverse class of cells intimately involved in many specific and nonspecific aspects of host defense. Phagocytes are distributed widely throughout the organism: they are found in the blood, bone marrow, liver, lymphoid tissue, connective tissue, nervous system, and serous cavities. The earliest recognizable precursor of the phagocytic cell is the promonocyte, which is found in greatest numbers in the bone marrow. Promonocytes are radiosensitive, rapidly dividing cells that after further differentiation enter the blood and become monocytes. Monocytes then circulate in the blood for a short period of time (24–48 hours), after which they can be shown to migrate to different tissues and to mature into macrophages. The tissue-localized macrophages are highly phagocytic and contain numerous lysosomes and endocytic vesicles. They infrequently divide and are relatively radioresistant. The factors that regulate their entrance and exit from tissues are not well understood.

Morphologically, monocytes and macrophages are recognized by a horseshoe-shaped, indented nucleus, adjacent to which are centrioles, Golgi apparatus, numerous

small vesicles, and dense granules. In the peripheral cytoplasm there are rough endoplasmic reticulum and mitochondria. Many of the dense granules can be shown to be lysosomes containing a number of hydrolytic enzymes that are intimately involved in the function of macrophages, including the degradation of protein, carbohydrate, and nucleic acid molecules. These lysosomes become more numerous as the cell matures or becomes activated.

PHAGOCYTIC FUNCTION OF MACROPHAGES

Some of the more important functions of the macrophages are listed in Table 1. The most primitive, but perhaps one of their most important functions, is their capacity to phagocytose and pinocytose foreign materials. Thus, these cells provide a clearing mechanism for ridding an organism of not only microorganisms and tumor cells but, in addition, other particulate matter, including antigen–antibody complexes. Defects in phagocytic mechanisms can be an important factor not only in the defense against infectious disease processes and tumors but also in the development of circulating immune complex diseases.

It is important to emphasize that macrophages have specific receptors on their cell surface that binds to the Fc portion of certain immunoglobulins (Fc receptors) and to the third component of complement after its activation (C3 receptors). These receptors can facilitate the phagocytic function of macrophages. Thus, although serum immunoglobulins can bind to the Fc receptor of macrophages, they usually rapidly dissociate from its surface. In circumstances in which foreign antigen is coated with antibodies, however, the binding of the Fc portion of the antibody molecule to the Fc receptor is more stable. For example, when bacteria are coated with antibacterial antibody, the binding of antibody to the Fc receptor is stabilized. Similarly, foreign material coated with complement or antibody and complement are stabilized at the macrophage surface.

Not all immunoglobulin classes have a binding site on the macrophage surface. IgG1 and IgG3 subclasses bind most strongly to macrophage surfaces, whereas IgG2 binds weakly and IgG4 binds poorly, if at all. Following the binding of antigen and/or antigen–antibody complement components to the cell surface of macrophages, the cell is triggered to ingest the material by the

Table 1
Macrophage Functions

Phagocytosis of particulate and/or insoluble substances
Degradation of antigens and particles
Antigen processing for immunospecific lymphocytes
Synthesis and secretion of enzymes, including lysozyme, plasminogen activators, collagenase, elastase, and complement components
Synthesis and release of immunoregulatory molecules
Microcidal activity and bacteriostasis
Protection from intracellular parasites

processes of pinocytosis and phagocytosis. In addition to Fc and C3 receptors, macrophages have receptors for a variety of T cell factors that have the capacity to activate macrophages to perform a variety of functions, including phagocytosis. Since macrophages do not have specific receptors for antigen, the presence of receptors for products of immunocompetent T cells that do have antigen receptors allows macrophages to participate actively in specific immune responses at the effector level.

MACROPHAGE SECRETIONS

In addition to the phagocytic functions of macrophages, another set of functions are the capacity of these cells to secrete an extraordinarily wide variety of molecules with diverse effects. One class of secretory products of the macrophages are enzymes capable of interacting with extracellular proteins. For example, macrophages secrete two molecular species of plasminogen activators of 28,000 and 48,000 daltons. These plasminogen activators are serine proteases that convert plasminogen into plasmin. Subsequently, plasmin is involved in the lysis of fibrin, and thus macrophage products become intermittently involved in the fibrinolytic system of homeostasis.

Other enzymes released from macrophages include the lysosomal proteases, acid phosphatase, β-glucuronidase, collagenase, and elastase, all of which are secreted into the extracellular environment. Collagenase is a particularly interesting metalloprotein capable of cleaving tropocollagen into fragments that are one-fourth and three-fourths of the original collagen chain length; it is also important in the process of collagen deposition in the extracellular space. More recently, it has been observed that macrophages also influence collagen homeostasis by releasing a collagenase-stimulating factor, a protein of 14,000 daltons. This molecule has the capacity to interact with synovial cells and stimulate the further release of collagenase by these cells. Since macrophages can be triggered by products of activated T cells (see below), the synthesis and release of molecules such as collagenase and collagenase-stimulating factor by macrophages allows one to envision mechanisms by which immune phenomena can have diverse effects, including alteration of extracellular components.

Other products of macrophages are more directly involved in the nonspecific mechanisms of host defense against bacteria and viruses. For example, activated macrophages release lysozyme, a well-characterized protein of 14,000 daltons, which is active against the peptidoglycan of bacterial cell walls. Lysozyme specifically hydrolyzes the 1–4 glycocytic linkages between N-acetylnuerominic acid and N-acetylglucosamine and contributes significantly to the bacteriocidal properties of macrophages.

Furthermore, macrophages release interferon, a protein of 45,000 daltons, which directly inhibits the cell-dependent replication of a wide variety of viruses. In addition, upon activation, macrophages synthesize and secrete components of the complement sequence, including C2 and C4. It is of interest that both of these complement proteins are genetically controlled by genes in the major histocompatibility complex (MHC). The evidence that macrophages have a number of other functions related to MHC gene products will be discussed below.

Other, less well-characterized biochemical products of macrophages include a number of molecules that influence the differentiation of thymocytes into T cells and, in addition, have immunoregulatory properties. These immunoregulatory molecules are not antigen specific and appear to modulate immune response by both amplification and suppression. The precise significance of these molecules remains to be further elucidated.

MACROPHAGE "ANTIGEN PRESENTATION"

In addition to the role of phagocytes and macrophages in nonspecific host defense mechanisms, these cells play a critical role in specific immune responses of immunocompetent T and B lymphocytes. In fact, it is becoming increasingly clear that macrophages may be central to many, if not all, humoral and cellular immune responses. The precise mechanism by which macrophages influence specific immune responses has only recently been delineated. It has been known for some time that phagocytes can concentrate and trap antigen molecules in lymphoid organs such as lymph nodes and spleen. Within the peripheral lymphoid organs macrophages subsequently present antigen to immunocompetent cells.

This "antigen presentation" function of macrophages refers to the inherent capacity of phagocytes after antigen uptake to deliver an immunogenic signal to specific receptors on lymphocytes, in particular T lymphocytes. The molecular events important in antigen presentation are not precisely understood, but it is known, for example, that macrophages can pinocytose, phagocytose, and partially degrade antigens and subsequently put out antigen fragments that bind to molecules on the plasma membranes. It is now apparent that macrophage surface membrane determinants themselves also contribute to the specificity of antigenic signals delivered to immunocompetent cells. Thus, immunocompetent T cells, and specifically the receptors on T cells, recognize antigen in association with surface molecules on the macrophage membrane.

The determinants recognized on the surface of macrophages, in addition to antigens and/or their fragments, are coded for by genes of the MHC. Particularly important are the molecules coded for by the immune response (Ir) region of the MHC. This genetic region in man is closely linked to HLA-D and codes for Ia antigens found on the surface of macrophages. As we shall see in subsequent chapters, the interaction of specific antigens with MHC gene products may be a general phenomenon involved in immune recognition and may explain, in part, the function of immune response genes in the specificity and control of both humoral and cellular immune reactions.

T LYMPHOCYTES: DIFFERENTIATION AND FUNCTIONS

T lymphocytes are small to medium size mononuclear cells found in the blood, bone marrow, and lymphoid organs of mammals; they are the predominant immunocompetent cells responsible for cell-mediated immune reactions and for regulating the different expressions of both humoral and cellular immune responsiveness. They are morphologically indistinguishable from other lymphocytes but can be identified by surface antigens and receptors on their plasma membrane. For example, human T cells have receptors for sheep erythrocytes (E receptors) but do not have either surface-membrane immunoglobulin or complement receptors, which are found on B lymphocytes. In contrast, B lymphocytes do not have E receptors.

DIFFERENTIATION

The T lymphocytes are derived from the only primary lymphoid organ in mammals, the thymus gland. The thymus is made up predominantly of lymphocytes and a few reticular cells and macrophages. It is organized into lobules, each composed of a cortex and medulla; the cortex is represented by a very dense accumulation of lymphocytes, whereas the medulla has more concentrated reticular cells.

Lymphocytes destined to differentiate in the thymus derive during embryonic life from stem cells, predominantly in the fetal liver and bone marrow. The mechanisms by which stem cells in the bone marrow become genetically programmed to migrate to and differentiate in the thymus gland are unknown. It is clear, however, that during their stay in the thymus a number of discrete differentiation events occur which culminate in the elaboration from the thymus gland of fully mature functionally competent T lymphocytes.

It is of interest that during differentiation in the thymus gland, T cells acquire distinct alloantigens on their surfaces which distinguish them from both prethymic T cells and from T cells that eventually populate the peripheral lymphoid organs. For example, there is a surface antigen, TL, that is present only on thymocytes and not on peripheral T cells or bone marrow cells. The designation "TL" comes from the observation that these antigens become reexpressed on circulating leukemic cells that originate from the thymus gland. In acute lymphatic leukemia of childhood approximately 20 percent of patients have blast cells bearing the TL antigen.

During thymic differentiation T cells also acquire cell surface markers that are subsequently found on all mature T cells. In the mouse this T cell marker is called theta (θ), and similar antigens are found on human thymocytes and T cells. Human T cells, in addition, acquire E receptors, which are subsequently found on all T lymphocytes. In addition to the TL antigen, θ antigens, and E receptors acquired during differentiation in the thymus, T cells acquire other differentiation antigens on their cell surfaces that are found on thymocytes and are preserved during further differentiation only on subclasses of peripheral T lymphocytes. This finding is of great importance since these alloantigens that are present on one set of peripheral T cells but not others (see below) have become a critical means of defining functionally unique subclasses of peripheral T cells.

Although the precise mechanisms of differentiation of T cells within the thymus is unknown, there is substantial evidence suggesting that hormones and other molecules synthesized and secreted from reticular and epithelial cells within the thymus play an important role in this differentiation process. In addition to acquiring cell surface alloantigens and specific functions while in the thymus, T lymphocytes also acquire the capacity to recognize MHC self-antigens and distinguish them from nonself MHC determinants. During later stages of differentiation this process becomes essential to many of the important functions of T lymphocytes.

FUNCTIONS

Some of these functions of T cells are listed in Table 1. Historically, the first group of functions associated with T lymphocytes were those characterized as cell-mediated immunologic reactions. This type of immune response is recognized by certain common histopathologic features. These lesions uniformly begin with perivenous infiltration of lymphocytes and monocytes. With time (24–48 hours), neutrophils, basophils, and eosinophils aggregate at the site of inflammation. In the zone of infiltration, one observes a variety of different types of parenchymal damage of varying degree, depending, at least in part, on the cellular make-up of the involved tissue; in addition, one observes vascular damage varying from barely perceptable changes in the permeability of vessels to complete vascular necrosis. This type of cell-mediated immunologic reaction is seen in a variety of situations, including allograft rejection, graft-versus-host reactions, tumor rejection, and delayed-type hypersensitivity reactions of the skin to soluble protein antigens.

The mechanisms involved in the pathogenesis of

Table 1
Functions of T Lymphocytes

In Vivo Function	In Vitro Correlate
Delayed hypersensitivity and lymphokine production	Proliferation, measurement of migration inhibition factor, leukocyte inhibition factor, mitogenic factor, etc.
Graft rejection and graft-versus-host reactions	Specific cytotoxicity of allogeneic targets
Helper function	Effect on antibody synthesis
Suppressor function	Effect on antibody synthesis
Control of viral infection	Specific cytotoxicity of virus-infected targets
Control of neoplastic cells	Specific killing of tumor cells
Control of intracellular parasites including mycobacteria	T cell–macrophage interactions including mediator production (see the first item)

these cellular reactions are complex and vary to some
extent with the nature of the antigen involved. The entire
process, however, is initiated by the triggering of immunospecific T cells by antigen presented on macrophage
surfaces. Interaction of the antigen complex with specific
receptors on the surface of T cells then results in a
number of biosynthetic changes which culminate in the
proliferation of responding T cells and the production and
release of a group of mediators, designated lymphokines.
The first of these mediators to be discovered was a
glycoprotein of 23,000 daltons which has the capacity to
inhibit the migration of macrophages and has been
termed *migration inhibition factor*. Furthermore, inhibitors of leukocyte migration (leukocyte inhibition factors)
are released. Other mediators released from sensitized
lymphocytes upon contact with antigens include chemotactic factors for macrophages, neutrophils, and
eosinophils.

Also of importance is the T cell release of mitogenic
factor, a molecule with the capacity to trigger the proliferation of lymphocytes not specific for the inducing antigen. The lymphocytes triggered by mitogenic factor subsequently release the same wide range of mediators
initially induced by the specific antigen. These molecules
account for the attraction and involvement of a large
number of inflammatory cells at the site of cellular immune reactions. By means of chemotactic mechanisms
that draw cells to the inflammatory site and subsequently
inhibit migration from the site, a variety of cells are held
in close proximity to the inciting antigen.

Other mediators released from sensitized T lymphocytes have the capacity to activate macrophages (macrophage-activating factors) such that their phagocytic, bacteriocidal, and cytolytic properties are enhanced. The
activation of macrophages by mediators released by anti-
gen-triggered T cells also results in the synthesis and
release by macrophages of the wide spectrum of molecules discussed above. These mechanisms are thought to
be particularly important in the immunity to infection
with organisms that can survive and multiply intracellularly. These infectious organisms include pathogenic mycobacteria, *Brucella, Salmonella, Listeria*, and a variety
of fungal and parasitic agents. These mechanisms also
play a role in host response to tumors.

In addition to proliferating and releasing soluble mediators upon contact with antigen, T lymphocytes, when
triggered by antigens on the surface of either autologous
or foreign cells, differentiate into cytotoxic lymphocytes
with the capacity to lyse target cells bearing surface
determinants in common with the triggering cell. This
cytotoxic response is known to be important in the rejection of allografts and in graft-versus-host disease; in addition, it is involved in the cellular destruction of tumor
cells bearing tumor-specific transplantation antigens. It
has also recently been demonstrated that virally infected
cells that express surface antigens unique to the infecting
virus can efficiently trigger T lymphocytes into becoming
specifically cytotoxic cells. These virus-specific killer T

cells provide one mechanism for the control of viral
infection and may also be important in some immuno-
pathogenic mechanisms associated with chronic tissue
destruction resulting from viral infection.

During the past decade it has been established that
the role of T cells in the immune response is not limited to
the class of cell-mediated immunologic reactions discussed above. In fact, it is clear that T lymphocytes play
an additional and critical role in the specific regulaton of
all types of immune responses, including the humoral
antibody response.

For example, T cells play an obligatory role with
respect to most antigens (T-dependent antigens) in the
differentiation of B cells into antibody-forming cells. This
role of T cells in augmenting B cell differentiation has
been called the "helper" function of T cells. In addition,
T cells can modulate B lymphocyte differentiation in a
negative mode; that is, T cells have the capacity to
suppress the differentiation of B cells into antibody-forming cells. The mechanisms and cell interactions that are
important in helper and suppressor functions of T cells
will be discussed in more detail below. The helper and
suppressor functions of T cells are not restricted to the
differentiation of B lymphocytes into antibody-forming
cells. The evidence is very substantial that both helper
and suppressor T cells modulate other T cell functions as
well, such as the differentiation of T cells into specifically
cytotoxic killer cells.

CLASSIFICATION

Cells undergoing thymus-dependent differentiation
mediate a wide range of immunologic activities. Until
very recently, these diverse functions of T cells—including their capacity to exert helper or suppressor effects,
generate killer cell activity, and elaborate mediators that
induce cellular inflammatory responses—have been attributed to a single pleuripotent mature T cell. It has been
shown, however, that T cells become programmed during
thymus-dependent differentiation to express not all, but
only a limited range of functions. For example, distinct
subclasses of T cells are programmed to express either
helper activity or suppressor function but not both. Similarly, T cell subclasses genetically programmed to release
soluble mediators after contact with antigens are distinct
from T cells that express killer cell activity in cell-mediated lympholysis.

The different T cell subclasses are distinguished not
only by their separate functions but also by the presence
of specific surface differentiation antigens on the plasma
membrane. For example, cells genetically programmed
during differentiation to express helper cell activity have
surface antigens quite distinct from those cells programmed to express suppressor and cytotoxic functions.
The presence of these differentiation antigens unique to
the surface of functionally distinct subclasses of T cells
have allowed the identification and preparation of both
alloantibodies and heteroantibodies to these differentiation antigens. These antibodies have been utilized specifically to isolate or deplete functionally unique subclasses

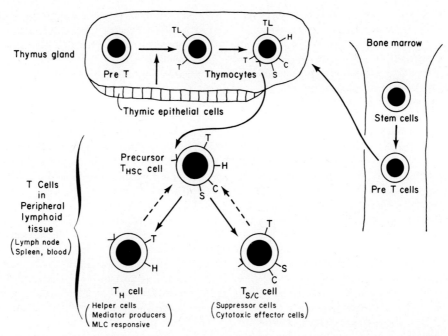

Fig. 1. Schematic model of T cell differentiation. Three types of fully differentiated T cells are depicted. The T_{HSC} is analogous to the $Ly_{1,2,3}$ cell in the house, whereas the T_H and $T_{S/C}$ cells are analogous to the Ly_1 and $Ly_{2,3}$ T cells, respectively. The antigen T, depicted on thymocytes and peripheral T cells, represents the theta antigen in mice and determinants analogous to the sheep cell (E) receptor on human T cells.

of cells and have allowed detailed studies of the cellular interaction that occurs between distinct T cells. In addition, by utilizing these antibodies to differentiation antigens, it has been possible to demonstrate that subclasses of T lymphocytes are already predestined to express distinct T cell functions prior to contact with antigen.

Four distinct subclasses of T lymphocytes have been definitively identified in mice on the basis of three antigens designated Ly_1, Ly_2, and Ly_3. One subclass, the thymocyte, expresses all three distinct lymphocyte differentiation antigens ($Ly_{1,2,3}$) on the cell surface as well as the TL and θ antigens. This subclass of thymocytes is found almost exclusively in the cortex of the thymus and is not found in the peripheral lymphoid tissue. They are considered to be immature cells and probably the precursors of all T lymphocytes. The second subclass of T lymphocytes expresses all Ly antigens ($Ly_{1,2,3}$) but during differentiation has lost the TL antigen. This $Ly_{1,2,3}$ T cell is the most abundant peripheral T cell. During early neonatal existence two additional T cell subclasses appear. One expresses exclusively the Ly_1 antigen and another expresses the Ly_2 and Ly_3 antigens.

Adult animals have the following distribution of peripheral T cell subclasses with respect to these differentiation antigens: $Ly_{1,2,3}$, about 50 percent; Ly_1, about 30 percent; and $Ly_{2,3}$, about 5–10 percent. The Ly_1 T cell has the following functional repertoire genetically programmed: (1) it is the helper cell for T cell–B cell interactions; (2) it is the cell that proliferates in response to allogeneic cells in mixed lymphocyte culture (MLC); (3) it is both necessary and sufficient for producing delayed-type hypersensitivity reactions, including the release of mediators important in these reactions; and (4) it is the cell that, in addition to helping B cells, can collaborate with T cells in inducing, for example, cytotoxic lymphocytes. $Ly_{2,3}$ T lymphocytes have none of the functions attributed to Ly_1 cells but they are the cells programmed to suppress both antibody and cell-mediated immune responses. In addition, $Ly_{2,3}$ T cells are the effector cells that mediate specific killer cell activity. The precise function of $Ly_{1,2,3}$ T cells is unknown, but these cells can be triggered by antigen to further differentiate into more mature Ly_1 or $Ly_{2,3}$ cells.

The evidence is rapidly accumulating that the pattern of T cell differentiation with respect to Ly antigens and functions is preserved during evolution. For example, human T cells can be divided into subclasses of cells programmed to perform special functions. Thus, human helper T cells can be distinguished from suppressor and cytotoxic T cells by virtue of cell surface antigens and receptors. Although the precise mechanisms and biologic significance of these modes of T cell differentiation in man remain to be fully understood, the evidence suggests that these pathways may have evolved, on one hand, to control the immune response homeostatically and, on the other hand, to adapt efficient mechanisms of recognition of self and nonself determinants. A schematic view of functional T cell differentiation is shown in Figure 1.

B LYMPHOCYTES: DIFFERENTIATION AND FUNCTIONS

The B lymphocytes can be defined as those small to medium size mononuclear cells found in peripheral blood and lymphoid organs that are programmed to differentiate into antibody-forming cells. These cells are indistinguishable from T cells by light or electron microscopic criteria but can be identified by the presence of surface membrane immunoglobulin. They can also be distinguished from T cells because they lack the alloantigens and receptors (θ antigens and E receptors) characteristic of T cells.

DIFFERENTIATION

In man and other mammals the B lymphocytes arise from hemopoietic stem cells in the bone marrow and further mature in the bone marrow (independent of the thymus gland) as well as in peripheral lymphoid organs. During ontogeny, progenitors of B cells are found in the fetal spleen, and after birth the bone marrow becomes a major source of B cells. Different stages of the differentiation process of B cells have now been identified.

The first cells, pre-B cells, are irrevocably committed to B lymphocyte development but do not yet express clear-cut B cell features such as surface membrane immunoglobulin or reactivity to antigens. These cells, found in the fetal liver and in adult bone marrow, are relatively large lymphocytes that are actively dividing. Although these cells do not bear surface-membrane immunoglobulin, IgM can be found in the cytoplasm of these cells. It is

thought that these pre-B cells then give rise to immature B cells which express surface IgM. These immature B cells appear to play a pivotal role in subsequent B cell differentiation.

During further development, the other immunoglobulin isotypes, IgG, IgA, IgE, and IgD, are synthesized and incorporated in the cell membrane. It is of interest that at one stage in B cell development doublets including both IgM and IgG, IgM and IgA, or IgM and IgD are found on the cell surface of B lymphocytes. It is of interest that the predominant doublet found in the peripheral lymphoid tissues of both mouse and man is IgM plus IgD. This is surprising since very little serum IgD is usually detectable. The precise role of IgD on the surface of B lymphocytes remains unknown.

The end stage of B cell differentiation is the plasma cell that contains abundant cytoplasm, rich in endoplasmic reticulum, and has a much smaller nuclear-to-cytoplasmic ratio than more immature B lymphocytes. Plasma cells synthesize immunoglobulin molecules at a higher rate than do B lymphocytes, and, in contrast to B cells, they do not divide and they have a life history of only 2–3 days. A schematic view of B cell differentiation is shown in Figure 1.

FUNCTIONS

In addition to surface immunoglobulins, which function on B lymphocyte membranes as receptors for antigen, there are a number of different surface macromolecules on B lymphocytes that are of particular interest. For example, most B cells have an Fc receptor, that is, a

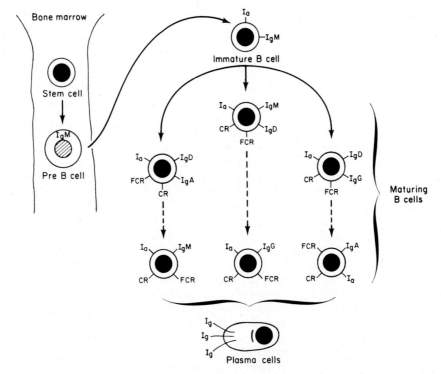

Fig. 1. Schematic model of B cell differentiation.

surface structure that specifically binds to the Fc region of IgG molecules. The precise function of the Fc receptor on the surface of B lymphocytes is unknown. In addition to Fc receptors, a subclass of B cells possess receptors for the complement component C3 which enable them to bind antigen–antibody–complement complexes. It is thought that the presence of the C3 receptors on a fraction of B lymphocytes indicates a more mature B cell population. However, the precise function of the C3 receptor remains to be determined.

In addition to immunoglobulins, Fc receptors, and C3 receptors, the majority of B cells also have unique macromolecules on their surfaces which represent MHC gene products selectively expressed on B cell surfaces but not on T cell surfaces. These gene products are coded for by the HLA-D region of the human MHC and have been termed *Ia antigens,* since the HLA-D region in man is analogous to the I region of the murine MHC. Ia antigens appear early in the differentiation of B lymphocytes and are expressed on the majority of B lymphocytes. These Ia antigens are believed to play an important role in B cell interactions with T cells. It is important to emphasize, however, that Ia molecules, although present on B cells and not T cells, are not restricted to B cell surfaces. As discussed above, Ia molecules are found on the surface of approximately 50 percent of macrophages and they are also present on epidermal cells and sperm cells. The precise function of these molecules is not clear but recent evidence suggests that they play critical roles in a variety of cell–cell interactions important in differentiation.

NULL LYMPHOCYTES

There is a class of lymphocytes, present in bone marrow and peripheral lymphoid organs (including blood), that lack the classic surface properties and functions of both T and B lymphocytes. In human peripheral blood these cells can be defined as those lymphocytes that lack surface E receptors and surface membrane immunoglobulins. However, a fraction of these cells are known to contain other surface determinants found on either T or B cells, including Ia antigens, C3 receptors, and Fc receptors. It is known that this population of cells, which accounts for approximately 5–10 percent of human peripheral blood lymphocytes, is extraordinarily heterogeneous. The null cells contain precursors of both B and T lymphocytes, as well as precursors of monocytes and other hemopoietic cell types.

From a functional point of view, this population contains effector cells capable of killing tumor cells and antibody-coated cells by mechanisms quite distinct from T cell-mediated processes. Because these killer cells are present in the null cell population, these cells are sometimes referred to as K cells. The precise role of these cells in host defense mechanisms remains to be established; however, evidence suggests that null cell killing mecha-

nisms may operate in the immune response to tumors and in the destruction of autologous tissue coated with antibody molecules.

REGULATION OF IMMUNE RESPONSES BY T LYMPHOCYTES

In the preceding chapters the differentiation history and functions of the major classes of lymphocytes and macrophages have been outlined. The compartmentalization of immunocompetent cells into two major classes, T cells and B cells, concerned with cellular and humoral immunity, respectively, has been a critical conceptual development in our understanding of lymphocyte function. The recognition during the past decade of highly sophisticated mechanisms for the regulation of immune responses by T cells has added substantially to our understanding of the cell–cell interactions involved in the generation and control of immune responses. The evidence that thymus-derived cells play a critical role in antibody formation was generated by experimental studies showing that neonatally thymectomized animals not only are markedly deficient with respect to cellular immunity (as demonstrated, for example, in allograft rejection) but also are quite deficient in their capacity to synthesize antibodies to a wide variety of cellular and protein antigens. Similarly, children congenitally deficient in thymic function not only have defects in cellular immunity but, in addition, do not have normal antibody responses.

Furthermore, it is known that irradiated animals (including man) can be spared the lethal effects of irradiation by the transfer of bone marrow cells. However, the capacity to recover full immunocompetence in terms of both cellular and humoral immunity requires the presence or adoptive transfer of thymocytes and/or T cells. Thus, such animals develop normal antibody-forming capacity only when treated with both thymocytes and bone marrow cells. Further studies have demonstrated that upon contact with antigen, the cells derived from the thymus gland are stimulated by the antigen to undergo cell division but are incapable of secreting antibodies. B lymphocytes derived from the bone marrow have been shown to be the precursors of antibody-forming cells but require interaction with thymus-derived cells for antibody production.

Additional mechanisms important in the T cell–B cell collaborative interaction have been uncovered. Perhaps the most important finding has been that T lymphocytes influence the differentiation of B cells into antibody-forming cells not only from the point of view of helper activity or amplification mechanisms, but also with respect to suppression. Moreover, these helper and suppressor effects of T lymphocytes on B cell differentiation are carried out by distinct subclasses of T cells which have differentiated prior to interaction with antigen. The critical point to emerge recently has been that these different subclasses of T cells do not carry out their

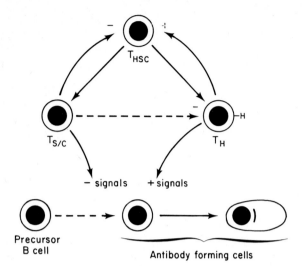

Fig. 1. Relationship of antibody production by sublclasses of T cells.

separate functions independently of one another. The helper and suppressor functions of the T cell subclasses seem to be precisely interlocked. Thus, helper cells not only have the capacity to induce B lymphocytes to secrete antibody molecules, but the same T cell helper subclasses also can interact with precursors of suppressor cells and with suppressor T cells themselves to amplify suppressor mechanisms. Similarly, suppressor cells not only interact with B cells but, in addition, they can also operate on helper T cells subclasses to dampen helper signals. This interlocking aspect of the cellular immune control mechanisms, schematically depicted in Figure 1, accounts for a highly ordered network of cell interactions controlling the immune response.

The underlying mechanisms by which T cell subclasses exert their regulatory influences on B cells and other T cells is only partially understood. Recent evidence suggests that after antigen presentation to T cells, biologically active, soluble regulating molecules are synthesized. Both helper and suppressor types of regulatory molecules have now been identified and isolated from T cells. Many of these immunoregulatory molecules interact with T cells as well as with B cells. These molecules can regulate immune responses in an extraordinarily specific manner. In fact, it is known that helper and suppressor molecules can interact specifically with antigen and, therefore, must have combining properties of conventional immunoglobulins. However, these molecules do not resemble immunoglobulin molecules chemically.

Both helper and suppressor molecules are proteins with molecular weights in the range of 40,000–50,000 daltons, and thus they are considerably smaller than conventional immunoglobulins. In addition, they lack antigenic determinants of the constant region of immunoglobulin molecules. Whether the combining sites of these specific regulatory molecules have antigenic determinants in common with variable region sequences of im-

munoglobulins remains to be established. The evidence to date indicates that these molecules are related, at least in part, to gene products of the MHC. The precise region of the MHC controlling the synthesis of these regulatory molecules is the Ir region.

Furthermore, the genes controlling helper molecules are distinct from the genes controlling suppressor molecules, although they both reside within the Ir region. The genetic control of these regulatory molecules is of more than theoretical biologic interest. The gene regions most intimately associated with a variety of autoimmune diseases in man, including rheumatoid arthritis, systemic lupus erythematosus, myasthenia gravis, and multiple sclerosis, are closely linked to HLA-D, that portion of the human MHC analogous to the murine Ir region. It is probably not by chance alone that genes controlling normal regulatory function of the immune system are associated with the expression of autoimmunity. Evidence is accumulating that suppressor and/or helper cell functions may be abnormal in patients with a number of autoimmune states. Whether the association of some of these diseases with HLA-D implies that disorders in the biosynthesis of immunoregulatory molecules may be found remains to be established.

Any discussion of the regulatory function of T cell subclasses and their interactions with B cells would not be complete without considering macrophage–T cell interactions in this context. As noted above, macrophages present antigens in association with MHC gene products on their cell surfaces to lymphocytes in order to initiate specific immune responses. The MHC gene products most important in this regard are the Ia antigens. In particular, it is those T cells that have been programmed during differentiation to express helper cell function that possess receptors that recognize Ir gene products on macrophages in conjunction with specific antigen. This subclass of T cells is also important in lymphokine production and MLC responsiveness. Both of these functions, as is the helper function, are triggered quite readily by Ia determinants in association with foreign antigens on the surface of macrophages. The T cells programmed to express suppressor or cytotoxic functions do not have receptors for Ia antigens; however, this subclass of T cells appears to recognize cell surface determinants coded for by MHC genes controlling serologically detected surface determnants, including HLA-A, B, and C (see below).

CELLULAR CYTOTOXIC INTERACTIONS

An important function of the immune response is to recognize foreign or altered determinants on the surface of cells and, as a consequence of this recognition, to generate effector mechanisms that result in cytolysis. One mechanism for the destruction of foreign cells is clearly to produce specific antibodies with specificity for the foreign or altered cells and, in the presence of comple-

Table 1
Mechanisms of Cell-mediated Destruction of Foreign Cells

Class of Killing	Effector Cell	Specificity	Targets	Role of MHC
T cell–mediated lysis	Cytotoxic T cells	Exquisitely specific, antigens recognized by T cells	Allogeneic cells or cells altered by viral, tumor, or chemically induced antigens	Critical
Macrophage-mediated cytotoxicity	Macrophages activated by T cells	Nonspecific	Tumor cell preference, intracellular parasites	None
Antibody-dependent cellular cytotoxicity	Null lymphocytes, granulocytes, monocytes	Specific, antigens recognized by antibody not by effector cells	Any nucleated cell, as well as red cells	None
Natural killing	Null lymphocyte	Nonspecific for tumor cells	Tumor cells	None

ment, to initiate cytolysis. In addition to direct antibody and complement-mediated cellular destruction, however, the lymphoid cells may utilize a variety of other mechanisms for the destruction of foreign target cells. These mechanisms, referred to as *cell-mediated cytotoxic mechanisms,* require intimate contact between two cells: a cell that can be damaged or killed (the target cell) and a cell that is capable of administering such damage (the effector cell).

Cell-mediated cytotoxic mechanisms are important in graft rejection, infected autologous tissue destruction, tumor cell rejection, and some autoimmune phenomena. Four types of cellular cytolytic effector mechanisms have been clearly distinguished (Table 1). T lymphocytes are triggered by antigens on the surface of foreign cells to proliferate and differentiate into killer cells that have the capacity to lyse target cells that have surface determinants in common with the sensitizing cell. In addition, macrophages are triggered by factors released from T lymphocytes to destroy foreign tissues. Unlike cytotoxic T lymphocytes, however, activated macrophages lyse cells nonspecifically; that is, once activated, macrophages will kill a variety of cell types independent of the original triggering foreign cell.

In addition to T cell and macrophage cytotoxic mechanisms, null lymphocytes bearing Fc receptors, upon contact with IgG-coated target cells, will lyse the target cells in question. This mechanism, called *antibody-dependent cellular cytotoxicity,* can also be performed by other cells bearing Fc receptors, such as granulocytes and monocytes. Finally, null lymphocytes have the capacity to lyse tumor cells, but not normal tissues, in the absence of antibody or complement. This phenomenon has been termed *natural killer (NK) cell activity.* The precise determinants that NK cells recognize are not clearly understood. It is thought that NK activity, however, may be important in the destruction of small numbers of tumor cells which might arise endogenously in the host; thus, these cells may perform a valuable surveillance or screening service.

Of all the cytotoxic mechanisms discovered, the generation of immunospecific cytotoxic T lymphocytes

(CTL) are the best understood. Our knowledge of the generation of CTL stems largely from detailed analysis of the allograft response leading to the rejection of grafts. It is known that a critical pathway in the allograft response involves the sensitization and subsequent differentiation of CTL. These potent and highly specific effector cells are triggered by and subsequently recognize foreign cell surface determinants that are genetically controlled, in large part, by the MHC antigens of the foreign cell.

The generation of these CTL requires the cooperative interaction of two distinct T cell subclasses cytotoxic precursor cells and helper cells. Thus, although specific clones of cytotoxic lymphocytes are activated by interaction with HLA-A, B, and C serologic determinants on foreign cells, their differentiation into killer cells requires the participation of helper T cells that recognize and proliferate in response to distinct MHC determinants coded for by the HLA-D region. As a consequence of the interaction between helper T cells and precytotoxic cells, each recognizing different products of the MHC, CTL are generated during the allograft phenomenon; the CTL may be detected in draining lymph nodes, spleen, peripheral blood, and are recoverable from the site of graft rejection. In the absence of this CTL response, allogeneic graft rejection does not occur.

It is obvious that the precise interactions of T cell subclasses involved in the generation of CTL could not have evolved exclusively to mediate destruction of allografts. More recently, insight into the evolutionary and biologic significance of the generation of cytotoxic lymphocytes has come from studies showing that CTL can be generated that are specific for autologous or syngeneic cells displaying non-MHC surface structures, including tumor-associated antigens, chemicals, and virus-associated cell surface determinants. An important aspect of these studies has been the demonstration that CTL generated to neoantigens on the surface of autologous cells lyse targets bearing the neoantigens (viral, tumor, etc.) only in association with self-MHC surface determinants. The same neoantigens, when presented on cells not sharing MHC structures, are not lysed. Based on this evidence, it is clear that CTL reactive with modified autologous cells recognize not only the neoantigen but also self-MHC structures. The MHC gene products recognized by CTL are the serologically defined HLA-A, B, and C determinants present on all cells.

These recent insights provide, for the first time, a clearer understanding of the function of MHC gene products not involved in immunoregulation. These molecules, HLA-A, B, and C, may serve as surface structures critical to recognition of altered-self determinants. When neoantigens appear on the surface of autologous cells, they form a complex with MHC products on that cell membrane. This neoantigen–MHC complex is subsequently recognized by T cell receptors as altered self. Whether T cells have two distinct receptors, one for the neoantigen and one for self (dual receptor hypothesis) or whether a single receptor exists which recognizes specific alteration of HLA molecules (altered-self hypothesis) is unknown.

Nevertheless, the function of these molecules as altered-self recognition structures explains, in part, why they must be present on all tissues in the body, since viral infections or neoplastic processes may occur in any tissue.

From a clinical point of view, CTL reactive with altered-self determinants may not only be important with respect to viral infection and neoplasia, but these cells may also be involved in autoimmune phenomena. For example, it is known that the CTL reactive with altered

self can initiate a number of autoimmune diseases in experimental animals, including autoimmune leukoencephalomyelitis and autoimmune orchitis. In man, evidence exists that CTL may be involved in the pathogenesis of such diverse diseases as chronic active hepatitis and polymyositis. Clearly, as we accrue knowledge concerning the function and regulation of these T lymphocytes, our capacity to understand the complex phenomena associated with autoimmunity will increase considerably.

REFERENCES

Benacerraf B: in Katz DH, Benacerraf B (eds): Role of Products of the Histocompatibility Gene Complex in Immune Responses. New York, Academic Press, 1976, p 225

Cantor H, Boyse EA: Lymphocytes as models for the study of mammalian cellular differentiation. Immunol Rev 33:105, 1977

Chess L, Schlossman SF: Human lymphocytes subpopulations. Adv Immunol 25:213, 1977

Remold HG, David JR: Migration inhibition factor and other mediators in cell-mediated immunity, in McCluskey RT, Cohen S (eds): Mechanisms of Cell-Mediated Immunity. New York, Wiley, 1974, pp 25–42

Shearer G, Schmitt-Verhulst A: Major histocompatibility complex restricted cell-mediated immunity. Adv Immunol 25:55, 1977

Unanue E: Symposium: Macrophage functions in immunity. Fed Proc 37:77, 1978

Mechanisms of Inflammation

Peter A. Ward

MEDIATORS OF INFLAMMATION

Over the past two decades dramatic improvements have been made in our understanding of the inflammatory system. We have increased our knowledge regarding mediators of inflammation, the mechanisms by which these factors work, and defects involving mediator production or abnormalities in the responses of tissues and cells to these mediators. Diseases featuring abnormalities in the inflammatory response involve depressed inflammatory responses or unremitting inflammatory reactions in tissues. In order to understand defects of the inflammatory system, it is first essential to understand the mediators and their control.

With the development of highly sensitive and quantitative techniques to measure the various factors, inflammatory mediators are divided into two separate and distinct categories: *vasopermeability mediators* and *chemotactic mediators*. By and large, the mediators in these two categories are chemically distinct and work independently of one another.

The vasopermeability factors, regardless of origin, seem to work by an effect on the contractile elements within endothelial and periendothelial cells, causing a

reversible opening of junctions between endothelial cells. Furthermore, the vasopermeability factors seem to have an effect that is geographically localized to the postcapillary venules of the vascular bed. With only a few exceptions, vasopermeability mediators in physiologic concentrations do not cause the in vitro movement or the in vivo accumulation of leukocytes.

The leukotactic factors increase both random and directed, or chemotactic, migration of leukocytes. They do so at very low concentrations (about 10^{-9}–10^{-12} M) and have been shown to interact with receptors on leukocytes. This interaction activates the cell membrane $Na^+K^+ATPase$, causes a transmembrane flux of Ca^{2+}, K^+ and Na^+, results in activation of the pentose shunt, and leads to cell swelling, membrane depolarization, leukocytic aggregation, and, finally, cell movement, The precise biochemical events that lead to cell movement are not known at the present time.

VASOPERMEABILITY MEDIATORS
Vasoactive Amines

Histamine and serotonin are the well-known factors in this class. They are among the few preformed mediators contained within intracellular stores in mast cells, basophils, and platelets. Active secretion is the most important mechanism related to their release. The secretory mechanisms involving basophils and mast cells include anaphylactic (IgE-mediated) release and anaphylatoxin-induced release (see below). Platelet secretion of serotonin is induced by a variety of complement-dependent mechanisms as well as by the platelet-activating factor (PAF), a substance released from basophils and probably also from mast cells.

Basic Peptides of Leukocytic Lysosomal Granules

Contained within lysosomal granules of neutrophils are preformed cationic peptides that increase vascular permeability either by inducing histamine release from basophils and mast cells, or by a histamine-independent reaction. The relative biologic importance of these peptides is not presently known.

Anaphylatoxins (C3a, C5a)

C3a and C5a are highly cationic peptides with molecular weights of approximately 9000 and 11,000, respectively; they are derivatives of the complement system. Each peptide is cleaved from the amino-terminal end of the α chain of the respective parent protein. This cleavage can be induced either by complement activation (via the classic or the alternative pathway), or by non-complement-related enzymes such as trypsin. C3a and C5a are potent inducers of vasopermeability, primarily through their ability to cause release of histamine from mast cells and basophils. Either or both anaphylatoxins has been considered to play a role in the diffuse capillary leakage seen in the dengue shock syndrome. The anaphylatoxins are active in concentrations in the range of 10^{-10} M. C5a has another important biologic function, namely, chemotactic activity for both monocytes and neutrophils (see below). C5a is probably not the exclusive C5 fragment with chemotactic activity.

Kinins

Kinins represent some of the more well-studied vasopermeability factors. The nonapeptide bradykinin is the best known kinin, although several others are also known, including lysylbradykinin (kallidin I) and methionyl-lysylbradykinin (kallidin II). Another group of kinins, which, in contrast to bradykinin, are acidic in nature, includes the so called *leukokinins*, which are produced by the action on a serum substrate of an enzyme from lysosomal granules of leukocytes and other cells. Bradykinin is produced by the enzyme kallikrein, which interacts with its substrate in plasma, kininogen. Kallikrein is converted from its precursor form by activated Hageman factor of the intrinsic clotting system. Thus, whenever Hageman factor activation occurs, one can anticipate the downstream production of bradykinin. Because there is a potent inactivator in serum, one rarely is able to measure by functional means the presence of bradykinin in human plasma or other biologic fluids.

Prostaglandins (PG)

Much has been learned about the PG system over the past decade. Figure 1 briefly outlines the biosynthetic pathways, which probably are initiated by activation of a membrane-associated phospholipase; this leads to the production of arachidonic acid, which, in turn, is converted by a lipoxygenase or a cyclooxygenase into a series of unstable compounds. HETE (12-L-hydroxy-5,8,10,14 eicosatetraenoic acid) is chemotactically active for leukocytes. The other PG have varying degrees of vasopermeability-inducing activity. Structurally they are designated according to the scheme in Figure 1.

Prostacyclin (PGI_2) is produced by an enzyme present in endothelial cells. PGI_2 has effects that seem to antagonize the effects of PGA_2 and thus prevent the aggregation of platelets along endothelial cell surfaces

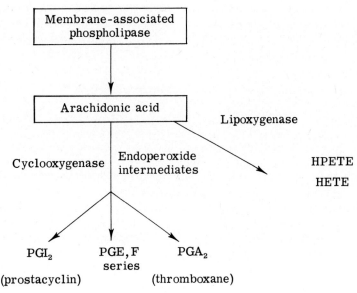

Fig. 1. Biosynthetic pathways in the prostaglandin system.

and the subsequent release of their vasoactive mediators. PGE₁ and PGE₂ have vasopermeability-inducing activity and limited chemotactic activity; they cause intracellular elevations in levels of cAMP. PGA₂, also known as thromboxane, is derived from platelets and causes their aggregation.

A large number of highly unstable PG intermediates are known. These poorly understood PG have a variety of different effects, including changes in peripheral vascular resistance, pulmonary artery pressure, etc. Determination of the relative effect of any or all of the PG is not possible at the present time. Whether the antiinflammatory effects of aspirin and indomethacin can be related to the blocking of virtually all PG biosynthetic pathways is not known at this time.

Other Permeability Factors

Slow-reacting substance of anaphylaxis (SRS-A), lymph node permeability factor, and several other vasopermeability mediators have been described, but their roles in biologic reactions have not been defined. It has been suggested that both PAF and SRS-A may be prostaglandins, but this remains to be proven.

CHEMOTACTIC MEDIATORS
Complement Chemotactic Factors

The complement-derived chemotactic factors include C3 fragments, C5 fragments (including C5a), and the trimolecular complex C$\overline{567}$. These mediators may be produced by enzymatic activities emanating either from within the complement system (via both the classical and the alternative complement pathways) or from other sources (Fig. 2). For instance, most tissues contain a neutral protease that cleaves a chemotactic fragment from C3, and leukocytes, especially neutrophils, contain a neutral protease (identified as elastase) that produces chemotactic fragments from C5. The biologic importance of these facts is discussed below.

Plasma Enzymes

It has been reported that certain enzymes of the alternative complement system, as well as kallikrein and plasminogen activator, are chemotactic. However, the inability to generate chemotactic activity in serum or plasma that is deficient in C5 under conditions in which the enzymes listed above should be activated suggests that they play a relatively minor role.

Products of Tissues

In contrast to Menkin's theory, few breakdown products of tissues are directly chemotactic. Collagen breakdown peptides, however, have chemotactic activity for neutrophils, monocytes, and fibroblasts. Most normal tissues contain neutral proteases that will cleave C3 and/or C5, thereby producing chemotactic fragments. An example of the C3-cleaving enzyme and the role of this fragment in the acute inflammatory reaction to a myocardial infarct are described subsequently (refer to Figures 3 and 4).

Bacterial Chemotactic Factors

It has been known for some time that bacteria produce chemotactic factors during the log phase of growth. The production of these factors seems to reflect the bacterial replicative cycle rather than the specific bacterium per se. Furthermore, no correlation has been shown between pyogenic bacteria and those that produce chemotactic factors in vitro. However, this finding may simply reflect the artificiality of in vitro cultivation conditions.

As a result of attempts to characterize the bacterial chemotactic factors, synthetic formylated peptides have been discovered that have very high specific activity. Most work has been done with formyl–Met–Leu–Phe, which is active for human neutrophils at a concentration of 10^{-10} M. The synthetic oligopeptides have been extremely useful in the study of structure–activity relationships and receptors on the surfaces of leukocytes, even though these peptides appear not to be structurally related to the naturally occurring factors (at least those from the complement system).

CONTROL OF INFLAMMATORY MEDIATORS

In general, there are three ways in which control of inflammatory mediators is achieved: activation or production of mediators with opposing actions, inactivators of the mediators, and inhibitors of the enzymes responsible for generation of the mediators. There is considerable

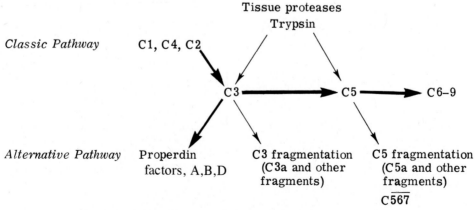

Fig. 2.   Production of chemotactic factors from the complement system.

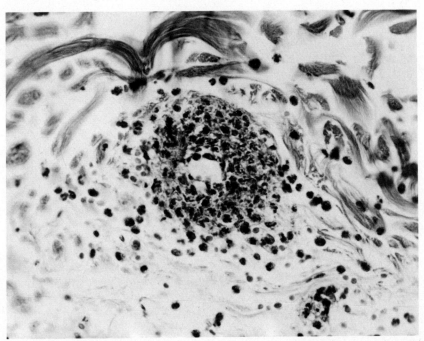

Fig. 3. Experimentally induced acute immune complex–induced vasculitis. The vessel wall is infiltrated with a large number of neutrophils. H & E. ×300.

interest in the opposing ways in which certain mediators may interact (for example, the effects of catecholamines and cholinergic agents in the vascular capillary network). While this concept is of theoretical interest, there is little direct evidence available to support it. Probably the clearest example of a control mechanism is the series of inactivators that destroy the biologic activity of pre-formed inflammatory mediators.

Regulators of the complement system have been studied rather intensively. There are three separate inhibitors of complement products: the C3b inactivator, the anaphylatoxin inactivator, and the chemotactic factor inactivator. C3b is important because of its role as an opsonic factor and because of its ability to activate the alternative complement pathway. The presence of the C3b inactivator prevents unfettered triggering of the complement system by C3b via activation of the alternative complement pathway. The absence of this inhibitor in vivo leads to consumptive depletion of the complement system, with virtually total disappearance of C3. Patients afflicted with this abnormality have greatly increased susceptibility to bacterial infections.

The anaphylatoxin inactivator of human serum is a B-type carboxypeptidase that not only inactivates C3a and C5a, but also bradykinin, because all three peptides have a susceptible C-terminal arginyl residue. Loss of this amino acid results in loss of biologic activity in each peptide. Abnormalities in levels of this inactivator have not been described.

The chemotactic factor inactivator (CFI) of human serum irreversibly inactivates C5 chemotactic peptides. While CFI levels in normal serum are quite low, they may rise several-fold above the usual level. Under such cir-

cumstances individuals with high serum levels of CFI manifest evidence of depressed inflammatory responses. This association has been noted in patients with Hodg-kin's disease, sarcoidosis, advanced hepatic cirrhosis, and lepromatous leprosy. CFI, which has been purified from human serum, also has potent antiinflammatory activity in vivo in experimental animals with immune complex–induced tissue injury (see below).

COMPLEMENT CHEMOTACTIC FACTORS IN EXPERIMENTAL AND CLINICAL INFLAMMATION

Complement-derived chemotactic factors have been demonstrated in experimental and clinical inflammatory states. In the former, immune complex–induced vasculi-tis is associated with the presence of C5 chemotactic factors in the developing inflammatory reaction (Fig. 3).

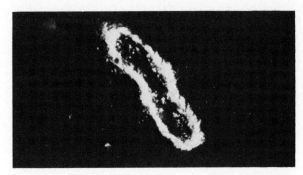

Fig. 4. Frozen section of vessel shown in Figure 3, stained for the presence of C3. Other reactant proteins also present are IgG and antigen; all are indicative of immune complexes. ×300.

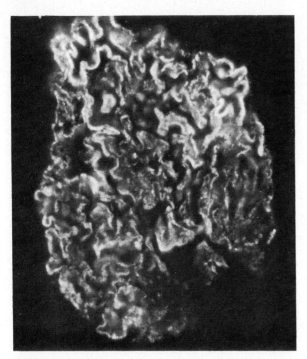

Fig. 5. Immunofluorescent stain for C3 in renal glomerulus of patient with immune complex nephritis (systemic lupus erythematosus). IgG was also demonstrated. The deposits are characteristically granular and within the basement membrane. ×200.

Complement proteins can be seen fixed in the walls of these vessels (Fig. 4), and tissue extracts reveal the presence of C5 chemotactic fragments and C$\overline{567}$. If the complement system is blocked, these mediators are not generated and no inflammatory reaction develops. In experimentally induced myocardial infarcts in rats, the inflammatory response is mediated by a C3 chemotactic peptide.

C5 chemotactic factors have been found in the synovial fluid of humans with rheumatoid arthritis. In many patients with inflammatory nonrheumatoid arthritis, synovial fluids contain C3 chemotactic peptide. Although C3 is often found by immunofluorescence in renal biopsy material of patients with nephritis (Fig. 5), whether complement-derived chemotactic and other phlogistic products of the complement system are present in the tissue, and whether any such factors as primary or secondary mediators of the inflammatory response play a role is little understood.

REFERENCES

Becker EL, Ward PA: Chemotaxis, in Parker C (ed): Clinical Immunology, vol. 1. Philadelphia, Saunders, 1978

Ward PA, Becker EL: Biology of leukotaxis. Rev Physiol Biochem Pharmacol 77:125, 1976

Wilkinson PC: Chemotaxis and Inflammation. Edinburgh, Churchill Livingston, 1974

CLINICAL DEFECTS IN THE INFLAMMATORY SYSTEM

Problems in host defense mechanisms in humans involving phagocytic and chemotactic responses have been carefully studied (Table 1). Defects in phagocytosis are often concomitantly associated with chemotactic abnormalities.

DEFECTS IN PHAGOCYTOSIS

Defects in the phagocytic system that are most commonly recognized relate to the inability of the leukocyte to internalize and, subsequently, kill ingested microorganisms. Although cellular defects are most often seen in metabolic disorders (diabetes mellitus, uremia) and leukemic diseases, they also occur in a variety of other conditions. Most of these conditions represent acquired cellular defects. Familial, genetically determined disorders of phagocytosis are rare; the only clearly recognized examples include the Chediak-Higashi and the actin-dysfunction syndromes. Chronic granulomatous disease, which shows an autosomal recessive pattern of inheritance, is not a disorder of phagocytosis per se, but rather a defect involving the lack of activation of the hexose monophosphate shunt, which results in ingested bacteria not being killed.

Defects of phagocytosis involving opsonic factors are best demonstrated in familial agammaglobulinemia, in which heat-stable opsonic factors (IgG) are deficient. Acquired or genetic deficiencies of complement components represent deficiencies of the heat-labile opsonins. The clinical manifestations vary depending upon which complement component is reduced, because susceptibility to a given microorganism depends on which pathway (classic or alternative) in the complement system is usually activated by that microorganism.

DEFECTS IN CHEMOTAXIS

Defects in chemotaxis are frequently seen. They may be due to cellular defects or serum abnormalities. The cellular defects may be genetic or acquired. Situations in which a genetic basis has been established include the Chediak-Higashi and actin-dysfunction syndromes. Much more commonly, the chemotactic defect is an acquired one, as is seen in metabolic diseases (diabetes mellitus, uremia, hypophosphatemia), acute viral infections (influenza), neoplastic states (malignant tumors), and in association with many other diseases. The ac-

Table 1
Phagocytic and Chemotactic Abnormalities in Humans

Phagocytosis
Cellular defects
Opsonic defects
Chemotaxis
Cellular associated defects
Serum inhibitors
Deficiencies of serum factors

quired cellular defects are usually reversible if the underlying disease is corrected.

Serum inhibitors represent another important cause of chemotactic defects. There are two types of inhibitors that are present in normal serum in low concentration. Both of these inhibitors, CFI (described in the preceding chapter) and the cell-directed inhibitor, appear to be natural regulators of the inflammatory system. The latter inhibitor is found frequently, although not exclusively, in sera from patients with malignant neoplasms. The presence of either inhibitor is associated with a spectrum of clinical manifestations ranging from anergic responses in skin testing to recurrent bacterial infections and the presence of unusual infectious agents, such as *Listeria*.

A likely, but largely unstudied, additional cause of defects in the chemotactic system is related to the fact that stimulated lymphocytes produce lymphokines, which include the monocyte/macrophage chemotactic factor, migration inhibitory factor, and a variety of macrophage-activating factors. If lymphocytes are absent or unable to respond to antigenic stimuli, it is likely that defects in the inflammatory response will be seen, not only because the source of the chemotactic mediators is missing, but also because monocytes and macrophages will not be exposed to factors that maximize their efficient function.

Another source of inhibitors is drugs that have antiinflammatory activity. The corticosteroid antiinflammatory drugs, such as hydrocortisone and methyl prednisolone, are potent reversible suppressors of chemotactic responses of leukocytes. The nonsteroidal antiinflammatory drugs, such as aspirin and indomethacin, have no such inhibitory effects.

Finally, there is evidence that chemotactic defects are found in some individuals who lack a factor in their serum that enhances leukocyte chemotactic responses.

A detailed understanding of the inflammatory mediators, the diverse reactions in which they may be generated, their regulation, the interactions between components of various mediator systems, and defects in the phagocytic–chemotactic system has provided us with an appreciation of the enormous complexity of the inflammatory response. At the same time, however, we stand on the threshold of developing exciting, novel, and highly specific approaches to the control of the inflammatory response.

REFERENCES

Gallin JI, Quie PG: Leukocyte Chemotaxis. New York, Raven Press, 1978

Ward PA: Leukotactic factors in health and disease. Am J Pathol 64:521, 1971

Complement

Michael M. Frank and Stephen W. Hosea

CLASSIC AND ALTERNATIVE COMPLEMENT PATHWAYS

The complement system is comprised of a complex series of interacting proteins that mediate many features of the inflammatory response and play an integral role in host defense against invading microorganisms. Because of its ability to become activated by immunologic mechanisms and foreign substances, complement is often also involved in the pathophysiology of immunologic and autoimmune diseases. In this case, inflammation mediated by complement acts to damage cells and tissues rather than an invading microorganism. Thus, antibody to a tissue antigen can bind to that antigen, activate complement, and mediate inflammation and tissue damage. Similarly, circulating antigen–antibody complexes can be deposited in tissue sites, activate complement, and cause tissue injury. Research in the past 10 years has underscored the vast complexity of the complement system. Nevertheless, the basic features of the complement cascade are now clearly outlined and will be discussed.

CLASSIC COMPLEMENT PATHWAY

Nomenclature

In general, the complement proteins circulate as inactive precursors in serum (Table 1). They are activated by precise biochemical mechanisms and the protein components have a very definite order of interaction. Each of the proteins of the classic complement sequence is designated by a capital "C" followed by a number. The early components were numbered in order of discovery and the later components, identified at a later time, were num-

Table 1
Physicochemical Characteristics of Complement Components

Component	Serum Concentration (μg/ml)	Molecular Weight	Electrophoretic Mobility
C1q	200	400,000	$\gamma 2$
C1r	180	168,000	β
C1s	22	79,000	$\alpha 2$
C2	30	117,000	$\beta 1$
C3	1200	180,000	$\beta 1$
C4	400	240,000	$\beta 1$
C5	75	185,000	$\beta 1$
C6	60	125,000	$\beta 2$
C7	60	120,000	$\beta 2$
C8	10	150,000	$\gamma 1$
C9	Trace	79,000	α
C1 INH	25	90,000	$\alpha 2$
Properdin	20	190,000	γ
Properdin B	225	100,000	β
Properdin D	Trace	25,000	

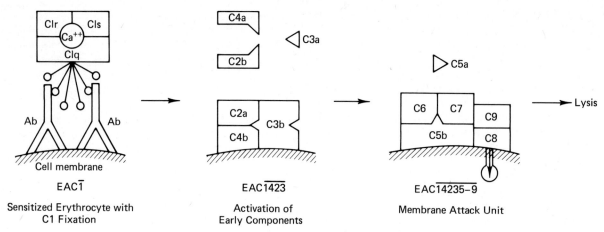

Fig. 1. Schematization of complement activation.

bered according to their sequence of action. The activated protein is indicated by the presence of an overbar. Thus the first component of complement discovered is designated as C1 and the activated protein as C̄1. Erythrocytes are designated "E" and antibody "A." Activation of C1 following its binding to sensitized erythrocytes leads to the formation of the cell-complement intermediate, EAC̄1. The fact that activated complement proteins often act as enzymes accounts for the amplification which occurs as one proceeds through the series of complement interactions. For example, activation of one C1 molecule on a bacterium or tissue site leads to the subsequent activation of many molecules of C4, and this interaction eventually leads to activation of hundreds or thousands of C3 molecules. This cascade effect allows for considerable tissue damage to be produced at limited numbers of complement-activating sites.

Complement Cascade

The most sophisticated studies of complement activation have examined the interaction of the components on the surface of red cell membranes. When erythrocytes are sensitized by specific antibody and interact with fresh serum as a source of complement, a specific series of reactions occurs, leading to opsonization (preparing for phagocytosis) or lysis of the erythrocytes (Fig. 1). This interaction is now understood in considerable detail, and the early steps form the basis of the so-called "classic" complement pathway. There are two major classes of antibody associated with activation of the classic complement pathway, IgM and IgG. A single molecule of IgM antibody, complexed to antigen on the surface of an erythrocyte, can bind or "fix" the first component of the complement system, C1, and initiate activation of the complement sequence. Two molecules of IgG, side by side, are required to form a site with sufficient binding affinity with C1 to produce activation of the classic complement pathway. Hundreds or thousands of IgG molecules combined with antigens on an erythrocyte surface may be required before two are placed sufficiently close together to activate and initiate the complement cascade. Thus, IgM may be 100- to 1000-fold more efficient than

IgG in activating the classic complement pathway. In human plasma the subclasses of IgG capable of activating the classic complement pathway are subclasses 1, 2, and 3. Subclass 4 of IgG does not appear to bind to C1 and does not initiate the classic complement cascade.

The steps in this classic complement cascade are shown in detail in Figure 2A. The system is highly complex. Some of the enzymes formed by complement activation are unstable and decay with loss of activity (Fig. 2A, step 3). There are several inhibitors in the sequence. It is clear that it is important to control activation of this system under inappropriate circumstances and thereby limit damage to normal tissues.

The component of the classic complement pathway that interacts with antibody is designated C1. This component is a three-part molecule with subcomponents termed C1q, C1r, and C1s. C1q is of particular interest because this subcomponent has been isolated from serum and radiolabeled. Its interaction with antigen–antibody complexes forms the basis of one of the more commonly performed tests for the presence of soluble antigen–antibody complexes in serum, the C1q-binding assay. There are six binding sites on the C1q subcomponent for the Fc fragment of the antibody's molecule. The binding of the C1q portion of C1 to the antigen–antibody complex is followd by C1 activation. This activation is associated with cleavage of protein chains within the subcomponents C1r and C1s and is followed by the appearance of an active, enzymatic site on the C1s subunit of the molecule (Fig. 2A, step 2). This is most easily shown by the fact that C1 develops esterase activity in vitro. The development of esterase activity on the C1 molecule allows it to interact with and activate the second component in the pathway, designated as C4.

There is a regulatory protein in serum, the C1 esterase inhibitor, which, given sufficient time, can bind to C̄1 esterase, preventing its interaction with C4. Active C1 enzyme interacts with the intact C4 protein, leading to cleavage of the C4 molecule into two fragments. The larger of these two fragments is capable of attaching to the membrane of a sensitized erythrocyte. The smaller

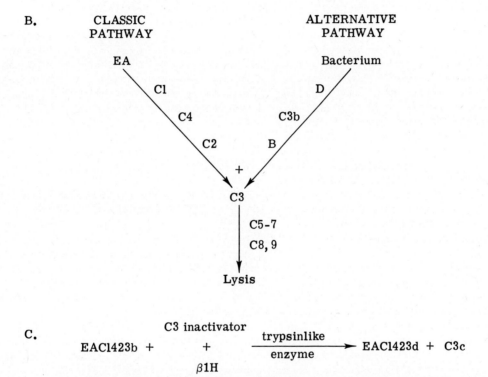

Fig. 2. **A.** Steps in classic complement cascade. **B.** Interaction of classic and alternative pathways. **C.** Cleavage of C3b. E, erythrocyte; A, antibody. Complement fragments designated by a letter are only indicated when they first occur.

fragment is released into the supernatant fluid surrounding the cell. This pattern of attachment of the large fragment of a complement protein to the cell membrane with release of a small fragment into the supernatant is characteristic of many of the early interactions of the complement sequence, as will become clear. Unlike C1, which is bound to the antibody molecule by rather weak ionic linkages, the C4 molecule is bound to the cell membranes by firm, covalent bonds.

The combination of $C\overline{1}$ and C4 on the erythrocyte surface leads to the formation of a new enzyme, $C\overline{14}$. In the presence of magnesium ion, the $C\overline{14}$ enzyme becomes capable of efficiently interacting with and cleaving the next component in the complement sequence, C2. The interaction of C1 and C4 with C2 again leads to

cleavage of C2 into two fragments, a large fragment that attaches and a smaller protein fragment that is released into the supernatant. In this case, it appears that the larger fragment of C2 attaches directly to the C4 molecule on the cell membrane. This interaction leads to the production of a new enzyme that is formed from a portion of C4 and a portion of C2, the $C\overline{42}$ enzyme, or C3 convertase. This enzyme is not stable and over a period of time will decay with release of the C2 fragment that had been attached to the C4 into the supernatant fluid. This release of a $C\overline{2}$ fragment leads to the loss of enzymatic activity and, in fact, the C4 is capable of receiving a new C2 molecule and reforming the $C\overline{42}$ enzyme (Fig. 2A, step 3).

The $C\overline{42}$ enzyme is now capable of interacting with the next component of the complement cascade, C3. Again, C3 is cleaved into two fragments, the larger of which, C3b, is capable of attaching to the cell membrane and the smaller of which, C3a, is released into the supernatant. The interaction of C3 with the $C\overline{42}$ enzyme has been studied in great detail and has been shown to have major biologic importance. As in the other enzymatic steps of the complement cascade, the $C\overline{42}$ enzyme is capable of cleaving many C3 molecules before its activity is lost. Thus, a limited number of antibody-activating sites on the cell surface can lead to the membrane deposition of tens of thousands of C3 molecules by the time this step in the interacting complement sequence is reached. As discussed in the next chapter, these fragments are potentially of great biologic importance.

In plasma, the C3b site on the erythrocyte surface is not stable, just as the $C\overline{42}$ site has only limited stability. In this case, intrinsic decay does not occur; however, other serum proteins are capable of interacting with the C3b site and destroying its activity. Two proteins that interact with this site, β1H and the C3 inactivator, have been studied in detail. In the presence of these two proteins, C3b is cleaved into two fragments. Following a further proteolytic step, a portion of C3b (termed C3c) is released from the cell membrane, and a small cleavage fragment of C3b (termed C3d) remains on the cell membrane (Fig. 2C). C3b, in the presence of the $C\overline{42}$ complex, forms yet a new enzyme capable of cleaving C5 (Fig. 2A, step 5). Again, C5 is cleaved into two fragments, the larger of which, C5b, attaches to the cell surface and the smaller of which, C5a, is released into the fluid surrounding the cell.

The steps following the interaction of C5 with the cell membrane have not been analyzed in as great detail as the earlier steps. It appears, however, that the next two components, and perhaps all of the remaining components, are not cleaved in their interaction with the complement enzymes. The activation of these components has not been studied in the same detail as that of the earlier components, but C6 and C7 are capable of interacting with C5b on the cell membrane to continue the complement cascade. This interaction appears to be associated with insertion of these proteins into the membrane of the cell. After these two components, C6 and C7, have interacted with C5b, a new, stable site is formed on the erythrocyte surface, termed EAC1-7. A cell containing this site is quite stable, but in the presence of the next component of the complement system, C8, it will sustain gradual lysis. In the presence of the final component of the complement cascade, C9, rapid lysis will ensue.

ALTERNATIVE COMPLEMENT PATHWAY

In the past 10 years, it has become clear that many microorganisms are capable of interacting with complement via a mechanism that is somewhat different from that outlined above. One of the important differences in this alternative complement pathway is the fact that this pathway does not require specific antibody for its activation. Materials with repeating polysaccharide subunits, such as zymosan or inulin, may activate the pathway and initiate the sequence of reaction, leading to either opsonization or cell lysis.

As shown in Figure 2B, the interaction of the components of the alternative pathway is similar to that of the classic pathway. It appears that activation of the alternative complement pathway depends upon the interaction of a series of proteins that are quite analogous to those of the classic pathway. The interaction of factors B and D, properdin, and C3 leads to the generation of C3b in a rather inefficient and slow manner. Once a small amount of C3b is generated, this C3 fragment interacts with components B and D of the alternative pathway in much the same way as C4 interacts with C1 and C2 of the classic pathway. Although the details differ, an enzyme formed from C3b and a cleavage product of B can lead to a C3-cleaving enzyme very similar to the enzyme formed from the interaction of C4 and C2. Thus, the alternative complement pathway, utilizing a series of proteins that differ from those of the classic complement pathway, forms a C3-cleaving enzyme which then continues the complement cascade in much the same way as the classic pathway C3-cleaving enzyme. The convergence of the alternative and classic pathways at C3 underscores the biologic importance of this protein.

BIOLOGIC ACTIVITY ASSOCIATED WITH COMPLEMENT ACTIVATION

As discussed in the preceding chapter, the complement system is responsible for many of the features of inflammation and plays an important role in host defense mechanisms. Many steps in the complement system have been shown to be associated with the generation of important biologically active proteins.

ACTIONS OF SPECIFIC COMPONENTS

The association of C1 with antigen–antibody complexes is followed by the stabilization of such antigen–antibody complexes (Table 1). The mechanism for this stabilization appears to reside in the multiple binding sites of the C1q molecule. Presumably, by cross-linking many antibodies in the antigen–antibody complex, the complex is stabilized.

The activation of the next component in the complement sequence, C4, is also associated with biologic importance. If the particle on which the complement is activated is a virus particle, the attachment of many C4 molecules to the envelope of the virion may be associated with neutralization of the virus. Presumably, the viral particle, because of steric hindrance, cannot attach to the membrane of the cell to be infected and the virus is no longer infectious.

Activation of the next component in the complement system, C2, is believed to be associated with the formation of a C2 cleavage fragment that has kininlike activity, termed C2 kinin. It is the generation of this kininlike molecule that is thought to account for the presence of swelling in patients with hereditary angioedema.

Table 1
Biologic Activities of Complement Activation

Component	Biologic Activity
C1	Increases affinity of some antibodies for antigens; binds directly to RNA tumor viruses
C1q	Aggregation of antigen–antibody complexes
C4	Neutralization of viral infectivity
C2	Cleavage products may have kininlike activity
C3a	Anaphylatoxin
C3b	Opsonization of particles (bacteria for phagocytosis or erythrocytes for clearance); receptors for C3b on surface of B lymphocytes, polymorphonuclear leukocytes, macrophages, and erythrocytes
C3d	Receptor for C3d on lymphocytes and macrophages
C5a	Chemotactic factor, anaphylatoxin
C5–7	Chemotactic factor
C8, 9	Insertion into lipid bilayer results in lysis of cells

C3 plays a key role in host defense mechanisms associated with complement activation. The cleavage fragment of C3, C3a, clearly serves as an anaphylatoxin. In the presence of this molecule, mast cells release histamine by a mechanism that is similar to that mediated by IgE; that is, the release occurs in the absence of cellular cytotoxicity. Following the release reaction, the mast cell regenerates its granules and can again be triggered to release mediators at a later time.

The larger fragment of C3, C3b, also has important biologic activity. As described in the preceding chapter, C3b promotes the activation of the alternative complement pathway. C3b has other activities. It can interact with C3b receptors present on a wide variety of cells. C3b receptors exist on polymorphonuclear neutrophils, macrophages, and B (bursa equivalent) lymphocytes as well as on other tissue sites, such as those on renal glomerular epithelial cells. The presence of these receptor sites allows for firm binding of particles coated with C3b. A red cell or bacterium coated with C3b can be bound by phagocytic cells via the C3b receptors, which, in turn, promotes the phagocytic process. It is believed that the attachment of antigen–antibody C3b complexes to the surface of B lymphocytes may be important in promoting the immune response to certain antigens. However, the mechanism by which this occurs is not at all clear.

C5 resembles C3 in many of its chemical and biologic properties. Clearly, particles coated with C5 as well as C3 bind firmly to phagocytic cells, although a true C5 receptor has not yet been described. The small fragment of C5, C5a, like C3a, has anaphylatoxic activity. Moreover, it acts as the principal chemotactic factor in serum. In the presence of C5a, phagocytic cells show directed migration toward the C5a source. Similarly, a complex composed of C5b, C6, and C7 has been said to demonstrate chemotactic activity. The product formed by the interaction of C5b and C6 is particularly of interest in that this product can dissociate from the cell membrane of a sensitized erythrocyte and reattach to the membrane of an unsensitized cell. In the presence of C7, C8, and C9, this unsensitized cell, now coated with C5b6, can sustain the damage-producing complement sequence and can be destroyed. After the reaction with C5–C9, lysis of erythrocytes or bacterium ensues. The mechanism of this lytic reaction has been studied in increasing detail over the past several years and appears to be associated with the insertion of the component proteins into the lipid bilayer of the membrane leaflet, leading to a disruption of the lipid bilayer and the formation of a channel that allows free communication between the intracellular and the extracellular milieu of the cell. The cell or bacterium can no longer maintain its osmotic equilibrium and therefore swells and lyses.

COMPLEMENT ACTIVATION IN THE INFLAMMATORY RESPONSE

It should be clear that many features of the inflammatory response can be manifest by activation of the complement system. If a bacterial infection develops, the bacterial surface can interact with components of the alternative complement pathway in the absence of antibody. In the presence of specific antibody, components of the classic pathway can interact with the bacterium as well. This interaction, in turn, can lead to the generation of complement fragments with anaphylatoxic activity that cause smooth muscle contraction, histamine release, and increased blood flow to the area of infection. In the presence of the C5a chemotactic factor, polymorphonuclear neutrophils and other phagocytic cells leave the blood vessel and migrate into the area of inflammation.

Although not discussed above, other fragments of complement proteins are thought to have biologic activity, although the data are not as widely accepted. For example, it is reported that a fragment of C3 causes white cells to be released from the bone marrow into the circulation—yet another feature of the inflammatory response. When complement is activated at the bacterial surface, C3b may coat the surface, thus promoting opsonization and phagocytosis of the bacterium. Following the interaction of all of the complement proteins with the bacterial surface, a bactericidal reaction may occur with lysis and death of the bacterium. Thus, many features of the host defense mechanism are associated with activation of the complement cascade.

REFERENCES

Atkinson J, Frank MM: Complement, in Parker CW (ed): Clinical Immunology. Philadelphia, Saunders (in press)

Frank M: Complement, in: Current Concepts. Scope Monograph, Upjohn, 1975

Frank M, Atkinson J: Complement in clinical medicine. DM (Jan.) 1975

Osler AG, Sandberg AL: Alternate complement pathways. Prog Allergy 17:51, 1973

Pillemer L, Blum L, Lepow IH: The properdin system and immunity. I. Demonstration and isolation of a new serum protein, properdin, and its role in immune phenomena. Science 120:279, 1954

Immune Complexes

William P. Arend and Mart Mannik

IMMUNE COMPLEX FORMATION

Immune complexes induce tissue damage in a variety of human illnesses, including most forms of glomerulonephritis, certain rheumatic diseases, endocrine disorders, and some complications of infections and malignancies. The pathogenic immune complexes usually consist of IgG antibodies and of antigens derived from autologous tissues, tumors, drugs, or infectious organisms. Complexes may form in the circulation and then become localized along basement membranes, or they may form in closed body cavities and the interstitium of various organs. The immune complexes deposited from the circulation or formed locally initiate the inflammatory response by the activation of complement and generation of chemotactic factors. The influx of phagocytic cells culminates in tissue damage. Common clinical manifestations of the deposition of immune complexes include vasculitis, glomerulonephritis, skin lesions, arthritis, and peripheral neuropathy.

The antibody response usually serves a protective role by expediting the removal of foreign or altered substances from the host. During this process circumstances may arise that lead to tissue deposition of immune complexes, inflammation, and organ damage. The pathogenic immune complexes fix complement and bind to specific receptors on phagocytic cells. These properties of immune complexes depend on the characteristics of the antigens and antibodies and on the nature of their interactions, particularly the lattice formation. Lattice formation is defined as the spatial arrangement and numbers of antigen molecules cross-linked by antibody molecules to form soluble or insoluble aggregates.

CHARACTERISTICS OF ANTIGENS

The size of the antigen molecule and the density of antigenic determinants influence the formation of lattice work in the immune complexes. Very small antigens and those with only one antigenic determinant cannot be cross-linked by antibody molecules. Immune complexes generated with such antigens contain one or two antigen molecules combined with one IgG molecule. Such small-latticed immune complexes are ineffective in complement fixation and in interaction with cell receptors. Antigen molecules of sufficient size may possess repeating identical or multiple different antigenic determinants. These multivalent antigens can be cross-linked by bivalent IgG molecules to form large-latticed immune complexes or immune precipitates.

Nearly all of the antigens in pathogenic immune complexes in human diseases are inadequately characterized in terms of valence and even physical size. Thus, very little information is available on the latticework of immune complexes in human disorders.

The availability of antigen influences the extent and duration of immune complex formation and tissue deposition. A single exposure to antigen predisposes to transient, acute disease. The continuous or intermittent presence of exogenous or endogenous antigen produces recurrent immune complex formation and deposition, thus leading to chronic tissue damage.

CHARACTERISTICS OF ANTIBODIES

The formation of injurious immune complexes also is influenced by characteristics of the IgG antibodies. The subclass of the IgG molecules in the soluble immune complexes affects their biologic properties. Human IgG subclasses 1 and 3 are effective in complement fixation and in adherence to phagocytic cells; these properties are weakly exhibited by IgG2 and are absent in IgG4 molecules. IgA and IgM antibodies are able to cross-link antigen molecules, but the role of immune complexes with these classes of antibodies has not been investigated in human diseases. The rate of synthesis and the concentrations of IgG antibodies in serum or other body fluids, relative to those of antigen, are important since the antigen–antibody ratio affects the lattice of formed complexes (see below). The quality of the immune response is influential, as low-affinity antibodies predispose to the formation of small-latticed complexes that do not bind avidly to phagocytic cells or activate complement. The effects of low-affinity antibodies on pathogenetic events in human immune complex diseases have not been clearly determined.

ANTIGEN–ANTIBODY RATIO

The degree of lattice formation is affected by the relative amounts of antigens and antibodies present. These relationships can best be illustrated through analysis of the precipitin curve. When serially increasing amounts of antigens are added to a constant amount of antibodies the degree of precipitate formation reaches a maximum at a critical ratio of both materials. This ratio will vary for each antigen–antibody system and is known as the point of equivalence, where nearly all available antigens and antibodies are precipitated. In the zone of antibody excess all available antigen is precipitated and usually no soluble complexes are formed. As more antigen is added, more precipitate is formed, until equivalence is reached. The addition of antigen beyond the point of equivalence leads to the formation of soluble complexes due to limited cross-linking and less lattice formation.

The soluble complexes vary in size depending on the existing degree of antigen excess and on the concentrations of both antigen and antibody. Large-latticed complexes result when antigen is present in up to 10- to 20-fold excess from the point of equivalence. Small-latticed complexes, containing one or two antibody molecules per complex, predominate when antigen is added at even greater excess. In addition to the relative degree of antigen excess, the absolute amounts of antigens and antibodies influence the lattice of immune complexes. A high concentration of reactants results in the formation of a greater proportion of large-latticed complexes than occurs in dilute solutions, even when the antigen–antibody ratio remains constant.

Thus, the nature of formed immune complexes is influenced by many factors. The soluble complexes possessing three or more antibody molecules per complex are thought to be responsible for the induction of tissue damage. The extent of formation of these pathogenic complexes in vivo depends on the availability of antigens and rate of synthesis of antibodies. Variations in the amounts of antigens and antibodies present may lead to intermittent immune complex formation, possibly explaining the waxing and waning course of human diseases.

REFERENCES

Haakenstad AO, Mannik M: The biology of immune complexes, in Talal N (ed): Autoimmunity: Genetic, Immunologic, Virologic and Clinical Aspects. New York, Academic Press, 1978, p 277

IMMUNE COMPLEX DEPOSITION

Immune complex formation occurs in the intravascular compartment or locally in tissues. Circulating complexes may deposit along basement membranes of blood vessels, renal glomeruli, or the choroid plexus. Local formation of complexes results from the union of antigens derived from the tissues and antibodies either synthesized locally or derived from the circulation.

CIRCULATING IMMUNE COMPLEXES

The fate of circulating immune complexes is determined by their biologic properties, and thus by their degree of lattice formation. Large-latticed soluble complexes are effectively removed from the circulation by Kupffer cells under normal circumstances. Small-latticed immune complexes are not rapidly removed by Kupffer cells and therefore remain in circulation longer.

Studies in experimental animals indicate that the hepatic clearance mechanism can be saturated. The circulation of large-latticed immune complexes is thereby prolonged, resulting in enhanced localization in other organs, including the kidneys. A similar situation may exist in human disorders characterized by the persistence of soluble complexes in the circulation. Studies in patients with active systemic lupus erythematosus suggest that the clearance function of the mononuclear phagocyte system for IgG-coated red blood cells is impaired.

The intravascular compartment was first recognized as the site of formation of soluble immune complexes during studies on serum sickness in rabbits. A single injection of a foreign protein (e.g., bovine or human serum albumin) into normal rabbits produces a transient syndrome of vasculitis, arthritis, and glomerulonephritis. The manifestations of disease appear 8–10 days after the initial injection, during the immune clearance of the antigen caused by the immune response. At this time soluble immune complexes are formed in the circulation; most of these complexes are removed from the circulation by Kupffer cells, but some complexes deposit in arteries and glomeruli. Only about 0.04 percent of the injected antigen is found in the kidneys, as a result of immune complex deposition. Thus, only a very small fraction of formed complexes are deposited in the glomeruli, but this is sufficient to initiate the inflammatory cycle leading to tissue damage.

Repeated injections of antigen lead to a chronic immune complex glomerulonephritis without arteritis in those rabbits in which the persistent conditions of excess antigen are maintained. If the repeated doses of antigen are varied to permit the continued presence of excess antigen, virtually all animals develop immune complex renal disease. If the doses of antigen are kept constant, kidney disease develops only in those rabbits that are weak to moderate antibody formers. Presumably a strong antibody response leads to the formation of precipitates or very large-latticed complexes that are quickly cleared from the circulation. Rabbits that develop chronic immune complex glomerulonephritis have soluble complexes in their circulation; the size of these complexes is between IgG and IgM or larger than IgM. IgG and complement components can be identified in the tissue lesions by immunofluorescent techniques.

The mechanisms whereby circulating complexes are deposited in organs have been characterized in the serum sickness model in rabbits. Complexes with sufficient degrees of lattice work are more likely to deposit in vessel walls where the integrity of the endothelium has been damaged by turbulent blood flow or by previous injury. The deposition of complexes along the basement membranes in arterial walls or in glomeruli also is enhanced under local conditions of increased vascular permeability. These conditions may result from the release of vasoactive amines by a mechanism involving antigen, IgE-sensitized basophils or mast cells, and platelets.

Human diseases characterized by the presence of circulating immune complexes are listed in Table 1. The presence of immunoglobulins and complement components along the basement membranes in vascular or glomerular lesions in these diseases has indicated the involvement of immune complexes. Further evidence incriminating complexes has come from the identification of specific antigens and antibodies in the eluates from glomeruli. For example, such studies in systemic lupus erythematosus have indicated the presence of immune complexes containing double-stranded DNA and IgG antibodies to double-stranded DNA. The kidneys of patients with malignancies and nephrotic syndrome may contain tumor-specific antigens and antibodies. In the vasculitis and glomerulonephritis seen with chronic hepa-

Table 1
Examples of Human Immune Complex Diseases

Intravascular immune complex formation
   Systemic lupus erythematosus
   Serum sickness
   Mixed cryoglobulinemia
   Hypergammaglobulinemic purpura
   Hepatitis B antigen–associated vasculitis and nephritis
   Vasculitis associated with rheumatoid arthritis
   Poststreptococcal glomerulonephritis
   Glomerulonephritis associated with:
      Bacterial infections (subacute bacterial endocarditis or
        infected shunts)
      Viral diseases (infectious mononucleosis)
      Other infections (syphilis, malaria, leprosy, schistosomiasis,
        or toxoplasmosis)
      Tumors (lymphomas, leukemias, or carcinomas)
      Endocrine disease (thyroiditis)
      Drug reactions (gold or penicillamine)

Local immune complex formation
   Synovitis of rheumatoid arthritis
   Arthritis associated with hepatitis B antigen disease
   Renal tubulointerstitial disease
   Acute thyroiditis
   Hypersensitivity pneumonitis

titis B virus infection, viral antigens and antibodies have been identified in both the vascular and renal lesions. Bacterial antigens have been found in the renal deposits of some patients with subacute bacterial endocarditis and glomerulonephritis.

The mechanisms of deposition of circulating complexes in human disorders are not known, but they are presumed to be similar to those described in animal models. Platelets are commonly found early in tissue lesions of human immune complex diseases and may be responsible for the induction of increased vascular permeability.

LOCAL IMMUNE COMPLEXES

Local immune complex disease is exemplified by the Arthus reaction in animals. In this model the local injection of antigen into the skin of actively or passively immunized animals leads to a vasculitis at the site of injection. Immune complexes are formed in the walls of small blood vessels, initiating an inflammatory response. Antigen-induced arthritis is a well-studied example of local immune complex disease. The intraarticular injection of antigen into the knee joint of rabbits previously immunized with the same antigen induces a similar local inflammatory response resulting in synovitis. In antigen-induced synovitis small amounts of immune complexes persist in the superficial layers of the articular cartilage and may contribute to the chronicity of inflammation observed in this model. Another animal model of local immune complex disease is experimental autoimmune thyroiditis in rabbits. Thyroid damage in this disease

results from the local formation of complexes between thyroglobulin and IgG antibodies.

The local formation of immune complexes is thought to be of pathogenic significance in a number of human diseases (Table 1). Immunoglobulins and complement have been found in the tissue lesions in these disorders and specific antigens have been identified in many. The synovitis of rheumatoid arthritis serves as an example. Local production of IgG- and IgM-rheumatoid factors has been documented in synovial tissues. The synovial fluid contains immune complexes formed by IgG-rheumatoid factors combining with normal IgG or by self-association of IgG-rheumatoid factors. The latter occurs where the specificity of these rheumatoid factors is directed to antigenic determinants that also exist on the Fc fragment of these molecules. IgG and complement, presumably representing immune complexes, are also found in the superficial layers of articular cartilage and in peri-articular collagenous tissues in rheumatoid arthritis.

Other human diseases in which the local formation of immune complexes appears important include autoimmune thyroid disease, tubulointerstitial renal disease, and hypersensitivity pneumonitis. In Hashimoto's thyroiditis the combination of IgG antibodies with thyroglobulin along the follicular basement membrane results in local inflammation and tissue damage. A similar mechanism may exist in the kidney, involving a tubular cell antigen with immune complex formation along the tubular basement membrane. In some forms of hypersensitivity pneumonitis, such as pigeon breeder's lung or Farmer's lung, inhaled antigens combine with IgG antibodies in the alveoli and initiate an inflammatory response.

REFERENCES

Cochrane CG, Koffler D: Immune complex disease in experimental animals and man. Adv Immunol 16:185, 1973

MECHANISMS OF TISSUE DAMAGE

COMPLEMENT ACTIVATION

In human immune complex diseases a common sequence of events leads to tissue damage, irrespective of the mechanisms of immune complex formation and deposition. Deposits of immune complexes activate complement via the classical pathway; split products are generated that increase vascular permeability and are chemotactic for phagocytic cells, particularly neutrophils. (For further details see the sections on Mechanisms of Inflammation and on Complement.)

The roles of complement and neutrophils in immune complex–induced tissue damage have been studied in experimental animals. The vascular lesions of acute serum sickness in rabbits are largely prevented by prior depletion of C3 with cobra venom factor or by induction of neutropenia with nitrogen mustard. In contrast, the glomerular lesions in one-shot serum sickness are only partially prevented by depletion of complement or neutrophils. Thus, mechanisms of renal damage appear to exist that are not totally dependent upon the complement system or the presence of neutrophils after the deposition of immune complexes.

ENZYME RELEASE

The disruption of normal tissue architecture in immune complex diseases probably results from the release of enzymes from phagocytic cells. Neutrophils release lysosomal enzymes to varying degrees after contact with different preparations of immune complexes. Soluble immune complexes induce the release of only small amounts of lysosomal enzymes from neutrophils. Immune precipitates in suspension, however, induce enzyme release to the exterior from premature extrusion of lysosomal contents into incompletely formed phagosomes.

Immune complexes on nonphagocytosable surfaces, however, are the most potent form of immune complexes in the induction of enzyme release from neutrophils. Neutrophils attach to the surface and attempt to interiorize the immune complexes. During this process lysosomal enzymes are discharged into the tissues without the formation of the phagosome. Some of the released lysosomal enzymes are active at neutral pH and are capable of degrading tissue proteins in the extracellular environment. The action of specific enzymes such as elastase and collagenase leads to a breakdown of structural molecules.

Macrophages also are involved in tissue destruction in immune complex diseases as these cells predominate in some chronic cellular infiltrates. For example, macrophages in the synovial pannus in patients with rheumatoid arthritis may interact with immune complexes enmeshed in the superficial layers of the articular cartilage. These cells secrete neutral proteases in a continuous fashion and normally are more active in the release of materials into the extracellular environment than are neutrophils. The mechanisms by which macrophages release enzymes in response to stimulation by different types of immune complexes have not been established. Other cells also may contribute to the process of tissue destruction; for example, the synovial cell most important in the synthesis of collagenase appears to be a fibroblastlike cell. In addition, cellular immunity may be operative in the chronic synovitis of rheumatoid arthritis, particularly in the attraction and activation of macrophages.

CLINICAL, PATHOLOGIC, AND LABORATORY FEATURES OF IMMUNE COMPLEX DISEASES

Human complex diseases are characterized by many common features. They will be reviewed briefly here and will be discussed more thoroughly in the section on Vasculitis and Immune Complex Disease in the fascicle on the Differential Approach to Major Immunologic Syndromes. Detailed clinical descriptions of each of the diseases mediated by immune complexes can be found in the fascicle on Specific Immunologic Diseases.

CIRCULATING IMMUNE COMPLEX DISEASES

Human diseases caused by the intravascular formation of immune complexes are characterized clinically by various combinations of vasculitic skin lesions, glomerulonephritis, synovitis, and peripheral neuropathy. The inflammatory events in each of these organs are initiated by the deposition of complexes in vessel walls, along the glomerular basement membrane, in the synovial capillaries, and in the small nutrient blood vessels in the vasa nervosum. The spectrum of clinical manifestations of immune complex diseases includes the following: palpable petechiae, purpura, urticaria, and skin microinfarcts; an active urinary sediment with or without renal insufficiency; arthralgias or arthritis; and mononeuritis multiplex or a diffuse peripheral neuropathy.

The pathologic abnormalities in immune complex diseases include the deposition of immunoglobulins and complement components along the basement membranes of the arterioles or glomeruli. In the vascular lesions, the deposition of complexes is followed by the infiltration of first neutrophils, then macrophages, lymphocytes, and plasma cells. The immune complex deposits in the glomeruli may be mesangial, subendothilial, or subepithelial in distribution. Immune complexes deposited in the glomeruli may lead to the infiltration of neutrophils and macrophages. The tissue destruction in arterioles and glomeruli induced by the subsequent release of enzymes is accompanied by fibrin formation and basement membrane thickening. A tissue biopsy of an involved organ is important in establishing the diagnosis and in implicating the involvement of immune complexes.

The laboratory abnormalities seen in patients with circulating complexes include hypocomplementemia, anemia, thrombocytopenia, elevated erythrocyte sedimentation rate, cryoglobulinemia, hematuria, and proteinuria. Assays for immune complexes in serum may be positive, as discussed below. Serologic testing for particular antigens, such as hepatitis B viral antigens or tumor-specific antigens, may clarify the etiology of the immune complex disease. Determination of the presence of specific antibodies may also assist in the diagnosis; these include antibodies to hepatitis B viruses, antinuclear antibodies, and rheumatoid factors (antiglobulins).

LOCAL IMMUNE COMPLEX DISEASES

The local formation of immune complexes leads to inflammatory disease within the specific involved organ. Thus, immune complexes formed in the joints, thyroid, or kidneys result in clinical arthritis, thyroiditis, or nephritis, respectively. Histologic examination of inflammed joints shows an initial infiltration of neutrophils with later predominance of lymphocytes, plasma cells, and macrophages in synovial and subsynovial distributions. Immunoglobulins and complement components may be found within the infiltrating phagocytic cells by immunofluorescent techniques. The hypertrophic synovium may grow over the articular cartilage, with enzyme release leading to the destruction of cartilage and periarticular collagenous structures.

DETECTION OF CIRCULATING IMMUNE COMPLEXES

ASSAYS

The finding of tissue deposits of immune complexes in an increasing number of diseases has led to extensive efforts to measure these complexes in the circulation. All of the many assays for circulating complexes have limitations and the patterns of positivity in diseases vary with different assays. The methods of immune complex detection can be classified into four categories: (1) physical separation of the complexes; (2) complement fixation or the binding of C1q by complexes; (3) interaction of antiglobulins with complexes; and (4) adherence of complexes to specific cell-surface receptors (Table 1).

Physical Separation Methods

Physical separation methods such as analytical ultracentrifugation, sucrose density gradient ultracentrifugation, and gel filtration chromatography have been used to detect circulating immune complexes. Intermediate complexes (between IgG and IgM in size) are detected by analytical ultracentrifugation in the sera of some patients with rheumatoid arthritis and in the sera of patients with hypergammaglobulinemia purpura of Waldenström. Large complexes (22 S) can be found in the sera of some patients with rheumatoid arthritis. These techniques require relatively large amounts of complexes for detection and are impractical for application to large numbers of patients.

Cryoglobulin formation is another method of physical separation of material from serum, probably representing precipitation of soluble immune complexes. Cryoglobulins exist in numerous conditions. IgM, IgG, and hepatitis B surface antigen are present in the cryoprecipitate found in the syndrome of mixed cryoglobulinemia, with the IgM possessing rheumatoid factor activity. IgM, IgG, IgA, C1q, C3, C4, and DNA have all been described in the cryoglobulins from the sera of patients with systemic lupus erythematosus. The cryoglobulins from the sera of some patients with hepatitis B virus infection and vasculitis contain hepatitis B surface antigen and specific antibodies. Similar components are present in the sediment from ultracentrifuged plasma from these patients. Cryoglobulin formation as a means of detection of immune complexes is relatively insensitive, may detect only a subset of complexes, and does not permit the determination of the size of the circulating complexes.

Complement Binding by Complexes

Complexes that have the capability of fixing complement can be detected by reaction with C1q in vitro. The first assay described the formation of a precipitin line in agar upon diffusion of purified C1q against immune complex–containing sera. Numerous quantitative assays have been developed that measure the amount of IgG-containing material in serum either by direct binding to radiolabeled C1q or by inhibition of binding of C1q to preparations of IgG aggregates or complexes.

The most widely used assay is the C1q-binding assay, which determines the percentage of a standard amount of radiolabeled C1q that is bound by a constant amount of test serum. The unbound C1q is separated by precipitation of bound C1q with polyethylene glycol. The assay is standardized using heat-aggregated IgG; its sensitivity is 50 to 100 μg equivalents of aggregated human IgG per milliliter of serum. This assay detects large-latticed complexes to a greater degree than small-latticed complexes; thus it underestimates the concentration of the latter. A higher percentage of positive results has been obtained with the C1q-binding assay when the serum samples are not preheated to inactivate complement.

Antiglobulin Binding to Complexes

Another early test for the detection of circulating complexes was the formation of a precipitin line in agar between purified monoclonal rheumatoid factor and complex-containing sera. Adaptations of this interaction have led to the development of sensitive radioimmunoassays for complexes. These assays are all dependent upon the fact that rheumatoid factor binds more firmly to complexes or aggregated IgG than to monomeric IgG. Monoclonal rheumatoid factor gives better results than polyclonal rheumatoid factors. The most widely utilized assay quantitates immune complexes by their ability to inhibit

---

Table 1

Assays for the Detection of Circulating Immune Complexes

Physical methods
    Ultracentrifugation, analytical, or sucrose density gradient
    Gel filtration chromatography
    Cryoglobulin formation

Complement binding by complexes
    Anticomplementary activity
    Direct binding of C1q
    Inhibition of C1q binding to IgG-coated particles

Antiglobulin binding to complexes
    Inhibition of binding of aggregated IgG to solid phase monoclonal rheumatoid factor
    Inhibition of binding of monoclonal rheumatoid factor to IgG-coated particles
    Similar assays with polyclonal rheumatoid factor

Complexes binding to cells
    Direct binding to Raji cells
    Inhibition of macrophage uptake of aggregated IgG
    Inhibition of K lymphocyte toxicity
    Aggregation of platelets

the binding of radiolabeled, heat-aggregated IgG of a defined size (25 S) to monoclonal rheumatoid factor coupled to a solid-phase carrier. Thus the concentration of complexes is expressed as microgram equivalents of aggregated human IgG per milliliter of serum. The monoclonal rheumatoid factor–inhibition assay appears to detect all sizes of immune complexes in the sera of patients with rheumatoid arthritis. Polyclonal rheumatoid factor in the samples does not interfere with the monoclonal rheumatoid factor–inhibition assay. This assay detects complexes at a level of 5 μg equivalents of aggregated IgG per milliliter of serum.

Complexes Binding to Cells

Another type of assay for the detection of immune complexes is dependent upon their interaction with receptors on cell membranes. Specific receptors for complement components and for the Fc portion of the IgG molecule are present on macrophages, polymorphonuclear neutrophils, platelets, and some lymphoblastoid cell lines. The most widely applied assay detects complexes that bind complement and then interact with receptors for complement components on the membrane of Raji cells, a B lymphocyte line maintained in tissue culture. The amount of immune complexes bound to the cells is detected with a radiolabeled anti-human IgG antibody prepared in rabbits. The assay is standardized with known amounts of heat-aggregated human IgG. Thus the results are expressed in terms of microgram equivalents of aggregated human IgG per milliliter of test serum. This assay detects complexes of a wide range of sizes but may underestimate the amounts of small-latticed complexes. Antilymphocyte antibodies also may contribute to positive results in the Raji cell assay. This assay is more sensitive than the C1q-binding assay and is almost as sensitive as the monoclonal rheumatoid factor assay, detecting complexes at a concentration of 10 μg equivalents of aggregated IgG per milliliter of serum.

RESULTS IN SYSTEMIC LUPUS ERYTHEMATOSUS AND RHEUMATOID ARTHRITIS

As examples of the application of these assays to the study of human diseases, results of analyses of serum samples from patients with systemic lupus erythematosus or rheumatoid arthritis will be discussed briefly.

Study of sera from patients with systemic lupus erythematosus yields positive results with both the C1q-binding assay and the Raji cell assay in 90 percent of analyzed specimens. A high level of complexes detected in lupus sera by the assays correlates with increased disease activity, high antibody titers to native DNA, and low serum complement levels. The assay for complexes utilizing reaction with rheumatoid factor is positive in less than 20 percent of lupus sera. The nature of the immune complexes detected by these assays in lupus sera is not known.

Many assays appear to detect complexes in the sera and synovial fluids of patients with rheumatoid arthritis.

Positive results are obtained with the C1q-binding assay in over 75 percent of sera or synovial fluids from rheumatoid factor–positive patients. This assay shows positive results in 70 percent of serum and 50 percent of synovial fluid samples from rheumatoid arthritis patients who are rheumatoid factor negative. The levels of C1q-binding complexes in rheumatoid sera do not correlate with the rheumatoid factor titers but are correlated with the presence of extraarticular manifestations, such as vasculitis. The reactive complexes in the rheumatoid sera and synovial fluids are primarily intermediate (i.e., between IgG and IgM), but larger complexes are frequently seen.

The monoclonal rheumatoid factor–inhibition assay is positive in 50–70 percent of rheumatoid sera and 25 percent or more of synovial fluid samples. The levels of complexes in the rheumatoid synovial fluids are often greater than those in the corresponding sera. The presence of monoclonal rheumatoid factor–reacting complexes in rheumatoid sera correlates with functional and anatomic parameters of disease activity.

The Raji cell assay gives positive results for the presence of complexes in 70 percent of rheumatoid sera, with particularly high levels in patients with rheumatoid vasculitis. The nature of the immune complexes in rheumatoid sera and synovial fluids that are detected by these three assays has not been determined, but probably includes IgG–anti-IgG complexes.

Lambert et al. utilized all three of the above assays for immune complexes on the same set of serum samples. Correlations were obtained between the Raji and C1q-binding assays with sera from either rheumatoid arthritis or systemic lupus erythematosus patients. The monoclonal rheumatoid factor–inhibition test, however, appeared to detect complexes of different characteristics that may be unique to rheumatoid arthritis. These assays for immune complexes have not been applied extensively to sera from patients with other rheumatologic diseases. Some patients with unidentified forms of vasculitis show positive results, as do some patients with inflammatory bowel disease, glomerulonephritis, sarcoidosis, or neoplasms.

REFERENCES

Gabriel A Jr, Agnello V: Detection of immune complexes. The use of radioimmunoassays with C1q and monoclonal rheumatoid factor. J Clin Invest 59:990, 1977

Lambert PH, Dixon FJ, Zubler RH, Agnello V, Cambiaso C, Casali P, Clarke J, Cowdery JS, McDuffie FC, Hay FC, MacLennan ICM, Masson P, Müller-Eberhard HJ, Penttinen K, Smith M, Tappeiner G, Theofilopoulos AN, Verroust P: A collaborative study for the evaluation of eighteen methods for detecting immune complexes in serum. Clin Exp Immunol (in press)

Luthra HS, McDuffie FC, Hunder GG, Samayoa EA: Immune complexes in sera and synovial fluids of patients with rheumatoid arthritis. Radioimmunoassay with monoclonal rheumatoid factor. J Clin Invest 56:458, 1975

Theofilopoulos AN, Wilson CB, Dixon FJ: The Raji cell radioim-
    mune assay for detecting immune complexes in human sera.
    J Clin Invest 57:169, 1976
Woodroffe AJ, Border WA, Theofilopoulos AN, Götze O, Glas-
    sock RJ, Dixon FJ, Wilson CB: Detection of circulating
    immune complexes in patients with glomerulonephritis.
    Kidney Int 12:268, 1977

Zubler RH, Nydegger U, Perrin LH, Fehr K, McCormick J,
    Lambert PH, Miescher PA: Circulating and intra-articular
    immune complexes in patients with rheumatoid arthritis.
    Correlation of ^{125}I–C1q binding activity with clinical and
    biological features of the disease. J Clin Invest 57:1308, 1976
Zubler RH, Lambert PH: Detection of immune complexes in
    human diseases. Prog Allergy 24:1, 1978

Immunogenetics

J. Claude Bennett

NATURE OF THE MAJOR HISTOCOMPATIBILITY COMPLEX

An association of genetic predilection, intrinsic immune response capabilities, and some environmental factors have been apparent in studies on the etiology and pathogenesis of the rheumatic diseases. This association continues to be the subject of intensive research. Over the past two decades there have been significant advances in our fundamental understanding of the way in which these factors interact. Perhaps the focus that has become most clearly visible has been the association of certain rheumatic diseases with products of the major histocompatibility complex (MHC). An understanding of the nature of this association and the role that it plays in specific disease susceptibility is one of the most challenging and intriguing problems in modern medicine.

This chapter will deal with the nature of the MHC, the importance of various subsets of genes within this complex and, particularly, the potential significance of the immune response genes relative to human disease. It is of significance that the information that has accrued from studies on two species, humans and mice, forms a basis for two distinctly different types of data. The studies on man, comprising an outbred population, provide us with the necessary stimulus of disease occurrence and MHC association. The genetic mechanisms that are thought to play a role in this association can be approached best through detailed genetic crosses involving defined inbred mouse strains. Hopefully, an analytical comparison of these data will help us to understand better the nature of the MHC, the nature of control of the immune response, and the role they might play in the pathogenesis of disease.

TERMINOLOGY

As in many areas of science that are rapidly advancing, immunogenetics has developed its own terminology, elucidated below.

Gene: A segment of DNA that directs the synthesis of a given messenger RNA, which in turn directs the synthesis of a given polypeptide chain. The gene is the basic unit of inheritance.

Locus: The position of a gene on a chromosome.

Allele: An alternative form of the same gene, usually having arisen by some mutational event. Within the MHC each locus possesses multiple alleles. When this occurs with appreciable frequency within a given population it is said to present *polymorphism.*

Phenotype: The characteristics of an individual that reflect the summation of all his genes and give him a descriptive identity.

Genotype: The genetic description that forms the basis for the observed phenotype. Generally, the genotype may be deduced from the inheritance pattern among the offspring of a given family.

Major histocompatibility complex (MHC): The MHC is a chromosomal region containing the loci that are responsible for the gene products that we define as the transplantation antigens and associated immune response gene products. The MHC of man is referred to as the HLA complex. In the mouse the analogous region is called the H-2 complex. The HLA loci are given letter names such as HLA-A, HLA-B, HLA-C, and HLA-D. Similarly, in the mouse, they are H-2K and H-2D.

Haplotype: A combination of closely linked HLA genes on the same chromosome. Two haplotypes (one from each parent) give rise to the genotype of the offspring. Thus, in the HLA system a haplotype would be

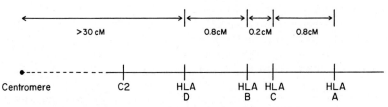

Fig. 1. Map of human chromosome No. 6 showing the relationship of regions within the MHC. Approximate map distances are given in centimorgans (cM).

Table 1
Currently Identified Alleles of the Four HLA Loci

HLA-A			HLA-B		HLA-C	HLA-D	HLA-DR*
1	26	w4	w18	w44	w1	w1	w1
2	28	w5	w21	w45	w2	w2	w2
3	29	w6	w22	w46	w3	w3	w3
9	w30	7	27	w47	w4	w4	w4
10	w31	8	w35	w48	w5	w5	w5
11	w32	12	37	w49	w6	w6	w6
w19†	w33	13	w38	w50		w7	w7
w23	w34	14	w39	w51		w8	
w24	w36	15	40	w52		w9	
25	w43	w16	w41	w53		w10	
		17	w42	w54		w11	

*HLA-DR refers to serologic identification of D loci antigens. The numerical assignments of D and DR are not necessarily related.

†The "w" in some of the allele designations refers to the fact that it is a working assignment, which has not yet received full recognition.

defined by components from each of the loci (A, B, C, and D).

Linkage: The tendency of related genes on the same chromosome to segregate together.

Linkage disequilibrium: The term used by geneticists to describe the observation that some alleles and closely linked loci occur together in the same haplotype more frequently than would be expected by chance alone.

HLA SYSTEM

The HLA region has been localized to chromosome No. 6, based on family studies and chromosome mapping using interspecies somatic cell hybrids. The relationships among the various loci are presented in Figure 1. The four closely linked loci, A, B, C, and D, thus far have been found to have 20, 33, 6, and 11 alleles, respectively (Table 1). In the case of the A, B, and C loci, the alleles are defined by serologic techniques, primarily microcytotoxicity assays. In the case of the D locus, allele definition has been by cell–cell interactions, involving the mixed lymphocyte culture test using homozygous typing cells. Those more recently described loci (C and D) have fewer known alleles, but clearly the number will increase as further studies are performed. Considering all of the known HLA alleles, a very large number of potential phenotypes could result from possible combinations. Therefore, each individual is likely to be distinct with respect to his HLA type. Because there is such an extraordinary scope of phenotypic possibilities, when a marked deviation from the normal frequency for a given allele or haplotype is found, as in disease associations, vigorous study of the etiologic relationships is likely to

lead to some understanding of the role of a particular MHC haplotype in disease susceptibility.

It should be noted that properdin factor B is linked to the HLA system, although the exact map position is somewhat uncertain. It has also been shown that deficiency of the second complement component (C2) is linked to HLA (see Fig. 1), and that the levels of C4 are similarly linked. The evidence is growing that the MHC plays a major role in the genetic control of the complement system, particularly of those components involved in the early stages of the complement cascade.

H-2 SYSTEM

A schematic genetic map of the H-2 gene complex in the mouse is presented in Figure 2. There are four major, discrete regions that determine the antigenic products of this portion of the 17th chromosome of the mouse. The K and D regions determine the classic transplantation antigens. These gene products are the principal antigenic targets for cell-mediated cytotoxicity in graft rejections, and they were the first products of the mouse MHC to be detected serologically. The I region determines those factors that are primarily responsible for the mixed leukocyte reaction. It also controls a variety of functions relating to the immune responses, particularly those functions that involve antigenic recognition and interactions between lymphoid cells. The S region determines components of the serum complement system. A fifth region, G, defines a locus whose product is recognized as an erythrocyte antigen.

Although, as seen in Figure 2, the terms *loci* and *regions* of the H-2 complex refer to the same chromosome areas, the terms are used to indicate slightly differ-

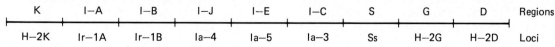

K	I—A	I—B	I—J	I—E	I—C	S	G	D	Regions
H–2K	Ir–1A	Ir–1B	Ia–4	Ia–5	Ia–3	Ss	H–2G	H–2D	Loci

Fig. 2. Map of mouse chromosome No. 17 showing the relationship of loci and regions within the MHC.

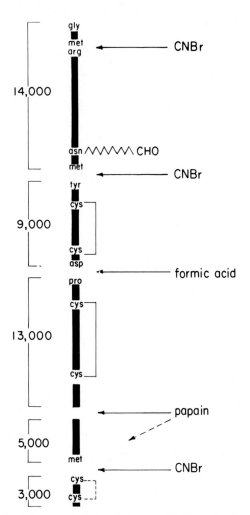

Fig. 3. Glycoprotein heavy chain of an HLA-B molecule. Molecular weights of the peptides do not add up precisely to the weight of the intact chain due to inexactness in the experimental determination of peptide molecular weights.

ent concepts. The genetic *loci* are single genetic units, defined in terms of specific gene products. *Regions* are defined as segments of chromosomes, identified from crossover experimentations that have separated the various marker loci. The implication of these distinctions is that a given genetic region could be quite large and might possibly include many genes in addition to the one that defines a given marker.

Many H-2 alloantigenic specificities have been defined as the gene products of H-2K and H-2D alleles. These alloantigenic specificities are determinants defined on the protein product of a given allele by the use of a specific *alloantiserum*. For example, the H-2^b haplotype is found to have 33 specificities in the H-2K region, as defined by alloantisera, and two in the H-2D region; and H-2^k is found to have 23 specificities in the H-2K region and 32 in the H-2D region. As in the studies of the HLA complex in man, the antisera that have been used in defining these specificities are extremely useful reagents

for the isolation, classification, and characterization of the products of the MHC region.

NATURE OF HLA ANTIGENS

HLA antigens are found to occur on the surface membranes of most cell types. They tend to be expressed early in fetal life, usually by the sixth week, and persist throughout the life of a cell. They amount to perhaps 1–2 percent of the total membrane protein, but may be shed into plasma and other body fluids. HLA-A and HLA-B consist of two polypeptide chains, a glycoprotein heavy chain of approximately 45,000 daltons, and a protein light chain, which has been identified as β_2 microglobulin, at 12,000 daltons. These molecular weights and chain associations are found in an exactly analogous arrangement in the H-2K and H-2D gene products of the mouse.

HLA molecules solubilized from membrane fractions by detergents contain both the 45,000-dalton glycoprotein component and the associated β_2 microglobulin. The enzyme papain cleaves the higher molecular weight glycoprotein chain in two steps. A 39,000-dalton fragment is first produced, which is then cleaved to the final product of 34,000 daltons (Fig. 3). The small peptides cleaved by papain are at the C-terminal end of the polypeptide chain. Since predominately hydrophobic amino acid residues are located in the second peptide released by papain, it has been proposed that this peptide (5000 daltons) is the one that is inserted into the membrane. This arrangement would suggest that the hydrophylic C-terminal peptide (3000 daltons) may extend though the membrane and into the interior of the cell.

At least a part of the interest in the structure of HLA molecules stems from the fact that they may have some structural analogy to the immunoglobulin molecules. Until recently, the only structural evidence implicating homology with immunoglobulins had been the demonstration that β_2 microglobulin has sequence homology with the C-3 domain of the immunoglobulin heavy chain. No homology between the heavy chain of HLA and any immunoglobulin has been found in the N-terminal sequences determined thus far. However, recent studies on the HLA-B7 molecule indicate that significant homology is found within the 13,000-dalton fragment (Fig. 3), near the third cysteine residue, when compared with the amino acid sequence around the second cysteine in the variable region of immunoglobulins. This fragment was obtained by cleavage of an aspartic acid–proline bond within the papain fragment of HLA-B7 by mild acid. hydrolysis. It is striking that 5 of the 17 residues in this area were identical with immunoglobulin sequences around the half-cysteine in the variable region if only one deletion was permitted in the sequence.

Fragments of HLA antigens, presumably produced by proteolysis of the surface molecules, are found in the urine and are also present in the serum in association with high-density lipoprotein.

The function of HLA-A, HLA-B, and HLA-C in humans, and of H-2K and H-2D in mice is by no means clear. However, some very important observations, made initially by Zinkernagel and Doherty in 1974, suggest that these molecules may be directly involved in certain cellular mechanisms. These workers found that effective cell-mediated killing reactions against virus-infected cells, which expressed on their membranes virus-induced surface antigens, required specific H-2 compatibility; that is, immune cells of a given haplotype would not kill infected cells expressing virus antigens unless those target cells were of the same H-2 haplotype. The implication is that the H-2–determined products are required for some sort of obligatory cell–cell interaction, in addition to recognition of the unusual viral antigen present on the surface of the target cell. It would seem, therefore, that the H-2 product makes a direct contribution to the antigenic site that is recognized by the receptor on a cytotoxic lymphocyte. This "altered self" concept relative to host expression of immune surveillance will be the subject of much future study. These observations stimulate a new awareness of mechanisms by which these molecules might contribute to MHC-associated host resistance phenomena.

IMMUNE RESPONSE GENES

Following the demonstration that there was genetic variation in the immune response to a synthetic polypeptide polymer, it was shown that this variation is controlled by a single genetic unit closely associated with the H-2 complex. Genes within this region control not only specific immune responses but also a variety of other activities of the immune system, including the mixed lymphocyte reaction, graft-versus-host reaction, delayed hypersensitivity, antigen-induced lymphocyte proliferation, T cell–B cell interaction, T cell–macrophage interaction, T cell helper function, and T cell suppressor function. Each of these functions is not necessarily controlled by a discrete gene. Nevertheless, it is clear that the I region genes and gene products are involved in some level of control of the major events of cellular immunology. There is now evidence to suggest that in several instances two I region genes collaborate in order to initiate a high response to a particular antigen. It is of interest that within subregions of the I region (Fig. 2) there are demarcations of specialized function. Subregions I-A and probably I-C, and their respective products, appear to be involved primarily in helper type functions. In contrast, the I-J subregion may code for a suppressor molecule. The product of I-J, designated Ia4, has been found only on suppressor T cells and in association with solubilized suppressor factors.

It has been possible to produce specific antisera that detect protein products of the I subregions by appropriate immunizations among mouse strains involving recombinant H-2 haplotypes. These Ia antigens, which are associated with the immune response genes, can be detected with alloantisera that contain no specificities against either H-2K or H-2D antigens. They are found on most B cells, but on only certain subpopulations of T cells. They are also present on sperm and epidermal cells, but are not present on platelets or erythrocytes. These molecules, at

Table 2
Traits of the Immune System Localized to Subregions of I

Property	I-A	I-B	I-J	I-E	I-C
Immune response	+	+	+	+	+
Ia antigens	+		+	+	+
Helper factors	+				
Suppressor factor(s)			+		
Cellular interaction	+	+	+	+	
MLR* antigens	+			+	+

*MLR: mixed leukocyte reaction.

least as isolated from B cells, are glycoproteins of approximately 58,000 daltons. They are comprised of two polypeptide chains of 25,000 and 33,000 daltons. They do not contain β_2 microglobulin. The alloantigenic properties reside within the polypeptides and are not associated with the carbohydrate moiety. Antibodies against Ia antigens have proved to be useful probes for the study of the function of the I region. Most of this work is based on a variety of assays that show the capacity of these antisera to inhibit known lymphocyte functions. Presumably, these inhibitions involve some sort of steric interference with the normal biologic functions of Ia molecules. Results from these studies indicate that anti-Ia can inhibit B cell receptors for T helper factors, Fc components of immunoglobulins, and lipopolysaccharide stimulants. They also inhibit antigen-induced T cell proliferation and macrophage function, and will bind to soluble mediators from T cells and macrophages. Table 2 summarizes the traits of the immune system that have been localized to the various subregions of the I region.

REFERENCES

Dausset J, Svejgaard A (eds): HLA and Disease. Copenhagen, Munksgaard, 1977
Fudenberg HH, Pink JRL, Wang AC, Douglas SD: Basic Immunogenetics (ed 2). New York, Oxford University Press, 1978
Götze D (ed): The Major Histocompatibility System in Man and Animals. Berlin, Springer, 1977

DISEASES ASSOCIATED WITH THE HLA SYSTEM

RHEUMATIC DISEASES

Although more than 40 diseases have been found to have a definite association with the HLA system, none is so dramatic as that with certain of the rheumatic diseases (Table 1). The most striking associations are found with HLA-B and HLA-D antigens. It is of particular note that none of the associations is absolute. Although 90 percent of patients with ankylosing spondylitis may be HLA-B27 positive, less than 25 percent of all people who carry B27 actually develop the disease. Hence, the presence of B27 is not the sole determinant in causing the disease; it must be influenced by other factors. Numerous mechanisms

Table 1
Rheumatic Diseases and HLA Association

Diseases	Racial Group	HLA Type	Antigen Frequency (%)		Relative Risk
			Patients	Controls	
Ankylosing spondylitis	Whites	B27	89.8	8.0	87.8
	Japanese	B27	66.7	0.0	305.7
	Haida Indians	B27	100.0	50.0	34.4
	Bella Coola Indians	B27	100.0	20.2	20.2
	Pima Indians	B27	36.0	18.0	2.6
Reiter's syndrome	Whites	B27	78.2	8.4	35.9
Yersinia arthritis	Whites	B27	79.4	9.4	24.3
Salmonella arthritis	Whites	B27	66.7	8.6	17.6
Psoriatic arthritis	Whites	B13	19.8	5.5	4.8
		B27	40.2	8.7	8.6
Central joints		Bw17	11.6	5.5	2.5
		Bw38	22.7	2.9	9.1
Peripheral joints	Whites	B13	9.9	5.5	2.3
		B27	15.5	8.7	2.5
		Bw17	24.8	5.5	5.8
		Bw38	12.6	2.9	4.5
Rheumatoid arthritis	Whites	Dw4	42.2	15.7	3.0
Sjögren's syndrome	Whites	B8	50.6	24.0	3.2
		Dw3	53.0	17.0	5.2
Chronic active hepatitis	Whites	A1	41.6	28.4	1.8
		B8	44.2	20.3	3.0
		Dw3	60.0	21.7	7.2
Behcet's disease	Whites	B5	35.1	11.1	4.3
	Japanese	B5	75.0	30.8	6.5

Adapted from McDevitt and Engleman: Arthritis Rheum 20:S9, 1977.

have been suggested for the association of HLA antigens with various diseases (Table 2).

The association of certain diseases with the D locus is of particular significance in view of the fact that HLA-D is the presumptive human analog of the mouse I region. Hence, the finding of an association between a disease and a D locus allele would support the concept that an immune response gene-like product is involved in the pathogenesis of that disease. The association of HLA-B and HLA-D with autoimmune disorders is striking. There are some in which the association with HLA-B and HLA-D is much greater than with HLA-B alone. It may be that as more and more D alleles are defined, association with disease will become even more clearly delineated. The

recent discovery of the association of HLA-Dw4 with rheumatoid arthritis in the absence of any apparent association with HLA-A or HLA-B is striking. This provides a major implication of the possible role of the immune response genes in disease. The finding in rheumatoid arthritis is that approximately 40 percent of patients with classic rheumatoid arthritis carry the Dw4 marker, as defined by mixed lymphocyte reactions. Another marker, Dw7, is also found in some patients with rheumatoid arthritis. Perhaps with more finely honed detection methods, especially with serologic technics to define the related surface antigens, a much higher association between the products of this genetic region and rheumatoid arthritis will become apparent.

B LYMPHOCYTE ALLOANTIGENS

Recent elegant work in multiple sclerosis would indicate that a very high number of such patients carry serologically defined B cell alloantigens. These may be considered to be indicative of HLA-D markers (the latter defined in mixed lymphocyte cultures), which are presumed to be the human counterpart of Ia antigens. Consequently, experimental approaches to define new B cell alloantigens in rheumatoid arthritis, systemic lupus erythematosus, and other rheumatic diseases will be of great importance for future research efforts. It may be that the definition of single specificities in this region will give us an exquisite diagnostic tool and will open new doors for research into the etiology of these diseases.

Human B lymphocyte alloantigens have a structure

Table 2
Possible Mechanisms for HLA and Disease Association

1. HLA antigen might serve as a receptor for a virus or environmental toxin.
2. HLA antigen might be structurally related to a bacterial or viral antigen (i.e., molecular mimicry).
3. HLA antigens might be involved in the formation of "new" or "altered self" antigenic determinants.
4. There may be a linkage disequilibrium with other genes, controlling a specific immune response or regulation (helpers or suppressors) of such response.
5. There may be a deficiency of a complement system component.

similar to that of the mouse Ia antigen—a bimolecular complex consisting of two chains of approximately 25,000 and 33,000 daltons. These molecules are expressed primarily on B lymphocytes, but also occur on monocytes and myeloblasts. The utilization of pregnancy or transplantation sera to identify these antigens has progressed rapidly. The B cell alloantigen system perhaps accounts for the majority of B cell–specific surface antigens and it may provide the best tool for identifying specific diseases. For example, sera have been found by Winchester which relate to both the Dw4 and Dw7 markers. Combinations of such antisera with specificity for human B lymphocytes give a reaction incidence of 79 percent with lymphocytes from patients with rheumatoid arthritis, as opposed to 24 percent with those of normal control subjects. It seems clear that the utilization of these techniques to define further the HLA-D locus sero-logically will be essential in relating immune reactivity of the host and disease associations.

SUMMARY

Recent developments in immunogenetics, utilizing both cellular and serologic technics to define antigens, have uncovered an array of MHC disease associations. These associations will become much more clearly defined as we develop better tools to uncover specific markers. Perhaps the most dramatic advance in all of medicine in the past decade has been the realization of disease association with products of the major histocompatibility locus.

REFERENCES

McDevitt HO, Engleman EG: Association between genes in the major histocompatibility complex and disease susceptibility. Arth Rheum 20:S9, 1977

Immunosuppressive Drugs

Robert S. Schwartz

EFFECTS OF IMMUNOSUPPRESSIVE DRUGS ON IMMUNITY

Immunosuppressive drugs may be classified into two categories: a relatively small group of compounds that are administered with the purpose of inhibiting one or more aspects of the immune system, and a larger group of agents with secondary, or unintended effects on immunologic functions. These two categories may be termed *primary* and *secondary immunosuppressants* (Table 1). Almost all primary immunosuppressants can also be secondary immunosuppressants; the classification thus depends on clinical intention.

The immunosuppressants listed in Table 1 may affect numerous aspects of immunologic function. The clinical effect depends mainly on dosage and duration of administration. All of the chemical compounds and x-rays are cytotoxic and they influence immunity by killing or inactivating lymphocytes, monocytes, macrophages, and granulocytes or their precursors. As a result, the acquisition of new immune responses, the expression of previously acquired immunity, and the generation of immunologically mediated inflammation can be impaired or obliterated during treatment with these compounds. Relevant clinical examples of these three major effects are (1) suppression of immunity to alloantigens in recipients of renal allografts (blocked acquisition of new immunity), (2) activation of latent herpesvirus infection during chemotherapy (impaired expression of preexisting immunity), and (3) amelioration of vasculitis by corticosteroids (inhibition of inflammatory reactions).

The vast literature on the immunosuppressive effects of cytotoxic drugs deals mainly with modifications of immune responses to defined antigens in experimental animals. In a typical example the effects of a compound such as cyclophosphamide on the production of antibodies by mice challenged with a single injection of sheep erythrocytes are determined. By and large, such experiments are irrelevant to clinical problems because (1) the patient usually seeks medical help long after the immune response has been initiated, (2) the nature of the antigenic stimulus in most autoimmune diseases is unknown, (3) as a rule there is a continuous antigenic stimulation of the

Table 1
Primary and Secondary Immunosuppressants

Primary immunosuppressants
Corticosteroids
Azathioprine
Cyclophosphamide
Methotrexate
Antilymphocyte (antithymocyte) serum
Total-body x-irradiation
Secondary immunosuppressants
Corticosteroids
Alkylating agents
Cyclophosphamide
Nitrogen mustard
Phenylalanine mustard
Chlorambucil
Thiopurines
6-Mercaptopurine
Thioguanine
Cytosine arabinoside
5-Fluorouracil
L-Asparaginase
Procarbazine
Phenothiazines
Chloramphenicol

patient, and (4) unlike inbred mice, human beings are genetically heterogeneous and the responses to therapy, as well as those to the disease, can be highly variable.

In a real life clinical situation the use of primary immunosuppressants raises two problems: *What are the risks? What can be achieved?* The physician must decide upon answers to these questions before recommending the treatment. Several facts, obtained initially in animals and subsequently confirmed in human subjects, can serve as guidelines:

1. Dividing cells are more susceptible to cytotoxic drugs than are nondividing cells. This means that proliferating lymphocytes (i.e., those actually engaged by antigen) are more susceptible to the drugs than non-dividing lymphocytes. Moreover, mature cells (e.g., polymorphonuclear leukocytes, monocytes, and plasma cells) are less likely to be affected than their immature precursors. Therefore, granulocytopenia or monocytopenia must entail an effect on the bone marrow, except in the case of corticosteroids (see below).

2. The inflammatory (efferent) phase of immunity is more sensitive to immunosuppressive drugs than the afferent phase. It is therefore often possible to block the peripheral expression of an immune response without (or before) the inhibition of antibody synthesis or the acquisition of cell-mediated immunity. In human beings, corticosteroids exert their effects on inflammation not by killing inflammatory cells, but by impeding their migration from the vascular tree. This effect is relatively rapid and occurs at doses of corticosteroids that are much lower than those needed to impair the synthesis of antibodies.

3. A preexisting immune response can be inhibited by cytotoxic drugs, but relatively high doses of the agent, chronic treatment (e.g., weeks to months), or both may be needed before an effect is seen. This requirement is due to two factors: the relative resistance of "primed" lymphocytes to immunosuppressants, and the metabolic half-life of preexisting antibodies (in humans this is about 1 month for IgG).

4. Cells that produce IgG antibodies are more sensitive to cytotoxic drugs than are cells that produce IgM antibodies.

5. Immunosuppressive therapy may *increase* the production of antibodies, presumably by toxic inhibition of suppressor cells. This effect occurs irregularly in human beings.

6. The actions of primary immunosuppressants on subpopulations of human T cells and B cells remain unpredictable. Chronic therapy often results in severe lymphocytopenia, thus the ratio of T cells to B cells within the relatively few remaining lymphocytes may have little clinical significance.

7. Certain immunosuppressive agents are more or less potent than others in animal tests. Some of this variability is related to metabolic peculiarities of certain species (e.g., the rabbit is resistant to methotrexate, whereas the guniea pig is susceptible). There are, however, very few (if any) proven instances of clinical "supe-

riority" of one immunosuppressant over another. The selection of an agent in a clinical setting is therefore based on toxicology (e.g., methotrexate is contraindicated by impaired renal function), side effects (cyclophosphamide causes sterility), convenience (antilymphocyte serum must be given parenterally), or some arbitrary factor ("experience").

8. It is an unproven assumption that the production of *autoantibodies* has the same basis as that proposed for antibodies generated during normal immune responses. The mechanism that leads to pathologic autoantibodies may differ radically from that of the normal immune response. For example, the primary defect in some autoimmune diseases may involve abnormal B cells that (1) produce secondary effects on T cells and (2) are more susceptible to immunosuppression that normal B cells. Evidence in support of this idea is scarce, but two observations in patients with systemic lupus erythematosus (SLE) merit attention: (1) anergy is common in patients during active SLE, but when the disease is controlled by treatment, cutaneous delayed hypersensitivity reactions return to normal; and (2) therapy (with either corticosteroids or cytotoxic drugs, or both) often causes a reduction or disappearance of autoantibodies, yet levels of "normal" antibodies (antibacterial antibodies, isoagglutinins) generally do not change drastically.

REFERENCES

Bach JF: The Mode of Action of Immunosuppressive Agents. Amsterdam, North Holland, 1975

Baxter JD, Forsham PH: Tissue effects of glucocosteroids. Am J Med 53:573, 1972

RISKS OF IMMUNOSUPPRESSIVE THERAPY

CORTICOSTEROIDS

There is general agreement that all steroid hormones bind to cytoplasmic receptors and that the receptor–hormone complex enters the nucleus, where it interacts with DNA to induce the transcription of certain proteins. The physiologic effects of the hormones are mediated by these newly induced proteins. The nature of the protein varies with the target tissue and the chemical structure of the corticosteroid. For instance, cortisone, a potent mineralocorticoid, may induce an enzyme, Na^+ permease, that alters the entry of Na^+ into certain cells. The function of lymphocytes is affected by a corticosteroid-induced protein that blocks the cellular uptake of glucose, and glycogenesis and gluconegenesis are simulated in the liver. Some of the actions of corticosteroids may be mediated by the cyclic adenosine 3′,5′-monophosphate (cAMP) system by inhibition of cAMP phosphodiesterase. The effects of corticosteroids are widespread because virtually all tissues possess receptors for these hormones (the bladder, uterus, prostate, and seminal vesicles are notable exceptions).

In most instances the toxicity of corticosteroids is a

function of dosage and duration of treatment. Among the most serious and common side effects are increased susceptibility to infection, osteoporosis, diabetes, psychiatric disturbances, myopathy, hypertension, and suppression of adrenal cortical function, even long after therapy has been stopped. Avascular necrosis of bone and posterior subcapsular cartaracts are less common. The induction of fetal abnormalities by corticosteroid therapy during pregnancy is possible, but the magnitude of this risk is unclear. There is a general belief that a high risk of peptic ulcer complicates corticosteroid therapy. Indeed, it is routine clinical practice to prescribe antacids for patients treated with corticosteroids. This view has been challenged on the basis of a restrospective analysis of a large number of controlled therapeutic trials of corticosteroids. Peptic ulcer was observed in about the same frequency (1 percent) in both the corticosteroid- and placebo-treated groups. The connection between peptic ulcer and corticosteroid therapy requires further study.

The activation of healed tuberculosis in patients treated with corticosteroids has also been challenged. It is common practice to administer isoniazid to all patients with a positive tuberculin test or x-ray evidence of healed tuberculosis who receive corticosteroids. In one report of 132 asthmatics who were treated chronically with corticosteroids, most of the patients had positive tuberculin tests. Evidence of active tuberculosis was not found in any of the patients, even after prolonged therapy with corticosteroids. The authors argue that the incidence of isoniazid-induced hepatitis is higher than that of tuberculosis in corticosteroid-treated asthmatics. Whether their recommendations against isoniazid prophylaxis should extend to all patients is an open question. Our own practice is to individualize the decision. It seems reasonable to administer isoniazid to any patient given corticosteroids who has a documented history of tuberculosis. Alarming evidence has been uncovered that chronic corticosteroid therapy accelerates cardiovascular disease, especially hypertensive heart disease and arteriosclerosis. This might be related to the effects of corticosteroids on lipid metabolism.

The introduction of alternate-day corticosteroid therapy is an important advance. This technic reduces or avoids many of the side effects of chronic treatment, including the physical signs of Cushing's syndrome, suppression of adrenal cortical function, inhibition of growth in children, cutaneous anergy, and perhaps hyperglycemia and osteoporosis. Alternate-day therapy seems as clinically effective as daily treatment for many conditions, including asthma, nephrotic syndrome, ulcerative colitis, lupus nephritis, and dermatoses. The technic is simple. The total 48-hour dosage is given as a single dose every other day. In some patients with active disease, treatment should begin with the daily administration of conticosteroids; once there is evidence that the inflammation or the immunologic abnormality is subsiding, maintenance treatment may continue with the alternate-day technique. In a patient with active SLE, for example, treatment may begin with 80 mg of prednisone daily; if, after 3 weeks, improvement occurs, the shift from daily to alternate-day therapy can be achieved by reducing the dose by 5 or 10 mg every second or fourth day. Dosage schedules are highly variable and often depend on clinical circumstances.

THIOPURINES

Although 6-mercaptopurine (6-MP) was synthesized in 1952, the details of its antimetabolic effects remain unclear. The drug is anabolized to a ribonucleotide, which in turn inhibits the initial steps of purine synthesis by a negative feedback effect. The conversion of inosinic acid to adenylic acid, a key step in the elaboration of purines, is highly sensitive to this inhibitory process. Some 6-MP is converted to a sister compound, thioguanine, which is ultimately incorporated into DNA. The substitution of thioguanine for guanine in DNA could impair its function or structure, or both. The locus of the major effect of 6-MP remains unclear: feedback inhibition of purine synthesis, or interference with DNA via thioguanine. 6-MP is a substrate for xanthine oxidase, which converts the drug to inactive thiouric acid. The enzymatic attack on the drug can be inhibited by attachment of a nitroimidazolyl ring to the sulfur atom of 6-MP. The resulting compound, azathioprine (Imuran), ultimately converts to 6-MP in the liver. Thus, azathioprine is a "slow-release" form of 6-MP. Whether it is clinically more efficacious than 6-MP as an immunosuppressant has not been demonstrated.

The short-term toxic effects of thiopurines are those anticipated from cytototic immunosuppressants: suppression of the bone marrow and increased susceptibility to infection. Hepatitis is less common and laboratory signs of abnormal liver function generally disappear after cessation of therapy. Continued treatment in the face of abnormal liver function may cause fatal hepatitis. The toxic effects of thiopurines on the liver must be distinguished from viral hepatitis, which may develop as a consequence of immunosuppression. Fetal abnormalities may occur, but in the majority of recorded cases of azathioprine therapy during pregnancy normal infants were born.

The risk of infection caused by azathioprine is difficult to assess because most patients receive corticosteroids simultaneously. The general experience among recipients of renal transplants, almost all of whom receive azathioprine and prednisone, is that the lower the dose of prednisone, the lower the risk of infection. Unusual infections may occur. Problems in the diagnosis and treatment of infection by *Pneumocystis carinii, Nocardia, Aspergillus,* and *papovaviruses* have been commented on frequently. Nevertheless, infection of these patients by a common organism is common. Atypical clinical signs of infection may occur because of impaired inflammatory responses. It would be a pity to miss a treatable case of pneumococcal pneumonia while seeking an obscure fungus because the patient has been treated with immunosuppressants.

Suppression of the bone marrow should be avoided in most patients. The intent of primary immunosuppression is different from that of secondary immunosuppression: the latter almost always involves myelosuppression, but there is no evidence that primary immunosuppression requires myelosuppression.

CYCLOPHOSPHAMIDE

Cyclophosphamide (Cytoxan) is an alkylating agent and therefore contains the characteristic grouping N-(CH_2CH_2)-Cl_2. This chemical moiety undergoes internal cyclization in vivo and the resulting compound attacks electron-rich regions in cellular macromolecules. Cyclization of cyclophosphamide does not occur until its ring structure is metabolized, a process that occurs principally in the liver. DNA is the most sensitive of all cellular macromolecules to alkylation. The effects of cyclophosphamide on DNA include alkylation of its bases, the formation of intra- and interstrand cross links, and actual rupture of the strands of the double helix. The damage at the molecular level includes interference with replication or transcription, or both, of DNA. The effect on the cell is lethal.

The major toxic effects of cyclophosphamide are similar to those of the thiopurines. Clinically, there are additional toxic actions: alopecia, hemorrhagic cystitis, fibrosis of the bladder, and infertility. The effects on the bladder are related to the cumulative dose of the drug. Impaired gonadal function is an important consequence of cyclophosphamide therapy. Virtually all males treated with this drug develop azoospermia, which may be permanent. After cessation of treatment, several years may be required before spermatogenesis improves. Amenorrhea and impaired ovarian function are also common, especially with chronic therapy. Cyclophosphamide is secreted into human milk and may thereby affect the nursing infant. The effect of cyclophosphamide on DNA renders it teratogenic; therefore, it should be avoided during pregnancy.

METHOTREXATE

Tetrahydrofolic acid is a cofactor in the synthesis of thymidylic acid, an essential component of DNA. The vitamin converts uridylic acid to thymidylic acid by provision of a methyl group. Tetrahydrofolic acid arises from the reduction of folic acid by dihydrofolic reductase. Methotrexate binds directly and tightly to this enzyme, thereby nullifying its action. The result is a depletion of usable cellular stores of tetrahydrofolic acid. The impoverished cell cannot synthesize DNA, fails to divide, and ultimately dies. Two facts support this interpretation of the action of methotrexate: cells acquire resistance to the drug by synthesizing very large amounts of dihydrofolic reductase, and methotrexate is the only antimetabolite with a specific antidote (tetrahydrofolic acid).

Methotrexate, like the other cytotoxic immunosuppressants, kills immature cells in the bone marrow. It may cause stomatitis, especially when high doses are given. The prolonged use of methotrexate, as in patients with psoriasis, may lead to a form of hepatitis that culminates in cirrhosis. The risk of hepatitis seems lower when the drug is given intermittently (e.g., by weekly intravenous injections) than when it is given daily. Liver biopsies done before treatment with methotrexate may give misleading information because fatty liver is often found in persons sick from a variety of diseases. Fatty liver is probably not a contraindication to methotrexate therapy. High doses of methotrexate can cause a transient interstitial pneumonia. Methotrexate is filtered by renal glomeruli and actively secreted by renal tubules. The kidney is the major portal of exit of the drug from the body: 50–90 percent of each dose is excreted unchanged into the urine. Therefore, impaired renal function greatly increases the toxicity of the drug. It should be used only with extreme caution, if at all, in patients with abnormal renal function.

RISK OF NEOPLASMS

An increasing number of case reports of malignancies that developed in patients treated with immunosuppressive agents has appeared. There seems little doubt that second malignancies arise with an increased frequency in patients treated for cancer with aggressive chemotherapy or chemotherapy combined with radiotherapy. This finding has been documented in Hodgkin's disease, multiple myeloma, and ovarian carcinoma. An increased risk of cancer has also been shown in recipients of renal allografts. The extent of this risk in patients with immunoinflammatory disease who are treated with immunosuppressive drugs is not clear because the number of patients "at risk" is unknown. Moreover, there is some evidence that untreated (or minimally treated) patients with SLE have a slightly higher incidence of cancer than matched controls. This is certainly so in Sjögren's syndrome, autoimmune hemolytic anemia, and chronic ulcerative colitis. Hematologic neoplasms—lymphoma and acute myelogenous leukemia (AML)—dominate the types of malignancies that develop in these patients. This is unusual because these forms of cancer are otherwise relatively rare. A form of lymphoma, immunoblastic sarcoma, is characteristic in recipients of renal allografts. The development of acute myelogenous leukemia seems to be associated with the use of alkylating agents. We therefore caution against chronic therapy (i.e., longer than 1 year) with alkylating agents. As in every clinical decision, the risks of the treatment must be balanced against possible benefits.

REFERENCES

Anderson RJ, Schafer LA, Olin JB, et al: Infectious risk factors in the immunosuppressed host. Am J Med 54:453, 1973

Buckley BH, Roberts WC: The heart in systemic lupus erythematosus and the changes induced in it by corticosteroid therapy. Am J Med 58:243, 1975

Conn HO, Blitzer BL: Nonassociation of adrenocorticosteroid therapy and peptic ulcer. N Engl J Med 294:473, 1976

Louie S, Schwartz RS: Immunodeficiency and the pathogenesis of lymphoma and leukemia. Prog Hematol 15:117, 1978

Schatz M, Patterson R, Kloner R, Fald J: The prevalence of tuberculosis and positive tuberculin skin tests in a steroid-treated asthmatic population. Ann Intern Med 84:261, 1976

CLINICAL APPLICATIONS OF IMMUNOSUPPRESSIVE DRUGS

Immunosuppressive drugs have been used in the treatment of a great variety of diseases from multiple sclerosis to ulcerative colitis. Debates over their efficacy continue, even in the case of renal allografts. The results of prospective, controlled clinical trials have failed to settle any important issues for the following reasons: patients with end-stage disease have been selected, in whom no medication could possibly lead to improvement; relatively small groups of patients have been treated, with statistically significant but clinically dubious results; treated and control groups have not been standardized, especially in nephritis, where the prognostic importance of the histology of the renal lesion has often been neglected; and different trials involving the same disease have not been standardized, thus rendering comparisons impossible. As a result, elements of dogmatism have become inevitable.

There are, nevertheless, some guidelines that can be useful in clinical practice. The use of immunosuppressants (especially thiopurines, alkylating agents, and methotrexate) is absolutely or relatively contraindicated in the following:

1. pregnant or nursing women (with the possible exception of recipients of allografts)
2. active viral, bacterial, fungal, or parasitic infection
3. preexisting hypoplasia of the bone marrow (with the possible exception of certain cases of aplastic anemia and pure red cell anemia, currently thought to be due to autoimmunization)
4. preexisting neoplasms or preneoplastic conditions (except where treatment is directed primarily against the neoplasm)

The institution of immunosuppressive therapy obliges the physician to monitor with care the clinical and laboratory results. Before embarking on this form of treatment, all secondary or complicating features must be eliminated: for instance, hypertension that aggravates impaired renal function in lupus nephritis should be brought under control by appropriate antihypertensive drugs; the ingestion of aspirin by the thrombocytopenic patient must be stopped; and the possibility of infection in an inflamed joint of the patient with rheumatoid arthritis must be excluded. These ordinary standards of medical care are occasionally forgotten and failure to improve or inevitable complications are blamed on the treatment.

Table 1 is a list of most of the diseases in which immunosuppressive treatment has been tried. The categories that describe the possibilities of benefit are deliberately *subjective*. The term "moderate" means that for some patients a trial of immunosuppressive therapy would be a reasonable step. The term "definite" implies that patients with the stated disease will improve. "None" and "slight" are self-explanatory. Not everyone will agree with this list and it cannot be taken as authoritative or final.

The Hematology Division of the Tufts-New England

Table 1
Possibilities of Benefit of Immunosuppressive Treatment in Various Diseases

None
  Asthma
  Urticaria
  Primary biliary cirrhosis

Slight
  Scleroderma
  Pericarditis
  Myasthenia gravis
  Multiple sclerosis
  Nephritis not due to SLE

Moderate
  SLE (A,C)
  Rheumatoid arthritis (A,C)
  Inflammatory bowel disease (A)
  Chronic active hepatitis (A)
  Immunothrombocytopenia (A,C)
  Autoimmune hemolytic anemia (A,C)
  Circulating anticoagulant (A,C)
  Pure red cell aplasia (C)
  Bullous pemphigoid (A)
  Uveitis (A,C)

Definite
  Wegener's granulomatosis (A,C)
  Corticosteroid—responsive nephrotic syndrome (C)
  Psoriatic arthritis (M)
  Dermatomyositis/polymyositis (M)
  Allograft rejection (A)

A, azathioprine; C, cyclophosphamide; M, methotrexate.

Medical Center evaluates patients on an individual basis. Candidates for immunosuppressive treatment usually fall into two categories: those with corticosteroid-resistant disease or those with severe toxicity from corticosteroid therapy. Unless there are unusual circumstances, we do not use immunosuppressive treatment unless there has been a previous trial of corticosteroids. The need for *any* immunosuppressive treatment must be documented by clinical and laboratory observations.

The duration of corticosteroid treatment prior to the institution of immunosuppressive drugs depends on circumstances. For instance, a patient with aggressive dermatomyositis who has involvement of pharyngeal and intercostal muscles should, in our opinion, receive methotrexate without undue delay. By contrast, we would recommend that all alternative forms of treatment should be given before a trial of cyclophosphamide in a patient with rheumatoid arthritis. In SLE, the prime indications for azathioprine or cyclophosphamide therapy in our clinic are active diffuse glomerulonephritis, uncontrollable autoimmune hemolytic anemia or thrombocytopenia, and uncontrollable systemic symptoms. The word "uncontrollable," as used here, is often difficult to quantitate and clinical judgment is an important element in making decisions. Patients with active disease who have developed disabling complications of corticosteroid therapy (e.g., psychosis, osteoporotic fractures, diabetes, or my-

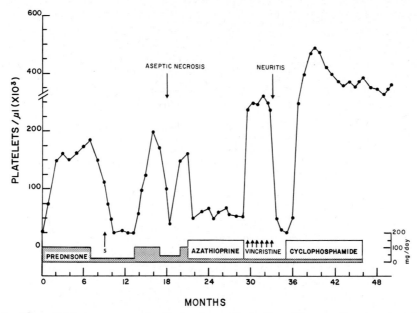

Fig. 1. Sequential immunosuppressive therapy in a patient with autoimmune thrombocytopenic purpura. Relatively high doses of corticosteroids were required to maintain a normal platelet count. Splenectomy and azathioprine failed to alter the disease. Vincristine had only a transient effect. Cyclophosphamide was associated with a prolonged remission.

opathy) are prime candidates for alternative forms of therapy. In these cases the possible benefits of azathioprine, cyclophosphamide, or methotrexate overshadow the risk factors. It is often more difficult to decide if alternative immunosuppressants should be instituted before the crippling effects of corticosteroids appear.

If a remission is induced or objective improvement occurs, every effort should be made to reduce and finally discontinue the immunosuppressive agent. We and others are now beginning to observe sustained remissions after discontinuation of all treatment. This has been noted in Wegener's granulomatosis, immunothrombocytopenia, steroid-dependent nephrotic syndrome, autoimmune hemolytic anemia, and SLE. The period of treatment can range from 2 months (nephrotic syndrome) to 1 year (Wegener's granulomatosis) before the drug can be safely stopped. If one immunosuppressant fails, another may succeed, as shown in Figure 1. The sequential application of different immunosuppressants or the use of combined immunosuppressive treatment has barely been

explored. Immunosuppressive treatment combined with plasmapheresis is a new approach that seems promising in certain diseases.

REFERENCES

Ackerman GL: Alternate-day steroid therapy in lupus nephritis. Ann Intern Med 72:519, 1970

Gershwin ME, Goetzl EJ, Steinberg AD: Cyclophosphamide: Use in practice. Ann Intern Med 80:531, 1974

Jones JV: Plasmapheresis: Great economy in the use of horses. N Engl J Med 297:1173, 1977

MacGregor RR, Sheagren JN, Lipsett MV, Wolff SM: Alternate-day prednisone therapy. N Engl J Med 28:1427, 1969

Rosman M, Bertino JR: Azathioprine. Ann Intern Med 79:694, 1973

Skinner MD, Schwartz RS: Immunosuppressive therapy of immunoinflammatory diseases. Rheum (Basel) Annu Rev 5:1, 1974

Steinberg AD, Plotz PH, Wolff SM, et al: Cytotoxic drugs in treatment of nonmalignant diseases. Ann Intern Med 76:619, 1972

Immunoglobulin E–Mast Cell–Mediator System

Robert A. Lewis and Stephen I. Wasserman

INTRODUCTION

Atopic (allergic) individuals are thought to exhibit their antigen-induced syndromes as a result of the tissue effects of mast cell and/or basophil-derived molecules, termed *mediators of immediate hypersensitivity*. The mediators include both granule-associated preformed molecules secreted by the cells as well as several newly synthesized products with varied biologic activities. The knowledge that mediators are active in disease follows from the in vitro definition of their biologic activities that relate to the pathophysiology of allergic diseases. The demonstration of non-IgE–mediated mechanisms of mediator release does not diminish the primacy of IgE-dependent events in allergy, but yields additional information on the potential influences modulating the allergic events.

As the relevance of these biologic mediators to specific diseases is discussed in the fascicle on Specific Immunologic Diseases, the present discussion will be confined to the basic biology of the initiating and effector events that provide the basis for the clinical allergic disorders.

The ordered interaction of several components is required to release the preformed mediators of immediate hypersensitivity in vitro and to generate the newly synthesized products. Included among these components are IgE, target cells (mast cells or basophils), antigen, ionic calcium, and an energy source (glucose).

ACTIVATION AND DEGRANULATION OF TARGET CELLS

IgE molecules belong to an immunoglobulin class defined by its activity in mediating allergic disease and by characteristic physicochemical properties. It has a molecular weight of 190,000 and is composed of two heavy and two light chains linked by disulfide bridges. IgE is incapable

of forming precipitates with specific antigen or of fixing complement, and it is uniquely heat labile. Its serum concentration is under genetic control and tends to be higher in atopic individuals than in normals. Papain digests IgE into three fragments, two of which (Fab) bind specific antigen, and the third (Fc) of which binds to specific surface receptors on mast cells and basophils (Fig. 1).

Mast cells and basophils possess 50,000–300,000 receptors for IgE and contain granules that stain metachromatically. The basophil is a circulating granulocyte with definable bone marrow precursors, whereas the mast cell is a tissue cell derived from an uncertain precursor. Mast cells are found along blood vessels of organs containing loose connective tissue and are numerous in lung, skin, serosa, and the mucosa of the respiratory and gastrointestinal tracts. It is relevant to their role in atopic disease that mast cells are abundant in nasal submucosa, the nasopharynx, and the peribronchial and perivascular connective tissue and mucosal surfaces of human lung; they may also be observed free in the bronchial lumen.

The IgE-dependent degranulation of mast cells and basophils is initiated by the bridging of pairs of cell-bound IgE molecules by antigen (Fig. 1). Mast cell degranulation is rapid and terminates in 2 minutes, whereas IgE-dependent basophil degranulation requires 30 minutes. The initial bridging results in an alteration of the cell mem-

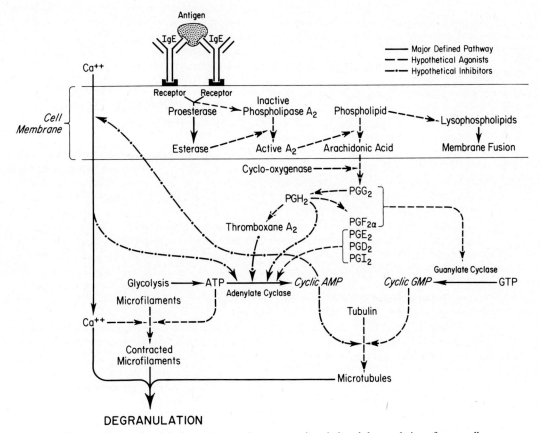

Fig. 1. Proposed metabolic pathways relevant to antigen-induced degranulation of mast cells.

brane which probably activates a surface membrane esterase. The cell membrane perturbation initiated by bridging is also reflected by increased energy-dependent calcium entry into the cell. The calcium requirement for degranulation is related to the activation of the membrane serine esterase, and perhaps also to functional requirements for the expression of phospholipase A activity, microfilament contraction, and subsequent membrane fusion. In addition, degranulation requires glucose and an intact glycolytic pathway. Finally, both ATP and calcium are required by a calcium-dependent ATPase which activates the contractile proteins of microfilaments. Following the ordered completion of these processes the perigranular membranes fuse with each other and with the cell membrane, and the granules are extruded (Fig. 1).

MODULATION OF DEGRANULATION

Several components of the reaction sequence have been defined that may act to modulate degranulation. Thus a fall in intracellular cyclic adenosine $3',5'$-monophosphate (cAMP) or a rise in cyclic guanosine $3',5'$-monophosphate (cGMP) enhances mast cell degranulation by IgE-dependent mechanisms. Increases in cAMP levels inhibit degranulation of both mast cells and basophils. Direct increases in cAMP may be induced by β-adrenergic agents, prostaglandin E_1 (PGE$_1$), and histamine. In the mast cell, falls in cAMP are a consequence of α-adrenergic stimuli, while cholinergic agonists are felt to induce increases in intracellular cGMP. The opposing actions of the cyclic nucleotides may reflect competition for a protein kinase that regulates the state of microtubule assembly. Both these structures and microfilaments have been demonstrated morphologically in rat peritoneal mast cells, but only the latter have been found in human mast cells.

Colchicine prevents microtubular aggregation and inhibits mediator release from human lung fragments and basophils, but it is a poor inhibitor of degranulation of rat mast cells. In contrast, cytochalasin B inhibits the contraction of microfilaments and suppresses immunologic degranulation of rat mast cells, but augments histamine release from human lung fragments and has little effect on basophils. These observations are suggestive of a role for these structures in degranulation, but the disparity of effects between cell types prevents clear delineation of their function. Another pharmacologic agent, cromolyn sodium, inhibits mast cell calcium uptake and subsequent histamine release but does not affect human basophils.

These differences between basophils and mast cells in modulation of mediator release may relate to the differences in granule extrusion; the basophils slowly degranulate in a piecemeal granule-by-granule fashion, whereas there is rapid fusion of multiple perigranular membranes in the mast cell.

NON-IgE–MEDIATED DEGRANULATION

A select number of agents apparently act to degranulate mast cells and basophils by interaction with receptors on their suface. Low-affinity IgG homocytotropic substances have been defined in rodents and rabbits. Rat IgGa competes with IgE in homologous mast cell degranulation, although not necessarily for the same receptors. The anaphylatoxins, C3a and C5a—products of complement activation derived from C3 and C5—degranulate both mast cells and basophils, cause wheal and flare reactions when injected intradermally in concentrations of 2×10^{-12} and 10^{-15} M, respectively, and act independently of IgE receptors.

Degranulation of both mast cells and basophils may also be induced by nonimmunologic stimuli. The enzymes chymotrypsin and cobra venom phospholipase A degranulate mast cells, probably by replacing the requirement for endogenous membrane enzyme activation. Sialidase, pronase, and phospholipase C are the only other enzymes that have been shown to degranulate rat mast cells. Sialidase removes the negatively charged cell surface sialic acid residues and thus theoretically decreases repulsion between membrane leaflets and enhances membrane fusion. Phospholipase C action on its preferred substrate, produces a transmembrane calcium transporter (ionophore). Ionophores are known to induce mast cell degranulation; synthetic examples include A23187, which has specificity for divalent cations, and the less specific X537A.

Polycationic amines and proteins such as compound 48/80, polymyxin B, neutrophil band 2 protein, protamine, and bee venom mellitin may effect mast cell mediator release by altering membrane electrostatic charges and secondarily increasing calcium influx. ATP-induced mast cell degranulation is calcium dependent and may involve a combined effect on microfilament contraction.

MEDIATORS OF IMMEDIATE HYPERSENSITIVITY

Rat mast cells contain several biologically active substances (preformed mediators) and a number of enzymes associated with their metachromatic granules, including the following: histamine, eosinophil chemotactic factors of low (about 450 daltons) and intermediate (1200–2500 daltons) molecular mass, a high molecular mass neutrophil chemotactic factor (NCF), serotonin, heparin in a macromolecular storage form, and the enzymes N-acetyl-β-D-glucosaminidase, arylsulfatase, and chymase (a chymotryptic enzyme). It is likely that most of these activities (except serotonin) will eventually be identified in the human mast cell.

Human basophils contain histamine, eosinophil and neutrophil chemotactic factors, arylsulfatase, and an arginine esterase called basophil kallikrein. As a consequence of IgE-mediated degranulation, each of these cell types also participates in the generation of newly formed lipid mediators, including slow-reacting substance of anaphylaxis (SRS-A), platelet activating factors (PAF), and the products of arachidonic acid metabolism (Table 1, pages 418–419).

BRONCHOSPASTIC AND VASOACTIVE MEDIATORS

Histamine, the product of decarboxylation of the amino acid histidine, is associated with mast cell and basophil granules. It is thought to be ionically bound to the proteoglycan–protein backbones of these granules and is displaced by sodium exchange in the extracellular fluid. Histamine is catabolized by either oxidative deamination or combined methylation and oxidative deamination. When histamine is given intravenously, its pulmonary effects are expressed as smooth muscle constriction of both large and small airways, thereby increasing airway resistance and decreasing compliance. It also dilates small radicles of the pulmonary vascular tree and increases the distance between endothelial cells of the venules, thereby increasing the potential for transudation of serum and for extravasation of leukocytes.

The biologic activities of histamine are expressed when the mediator stimulates either of two specific classes of receptors on target cells. Those receptors designated H_1 predominate in skin and smooth muscle and are blocked by classic antihistamines, while H_2 receptors, such as those in gastric mucosa, are selectively blocked by a recently developed group of compounds, including the thiourea derivatives, buramimide and metiamide. Pulmonary bronchoconstriction and vasodilation are H_1 effects, while H_2 effects include inhibition of both human lymphocyte-mediated cytotoxicity and IgE-mediated histamine release. Histamine also inhibits chemotaxis through H_2 receptors, presumably by stimulating adenylate cyclase and increasing cAMP. Patients undergoing systemic anaphylaxis, allergic asthmatics with significant pulmonary responses to antigen-inhalation challenge, and cold urticaria patients challenged locally with ice water release histamine into the systemic circulation in detectable quantities.

Slow-Reacting Substance of Anaphylaxis (SRS-A)

Although SRS-A remains structurally undefined, it is known to be an unsaturated acid sulfur–containing lipid of 300–500 daltons. It is active as a constrictor of peripheral airways to a much greater extent than of central airways, and causes vasodilation. SRS-A is generated in vivo in guinea pigs undergoing systemic anaphylaxis. Although SRS-A has not yet been demonstrated in vivo in the human, lung tissue, dispersed pulmonary cells, nasal polyps, and peripheral leukocytes generate SRS-A during IgE-dependent immunologic reactions.

The generation of this mediator subsequent to mast cell or basophil degranulation does not identify its cell source(s). The facts that decreasing amounts of SRS-A are generated by increasingly pure human lung mast cell preparations and that a calcium ionophore has the capacity to initiate SRS-A generation in other cell types imply the possible involvement of another cell type in its generation.

Presently the only acceptable assay for SRS-A employs the antihistamine-treated guinea pig ileum, but it is not specific for this mediator. Therefore, SRS-A must be further identified by its solvent elution profile from lipophyllic columns, its susceptibility to inactivation by arylsulfatases, and its decreased assayability in the presence of a semispecific blocker, FPL55712.

Bronchospastic Arachidonic Acid Metabolites

In the human, products of arachidonic acid metabolism constitute the vast majority of prostaglandins and related compounds. Arachidonic acid is mobilized from cell membrane phospholipids in a number of mammalian cells by the action of phospholipase A_2. It is then either metabolized to prostaglandins and thromboxanes by a series of enzymatic steps beginning with cyclooxygenase, or converted by a lipooxygenase to 12-L-hydroxy-5,8,-10,14 eicosatetraenoic acid (HETE), and related compounds (Fig. 1, page 420). Several of these products have been described in vitro subsequent to anaphylactic challenge of lung tissue and rat mast cells. Guinea pig central airway smooth muscle is constricted by $PGF_2\alpha$, thromboxane A_2, and both cyclic endoperoxides PGG_2 and PGH_2. In the anesthetized dog, $G_2\alpha$ and D_2 both constrict central and peripheral airways. While prostaglandins of the E and F series may be identified by radioimmunoassay, other arachidonic acid products must be isolated and measured by thin-layer chromatography or gas chromatography—mass spectroscopy.

Arginine Esterase

A preformed enzyme termed *argenine esterase* (basophil or lung kallikrein) is released subsequent to antigen challenge of IgE-sensitized human basophils or lung fragments. This activity can cleave kininogen to yield bradykinin and/or lysylbradykinin. The products may contract bronchial smooth muscle and increase vascular permeability. Kinins have also been noted to induce bronchospasm when inhaled by asthmatic humans and have been detected in the serum of a single patient sustaining an acute asthma attack. The smooth muscle–constricting potential of these products allows their biologic assay by dose-related constriction of a variety of mammalian tissue preparations in organ bath.

Platelet-Activating Factors (PAF)

Although PAF are themselves neither bronchospastic nor vasoactive, they induce platelet aggregation and subsequent release of serotonin (5-hydroxytryptamine; 5-HT). This monoamine has contracting activity on several smooth muscle preparations and induces pulmonary venular transudation in the rat, but it is without apparent bronchospastic effect on the human lung. PAF are immunologically generated subsequent to IgE-mediated reactions in both human lung and peripheral leukocytes, as well as in rabbit lung and leukocytes, and by IgGa-dependent mechanisms in the rat peritoneal cavity. The best chemically described PAF are apparently phospholipids, susceptible to inactivation by phospholipases. PAF from different sources are not identical, as shown by the inability of rabbit PAF from two sources to deactivate platelets to the biologic effects of each other and by the somewhat different phospholipase inactivation profiles of rabbit leukocyte and rat peritoneal PAF.

Table 1
Mediators of Immediate Hypersensitivity

Mediator	Structural Characteristics	Function	Inhibition	Inactivation
Bronchospastic and vasoactive activity				
Histamine (preformed)	β-imidazolylethylamine MW 111	Contraction of smooth muscle; increase of vascular permeability; elevation of cAMP; stimulation of suppressor T lymphocytes; generation of prostaglandins; enhancement (H_1) or inhibition (H_2) of chemotaxis	H_1 classic H_2 thiourea	Histaminase (diamine oxidase); histamine N-methyl transferase
SRS-A (newly generated)	Acid hydrophilic sulfur-containing lipid MW 400	Contraction of smooth muscle; increased vascular permeability; synergistic with histamine; generation of prostaglandins	FPL-55712	Arylsulfatases A and B
Serotonin (preformed)	5-hydroxytryptamine MW 176	Contraction of some smooth muscle; increased vascular permeability	Hydroxyrine cyproheptadine; lysergic acid	Monoamine oxidase
PAF(s) (newly generated)	Lipidlike MW 400–1000	Release of platelet amines; platelet aggregation; sequestration of platelets	Unknown	Phospholipase D (rat) or A/C (rabbit)
Arachidonic acid metabolites (newly generated)	C-20 fatty acids (HHT C-17 fatty acid)	Contraction of smooth muscle (PGD_2, $PGF_2\alpha$, TxA_2, PGG_2, PGH_2); relaxation of smooth muscle (PGE_2); elevated cAMP (PGE, PGD, PGI); elevated cGMP ($PGF_2\alpha$, PGG_2); dose-dependent chemotactic attraction of eosinophils or neutrophils (HETE or HHT)	Unknown	Specific dehydrogenases
Chemotactic activity				
ECF-A (preformed)	Val/Ala–Gly–Ser–Glu MW 360–390	Chemotactic attraction and deactivation of eosinophils and neutrophils	Val/Ala–Gly–Ser; Gly–Ser–Glu	Aminopeptidase Carboxypeptidase A
ECF-oligopeptides (preformed)	Peptides MW 1300–2500	Chemotactic attraction and deactivation of eosinophils and neutrophils	Unknown	Unknown

CHEMOTACTIC MEDIATORS
Eosinophil Chemotactic Factor of Anaphylaxis (ECF-A)

The first mast cell–associated chemotactic factor described, ECF-A, was identified in the anaphylactic supernatant of challenged guinea pig lung fragments and subsequently in the analogous human tissue and rat mast cells. This factor is preferentially chemotactic for eosinophils. It also deactivates this cell type to further chemotactic migration. A small peptide of about 400 daltons, ECF-A has also been identified preformed in purified rat mast cell granules and human lung. This mediator from

Table 1 *continued*

Mediator	Structural Characteristics	Function	Inhibition	Inactivation
NCF (preformed)	Neutral protein MW > 750,000	Chemotactic attraction and deactivation of neutrophils	Unknown	Unknown
Lipid chemotactic factors (newly generated)	? HHT; ? HETE; ? other lipids	Chemotactic attraction of neutrophils and eosinophils; chemokinesis of neutrophils; deactivation of neutrophils	Unknown	Unknown
Histamine (preformed)	β-imidazolylethylamine MW 111	H_1 chemotactic and chemokinetic activation of eosinophils	H_1 classic	Histaminase (diamine oxidase);
		H_2 chemotactic and chemokinetic inhibition of neutrophils and eosinophils	H_2 thiourea	Histamine N-methyl transferase

Structural components

Mediator	Structural Characteristics	Function	Inhibition	Inactivation
Heparin (preformed)	Proteoglycan MW ~750,000 (rat mast cells), N and O sulfated	Anticoagulation; antithrombin III interaction; inhibition of complement activation	Protamine	Heparinase
Chondroitin 6-sulfate (preformed)	Proteoglycan (guinea pig basophils)	Unknown	Unknown	Chondroitinase
Dermatan sulfate (preformed)	Proteoglycan (guinea pig basophils)	Unknown	Unknown	Chondroitinase

Enzymes

Mediator	Structural Characteristics	Function	Inhibition	Inactivation
Chymase (preformed)	Protein MW 29,000	Proteolysis with chymotryptic specificity	Serotonin; heparin; chymotrypsin inhibitors	Unknown
Arylsulfatase (preformed)	Protein MW 116,000 (A) or 50,000 (B)	Hydrolysis of SRS-A and various sulfate esters	PO_4; SO_4; product, substrate	Unknown
N-acetyl-β-D-glucosaminidase (preformed)	Protein MW 158,000	Cleavage of glucosamine residues	Product	Unknown
Basophil (lung) kallikrein of anaphylaxis (preformed)	Protein MW 400,000	Cleavage of kinin from kininogen, tryptic specificity	Trypsin inhibitors	Unknown

Abbreviations: MW, molecular weight; SRS-A, slow-reacting substance of anaphylaxis; PAF(s), platelet-activating factor(s); HHT, 12-L-hydroxy-5,8,10 heptadecatrienoic acid; PG, prostoglandins; TxA_2, thromboxane A_2; HETE, 12-L-hydroxy-5,8,10,14 eicosatetraenoic acid.

human lung has been structurally characterized as two acidic tetrapeptides with the amino acid sequence Val/Ala–Gly–Ser–Glu.

Intermediate Molecular Weight Eosinophil Chemotactic Peptides

Sephadex G-25 chromatograms of eosinophilotactic activities extractable from rat mast cells and human lung fragments consistently demonstrate peptides of 1200–2500 daltons in addition to ECF-A. These activities are immunologically releasable and capable of deactivating their target cells.

Neutrophil Chemotactic Factors (NCF)

Originally noted in the released material from ionophore-stimulated leukemic human basophils, NCF activities excluded on Sephadex G-25 have been described in rat mast cells, human lung fragments, and the serum of

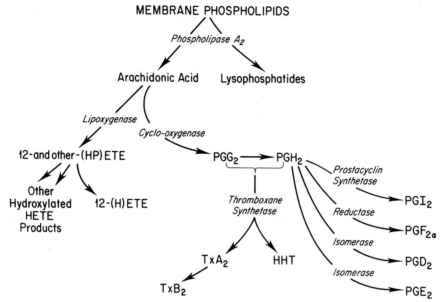

Fig. 1. Pathway for generation of oxidative products of arachidonic acid.

asthmatic patients following inhalation challenge with specific antigen. NCF has also been characterized as a 750,000-dalton neutral protein from the venous effluent of ice water–challenged extremities of cold urticaria patients. These factors attract and deactivate neutrophils in vitro.

Histamine

In addition to its smooth muscle and vasoactive effects, histamine is a weak chemotactic factor for eosinophils. It also enhances random eosinophil and neutrophil motility and augments chemotactic response by these cells by an H_1 mechanism. Histamine may also inhibit eosinophil and neutrophil leukocyte chemokinesis (nondirected migration) and chemotaxis via an H_2 effect.

HETE and Other Lipid Chemotactic Factors

The lipooxygenase product of arachidonic acid, HETE, has an ECF-A–like spectrum of activity. Unlike ECF-A, however, it also increases eosinophil chemokinesis. Equivalent effects on neutrophils have recently been described for the cyclooxygenase product 12-L-hydroxy-5,8,10-heptadecatrienoic acid (HHT). A possibly related factor, extractable from rat peritoneal anaphylactic exudate, is a nonpolar lipid with chemotactic activity mainly for neutrophils.

Heparin and Mast Cell Granule-Associated Enzymes

The rat peritoneal mast cell granule has a latticelike structure on electron photomicrographs and consists of sulfate proteoglycans and proteins. The former material is responsible for the metachromatic staining of the granules and, in the rat, is predominantly heparin. The granule protein consists, at least in part, of several enzymes: one with chymotrypsinlike proteolytic specificity, termed

chymase, N-acetyl-β-D-glucosaminidase, arylsulfatase, and possibly a tryptase.

The heparin in the rat mast cell granule is stored as a high molecular weight (about 750,000 daltons) proteoglycan which is released immunologically with histamine during degranulation. This heparin has only 10–20 percent of the anticoagulant activity of commercial heparin on a molar basis. In addition to its anti-thrombin III cofactor activity, heparin interferes with the formation of the alternative complement pathway convertase. Heparin is also present in mast cell–rich fractions of dispersed human lung cells. Glycosaminoglycans of the basophil have been defined only for the guinea pig; in that cell they consist of chondroitin and dermatan sulfates rather than heparin.

Arylsulfatases A and B have been identified in both mast cells and leukemic basophils of the rat; an uncharacterized activity has been identified in mast cell–rich dispersed human lung cells and leukemic basophils. These enzymes inactivate SRS-A, as do arylsulfatases from other sources. Furthermore, arylsulfatase A is immunologically released with the mast cell granule in the rat.

Chymase has been isolated from the mast cell of the rat but has been identified only histochemically in the human mast cell. This enzyme is minimally active as a protease while stored in the granule, probably due to active site inhibition by serotonin and masking of the active site by heparin. Once freed, its specific activity is comparable to that of pancreatic α-chymotrypsin. Chymase may be physically reassociated with macromolecular heparin in vitro.

The N-acetyl-β-D-glucosaminidase and tryptase activities noted in rat mast cell granules have yet to be defined in the human. Finally, the kininogen-cleaving activities immunologically released from human lung and leukocytes (designated, respectively, lung and basophil kallikrein of anaphylaxis) have an undefined relationship with the rat mast cell granule proteases.

RELATIVE MEDIATOR RELEASE

Since the preformed mediators of immediate hypersensitivity are granule associated, they are released from the mast cell when fusion of cell membrane and perigranular membranes produces open channels between granule contents and the extracellular fluid. Histamine and ECF-A are released from the granule by ion exchange and may be found in the extracellular milieu in the absence of degranulation, whereas heparin and chymase are tightly granule bound and their liberation occurs only after actual granule extrusion. This implies that the quantities, rates of release, and biologic activities of different preformed mediators are regulated not only by the degree of mast cell activation but also by the avidity with which they are granule associated. An example of such regulation is the increase in proteolytic activity of rat mast cell chymase following granule solubilization. The prolonged kinetics of basophil histamine release which relate to the piecemeal (granule-by-granule) extrusion and delayed contact between granule contents and extracellular fluid represents another type of regulation of mediator release.

The relative quantities of preformed and newly generated mediators released also vary and may reflect differences in the intensity of the immunologic stimulus. Thus intracellular SRS-A accumulates after immunologic stimuli that are too slight to elicit its release or that of histamine despite the fact that the intracellular accumulation of SRS-A begins within seconds of immunologic challenge and increases in parallel with histamine release. However, SRS-A release begins only after histamine release is essentially complete. Experimentally, SRS-A release is suppressed by some chemical additives, such as isoproterenol in the presnce of carbamylcholine and the cytochalasins A and B, which either enhance or do not affect histamine release. Furthermore, doses of indomethacin which do not alter histamine release enhance SRS-A generation and release. Finally, human lung fragments from different patients release quantities of SRS-A that are totally independent of the maximal degree of histamine release.

MEDIATOR INTERACTIONS

Although the mediators of immediate hypersensitivity are assayed for their isolated effects in vitro, their effects in vivo may be modified by competition or synergism; thus the constricting effects of histamine upon the guinea pig ileum in vitro are potentiated by SRS-A. Both SRS-A and histamine are known to induce release of prostaglandins from lung tissue, thereby modifying their own spasmogenic activity.

A greater number of observations have been made regarding chemotactic mediator interactions. Histamine in high doses inhibits and in low doses facilitates eosinophil chemotaxis induced by ECF-A tetrapeptides. Imidazole acetic acid, a catabolic product of histamine, is also chemotactic for eosinophils. The N-terminal tripeptide degradation product of the ECF-A tetrapeptides is a reversible stimulus-specific inhibitor of eosinophil chemotaxis toward the ECF-A tetrapeptides, while the C-terminal tripeptide is a cell-directed irreversible inhibitor. This observation anticipates demonstration of ECF-A catabolism by circulating peptidases and related mast cell and granulocyte enzymes. Finally, PGE_1 inhibits neutrophil chemotaxis by increasing cellular cAMP, while $PGF_2\alpha$, via cGMP, has the opposite effect.

EFFECTOR TISSUE RESPONSIVENESS

The dose-dependent action of the mediators of immediate hypersensitivity may be altered by adrenergic and cholinergic influences on the effector tissues. Airway constrictor responses to histamine, $PGF_2\alpha$ and PGD_2 are inhibited by atropine, as is histamine-induced bronchospasm in the asthmatic or respiratory virus–infected human. β-adrenergic agents directly relax respiratory smooth muscle in asthmatic humans, thus quantitatively altering respiratory responses to bronchospastic mediators. The demonstrated innervation of mammalian airway smooth muscle underlies the physiologic relevance of these pharmacologic observations.

MEDIATOR INACTIVATION

Effective tissue response to the mediators of immediate hypersensitivity is time limited even in untreated patients with atopic disease. While this phenomenon reflects both a limited availability of all mediators, probable tachyphylaxis to some, and mediator clearance by excretion, it is also presumably affected by enzymatic inactivation of these biologic activities. As many mast cell–derived chemotactic mediators are eosinophilotactic, the eosinophil content of mediator-inactivating enzymes may provide a feedback control of mediator effects. Notably, the eosinophil contains histaminase, arylsulfatase, and phospholipase D, which inactivate histamine, SRS-A, and PAF, respectively. SRS-A is inactivated not only by extracted eosinophil arylsulfatase, but also by the enzyme-rich resting granulocyte, presumably after cellular uptake of the mediator.

Some other cells also contain mediator-inactivating enzymes. Neutrophils contain histaminase, and at least one mononuclear cell population is rich in histamine methyltransferase. Interestingly, both mast cells and basophils contain arylsulfatase.

Inactivation of arachidonic acid metabolites is complicated, as some intermediate metabolic products are biologically active. Thus PGD_2 and thromboxane A_2 derived from the cyclic endoperoxides are potent bronchoconstrictors. However, most stable catabolic end products of arachidonic acid metabolism, such as thromboxand B_2 (from thromboxane A_2) and 6-keto-PG-$F_1\alpha$ (from PGI_2) have little or no defined biologic activity.

CONCLUSION

The mast cell and basophil-derived preformed and newly generated mediators of immediate hypersensitivity are released by IgE-dependent mechanisms and are biologically available during allergic events. The relevance of these mediators to allergic disease has been derived from studies of the pathophysiologic alterations induced by the individual mediators, identification of the mediators in tissue or biologic fluids of patients experiencing allergic reactions, and the known pathophysiology of the various atopic diseases.

Mediators of immediate hypersensitivity not only possess the ability to induce immediate tissue responses such as a wheal and flare, anaphylaxis, or rapid-onset brief-duration alterations in pulmonary function, but may also mediate a prolonged inflammatory response. The fact that IgE and mast cells are relevant to prolonged inflammatory events has been documented by passive transfer, with isolated IgE, of delayed (4–12 hours) inflammatory responses in skin and by the dependence upon IgE antibody for similar delayed alterations in lung mechanics following inhalation of antigen. In lung, these delayed responses are prevented by pretreatment with disodium cromoglycate, which supports the central role

of the mast cell. Histopathologic assessment of delayed responses reveals an influx of neutrophils, eosinophils, basophils, lymphocytes, and mononuclear leukocytes, the deposition of fibrin, and vascular abnormalities which may progress to frank vasculitis. Although some of the mediators responsible for the early and later phases of the IgE–mast cell reaction can be surmised from the kinetics of their in vitro effects, their absolute identification and participation in atopic disease requires further definition.

The postulated role of the mast cell and its mediators in inflammation may provide insight into the clinical evolution of some allergic disorders such as progression of seasonal to perennial asthma. Although much remains to be clarified, the rapidly expanding understanding of target cell activation together with the identification of mast cell and basophil-derived mediators provides a framework for definition of the complex processes that lead to atopic diseases.

Lysosomes

Robert B. Zurier

NATURE OF LYSOSOMES

LYSOSOMES AS ORGANELLES

The study of cellular organelles, while a collaborative effort, usually begins with the morphologic observations of the cell anatomist followed by the biochemist's analysis of the isolated organelles and their molecular components. The pattern was reversed for lysosomes, whose nature and function were not recognized until they had been characterized chemically. In 1949 deDuve and his colleagues, using the then newly developed technic of centrifugal fractionation of cells, isolated a class of subcellular particles from rat liver having centrifugal properties intermediary between those of mitochondria and microsomes. These particles were found to have a high content of acid phosphatase and other hydrolytic enzymes. By centrifugation it was calculated that the size of the particles was 0.2–0.8 μm.

It was also determined that these enzymes were inactive toward their potential substrates if the fraction was carefully prepared to avoid disruption of the organelles. However, preparation of the fraction without regard to cellular organization, or exposure of the fraction to decreased osmotic pressure (distilled water), blendorization, or surface-active agents (detergents) resulted in a considerable increase in enzyme activity. This special relationship between particle and enzymes whereby disruption of the organelle is required for maximum enzyme activity is termed *structure-linked latency*, and its establishment led to the hypothesis that the acid hydrolases are packaged together in a previously undescribed, mem-

brane-bound organelle. Because of its cargo of hydrolytic enzymes the particle was called a lysosome (Greek: *lysis,* dissolution; *soma,* body).

In 1955, Novikoff obtained the first electron micrographs of deDuve's cell fractions containing partially purified lysosomes. Particles morphologically distinctive from mitochondria were seen which gave a positive staining reaction for acid phosphatase. Thus, the cytochemical definition of lysosomes as particles that are bound by a single unit membrane and yield a positive staining reaction for acid phosphatase may be considered for most practical purposes as equivalent to the biochemical definition.

The isolation and characterization in the 1960s of lysosomal granules from polymorphonuclear leukocytes opened an era of intensive research during which the origin, composition, and function of these polymorphic organelles have been elucidated. Two types of granules, elaborated at different stages of differentiation and originating from opposite faces of the Golgi complex, have been described. Azurophil granules appear early, arise from the concave surface of the Golgi complex, and are rich in acid phosphatase and peroxidase. Smaller specific granules appear later in myelocyte maturation, arise from the convex side of the Golgi, and are rich in alkaline phosphatase. Particles of lower density containing the remainder of acid hydrolases are heterogeneous.

There are four principal varieties of lysosome: the storage granule, the heterophagic vacuole, the autophagic vacuole, and the residual body. The first is a primary, or pure lysosome; the other three are secondary lysosomes.

The primary lysosome is a membrane-limited structure containing newly synthesized acid hydrolases that have not as yet participated in acts of digestion. Electron microscopic observations led to the conclusion that lysosomal enzymes are synthesized by ribosomes, accumulate in the rough-surfaced endoplasmic reticulum, enter the cisternae of the endoplasmic reticulum, and then are transported to the smooth endoplasmic reticulum, where small vesicles containing the hydrolases bud and pinch off. These vesicles merge with elements of the Golgi complex which serve to concentrate their contents by removal of water and low molecular weight constituents.

VACUOLAR SYSTEM

It is now recognized that rather than referring to a particular "soma," the term *lysosome* encompasses all the various forms of vesicles, granules, and pockets of the vacuolar system or apparatus, the role of which involves the intracellular digestion of endogenous and exogenous substrates. The vacuolar apparatus is a dynamic system that enables materials to move into, through, and out of the cell while remaining at all times screened from the cytoplasm. Materials enter the cell by a process termed *endocytosis,* a word which represents all the cell's engulfing properties, including phagocytosis, pinocytosis, and micropinocytosis. A portion of the cell membrane first attaches itself to the material to be ingested and then appears to be sucked inward to form an internal pocket containing the material. The pocket pinches free from the cell membrane and is now a phagosome.

The initial phagosome, an enclave of external milieu separated from the cytoplasm by a bit of plasma membrane, rapidly leaves the periphery where it was formed and moves toward the center of the cell. During that migration it may become fragmented by budding or may merge with other phagosomes, and then it fuses with the membrane of a primary lysosome. The lysosomal enzymes are discharged in an explosive fashion into the phagosome, there to degrade the ingested material. The new vacuole is a phagolysosome, or heterophagic vacuole. The merger of phagosome with primary lysosome is generally assumed to occur by fusion of the phagosomal membrane with that of the lysosome. It is not clear why lysosomal membranes fuse only with those of phagosomes or plasma membrane but not with mitochondrial or nuclear membranes.

When a cell must sacrifice a portion of its own cytoplasm as a result of sublethal injury (irradition, anoxia), starvation, or active catabolism, an autophagic vacuole forms that is bounded by a single or double membrane and encloses such structures as mitochondria, Golgi vesicles, and endoplasmic reticulum. Autophagy may be the process whereby the normal wear and tear of organelles is controlled by what amounts to physiologic focal autolysis.

When lysosomes have completed digestive functions as either hetero- or autophagic vacuoles, they appear filled with debris. The resultant structures are the residual body form of lysosomes.

REFERENCES

deDuve C: Lysosomes, a new group of cytoplasmic particles, in Hiyashi T (eds): Subcellular Particles. New York, Ronald Press, 1959, p 128

deDuve C, Wattiaux R: Functions of lysosomes. Ann Rev Physiol 28:435, 1966

Novikoff AB: Lysosomes and related particles, in Brachet J, Mirsky AE (eds): The Cell, vol. 2. New York, Academic Press, 1961, pp 423–488

LYSOSOMES AND TISSUE INJURY

Lysosomes and the extracellular release of lysosomal enzymes are important to both natural immunity and acute inflammation, and their study has helped in the understanding of the pathogenesis of joint tissue injury that occurs in the rheumatic diseases. An important property of lysosomes is their stability in living cells. Among the first suggestions relating the lysosome concept to pathology was the possibility that lysosomal membranes might rupture and that an excessive or inappropriate release of enzymes into the cell sap or surrounding medium would cause cell and tissue damage. It is now clear that although lysosomes are suitably equipped for this role, the circumstances under which they act as "suicide sacs" are rare (one of these is the loss of integrity of lysosomal membranes with escape of enzymes and cell death which follows uptake of monosodium urate crystals by polymorphonuclear leukocytes during an attack of gouty arthritis). However, by a variety of mechanisms which resemble secretory processes in other cells, polymorphonuclear leukocytes and macrophages are able to release lysosomal enzymes in a sort of reverse endocytosis without incurring cell damage. Enzyme release (secretion) appears to be regulated by cellular cyclic nucleotides, transmembrane divalent cation movement, and rapid alterations in the cytoskeleton (microtubules and microfilaments).

ACUTE JOINT INFLAMMATION

There is substantial evidence that lysosomes can mediate, in part, acute and chronic inflammation in joints. The local lesions of rheumatoid arthritis—the appearance in synovial fluid of neutrophils, hypertrophy and hyperplasia of synovial lining cells, clusters of lymphocytes in the synovium, pannus formation, and cartilage degradation—all develop in laboratory animals injected with lysates of purified lysosomes. Synovial fluid from patients with rheumatoid arthritis is rich in lysosomal enzymes and their synovial cells contain residual bodies indicative of lysosomal activity. During phagocytosis of immune complexes, neutrophils and phagocytic synovial cells release lysosomal enzymes into the joint space, a process that helps initiate and perpetuate inflammation and tissue injury.

The major macromolecules of cells and extracellular materials such as collagen, protein, polysaccharides, nucleic acids, etc. can be broken down by lysosomal enzymes. Neutral and acid proteases ordinarily contained within lysosomes can split molecules whose biologic function is to initiate and propagate inflammation. They can cleave complement components to subfractions that are chemotactic for polymorphonuclear leukocytes. They can disrupt mast cells, with a resultant release of vasoactive amines, and they can cause increased vascular permeability. In short, they can help initiate acute inflammatory reactions.

CHRONIC JOINT INFLAMMATION

Lysosomes are also important to chronic inflammatory responses. The uptake and processing of antigen by the vacuolar system of macrophages helps initiate the immune response. Lysosomes may also be relevant to lymphocyte function. When lymphocytes are stimulated by antigen to transform, immediately prior to cell division there is an increase in the number of lysosomes as well as enzyme release to the surrounding media. Many of the lymphocytes that appear as follicular clusters in rheumatoid arthritis synovium resemble lymphocytes stimulated by specific antigen. Such cells are therefore equipped with an augmented complement of lysosomal hydrolases. Lysosomal enzymes may alter tissue constituents and render them antigenic. These degraded substances stimulate formation of antibodies that can react with both altered and normal tissue constituents. An environment may then be created for persistent immune response and inflammation.

REFERENCES

Weissmann G: Lysosomal mechanisms of tissue injury in arthritis. N Engl J Med 286:141, 1972

Zvaifler NJ: The immunopathology of joint inflammation in rheumatoid arthritis. Adv Immunol 16:265, 1973

DIFFERENTIAL APPROACH TO MAJOR IMMUNOLOGIC SYNDROMES

Hypergammaglobulinemia

Edward C. Franklin

DIFFERENTIAL DIAGNOSIS OF DIFFUSE HYPERGAMMAGLOBULINEMIA

The concentration of the aggregate of normal immunoglobulins, regardless of type and function, is most readily estimated by electrophoretic techniques, which give a rather accurate quantitation of the sum of all classes and subclasses of immunoglobulins. Heavy chain–related classes can be readily quantitated by a variety of methods, but the difficulties in producing appropriate specific antisera to subclasses preclude this type of analysis for routine clinical use even though their concentrations may on occasion be of clinical interest.

Increased levels of gamma globulins are, in all instances, due to synthesis of excessive amounts of immunoglobulins since there are no diseases associated with a decrease in catabolism. There are two major types of hypergammaglobulinemia. The first of these is a diffuse heterogeneous increase of all immunoglobulins, which is associated with a variety of inflammatory, infectious, and neoplastic diseases, as well as chronic diseases of the liver (Table 1). This type of hypergammaglobulinemia, even if analyzed in as detailed a manner as possible, is generally of very little diagnostic value and does not really warrant the effort and expense involved in attempting to determine the contribution of the various classes and subclasses of immunoglobulins to the increase in gamma globulin. Nevertheless, the finding of a diffuse increase in immunoglobulins points toward the types of diseases listed in Table 1 and can be interpreted only in the light of the clinical findings.

In diseases associated with a diffuse increase of immunoglobulins, a search for specific antibodies may, however, be of some value. For example, the finding of high titers of antinuclear antibodies, rheumatoid factors, antibodies to thyroglobulin and other thyroid antigens, and antibodies to certain tissue constituents, such as mitochondria and other structures, can obviously point in the direction of some of the connective tissue diseases, rheumatoid arthritis, thyroid abnormalities, biliary cirrhosis, etc.; tests attempting to detect specific antibodies should definitely be initiated. In addition, in many bacterial and viral infections, some of which may be associated with a diffuse increase in gamma globulins, and in some of the complications caused by the presence of immune complexes, the finding of a specific antibody to a certain bacterial or viral substance may point to a causal role for that agent, which may sometimes be difficult or impossible to culture. In certain instances, for example, in acute rheumatic fever, acute poststreptococcal glomerulonephritis, and other similar diseases that are diagnosed long after the subsidence of the acute infection, the finding of a change in antibody titer may be very significant in establishing the diagnosis.

Thus, in disorders associated with a diffuse increase in gamma globulins, a great deal of information can be obtained by identifying the responsible antibody. It should be remembered that in many of these diseases the marked increase in gamma globulin is due to the augmentation of a variety of different immunoglobulins, only a few of which are measured when one identifies a single antibody type.

Table 1
Diseases Associated with Hyperglobulinemia

Polyclonal*
  Infections: bacterial, viral, fungal, or parasitic, especially in the chronic stage
  Liver disease: various types of cirrhosis and hepatitis
  Connective tissue diseases: rheumatoid arthritis, systemic lupus erythematosus, polyarteritis, scleroderma, Sjögren's syndrome, etc.
  Chronic granulomatous diseases: sarcoidosis, ulcerative colitis, granulomatous ileitis
  Hematologic malignancies: certain rare instances of lymphoma, Hodgkin's disease, leukemia
  Endocrine: thyroiditis
  Miscellaneous: hypergammaglobulinemic purpura, amyloidosis, certain carcinomas

Monoclonal
  Multiple myeloma
  Macroglobulinemia
  Benign monoclonal gammopathy
  Heavy chain diseases and other immunoglobulin variants

*On rare occasions, many of these diseases can have monoclonal components.

Table 1
Features of Monoclonal Hypergammaglobulinemic Disorders

| Test | Multiple Myeloma | Macroglobulinemia | Benign Monoclonal Gammopathy | Heavy Chain Diseases | | |
				γ	α	μ
Clinical	Bone lesions	Lymphadenopathy	None	Lymphadenopathy	Intestinal lymphoma	Chronic lymphocytic leukemia
	Anemia	Hepatosplenomegaly		Hepatosplenomegaly	Malabsorption	Lymphadenopathy
	Infections			No bony lesions		Hepatosplenomegaly
Bone marrow	Plasma cellular infiltrates (sheets)	Lymphocytosis or lymphocytoid plasma cells	Moderate plasmacytosis (<10%)	Plasma cells or lymphocytoid plasma cells	—	Lymphocytosis or lymphocytoid plasma cells with vacuoles
Electrophoresis Serum	(−)					(+)
Urine	20%	10%	Rare	Common	Rare	Common
Immunoelectrophoresis Serum	One type of heavy chain (γ, λ, δ, or ϵ)	μ chain	One type of heavy chain (γ, λ, δ or ϵ)	γ chain	α chain	μ chain
	One type of light chain (κ or λ)	One type of light chain (κ or λ)	One type of light chain (κ or λ)	No light chain	No light chain	Free κ or λ in two-thirds
Urine	κ or λ	κ or λ	Rare κ or λ	—	—	κ or λ in two-thirds

DIFFERENTIAL DIAGNOSIS OF MONOCLONAL HYPERGAMMAGLOBULINEMIA

Electrophoresis and immunoelectrophoresis are used for the precise characterization of immunoglobulins in diseases that are accompanied by the production of a single monoclonal homogeneous immunoglobulin (see Table 1 in preceding chapter) and in immunodeficiency states. The predominant clinical features as well as the characteristic electrophoretic patterns that might be encountered are summarized in Table 1.

Multiple Myeloma

Approximately 98 percent of patients with multiple myeloma have an abnormal homogeneous protein in the serum, the urine, or both. The important feature of the electrophoretic pattern is the presence of a monoclonal homogeneous protein with a mobility ranging from the slow gamma to the alpha globulins. The homogeneity and narrowness of the peak is more important than the absolute concentration. In all instances in which such a monoclonal protein is seen, routine electrophoretic analysis alone, with rare exceptions, does not allow a more precise definition of the class of immunoglobulin involved. In order to do this, immunoelectrophoresis or immunoglobulin class and subclass quantitation are required. All types of multiple myeloma give a homogeneous monoclonal spike with the exception of certain IgA myelomas, which tend to give a broad heterogeneous peak in the beta or alpha$_2$ globulin region, largely due to the fact that these proteins exist in the serum as a series of polymers and also vary significantly in carbohydrate content.

Approximately 20 percent of patients with myeloma produce a Bence Jones protein in addition to a serum myeloma protein. Comparison of the serum and urine of patients that have both a Bence Jones protein and a myeloma protein generally shows the two proteins to have different electrophoretic mobilities. If the mobilities are identical, it is purely coincidental or it may indicate, especially if large amounts of albumin or other lower molecular weight protein are present, the loss in the urine of the myeloma protein.

In patients with multiple myeloma, quantitation of immunoglobulins generally reveals a marked increase (usually greater than 2.5–3 g/dl) in one class of immunoglobulin, often associated with a concomitant depression of the other classes of immunoglobulins. This depression of background immunoglobulins is important in the diagnosis of myeloma and helps to distinguish it from benign monoclonal gammopathy. In general, regular inspection of the electrophoretic pattern suffices for routine follow-up as it allows the ready detection of changes in the myeloma protein and the remaining gamma globulin; more accurate quantitation is usually unnecessary. Examination of the urine is carried out most easily by the heat test for Bence Jones proteins, but more accurately by electrophoretic and immunoelectrophoretic analyses. It should be remembered that Bence Jones proteins are often missed by the usual Albustick test used to detect protein in the urine. In general, early in the disease, only the Bence Jones protein is visible. As renal damage occurs, the Bence Jones protein can be obscured by other serum proteins that spill in the urine, and, in many instances, even the myeloma protein may occur in very large amounts. It should be noted that Bence Jones proteins can often be produced in the absence of an intact myeloma protein.

Benign Monoclonal Gammopathy (Monoclonal Gammopathy of Undetermined Significance)

Benign monoclonal gammopathy, which is closely related to multiple myeloma, can involve any of the immunoglobulins with the exception of IgM. The diagnosis of benign monoclonal gammopathy is usually one of exclusion; e.g., this diagnosis may be made in a patient who demonstrates a monoclonal spike in whom the diagnosis of multiple myeloma cannot be made definitively on clinical grounds or bone marrow examination. In general, the concentration of the abnormal protein is lower than in multiple myeloma, usually less than 2–2.5 g/dl, and in most instances there is no associated depression of the other classes of immunoglobulins. The production of Bence Jones proteins is rare, although a few instances have been reported.

Aside from the fact that the concentration of the monoclonal protein is generally low and the background immunoglobulins are generally normal, it is not possible to distinguish monoclonal gammopathy from multiple myeloma simply on the basis of biochemical analyses. The differential diganosis is ultimately dependent upon clinical features and the absence of a characteristic diffuse bone marrow infiltratation by plasma cells.

Macroglobulinemia of Waldenström

On the basis of electrophoretic analysis of serum, this disease is indistinguishable from multiple myeloma. In about 75 percent of the patients the monoclonal protein is water insoluble, as indicated by a positive Sia water test. However, this sign is neither universally present nor specific since a number of myeloma proteins are also water insoluble. The diagnosis of macroglobulinemia of Walderström is therefore made on the basis of immunoelectrophoretic analysis and/or immunoglobulin quantitation by radial immunodiffusion. The following additional tests should be carried out in any patient suspected of having macroglobulinemia of Waldenström. Serum viscosity should be tested because the incidence of hyperviscosity syndrome is very high in patients with macroglobulinemia, and the diagnosis should be made early so that appropriate therapy can be initiated. A search for cold agglutinins should be made because a fair percentage of macroglobulins have antibody activity to the big I or occasionally the little i antigen. If cold agglutinins are present, the patients frequently have evidence of hemolysis, often precipitated by exposure to the cold. Rheumatoid factor tests should also be carried out in patients with macroglobulinemia since many macroglobulins are positive for rheumatoid factor activity. As is the case in multiple myeloma, patients with macroglobulinemia can, on occasion, also produce Bence Jones proteins, which are then diagnosed in a manner similar to those in multiple myeloma.

Sera in all three of these diseases should be carefully examined for the presence of cold-insoluble proteins, i.e., cryoglobulins. Cryoglobulins in patients with palsma cell or lymphoid neoplasms are frequently asymptomatic and are discoveed accidentally in the performance of a routine laboratory procedure. By definition, a cryoglobulin has to precipitate in the cold and can go back in solution when the serum is heated. Precipitation usually occurs between 20°C and 4°C but occasionally a serum has to be cooled to 0°C so that the protein will precipitate. In general, if a cryoglobulin is present, part or almost all of the homogeneous protein is cold insoluble and an analysis of the supernatant serum will allow a good estimate of the amount of cryoglobulin present.

Heavy Chain Diseases

Heavy chain diseases provide rather characteristic electrophoretic or, at times, immunoelectrophoretic patterns and thus can be readily recognized in the laboratory.

γ heavy chain disease. γ heavy chain disease is invariably associated with the presence in the serum and usually also in the urine of a heterogeneous spike most often having the mobility of the beta globulin, but occasionally also residing in the gamma globulin region. The amount of protein present in the serum and in the urine can vary from trace amounts to up to 15 g/day in the urine and 3–4 g/dl in the serum. In many instances, however, the quantities present both in serum and urine are significantly smaller. γ heavy chain disease can be suspected on clinical grounds and the diagnosis has to be confirmed by immunoelectrophoretic analysis.

The salient features are as follows: (1) electrophoretic mobility of the serum and urine protein are identical and the protein bands are usually broad and heterogeneous, and (2) immunoelectrophoretic analysis demonstrates a reaction with antisera to the Fc fragment of the heavy chain and no reaction with antisera to light chains. Further analysis of the proteins usually shows them to be deleted heavy chains with a molecular weight ranging from 30,000 to 40,000 for the monomer or 60,000 to 80,000 for the dimer. The nature of these proteins has been clearly described in several recent reviews.

α heavy chain disease. α heavy chain disease is marked by the presence of a relatively broad heterogeneous spike in the β or alpha globulin region. Again, the quantity can vary from an easily detectable component to one which requires immunoelectrophoretic analysis for its detection. The amount of protein present in the urine is generally not very great and it is sometimes not present at all. Because the lymphomatous involvement is largely in the intestine, α chain disease patients frequently show the same abnormal protein in the intestinal fluids. The diagnosis, as was the case with γ heavy chain disease, is based on immunoelectrophoretic analysis and the demonstration of a spike in the serum and urine reactive with antisera to IgA and unreactive with antisera to light chains.

μ heavy chain disease. μ heavy chain disease is generally difficult to diagnose because the amount of protein produced is usually small and therefore not readily detectable on routine cellulose acetate or on paper electrophoresis. The diagnosis is generally dependent upon immunoelectrophoretic analysis of the serum, which shows a protein reactive only with antisera to μ chains in the alpha$_2$ to alpha$_1$ globulin region. Unlike patients with γ and α chain disease, patients with μ chain disease frequently continue to produce light chains which fail to assemble to the deleted μ chain. As a consequence, the serum often contains a Bence Jones protein which has a different mobility from the μ chain fragment. Since the μ chain fragment generally exists in the serum as a polymer, it is rarely, if ever, found in the urine. However, large amounts of free light chains, usually of the κ type, are often encountered.

Other Immunoglobulin Variants

To date it is not possible to recognize distinctly other immunoglobulin variants on the basis of characteristic electrophoretic or immunoelectrophoretic features. In most instances, these variants are readily detected by additional analytical procedures such as molecular weight determinations, examination of the protein under dissociating conditions, etc. These are relatively sophisticated laboratory techniques that are not yet in general clinical use.

The work-up of a patient suspected of having a monoclonal protein should procede somewhat along the following lines: (1) Initially, electrophoretic analysis should be carried out. Any one of the standard supporting media such as cellulose acetate, paper, agarose, or any other can be used. By this procedure it is possible to detect the presence of a monoclonal homogeneous band in the serum and in the urine. (2) When such a monoclonal band is found, immunoelectrophoretic analysis is performed using specific antisera to the major classes of immunoglobulin heavy chains and to κ and λ light chains. This type of analysis allows one to clearly define the abnormal component in virtually all instances. It should be remembered that certain macroglobulins and IgA myelomas have nonreactive light chains, so that it is difficult to classify precisely the nature of the associated light chains. It is usually advisable, in part to confirm the immunoelectrophoretic analysis, and in part to help distinguish the benign form from the more malignant ones,

to quantitate the immunoglobulin levels by radial immunodiffusion with specific antisera.

Treatment and progress of the disease can be followed most easily by simply repeating electrophoresis since the major part of the immunoglobulin band happens to be the monoclonal protein. If one wishes to be more precise, it is of value to quantitate the immunoglobulin levels to detect a return of the background immunoglobulins to normal.

Examination of the urine proceeds along the following lines. Initially the test for Bence Jones proteins is usually carried out at pH 4 and pH 7. It should be remembered that many Bence Jones proteins do not register on the usual dip stick test. In order to confirm or more clearly define the nature of the Bence Jones protein, electrophoresis and immunoelectrophoresis should be carried out. In all instances, it is important to use appropriate specific antisera.

The following additional studies should be carried out on all patients with monoclonal proteins: (1) cryoglobulins; (2) serum viscosity; and (3) cold agglutinins. The latter two are most important if there is a clinical indication or if the patient has macroglobulinemia of Waldenström.

It should be mentioned at this point that the diagnosis of each of these conditions is largely dependent on histologic studies of the bone marrow or lymphoid tissues; analysis of the serum and urine proteins is not sufficient to permit a clear-cut differential diagnosis.

REFERENCES

Franklin EC (ed): Immunoglobulin diseases, parts I and II. Semin Hematol 10 (January, April), 1973

Franklin EC, Buxbaum J: Immunoglobulin structure, synthesis, secretion, and relation to neoplasms of B cells. Clin Haematol 6:503, 1977

Franklin EC, Frangione B: Structural variants of human and murine immunoglobulins. Contemp Top Mol Immunol 4:89, 1975

Kyle RA: Monoclonal gammopathy of undetermined significance. Am J Med 64:14–826, 1978

Ritzmann SE, Daniels JC: Serum Protein Abnormalities: Diagnostic and Clinical Aspects. Boston, Little, Brown, 1975

B and T Cell Immunodeficiencies

Thomas A. Waldmann

INITIAL EVALUATION OF B AND T CELL IMMUNODEFICIENCIES

Primary immunodeficiency disorders with a profound defect of either B or T cell function are characterized clinically by an increased incidence of infections. In patients with B cell defects these infections are usually caused by encapsulated highly virulent bacterial organisms, whereas in patients with T cell defects and impaired

cell-mediated immunity the patients may develop infections with a variety of agents, including viruses, fungi, and protozoa. Ordinarily benign agents such as varicella, measles, herpes simplex, or cytomegalovirus may develop into fatal diseases or progressive and fatal disease may follow immunizations with live virus vaccines or bacillus Calmette-Guerin (BCG). In addition, the patients with T cell defects may develop graft-versus-host disease after receiving viable allogeneic lymphocytes via blood transfusions since they lack the ability to reject histoin-compatible cells.

Similar clinical patterns may be associated with different pathogenic mechanisms and with defects at distinct points in the maturation sequence from stem cells into mature T or B cells. A series of screening tests as well as more advanced procedures have been developed to define the position of the defect in the events of cellular maturation and regulatory cellular interactions that lead to these immunodeficiency states. The application of these tests to the study of patients with primary immunodeficiency diseases as well as those with secondary immune abnormalities associated with allergic, autoimmune, and neoplastic states is of importance in understanding the basic immune defects associated with these disorders. Finally, the concepts derived from the study of patients with immunodeficiency are leading to the development of more rational strategies for the therapy of patients with these disorders.

Initial screening studies for disorders of antibody-mediated immunity include the quantitation of the levels of circulating IgG, IgM, and IgA, Schick tests measuring specific antibody response following immunization for diphtheria, pertusis, and tetanus (DPT), and the determination of isohemagglutinin (anti-A and anti-B) titers to measure predominantly IgM function. A more thorough evaluation of humoral immunity involves the assessment of the patient's ability to produce specific antibody following antigenic challenge, the quantitation of the number of circulating B cells, the determination of immunoglobulin levels and secretory piece in the external secretions, and the determination of the number of pre-B cells in the marrow. In addition, a series of in vitro immunoglobulin biosynthesis studies have been developed that permit an analysis of B cell–plasma cell function as well as an evaluation of immunoregulatory T cell (helper T cells and suppressor T cells) activity in patients with hypogammaglobulinemia.

Initial screening evaluation of cell-mediated immunity would include the white blood cell count and differential in order to measure the total lymphocyte number and tests of the delayed-type skin test responses to recall antigens in order to measure specific T cell and macrophage response. Two broad categories of tests are commonly employed for further evaluation of T cell immunity, including (1) tests enumerating circulating T cells and T cell subpopulations and (2) in vivo and in vitro tests of T cell function, including delayed-type skin tests to administered antigens such as dinitrochlorobenzene and keyhole limpet hemocyanin, tests of the ability of lymphocytes to proliferate and release soluble products in vitro, and tests of T cell killer, helper, and suppressor function.

REFERENCES

Fudenberg H, Good RA, Goodman HC, Hitzig W, Kunkle HG, Roitt IM, Rosen FS, Rowe DS, Seligmann M, Soothill JR: Primary immunodeficiencies. Report of World Health Organization Committee. Pediatrics 47:927, 1971

Rose NR, Friedman H: Manual of Clinical Immunology. Washington, DC, American Society for Microbiology, 1976

ASSESSMENT OF CAPACITY TO SYNTHESIZE IMMUNOGLOBULINS AND ANTIBODIES

MEASUREMENT OF SERUM IMMUNOGLOBULIN CONCENTRATION

A variety of methods are available for measuring serum immunoglobulin concentrations. With the exception of electrophoresis, all depend on the use of specific antisera; they include single radial diffusion, double diffusion in agar gel, immunoelectrodiffusion, radioimmunoassay, and automated nephelometry. The single radial diffusion assay is the most widely used procedure. In this procedure antibody is added and uniformly distributed in a layer of agar or agarose gel, followed by the introduction of standard sera or the sera to be assayed for immunoglobulin levels into wells punched into the gel. The agent being assayed diffuses rapidly into the gel antibody mixture, forming a visible ring of precipitate at a point dependent on antigen–antibody stoichiometry. The IgG, IgA, and IgM levels in sera can be obtained after 24 hours of diffusion by comparing the diameter of the rings obtained with the unknown serum with values derived from dilutions of standard solutions on the same plate.

Gel diffusion methods are sensitive to differences in diffusion constants and thus molecular size. Therefore, one cannot measure the concentration of immunoglobulin in a biologic fluid unless the size of the molecules measured in this fluid is the same as those in the standard. Thus, reliable measurements cannot be made of such proteins as low molecular weight IgM in abnormal plasmas or IgA in external secretions where it appears as a dimer rather than as the monomer present in standard sera unless special standard preparations containing immunoglobulins of the same size are used. Another problem may occur if goat or sheep antisera are used in the gel diffusion assay because spuriously high estimates for serum IgA concentrations may be obtained in the study of patients with selective IgA deficiency. This occurs because these patients frequently have circulating antibodies to bovida IgA proteins that precipitate these proteins present in the antisera distributed in the agar. IgA levels in such patients should be assayed with antisera produced in nonbovida species such as the rabbit or horse.

Radioimmunoassay methods, including both double-antibody procedures and solid phase radioimmunoassays, can detect serum immunoglobulin levels at concentrations of the order of 1 ng/ml. They depend on the capacity of the immunoglobulin in the test serum to inhibit the interaction of purified radiolabeled immunoglobulin with antisera specifically directed toward the protein being studied. Such radioimmunoassays are of special value in estimating the serum level of immunoglobulins, such as IgE, that are present in serum at very low levels or in estimating the levels of immunoglobulins in body fluids, such as cerebrospinal fluid or amniotic fluid, in which the levels may be too low to be accurately quantitated by other conventional methods.

Concentrations of immunoglobulins in the sera of normal individuals vary with age and environment and from individual to individual. Normal levels have been reported to be 12.6 ± 2.6 mg/ml for IgG, 2.6 ± 1 mg/ml for IgA, 1.4 ± 0.6 mg/ml for IgM, and 100 ng/ml (90 percent confidence interval 15–742 ng) for IgE. Although no rigid standards for the diagnosis of immunoglobulin deficiency exist, a value of 2 mg/ml or less of IgG may constitute a practical threshold value for identifying patients who require gamma globulin therapy.

Immunoglobulins can also be measured in the body secretions, i.e., saliva, tears, milk, etc. In patients with respiratory infections or with diarrhea, the presence or absence of 11 S IgA and secretory component may be detected in normal secretions by single radial diffusion or by radioimmunoassay with an antiserum specific for this component.

Since the concentration of the immunoglobulin is the net result of synthesis, breakdown, and distribution, the interpretation of an immunoglobulin level must consider not only the normal values described above but also these metabolic factors. Metabolic turnover studies employing intravenously administered purified radioiodinated immunoglobulins may be used to differentiate syndromes with hypogammaglobulinemia due to diminished synthesis from those associated with a short immunoglobulin survival due to either increased endogenous catabolism or excessive loss of immunoglobulins into the urinary or gastrointestinal tracts.

ASSESSMENT OF ANTIBODY FORMATION FOLLOWING IMMUNIZATION

Antibody responses may be studied by means of tests for antibodies to antigens to which the population is commonly exposed or by tests that quantitate antibody formation following active immunization with protein or polysaccharide antigens. Live vaccines should never be given to a patient suspected of severe primary or secondary immunodeficiency. The following tests are recommended: (1) determinations of natural antibodies to blood groups A and B and of bactericidal antibodies against *Escherichia coli* are useful for screening; (2) diphtheria and tetanus vaccine, killed poliomyelitis vaccine, *Hemophilus influenzae* polysaccharide, pneumococcal polysaccharides, Vi antigen of Enterobacteriaceae, keyhole limpet hemocyanin, and *Brucella abortus* antigens may be used in immunization schedules. Blood is taken prior to the immunization and 2 weeks following injection, and the antibody levels are determined by standard approaches.

B LYMPHOCYTE ENUMERATION

B lymphocytes can be identified and enumerated by the presence of several surface receptors not found on T lymphocytes. These include membrane-bound immuno-globulin synthesized by B cells themselves, a receptor for aggregated immunoglobulin (Fc receptor), a receptor for the C3 complement component, and a receptor for the Epstein-Barr virus. The detection of surface immunoglobulin is most frequently used to quantitate B cells since other cell populations have surface C3 and Fc receptors.

Mononuclear cells isolated by means of Ficoll–Hypaque density gradients are incubated at 37°C for 45 minutes and then reacted with goat or with (Fab')$_2$ fragments of heterologous rabbit antibodies to each of the heavy or light chain determinants to be studied. Fluorescein- or rhodamine-labeled antisera are commonly used. After the lymphocytes are washed in a protein solution they are examined under a fluorescence microscope, preferably one equipped with epielumination. Fluorescent spots or crescents on lymphocytes indicate the presence of surface immunoglobulins in high density. If initial incubation at 37°C is not performed or if complete rabbit antibodies are fluoresceinated, spuriously high estimates for the B cell percentage may be obtained due to IgG binding by the Fc receptors of other cell types. Evidence confirming that the surface immunoglobulins identified are made by B lymphocytes may be obtained by removal of surface immunoglobulin by trypsinization followed by a 6-hour incubation in culture media and restaining to detect newly synthesized surface membrane immunoglobulin. Normally, 8–25 percent of the circulating lymphocytes have detectable surface immunoglobulin.

Purified antibodies (preferably labeled with rhodamine because of its slow quenching) are used to identify pre-B cells among bone marrow cells; these lymphocytes do not have easily demonstrable surface immunoglobulins but have small quantities of cytoplasmic IgM. Patients with hypogammaglobulinemia may have defects at varying levels along the pathway of maturation from stem cells to plasma cells. Patients with severe combined immunodeficiency disease of the Swiss type and those with thymoma and associated hypogammaglobulinemia do not have demonstrable pre-B cells; patients with X-linked agammaglobulinemia usually have pre-B cells but cannot produce B cells; and most patients with common variable immunodeficiency can produce B cells but these cells do not mature into immunoglobulin-synthesizing and *secreting plasma cells*.

Further insights into the nature of the defects in immunoglobulin production may be obtained by the use of in vitro immunoglobulin biosynthetic studies. A variety of such procedures have been developed to study defects in B cell maturation into immunoglobulin-secreting plasma cells. Peripheral blood mononuclear cells from the patient to be studied are cultured with a polyclonal activator of B cells such as pokeweed mitogen. Immunoglobulins synthesized and secreted by the plasmacytoid cells generated may be determined by specific radioimmunoassay of the supernatant fluid on the 7th–12th day of culture or by quantitation of the labeled precursor amino acid taken up into intracellular immunoglobulin during the final 4–18 hours of the 7-day culture. The generation of immunoglobulin-containing cells can also be identified by demonstration of immunoglobulin in the cytoplasm of the cultured cells on the 7th day with fluoresceinated antisera.

REFERENCES

Bach FH, Good R: Clinical Immunobiology, Vol 3. New York, Academic Press, 1976

Fudenberg H, Good RA, Goodman HC, Hitzig W. Kunkle HG, Roitt IM, Rosen FS, Rowe DS, Seligmann M, Soothill JR: Primary immunodeficiencies. Report of World Health Organization Committee. Pediatrics 47:927, 1971

Rose NR, Friedman H: Manual of Clinical Immunology. American Society for Microbiology, Washington, DC, 1976

Vyas GN, Stites DP, Brecher G (eds): Laboratory Diagnosis of Immunological Disorders. Grune & Stratton, 1975

ASSESSMENT OF CELL-MEDIATED IMMUNITY

T LYMPHOCYTE ENUMERATION

The most commonly used method for determining the number of circulating thymic-dependent lymphocytes (T cells) in man is to enumerate the cells that form spontaneous rosettes with sheep red blood cells. Normally, more than 75 percent of the lymphocytes in the peripheral blood form spontaneous rosettes with sheep red blood cells when the red cells have been pretreated with neuraminidase. Normal values reported for the absolute number of circulating T cells determined by this approach are 1620–4320/mm³ for the first week to 18 months of life and 590–3090/mm³ following 18 months of age.

The numbers of circulating T cells and T cell subpopulations have also been determined by using antisera specific for T cells. This antisera is obtained by using human fetal thymocytes, monkey thymocytes, peripheral blood lymphocytes from patients with X-linked agammaglobulinemia, T leukemia cells, or T lymphoid lines as the source of the T cell antigen. The number of T lymphocytes in the peripheral blood may then be determined with absorbed antisera. In general, cytotoxicity assays must be used since in most cases these absorbed antisera have not been specific when assessed by immunofluorescence.

In Vitro Stimulation of Lymphocytes

Small peripheral blood lymphocytes enlarge and are converted to blastlike cells that synthesize DNA and incorporate thymidine after an appropriate stimulation in vitro. This process is called *lymphocyte blastic transformation*. Stimulating substances can be divided into three groups: (1) nonspecific mitogens such as phytohemagglutinin (PHA), pokeweed mitogen (PWM), or concanavalin A (Con A); (2) antigens such as *Candida,* purified protein derivative (PPD), streptokinase-streptodonase (SK-SD), tetanus, and diphtheria, which require that the patient have prior encounter with the antigen; and (3) allogeneic

cells, which are used in the one-way mixed lymphocyte culture (MLC), in which the cells of the stimulating panel are irradiated or treated with mitomycin C prior to culture.

To assess lymphocyte stimulation in vitro, the patient's lymphocytes should be challenged with PHA, PWM, PPD, *Candida,* SK-SD, and a panel of allogeneic cells from donors with known HLA type. To perform these in vitro lymphocyte blastogenesis studies peripheral blood mononuclear cells are isolated from heparinized blood by Ficoll–Hypaque gradient centrifugation. Then $1–2 \times 10^5$ lymphocytes are cultured in a microtiter culture system with the lectin to be studied in medium supplemented with 10–20 percent serum pooled from normal donors. Optimal mitogenic concentrations of the lectin should always be established. In the MLC test, the ratio between responder cells and stimulatory cells should be 1:1. Cultures with lectin are assayed at 72–96 hours and those with specific antigens or allogeneic cells are assayed at 120–144 hours of culture.

The cell responses are assayed by ³H- or ¹⁴C-labeled thymidine incorporation during either the 4 hours or 16–24 hours prior to termination of the culture. Data on unstimulated cultures and stimulated cultures from the patients should always be provided. Cells from at least two normal people should be tested simultaneously as controls. The interpretation of mitogenic responses to various stimuli must be made with caution as to the type of responding cell. Soluble PHA and Con A stimulate T cells but may also stimulate B cells when bound to particulate matter. PWM stimulates a response in both T and B cells, although T cells must be present for the B cells to be stimulated. The MLC reaction is the result of T cell reactivity to antigens displayed on B cells and monocytes. It should be noted that the T cells in the populations of normal irradiated or mitomycin C–treated lymphocytes used as the stimulators may secrete factors that induce blastogenesis by the patient's lymphocytes. This may be quite misleading; therefore, it is preferable to use B cell lines or T cell–depleted normal cells as the stimulators.

Numerous soluble products (lymphokines) have been described, including migration inhibition factor (MIF), interferon, and lymphotoxin. However, since B cells as well as T cells release many of these lymphokines, assays for the production of these lymphokines are not reliable tests of T cell functions unless purified T cell populations are used.

DELAYED-TYPE SKIN TESTS

The ability of patients to manifest preexisting T cell immunity has been evaluated in vivo using a series of recall skin test antigens such as mumps, *Trichophyton,* PPD, *Candida,* and SK-SD. In those patients with an immunodeficiency disease who do not respond to any recall antigens, 2-4-dinitrochlorobenzene or keyhole limpet hemocyanin may be used as active sensitizing agents. When these agents are used, the skin test response is assayed 2 weeks after the initial sensitizing dose.

MEASUREMENT OF T CELL
REGULATORY FUNCTIONS

The normal immune response is regulated in both a positive and negative fashion by subsets of helper and suppressor T cells, respectively. Assays for an increase or decrease in activity of these subsets of T cells have been utilized in attempts to define the primary or associated defects in patients with immunodeficiency diseases.

Assays for Helper T Cell Activity

A modification of the method of analysis of in vitro PWM-stimulated B lymphyocyte immunoglobulin synthesis discussed above may be used to assess a deficiency of helper T cell function. This takes advantage of the observation that PWM-stimulated B cells require the cooperation of helper T cells in order to synthesize immunoglobulin. For this assay, normal peripheral blood B cells and monocytes are freed of T cells by a double purification procedure and then cocultured with PWM and the cells to be assayed for helper activity. Immunoglobulin synthesis by the B cells cultured alone and following addition of the T cells to be assessed for helper activity is determined as discussed above.

Assay for Increased Suppressor T Cell
Activity

The in vitro PWM-stimulated lymphocyte immunoglobulin synthesis system may also be used to detect excessive numbers of activated suppressor T cells. Peripheral blood mononuclear cells or purified T cells from the patient with immunodeficiency are cocultured with normal peripheral blood cells and PWM and the immunoglobulin synthesis is assessed. The immunoglobulin synthesis in the cocultures is related to that expected from the immunoglobulin synthesis of the two populations of cells cultured alone. Profoundly increased suppression is present if there is an 80–100 percent suppression of immunoglobulin synthesis of a panel of normal cells when cocultured with the patient's cells. The suppression should occur at low T cell to B cell ratios (4:1 or preferably 1:1) when PWM is used as the stimulator since even normal T cells may be activated by PWM to act as suppressors when high T cell to B cell ratios are utilized.

Assay for Decreased Suppressor T Cell
Activity

Diminished T suppressor cell activity is considered in patients with autoimmunity, including those with autoimmunity in association with a primary immunodeficiency disease. Precursors of suppressor T cells in normal peripheral blood can be activated by incubation with Con A for 48 hours. The cells are then washed free of their lectin and cocultured with normal target cells. Either suppression of PWM-induced immunoglobulin synthesis or Con A mitogen–induced blastogenesis is observed when normal cells are pulsed to become suppressors with Con A, whereas such mitogen-inducible suppressors may not be present in the blood of certain patients with immunodeficiency and autoimmunity.

Conclusion

These in vitro functional tests of T cell regulatory activity must be interpreted cautiously since most are not antigen specific and many involve the coculture of cells from individuals who differ at the major histocompatibility locus. However, the present procedures have provided significant insights into disorders of T cell function in immunodeficiency.

REFERENCES

Bloom BR, David JR: In Vitro Methods in Cell Mediated and Tumor Immunity. New York, Academic Press, 1976

Waldmann TA, Blaese RM, Broder S, Krakauer RS: Disorders of suppressor immunoregulatory cells in the pathogenesis of immunodeficiency and autoimmunity. Ann Intern Med 88:226, 1978

Hypocomplementemia

Stephen W. Hosea and Michael M. Frank

GENERAL CONSIDERATIONS

The differential diagnosis of hypocomplementemia can best be approached by considering the pathophysiology of complement activation and the factors that influence the level of any circulating protein. The proteins that comprise components of the complement cascade circulate in inactive form. Activation of the complement sequence leads to utilization of the components and a fall in their level in the blood. The blood level, however, is the sum of the rates of synthesis, degradation, and utilization of the components. Thus, the blood level is a static measurement that one uses as a guide to indicate whether the complement system has been activated by an immunologic and/or pathologic mechanism. Because this level is a static measurement of a dynamic process, it must be kept in mind that the blood levels may be perfectly normal in a number of situations in which complement is utilized. For example, in the disease primary biliary cirrhosis, the serum C3 level is usually elevated. As is true of most of the complement proteins, C3 acts as an acute phase reactant and the presence of an inflammatory disease process within the liver leads to elevated serum levels of C3. If turnover studies are performed, however, it is found that the C3 turnover rate is actually markedly increased. Thus the data obtained from static measurements of blood levels lead to an incorrect conclusion about complement activation in this particular disease.

Complement proteins may be very efficient in mediating certain biologic functions. Therefore complement activation can be involved in a disease process in the presence of normal serum levels of the individual components. For example, complement acting on a cell membrane may be quite efficient in molecular terms. Thus, relatively few molecules on a cell surface may mediate either opsonization or cytotoxic destruction of the cells. When one considers serum complement levels in terms of the number of available component molecules, it becomes clear that an efficient molecular process leading to cell destruction may not lower the titer of a component below the normal range. Thus, certain cytotoxic or opsonic mechanisms may be associated with very little lowering of the complement titer, even though complement is mediating the damage. Examples of this situation would include a number of the hemolytic anemias associated with complement activation, red cell sequestration in the reticuloendothelial system, and red cell destruction. In these cases, complement plays a major role in the destruction of the red cells, although the serum titer may not be below the normal range. In normotensive patients with bacterial sepsis, the presence of cleavage products of activated complement proteins may be the only indication of complement activation.

The various body compartments may be isolated from one another with respect to transport of complement components. Thus, complement may be activated in the joint space in patients with rheumatoid arthritis, but this may not be reflected in an abnormality in serum complement. The blood–brain barrier prevents access of the complement proteins to the brain, except in inflammatory states and, again, the compartmentalization of these rather large protein components may be important in determining whether or not the titer is lowered.

APPROACH TO INTERPRETATION

Let us begin our consideration of the differential diagnosis of hypocomplementemia by considering complement in a static fashion. The components of the complement sequence can be considered in groups (see the chapter on Classic and Alternative Complement Pathways in the section on Complement in the fascicle on Immunology): (1) the classic complement pathway, with its early components C1, C4, and C2; (2) the components of the alternative pathway, properdin factors D and B, properdin, and C3NeF; and (3) the later components of the complement sequence, C3–C9. If the classic complement pathway is efficiently activated, one would expect utilization of the components C1, C4, C2, and C3–C9 and a lowering of the titers of these components as they are "fixed" by antigen–antibody aggregates. If the alternative pathway is activated alone, one would expect a marked lowering of properdin factor B, properdin, and other components of the alternative pathway, as well as a fall in the levels of C3–C9, the late acting complement components.

Therefore, it is useful to study a serum sample for its levels of the following components: C4, a component of the classic pathway; properdin factor B, a component of the alternative pathway; and C3, a component of both pathways. If C4 and C3 are low and properdin factor B is normal, as is often found in patients with lupus erythematosus, one may suspect that the classic complement pathway has been activated. If, on the other hand, one finds low levels of properdin factor B and C3, one may suspect that the alternative pathway plays the prime role in complement activation. Such is often the case in membranoproliferative glomerulonephritis.

As mentioned earlier, the complement level, however, is the result of a number of dynamic interactions. A low C3 level can be the result of decreased synthesis or increased catabolism. In some but not all patients with glomerulonephritis, the low C3 levels are due to a decrease in synthesis of C3 rather than an increase in utilization, as had been postulated. In fact, in a number of disease states associated with low levels of complement components, decreases in synthesis have been observed rather than the expected increases in catabolism. The reasons for this effect are still not clear. The first postulate, and one which may indeed still be correct, is that complement degradation products feed back to regulate the rate of synthesis of component proteins. Thus far, it has not been possible to prove that such is the case and, in fact, we know little about the factors that govern the levels of complement protein in serum and their rates of synthesis.

The complement proteins themselves turnover very rapidly, even in the resting state. The turnover of most of the components that have been examined (C1q, C4, C3, C5, properdin factor B, and properdin) is on the order of about 2 percent/hr or about 50 percent/day.

It is clear that regulatory factors in the blood contribute to regulating this turnover of proteins. Patients who are missing the regulatory protein, C3 inactivator, have very low levels of C3 in their circulation. It would appear that small amounts of C3 are cleaved during the course of normal physiologic functioning and, thereby, small amounts of C3b are generated. In the presence of C3b inactivator, this C3b is cleaved and inactivated (see the chapter on Classic and Alternative Complement Pathways in the section on Complement in the fascicle on Immunology). In the absence of C3b inactivator, however, the C3b is not destroyed and is capable of interacting with components of the alternative pathway to mediate greatly increased C3 cleavage. Thus, the absence of a regulatory protein, the C3 inactivator, leads to marked C3 cleavage via activation of the alternative pathway and low serum C3 levels.

ASSAYS

There are a number of different types of assays that may be chosen in testing for hypocomplementemia, and the type of test chosen will markedly influence the type of information obtained (Table 1). Most hospital laboratories have tests available for C3 (β-1C). In some hospital laboratories, C4 can also be assayed (β-1E). These tests, available in commercial kits, evaluate the level of a component by means of radial immunodiffusion. A glass plate coated with agar gel is impregnated with antibody to the

Table 1
Assays of Complement Components

Method	Sensitivity	Use
CH_{50}	Fair	Good screen for complement deficiency or gross activation of complement
Radial immunodiffusion	Good	Standard for C3, C4, and factor B determinations
Hemolytic assay of components	Excellent	Exquisite sensitivity for individual complement components but use limited to research laboratory
Immunoelectrophoresis of activated complement	Excellent	Factor B, C4, and C; may be positive with normal component levels
Immunofluorescence	Good	Demonstration of complement components in tissue

specific component under study. The patient's serum or plasma is placed in a hole in the gel layer and the plate is incubated for 24–48 hours. After incubation, a ring of precipitation is formed that reflects the formation of antigen–antibody complexes in the gel. The diameter of the ring is directly proportional to the concentration of the serum protein.

This antigenic analysis is most useful in following patients with diseases in which complement activation plays a role. For example, following the levels of C3 or C4 by this assay is of great value in evaluating disease activity in patients with systemic lupus erythematosus. In general, falls in component levels often indicate a worsening of the pathophysiologic process. Antigenic analysis of this type gives no information as to the functional activity of the protein under study. If a patient were to be found with a nonfunctioning C3 or C4, such a test would miss this abnormality. Nonfunctioning complement proteins have not been discovered thus far; however, a nonfunctioning inhibitor of one of the complement components, C1 esterase, has been identified and is of great importance in patients with hereditary angioedema. In this situation, about 15 percent of patients have nonfunctioning C1 esterase inhibitor present in normal or supranormal amounts. Such a nonfunctining protein would be missed if one were evaluating only the level of C1 esterase inhibitor in serum by antigenic analysis.

Functional assays allow one to determine whether the protein is present and whether it has normal functional activity. These assays are considerably more difficult to perform, and therefore they are generally less available than antigenic analyses. Tests for specific components are considerably more sensitive than antigenic analyses and often are able to detect components at high dilutions of serum or other body fluids. The most commonly utilized functional analysis of complement activity is the CH_{50}. This test examines the ability of fresh serum to lyse sensitized sheep erythrocytes. Thus it reflects activity of all of the numbered components, C1–C9. The test, however, is relatively insensitive. Normal values obtained vary considerably according to the actual technic followed and may range in various laboratories from 20 to in the range of 300. In general, functional titers obtained for individual components are much higher. Nevertheless, if one is dealing with a genetically controlled total deficiency of any one of the numbered components, one finds a CH_{50} titer approaching 0. If such is found, the serum titer should be repeated and the serum examined in further detail.

The examination of freshly obtained EDTA plasma by antigenic analysis for the presence of cleavage fragments of complement proteins has been gaining interest as a method of determining whether complement is activated in vivo. There are now technics for the identification of cleavage fragments, C3, and properdin factor B, as well as other components; and the presence of these cleavage fragment suggests activation of complement, even in the absence of lowered complement titers.

INTERPRETATION OF HYPOCOMPLEMENTEMIA

COMPLEMENT ACTIVATORS

The presence of depressed levels of several components of the classic and/or alternative pathway suggests that complement is being activated in serum. Many factors can activate the complement cascade. Such nonspecific activators as proteolytic enzymes released from dying cells, from phagocytic cells during phagocytosis, and from metabolizing bacteria have all been shown to activate the complement sequence in the absence of true, immunologic recognition. Nevertheless, when one finds depressed levels of complement components, one thinks of an ongoing, immunologic process leading to utilization of components and depression of complement levels. In many cases, depressed component levels are associated with the presence of circulating immune complexes.

There are other factors that may activate complement and lower complement levels by nonimmunologic mechanisms. It has also been clearly shown that certain polyanions, such as heparin or heparin protamine complexes, can activate complement. Even C-reactive protein binding to its substrate on the C-polysaccharide of pneumococci can activate the complement cascade. Various exogenous factors, such as the dialysis membrane in an artificial kidney, may activate complement directly via the alternative pathway. For these reasons, it is impossible to be certain of immunologic activation when one observes depressed levels of complement components. The alternative pathway can be activated in the absence of specific antibody acting as a recognition factor (see the chapter on Classic and Alternative Complement Pathways in the section on Complement in the fascicle on Immunology). Antigen–antibody complexes of many classes, however, including IgA and IgE, can activate the alternative pathway, although in general large quantities of complexes are required. Many infectious organisms can interact directly with the proteins of the alternative pathway and mediate depressed levels of complement components (Table 1).

COMPONENT INTERACTIONS

If one finds depression in the level of a component either by antigenic analysis or by CH_{50}, the first reasonable question to ask is, "Does this finding represent the absence or depression of an individual component or of all of the components of the pathway?" Many of the

Table 1
Pathway Primarily Activated in Hypocomplementemias

Disease	Alternative	Classic
Infectious		
Bacterial		
Gram-negative sepsis	+++	+
Pneumococcal sepsis	++	++
Viral		
Dengue fever		+++
Hepatitis B		+
Fungal		
Disseminated		
cryptococcosis	++	
Parasitic		
Malaria paroxysm		++
Trypanosomiasis	++	++
Rheumatology		
Systemic lupus erythematosus (active)	+	+++
Rheumatoid arthritis (joint fluid)		++
Serum sickness		++
Vasculitis		+
Hematology		
Transfusion reaction		++
Neutropenia of dialysis	++	
Nephrology		
Membranoproliferative (with C3Nef)	+++	
Post-streptococcal	++	
Miscellaneous		
Hereditary angioedema		++++
C3 inactivator deficiency	++++	
Urticaria		+

Symbols: +, described; ++, occasional; +++, frequent; ++++, usually. This list is not meant to be all inclusive since complement levels have been measured in only a few disease states. There also may be a wide range of complement levels in an individual pathologic entity. For instance, complement levels are more apt to be lowered in shock than in normotensive patients with gram-negative sepsis.

Table 2
Hereditary Deficiencies of Complement

Component	Clinical Findings
C1q	Combined immunodeficiency
C1r	SLE, glomerulonephritis
C1s	SLE
C4	SLE
C2	Most common hereditary deficiency: spectrum ranges from normal to SLE, DLE, vasculitis, glomerulonephritis, anaphylactoid purpura
C3	Recurrent infections
C5	SLE
C6	Normal to repeated *Neisseria* infections
C7	Normal, Raynaud's syndrome, *Neisseria* infections
C8	SLE, *Neisseria* infections
C9	Not reported
C1EI	Hereditary angioedema
C3b INA	Repeated infections

Abbreviations: SLE, systemic lupus erythematosus; DLE, discoid lupus erythematosus.

factors that regulate the interaction of components are still unknown. Thus, patients with hereditary angioedema, missing C1 esterase inhibitor, have unopposed activation of C1, which cleaves C4 and C2. Nevertheless, their C3 level is normal, as is the level of all of the later components. Other disease processes stop with the activation of C3 and/or C5. Therefore, it is not surprising to observe lowered titers of several, but not all, components of a pathway. As an example, it has been reported that patients with membranoproliferative glomerulonephritis tend to have low levels of properdin factor B, but relatively normal levels of properdin. On the other hand, many patients with post-streptococcal glomerulonephritis have very low levels of properdin, but relatively normal levels of properdin factor B. The reasons for this difference in the amount of activation of components of a pathway are totally unknown. Certain situations have been described in which complement is activated by abnormal cells. In particular, certain kinds of tumors, including lymphoid malignancies and adenocarcinomas, have activated C1, leading to cleavage of C4 and C2 and the general symptom complex of hereditary angioedema.

SUMMARY

If a single component is lowered, it is reasonable to question whether the patient has a genetically controlled defect (Table 2). Studies of family members may be in order. If most of the components of a pathway are lowered, a reasonable supposition is that complement is being activated; we then turn to a consideration of the factors that may activate complement. When hypocomplementemia is associated with a fall in titer of several components, it is often possible to determine whether the classic or alternative pathway is the major pathway being activated; this, in turn, may suggest certain diagnoses and rule out others (Table 1). Thus, a consideration of the pathophysiology of the complement system and of the factors that activate complement leads to a general approach to hypocomplementemic disorders.

REFERENCES

Atkinson A, Frank MM: Complement, in Parker CN (ed): Clinical Immunology. Philadelphia, Saunders (in press)

Frank M: Complement, in: Current Concepts. Scope Monograph, Upjohn, 1975

Frank M, Atkinson J: Complement in clinical medicine. DM 1975

Ruddy S, Carpenter CB, Chin KW, Knostman JN, Soter NA, Gotze O, Muller-Eberhard JH, Austen KF: Human complement metabolism: An analysis of 144 studies. Medicine (Baltimore) 54:165, 1975

Ruddy S, Gigli I, Austen KF: The complement system of man. N Engl J Med 287:489, 545, 592, 642, 1972

Vasculitis and Immune Complex Disease

William P. Arend and Mart Mannik

CLASSIFICATION AND MANIFESTATIONS

The presence of an immune complex disease should be suspected in any patient presenting with vasculitis or glomerulonephritis. These are the two primary clinical manifestations of tissue damage secondary to the deposition of circulating immune complexes. The purpose of this chapter is to assist the physician in arriving at a specific diagnosis in the evaluation of patients with suspected immune complex disease or vasculitis. Detailed descriptions of clinical manifestations are given in the fascicle on Specific Rheumatic Diseases. A differential approach to the patient who manifests only glomerulonephritis will not be included in this chapter as this topic will be discussed in the volume on nephrology.

CLASSIFICATION

The classifications of immune complex diseases and vasculitis syndromes are inadequate at this time as the concepts of these disorders have evolved from morphologic descriptions, to pathogenic categorization or etiologic diagnoses. The designation of immune complex disease should be restricted to those conditions in which immune complexes have been demonstrated to be the pathophysiologic agent in the induction of tissue damage. Such proof is available for many of the clinical disorders to be discussed in this chapter, but conclusive evidence of the involvement of immune complexes in some forms of vasculitis is lacking. Other mechanisms not involving immune complexes may also be active in these disorders. The detection of circulating immune complexes is not an adequate sole criterion for making the diagnosis of immune complex disease. Recently developed assays may detect immune complexes in a variety of normal situations (e.g., in pregnancy and in the response to infections). In addition, circulating immune complexes may be present episodically in many diseases and may not be detected in the serum at a time when tissue damage is continuing.

Previous systems of classification of the vasculitides have emphasized histologic features and anatomic predilections. In evaluating a patient with suspected immune complex disease or vasculitis it is useful to categorize patients initially accordng to the presence or absence of glomerulonephritis and secondarily by the size of the involved vessels. Table 1 presents such a classification system, which will be utilized as a framework for this chapter.

CLINICAL AND LABORATORY FINDINGS
Diseases Accompanied by Glomerulonephritis

The presence of an immune complex disease or vasculitis should be suspected in any patient with symptoms and signs involving the skin, joints, central or peripheral nervous system, lungs, arteries, and kidneys. Disorders manifesting both vasculitis and glomerulonephritis are the most common form of immune complex disease and should be considered first in the differential diagnosis of all patients. The clinical manifestations of these disorders vary, depending primarily on the size of the vessels involved. The absence of hematuria, proteinuria, or renal dysfunction when the patient is first seen, however, does not rule out the presence of glomerulonephritis, as this pathologic process may be subclinical or may not appear until later in the course of the disease.

Characteristics of skin lesions can be helpful in differential diagnosis. The types of skin lesions seen with small vessel vasculitis include palpable petechiae, purpura, urticaria, morbilliform erythematous rashes, small maculopapular lesions, and livedo reticularis. These lesions result from inflammation in venules, capillaries, and small arterioles and occasionally progress to bullous formation and superficial dermal necrosis. On the other hand, mucosal or digital ulcerations, microinfarcts, painful nodules, large necrotic or bullous lesions, and poorly healing peripheral ulcerations all suggest the involvement of more medium-sized muscular arterioles or arteries. Lesions of both small and medium vessels may be more prominent in the lower extremities. The skin lesions may appear in recurrent crops or the lesions may be present continuously in various stages of maturation. Any suspicious skin lesion should be biopsied to confirm the diagnosis of vasculitis and to identify the sizes of the involved vessels (see below).

Small vessel lesions are the most common manifestation of vasculitis and glomerulonephritis. Single or recurrent episodes of skin lesions of small vessel vasculitis and nonprogressive glomerulonephritis may accompany the immune response to an extrinsic agent. The diagnosis of hypersensitivity angiitis is suggested by the temporal onset of disease following ingestion or injection of a drug, exposure to an environmental allergen, or a viral illness.

Table 1
Approach to Immune Complex Diseases and Vasculitides

Category	Presentation	Diseases
Immune complex disease or vasculitis usually with glomerulonephritis	Vasculitis of small vessels	Hypersensitivity angiitis Serum sickness Henoch-Schönlein purpura

	Vasculitis of small and/or medium vessels	Systemic lupus erythematosus
		Mixed cryoglobulinemia
		Periarteritis nodosa
		Allergic granulomatosis
		Wegener's granulomatosis
		Vasculitis and glomerulonephritis associated with
		  Viral infections (hepatitis B or infectious mononucleosis)
		  Bacterial infections (post-streptococcal, subacute bacterial endocarditis, infected arteriovenous shunt, or tissue infections)
		  Malignancies (lymphomas, leukemias or carcinomas)
		  Drugs (amphetamines, heroin, etc.)

Immune complex disease or vasculitis usually without glomerulonephritis	Vasculitis of small vessels	Hypergammaglobulinemic purpura Dermal vasculitis (no other organ involvement)
	Vasculitis of small and/or medium vessels	Rheumatoid vasculitis
	Vasculitis of medium and large arteries	Giant cell (temporal) arteritis Takayasu's arteritis or aortic arch syndrome
Immune complex glomerulonephritis without vasculitis*		
Immune complex disease without vasculitis or glomerulonephritis		Drug-induced anemia or thrombocytopenia Diseases with local immune complex formation

*See the volume in this series on nephrology.

These patients also may experience transient arthralgias or arthritis, fever, and myalgias. Serum sickness is a similar syndrome following injection of a foreign serum protein. The diagnosis of Henoch-Schönlein purpura is suggested by the appearance of skin lesions of small vessel vasculitis in association with abdominal pain, joint symptoms, and glomerulonephritis. This disease is more common in children and often follows a viral upper respiratory infection. Serologic testing usually is not of value in differentiating between these diagnoses. Skin and renal biopsies may be helpful as patients with Henoch-Schönlein purpura often possess deposits of IgA and C3 in dermal capillary walls and in the glomerular mesangium.

The presence of skin lesions of both small and medium vessel vasculitis in a patient with glomerulonephritis suggests one of the six diagnoses listed on Table 1. Each of these disorders involves particular findings that are of assistance in differential diagnosis.

Systemic lupus erythematosus. Systemic lupus erythematosus is the prototype of a multisystem immune complex disease with vasculitis and glomerulonephritis. Skin lesions are common in this disorder and include manifestations of small vessel vasculitis, photosensitive and atrophic lesions in a malar distribution, and occasionally digital infarcts or necrosis. Joint, renal, hematologic, lung, and peripheral or central nervous system involvement are all seen in this disease in various combinations. A history of repeated episodes of pleurisy or pericarditis, a nondeforming arthritis, cranial nerve abnormalities, seizures, or functional mental disorders should suggest the diagnosis of systemic lupus erythematosus in a patient with vasculitic skin lesions or glomerulonephritis. Antibodies to nuclear antigens (particularly to native DNA), low titers of rheumatoid factor, anemia, leukopenia, and thrombocytopenia are all common in systemic lupus erythematosus.

Mixed cryoglobunemia. The diagnosis of mixed cryoglobulinemia is suggested by the presence of large amounts of serum cryoglobulins in a patient with vasculitis and glomerulonephritis. Small amounts of cryoglobulins, however, are commonly found in many other forms of immune complex disease. High titers of rheumatoid factor are also present in mixed cryoglobulinemia. Over one-half of patients with mixed cryoglobulinemia have positive serologic tests for hepatitis B antigen or antibodies.

Periarteritis nodosa. Patients with periarteritis nodosa may have tender, subcutaneous nodules, representing inflamed arteries, in association with the sudden onset of neuropathy involving single or multiple large peripheral nerves (mononeuritis multiplex). Abdominal pain, intestinal bleeding, testicular inflammation, gangrene of digits, and coronary artery disease also may be seen in periarteritis nodosa. Hepatitis B antigen or antibodies may be present in 30–40 percent of patients with periarteritis nodosa. The demonstration of microaneurysms by angiography of mesenteric, coeliac, or peripheral vessels establishes this diagnosis.

Allergic granulomatosis. Allergic granulomatosis has clinical findings similar to those of periarteritis nodosa but these patients often have a history of asthma and present with diffuse pulmonary disease and eosinophilia.

Wegener's granulomatosis. The diagnosis of Wegener's granulomatosis should be suspected in any patient with undiagnosed nodular or infiltrative lung lesions, particularly in the presence of vasculitis or glomerulonephritis. Chronic otitis media or sinusitis are other frequent features of this disease. Some patients are thought to have Wegener's granulomatosis limited to the lung but many of these patients have subclinical renal disease and later may develop clinical skin, joint, or renal involvement. Serologic tests are not helpful in the diagnosis of Wegener's granulomatosis and open-lung biopsy is usually necessary to establish the diagnosis.

Other syndromes. Many syndromes of small or medium vessel vasculitis seen with glomerulonephritis are associated with viral infections, bacterial infections, malignancies, or drugs (Table 1). Syndromes associated with hepatitis B virus infection are being recognized with increasing frequency and can take two forms. An acute, transient episode of vasculitic skin lesions, fever, myalgias, arthralgias, or arthritis tends to occur prior to the appearance of jaundice and overt liver disease. Patients with persistent hepatitis B virus infection, on the other hand, may develop a chronic syndrome of fever, vasculitis, neuropathy, arthritis, and glomerulonephritis. Many patients diagnosed as having mixed cryoglobulinemia or periarteritis nodosa may actually have chronic infections with hepatitis B virus. The differential diagnosis of vasculitis and glomerulonephritis in association with viral or bacterial infections, malignancies, or drugs is aided by a careful history and physical examination for evidence of the underlying disease. Specific serologic tests are useful in viral infections (hepatitis B antigen or antibodies, heterophil agglutination test), bacterial infections (antistreptococcal antibodies, blood cultures), and tumors (carcinoembryonic antigen, α-fetoprotein). The use of any intravenous drug may result in vasculitis and glomerulonephritis, although amphetamine and heroin abuse has been particularly incriminated. It is not known whether the drugs per se or contaminants in the preparations cause the disease.

Diseases Usually Not Associated with Glomerulonephritis

If glomerulonephritis is absent and all of the above diagnoses are considered unlikely, the patient may have a form of immune complex disease in which renal involvement is uncommon. The differential diagnosis of those patients presenting with small vessel vasculitis of the skin is limited to three disorders (Table 1).

Hypergammaglobulinemic purpura and dermal vasculitis. Hypergammaglobulinemic purpura is suggested by the presence in females of slowly progressive purpura of the lower extremities, enhanced by constricting garments or by prolonged standing or walking. This diagnosis is further suggested by the finding of increased levels of gamma globulin on serum protein electrophoresis. Intermediate complexes, sedimenting between IgM and IgG, are present in the serum by analytical ultracentrifugation. Some patients may have small vessel vasculitis of the skin, with or without hypocomplementemia, in the absence of any evidence of other organ involvement. Patients with hypergammaglobulinemic purpura or with vasculitis apparently limited to the skin may develop features of other immunologic diseases, such as Sjögren's syndrome or systemic lupus erythematosus.

Rheumatoid vasculitis. Lesions of both small and medium vessel vasculitis are seen in patients with rheumatoid vasculitis. These patients have established rheumatoid arthritis, usually with destructive joint disease, skin nodules, and a high titer of rheumatoid factor. A mild sensory–motor neuropathy in a stocking and glove distribution is a common manifestation of vasculitis in rheumatoid arthritis. A small percentage of patients have a more malignant form of vasculitis with skin infarcts, monomeuritis multiplex, coronary arteritis, and mesenteric ischemia or infarction.

Giant cell arteritis and Takayasu's arteritis. Two syndromes characterized by vasculitis of medium and large vessels in the absence of glomerulonephritis are giant cell (temporal) arteritis and Takayasu's arteritis (Table 1). Systemic manifestations common in these two disorders include weight loss, malaise, myalgias, and fever. Patients with temporal arteritis may have proximal muscle pain made worse with exertion, suggestive of polymyalgia rheumatica. Temporal arteritis occurs in older individuals, whereas Takayasu's arteritis is more common in young females of Far Eastern origin. Symptoms of cerebral vascular insufficiency such as dizziness, headaches, visual blurring, or transient loss of vision signify the involvement of large arteries in the neck or leading from the aortic arch in both of these diseases. Segmental inflammation of iliac or femoral vessels may occur in either of these disorders, producing symptoms of peripheral claudication. Bruits may be heard over the involved segments of arteries and local tenderness may be present. Patients with these two forms of vasculitis have very high erythrocyte sedimentation rates during the active inflammatory stage of the diseases. The diagnosis of giant cell arteritis may be made by biopsy of a

Table 2
Radiologic Abnormalities in Patients with Immune Complex Disease
or Vasculitis

X-ray	Abnormalities	Diseases
Chest	Interstitial fibrosis; bilateral, more often in lower lobes	Systemic lupus erythematosus Rheumatoid arthritis Hypersensitivity pneumonitis Periarteritis nodosa Allergic granulomatosis
	Single or multiple nodules	Rheumatoid arthritis Wegener's granulomatosis
	Patchy parenchymal infiltrates	Allergic granulomatosis Wegener's granulomatosis Periarteritis nodosa Hypersensitivity angiitis Systemic lupus erythematosus
	Consolidated parenchymal lesions	Allergic granulomatosis
	Pleural effusions	Rheumatoid arthritis Systemic lupus erythematosus Wegener's granulomatosis
Sinus	Chronic mucosal thickening, with or without necrosis of adjacent bone	Wegener's granulomatosis
Arterial angiography	Segmental narrow of multiple vessels leading from the aorta	Takayasu's arteritis Giant cell arteritis
	Microaneurysms in mesenteric or peripheral arteries	Periarteritis nodosa

temporal artery and Takayasu's arteritis is diagnosed by arteriography or biopsy.

Immune complex diseases not associated with vasculitis or glomerulonephritis. Some forms of immune complex disease lack any manifestation of vasculitis or glomerulonephritis. Drugs may participate in immune complex formation with secondary attachment to red blood cells or platelets and fixation of complement. These cells are removed from circulation by the fixed-tissue macrophages in the liver and spleen, resulting in hemolytic anemia or thrombocytopenia. Quinidine is the most common drug producing these abnormalities. The induction of neutropenia by an immune complex mechanism is suspected in several diseases, including rheumatoid arthritis, but has not been proven.

Diseases with primarily local formation of immune complexes, such as hypersensitivity pneumonitis, usually do not exhibit vasculitis or glomerulonephritis. Exceptions to this generalization do exist, however, as patients with autoimmune thyroiditis may develop glomerulo-nephritis with thyroglobulin present as the antigen in the immune complexes. Patients with tubulointerstitial renal disease may develop glomerulonephritis secondary to the deposition of immune complexes containing renal tubular cell antigens. Furthermore, the synovitis of rheumatoid arthritis is characterized by intraarticular formation of immune complexes but circulating complexes are common in this disorder.

RADIOLOGIC AND LABORATORY STUDIES

A chest x-ray should be obtained for every patient with suspected immune complex disease or vasculitis, as findings indicating a specific diagnosis may be present. X-rays of other organs or arterial angiography may be of diagnostic value in selected patients. A summary of the radiologic abnormalities in these disorders, including features helpful in differential diagnosis, is presented in Table 2. The nodular or infiltrative lesions in Wegener's granulomatosis often are transient or rapidly changing. The presence of cavitation in a nodular lesion suggests

Table 3
Results of Tissue Biopsies in Immune Complex Disease or Vasculitis

Organ	Histologic Features	Diseases
Skin	Small vessel vasculitis: intimal proliferation, infiltration with neutophils throughout the wall and surrounding capillaries, venules, and small arterioles	Diseases with small vessel vasculitis, with or without glomerulonephritis (Table 1)
Skin or muscle	Medium vessel vasculitis (nongranulomatous): same features as above in arterioles and arteries, with disruption of internal elastic lamina without giant cells or granulomata	Systemic lupus erythematosus Rheumatoid vasculitis Mixed cryoglobulinemia Hepatitis B virus syndromes Periarteritis nodosa
	Medium vessel vasculitis (granulomatous): same features as above in arterioles and arteries, with disruption of internal elastic lamina with giant cells and granulomata	Allergic granulomatosis Wegener's granulomatosis
Artery	Arteritis of larger vessels with giant cells, but without granulomata or neutrophils	Giant cell arteritis Takayasu's arteritis
Lung	Granulomas with giant cells and vasculitis, without eosinophils	Wegener's granulomatosis
	Granulomas with giant cells and vasculitis, with eosinophils	Allergic granulomastosis
	Interstitial fibrosis, with or without lymphocytes	Rheumatoid arthritis Systemic lupus erythematosus Hypersensitivity pneumonitis Periarteritis nodosa Allergic granulomatosis

Wegener's granulomatosis. The diagnosis of lung carcinoma, however, must always be considered in a patient with lung lesions and glomerulonephritis.

Routine laboratory tests are often abnormal in patients with these disorders but usually they are not particularly helpful in differential diagnosis. Mild elevations in the white blood cell count or erythrocyte sedimentation rate commonly are seen as a response to inflammation in most of the diseases listed in Table 1. A fall in these abnormalities usually follows a clinical response to treatment. A persistent leukocytosis with the presence of immature cells should suggest the possibility of infection as a cause of the vasculitis. A mild hypoproliferative anemia often is seen secondary to the inflammation in many forms of immune complex disease or vasculitis. An iron-deficient anemia may be secondary to intestinal blood loss from vasculitis or drug-induced mucosal irritation. Hemolytic anemia often occurs in systemic lupus erythematosus, but it also may be seen in rheumatoid arthritis or secondary to drugs. Proteinuria, hematuria, and white blood cell or granular casts are all seen in many forms of renal disease but red blood cell casts are virtually diagnostic of glomerulonephritis. These and other aspects of renal involvement seen with immune complex diseases or vasculitis are discussed in the volume on nephrology.

Special serologic tests are of some use in differential diagnosis. Antibodies to nuclear antigens are present in virtually all patients with systemic lupus erythematosus. They also are found in 20–30 percent of patients with rheumatoid arthritis and in normal old individuals, and they may be found secondary to many drugs. The presence of elevated titers of antibodies to native DNA, as detected by the DNA-binding assay, is almost limited to systemic lupus erythematosus. Low serum complement levels are also found in many forms of immune complex disease or vasculitis; this topic is discussed in detail in the section on the Differential Diagnosis of Hypocomplementemia.

The results of assays for immune complexes in the serum are discussed in the chapter on the Detection of Circulating Immune Complexes in the fascicle on Immunology. These assays frequently are positive in patients with systemic lupus erythematosus or rheumatoid arthritis; they are positive in a lower percentage of patients with various vasculitides, glomerulonephritis, or malignancies.

TISSUE BIOPSY

A histologic evaluation is helpful in establishing the diagnosis and in clarifying the type of vasculitis present (Table 3). Any skin lesion suspected of being vasculitic should be biopsied. The term *leukocytoclastic vasculitis* often is applied when the biopsy reveals cellular fragments phagocytosed within neutrophils in the lesions of small vessel vasculitis. This term is nonspecific, however, as this histologic feature does not distinguish between the diagnoses listed in Table 1 where small vessels are involved. The types of cells present in the skin lesions (neutrophils or lymphocytes), a depression in the serum complement level, and other evidence of systemic vasculitis are variable features in some patients with small vessel vasculitis. This variability may reflect stages in the evolution of the disease process in some cases and different diseases in others. Granulomatous changes and giant cells usually are not seen in the small vessels sampled on skin biopsy. A muscle biopsy is more likely to show these abnormalities in arterioles and small arteries.

Immunoglobulins and complement components may be searched for using immunofluorescent techniques but are inconsistently present in vasculitic lesions in skin or muscle biopsies. This variability may be due in part to the age of biopsied lesions as immune complexes in inflamed lesions may not persist more than 1–3 days due to removal by infiltrating neutrophils. Immunoglobulins and complement may be present, however, along the dermal–epidermal junction of normal or diseased skin in patients with systemic lupus erythematosus.

Any patient suspected of having giant cell arteritis should have a temporal artery biopsy; serial sections should be made for histologic examination since the disease is segmental in distribution. A transbronchial or open-lung biopsy usually is necessary to make the diagnosis of granulomatous arteritis (Wegener's or allergic) as characteristic histologic features often are not found in skin, muscle, or kidney biopsies. The indications for and interpretation of renal biopsies in the evaluation of patients with possible immune complex disease or vasculitis are discussed in the fascicle on Specific Rheumatic Diseases and in the volume on nephrology.

REFERENCES

Alarcon-Segovia D: The necrotizing vasculitides. A new pathogenetic classification. Med Clin North Am 61:241, 1977

Christian CL, Sergent JS: Vasculitis syndromes: Clinical and experimental models. Am J Med 61:385, 1976

Chumbley LC, Harrison EG Jr, DeRemee RA: Allergic granulomatosis and angiitis (Churg-Strauss syndrome). Report and analysis of 30 cases. Mayo Clin Proc 52:477, 1977

Conn DL, McDuffie FC, Holley KE, Schroeter AL: Immunologic mechanisms in systemic vasculitis. Mayo Clin Proc 51:511, 1976

Duffy J, Lidsky MD, Sharp JT, Davis JS, Person DA, Hollinger FB, Min K-W: Polyarthritis, polyarteritis and hepatitis B. Medicine (Baltimore) 55:19, 1976

Fauci AS, Haynes BF, Katz P: The spectrum of vasculitis. Ann Intern Med 89:660, 1978

Gilliam JN, Smiley JD: Cutaneous necrotizing vasculitis and related disorders. Ann Allergy 37:328, 1976

Sams WM Jr, Thorne EG, Small P, Mass MF, McIntosh RM,
Stanford RE: Leukocytoclastic vasculitis. Arch Dermatol 112:219, 1976

Zeek PM: Periarteritis nodosa: A critical review. Am J Pathol 22:777, 1952

PRINCIPLES OF TREATMENT

The objectives to treatment of immune complex diseases or vasculitis include the following: (1) elimination of the exogenous or endogenous source of antigen; (2) suppression of the inflammatory mechanisms of tissue damage by antiinflammatory medications; and (3) removal of injurious immune complexes from the body.

Pursuit of the first objective would include appropriate treatment of specfic bacterial or viral infections (e.g., bacterial endocarditis or tissue infections), discontinuation of drugs to which the patient may be sensitized, avoidance of contact with extrinsic allergens, or removal of tumors associated with immune complex glomerulonephritis. In most forms of immune complex disease or vasculitis, however, the antigen is not known or cannot be eliminated.

Most current forms of treatment for these disorders are directed toward the second objective. Specific diagnoses should be established since the prognoses vary, antiinflammatory medications possess less or greater side effects, and some diseases respond better to particular therapeutic agents. Salicylates or nonsteroidal antiinflammatory agents are indicated for symptomatic relief of joint involvement in most of these disorders. Glucocorticoids in low dosage may be of value in the treatment of skin, joint, or renal disease, particularly when the latter is non-life threatening. Treatment with high doses of glucocorticoids or immunosuppressive drugs should be limited to patients with potentially life-threatening disease. Further details on the use of antiinflammatory agents can be found in the fascicle on Specific Rheumatic Diseases.

The third objective in treatment, to remove injurious immune complexes from the body, requires modalities that are still experimental. Plasmapheresis has been utilized successfully in some patients with transient immune complex disease but its applicability in chronic disorders is unknown. Removal of specific antigens or immune complexes from circulation by solid-phase immunoabsorbents or extracorporeal circulation has been tried in animal models of immune complex disease; much more experimental work is required prior to application to human diseases.

REFERENCES

Pirofsky B, Bardana EM Jr: Immunosuppressive therapy in rheumatic disease. Med Clin North Am 61:419, 1977

Roe RL: Drug therapy in rheumatic disease. Med Clin North Am 61:405, 1977

SPECIFIC IMMUNOLOGIC DISEASES

Primary Immunodeficiency Diseases

Thomas A. Waldmann

T CELL AND COMBINED T CELL–B CELL IMMUNODEFICIENCY DISEASES

The immunologic deficiency diseases may be broadly categorized either as disturbances in the synthesis of the various components of the immunologic system or as abnormalities of the endogenous breakdown or external loss of these components. These defects lead to specific abnormalities in the complex pathways of cellular maturation and regulatory cellular interactions that are required for a normal immune response (Fig. 1). Normally, precursor cells destined to subserve immunologic functions arise from various hematopoietic tissues (yolk sac, fetal liver, and bone marrow in the fetus and bone marrow postpartum) and then migrate to other lymphoid organs where they undergo further differentiation.

One population of such cells, the progenitors of T cells, is induced to differentiate by thymic epithelial cells and their humoral products into thymus-derived lymphocytes or T cells. These cells bear specific surface markers and are responsible for a series of cell-mediated immune functions including delayed hypersensitivity, allograft rejection, cytotoxic reactions, and helper and suppressor regulation of the immune response. Distinct subpopulations of T cells have been identified that differ in their functional capacities and surface developmental antigens. For example, one population of T cells functions as helper cells to other lymphoid cells in the development of their functions, whereas a second group of T cells is programmed for suppressor and cytotoxic functions.

A second major population of cells differentiates into B cells and plasma cells. The first step in the differentiation of this group of cells is from lymphoid stem cells into pre-B cells, that is, into cells that have a small quantity of IgM in their cytoplasm but no immunoglobulin easily demonstrable on their surface. These pre-B cells mature into B cells that can be identified in the peripheral blood as lymphocytes with a number of receptors on their surface, including membrane-bound immunoglobulins acting as receptors for antigen, receptors for the third component of complement, receptors for antigen-antibody complexes, and receptors for the Epstein-Barr virus. The union of appropriately presented antigen with the immunoglobulin membrane receptors triggers second-stage events which include B cell proliferation and terminal differentiation into antibody-secreting plasma cells. The maturation of B cells is carefully regulated both positively and negatively by separate series of cells. Specifically, many antigens require the presence of both helper lymphocytes of thymic origin (helper T cells) and macrophages as well as B cells to induce a full antibody response. More recently it has been recognized that a separate class of thymus-derived cells, suppressor T cells, act as negative regulators of B cell maturation, inhibiting this process.

Two major classes of immunodeficiency diseases are recognized: (1) T cell or combined T cell–B cell immunodeficiency disorders that lead to abnormalities of cell-mediated immunity and (2) B cell–plasma cell disorders that are associated with humoral immune defects. The T cell disorders include errors at the distinct steps along the maturation sequence from hematopoietic stem cells to the mature T lymphocytes. Certain disorders reflect a failure of the generation of stem cells, whereas others reflect biochemical abnormalities, especially those of the purine salvage pathway that lead to failure of the T cell and, to a lesser extent, the B cell system. Another major pathogenic mechanism leading to T cell immunodeficiency is failure of the development or the function of the thymus, the central lymphoid organ required for the expansion of stem cell precursors into functionally effective T cells. Finally, there are disorders that do not reflect abnormalities of the production of T cells but are abnormalities in the host environment which either alter the survival or functional capacity of T cells, such as occurs in patients with antibodies to T cells or in patients with a short survival of T lymphocytes due to gastrointestinal loss.

Defects of humoral immunity also reflect a variety of errors in the maturation and regulatory interactions of the cells of the immune system. In some disorders there is a failure of the development of pre-B cells from lymphoid stem cells; in others there is a failure of the maturation of pre-B cells into mature B cells; and in still others there is a failure of terminal maturation of B cells into plasma cells. In other patients with defects of humoral immunity there is an abnormality of an immunoregulatory T cell subpopulation, that is, a deficiency of helper T cells or an excessive number of functionally active suppressor T cells that regulate B cell maturation into plasma cells. In

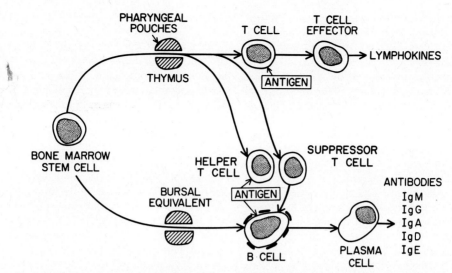

Fig. 1. Normal T cell and B cell immune response. (Reproduced with permission from Waldmann TA, Blaese RM, Broder S, Krakauer RS: Ann Intern Med 88:226, 1978.)

another category of immunodeficiency disease the effectors of the cellular and humoral systems are present but there are profound abnormalities of specific antibody and cell-mediated immune responses that may be due to defects in the afferent loop of immunity, that is, defects in antigen processing and recognition. These varied defects in the maturation and in the interactions of lymphoid cells may have different clinical presentations and require different approaches for rational therapy.

SEVERE COMBINED IMMUNODEFICIENCY DISEASE

Severe combined immunodeficiency disease (SCID) encompasses a series of different diseases defined by gross functional impairment of both humoral and cell-mediated immunity that is usually congenital and frequently genetic. Affected individuals have rampant infections with a whole range of microorganisms, including bacteria, fungi, and viruses such as measles virus resulting in giant cell pneumonia or cytomegalovirus. *Pneumocystis carinii* infection is present in the majority of infants at the time of death. Fatal bacillus Calmette-Guerin sepsis following inoculation and progressive vaccinia following smallpox vaccination have been documented in many patients.

The patients have skin lesions that vary in etiology and location. *Candida* infection of the mucous membranes and skin is almost always present and may be the first sign of the disease. Bronchial pneumonia is a repetitive event and nearly all patients have diarrhea with loose watery stools from an early age. As these patients lack T cell immunity they are susceptible to graft-versus-host reactions following the infusion of viable cells in the form of blood transfusions or attempts at immunotherapy. This syndrome can result from a diverse number of pathogenic mechanisms with different inheritance patterns that lead to defects at different levels of cellular differentiation.

SCID with Generalized Hematopoietic Hypoplasia (Reticular Dysgenesis)

The most severe form of SCID, termed *reticular dysgenesis,* is a disease in which there is a basic cellular defect in the development of hematopoietic stem cells. Patients with this disorder have a virtual absence of T cells, B cells, and granulocytes and have died within the first few hours or days of life as a consequence of the failure of both specific and nonspecific protective mechanisms against infections.

"Swiss Type" SCID with Failure of Lymphoid Stem Cell Development

The "Swiss type" of SCID appears to represent a failure of lymphoid stem cell development with a consequent reduction in the numbers of circulating lymphocytes that bear either T or B cell markers. This disorder may be inherited in an autosomal recessive fashion or may occur sporadically. Patients with this disorder have an inability to manifest either cell-mediated or antibody responses to antigenic challenge and die within the first years of life unless treated. This defect has been repaired by transplantation of bone marrow from an HLA-matched sibling or in certain cases by transplantation of fetal liver.

SCID with Adenosine Deaminase Deficiency

A pattern of severe combined immunodeficiency inherited as an autosomal recessive defect may occur in association with a deficiency of adenosine deaminase (ADA). These patients have clinical manifestations that are similar to those seen with other forms of SCID; however, they also have characteristic radiologic abnormalities, including concavity and flaring of the anterior ribs and an abnormal bony pelvis. At the onset, these patients may have some lymphoid development of the thymus, may have circulating lymphocytes that proliferate on culture with nonspecific mitogens, and may be able to synthesize IgM. With time, there is thymic atrophy. The involuted thymus with Hassall's corpuscles observed in these patients differs in pathologic appearance from the thymus in other forms of SCID in which there is an embryonic appearing thymus with no or only rudimentary Hassall's corpuscle formation. With time, the patients develop severe lymphocytopenia and a failure of lymphocyte mitogen responsiveness.

Some patients have a profound reduction of B cell development and immunoglobulin synthesis, whereas others continue to have substantial numbers of B cells. The enzyme ADA, which catalyzes the conversion of adenosine to inosine, appears to be necessary for the maintenance of normal function of lymphocytes, especially T cells. The suppression of lymphocyte function appears to be due to toxicity of increased intracellular adenosine or adenosine deoxynucleotides. It has been shown that the erythrocytes of ADA-deficient patients contain 100-fold higher concentrations of deoxyATP than do normal erythrocytes, and it has been proposed that this compound is cytotoxic by virtue of its ability to inhibit ribonucleotide reductase and thus inhibit the synthesis of all deoxyribonucleotide precursors of DNA.

The immunologic defects in SCID patients with ADA deficiency have been corrected by transplants of either fetal liver or histocompatible bone marrow as sources of healthy stem cells capable of ADA production. In some but not all patients, the transfusion of irradiated red blood cells from individuals with normal ADA activity has led to the development of a visible thymus shadow, normal T lymphocyte responsiveness, and normal immunoglobulin levels.

SCID Associated with Absence of T Lymphocytes

Another form of severe combined immunodeficiency is associated with the absence of T lymphocytes but normal or near normal numbers of circulating B lymphocytes. Such patients do not have lymphocytopenia, and immunoglobulin is demonstrable on virtually all of their lymphocytes. These patients usually have some circulating IgM but very low levels of IgG and IgA. The cells of two such patients synthesized IgM but essentially no IgG or IgA when cultured in the in vitro immunoglobulin biosynthesis system in which B cell maturation was stimulated by the thymic-dependent lectin, pokeweed mitogen. However, when cultured with T cells from another individual that could fulfill normal helper function, the B cells of the patients synthesized normal or even increased quantities of all classes of immunoglobulins.

These observations imply that the B lymphocytes may have developed normally in these patients with this phenotypic form of severe combined immunodeficiency but lack the required T cell help and therefore are not triggered normally by antigens. Theoretically, two cellular defects may lead to this phenotypic form of severe combined immunodeficiency. Such patients may have a failure of stem cells required for the development of T cells. In accord with this view, there has been lasting correction of at least one such patient with histocompati-

ble bone marrow. On the other hand, some patients might have a faulty development of the thymic epithelium or production of thymic humoral factors. This mechanism is supported by the observation that certain patients with SCID had a reconstitution of not only T cell but also B cell function following transplantation of fetal thymus or cultured thymic epithelium. In addition, the cells from the bone marrow of an affected boy acquired T cell characteristics when cultured on normal thymic epithelium.

THYMIC HYPOPLASIA (DiGEORGE SYNDROME)

Thymic hypoplasia (DiGeorge syndrome) is a disorder of the development of the structures derived from the third and fourth pharyngeal pouch during embryonic life which leads to abnormalities of the ear and facial structures, congenital heart disease, abnormalities of the parathyroids with consequent hypocalcemic tetany, and aplasia or hypoplasia of the thymus with an associated cellular immunodeficiency state.

Pathogenesis

The thymus develops during the 6th–8th week of embryonic life from the third and fourth pharyngeal pouches and migrates caudally to the anterior mediastinum by the 12th week. The parathyroids and certain aortic arch structures also arise from the third and fourth pharyngeal pouches. The DiGeorge syndrome is not genetically determined; it seems likely that some intrauterine insult occurring early in gestation leads to abnormal embryogenesis of structures derived from the third and fourth pharyngeal pouches.

Clinical Manifestations

The following are typical clinical features of the DiGeorge syndrome: (1) facial abnormalities, including micrognathia, hypertelorism, blunted nose, low-set ears with notched ear pinnae, short philtrum of the lip, and antimongoloid slant of the eyes; (2) hypoparathyroidism with hypocalcemic tetany and seizures during the first week of life; (3) cardiovascular defects including a right-sided aortic arch, a double aortic arch, or tetralogy of Fallot; and (4) a T cell immunodeficiency state associated with increased susceptibility to infections manifested by chronic rhinitis, recurrent pneumonia (including *Pneumocystis carinii* pneumonia), candidiasis, and diarrhea.

Immunologic Defect

The DiGeorge syndrome is a classic example of an isolated T cell immunodeficiency disease associated with thymic hypoplasia. It should be noted, however, that the thymic abnormality and the defects of cell-mediated immunity are quite variable. Although most patients do not have a thymus demonstrable on lateral x-ray of the mediastinum, the majority have one or more histologically normal but unusually small thymus glands in an ectopic location. The absolute lymphocyte count is usually normal or at times moderately decreased. However, the percentage of B cells demonstrable by membrane immunofluorescence studies is increased and the percentage of T cells is markedly reduced.

Patients with the complete DiGeorge syndrome have profound defects of T cell function with decreased or absent lymphocyte response to stimulation in vitro with nonspecific mitogens, specific antigens, or the allogeneic lymphocytes. Skin tests with recall antigens are usually negative and there may be a failure of sensitization with dinitrochlorobenzine and a prolonged skin graft survival. At the other extreme, certain patients have been described with the nonimmunologic manifestations of the DiGeorge syndrome but with normal T cell function. Humoral immunity has been relatively normal in most of the patients studied, although occasionally patients had reduced immunoglobulin levels and poor antibody production following antigenic challenge.

Incubation of bone marrow cells from patients with the DiGeorge syndrome with thymic humoral factors has led to a marked increase in the number of cells that bear surface antigens recognized by antithymocyte antibodies. These observations support the view that the defect in the patients with the DiGeorge syndrome is not at the level of the precursor T stem cell but is in the development of the thymus, the organ required for differentiation of stem cells into functioning T cells.

Treatment

Initial treatment is directed toward controlling the hypoparathyroidism by intravenous calcium gluconate, following by orally administered calcium in conjunction with large doses of vitamin D to prevent hypocalcemic seizures. Congenital heart disease frequently results in congestive heart failure that may require immediate surgical correction. In three of the four patients studied, repair of the T cell deficiency quickly followed the transplantation of a fetal thymus. In the fourth patient there was a more gradual improvement.

PURINE NUCLEOSIDE PHOSPHORYLASE DEFICIENCY

Purine nucleoside phosphorylase (PNP) deficiency is an autosomal recessive disorder characterized by deficiency of the enzyme purine nucleoside phosphorylase and deficient T cell function.

Clinical Presentation

Three of the five patients reported with PNP deficiency developed generalized vaccinia, which led to the death of two of the patients. Recurrent pneumonia, otitis media, and pharyngitis have been reported in these patients. Isolated patients have had diarrhea, anemia with megaloblastic changes in the marrow, lymphosarcoma, and mild spastic paresis.

Immunologic Defects

B cell function is normal, including normal to elevated serum immunoglobulins and normal antibody responses. There is a progressive decline in lymphocyte numbers, leading to significant lymphocytopenia, decreased total number of T cells, absent cutaneous delayed reactivity, and depressed in vitro proliferative responses to phytohemagglutinin (PHA) or allogeneic cells.

Pathogenesis

Patients with PNP deficiency show less than 1 percent of the normal level of purine nucleoside phosphorylase in their red cells, lymphocytes, and fibroblasts. The parents of the patients have, in general, shown approximately one-half of the normal enzyme level, thus supporting an autosomal recessive inheritance for this disorder. PNP catalyzes the conversion of inosine to hypoxanthine, the step in the purine metabolic pathway beyond that catalyzed by ADA. Patients deficient in PNP excrete increased quantities of inosine, deoxyinosine, guanosine, and deoxyguanosine in their urine. Of these substrates, only deoxyguanosine is highly toxic to cultured T cells. Furthermore, only deoxyguanosine can be phosphorylated, and it accumulates as deoxyGTP. It has been suggested that deoxyGTP inhibits ribonucleotide reductase and thus leads to a depletion of deoxyCPT and deoxyTTP and, therefore, to diminished lymphocyte DNA synthesis with the consequent T cell immunodeficiency state.

ATAXIA–TELANGIECTASIA

Ataxia–telangiectasia is an autosomal recessive disorder characterized by cerebellar ataxia, oculocutaneous telangiectasia, recurrent sinopulmonary infections, a high incidence of neoplasia, and a variable immunodeficiency state involving the humoral or cellular immune system, or both.

Clinical Manifestations

Neurologic abnormalities dominated by cerebellar ataxia usually have their onset at 9 months to 4 years of age. Telangiectasia consisting of dilated venules usually appears between 2 and 8 years of age and occurs on the conjunctiva and exposed areas of skin. Other integumental abnormalities include vitiligo, cafe au lait spots, sclerodermoid changes, and gray hair. The patients frequently have significant retardation of growth. Abnormalities of endocrine function have been described, including abnormalities of ovarian histology in some cases and the absence of ovaries in others. Somewhat over half of the patients have an abnormality of carbohydrate metabolism consisting of glucose intolerance, elevated plasma insulin levels, failure of insulin to reduce blood sugar levels, and, in the two cases examined, anti-insulin receptor antibodies.

Recurrent infections, particularly of the sinopulmonary tract, occur frequently. They begin as multiple discrete episodes, and in about one-third of the patients they are persistent and chronic, leading to structural lung disease and pulmonary insufficiency. Malignancy is a frequent occurrence, appearing in at least 10 percent of the patients reported. Most of the neoplasms involved lymphoid tissue, but gastric carcinomas, malignancies of the central nervous system, and ovarian tumors have also been reported.

Immunologic Defect

The various clinical features are accompanied by a complex immunologic deficiency state involving both cellular and humoral immune responses. In the humoral area 70 percent of the patients have IgA deficiency and 80 percent have IgE deficiency. These deficiencies may frequently coexist but may also occur independently. A second humoral abnormality particularly common in those with IgA deficiency is the presence of low molecular weight (8 S) IgM in the serum. IgG is usually present in normal amounts. Metabolic turnover studies with radioiodinated purified immunoglobulins designed to determine the genesis of the various immunoglobulin abnormalities have shown that the primary factor in the reduced IgA and IgE levels was markedly decreased synthesis of these classes. In some patients, however, in addition to the decreased rate of IgA synthesis, there was a markedly reduced survival of IgA associated with circulating antibodies with IgA specificity.

Although patients with ataxia–telangiectasia frequently have no IgA or IgE detectable in their serum, they have normal or slightly increased numbers of circulating B cells with a normal class distribution on their surface. Most patients tested could make antibody responses to various antigens although the mean rise in antibody titer was significantly less in the patients than in the control group. The patients have quite poor antibody responses to viral antigens and, in addition, local secretory antibody responses have been relatively uniformly impaired.

Patients with ataxia–telangiectasia also have a variable disorder of cell-mediated immunity. One of the most striking and consistent pathologic features of the disease is that the thymus is absent or small and embryonic in appearance. The patients have defects in T cell functions, as demonstrated by the fact that only 15 percent of the patients manifested a positive delayed-type skin test to a battery of common skin test antigens and in some cases could not be sensitized to dinitrochlorobenzene. Delayed rejection of skin allografts was noted in over 80 percent of ataxia–telangiectasia patients studied. In addition, the patients frequently manifest a poor in vitro response to stimulants of lymphocyte blastogenesis. In an extensive analysis of a large group of these patients it was concluded that progressive respiratory infection occurs mainly in those patients who manifest both cellular and humoral defects.

Pathogenesis

The underlying defect in this disease has not yet been defined. One of the possibilities is a primary thymic abnormality wherein T cells are defective both in classic cell-mediated reactions and in their helper function required for IgA and IgE antibody responses. However, a primary thymic defect cannot explain all of the humoral immune defects of patients with ataxia–telangiectasia nor can it explain many of the nonimmunologic features of this disease.

An alternative explanation for some of the manifestations of the disease follows the recent observation that patients with ataxia–telangiectasia have a defect in DNA repair. They are exceedingly sensitive to x-rays and develop severe or even fatal reactions following x-ray therapy for cancer. The lymphocytes have a high frequency of spontaneous chromosomal breaks, most frequently among the group D chromosomes, especially chromosome 14. The fibroblasts of patients with ataxia have a markedly reduced colony-forming ability following x-irradiation. In addition, they have been shown to have a defect in DNA repair following x-irradiation under anaerobic conditions. These observations of a DNA repair defect in patients with ataxia–telangiectasia would provide one explanation for the high incidence of cancer and may also be of relevance to the immunodeficiency observed.

Another explanation for the defect in patients with ataxia–telangiectasia involves the concept of a defect in tissue differentiation. Normally the thymus, along with other organs, requires the interaction of a mesenchymal inducer and an entodermal anlage. An abnormality of a mesenchymal inducer could explain the embryonic appearance of the thymus. Waldmann and McIntire considered the possibility that a postulated defect in organ differentiation and maturation due to an abnormal mesenchymal inducer might lead to an abnormality of hepatic cell differentiation as well since this differentiation requires a similar interaction between entodermal and mesodermal germ lines. They demonstrated that α-fetoprotein, a protein produced by the fetal liver, was elevated in all 20 of the patients with ataxia–telangiectasia examined but not in patients with other immunodeficiency disorders. This observation is in accord with the view that a defect in organ differentiation occurs in patients with ataxia–telangiectasia.

Treatment

Specific therapy directed at immunologically reconstituting patients with ataxia–telangiectasia has been disappointing. Symptomatic treatment, including rapid control of infections, has resulted in an apparent increase in survival.

REFERENCES

Bergsma D, Good RA, Finstad J (eds): Immunodeficiency in Man and Animals. National Foundation–March of Dimes Original Article Series. Sunderland, Mass, Sinauer, 1975

DiGeorge AM: Congenital absence of the thymus and its immunologic consequences: Concurrence with congenital hypoparathyroidism, in Immunologic Deficiency Diseases in Man. New York, National Foundation, 1968, p 116

Fudenberg H, Good RA, Goodman HC, Hitzig W, Kunkel HG, Roitt TM, Rosen FS, Rowe DS, Seligmann M, Soothill JR: Primary immunodeficiencies. Report of a World Health Organization Committee. Pediatrics 47:927, 1971

Giblett ER, Anderson JE, Cohen I, Pollara B, Meuwissen HJ: Adenosine deaminase deficiency in two patients with severely impaired cellular immunity. Lancet 2:1067, 1972

Hitzig WH: Congenital thymic and lymphocytic deficiency disorders, in Immunologic Disorders in Infants and Children. Philadelphia, Saunders, 1973

Horowitz SD, Hong R: The pathogenesis and treatment of immunodeficiency. Monogr Allergy 10:1, 1977

McFarlin DE, Strober W, Waldmann TA: Ataxia–telangiectasia. Medicine (Baltimore) 51:281, 1972

Meuwissen HJ, Pickering RJ, Pollara B, Porter IH (eds): Combined Immunodeficiency and Adenosine Deaminase Deficiency. A Molecular Defect. New York, Academic Press, 1975

Stiehm ER, Fulginiti V: Immunologic Disorders in Infants and Children. Philadelphia, Saunders, 1973

B CELL IMMUNODEFICIENCY DISEASES

X-LINKED INFANTILE AGAMMAGLOBULINEMIA (BRUTON-TYPE AGAMMAGLOBULINEMIA)

Bruton-type agammaglobulinemia is characterized by an exceedingly low concentration of all classes of serum immunoglobulins, normal cell-mediated immune responses, recurrent bacterial infections, and X-linked inheritance.

Clinical Features

Patients with X-linked infantile agammaglobulinemia usually remain asymptomatic during the first 6 months of life while passively transferred maternal IgG protects these individuals. At 6 months to 3 years of age the patients develop severe recurrent infections with encapsulated highly pathogenic pyogenic organisms including pneumococcus, Staphylococcus aureus, meningococcus, Hemophilus influenzae, and, less often, β-hemolytic streptococcus and Pseudomonas aeruginosa. These patients have a high frequency of otitis media, pharyngitis, sinusitis, bronchitis, pneumonia, empyema, and pyoderma. The children usually handle most viral infections, with the exception of infectious hepatitis, normally.

From 20 to 40 percent of the patients develop a rheumatoid arthritis–like pattern with sterile effusions involving one or more joints. Rarely the patients may develop a slowly progressive neurologic disease accompanying a dermatomyositislike syndrome associated with prolonged shedding of an ECHO virus. Diarrhea and malabsorption with protein-losing enteropathy, frequently associated with infestation by Giardia lamblia, are noted in some patients.

Immunologic Defects

Patients with infantile X-linked agammaglobulinemia have a failure of the humoral immune system but normal cell-mediated immunity. The circulating IgG concentration is less than 1 mg/ml, and IgM, IgD, and IgE are usually undetectable. In the majority of patients, B lymphocytes with easily demonstrable immunoglobulin on their surface cannot be found in the blood and tissues. Recently, affected boys with X-linked agammaglobulinemia have been shown to have normal numbers of pre-B cells, that is, bone marrow lymphoid cells that contain intracytoplasmic IgM in small amounts but no easily detectable surface IgM. Thus, these patients may be viewed as having an arrest at a very early stage in the cellular differentiation along the B cell pathway.

It should be noted that a few patients have been reported with well-documented X-linked inheritance of panhypogammaglobulinemia and normal numbers of immunoglobulin-bearing lymphocytes, suggesting that there may be two distinct forms of X-linked agammaglobulinemia. Patients with X-linked hypogammaglobulinemia do not have natural antibodies such as isohemagglutinins and do not produce antibody on antigenic challenge. Their lymph nodes and spleens are devoid of germinal centers and plasma cells and their gut-associated lymphoid tissues, including tonsils and adenoids, are very poorly developed.

The total number of circulating lymphocytes, the number of circulating T cells, and T cell function as measured by the in vitro blastogenic responses are normal. Suppressor T cells that inhibit the maturation of cocultured normal B cells in in vitro pokeweed mitogen–stimulated cultures have been identified in the circulation of some patients.

Pathogenesis

This disease is an X-linked disorder characterized by an arrest at a very early stage in cellular differentiation along the B cell pathway. This may reflect an intrinsic defect in the cells of the B cell–plasma cell series or may reflect the lack of a microenvironment required for the differentiation of primitive pre-B cells into B cells. An analogous disorder may be produced in birds by the removal of the bursa of Fabricius prior to hatching.

Treatment

The most important aspect of treatment is replacement therapy with human immune serum globulin. The patients are treated with 0.6 ml/kg/month or 0.3 ml/kg/2 weeks of a 16.5 percent solution of gamma globulin. Gamma globulin is given by deep intramuscular injection since intravenous injection causes severe reactions. Some patients have been treated with plasma infusions from a single donor, but this method carries the risk of hepatitis.

TRANSCOBALAMIN II DEFICIENCY

Hitzig and co-workers have described one kindred in which transcobalamin II deficiency was inherited as an autosomal recessive trait. The deficiency of this protein involved in the transfer of vitamin B_{12} was associated with profound hypogammaglobulinemia, megaloblastic anemia, and diarrhea in the propositus. The child had normal T cell function and B lymphocyte numbers were normal. Following the administration of 1000 μg of vitamin B_{12} immunoglobulin levels increased to normal levels and the patient made antibodies to antigens used for sensitization prior to the vitamin B_{12} therapy. The disease manifestations were thought to be due to B_{12} deprivation of hematopoietic, intestinal mucosal, and lymphoid tissues, the three most rapidly replicating tissues.

COMMON VARIABLE IMMUNODEFICIENCY

Common variable immunodeficiency is a term applied to a heterogeneous group of syndromes characterized by hypogammaglobulinemia, decreased ability to produce antibody following antigenic challenge, and increased incidence of infections but variable times of onset, variable patterns of clinical manifestation, and variable basic pathophysiologic defects.

Clinical Features

Generally speaking, patients with common variable immunodeficiency have clinical features that are similar to those discussed above for patients with X-linked agammaglobulinemia. They have a high incidence of recurrent pneumonia, chronic sinopulmonary disease, bronchiectasia, otitis media, septicemia, and meningitis. These patients differ from those with X-linked agammaglobulinemia in that they manifest a higher incidence of gastrointestinal disorders with malabsorption, diarrhea, and protein-losing gastroenteropathy. These manifestations may be due to specific gastrointestinal bacterial infections but more frequently are associated with infestation with *Giardia lamblia* or with an inability to deal with microflora normally present in the alimentary tract. Pathologically the gastrointestinal tract may show nodular lymphoid hyperplasia or a spruelike pattern with blunted intestinal villi.

Autoimmune disease is also a common feature in patients with acquired hypogammaglobulinemia. Many develop a rheumatoid arthritis syndrome, systemic lupus erythematosus, idiopathic thrombocytopenic purpura, neutropenia, pernicious anemia, or Coombs'-positive hemolytic anemia. Hepatosplenomegaly is observed in 20–60 percent of patients.

Immunologic Defects

Common variable hypogammaglobulinemia invariably involves an immunoglobulin defect, but the classes involved and degree of reduction are variable. The most common pattern is a marked reduction in all major classes of immunoglobulin molecules. These patients have a low level of natural antibodies with low or absent isohemagglutinin titers. In addition, they have a markedly reduced capacity to produce antibodies following antigenic challenge. Approximately one-fourth of the patients have normal or increased numbers of circulating B cells; approximately one-half have slightly or moderately reduced numbers of circulating B cells; and the remaining one-fourth have a markedly reduced number of these immunoglobulin-bearing lymphocytes.

A high percentage of patients with common variable immunodeficiency have an associated abnormality of delayed hypersensitivity. Over 30 percent of the patients are cutaneously anergic and are unable to respond to a battery of common recall antigens. A significant number cannot be sensitized to dinitrochlorobenzene, and, in some, skin allograft rejection is abnormally delayed. In the majority of but not all studies, the lymphocyte transformation response to PHA was depressed. Thus, patients with common variable immunodeficiency frequently have a significant disorder of cell-mediated immunity.

Pathogenesis

Common variable immunodeficiency was considered to be a truly sporadic or acquired defect. However, the observation that there was a high incidence of immunoglobulin disorders and autoimmune phenomenon in family members of certain patients with common variable immunodeficiency supports the view that genetic mechanisms are involved at least in some cases of this syndrome. In certain cases common variable immunodeficiency has followed intrauterine infection with rubella virus or postnatal infection with Epstein-Barr virus.

As noted above, patients with common variable immunodeficiency are heterogeneous in terms of the site of the block in cellular differentiation and in terms of the basic defect that leads to the reduced immunoglobulin synthesis. The majority of patients appear to have a defect in the maturation of stem cells into plasma cells due to an intrinsic defect of the B cell–plasma cell system. In some, there are virtually no circulating B cells with an apparent failure of maturation of stem cells into B cells. In others, representing the majority, there are normal numbers of B cells but a defect in the terminal maturation of these cells into plasma cells. A small subgroup of these patients has been shown to be able to synthesize immunoglobulins but is unable to secrete these molecules. The patients of this last group do not glycosylate immunoglobulins normally and do not have the receptor for Epstein-Barr virus on the surface of their B cells. In other patients, there are defects extrinsic to the B cell–plasma cell system. Certain patients have been shown to have a failure of maturation of B cells associated with a circulating inhibitor. The lymphocytes of such patients are able to synthesize immunoglobulin in in vitro studies when cultured in fetal calf serum but not when cultured in the patient's plasma.

Finally, hypogammaglobulinemia in some patients has been shown to be associated with an abnormal number of activated suppressor T cells which act to suppress B cell maturation and antibody production. The T cells from such patients suppress immunoglobulin synthesis of normal lymphocytes when they are cocultured with them in the presence of the B cell activator pokeweed mitogen. In a significant number of patients with common variable hypogammaglobulinemia there is a primary B cell defect, and the increased numbers of suppressor T cells appear to be a secondary factor but one that is of importance in the perpetuation of the hypogammaglobulinemia. In other cases, however, it has been shown that the suppressor T cell defect is a more primary pathogenic factor. In these cases, the B cells of the patients largely freed of their T cells in vitro synthesize immunoglobulins. These observations suggest that a subset of patients with common variable hypogammaglobulinemia has a disorder of suppressor T cells that inhibits the maturation of B cells into immunoglobulin-synthesizing plasma cells.

Treatment

The primary therapy is the same as for patients with X-linked agammaglobulinemia; intramuscular injections of gamma globulin or intravenous infusions of plasma are the primary approaches to therapy.

IMMUNODEFICIENCY ASSOCIATED WITH A THYMOMA

At least 50 patients have been identified who had a benign thymoma, usually of the spindle cell variety, and associated hypogammaglobulinemia. Such patients have a reduction in the serum concentration of all classes of immunoglobulin molecules, are unable to produce antibody to antigenic challenge, and have clinical features similar to those of patients with common variable immunodeficiency. These patients also have certain additional features, including extreme eosinopenia in the majority and pure red cell aplasia or pancytopenia in a significant minority of cases. The level of the immunologic defect also appears to differ from that in certain other forms of hypogammaglobulinemia.

The patients with thymoma and hypogammaglobulinemia have an extreme reduction or absence of lymphocytes bearing surface immunoglobulin, in contrast to the majority of patients with common variable immunoglobulin deficiency. In addition, they lack marrow pre-B cells, in contrast to patients with X-linked agammaglobulinemia, who have normal numbers of such cells. It should be noted that an excessive number of activated suppressor T cells has been demonstrated in several patients with thymoma and hypogammaglobulinemia. It is not clear whether such suppressor cells act to prevent the emergence of cells of the B cell–plasma cell series in these patients or, more likely, they represent the secondary development of activated suppressor T cells in patients with a fundamental B stem cell defect. In no instance has the removal of the thymoma resulted in a reversal of the immunodeficiency. This is in contrast to pure red cell aplasia and myasthenia gravis, disorders which may improve following removal of a thymoma.

SELECTIVE IgA DEFICIENCY

Selective IgA deficiency is characterized by a serum IgA level of less than 5 mg/dl in an individual with normal levels of IgG and IgM. IgA deficiency associated with the ataxia–telangiectasia syndrome is considered separately.

Clinical Features

IgA deficiency occurs in 1 in 500 to 1 in 700 individuals of European ancestry. Individuals with selective IgA deficiency may be healthy, but as a group they have increased numbers of sinopulmonary infections, chronic diarrheal diseases, and autoimmune syndromes. Since IgA is the major immunoglobulin molecule of the external secretions, it may be viewed as a first line of defense of the secretory system. Patients with selective IgA deficiency have an increased incidence of sinopulmonary infections; however, in contrast to patients with agammaglobulinemia or those with ataxia–telangiectasia, these infections rarely lead to profound respiratory insufficiency. Respiratory tract allergy and pulmonary hemosiderosis are also more common in these patients. Gastrointestinal tract disorders, including gluten-sensitive enteropathy, diarrhea with intestinal nodular lymphoid hyperplasia, and, more rarely, ulcerative colitis or regional enteritis occur at an increased frequency in these patients. Patients with IgA deficiency states also have an increased incidence of autoimmune disorders and autoantibodies, including rheumatoid arthritis, systemic lupus erythematosus, and, to a lesser extent, dermatomyositis, pernicious anemia with anti-intrinsic factor and anti-parietal cell antibodies, thyroiditis, Coombs'-positive hemolytic anemia, Sjögren's syndrome, and chronic active hepatitis.

The most common clinically significant circulating antibodies in patients with selective IgA deficiency are anti-IgA antibodies. Patients with such antibodies may develop anaphylactic reactions upon receiving whole blood, plasma, or other biologic fluids containing IgA. Patients with IgA deficiency also have a high incidence of antimilk antibodies especially directed toward bovine IgM. In addition, they have an increased incidence of such antibodies as antinuclear antibodies, anti-DNA antibodies, and anti-basement membrane antibodies. Finally, surveys of atopic populations show a high incidence of selective IgA deficiency in comparison to the normal population.

Immunologic Defects

Patients with selective IgA deficiency have by definition a serum level of IgA of less than 5 mg/dl and normal or increased levels of IgG and IgM. In most patients, secretory IgA levels are also markedly depressed. Serum IgE levels may be increased in some patients with associated allergy. However, there is a greater than chance association of IgE deficiency in patients with selective IgA deficiency. Most patients with IgA deficiency are capable of forming normal amounts of antibody following parenteral immunization. The number of circulating B cells, including IgA-bearing B cells, is normal. Cell-mediated immunity is normal in most patients, although depressed numbers of T cells and diminished production of T cell interferon have been reported in a few.

Pathogenesis

Most commonly, IgA deficiency occurs sporadically; however, it has also been associated with an autosomal dominant or a recessive pattern of inheritance. Family members may have panhypogammaglobulinemia. IgA deficiency has been associated with abnormalities of chromosome 18. In addition, it has occurred following infections with rubella, cytomegalovirus, and *Toxoplasma gondii* organisms or after hydantoin therapy.

The pathogenesis of IgA deficiency appears to involve a defect in the terminal maturation of B cells since patients with this disorder have normal numbers of IgA-bearing B lymphocytes. In one study, the lymphocytes of some patients with IgA deficiency cultured with pokeweed mitogen could be induced to mature into plasma cells that secrete IgA. A deficiency of helper T cells was considered as a possible mechanism in these studies. In other studies a small subset of patients with IgA deficiency was shown to have IgA class-specific circulating suppressor T cells that developed as a primary or more probably a secondary event. The majority of patients with IgA deficiency, however, appear to have an intrinsic defect of the B cell–plasma cell system without associated abnormalities of helper or suppressor T cells.

Therapy

Patients with selective IgA deficiency should not be treated with gamma globulin since it contains IgA and these patients are capable of forming normal amounts of antibody of other immunoglobulin classes to this IgA. The use of gamma globulin in these patients increases the risk of development of anti-IgA antibodies and anaphylactic reactions with subsequent transfusions. If such patients require a blood transfusion, blood from an IgA-deficient donor should be used if available. If not, the use of frozen, washed red blood cells reduces the risk of developing anti-IgA antibodies.

IMMUNOGLOBULIN DEFICIENCY WITH NORMAL OR INCREASED IgM

A series of X-linked, autosomal recessive and sporadic immunodeficiency disorders have been described that are characterized by normal or increased concentrations of serum IgM but decreased or absent IgG and IgA. Patients with these disorders present with recurrent pyogenic infections, including otitis media, pneumonia, and septicemia. Some patients have cyclic or persistent neutropenia, hemolytic anemia, or thrombocytopenia. B cell lymphomas of the intestinal tract have been the cause of death in some of these patients. The patients have a normal to markedly increased serum IgM concentration with markedly reduced concentrations of the other immunoglobulin classes. Isohemagglutinin titers may be elevated and the patients may make antibody responses to some but not all antigens. In some forms of this disorder there are normal numbers of B cells with normal isotype diversity, that is, surface membranes with IgM, IgD, IgG, and IgA. In another group of patients there are no IgG- or IgA-bearing B cells demonstrable. The patients have not had lymphocytopenia and their cellular immune responses appear to be normal.

It has been postulated that in the normal individual there is a sequential development of immunoglobulins initiated by IgM production, with IgG and IgA produced subsequently. An arrest in the development of the immunoglobulin-producing cells after the formation of IgM-synthesizing cells would be a possible defect in this disorder. In one group of patients this defect would be at the level of pre-B or B cell isotype diversification, characterized by the production of B cells with IgM on their surfaces and by the failure of development of B cells with surface-membrane IgG and IgA. In the other group of patients, in whom all classes of immunoglobulin appear in normal frequency on B cells, there appears to be a failure of terminal differentiation of the B alpha and B gamma lymphocytes.

WISKOTT-ALDRICH SYNDROME

The Wiskott-Aldrich syndrome is an X-linked recessive disorder characterized by thrombocytopenia, eczema, multiple infections, and a high incidence of reticuloendothelial malignancies.

Clinical Features

The initial manifestations of the Wiskott-Aldrich syndrome are usually related to bleeding episodes, including petechiae, gastrointestinal bleeding, and even severe bleeding episodes into the brain secondary to thrombocytopenia. Eczema that is typical in its distribution develops during the first year of life. Another dominant feature of the disease is recurrent infections with an array of organisms, including bacteria, viruses (including cyto-

megalovirus), and the organisms such as *Pneumocystis carinii*. Otitis media, skin infection, pneumonia, and septicemia are frequent. Chronic herpes simplex infections of the eye may lead to chronic keratitis or, in some patients, to widespread lesions and death. Coombs'-positive hemolytic anemia, splenomegaly, hepatomegaly, and arthritis have been described in some patients. From 20 to 30 percent of the patients with the Wiskott-Aldrich syndrome develop a malignancy, usually of the reticuloendothelial system.

Immunologic Defects

The function of the cellular immune system is abnormal in the majority of patients. In general, they are unable to manifest delayed hypersensitivity responses to common recall antigens, to develop delayed hypersensitivity to new antigens such as dinitrochlorobenzene, and to reject skin allografts normally. Despite these functional defects of cell-mediated immunity the patients have normal numbers of circulating lymphocytes that transform normally when cultured in vitro with nonspecific mitogens such as phytohemagglutinin. Clearly responsive lymphocytes are present in these patients, but there is a defect in the ability of these cells to proliferate in response to specific stimuli, including antigens and allogeneic cells.

Immunoglobulin levels are normal or elevated. Serum IgG and IgD levels are normal, whereas IgA levels and IgE levels are significantly increased. On the other hand, the mean serum IgM level is decreased. Studies of the metabolism of serum immunoglobulins with radioiodinated serum proteins have shown that the survival of each of the immunoglobulins is significantly shortened as a result of an increased rate of endogenous catabolism of these proteins. Despite these normal immunoglobulin levels functional defects in the humoral system are a universal feature of this disorder. When immunized with complex particulate antigens such as typhoid or *Brucella* antigens, the patients produced some antibodies although not to normal levels. Responses to more purified simple protein antigens such as diphtheria and tetanus were also depressed. The most profound defect in antibody response, however, was found when the children were immunized with a variety of predominantly polysaccharide antigens. They made virtually no antibodies to the VI antigen of *Escherichia coli* or to pneumococcal polysaccharide antigens.

Pathogenesis

The basic defect in patients with the Wiskott-Aldrich syndrome has not been identified. It is clear, however, that the level of the immunologic defect is distinct from that in the primary immunodeficiency diseases discussed above in which there is a disorder of the effectors of the immune response. Patients with the Wiskott-Aldrich syndrome have normal thymus glands and normal numbers of circulating lymphocytes that respond to nonspecific mitogens; however, these patients are anergic and unable to make specific cell-mediated immune responses. Similarly, these patients have normal immunoglobulin levels and synthetic rates yet fail to produce specific antibody normally following immunization, especially with polysaccharide antigens. This combination of findings is consistent with a defect in the steps of antigen processing and recognition and initiation of the specific immune response, that is, a defect in the afferent limb of immunity.

Therapy

Fresh platelets and blood are administered for bleeding manifestations as necessary. Splenectomy is in general to be avoided unless it is absolutely mandated by extreme thrombocytopenia since it is usually followed by overwhelming sepsis within 1 year. Transfer factor has been advocated by some groups as therapy for patients with the Wiskott-Aldrich syndrome. However, other groups have not found it to be of benefit. Transplantation of marrow from an HLA MLC matched sibling has led to a complete reversal of the manifestations of the Wiskott-Aldrich syndrome.

REFERENCES

Ammann AJ, Hong R: Selective IgA deficiency: Presentation of 30 cases and a review of the literature. Medicine (Baltimore) 50:223, 1971

Bergsma D, Good RA, Finstad J (eds): Immunodeficiency in Man and Animals. National Foundation–March of Dimes Original Article Series. Sunderland, Mass, Sinauer, 1975

Blaese RM, Strober W, Brown RS, Waldmann TA: The Wiskott-Aldrich syndrome. A disorder with a possible defect in antigen processing or recognition. Lancet 1:1056, 1968

Cooper MD, Chase HP, Lowman JT, Krivit W, Good RA: Wiskott-Aldrich syndrome: Immunologic deficiency disease involving the afferent limb of immunity. Am J Med 44:499, 1968

Cooper MD, Seligmann MB: B and T lymphocytes in immunodeficiency and lymphoproliferative diseases, in Loor F, Roelants GE (eds): B and T Cells in Immune Recognition. London, Wiley, 1977, p 377

Geha RS, Schneeberger E, Merler E, Rosen RS: Heterogeneity of "acquired" or common variable agammaglobulinemia. N Engl J Med 291:1, 1974

Good RA, Kelly WD, Rotstein J, Varco RL: Immunological deficiency diseases: Agammaglobulinemia, hypogammaglobulinemia, Hodgkin's disease and sarcoidosis. Prog Allergy 6:187, 1962

Hitzig WH, Dohmann V, Pluss HJ, Vischer D: Hereditary transcobalamin II deficiency: Clincal findings in a new family. J Pediatr 85:622, 1974

Horowitz SD, Hong R: The pathogenesis and treatment of immunodeficiency. Monogr Allergy 10:1, 1977

Rosen FS, Janeway CA: The gamma globulins. III. The antibody deficiency syndromes. N Engl J Med 275:709, 1966

Stiehm ER, Fulginiti V: Immunologic Disorders in Infants and Children. Philadelphia, Saunders, 1973

Waldmann TA, Blaese RM, Broder S, Krakauer R: Disorders of suppressor immunoregulatory cells in the pathogenesis of immunodeficiency and autoimmunity. Ann Intern Med 88:226, 1978

Waldmann TA, Broder S, Blaese RM, Durm M, Blackman M, Strober W: Role of suppressor T cells in pathogenesis of common variable hypogammaglobulinemia. Lancet 2:609, 1974

Serum Sickness

Ross E. Rocklin

ETIOLOGY AND PATHOGENESIS

ETIOLOGY

Serum sickness is an immune complex disease that develops following the injection of foreign (usually equine-derived) serum or serum products; it is characterized by fever, arthralgia, skin eruptions, and edema. Drug allergy may also produce a clinical picture that simulates serum sickness. This condition may also occur following the transfusion of whole blood. This disease is not the medical problem it once was because serum has not been used for the treatment of microbial infections since the advent of antibiotics. At present, equine antisera (IgG) are used for the neutralization of toxins produced by microorganisms that cause tetanus, botulinus, rabies, diphtheria, as well as snake venom.

The incidence of this disease is directly related to the type and the amount of preparation administered. In general, 2–5 percent of patients administered tetanus antitoxin develop serum sickness. If the total amount of tetanus antitoxin injected is 5–10 ml, one may expect reactions in 10 percent. If the amount is as much as 80 ml, then one almost always finds the disease developing to some extent. Sixteen percent of patients who receive rabies antiserum develop serum sickness. The tendency to develop this disease increases with age, being minimal in childhood and reaching a maximal incidence in adults. A mild form of the disease lasting 1–4 days is observed in children, while a more severe disease lasting several weeks develops in patients over 15 years of age.

The method of production of various equine antisera may have a profound effect upon the ability of a given serum to induce a reaction. Most tetanus antitoxin preparations are digested by pepsin, which does not impair the antitoxic properties of the preparation but does destroy many of the irrelevant and potentially sensitizing proteins in the serum. In contrast, antirabies antiserum is not subjected to peptic digestion because of the great loss in antibody activity experienced with this form of treatment. While drugs are known to induce a serum sickness-like syndrome, the age and dose relationships that pertain to serum sickness do not strictly follow the same pattern

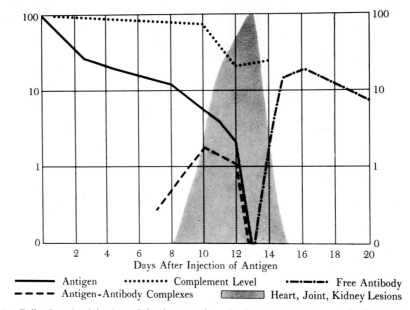

Fig. 1. Following the injection of foreign proteins, the host generates an antibody response. As detectable antigen–antibody complexes appear in the circulation, complement levels fall and lesions in the heart, joints, kidney, and blood vessels appear. Shortly after all antigen–antibody complexes are eliminated, free antibody appears in the circulation, and inflammatory lesions rapidly disappear.

as the syndrome induced by drugs. Since drugs are haptens and only become immunogenic by first combining with serum proteins, one must also take into account the genetic potential of the patients to metabolize the drug as well as to mount an immune response against the drug–protein conjugate.

PATHOGENESIS

The essential basis of this disease is antigen–antibody interaction and the effect of the products of this reaction on various organ systems. Shortly after treatment with the serum product has begun, circulating foreign protein (usually IgG) becomes detectable in the blood of patients. This protein is metabolized in a manner similar to that seen in the animal from which it was derived. This initial period is called the latent period and usually lasts 4–10 days.

During this time the patient also develops an immune response characterized by the appearance of antibody against the injected protein (drug–protein conjugate). As soon as antibody appears, it combines with the protein antigen to form soluble immune complexes. These complexes are disposed of in a variety of ways, depending upon their nature and the ratio of antigen to antibody in the complex. As shown in Figure 1, there is a point at which the soluble immune complexes form and are deposited, and the clinical manifestations of the disease become evident. Experimental studies in the rabbit have demonstrated that these complexes are deposited beneath the endothelium of blood vessels. Antibodies of the

IgM or IgG classes may initiate fixation and activation of the complement system with a lowering of complement levels (Fig. 1). With localization of the antigen–antibody complexes in the walls of blood vessels and the subsequent attachment of complement components, polymorphonuclear leukocytes are attracted to these sites and may injure the vessel by release of enzymes found in their lysozomal granules. The vascular injury that ensues may lead to thrombosis and hemorrhage, clinically characterized by the petecchial and ecchymotic rash of serum sickness.

In addition to the vascular damage induced by antigen–antibody complexes described above, there is also a release of vasoactive amines such as histamine, serotonin, bradykinin, and slow reacting substance of anaphylaxis. The release of these mediators may lead to vasodilation with leakage of protein and fluid from the vascular space into the tissues, resulting in edema. Whereas many of the studies performed in animals involving immune complex disease have illustrated significant renal damage due to the deposition of antigen–antibody complexes, little of this effect is observed in man, in whom renal disease is minimal if present at all. The vascular lesions that are produced by this mechanism are indistinguishable from those described for periarteritis nodosa.

Serum sickness is a self-limited disease because the antigen supply soon becomes exhausted. Unless the foreign proteins are readministered, the symptoms resolve within several days to 1 week. Perpetuation of the disease is therefore dependent upon a continual supply of antigen. The immune complexes that are formed are removed by the reticuloendothelial system. As they are removed and metabolized there is an increase in the titer of serum antibody directed against the foreign proteins. These antibodies can be detected in the patient's serum during convalescence and for long periods thereafter. Therefore, readministration of the same foreign protein will lead to the formation of immune complexes and renewed clinical manifestations of the disease.

MANIFESTATIONS AND TREATMENT

LABORATORY STUDIES

Laboratory studies usually provide little assistance in diagnosing serum sickness. One may find a leukocytosis, increased numbers of circulating plasma cells, a mildly elevated sedimentation rate (but it is usually normal), and occasionally a peripheral eosinophilia. The urine is usually normal but may contain excess amounts of protein, red blood cells, and occasional casts. Renal impairment, however, is minimal. Complement levels are decreased during the acute phase of the disease. There is also an increased titer of heterophil antibodies directed against sheep red blood cells. The diagnosis of this condition can usually be made from the history of a recent administration of serum or drugs, but without that evidence this illness may be mistaken for rheumatic fever.

CLINICAL MANIFESTATIONS

The patient first experiences a local reaction characterized by itching at the site of injection. This is soon followed by the development of systemic symptoms, including facial edema, an intensely pruritic urticarial or erythematous rash, arthalgia, and myalgia. Of particular concern is the potential development of neurologic signs (as a result of vasculitis), including weakness in the extremities, sensory deficit, and facial palsy. The patient may also experience abdominal pain with nausea and vomiting. The erythematous or urticarial rash develops in about 90 percent of the patients and facial edema is seen in about 30 percent.

On physical examination, lymphadenopathy may be found in the nodes draining the site of injection accompanied by a rash and tenderness at that site. Occasionally, cardiac arrhythmia or a pericardial friction rub may be heard. Splenomegaly is uncommon. Fever (100°–102°F) may begin 3–4 days after the development of symptoms, as can the gastrointestinal symptoms. The joints are involved 80 percent of the time and one can frequently observe tenosynovitis with the presence of effusion. The temporomandibular joints are often involved early in the development of symptomatology. In addition to the urticarial and erythematous rash, the skin reveals a petecchial or purpuric rash.

In contrast to the slowly developing reaction described above in patients with a first exposure to antigen, an acute reaction may occur within seconds following the readministration of the same foreign protein or drug. This reaction is characterized by a feeling of apprehension in the patient, violent itching, sneezing, coughing, bronchospasm, and generalized urticaria. Shortly thereafter, the blood pressure may fall, the pulse become weak, and the patient may go into shock. There may be a loss of consciousness with convulsions. Death can occur within 10 minutes following the initial injection. Patients who survive this acute reaction usually go on to exhibit the other symptoms that are seen with the disease.

TREATMENT

The most effective form of treatment for this condition is prevention, i.e., recognition of hypersensitivity in a patient prior to the administration of the serum. The physician must be alerted to a possible reaction in those patients with a history of atopy. All patients should be tested by both intradermal skin tests and conjunctival application before receiving the serum injection. The serum is administered intradermally in a 0.02-ml volume of a 1:10 dilution of the serum; 15–20 minutes later the presence of a wheal and flare reaction is observed. If the skin test is negative, then the same volume (0.02 ml) of a 1:100 dilution is applied to the conjunctiva and observed for a reaction. If either test is positive, the use of this material should be reconsidered. If it is absolutely necessary to treat the patient with the serum, then the patient should first be desensitized (in a setting equipped to treat anaphylaxis) by repeated injections of the material in increasing doses. Start with a 0.10-ml volume of a 1:100 dilution subcutaneously, wait 15 minutes for the reaction, and if none occurs proceed by doubling the dose until a total of 1 ml is given.

If an immediate or anaphylactic reaction occurs following an injection of serum, the first measure is to apply a tourniquet above the area of injection. This slows the absorption of the material. The patient should then be treated with 0.5 ml of epinephrine (1:1000 dilution) subcutaneously and the same volume at another site, followed by the parenteral administration of an antihistamine such as tripelinamine hydrochloride (50 mg every 4 hours) or brompheniramine (4 mg every 4 hours). This should be sufficient treatment for most mild cases. When severe reactions occur, the use of steroids may be required. Prednisone can be administered, 40 mg/day over a 4–5-day period, and then stopped. Salicylates can be used in mild cases in which joint symptoms are present.

In cases in which tetanus antitoxin must be adminstered and there is either a question of or proven hypersensitivity, human serum preparations should be administered instead of equine preparations. Furthermore, in patients who have experienced a serum sickness reaction with the antitoxin, it then becomes necessary to immunize the patient with tetanus toxoid since the serum treatment cannot be continued.

REFERENCES

Arbesman CE, Kantor S, Rose N, Witebsky E: Serologic studies following prophylactic tetanus antitoxins. J Allergy 31:257, 1960

Cochrane CG: Mechanisms involved in the disposition of immune complexes in tissues. J Exp Med 134:75s, 1971

Dixon FJ: The pathogenesis of glomerulonephitis. Am J Med 44:493, 1968

Kunkel HG: Symposium on immune complexes and disease. J Exp Med 134:1s, 1971

McCluskey RT, Benacerraf B, Potter JL, Miller F: The pathologic effects of intravenously administered soluble antigen–antibody complexes. J Exp Med 111:181, 1960

Vaughan JH, Barnett EV, Leadley PJ: Serum sickness: Evidence in man of antigen–antibody complexes and free light chains in the circulation during the acute reaction. Ann Intern Med 67:596, 1967

Drug Allergy

Ross E. Rocklin

INCIDENCE AND PATHOGENESIS

INCIDENCE

Drug allergy or hypersensitivity may be defined as a complex of symptoms resulting from sensitization either during or following the administration of various drugs. These symptoms bear no relationship to the pharmacologic properties of the drug concerned and may occur at low concentrations. Drug allergy must be distinguished from intolerance to a drug(s), which is an undesirable pharmacologic effect also occurring at low concentrations, and idiosyncratic reactions, which are based on biochemical alterations in the metabolism of a drug. The latter reaction is independent of the dose, does not require prior exposure, and is not a pharmacologic effect of the drug.

The ever-increasing number of prescription and nonprescription drugs, while alleviating suffering in many instances, have been attended by correspondingly greater numbers of adverse reactions. For example, hospitalized patients receive, on the average, 10 drugs during their hospital stay, and that number may be as high as 50–60 in some cases. It has been calculated that patients receiving less than 6 drugs have only a 5 percent chance of developing a drug reaction, while those receiving more than 15 drugs have a 40 percent chance of developing one.

Between 1 and 2 percent of hospitalizations are for drug-related illnesses. Drug-induced conditions that frequently require hospitalization include systemic anaphylaxis, Stevens-Johnson syndrome, erythema multiforme, exfoliative dermatitis, serum sickness, pneumonitis, interstitial nephritis, and cytotoxic drug reactions. While the vast majority of anaphylactic drug reactions are potentially serious, and in fact 2.7 percent end in fatality, prompt recognition of this condition along with the institution of immediate and proper therapy should help to reduce the sequelae.

The drug that most commonly induces allergic reactions is penicillin. Between 1 and 5 percent of patients receiving penicillin develop some allergic manifestations. The incidence approaches 1 percent in outpatient populations and 5 percent in hospitalized patients. Penicillin accounts for 90 percent of all allergic reactions to drugs.

Moreover, penicillin accounts for 97 percent of the approximately 300 yearly deaths caused by anaphylactic drug reactions. In addition to penicillin, the following drugs are also known to frequently induce allergic manifestations: aspirin; local anesthetics; opiates; hormones; heparin; streptomycin; diagnostic reagents such as bromsulphthalein, Congo red, and decholin; dextran; vitamins; tetracycline; cephalin; and organic iodine.

PATHOGENESIS

Patients may vary widely in the way they absorb, metabolize, and excrete drugs. Therefore, the administration of a standard dose of a drug to groups of individuals reveals blood levels that are high in some and low in others. Furthermore, measurement of the rates of absorption, metabolism, and excretion of a given drug will single out those in whom these functions are rapid or slow. Drugs having wide dose–response curves or large therapeutic to toxic dose ratios may produce the desired effect with little risk of toxicity in standard doses. These factors may influence the type of adverse reaction that develops.

There are also a number of drug properties that determine the likelihood inducing an adverse drug reaction: (1) chemical structure and reactivity of the drug (discussed below); (2) cross-reactivity between drugs (some drugs contain a similar basic structure, e.g., in penicillin and cephalin, the 6-aminopenicillenic acid nucleus); (3) amount of drug administrated (dose, duration of treatment, number of courses); (4) mode of administration (the oral route is less sensitizing than the parenteral route); (5) presence of contaminants, additives, or solvents (adjuvants to slow absorption may be undesirable because they can increase the chance of sensitization). Patient factors, such as a history of prior sensitivity, atopy, age, genetic factors controlling drug metabolism or immune response, or underlying diseases that affect metabolism or excretion (e.g., liver or kidney disease), can also determine whether an adverse drug reaction will occur. Patients who have experienced one adverse drug reaction have a predisposition to develop others. Furthermore, the number of different drugs being ingested at one time may also predispose a patient to develop a reaction since the simultaneous administration of several drugs may inhibit or enhance enzyme production or competition for serum binding, thus influencing the pharmacologic or other activity of a given drug.

Because of their small size (molecular weight less than 2000), drugs are incomplete antigens (haptens) and are by themselves unable to induce hypersensitivity. In order for them to become immunogenic, covalent binding to tissues or serum proteins must occur. In the latter form, they are recognized as "foreign" by the host. Thus, host immune responses, in the form of antibodies, are directed against the drug portion of the hapten–protein conjugate. Drugs that are highly reactive chemically are the ones that most often induce a state of sensitization. During the process of conjugation, the drug may undergo marked chemical rearrangement, resulting in an antigen that is different from the original drug. The latter finding may explain some of the difficulties experienced by investigators who utilize in vitro or in vivo tests to diagnose drug allergies (discussed below). One does not know which form of the drug has become immunogenic and the incorrect choice of a reagent may lead to false-negative responses in the patient as well as a false sense of security regarding the absence of allergy.

Since penicillin is the most common cause of allergic drug reactions and since much experimental evidence has been gathered concerning the nature of reactions with this drug, a more detailed discussion is presented. The penicillin group reacts with ϵ-amino lysine residues of proteins to form a penicilloyl–protein conjugate; 98 percent of all antipenicillin responses are directed against this form of the drug and it has appropriately been termed the *major determinant*. Alternatively, penicillin may slowly isomerize to form penicillenic acid, which then binds to endogeneous lysine groups to form the penicilloyl determinant. Penicillenic intermediates may also react in other ways to form the so-called *minor determinants*. The conjugation of penicillin groups to protein proceeds relatively slowly, thus the number of multivalent antigen forms are greatly outnumbered by free or unconjugated drug. The free hapten can competitively inhibit the binding of multivalent antigen to immunoglobulin on cell surfaces and therefore prevent the occurence of an immunologic reaction. Furthermore, the inhibition by unconjugated hapten explains the occurrence of negative skin tests with a simple chemical in the presence of unquestioned evidence of sensitivity to the drug.

Drug reactions may be classified as those having a proven allergic basis (immunologic reaction can be demonstrated, such as immediate hypersensitivity, drug–antibody complex, or delayed hypersensitivity) and those with a possible or suspected allergic basis. In the patient with a proven reaction one can demonstrate IgE antibodies as well as a positive immediate hypersensitivity skin test to the drug and the presence of drug–antibody complexes. IgE bound to mast cells will induce an immediate hypersensitivity reaction following interaction with drug–protein conjugate, characterized by the release of histamine or other allergic mediators resulting in vasodilation and smooth muscle contraction. Drug–antibody complexes induce an arthus-type reaction and/or a serum sickness-like syndrome. A delayed hypersensitivity reaction to drugs results in the release of lymphokines, and such factors can cause perivascular mononuclear cell cuffing. This type of reaction, however, is not always correlated with the presence of clinical symptomatology.

Cytotoxic reactions to drugs occur when the drug binds to the surface of cells and antibodies or lymphocytes cause destruction (e.g., penicillin-induced hemolytic anemia, and quinidine-induced thrombocytopenia). Drug–antibody complexes may also bind to the cell surface, initiating a complement-dependent cell lysis, the so-called "innocent bystander" phenomena. Drugs may also induce an immune response directed against certain tissues (e.g., α-methyldopa antibody against red blood cells).

Some drug reactions are suspected of being due to allergic (pseudoallergic) mechanisms, but the evidence is scanty (e.g., no IgE is detected to drugs), although the symptoms are indistinguishable from those reactions having an allergic basis. Some of the drugs that have been implicated in these reactions are aspirin, tartrazine, radioiodinated contrast agents, and ampicillin. Aspirin induces bronchospasm in nonatopic asthmatics who also may have nasal polyps.

Recent evidence suggests that aspirin intolerance involves an imbalance in the normal homeostatic mechanism of the prostaglandin system. The result is increased constrictor ($PGF_2\alpha$) tone instead of dilatation (PGE_2). Between 15 and 20 percent of patients who experience adverse reactions to aspirin also develop similar symptoms when they ingest chemically dissimilar drugs such as tartrazine, a yellow food additive, and indomethacin. The mechanism for the latter two drugs seems to be similar to aspirin intolerance. On the other hand, sodium salicylate, which is chemically similar to aspirin, does not cause symptoms when administered to these patients. Taken together, these observations support the hypothesis that pseudoallergic reactions to aspirin are not mediated by antigen–antibody interactions since antibodies that are directed against aspirin should also combine with structurally related compounds such as sodium salicylate.

Radioiodinated contrast agents are an example of drugs that cause anaphylactic symptoms (1.7 percent of patients) in which no allergic mechanism can be demonstrated with confidence. The drug itself or a metabolite may directly induce histamine release to account for the symptoms. It would appear that drug–antibody interaction is not necessary for this reaction to occur.

Ampicillin causes a maculopapular (nonpruritic) rash that looks like an allergic dermatitis but is not accompanied by systemic symptoms. Nine percent of patients ingesting ampicillin will experience this reaction, and the incidence increases to 50 percent if the patient has infectious mononucleosis. These patients will have negative skin tests to penicillin antigens, and of interest, will not develop this reaction if rechallenged with ampicillin at a future date. It is therefore important to distinguish this type of ampicillin rash from true urticarial lesions since the latter may signify an allergic reaction and more serious symptomatology may develop if rechallenge is attempted.

CLINICAL MANIFESTATIONS, DIAGNOSIS, AND TREATMENT

CLINICAL MANIFESTATIONS

Probably the most common clinical manifestation of drug allergy is the development of a mild systemic illness simulating serum sickness which is characterized by urticarial skin eruptions, arthralgias or arthritis, lymphadenopathy, and fever. These symptoms begin 6–12 days following the administration of a drug and may take several days to 1 week to subside following the cessation of the drug. Drugs that may cause these symptoms include pencillin, sulfonamides, chlortetracycline, streptomycin, aspirin, barbituates, diphenylhydantoin, thiouracil, and iodides. Drug-induced fever may occur alone or in combination with the above symptoms and develops during the second week of treatment. It is usually low grade in nature (100°–102°F) and the patient appears less ill than would be anticipated from the high temperature. The temperature decreases 1–2 days following cessation of the drug but may take longer if other organs are also involved.

Dermatitis, as a manifestation of drug allergy, may take several forms. A fine maculopapular rash appearing in the axillary line and on the extensor surfaces of the extremities and trunk may go unnoticed by the patient. Urticarial lesions are usually reported to the physician because they are accompanied by pruritis. The persistent administration of a drug that is causing maculopapular lesions may lead to confluent erythroderma and subsequent exfoliative dermatitis as well as eczema. Erythema multiforme-like lesions are characterized by the formation of sharply circumscribed areas that are symmetric in distribution and develop clear central areas. The latter forms an annular pattern with secondary and tertiary rings that evolve into a target or iris lesion. Lesions that simulate erythema nodosum may be caused by such drugs as penicillin, sulfonamides, and iodides. Fixed drug eruptions are erythematous and sharply defined lesions that recur at the same site and in the same form upon reexposure to the same drug. These lesions may be caused by barbituates, phenothiazine, bromide, iodides, and sulfonaides. Photosensitivity reactions to drugs are characterized by erythema, edema, and mild scaling and are sharply limited to areas exposed to light. They may be caused by sulfonamides and thiazides.

The hematopoietic system is frequently involved in drug reactions. Thrombocytopenic purpura may occur following the administration of quinine, quinidine, sedor-

mid, thiouracil, gold salts, and the hydantoin derivatives. Hemolytic anemia may occur with sulfonamides, thiouracil, and quinidine. Agranulocytosis may be caused by the latter drugs and aminopyrine and phenobutazone. Aplastic anemia, involving a loss of the formed elements, has been associated with the administration of chloramphenicol, gold, and the sulfonamides. This reaction usually occurs if the drug has been administered for 4 or more weeks.

Gastrointestinal symptoms are common adverse reactions to the administration of drugs but the mechanism of action is rarely allergic in nature. Nephritis may occur following the administration of sulfonamides and methacillin. A periarteritis nodosa syndrome may occur following the administration of sulfonamides, penicillin, iodine thiourea, and diphenylhydantoin derivatives. Liver damage has been attributed to treatment with heavy metals, thorazine, and sulfanamides, although the evidence supporting an allergic basis for these reactions is insufficient.

A lupus eythematosus-like syndrome has been described following the ingestion of hydralazine, procainamide, and the hydantoin derivatives. The manifestations may vary from mild, including a positive LE test, to the full-blown picture of fever, arthritis, polyserositis, and hematologic manifestations. Pneumonitis with eosinophilia, peripheral neuritis, and encephalitis have all been ascribed to allergic drug reactions and probably represent involvement of vasculature in the particular organs effected.

Generalized anaphylaxis is a serious manifestation of drug allergy that must be dealt with promptly by the physican in order to avoid a fatal outcome. The symptoms are usually initiated within minutes after the injection of the offending drug, although, rarely, orally administered tablets may produce this reaction. The symptoms begin as generalized pruritis or itching on the soles and palms associated with hyperemia of the skin, angiodema, laryngeal edema, and swelling of the eyelids. This may be followed by decreased plasma volume, resulting in hypotension, subsequent vascular collapse, and shock.

DIAGNOSIS

The following observations might suggest the presence of an allergic drug reaction: (1) the reaction does not resemble the pharmacologic action of the drug; (2) it may be elicited by minute doses of the drug; (3) it usually occurs after a period of days following the initial administration of the offending drug; (4) it includes symptoms that are generally associated with allergy; (5) it reappears on challenge with progressive shortening of the latent period before developing symptoms; (6) cross-reactivity occurs with structurally similar drugs. As stated previously, some of the criteria for establishing an immunologic origin of drug allergy include the detection of an immune response to the drug or its metabolities (such as the presence of IgE drug-specific antibodies) and demonstration of the drug-initiated immunopathologic event. On the other hand, the presence of other classes of antibodies or cell-mediated immunity does not necessarily correlate with immunopathologic mechanisms, i.e., there are frequently no symptoms evoked following rechallenge with the drug. Rechallenging a patient with a drug suspected of causing a reaction may have diagnostic implications but is not recommended because of the potential fatal sequelae that may develop.

Because of the problems associated with the in vivo readministration of drugs, many investigators have attempted to use in vitro tests. The suspected drug is mixed together with sensitized leukocytes from the patient and either basophil degranulation or histamine release, lymphocyte proliferation, or the release of lymphocyte mediators is measured. Because the correlation of a positive in vitro assay with a suspected clinical reaction is relatively poor, these techniques have not gained the status of routine clinical tests and therefore remain, for the most part, a research tool. A major drawback that in vitro assays must overcome is an inability to simulate in vivo conditions. Incubation of the intact drug in vitro with cells does not take into account the requirement for metabolism to occur before the drug can be converted into the relevant immunogenic form. Therefore, negative results with these assays may not be meaningful, as described above. One in vitro test that is gaining wide usage is a procedure that measures specific IgE antibodies to certain drugs such as penicillin. This test, termed the *radioallergosorbent test* (RAST), is highly specific and can detect minute quantities of IgE to the suspected drug. Because it is costly, however, it is not being as widely used at the present time as skin testing.

Penicillin skin testing, while not recommended for routine use, appears to be of practical value in selected cases. The penicillin skin test reagents include a synthetic penicillin derivative, penicilloyl polylysine (PPL), which measures sensitivity to the major determinant, and partially aged penicillin G itself, which contains many of the minor determinants. Studies on large numbers of patients have revealed the following observations. Only 21 percent of patients with a positive history of an allergic reaction to penicillin had a positive skin test to PPL; 13 percent with a positive history also reacted to penicillin G. Overall, therefore, approximately 75 percent of patients with a positive history of having had a previous reaction to penicillin had negative skin tests. When these patients were rechallenged with penicillin, only 1 percent had an immediate reaction. Therefore, skin testing may be more predictive of sensitivity than the history. On the other hand, patients with a negative history of a previous reaction to penicillin may have a positive skin test. In these instances, it may be dangerous to administer penicillin to these patients. It should be noted that false-negative skin tests to penicillin may occur during and for a short time after urticarial reactions, but later turn positive with retesting.

Patients with documented reactions to penicillin in the past should not be skin tested unless a life-threatening indication for therapy outweighs the potential anaphylactic reaction that may occur with skin testing. In this case,

one should begin scratch testing at a very dilute concentration and increase the dose if the reactions are negative. If the skin test is positive, a course of desensitization should be undertaken with the proper personnel and equipment present in case of a reaction.

The skin test data may be summarized as follows: Skin testing is of diagnostic value following a reaction because it is frequently positive in penicillin-induced urticaria and serum sickness reactions, although it is not useful in cases of morbilliform eruptions, drug fever, or anaphylaxis. It may be predictive for determining the current allergic potential for immediate or accelerated reactions but is not predictive for late cutaneous manifestations. Skin testing may eventually be used for screening purposes to identify the patient who may develop an allergic reaction among those who have a negative history of previous reactions, as well as to identify the patient with a "positive" history of reaction in whom penicillin may be safely used.

TREATMENT

Management of drug allergy begins with the suspicion that a drug reaction may occur at any time. The presence of unexplained rash, fever, lymphadenopathy, or wheezing should alert the physician to this possibility. As is the case with any allergic illness, the basic form of treatment is avoidance or removal of the offending agent from the environment. Therefore, the drug or drugs should be stopped when the reaction occurs. Symptoms due to drug allergy should subside within 1–2 days following cessation of drug therapy, although in some instances they may take as long as a week to subside. In severe cases, the physician may want to aid the elimination of the drug by administering large amounts of fluids, diuretics, or laxatives. In some instances in which a drug allergy is strongly suspected but the symptoms do not subside following cessation of drug therapy, the physician should be aware of the possibility that the patient may be receiving the offending drug in his food. Many animal food products contain hormones or antibiotics.

In general, treatment of the drug reaction should be directed against the altered physiology. With reactions involving the release of vasoactive substances that cause hypotension, use of a vasoconstrictor such as epinephrine may be lifesaving (0.5–1.0 ml of a 1:1000 dilution). Corticosteroids should be used after stabilization of the blood pressure. The latter drug has been shown to be of use in arthus-type reactions such as serum sickness and polyarteritis as well as in forms of delayed hypersensitivity reactions. Large doses (40–60 mg/day) of prednisone may be administered for several days. The drug may then be stopped without a prolonged course of withdrawal. Together with epinephrine, antihistaminics such as diphenhydramine (50 mg) or brompheniramine (4 mg) may also be administered orally or parenterally but should not be used intravenously.

Under some circumstances, if there is a life-threatening need to use a drug that is shown to be causing an allergic reaction in a patient, one may attempt to desensitize a patient and then use the drug. Desensitization should only be carried out in hospitalized patients under circumstances in which immediate attention can be given to the patient should a reaction occur. Patients have been successfully desensitized to penicillin, insulin, paraminosalicylic acid, isoniazid, penicillamine, tetracycline, nitrogen mustard, and streptomycin. After desensitization, the drug can be administered in full doses for as long as 6–8 weeks without allergic symptoms developing.

In the case of penicillin allergy, preliminary attempts have been made to utilize univalent haptens, such as formyl penicilloyl derivative, for the prevention or treatment of penicillin allergy. Univalent haptens can block penicilloyl or other hapten-specific allergic reactions and are based on sound immunologic principles. This reagent could be administered to patients in situations in which penicillin treatment is absolutely necessary. Further clini-

cal trials with this material are required before it can be accepted for general use.

REFERENCES

Ackroyd JF: Sedormid purpura: An immunological study of a form of drug hypersensitivity, in Kallos P: Progress in Allergy, vol 3. New York, Interscience, 1952, p 531

Cluff LE: Clinical Problems with Drugs. Philadelphia, Saunders, 1975

DeWeck AL: Drug reactions, in Samter M: Immunological Diseases (ed 3). Boston, Little, Brown, 1978 (in press)

Gardner P, Cluff LE: The epidemiology of adverse drug reactions: A review and perspective. Johns Hopkins Med J 126:77, 1970

Hansten PD: Drug Interactions. Philadelphia, Lea & Febiger, 1974

Levine BB: Immunochemical mechanisms of drug allergy. Ann Rev Med 17:23, 1966

Allergic Rhinitis

Edward K. Dunham and Albert L. Sheffer

PATHOGENESIS

DEFINITION

Allergic rhinitis is a reaction, focused in the upper respiratory tract, of reaginic hypersensitivity to airborn allergens; exposure of a patient to an allergen to which he has become sensitized causes itching, sneezing, rhinorrhea, and nasal obstruction. Sensitization requires exposure of a susceptible subject to an allergen and involves synthesis by plasma cells of antibody (of the IgE class), that becomes bound to the surface of mast cells. Subsequent challenge with allergen causes the antibody-sensitized mast cell to release chemical mediators of inflammation that act upon their target tissues to produce the characteristic manifestations of the illness.

Seasonal allergic rhinitis, commonly called "hay fever," recurs at the same season in successive years and is generally caused by the pollens of wind-pollinated plants or by mold spores. Perennial allergic rhinitis is a similar illness without a seasonal pattern. It may be chronic and caused by allergens to which the patient is continually exposed, (such as house dust or animal danders) or paroxysmal, occurring when the patient encounters an allergen to which he is sensitive but is usually absent from his environment. Symptoms of allergic rhinitis are commonly aggravated by nonimmunologic factors such as drafts, temperature changes, odors, aerosols, and emotion. *Vasomotor rhinitis* is a term often used for an illness indistinguishable from allergic rhinitis except that no immunologic mechanism can be demonstrated.

NASAL PHYSIOLOGY

Besides olfaction, normal functions of the nose include regulation of the temperature and humidity of the inspired air as well as removal of foreign particles and gases by physical, enzymatic, and immunologic means.

Entering the nares in an upward direction, the inspired air is first directed backward between the turbinates and the septum and then downward in the nasopharynx. With these changes in the direction of its flow, the airstream impinges on the mucous membranes, which are presented over a large surface area by the convolutions of the turbinates. Heat is taken up from the mucosal vasculature, moisture is added by evaporation from the fluid secretions lining the mucosal surface, and particulate matter is entrapped in the mucus and carried to the nasopharynx by mucociliary transport.

The tissues lining the nose are erectile and richly supplied with goblet cells and mucus glands. Their degree of engorgement and rate of secretion of mucus are influenced by neural, hormonal, and pharmacologic factors; they are capable of rapid response to environmental changes and to physical and emotional stress. The nasal secretions contain lysozyme, a potent though nonspecific defense against bacterial infection, which may also be important in allergic rhinitis, that acts by stripping the carbohydrate coats from pollen grains and releasing the protein allergens within. Immunoglobulins, chiefly IgA and smaller amounts of IgG, are also prominent constituents of nasal mucus; their concentrations are increased in patients with allergic rhinitis. In the presence of rhinitis, granulocytes and mast cells are found in the mucus. The clearance of the mucus from the nose posteriorly may be important in the initiation of immune responses because antigenic matter is thereby carried to the lymphoid tissue of the adenoids.

PREDISPOSING FACTORS

Allergic rhinitis is often familial and in many kindreds is associated with asthma and atopic dermatitis. Probably a number of genetic factors participate in its inheritance. There is evidence that in man the capacity to respond immunologically to ragweed pollen antigens is conferred by single autosomal dominant genes closely linked to the major histocompatibility locus, as is the case in a large number of experimental systems in animals, and it seems likely that such mechanisms govern responsiveness to other antigens. Certain inbred strains of mice have a greater proclivity than others to developing reaginic responses, and it may be that in man, genetic factors can lead to heightened synthesis of IgE in response to an antigen challenge and to heightened tissue responsiveness to the mediators released from the IgE-sensitized mast cell. Genetic considerations aside, it is found that repeated administration of small doses of antigen favors a reaginic response in mice, and this pattern of antigen administration mimics natural exposure to environmental aeroallergens.

ALLERGENS

Airborne pollens, mold spores, house dust, and animal epidermal products are the allergens most often implicated in the causation of alleric rhinitis. The pollens of chief importance are those of wind-pollinated plants, which generally bear inconspicuous flowers, rather than those of insect-pollinated ones, which often bear very showy flowers adapted to attract pollen-carrying insects; the latter are therefore more conspicuous in the environment but their pollen grains are in most cases not widely airborne. Thus, patients with ragweed hay fever often attribute their symptoms to goldenrod, whose conspicuous blossoms appear at the same time as the scarcely noticeable ones of ragweed; "rose fever," that is, allergic rhinitis occurring in the late spring, is usually due to grass pollen.

In the United States, the pollen causing allergic rhinitis in the largest number of patients is that of ragweed; this plant is very widely distributed and its pollen is carried great distances by the wind. In the northern half of the country, it pollinates in late August and September. Second in importance are the pollens of the ubiquitous grasses, which pollinate in the late spring and early summer, the exact times varying from place to place. One or another species of tree is generally the source of the earliest pollen of spring, with other species pollinating for several weeks each throughout the spring. The distribution of the various tree species is less uniform than that of ragweed and grasses, and the species of importance may vary even among nearby locales; a patient may have allergic rhinitis caused by the pollen of a single nearby tree which is not of an indigenous species. In general, the pollens of importance differ from one area to another, and the same pollen appears at different times in different places. Pollen is generally released early in the morning, and, as it is spread by wind, pollen hay fever is generally worse on dry, breezy days; on the other hand, pollen is fairly well cleared from the air by rain, which may therefore abate pollen hay fever.

Fungal spores abound in the air at most seasons except in the depths of winter, when frozen soil and snow cover inhibit their production and release by the molds of chief importance—those that live in the soil and on leaf surfaces and participate in the decomposition of dead organic matter. Spores from *Hormodendrum* are most prevalent in July and those from *Alternaria* in October, but high local concentrations of mold spores may be encountered at other times in the woods, in fields, in new mown grass, or near compost heaps or other aggregations of decaying matter. Indoors, quantities of mold spore sufficient to cause symptoms in a highly sensitive patient can result from a damp basement, from the potting soil of houseplants, or from mildew on walls, shower curtains, and books; they are often found at summer cottages near the water that are closed during the winter. In contrast to pollen grains, mold spores, because of their much smaller size, are very imperfectly cleared from the air by rain.

Even more important among indoor allergens, however, are house dust and animal danders. These two categories are appropriately considered together, as the allergenicity of house dust is likely to be due largely to the desquamated human epidermal cells that it contains as well as the dust mites of *Dermatophagus* species that feed on this human dander. In addition, it may contain allergenic vegetable fibers and particles from feathers, horsehair, wool, and mohair as well as dander from any domestic animals that may be present. Patients who react to house dust very often react to animal danders as well. Among these patients symptoms of rhinitis may be provoked not only by dust and by furred and feathered animals, but also by feather pillows, down quilts, horsehair mattresses, and occasionally by fur, wool, or silk garments. In dwellings infested by cockroaches, their emanations can be clinically significant allergens.

Although the allergens mentioned thus far account for the bulk of allergic rhinitis, others may be of importance in individual cases. Flour, food allergens made airborne in cooking, and enzymes in detergents and meat tenderizers have precipitated allergic symptoms, as have organic dusts and simple organic chemicals encountered in industry. In some of these cases, the allergens may be volatile and impossible to detect by conventional methods of environmental monitoring, which rely on morphologic identification of particulate matter.

The role of allergens not carried in the air is controversial. A few patients experience rhinitis after eating specific foods. In many such cases, the food has been found to have inherent vasodilator properties, (e.g., alcohol), which would be expected to aggravate any engorgement of the nasal tissues, or to have a pungent or irritating odor (e.g., pepper and the garlic family). In these cases the mechanism may involve direct and specific pharmacologic actions of constituents of the foods on the nasal tissues, or it may involve nonspecific responses, presumably neurally mediated, to irritants and odors rather than the IgE–mast cell mechanism clearly implicated in responses to airborne allergens. Patients with allergic rhinitis undergoing allergen injection therapy have, however, been observed to experience rhinitis as a reaction to an allergen injection, and it therefore seems probable that rhinitis can be caused by an immunologic reaction to an allergen introduced by other than the respiratory route. Therefore, the rôle of food allergens as precipitants of allergic rhinitis, while difficult to establish, cannot be ruled out.

IMMUNOLOGIC BASIS

The experimental model in which antigen causes the release of mediators of inflammation from IgE-sensitized mast cells (described in the chapter on the Immunoglobulin E–Mast Cell–Mediator System in the fascicle on Immunology) satisfactorily explains most of the manifestations of allergic rhinitis. Briefly, exposure to antigen leads to the synthesis of IgE. The major sites of synthesis are the lymphoid tissues of the respiratory and gastrointestinal tracts, and hence exposure by the respiratory route favors synthesis of this immunoglobulin class. In normal individuals, the concentration of circulating IgE rarely exceeds 100 IU/ml; in patients with allergic rhinitis, allergic asthma, atopic dermatitis, and parasitic infestations it regularly reaches that level and may attain several times that value. Conversely, an IgE concentration of less than 20 IU/ml is prima facie evidence against an allergic mechanism.

Although IgE has a short half-life in the circulation, the Fc portion of its molecule binds with very high affinity to specific receptors on the surface membranes of mast cells. Such tissue-fixed IgE can be detected up to 3 weeks. Mast cells are identifiable in the nasal mucus of patients with allergic rhinitis, and IgE-containing plasma cells have been demonstrated by immunofluorescence in the nasal mucosa of patients with allergic rhinitis but in that not of normals. Nasal polyp tissue removed surgically, sensitized in vitro with IgE, and challenged with specific antigen releases histamine, slow-reacting substance of anaphylaxis, and eosinophil chemotactic factor of anaphylaxis. In addition to these three mediators, nasal secretions of patients with allergic rhinitis have been found to contain eosinophils, prostaglandin E, and kinins.

MANIFESTATIONS

CLINICAL MANIFESTATIONS

The prevalence of allergic rhinitis has ranged in various surveys from 1 in 15 to 1 in 4 individuals. Because symptoms are often mild and because an attack may be mistaken for a "cold," the prevalence is likely to be underestimated, and the large figure is probably more accurate. The onset may come at any age but usually occurs in childhood or early adult life and is uncommon after age 40. Symptoms may remit in adolescence or middle age but recur later. Susceptible persons exposed for the first time to an allergen take time to become sensitized. Thus, an immigrant to the United States from Western Europe, where ragweed is practically nonexistent, rarely develops ragweed hay fever before his third season's exposure. Patients often protest that as they have lived with a pet for years it cannot be the cause of their allergic rhinitis; but it often is. It is not known why sensitization suddenly develops after years or decades of uneventful exposure to an allergen.

Allergic rhinitis varies in severity from a trivial annoyance to a disabling affliction. In the mildest form, only mild itching, watery rhinorrhea, or sneezing may be present. The itching, in a more severely affected patient, can be of consuming intensity and affect the eyes, throat, and external ear canal as well as the nose. A watery discharge issues copiously from the nose and eyes. With chronicity, the nasal discharge becomes thicker but remains mucoid, in contrast with the purulent aspect that large numbers of eosinophils can give to the bronchial secretions in asthma. Sneezing may come in uncontrollable paroxysms of scores of sneezes that last for minutes and leave the patient breathless and exhausted. With any but the mildest and most short-lived attacks there is a degree of nasal obstruction; in the severest cases such obstruction can progress to complete blockge of both nasal choanae. Pain, sometimes severe, is often felt over the frontal and maxillary sinuses, usually without any other evidence of sinus disease. Symptoms are usually worst on arising in the morning. This is the chief time when pollens are released into the air, but it remains the worst time for patients whose symptoms are due to allergens with no such diurnal peak, perhaps in part because it follows by a few hours the time when concentrations of circulating cortisol are lowest.

Eustachian tube obstruction is a common concomitant of allergic rhinitis, and patients often report that their ears "pop." Serous otitis media is an occasional complication, especially in children. It occurs most frequently after an airplane flight. A profound lassitude often accompanies allergic rhinitis even in the absence of sufficient symptoms to tire the patient and of treatment with antihistamines or other sedating drugs. An irritative cough may parallel the commonly experienced itch in the throat or may be a response to increased clearance of nasal mucus via the pharynx. Obstruction of the lower airways is often demonstrable in patients with allergic rhinitis who have no symptoms or other signs of asthma. The increased incidence of clinical asthma in patients with allergic rhinitis may simply be due to the fact that in many kindreds the two diseases are inherited together; the evidence is insufficient to demonstrate that allergic rhinitis per se causes asthma or that control of the rhinitis diminishes the risk of the subsequent emergence of asthma.

Patients with rhinitis, allergic or not, usually experience aggravation of their symptoms by aerosols (sprays, smokes), strong odors (including those not inherently unpleasant or irritating), drafts, and the dry air of winter. Exercise, by releasing catecholamines, and humidification, by diminishing the work of the nose in saturating the inhaled air with water, often alleviate symptoms.

PHYSICAL FINDINGS

Dark crescents under the eyes—"allergic shiners"—can suggest allergic rhinitis at a glance, as can the "allergic salute" in children—wiping the nose with a characteristic upward movement of the open palm, which may in time cause a crease across the nose just above the tip. There may be pallor and tachycardia, but fever, especially in an adult, must be taken as a warning of something other than allergic rhinitis. The blood pressure is often low in atopic individuals but it may be mildly elevated in the course of an attack. Despite the copious nasal discharge, the skin of the alae nasae is rarely reddened as it is in the common cold. If a cough is present, bronchitis and asthma should be excluded. In adults, allergic rhinitis does not cause an enlargement of lymphoid tissue; thus, enlargement of the tonsils, adenoids, or cervical lymph nodes should prompt a search for other disease.

The nasal mucosa is usually glistening with clear mucus, but in winter crusts may form and there may be bleeding from the anterior septal triangle. The mucosa of the turbinates is usually swollen and may take on a grossly boggy appearance. In uncomplicated allergic rhinitis it is usually pale or violaceous, but it may be red, as in vasomotor or irritant rhinitis and in the common cold. Occasionally, nasal polyps may be seen in the middle or upper meatus. The term *polyp* is misleading, as these are not neoplasms but grossly hypertrophied mucous glandular tissue; *mucocele* is a more descriptive term. The tympanic membranes should be inspected for retraction or fluid. The palpebral and scleral conjunctiva may be pale or injected and even show some degree of cobblestoning. The posterior pharynx may be reddened and may exhibit mucus draining from the nose. In uncomplicated allergic rhinitis, the remainder of the physical examination will disclose no abnormality.

LABORATORY FINDINGS

In allergic rhinitis, the predominant cell in the nasal discharge is the eosinophil, which is only seen in small numbers in other types of rhinitis. Peripheral blood eosinophila of a moderate degree (less than 1000/mm³) is common. A high concentration of total IgE suggests an allergic mechanism. X-rays of the paranasal sinuses are usually normal, even in the presence of pain simulating sinusitis, but thickening of the mucosa (sometimes interpreted as "chronic sinusitis") and mucoceles may be seen in the absence of any disease other than allergic rhinitis.

DIAGNOSIS

IDENTIFICATION OF CAUSAL ALLERGENS

The diagnosis of allergic rhinitis rests on the identification of the responsible allergens and the demonstration of IgE specific for them. The most important tool is the history. Any seasonal pattern of the patient's symptoms must be defined as precisely as possible and compared with the pollen seasons prevailing locally; as pollen seasos vary in timing and severity from year to year, it is helpful to know the experiences of other patients with known sensitivities in the years under consideration. As detailed as possible a catalog must be assembled of the patient's domestic, occupational, and recreational exposure to potential allergens and of the symptoms he has experienced in each of these different settings. Notice must be taken of any factors, whether allergenic or not,

that the patient has observed to precipitate or to exacerbate symptoms. With this information, the physician should be able to distinguish tentatively an allergic from a nonallergic illness and to identify the allergens most likely to be responsible.

The most generally useful means of demonstrating IgE specific for suspected allergens is skin testing using commercially available aqueous extracts of common inhalant allergens. These extracts are usually labeled as to potency according to one of two rather crude scales of measurement. The "weight per volume" method simply represents the ratio of the weight of crude allergen to the volume of extracting fluid. Thus, ragweed extract 1:50 would result from extracting 1 g of defatted ragweed pollen with 50 ml of fluid; a 200-fold dilution of this extract would be labeled 1:10,000. Alternatively, the concentration may be given in protein nitrogen units (PNU); 1 PNU represents 10 ng protein nitrogen as determined by Kjeldahl analysis of the extract itself. As the specific antigens relevant for a particular patient constitute but a small fraction of the protein and an even smaller one of the crude material, and as these fractions can vary substantially from one batch to another, neither method of labeling gives more than the crudest indication of allergenic potency.

Skin testing is carried out by intradermally injecting 0.01–0.02 ml of dilute allergen extract, by applying a drop of extract to a tiny scratch on the skin, or by pricking the skin with a needle through a previously applied drop of extract. In each case, a positive reaction is a wheal and flare 15 minutes after the test is planted. As skin testing is capable of provoking systemic anaphylaxis, facilities for dealing with such an emergency must be at hand, and if the history indicates a high degree of sensitivity to a particular allergen, that allergen should not be used or used only very dilute. It is prudent to put skin tests on an extremity so that a tourniquet can be applied proximal to them in case of a systemic reaction; injection of epinephrine into the test site will also retard absorption of the allergen.

False-negative skin tests are most often caused by antihistamines (which can suppress skin tests as long as 5 days after the last dose) and by sympathomimetic drugs, but they are also seen in young children and in disease of recent onset. Corticosteroids and methylxanthines do not suppress the immediate skin test response. Positive skin tests are often seen to allergens to which the patient is regularly exposed with complete impunity, and positive reactions in dermatographic patients may defy interpretation. In general, however, the immediate cutaneous reaction is a reliable, swift, inexpensive, and fairly innocuous way of demonstrating specific IgE, and for this purpose is at least as sensitive as any other method available for routine use.

The Prausnitz-Küstner reaction, in which the patient's serum is used to sensitize passively a site on a recipient's skin which is subsequently challenged with antigen, is rarely used because of the risk of transmitting hepatitis. The measurement of histamine released from peripheral blood leukocytes by antigen challenge is a recognized investigational method that is not yet practical for routine clinical use.

The radioallergosorbent test (RAST) employs allergen coupled to an insoluble support, usually a paper disk activated by cyanogen bromide, which is incubated with the serum to be tested. After being washed, the disk is incubated with radiolabeled antibody specific for human IgE; and after further washing the radioactivity remaining bound to the disk is measured as an index of the concentration of specific IgE in the serum. The RAST is commercially available for a number of common allergens and can in principle be set up for any antigen containing free amino groups. The results of the test correlate well with skin testing and leukocyte histamine release, but it is somewhat expensive and no more sensitive than skin testing. It can be useful in patients who cannot tolerate interruption of antihistamine therapy for skin testing or are dermatographic, or in whom a severe reaction to skin testing is feared. It may also be found to be useful in determining IgE specific for suspected allergens that by irritation or a direct histamime-releasing action on the mast cell cause false-positive skin tests in normal subjects.

DIFFERENTIAL DIAGNOSIS

Given typical symptoms, a family history positive for atopy, and agreement between allergens suggested by the history and those eliciting positive skin tests, a diagnosis of allergic rhinitis can be made with some confidence. On the other hand, atypical history and negative skin tests (absent factors causing false-negative skin tests) cast doubt on an allergic etiology. In such cases, the peripheral blood eosinophil count, the proportion of eosinphils in the nasal secretions, and the laboratory determinations of total and antigen-specific IgE may weigh the balance to one side or the other. In cases of doubt, one must consider the possibilities of chronic or recurrent infections and immunologic deficiencies predisposing to them, endocrine abnormalities such as myxedema, and anatomic problems such as marked septal deviation. Atrophic rhinitis may occasionally give rise to symptoms that can be confused with those of perennial allergic rhinitis; the presence of ozena should alert the physician to this diagnosis, which is readily confirmed or excluded by examination. The possible role of drugs must be kept in mind, especially aspirin and other agents affecting prostaglandin biosynthesis, topical vasoconstrictors, reserpine, and beta-adrenergic blocking agents.

TREATMENT

AVOIDANCE

In cases in which etiologic or contributing factors can be identified that it is possible to avoid, such avoidance should be stressed as the cornerstone of treatment. The commonest of these allergenic factors are pets, animal epidermal products such as feathers in pillows and quilts, horsehair in mattresses, and wool or mohair in upholstery, hangings, and floor coverings, and house dust. Although vacationing in a ragweed-free area is effective in avoiding ragweed hay fever, avoidance of pollens is seldom practical. A window air conditioner whose filter is frequently changed, however, can effect considerable amelioration in many cases of pollen hay fever. Masks can be useful against house and industrial dusts and against cold air. Air filtration systems and electrostatic precipitators are sometimes very effective, but patients should be warned against making a substantial financial commitment without an adequate trial, as results may be disappointing; electrostatic precipitators can give rise to irritating concentrations of ozone. Winter rhinitis is often dramatically relieved by adequate humidification, but the same caution must be applied, especially as humidifiers have occasionally been found to foster the growth of molds and of organisms causing hypersensitivity pneumonitis.

DRUG THERAPY

In cases in which control of the disease by avoidance of etiologic factors fails, drugs can often effectively suppress disease manifestations without regard to their cause. Antihistamines are the most generally useful drugs for this purpose. They are usually effective against rhinitis of moderate severity if side effects do not preclude administration of a sufficient dosage, but sedation, anticholinergic effects, and nausea are common. The susceptibility of individual patients to the side effects of antihistamines is notoriously unpredictable, and claims that one preparation or even one class of antihistamines has a higher therapeutic index than another should be viewed with skepticism. Tolerance to side effects and, less often, to therapeutic effects may develop with continued administration. Antihistamines are more effective in preventing rhinitis than in treating it once it has arisen. So-called sustained-release preparations are a convenience to many patients but may be poorly absorbed; antihistamines should not be abandoned as ineffective if only these preparations have been tried. Serious adverse reactions to antihistamines, such as agranulocytosis, solar sensitivity, and dystonic reactions, are very rare.

Sympathomimetic drugs are effective in rhinitis, and the central nervous system stimulation they cause can balance the sedation caused by antihistamines. The agents most commonly used—ephedrine, pseudoephedrine, phenylpropanolamine, and phenylephrine—all have significant alpha-adrenergic activity (which relatively contraindicates their use in the presence of hypertension). Pure beta-agonists, such as methylxanthines, have little effect in rhinitis, suggesting that their beneficial effect is due to actions on target organs (blood vessels and mucus glands) rather than on mast cell mediator release.

Anticholinergic drugs, although effective in drying nasal secretions, have been effectively supplanted by the antihistamines, (which of course have significant anticholinergic activity themselves), but they are still found in some combination preparations. Cromolyn sodium, which blocks the release of mediators from the mast cell by a mechanism distinct from those involved in the actions of sympathomimetics, anticholinergics, and methylxanthines, has been reported to be effective in the treatment of allergic rhinitis when applied topically as a 2 percent solution.

Glucocorticoids are the most effective drugs in relieving allergic rhinitis but carry risks of serious toxicity that cannot be ignored and interdict their use in all but the most disabling cases. A single injection of a long-acting preparation or a 1-week course of oral prednisone, tapering from an initial dosage of 30 mg/day, may, however, provide relief of incapacitating symptoms for an entire pollen season, and the risk of serious toxicity is very small with such brief treatment. Topical glucocorticoid treatment with an intranasal aerosol can afford relief of symptoms refractory to other classes of drugs. Continuous treatment carries a risk of irreversible atrophy of the nasal tissues and of rebound on withdrawal. Absorption from the nose is substantial, but the dosage required for control of rhinitis is not usually sufficient to suppress adrenal function. On the other hand, extranasal symptoms, particularly in the eyes, may not be controlled by intranasal glucocorticoids. Topical glucocorticoids in the eye, when indicated, are best prescribed by the ophthalmologist as there is a substantial risk of glaucoma, cataracts, or infection in susceptible individuals.

ALLERGEN INJECTION THERAPY

The practice of treating hay fever by injection of extracts of the causative pollens was instituted in 1911 by Noon, who viewed it as a way of raising protective antibodies against a putative toxin responsible for the symptoms. While long accepted, it is only lately that allergen injection therapy has been subjected to properly designed trials and some understanding has been gained of its mechanism of action. Whereas introduction of antigen via the respiratory tract in repeated small doses favors an IgE response, injection of larger doses favors an IgG response and blunts the IgE response; probably antigen introduced by the different routes reaches different populations of class-specific helper and suppressor T lymphocytes. The IgG synthesized in response to systemic introduction of the antigen may also serve a blocking role by combining with antigen before the latter reaches the IgE fixed on mast cell surfaces. Depletion of mediators from the mast cell may also be involved, as is suggested by the finding in leukocyte histamine-release studies that the response to other antigens is diminished as well as that to the antigen given in the injection therapy.

In controlled double-blind studies, allergen injection therapy has been shown to be effective in treating ragweed and grass pollen hay fever. Efficacy was correlated with the total dose administered and was demonstrated in terms of both clinical and immunologic observations. Results with house dust have been equivocal and tests with mold extracts have not been done. The studies have been carried out in patients with well-defined seasonal symptoms congruent with their positive skin tests and other indices of specific IgE. Clinical experience agrees that it is precisely such patients who respond best to allergen injection therapy. There is probably no indication for allergen injection therapy if the illness can be managed by avoidance and such relatively innocuous medications as antihistamines and sympathomimetics, as it involves a major investment of time and considerable expense and carries a small risk of a serious anaphylactic reaction. In patients with disabling symptoms that cannot be controlled by simpler measures, it can make a major contribution to the patients' well-being provided the identification of the causal allergens is clear.

REFERENCES

Holmes TH, Goodell H, Wolf S, Wolff HG: The Nose. Springfield, Ill, Charles C Thomas, 1950

Norman PS: Immunotherapy (desensitization) in allergic disease. Ann Rev Med 26:337, 1975

Proctor DF: The upper airways. I. Nasal physiology and defense of the lungs. Am Rev Resp Dis 115:97, 1977

Tennenbaum JI: Allergic rhinitis, in Patterson R (ed): Allergic Diseases. Philadelphia, Lippincott, 1972, p 161

Urticaria and Angioedema

Frank J. Twarog and Albert L. Sheffer

PATHOGENESIS AND ETIOLOGY

The clinical recognition of urticaria or angioedema rarely presents a significant problem. On the other hand, in its chronic form, identification of the precipitating factor(s) is often a perplexing, if not impossible, task. Urticarial lesions may occur on any area of the body and have raised erythematous serpiginous edges with blanched centers. Varying in size, such wheals are intensely pruritic. Angioedema, a similar process occurring in the deeper subcutaneous layers, presents as areas of colorless, well-demarcated edema, most frequently on the face (periorbital and perioral regions) and extremities. These lesions may be pruritic.

It is estimated that 20 percent of the population experiences at least one acute episode of urticaria or angioedema. Of these cases, only a small percentage progress to the chronic form, which is defined as recurrence of lesions over a 4–6-week period. The frequency of acute urticaria is slightly higher in an atopic population, but chronic urticaria occurs equally in all individuals regardless of hereditary background. Although urticaria or angioedema may develop at any age, the peak incidence for chronic urticaria is between the third and fourth decades. There is a preponderance of females affected

Urticaria and angioedema frequently coexist. In one large series, 49 percent of the patients had both urticaria and angioedema, whereas 40 percent suffered from urticaria alone and 11 percent from angioedema alone. Individual attacks may last from hours to days. However, it is not unusual for patients with chronic urticaria/angioedema to have recurrent episodes for years. Despite the fact that chronic urticaria/angioedema is generally not associated with a serious disease process, the tendency for it to recur and relapse may be very distressing to the individual plagued by this problem. Because of the long-term morbidity suffered by those whose attacks recur over a prolonged period, as well as the occasional association with a significant underlying disorder, complete evaluation of individuals with chronic urticaria should be undertaken.

PATHOGENESIS

The tissue changes characteristic of urticaria and angioedema may be caused by a number of mechanisms. A final common pathway for urticaria/angioedema of many causes is release of chemical mediators of immediate hypersensitivity. Through intensive investigation a large number of mediators produced by mast cells and basophils are being identified and characterized (see the section on Immunoglobulin E–Mast Cell–Mediator System in the fascicle on Immunology). The relative importance of each of these substances in the pathophysiology of urticaria and angioedema has not been clarified. However, increasing evidence suggests that histamine may be a primary mediator acting at secondary sites in preparation for the mediator release.

Release is an active process that may be initiated by a variety of stimuli. In the allergic reaction, interaction of antigen with IgE antibody fixed to the surface of mast cells or basophils causes mediator release. The anaphylotoxins C3a and C5a, which are formed following activation of complement, either directly or by an antigen–antibody reaction may also induce release. Substances such as curare, morphine, polymyxin B, and radiocontrast material cause direct release of mediators. Finally, it has been demonstrated that physical agents such as temperature, pressure, and vibration can also initiate release. An IgE mechanism has been demonstrated in several of the physical forms, including dermatographism, cold, cholinergic, and solar urticaria.

Study of individuals with physical urticaria has provided the primary source of in vivo information on mediator release. Transient elevations of histamine and eosinophil chemotactic and neutrophil chemotactic factors have been detected following appropriate challenge in individuals with vibratory and cold-induced urticaria.

Derangements in the in vitro release of histamine and eosinophil chemotactic factor of anaphylaxis (see the section on Immunoglobulin E–Mast Cell–Mediator System in the fascicle on Immunology) from leukocytes of patients with chronic urticaria have also been demon-strated. This may be a result of in vivo desensitization of the basophilic leukocyte following chronic mediator release. Whether the tissue-fixed mast cell will demonstrate similar abnormalities is not known.

In hereditary angioedema the absence of a functional $C\bar{1}$ inhibitor ($C\bar{1}$-INH) protein may result in uncontrolled activation of the early complement sequence. The angioedema manifested in this disease is probably not mediated by histamine, even though urine levels of histamine may be strikingly elevated late in an attack. A kininlike molecule has been identified in the plasma of individuals with hereditary angioedema. This kinin is a product of C2, one of the natural substrates of C1 esterase. $C\bar{1}$-INH is also important in regulating the generation of bradykinin by its ability to inhibit activated Hageman factor. In the acquired form of hereditary angioedema occuring in patients with malignancy, concentrations of C1 are decreased.

The pathogenesis of urticarial lesions in patients with vasculitis remains to be clarified. However, the frequent finding of hypocomplementemia in this group of individuals suggests that complement activation, probably mediated by immune complexes, may play an important role in forming these lesions. Activation of the alternative complement pathway through the C1 bypass mechanism may occasionally result in urticarial lesions as well.

Aspirin-intolerant individuals may develop urticaria, rhinitis, and/or asthma following ingestion of acetylsalicylic acid. In addition, nonsteroidal antiinflammatory drugs that are known to inhibit cyclooxygenase, an enzyme important in the synthesis of prostaglandins, have been reported to induce bronchoconstriction, urticaria, or angioedema in aspirin-intolerant asthmatics, thus implicating prostaglandins in the mediation of these reactions.

ETIOLOGY

Both acute and chronic types of urticaria and/or angioedema may be caused by a wide variety of factors, as should be evident from the different mechanisms implicated in initiating mediator release. It is difficult to estimate the frequency with which the etiology of acute urticaria is identified, since many individuals with mild acute episodes may not seek medical assistance. Of those patients evaluated with chronic forms of the disease, however, it has been estimated that an etiology is determined in less than 20 percent.

Due to the diversity of etiologies and mechanisms involved in this symptom complex, it is difficult to develop a rational classification; Table 1 therefore merely is a list of the known causes without attention to mechanism. One hopes that the identification of released mediators and/or altered immunologic pathways eventually will permit the development of a mechanistic classification.

Allergic

Inhaled allergens such as pollens and molds most frequently cause asthma or rhinitis in atopic individuals. Infrequently, especially when encountered in higher concentrations, these allergens may precipitate attacks of urticaria. Urticaria of this type may even occur repeatedly on a seasonal basis. Animal danders cause urticaria both by inhalation as well as contact.

Foods are frequently implicated in acute and/or recurrent attacks of urticaria and angioedema. Among the most common offenders are milk, eggs, chocolate, shellfish, fish, and nuts. Some food allergens, especially fish and peanut antigens, are extremely sensitizing and cause symptoms by inhalation as well as ingestion. Individuals with food hypersensitivity often suffer from associated symptoms such as abdominal pain. Foods, however, are not often associated with chronic forms of urticaria. Repeated ingestion may be associated with accentuation of symptoms or even life-threatening anaphylactic reactions.

Milk products are occasionally contaminated with penicillin and have been implicated in the etiology of urticaria in penicillin-sensitive individuals. Histamine-releasing factors have been identified in strawberries, shellfish, and other foods. Whether these ever play a role in food-induced urticaria is unclear. Finally, food dyes and preservatives are responsible for nonatopic urticaria, especially in aspirin-sensitive individuals. This may occasionally be interpreted as food allergy.

Physical

An interesting group of urticarias are those caused by physical agents. Among these is dermatographism, a wheal and flare reaction resulting from firm stroking of the skin. This is the most common form of physical urticaria and is present in approximately 5 percent of the normal population.

Pressure and vibration may also be responsible for urticaria in some individuals. Lesions develop immediately in the vibratory type, whereas they may be delayed for as long as 4–6 hours in some forms of pressure-induced urticaria. This etiology should be considered when angioedema or urticaria is prominent in areas under brassiere straps or belts.

Heat as well as cold may induce both immediate and delayed forms of urticaria. Acquired cold-induced urticaria is by far the most common form. Lesions may be limited to exposed areas or be generalized and often do not develop until reenterance into a warm environment following cold exposure. Edema of the mouth, tongue, or pharynx may occur with cold drinks and wheezing may develop during more serious attacks. Sudden, massive exposure to cold, such as occurs upon diving into cold water while swimming, may be fatal.

Familial cold urticaria is a dominantly inherited disorder and occurs in two forms. The immediate type develops within 30 minutes of cold exposure and is associated with erythematous burning lesions, often accompanied by fever, chills, arthralgias, and headache. Localized deep swelling occurs some 9–18 hours after cold exposure in the delayed form. The possibility of a cold hemolysin or cryoglobulinemia should be considered in acquired cold urticaria.

Solar urticaria is a rare form of urticaria caused by light exposure. Urticaria occurs only on exposed areas of the skin in this condition, but when large areas are uncov-

Table 1
Etiology of Urticaria and Angioedema

Allergic
  Atopic: inhaled allergens
  Anaphylaxis: ingested allergens (foods, drugs): or injected
    allergen drugs (e.g., penicillin, biologicals)
Physical
  Dermatographism
  Pressure induced
  Vibration induced
  Cold induced
  Heat induced
  Solar
  Aquagenic
  Cholinergic
Infections
Agents affecting prostaglandin synthesis
  Nonsteroidal antiinflammatory agents (aspirin)
   Azodyes and preservatives
Vasculitis
Hereditary angioneurotic edema
Drugs: serum products and mast cell–releasing agents
Neoplasms
Endocrine related
Psychogenic
Idiopathic

ered systemic symptoms such as wheezing and lightheadedness may develop. The wavelength of light eliciting this reaction varies between individuals, and classifications according to these criteria have been devised.

Urticarial lesions somewhat resembling cholinergic-type urticaria have been reported in rare individuals on exposure to water, regardless of the temperature. Very little is known concerning this condition, which has been called *aquagenic urticaria*.

Infections

Acute urticaria has been associated with a variety of infections. It is important, however, to eliminate the contribution of drugs, especially aspirin and penicillin, to the syndrome. Urticaria may precede overt clinical manifestations of infectious mononucleosis and viral hepatitis. It has been postualted that circulating immune complexes may be responsible for these lesions. Bacterial and parasitic infections have also been implicated in acute and chronic forms of urticaria.

Agents Affecting Prostaglandin Synthesis

Aspirin, nonsteroidal antiinflammatory agents, azodyes, and benzoate all may induce urticaria and angioedema. Aspirin is a frequent cause of acute and chronic forms of urticaria and angioedema. Individuals with aspirin intolerance also react to indomethacin, ibuprofen, and other nonsteroidal antiinflammatory drugs, all of which affect prostaglandin synthesis. Up to 20 percent of these patients also react to azodyes (especially tartrazine FD&C No. 5) and benzoate food preservatives. Some of these individuals have associated asthma and nasal polyps. The reactions are dose dependent; whereas 300 mg of aspirin may be well tolerated, violent reactions may be precipitated by 600 mg.

It has been postulated that 25–60 percent of cases of chronic idiopathic urticaria are related to one or more of these agents. This hypothesis has been substantiated by blind challenges with the substances in question. It should be noted that these dyes and preservatives are used in a wide variety of drugs.

Vasculitis

Biopsy of typical urticarial lesions in this group of patients reveals fibrinoid necrosis of vessels and infiltrate with lymphocytes and polymorphonuclear leukocytes. Such lesions occur most frequently in females during the third and fourth decades. Although the urticarial lesions are not unusual, palpable purpuric lesions may develop in the lower extremities. Nearly all of these patients complain of arthralgias, often occurring coincidental with the skin lesions. Approximately one-quarter also complain of episodic abdominal pains, nausea, vomiting, and diarrhea. Progression of the disease process may occasionally lead to glomerulonephritis. Suggestive laboratory data include elevated erythrocyte sedimentation rate and hypocomplementemia. Urticaria may also be asociated with systemic lupus erythematosus.

Hereditary Angioneurotic Edema

Hereditary angioneurotic edema (HAE) is an autosomal dominant disorder in which the $C\bar{1}$-INH is either deficient or nonfunctional. This results in recurrent episodes of well-demarcated swelling, particularly of the face and extremities. Involvement of the respiratory tract results in upper respiratory obstruction with the danger of asphyxiation due to laryngeal edema. Some individuals have primarily internal edema with a pattern of recurrent abdominal pain secondary to small bowel angioedema.

Urticaria is not seen in HAE, but an early eruption resembling erythema marginatum often occurs. Attacks of angioedema may begin at any age, but an accentuation of the frequency of such episodes is often associated with adolescence or young adulthood. When HAE is first diagnosed in an older individual, an acquired form associated with lymphoma must be considered.

Drugs

Drug-induced urticaria and angioedema may be mediated by IgE antibodies, antigen–antibody complexes resulting in serum sickness, direct histamine release, or a dye or preservative in the drug vehicle. Penicillin is the most important antibiotic associated with IgE-mediated urticaria. Among the agents causing direct mediator release are curare, opiates, tetracyclines, meperidine, and many others. Radiocontrast dyes probably act by direct mediator release as well. The list of pharmacologic agents implicated is much too extensive to review in detail here, but drugs, biologicals, etc., may be considered in the differential of all cases of acute and chronic urticaria.

Neoplasms

Although probably a rare cause of chronic urticaria, tumors must be considered a possibility. Proof of a direct causal effect has not been presented but the resolution of chronic urticaria coincident with removal of a malignant lesion suggests a relationship in some instances. Blood dyscrasias, such as polycythemia vera and leukemia, especially acute myelogenous leukemia, may be associated with chronic recurrent urticaria.

Endocrine Related

A variety of unusual endocrine-related disorders may result in urticaria and/or angioedema. Autosensitization to progesterone has been implicated as a cause of urticaria which waxes and wanes in women, associated with the menstrual period. Urticaria and pruritus have occurred with both hyperthyroidism and pregnancy. Contact with seminal fluid may rarely cause severe urticaria and angioedema in sensitized women.

Psychogenic

In one study psychologic factors were considered to be the major cause of urticaria in 11 percent of the cases. There is no question that psychologic stress may aggravate urticarial reactions, but since the majority of causes of chronic urticaria are unknown, it is difficult to implicate psychologic factors as the sole mechanism involved.

Idiopathic

Despite the many recognized or suspected causes of urticaria and angioedema, the etiology remains unknown in at least 80 percent of cases.

REFERENCES

Kaplan AP, Gray L, Shaff R, Horakova Z, Beaven MA: In vivo studies of mediator release in cold urticaria and cholinergic urticaria. J Allergy Clin Immunol 55:394, 1975
Samter M, Beers RF, Jr: Intolerance to aspirin. Ann Intern Med 68:975, 1968
Soter NA: Chronic urticaria as a manifestation of necrotizing vasculitis. New Engl J Med 296:1440, 1977
Szczeklik A, Gryglewski RJ, Czerniawska-Mysik G: Clinical patterns of hypersensitivity to non-steroidal anti-inflammatory drugs and their patrogenesis. J Allergy Clin Immunol 60:276, 1977

LABORATORY EVALUATION

Evaluation of individuals with urticaria or angioedema should be guided by the suspected etiology. Some useful procedures in this attempt are outlined in Table 1. Frequently a carefully obtained history and physical examination will obviate the necessity for extensive testing.

A screening including complete blood count, urinalysis, chest x-ray, and biochemical profile offers general background data. Erythrocyte sedimentation rate, complement assay, and immunoglobulins should be determined when vasculitis is suspected. If any of these results are abnormal, a skin biopsy may confirm the presence of a vascular lesion.

Because of the occasional association of cold urticaria with cryoprecipitins, blood should be drawn, separated (preferably at 37°C), and assayed for the presence of cryoglobulins and cryofibrinogen. A serologic test for syphylis is recommended as well. Appropriate cultures, stool examinations for ova and parasites, and radiologic examinations aid in pursuing an infectious pathogen.

Table 1
Laboratory Evaluation of Urticaria and Angioedema

Suspected Etiology	Procedures
General screening	Complete blood count, urinalysis, chemical profile
Vasculitis or complement related	Sedimentation rate, immunoglobulin analysis, antinuclear factor, quantitative complement (C3, C4, $\overline{C1}$-INH, CH_{50}), skin biopsy
Cold urticaria	Cryoglobulins, cryofibrinogens, serologic test for syphilis
Infections	Culture, x-ray, stool for ova and parasites, hepatitis-associated antigen
Atopic	Eosinophil count, IgE, skin testing and/or radioallergosorbent test for suspected allergen
Physical:	
Cholinergic	Mecholyl test, stress induced
Dermatographism	Firm stroking of skin
Cold	Ice cube application
Solar	Light exposure
Heat	Warm water immersion
Hereditary angioedema and acquired angioedema with lymphoma and other neoplasia	$\overline{C1}$-INH, C1q, CH_{50}, C4, C2

Skin testing for immediate hypersensitivity rarely is helpful in identifying the causal agent of chronic urticaria because atopy is infrequent and would usually be suspected from the history.

When physical urticaria is suspected, specific tests, such as the ice cube test, mecholyl skin test, and exposure to light of specific wavelengths, can be diagnostic.

Diagnosis of hereditary angioedema should be suspected with significant reduction in the concentration of C4 or C2. The diagnosis is then confirmed by establishing the absence of $\overline{C1}$-INH. As 10 percent of individuals with HAE have nonfunctional $\overline{C1}$-INH protein present, this substance must be assayed both quantitatively and functionally.

Finally, challenge under careful observation may be employed with the specific food, food additive, or other suspected trigger agent. Since an anaphylactic reaction is a distinct possibility, such tests should be performed in a hospital setting with appropriate facilities for treating anaphylaxis.

REFERENCES

Champion RA, Roberts OB, Carpenter RG, Roger JH: Urticaria and angioedema: A review of 554 patients. Br J Dermotol 81:588, 1969

Gigli I, Sheffer AL, Austen KF: Angioedema, in Samter M (ed): Immunological Diseases, 3rd ed. Boston, Little, Brown, 1978

Miller DA, Freeman G, Akers WA: Chronic urticaria: A clinical study of fifty patients. Am J Med 44:68, 1968

Sheldon JM, Matthews KP, Lovell RG: The vexing urticarial problem: Present concepts of etiology and management. J Allergy 25:525, 1959

Michaelsson G, Juhlin L: Urticaria induced by preservatives and dye additives in food and drugs. Br J Dermotol 88:525, 1973

Schatz M, Patterson R, O'Rourke J, Nickelsen J, Northup C: The administration of radiographic contrast media to patients with a history of previous reaction. J Allergy Clin Immunol 55:358, 1975

TREATMENT

If the urticaria or angioedema is associated with a specific ingested or inhaled substance, avoidance is obviously the preferred approach. With physical urticaria, avoidance of the precipitating factor, such as cold or sunlight, is advisable. Sun screen has been beneficial in solar urticaria.

Pharmacologic control in chronic recurrent idiopathic urticaria with H_1 antihistamines has been only partially effective. Studies currently underway suggest that the effect of combined H_1 and H_2 receptor antagonists may be more salutary. There is no significant difference in the efficacy of available antihistamines. Hydroxyzine has been particularly helpful in controlling cholinergic urticaria in certain instances, and other investigators suggest cyproheptadine for the control of cold urticaria. The recently developed Azatadine may obviate some of the adverse side effects of cyproheptadine on the pituitary gland. In hereditary angioedema, androgen therapy, specifically with oxymetholone (5 mg), has clearly prevented life-threatening attacks.

The treatment of acute episodes is of major concern. Recent studies suggest that the use of the purified $\overline{C1}$-INH protein, where available, would be lifesaving. A more practical approach would be the administration of 5 g epsilonaminocaproic acid (EACA) every 6 hours in conjunction with 10 mg oxymetholone every 6 hours until the reaction is controlled.

In chronic recurrent urticaria and angioedema unaffected by specific remedies, nonspecific additions, such as β-adrenergic stimulating agents, hydration of the skin, and, if necessary, steroid therapy, have been helpful. In most instances these entities can be clinically controlled with a salutary outcome. The life-threatening complications arise from disorders due to upper respiratory obstruction, as seen in anaphylaxis and in hereditary angioedema. Patients with chronic cutaneous vasculitis may progress to glomerulonephritis. Urticaria may also suggest a more serious underlying entity. For this reason, a detailed analysis is always prudent in assessing such disorders. Once the benign nature of the disorder has been established, reassurance is often the best therapy.

REFERENCES

Gigli I, Sheffer AL, Austen KF: Angioedema, in Samter M (ed): Immunological Diseases, 3rd ed. Boston, Little, Brown, 1978

Sheldon JM, Matthews KP, Lovell RG: The vexing urticarial problem: Present concepts of etiology and management. J Allergy 25:525, 1959

Anaphylaxis

Albert L. Sheffer and Stephen I. Wasserman

PATHOGENESIS, CLINICAL MANIFESTATIONS, AND PATHOLOGY

Anaphylaxis is the most emergent manifestation of allergic diseases. Often explosive in onset, it results from the antigen-induced release of biologically active materials from mast cells or basophilic leukocytes sensitized with specific IgE antibody (see the section on Immunoglobulin E–Mast Cell–Mediator System in the fascicle on Immunology). The sites of clinical expression include the skin, the respiratory and gastrointestinal tracts, and the cardiovascular system; these sites may be involved singly or in any combination. Similar syndromes may occur after direct mast cell degranulation or in association with alterations of the arachidonic acid–prostaglandin or complement pathways independent of IgE antibody. Such reactions may cause the release of the same active substances produced in IgE-dependent reactions.

EPIDEMIOLOGY

Age, race, sex, occupation, geographic location, and season of the year can be implicated in anaphylactic reactions only insofar as they might contribute to exposure to the eliciting agent. Reliable data on the incidence of reactions to a particular antigen in a sensitized population are generally lacking. Fatal anaphylaxis to penicillin has been estimated to occur with a frequency of 0.002 percent; however, the incidence of nonfatal reactions is unknown. Although high doses and the continuous rather than interrupted administration of therapeutic agents have been claimed to lower the risk of anaphylaxis, prevalent opinion suggests that risk increases with the length and frequency of encounters with an immunogen. The parenteral administration of an immunogen is more likely to precipitate a clinical reaction than is administration by the oral route. Although atopy is claimed to predispose individuals to an increased risk of anaphylaxis, recent data suggest that atopic individuals are not more susceptible to anaphylaxis.

PATHOGENESIS

Materials known to elicit specific IgE antibodies and subsequent anaphylactic reactions include proteins, polysaccharides, and haptens. The latter are small nonimmunogenic molecules that become immunogenic after they, or one of their metabolites, form a stable bond with a host protein. There are no common distinguishing features shared by antigens capable of eliciting an IgE response. The major immunogens encountered in clinical practice are haptens from nearly every class of diagnostic and therapeutic agent and *Hymenoptera* venoms. IgE-dependent reactions may follow the entry of antigen by any route.

CLINICAL MANIFESTATIONS

The initial manifestation of anaphylaxis is often a sensation of warmth, pruritus, or tingling that may progress to urticaria and/or angioedema with particular involvement of the face, oral cavity, or pharynx. A sensation of constriction of the throat or hoarseness may signal upper respiratory tract obstruction due to laryngeal edema. Respiratory tract involvement may also be characterized by chest tightness that may be accompanied by wheezing and dyspnea. Other clinical manifestations include lightheadedness, chest discomfort, abdominal distress, hypotension, and loss of consciousness. The various clinical manifestations can occur alone or in any combination.

PATHOLOGY

The anatomic findings in fatal systemic anaphylaxis in humans consist of acute pulmonary hyperinflation, laryngeal edema, and edema of the upper respiratory tract. In patients with acute hyperinflation, histologic studies show increases in bronchial secretions, occasional submucosal edema, peribronchial vascular congestion, and eosinophilic infiltration of the bronchial walls. Tissue eosinophilia in the splenic and liver sinusoids, within pulmonary capillaries, and within the vessels and lamina propria of the upper respiratory tract is prominent in individuals dying of systemic anaphylaxis. Histologic study of the urticarial lesions associated with anaphylaxis has not been reported.

ETIOLOGY

IgE-DEPENDENT ANAPHYLAXIS

A personal or family history of asthma, rhinitis, or eczema is often obtained from patients who have experienced an anaphylactic reaction, and such anaphylactic reactions are assumed to be IgE dependent. In clinical practice, however, anaphylaxis is rarely a manifestation of asthma, rhinitis, or eczema when these are induced by natural exposure to an offending antigen.

Definitive demonstration of IgE-dependent mechanisms in the pathogenesis of anaphylaxis has been accomplished in nonatopic as well as atopic individuals. Examples of specific antigens that provoke such reactions include the following: foods, such as shellfish, nuts, and chocolate; drugs and therapeutic agents, notably penicillin and immunotherapeutic extracts; and bee, wasp, yellow jacket, hornet, and fire ant venom.

REACTIONS TO ADMINISTRATION OF WHOLE BLOOD, SERUM, OR IMMUNOGLOBULINS

Anaphylaxis is an uncommon complication of the administration of blood, serum, or immunoglobulin. One mechanism for this reaction may be the transfusion of IgE of donor origin directed toward an antigen to which the recipient is then exposed; another mechanism is the transfusion of a soluble antigen present in the donor preparation into a previously sensitized recipient. Thus the transfer of antigens from silk, originally used in purification of immunoglobulin preparations, was deemed responsible for some IgE-dependent anaphylactic responses to human gamma globulin.

More commonly, however, reactions seen with transfusion of blood or serum or administration of IgG are the result of immune complex formation and complement activation leading to direct vascular and smooth muscle alterations, and indirectly, via anaphylatoxins, to mast cell–mediator release. This mechanism has been clearly delineated in reactions to blood, plasma, or immunoglobulin in patients with antibodies to IgA. Such antibodies occur frequently in patients with IgA deficiency, in patients who have received multiple blood transfusions, and in some normal adults. These patients lack skin test reactivity to erythrocytes, leukocytes, plasma, and IgA but possess IgG antibodies to IgA. Such antibodies form complexes with IgA and thereby activate complement. Inasmuch as IgA may comprise 0.5–4 percent of IgG preparations, such anti-IgA reactions may occur in patients receiving replacement immunoglobulin therapy.

Urticarial or anaphylactic reactions to the administration of serum or its products do not invariably involve antibody to IgA. Numerous reports have identified aggregates of immunoglobulin capable of fixing complement as responsible for such reactions. If such aggregates are removed, administration of the relevant material can then be tolerated. These data suggest the nonimmune nature of this form of anaphylactic reaction.

PRESUMED ABNORMALITIES OF PROSTAGLANDIN METABOLISM

Urticaria/angioedema and anaphylactic responses to aspirin and related nonsteroidal antiinflammatory agents have been estimated to occur in approximately 1 percent of individuals, and in some instances may have a familial basis. Intolerance to aspirin manifested as bronchospasm occurs primarily in asthmatic patients, whereas urticaria/angioedema occurs primarily in normal individuals or patients with rhinitis. The incidence of aspirin intolerance in patients with asthma ranges from 2 to 10 percent. Patients intolerant to aspirin also frequently react to a variety of nonsteroidal antiinflammatory agents; in addition, up to 15–20 percent of such patients react to azodyes, notably tartrazine, and to benzoates used as preservatives. Intolerance to aspirin, azodyes, and benzoates is often unrecognized and then can only be documented by challenge studies.

Clinical manifestations of intolerance to those agents may appear anywhere from 15 minutes to 2 hours after ingestion. In asthmatic patients the onset of the reaction is marked by profuse rhinorrhea and is often accompanied by a scarlet flush of the upper body. Bronchoconstriction, wheezing, and rarely cyanosis often begin within 30 minutes and may progress for several hours. Most asthmatic patients recover within hours, but excessive bronchial secretion may persist for days.

Reactions to aspirin do not occur following exposure to closely related compounds such as sodium salicylate or choline salicylate, whereas the structually unrelated nonsteroidal antiinflammatory agents and tartrazine do precipitate the clinical symptoms. Prick skin testing is of no diagnostic value, passive transfer reactions are negative, and neither IgG nor IgE antibodies correlate with clinical disease. Aspirin and the nonsteroidal antiinflammatory agents inhibit cyclooxygenase, an enzyme operative in the generation of prostaglandins from arachidonic acid, and the ability of these agents to induce bronchoconstriction appears to be related to their potency in inhibiting prostaglandin synthesis. Whether mediators other than prostaglandins play a role is unclear as minimal elevations in plasma histamine and depletion of serum complement factors have been noted after the ingestion of aspirin in some but not all patients after experimental challenge. The mechanism by which alterations in prostaglandin synthesis elicit the characteristic clinical manifestations is presumed to be an inherited or acquired abnormal sensitivity to normal metabolites or, less likely, the generation of an abnormal product.

DIRECT MAST CELL DEGRANULATING AGENTS

Anaphylacticlike syndromes have been attributed to a variety of therapeutic and diagnostic agents. As many as 8 percent of patients receiving radiocontrast media experience such reactions. Although an antibody to radiocontrast media has not been found and skin testing is not predictive, there is evidence that suggests that patients who have experienced adverse reactions are at increased risk for subsequent reactions to these agents. These media, as well as opiates, curare, d-tubocurarine, and highly charged antibiotics such as polymyxin B, can directly release histamine from mast cells and basophils. In addition, alterations in serum complement levels have been noted after administration of radiocontrast media. The pathobiologic mechanism by which these agents cause anaphylaxis, however, remains obscure.

LABORATORY EVALUATION AND TREATMENT

LABORATORY EVALUATION

IgE can be recognized in vivo by prick skin testing or by passive transfer to humans or monkeys. These tests have been of value in predicting anaphylactic sensitivity to protein antigens and pencillin analogs and metabolites but not to other drugs, and skin testing carries the hazard of anaphylaxis.

In vitro techniques to assess the presence of specific IgE antibodies include the radioallergosorbent test (RAST), which can quantitate nanogram quantities of specific antibody, the release of histamine from leukocytes of sensitive individuals upon antigen challenge, or the ability of patients' sera to passively sensitize normal tissues such as leukocytes for the subsequent antigen-induced release of mediators. RAST analysis has allowed the diagnosis of sensitivity to a variety of antigens, including foods, pollens, and *Hymenoptera* venom. However, as skin test-negative–RAST-positive and RAST-negative–skin test-positive individuals with anaphylactic sensitivity to hymenoptera venom have been identified, laboratory findings must be used with caution in the diagnosis and management of anaphylactic syndromes.

TREATMENT

Owing to its dramatic nature, the diagnosis of systemic anaphylaxis is usually apparent. In the diagnosis of sudden collapse in the absence of accompanying urticaria/angioedema, one must consider such causes of unconsciousness as cardiac arrhythmia, myocardial infarction, aspiration of a bolus of food, pulmonary embolism, and seizure disorders.

Factors to consider in the prevention and management of anaphylactic reactions are the sensitivity of the recipient, the amount of antigen, and the rate of its absorption. If there is a history of anaphylactic sensitivity to a particular immunogen, another noncross-reacting therapeutic or diagnostic agent should be employed if possible. In addition, attempts to avoid the relevant immunogens present in foods, proprietary drugs, and the environment should be undertaken.

A skin test should be performed before certain materials known to produce a high incidence of anaphylactic reactions, such as serum or immunotherapeutic extracts, are administered. Similarly, skin tests may prove helpful when there is a history of a previous reaction which was not clearly anaphylactic in onset and manifestation and for which testing in vitro is either unavailable or inadequate. For example, skin testing to determine the presence and haptenic specificity of IgE may be justified if penicillin is clearly the drug of choice. However, negative skin tests do not rule out anaphylactic sensitivity. Inasmuch as the minute amounts of antigen used in a skin test can produce a serious reaction, a scratch test should precede the intradermal skin test in patients who are in a high-risk situation. Skin testing must always be performed with appropriate precautionary measures, and therapeutic modalities for resuscitation must be immediately available.

If a therapeutic agent is to be used despite a history of anaphylactic signs and symptoms and/or a positive skin test, desensitization to the agent may be attempted. Precautionary measures should accompany desensitization and include access to the circulation for the administration of epinephrine and/or fluids in the event of vascular collapse. The success and persistence of desensitization cannot be predicted, and in several instances the parenteral injection of a therapeutic agent after a desensitization protocol has proved fatal. Through an unknown mechanism, desenitization may be induced by repeated injections of purified venom in the control of sensitivity to individual *Hymenoptera* species.

Early recognition of an acute anaphylactic reaction is mandatory, as death may occur within minutes. The interval between antigen insult and death in six fatal cases ranged from 16 to 24 minutes; however, in some instances of *Hymenoptera* sensitivity, death occurred after intervals as long as 96 hours. The maintenance of both a patent airway and an adequate systemic blood pressure level are essential. The therapeutic agent of choice for the control of the acute anaphylactic syndrome is epinephrine. Mild symptoms can be controlled by the subcutaneous injection of epinephrine. If the responsible immunogen was injected into an extremity, the rate of its absorption may be reduced by prompt application of a tourniquet proximal to the reaction area and by the administration of epinephrine directly into the site. Epinephrine should be administered in repeated doses as required and tolerated.

Severe symptoms such as vascular collapse should be treated by the administration of fluids and may require intravenous administration of epinephrine. Oxygen and methylxanthines may be useful in reducing airway obstruction and resulting hypoxia; in the advent of progressive hypoxia, and particularly in the event of laryngeal edema, intubation and mechanical ventilation may be required. Thus, the critical measures are to decrease the rate of antigen absorption, to support the circulation, and to prevent hypoxia. These are best accomplished by administration of epinephrine and establishment of an intravenous infusion; respiratory support must also be available.

The therapeutic efficacy of other agents is debated; antihistamines may be used if urticaria/angioedema are the predominant manifestations of the anaphylactic syndrome. Although the value of corticosteroid preparations in the therapy of anaphylaxis remains unproven, clinical experience suggests reversal of the acute reaction may be enhanced.

REFERENCES

Austen KF, Sheffer AL: Vascular responses, the anaphylactic syndrome, in Fitzpatrick TB, Arndt KA, Clark WH, Eisen AZ, VanScott EJ, Vaughn JH (eds): Dermatology in Internal Medicine. New York, McGraw-Hill, 1971, pp 1244–1261

James LP Jr, Austen KF: Fatal systemic anaphylaxis in man. N Engl J Med 270:597, 1964

Levine BB: Immunologic mechanisms of penicillin allergy. N Engl J Med 275:1115, 1966

Stechschulte DJ, Austen KF in Zweifach BW, Grant L, McCloskey RT (eds): Anaphylaxis, The Inflammatory Process, vol 3 (ed 2). New York, Academic Press, 1974, pp 237–276

Lysosomal Diseases

Robert B. Zurier

LYSOSOMAL DISEASES

The clearest form of a lysosomal disease is one in which a lysosomal enzyme is absent, consequent to which its substrate accumulates in tissues. In most of these deposition diseases there is a congenital defect of an acid hydrolase with subsequent accumulation of complex mucopolysaccharides and/or glycolipids. The chemical heterogeneity of the stored material is explained by the fact that lysosomal acid hydrolases do not display a high substrate specificity. The congenital defect of one acid hydrolase will therefore lead to storage in the vacuolar system of all substances for whose breakdown the missing enzyme is required. The abundance of each substance varies from tissue to tissue. The reticuloendothelial system is overloaded, and the brain, for example, contains a preponderance of lipid structures. It would appear that enzyme replacement therapy should cure these storage diseases, but clinical success in this regard has not been forthcoming.

MUCOPOLYSACCHARIDOSES

Mucopolysaccharides (glycosaminoglycans) are a family of molecules consisting of a protein core to which are attached long chains of repeating units of sulfated disaccharide. Mucopolysaccharidoses involve a distur-
bance in the lysosomal catabolism of two polymeric substances, dermatan sulfate and heparan sulfate, singly or in combination. These polymers are made up of alternating residues of sulfated hexosamine (glucosamine or galactosamine) and uronic acid (glucuronic or L-iduronic acid), and their major degradative pathway is by lysosomal enzymes (glycosidases and sulfatases that cleave the chain from the nonreducing terminus). Removal in sequence of each chemically distinct sugar residue or sulfate group requires a different enzyme. Thus, the concerted action of several enzymes may be required to degrade the chain. If any one enzyme is missing or malfunctioning the degradative sequence is altered, although limited degradation may occur by enzymes, such as hyaluronidase, that can cleave the chain into fragments. Normally, degradation of dermatan sulfate and heparan sulfate results in the formation of sulfate, which is excreted, and hexosamine and uronic acid, which are recycled. In contrast, degradation of dermatan sulfate and heparan sulfate in mucopolysaccharidosis patients results in fragments, some of which are excreted in urine, but most of which are retained in cells within lysosomes. Their storage is cumulative, which leads to abnormal cell function and clinical disease.

A series of in vitro cross-correction experiments

Table 1
Mucopolysaccharidoses (MPS)

Designation/Syndrome	Clinical Features	Excessive Urinary Mucopolysaccharides	Enzyme Deficiency
MPS IH/Hurler's	Early corneal clouding, coarse facial features, dwarfing, mental retardation, death before age 10	Dermatan sulfate Heparan sulfate	α-L-Iduronidase
MPS IS/Scheie's	Stiff joints, claw hand, aortic incompetence, corneal clouding, normal intelligence	Dermatan sulfate Heparan sulfate	α-L-Iduronidase
MPS II/Hunter's	Similar to Hurler's, but onset later and course slower; no corneal clouding, death before age 15 in severe (MPS IIA) and longer survival with mild (MPS IIB) syndrome	Dermatan sulfate Heparan sulfate	Sulfoiduronate sulfatase
MPS III/Sanfilippo's MPS IIIA/Sanfilippo A MPS IIIB/Sanfilippo B	IIIA and IIIB: same phenotype, coarse facies, hypertrichosis, minimal skeletal abnormalities, severe mental retardation, death in midtwenties	Heparan sulfate	Heparan sulfate sulfatase N-Acetyl α-D-glucosaminidase
MPS IV/Morquio's	Spondyloepiphyseal dysplasia, corneal clouding, aortic regurgitation; bone growth ceases at age 5	Keratan sulfate	Unknown
MPS VI/Maroteau-Lamy	Similar to but milder than Hurler's; normal intelligence	Dermatan sulfate	Maroteau-Lamy corrective factor from normal urine
MPS VII/β-glucuronidase deficiency	Hurler-like; late mental retardation, hepatosplenomegaly	Dermatan sulfate Chondroitin sulfate	β-Glucuronidase

Table 2
Sphingolipidoses

Designation	Clinical Features	Product Stored	Enzyme Deficiency
Gangliosidosis GM$_1$	Features similar to Hurler's; onset at birth, death by age 2	Ganglioside GM$_1$ in brain Visceral storage of mucopolysaccharides	GM$_1$ β-Galactosidase
Gangliosidosis GM$_2$			
Type I, Tay-Sachs	Onset at 4–6 months, progressive mental and motor deterioration, blindness, cherry redspot in macula, Jewish parentage	GM$_2$ ganglioside	N-Acetyl hexosaminidase A
Type II, Sandhoff's	Clinically same as Tay-Sachs; non-Jewish parentage	GM$_2$ ganglioside Globoside	N-acetyl hexosaminidase A & B
Type III, juvenile	Onset at 2–6 years, progressive weakness and spasticity, blindness without macular red spot, death by age 15	GM$_2$ ganglioside	Partial deficiency hexosaminidase A & B
Fabry's disease	Males have dark purple maculopapular rash, angiokeratoma corporis diffusum, death by age 40 due to renal failure or cardiovascular disease; females may have limited disease	Ceramide trihexoside	α-Galactosidase
Krabbe's leukodystrophy	Rapid motor and mental deterioration, death by age 2		β-Galactocerebrosidase
Metachromatic leukodystrophy	Onset at 1–4 years, progression to quadriplegia, mental deterioration; adult form rare, may mimic mental disorder	Galactosyl (SO$_4$) ceramide	Aryl sulfastase
Gaucher's disease	In acute infantile form, neurovisceral disorder with death by age 2; in adult form, progressive visceral disorder, hepatosplenomegaly	Glucocerebroside	β-Glucosidase
Niemann-Pick disease	Disease of infancy most common; massive hepatosplenomegaly, progressive neurologic deterioration		Spingomyelinase
Farber's disease (lipogranulomatosis)	Childhood onset, progressive arthropathy, psychomotor retardation	Ceramide	Ceramidase

helped define the enzymatic defect in many of these disorders and together with clinical correlation has allowed classification of the storage diseases. When fibroblasts from patients with mucopolysaccharidosis are grown in the presence of radioactive sulfate, they accumulate and store it as sulfated glycosaminoglycans. This is due to impaired degradation rather than increased synthesis. When mucopolysaccharidosis patient fibroblasts are cultured in the presence of normal fibroblasts the defect is corrected and degradation returns to normal. All the mucopolysaccharidoses are autosomally inherited,

except Hunter's syndrome, which is an X-linked disorder (Table 1).

SPHINGOLIPIDOSES

Complex molecules such as gangliosides, globosides, and sphingomyelin, constitute the means whereby the lipid moiety of myelin is bonded to polysaccharides. In the breakdown of these molecules intermediates are formed which, if not cleared from the cells, become segregated in lysosomes. Each pathway in the catabolism of these complex lipids has become the site of a genetic variant that leads to discrete clinical manifestations. All these disorders, except Fabry's disease, appear to be inherited as autosomal recessives (Table 2). Fabry's disease is an X-linked recessive disorder.

LIPID DISORDERS

Two disorders of simple lipids associated with deficient lysosomal enzymes have been described. Wolman's disease, or familial xanthomatosis with calcification of the adrenals and deposition of triglycerides and cholesterol esters in visceral organs, is due to a deficiency of lysosomal acid lipase. The same enzyme activity is missing in cholesterol ester storage disease.

MUCOLIPIDOSES

Several clinical entities share features of both lipid and mucopolysaccharide disorders and have been called *mucolipidoses*. In addition to four diseases usually classified as sphingolipidoses (gangliosidoses GM$_1$ and GM$_2$, metachromatic leukodystrophy, and Farber's disease), they include fucosidosis (a fucosidase deficiency), manosidosis (acid α-mannosidase deficiency), lipomucopolysaccharidosis, pseudo-Hurler polydystrophy, and I cell disease. I cell disease derives its name from the presence in cells of large inclusions ("I"). These are debris-packed lysosomes visible by phase microscopy. In this disorder there appears to be a defect in several enzymes that does not allow for their normal sequestration within lysosomal membranes.

SINGLE-ENZYME DEFECTS

Syndromes due to single-enzyme defects include the Nadler-Egan syndrome (familial deficiency of acid p-nitrophenyl phosphatase) and the acid maltase deficiencies: Pompe's disease (glycogen storage disease type II), the first disease to be attributed to the absence of a lysosomal hydrolase, acid α-1,4-glucosidase; adult acid maltase deficiency; and aspartyl glucosaminuria, which appears to be due to deficient N-aspartyl-β-glucosaminidase activity.

DISORDERS OF LYSOSOMAL FUNCTION

Chronic granulomatous disease is an X-linked recessive disorder that occurs mainly in male children and is characterized by repeated bacterial infections, including pneumonias, and death at an early age. The response to pyogenic infection is formation of granulomas. Cervical adenitis with suppuration, eczematoid skin lesions, hepatic abscesses, and osteomyelitis are common findings. The primary defect is absence from the leukocytes of the enzyme (nicotinamide adenine dinucleotide oxidase) responsible for hydrogen peroxide generation during phagocytosis. Thus bacteria that do not generate hydrogen peroxide (staphylococci, gram-negative bacilli) are not killed efficiently. Myeloperoxidase deficiency has also been described in a few patients vulnerable to certain fungal and bacterial infections.

The Chediak-Higashi syndrome is a rare autosomal recessive disorder characterized by partial oculocutaneous albinism, photophobia, nystagmus, frequent pyogenic infections, and the presence of giant irregularly shaped lysosomes in granule-containing cells. An accelerated (lymphomalike) phase develops, during which patients have hepatosplenomegaly and lymphadenopathy. Death usually occurs in childhood due to infection or hemorrhage. Although Chediak-Higashi syndrome has been considered primarily a lysosomal disease—and there is evidence that the giant lysosomes are bounded by a membrane more permeable than those which surround normal granules with which they coexist in the cell—a major defect in Chediak-Higashi neutrophils appears to be failure of microtubule assembly, which leads to poor degranulation and bactericidal activity. In a few patients, normal leukocyte function has been restored and recurrent infections prevented by treatment with vitamin C. It is not yet known if such treatment will prevent the accelerated phase of the disease.

CLINICAL IMPLICATION OF LYSOSOMES IN OTHER DISORDERS

The possible role of lysosomes in joint tissue injury has been discussed. In hepatitis and cholestatic jaundice the PAS-positive reacting structures noted in the liver are autophagic vacuoles. The hepatocellular pigments seen in Dubin-Johnson disease are deposited in lysosomes. It is thought that hepatotoxicity in Wilson' disease may be due to the failure of excess copper to remain localized in lysosomes. The numbers of autophagic vacuoles and residual bodies are increased in specimens of myocardium from patients with congestive heart failure, and atherosclerotic aortas contain higher concentrations of lysosomal enzymes than normal specimens. Many properties of lysosomes were first discovered or thoroughly investigated using kidney proximal tubule lysosomes. In renal disease large quantities of protein are absorbed in the proximal tubules by way of lysosomes (hyaline droplets). The lysosomes of the intercapillary cells degrade absorbed residues of filtration that could otherwise damage the glomerular basement membrane. The epithelioid cells of the afferent glomerular arteriole (juxtaglomerular apparatus) contain many large granules. These granules, which are lysosomes, secrete the protease renin and thus appear to play a role in the pathogenesis of hypertensive disease.

There is widespread interest in the possibility that lysosomes play a role in carcinogenesis. Agents known to be carcinogenic are found in lysosomes soon after uptake by cells. Lysosomal hydrolases can be involved in cell damage, and cell damage and carcinogenesis are often related. Deoxyribonuclease can be liberated from lysosomes and provoke DNA damage manifest as chromosome alterations. Finally, lysosomal enzymes may mediate induction or derepression of cell division. So little is known of the fundamental processes responsible for carcinogenesis that a possible role for lysosomes deserves further study.

REFERENCES

Hers HG, VanHoof F (eds): Lysosomes and Storage Diseases. New York, Academic Press, 1973

Hirschorn R, Weissmann G: Genetic disorders of lysosomes. Prog Med Genet 1:49, 1976

McKusick VA: The mucopolysaccharidoses, in: Heritable Dis-orders of Connective Tissue (ed 4). St Louis, Mosby, 1972, p 521

Neufeld EF: The biochemical basis for mucopolysaccharidoses and mucolipidoses. Prog Med Genet 10:81, 1974

Oliver JM, Zurier RB: Correction of characteristic abnormalities of microtubule function and granule morphology in Che-diak-Higashi syndrome. J Clin Invest 57:1239, 1976

INDEX